Textbook of Shoulder Surgery

Ian A. Trail • Lennard Funk
Amar Rangan • Matthew Nixon
Editors

Textbook of Shoulder Surgery

Springer

Editors
Ian A. Trail
Wrightington Hospital
Wigan
Lancashire
UK

Lennard Funk
Wrightington Hospital
Wigan
Lancashire
UK

Amar Rangan
Orthopaedic Surgery Department
The James Cook University Hospital
Middlesbrough
North Yorkshire
UK

Matthew Nixon
Trauma & Orthopaedics Department
Countess of Chester Hospital
Chester
Cheshire
UK

ISBN 978-3-319-70098-4 ISBN 978-3-319-70099-1 (eBook)
https://doi.org/10.1007/978-3-319-70099-1

Library of Congress Control Number: 2018957858

This Springer imprint is published by the registered company Springer Nature Switzerland AG
The registered company address is: Gewerbestrasse 11, 6330 Cham, Switzerland

Preface

Over the last 25 years, significant advances have been made in the understanding of the shoulder biomechanics and treatment of its pathologies. Arthroscopic techniques and instrumentation have enabled many conditions to be treated with low morbidity to the patient. There have been numerous advances in arthroplasty surgery since John Charnley developed the low-friction hip replacement. Improvements in trauma technologies mean patients can expect to return to near-normal function after complex injuries.

There are still many challenges to the modern shoulder surgeon. These include consolidating and comprehending the vast amounts of knowledge available, predicting the long-term outcomes of new technologies, and dealing with new complications (such as glenoid erosions and implant loosening after shoulder arthroplasty). Patients with shoulder problems understandably have higher expectations of returning to high-performance sports, older patients with complex medical co-morbidities demand effective pain relief and independent function, and children born with congenital abnormalities want near-normal shoulder development and function.

This textbook provides the most up-to-date information on shoulder surgery along with practical approaches for patient evaluation and treatment options. The book is divided into key parts, providing coverage on soft tissue disorders of the shoulder, arthritis of the shoulder, the paediatric shoulder and other miscellaneous topics relevant to treating this area. Its strong clinical focus will help practicing shoulder surgeons, residents and medical students to manage patients in a practical way, based on the most recent scientific evidence and the most effective surgical and non-surgical techniques. Thus, we hope it will become a valuable reference and resource for young doctors and students looking to increase their professional skills and knowledge when treating shoulder injuries and disorders in clinical practice.

Ian Trail is the senior upper limb surgeon at Wrightington Hospital. He has extensive experience of complex pathologies in the shoulder and is a leading authority on arthroplasty in the upper limb.

Lenard Funk is an experienced clinician, an expert in arthroscopic shoulder surgery and an authority on sports shoulder surgery in elite athletes. He is a highly regarded surgical trainer and educator for health-care professionals and patients.

Amar Rangan is a leading expert in shoulder conditions, particularly due to trauma. He is a key member on several national research councils and attracts many tertiary referrals for complex shoulder pathologies.

Matthew Nixon won the gold medal for the FRCS (Orth) exam and has since established himself as an authority on shoulder and upper limb pathologies in children. He runs a dedicated paediatric shoulder clinic dealing with congenital, neuromuscular, posttraumatic and tumour pathologies.

These editors, together, with carefully selected international experts aim to bring you a comprehensive review of what is known about shoulder pathologies, together with clinical pearls and operative techniques to help with their management.

Contents

Part I Trauma

1 **The Sternoclavicular Joint** 3
Graham Tytherleigh-Strong

2 **Clavicle Fracture** 17
Rajesh Nanda and Amar Rangan

3 **Acromioclavicular Joint Injuries** 45
Simone Cerciello, Felix Dyrna, Leo Pauzenberger, Jeremiah D. Johnson, Knut Beitzel, and Augustus D. Mazzocca

4 **Scapular fractures** 55
Jan Bartoníček, Michal Tuček, and Ondřej Naňka

5 **Proximal Humeral Fractures** 75
C. Spross and B. Jost

6 **Outcome Measures Following Upper Limb Trauma** 101
Ramsay Refaie and Amar Rangan

Part II Soft Tissue Disorders of the Shoulder

7 **Glenohumeral Joint Instability** 121
Paolo Paladini, Giovanni Merolla, and Giuseppe Porcellini

8 **Rotator Cuff Pathology** 131
Teruhisa Mihata

9 **Calcific Tendinitis** 145
Simon Boyle and Geoffrey C. S. Smith

10 **Long Head of the Biceps Tendon Complex: Pathology and Treatment Approach** 157
Brian B. Gilmer, Sarah D. Lang, and Dan Guttmann

11 **The Stiff Shoulder** 173
Richard S. Page and Goran Mitreski

12 **Muscle Ruptures of the Shoulder Girdle** 195
Ewan Bigsby and Alex A. Malone

Part III Arthritis of the Shoulder: I

13 **Design of Polyethylene Glenoid Components** 213
Ian A. Trail

14 **Design of Humeral Stems** 223
Emmet John Griffiths, Ian A. Trail, and Gilles Walch

15 **Results of Anatomical Shoulder Arthroplasty** 233
Clemens Abel and Frank Gohlke

16 **Complications in Anatomic Shoulder Replacement** 253
Ludwig Seebauer

Part IV Arthritis of the Shoulder: II

17 **Design Principles of Reverse Arthroplasty** 275
Anders Ekelund and Didier Poncet

18 **Results of the Reverse Total Shoulder Arthroplasty** 287
Ian A. Trail

19 **Complications of the Reverse Implant** 301
Daniel Mok, Francis Lam, and Ram Chidambaram

20 **Glenoid Bone Augmentation in Shoulder Arthroplasty** 323
Steve Bale

21 **Polyethylene Augmented Glenoid Components in Anatomic Total Shoulder Arthroplasty** 337
Jason C. Ho, Eric T. Ricchetti, and Joseph P. Iannotti

22 **Metal Augments in Shoulder Arthroplasty** 349
Ian P. Mayne and Peter C. Poon

Part V Arthritis of the Shoulder: III

23 **Complications of Shoulder Arthroplasty** 367
Michael Walton, Daoud Makki, and Steven Brookes-Fazakerley

24 **Revision Shoulder Arthroplasty** 383
Adam Seidl, Derek Axibal, Mikaël Chelli, and Pascal Boileau

Part VI Arthritis of the Shoulder: IV

25 **The Anatomic Stemless Humeral Prosthesis** 407
Nael Hawi and Peter Habermeyer

26 **Patient Specific Instrumentation** 421
Kyong S. Min, Henry M. Fox, and Jon J. P. Warner

27 **Rehabilitation Following Shoulder Arthroplasty** 441
Julia Walton, Sonya Spencer, and Michael Walton

Part VII The Paediatric Shoulder

28 Paediatric Trauma Around the Shoulder 453
Abdulaziz F Ahmed and Talal Ibrahim

29 Neuromuscular Shoulder Reconstruction in Children 473
Peter M. Waters and Carley Vuillermin

30 Paediatric Shoulder Instability 493
Mattthew F. Nixon and Allen Stevenson

Part VIII Miscellaneous

31 Nerve Problems Around the Shoulder 515
Chye Yew Ng, Dominic Power, and Sohail Akhtar

32 Tumours of the Shoulder 533
Roger M. Tillman and Scott Evans

33 Infection of the Shoulder Joint 545
Aravind Desai, Pratima Khincha, Robert Nelson, and Puneet Monga

34 History Taking and Clinical Assessment of the Shoulder 555
Simon Robinson, Nanette Oakes, and Shantanu Shahane

35 Radiological Evaluation 587
David Temperley

Index 611

Part I

Trauma

The Sternoclavicular Joint

1

Graham Tytherleigh-Strong

Anatomy

The sternoclavicular joint (SCJ) is formed by the articulation between the medial end of the clavicle and the sternal manubrium and plays a vital role in the attachment of the shoulder girdle to the body. In fact, it is the only true articular connection between the upper limb and the axial skeleton, as the scapulothoracic joint is not a true synovial joint.

The SCJ is a synovial joint with largely incongruent articular surfaces (Fig. 1.1). On the clavicular side the surface is saddle shaped with a concavity in the anteroposterior plane and convexity in the vertical plane [1, 2]. Between the articular surfaces lies a fibrocartilaginous disc, similar to the meniscus of the knee [3]. This separates the joint into a medial and lateral compartment and is attached to the capsule at its periphery, to the superior surface of the medial clavicle and the first costal cartilage inferiorly. Contrary to most classic anatomical texts, a recent anatomical study has shown that the superior part of the disc inserts into the superior third of the medial end of the clavicle. Articular cartilage only covers the lower two-thirds of the medial end of the clavicle [2]. Despite the incongruent articular surfaces and small surface area of the joint, the SCJ is extremely stable owing to the effect of strong static (both intrinsic and extrinsic) and dynamic soft tissue stabilizers (Table 1.1) [4].

The anterior and posterior sternoclavicular ligaments are formed by thickenings in the capsule and are the most important contributors to antero-posterior stability [5]. The intra-articular fibrocartilagenous disc resists medial translation of the clavicle [4]. As a result, the disc can be prone to shearing injury, usually as a degenerate tear but occasionally as an acute incident.

The interclavicular ligament passes between the medial ends of both clavicles via the posterior aspect of the sternal notch and resists clavicular superior translation from gravity or forceful depression of the upper limb [4, 6]. The costoclavicular ligament passes from the inferior aspect of the medial clavicle to the first rib and/or first costal cartilage [7]. It is an important restraint when the clavicle is elevated.

The dynamic stabilizers form a musculotendinous envelope around the joint. The sternocleidomastoid and pectoralis major tendons lie anterior and posterior to the SCJ respectively and play a role in anterior and posterior stability, whilst the subclavius passes from the inferior aspect of the clavicle to the first rib providing superior stability as well as an additional anterior/superior component.

Several vital structures lie posterior to the SCJ including the great vessels of the neck, oesophagus and the trachea. These are at potential risk follow-

G. Tytherleigh-Strong,
FRCS(Orth), DSportMed, FFSEM (✉)
Division of Orthopaedics, Addenbrooke's Hospital,
Cambridge University Hospitals Trust,
Cambridge, UK

I. A. Trail et al. (eds.), *Textbook of Shoulder Surgery*, https://doi.org/10.1007/978-3-319-70099-1_1

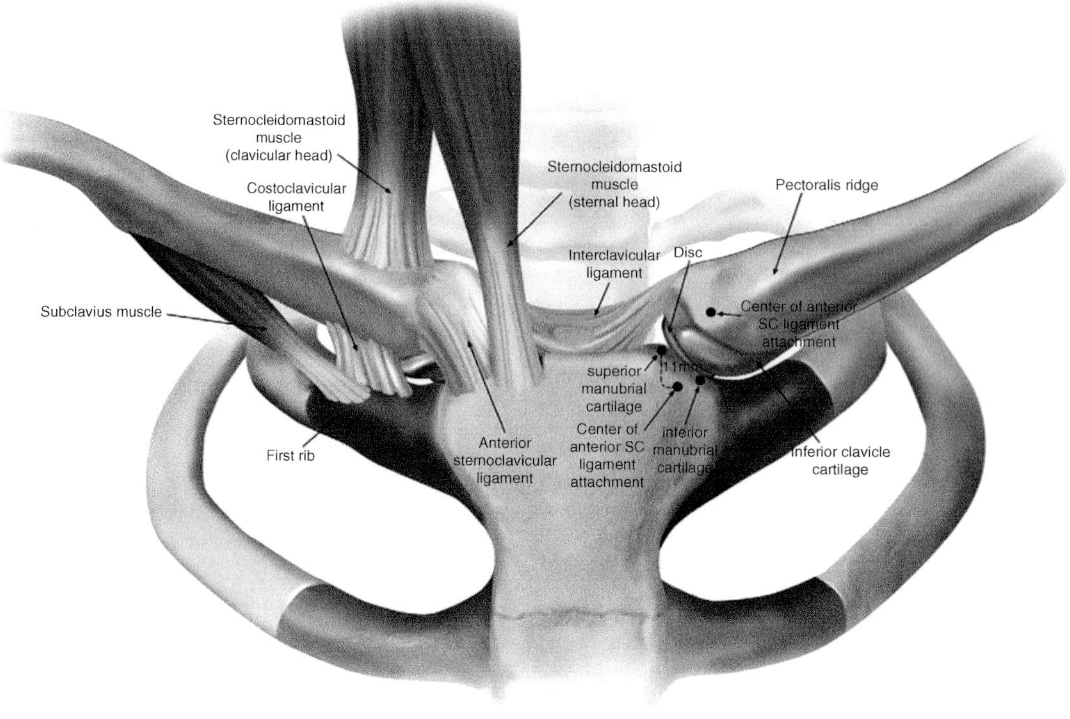

Fig. 1.1 Sternoclavicular joint

Table 1.1 Stabilisers of the SCJ

Static Stabilizers	Dynamic Stabilizers
Capsule	Subclavius muscle
	Sternocleidomastoid muscle
Intrinsic stabilizers Intra-articular disc ligament Anterior sternoclavicular ligament Posterior sternoclavicular ligament	Pectoralis major muscle
Extrinsic stabilizers Interclavicular Costoclavicular	

ing posterior dislocations. A layer formed by sternothyroid and sternohyoid muscles lies between these structures and the joint capsule [1, 2].

The epiphysis of the medial end of the clavicle is the first epiphysis to appear in utero and the last to close [8, 9]. This is of relevance because the physis at the medial end of the clavicle is weaker than the SCJ ligaments. Significant traumatic injuries before physeal closure, under the age of 25 years, may result in a fracture through the physis, Salter-Harris II fracture, rather than a true SCJ dislocation.

The SCJ moves in three planes: retraction/protraction, elevation/depression and rotation [10]. Movement at the SCJ and ACJ allows the scapula to move around the thorax to position the glenoid in the optimal location to maintain glenohumeral joint congruency for upper limb positioning.

History & Examination

As with any upper limb complaint, it is important to consider the age, handedness, sport, aspirations and occupation of the patient. An acute injury typically involves a high-energy mechanism and an SCJ injury may be missed in the presence of more dramatic components. Details of the exact mechanism of injury including direction of impact should be sought. Up to 30% of acute posterior dislocations develop mediastinal compromise, concerning features include dyspnoea, dysphonia, dysphagia, coughing and venous congestion of the ipsilateral arm and should be considered as a medical emergency. Patients usually present with pain over the SCJ in the presence of a deformity, a prominence of the medial clavicle in anterior dislocations and a defect lateral to the sternum in a posterior dislocation.

In patients presenting with more chronic problems a history of previous trauma or a change of activity preceding the onset of symptoms may be relevant. In younger patients complaints of pain, clicking, a feeling of instability or even recurrent dislocation in the absence of injury may suggest an atraumatic instability. A history of connective tissue disorders such as Ehlers-Danlos Syndrome maybe relevant. Older patients may present with a pain and restriction of movement associated with a swelling over the medial end of the clavicle, in keeping with osteoarthritis.

SCJ examination is predominantly based on comparison and any asymmetry between sides. This requires exposure of the upper trunk to allow for comparison of both shoulder girdles including the clavicles, glenohumeral joints and scapulothoracic movements. There may be obvious asymmetry between the patient's SCJs with a lump present on the affected side. It is important to determine whether this is soft, representing an effusion or synovitis secondary to an inflammatory arthropathy or infection, or hard which could represent either a chronic anterior dislocation of the medial end of the clavicle or an osteophyte secondary to osteoarthritis.

Movements at the SCJ are intimately related to the rest of the shoulder girdle, so that assessment of the ACJ, Glenohumeral joint and scapulothoracic movements are essential to identify any confounding pathology. Both the SCJs should be examined and compared in 3 planes of movement. External and internal rotation with the elbow bent at 90° and the arm at 90° of abduction, protraction/retraction with the arms in extension and elevation with the arms in maximal abduction. Whilst examining the range of motion it is important that the examiner places a hand over the anterior joint to feel for any abnormal movement and clicking. Clicking, popping, or crepitus at the joint during movement may suggest degenerative changes or, in a younger patient, a disc tear. The medial end of the clavicle may sublux or even dislocate anteriorly in patients with instability (Fig. 1.2). In this instance broader assessment of the stabilising soft tissue envelope, particularly looking at sternoclcidomastoid and the sternal part of Pectoralis Major, for muscle sequencing over activity should be undertaken.

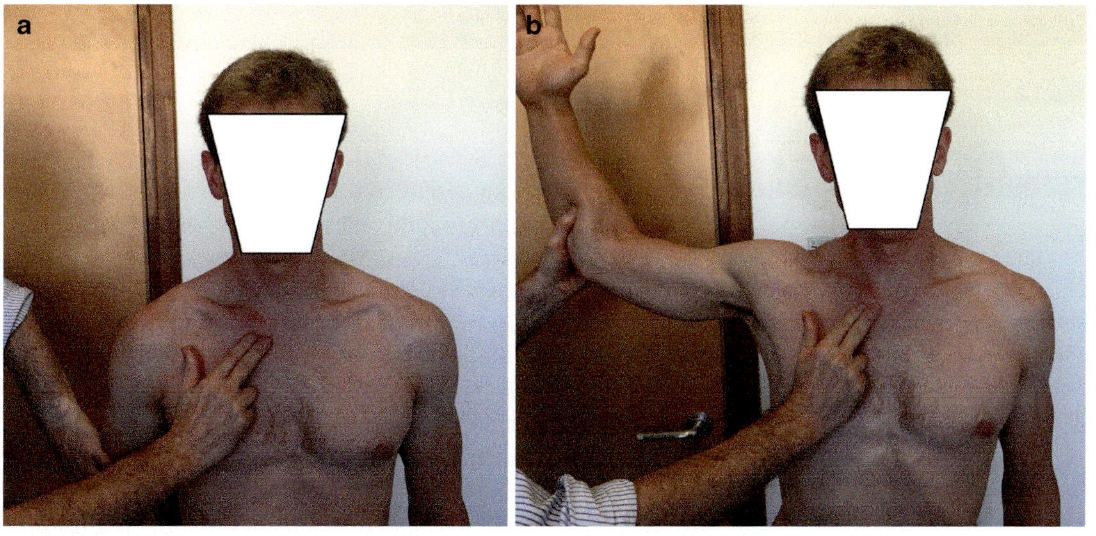

Fig. 1.2 Examination of the SCJ. (**a**) Palpation over the anterior joint line for pain and extruded disk. (**b**, **c**) Exterrnal & internal rotation: with the elbow bent at 90° and the arm at 90° abduction rotate the arm from external to internal rotation feeling for crepitus. (**d**, **e**) Protraction & retraction. (**f**) Elevation

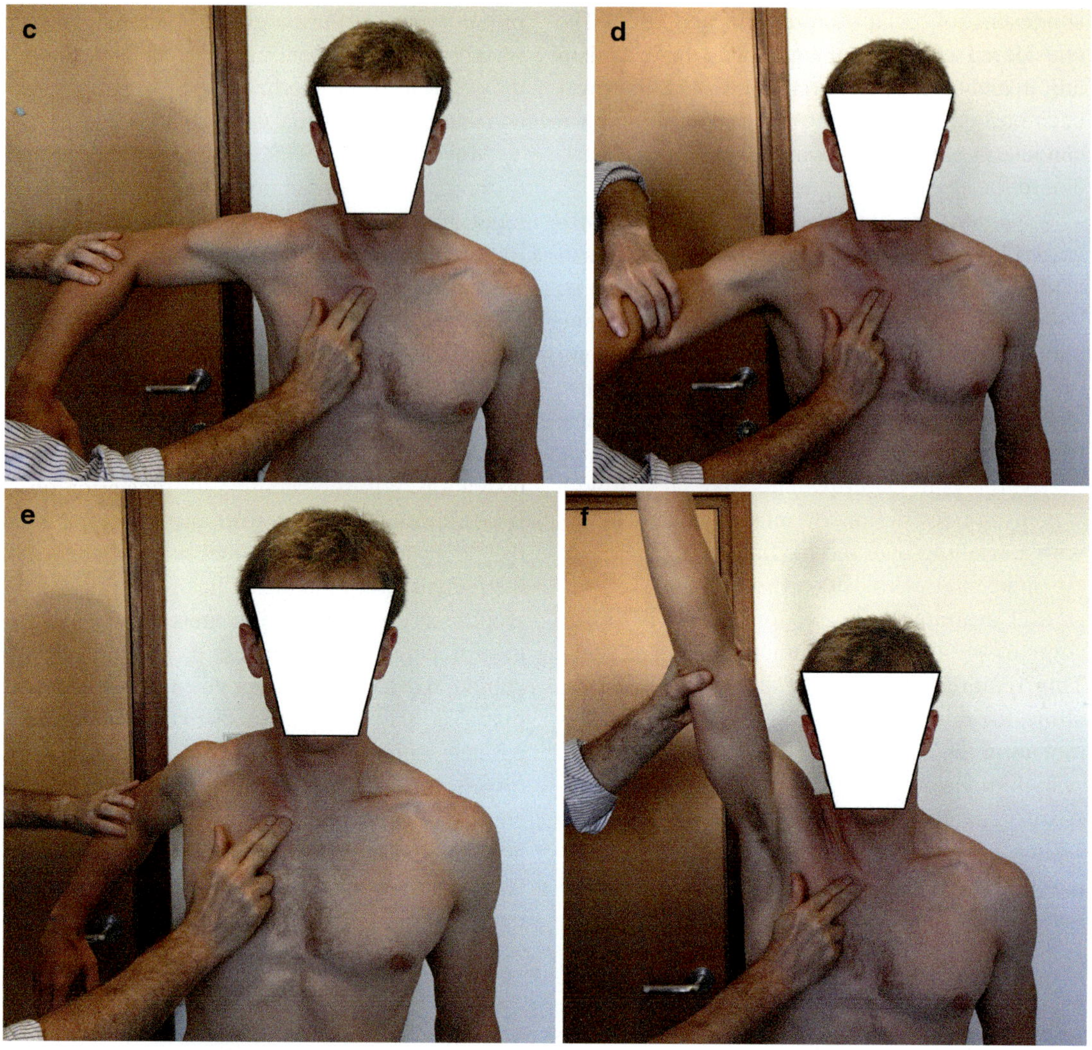

Fig. 1.2 (continued)

Sternoclavicular Joint Instability

Sterno-clavicular joint (SCJ) instability can be classified by direction (anterior or posterior), by severity (sprain, subluxation or dislocation – often referred to as type 1,2 or 3) or by whether it is acute, recurrent or persistent (chronic / unreduced). Whilst these classifications are descriptive none of them are able to take into account the traumatic or atraumatic nature of the instability. However, a classification system, that is a direct derivation of the Stanmore tri-polar instability triangle for the glenohumeral joint, has recently been described for the SCJ [11]. In the Stanmore SCJ instability classification there are three polar groups: type I traumatic structural, type II atraumatic structural and type III muscle patterning (neuromuscular) (Fig. 1.3). The type I traumatic structural group comprises traumatic subluxations and dislocations of the SCJ, as well as medial physeal fracture displacements. The type II atraumatic structural group comprises conditions which lead to laxity of the restraining ligaments, and includes connective tissue disorders (Marfan's, Ehlers Danlos), degenerative arthritis, inflammatory arthritis, infection and clavicular shortening secondary to previous malunion. The type III muscle patterning group can occur in isolation and is most commonly due to an over active or aberrant pectoralis major muscle but it can also develop secondary to a type I or type II disorder.

A continuum exists between the groups. Therefore, a patient with an initial type II instability can develop secondary muscle patterning (type III) over time; this patient would be then classified as type II/III. The effect of any treatment can also be monitored using the Stanmore SCJ instability classification system. Patients 'migrate' around the triangle, depending on the presenting pathology, and how that changes over time as their treatment progresses.

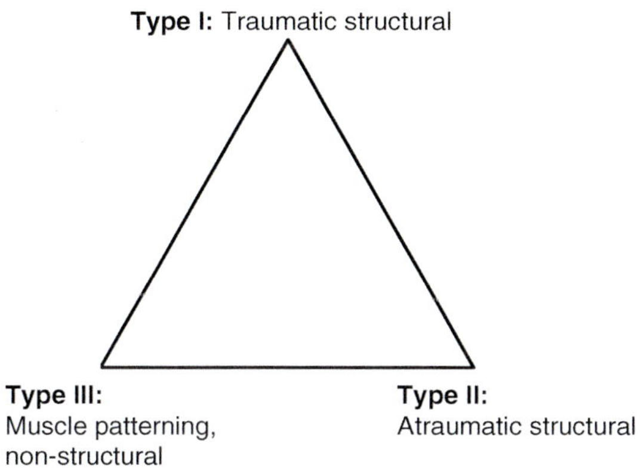

Fig. 1.3 Stanmore triangle

Type I Traumatic Structural

Traumatic SCJ dislocations are rare, accounting for less than 1% of upper limb injuries, and usually occur as the result of a high energy impact. The force is usually indirect and follows an impact either to the front or the back of the humeral head [12]. The force vector is then transferred along the clavicle resulting in disruption of the SCJ's restraining soft tissues. If the scapula is protracted at the time of impact a posterior dislocation is more likely and if the scapula is retracted it is more likely to dislocate anteriorly (Fig. 1.4). Less frequently a direct anterior blow to the clavicle can drive the medial end posteriorly into the mediastinum [13]. Biomechanical studies have shown that the force required to dislocate the SCJ posteriorly is 50% greater than that required to cause an anterior displacement [14].

A metanalysis of one hundred and forty adolescents with posterior SCJ dislocations reported that 71% occurred during sporting activities [15]. Although still rare this requires particular vigilance by pitch side sports physicians and physiotherapists as over 30% of patients following an acute posterior SCJ dislocation develop

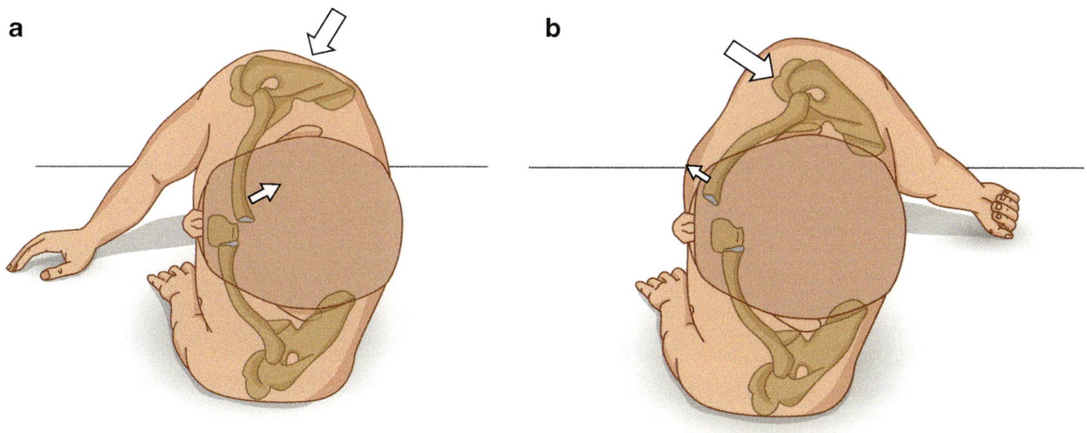

Fig. 1.4 Mechanism of injury. (**a**) Posterior dislocation: the scapula is protracted with an indirect force to the posterior shoulder. (**b**) Anterior dislocation: the scapula is retracted with an indirect force to the anterior shoulder

mediastinal pressure symptoms. Acute symptoms include dyspnoea (14%) and dysphagia (22.5%) due to pressure on the trachea and oesophagus and venous congestion or oedema of the ipsilateral arm due to compression of the vessels (14%). Less common complications of posterior dislocations include mediastinal hematoma, vessel laceration (leading to death), stroke, pneumomediastinum, pneumohemothorax, and venous thromboembolism (0.72–2.90%). As a result, an acute posterior SCJ dislocation should be treated as a medical emergency.

Patients presenting more chronically often complain of pain and deformity over the SCJ. In certain patients, as the medial clavicle has been pushed posteriorly, the whole of the shoulder girdle has rotated anteriorly and superiorly. As a result, the scapular tends to sit in a more superior and protracted position. Patients may complain of problems with glenohumeral function and of asymmetrical scapular protraction which, for example, can make sitting in high backed chairs uncomfortable as the medial scapula adopts a winged position (Fig. 1.5).

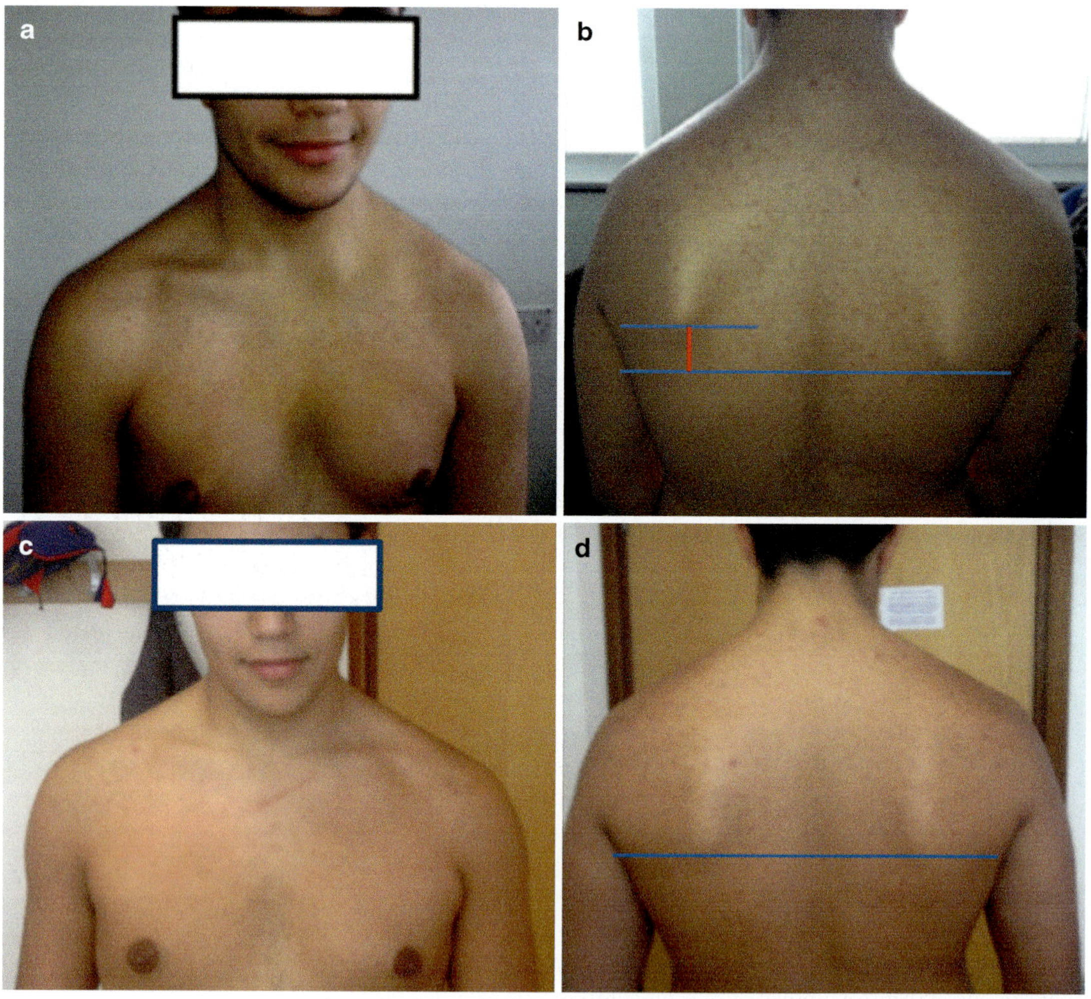

Fig. 1.5 Posterior dislocation. A 16 year old boy referred 4 weeks after sustaining a left posterior SCJ dislocation in a tobogganing accident. His CT scan confirmed an SCJ dislocation rather than an expected medial clavicular physeal injury. (**a**) Anterior view: note the asymmetry and loss of clavicular contour on the left. (**b**) Posterior view. Note the elevated and winged scapula on the left hand side. 3 months following open reduction and stabiisation using a figure of eight gracilis graft. (**c**) Anterior view: clavicular symmetry has been returned. (**d**) Posterior view: the left scapula has now returned to its normal position

On examination a patient with an anterior SCJ dislocation presents with an obvious forward displacement of the clavicle, while a patient with a posterior dislocation demonstrates asymmetry compared to the contralateral side, with diminution of the entire clavicular contour on the affected side. However, following an acute posterior dislocation, significant soft-tissue swelling often occurs over the first few days making a posterior deformity less obvious. It can also be difficult to clinically distinguish a medial clavicular physis fracture-dislocation from a true SCJ dislocation. A high clinical suspicion for medial clavicle physeal injury should remain for anyone under the age of 25 years.

Traditionally initial investigations following an SCJ injury include plain radiography using a Serendipity view. However, these are often difficult to interpret. A plain chest x-ray may be considered following an acute injury to check for an associated pneumothorax secondary to rib fractures. Currently the investigation of choice is a CT scan or, in the case of a posterior dislocation, a CT angiogram, this should be undertaken as a matter of urgency in the acute situation should there be any concern with regards to mediastinal compromise [16]. A CT scan can accurately assess the position of the medial end of the clavicle with regards to the sternum and the contralateral SCJ. It can also differentiate between a dislocation and a medial physeal injury. A CT angiogram additionally shows the arch of the aorta and great vessels in relation to the medial clavicle (Fig. 1.6). An MRI scan has poorer bony resolution than a CT scan but is able to more effectively demonstrate the ligamentous structures following subluxation and recurrent dislocation. It is also able to assess the intra-articular disc for injury and the condition of adjacent neurovascular anatomy.

Management of Type 1 SCJ instability depends on the severity of the injury, the direction of instability and the time from injury. Anterior and posterior undisplaced ligamentous sprains and subluxations of the SCJ (Grades 1 and 2) and minimally displaced medial physeal fractures can usually be treated with conservative measures. Initial reassurance, oral analgesia, and ice coupled with a short period of immobilisation

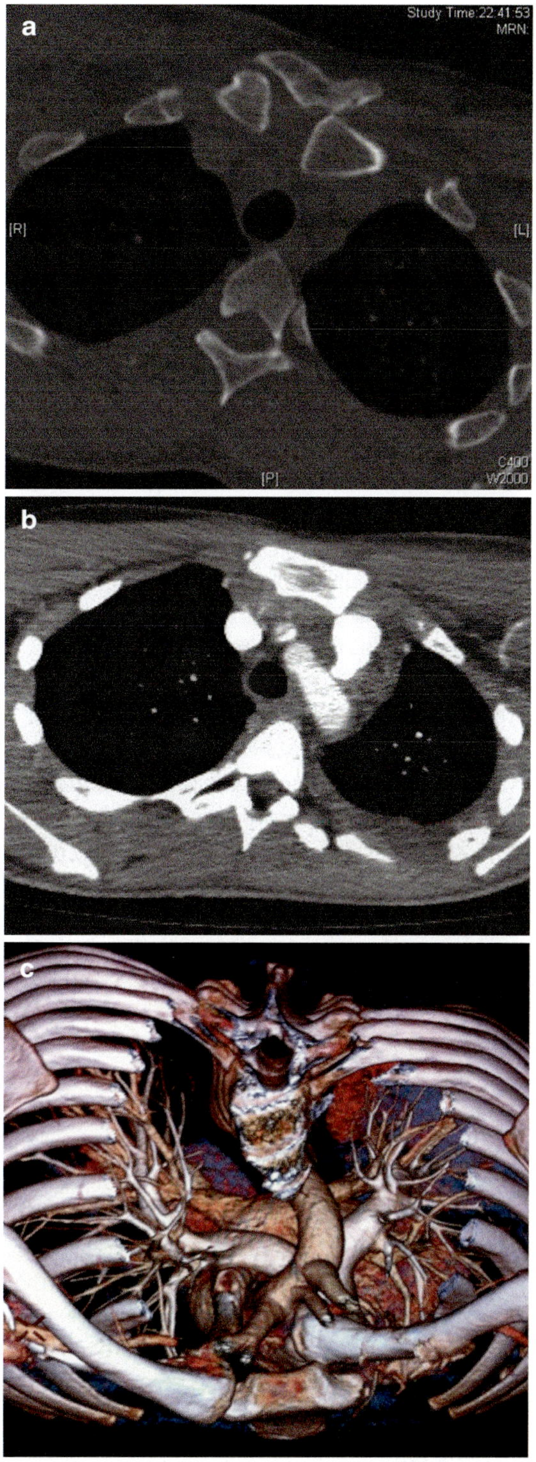

Fig. 1.6 CT scan (plain, angiogram and 3D reconstruction) of an acute posterior dislocation of the left SCJ. (**a**) Plain CT: axial view. (**b**) CT angiogram: axial view. The dislocated medial end of the left clavicle is abutting the arch of the aorta. (**c**) CT angiogram 3D reconstruction: the medial end of the clavicle is sitting on the arch of the aorta

in a sling is usually sufficient. The patient should be advised to avoid re-injury for 3 months and should avoid contact sports or other high-risk activities until there is a resolution of clinical symptoms [17]. There is no brace or support that will provide any extra protection to the SCJ on return to contact sports.

The management of SCJ dislocations (Grade 3 injuries) is dependent on the direction and the time after injury (<48 h or later). For anterior dislocations that are less than 48 h post injury, a closed reduction under sedation or general anaethetic can be attempted. With a bolster placed under the patient between their scapulaethe clavicle is pushed in a posterior direction. The SCJ usually reduces easily but sometimes traction to the arm is necessary to pull the clavicle laterally. The arm should then be kept in a sling for 4 weeks in internal rotation [11]. Unfortunately, in over 50% of cases the SCJ re-dislocates.

The majority of surgeons adopt a wait and see policy following an anterior dislocation. Over a period of 3 to 6 months many patients' symptoms settle with conservative management, including a combination of physiotherapy and time [14]. A recent study has described a surgical repair technique for the treatment of first time traumatic anterior dislocations of the SCJ in younger patients involved in contact sports. They undertook a repair and plication of the anterior capsule augmented with internal bracing in 6 patients following a first time anterior dislocation. At a median follow-up of 28.2 months (range 24–35 months) none of the patients had sustained a further dislocation and they had all returned to their pre-injury level of sport [18].

If a patient continues to experience significant symptoms, despite an adequate period of conservative management, or if they sustain further recurrent dislocations then surgical stabilisation may be considered. This would usually require reconstruction using an autograft, allograft or synthetic ligament [19].

For posterior SCJ dislocations there is a greater need to reduce and maintain reduction of the joint. In the acute situation, in the face of mediastinal compromise, this is particularly the case. A chronic posterior dislocation may affect shoulder girdle function due to protraction of the scapula and there are concerns of potentially developing erosion to the subclavian artery or thoracic duct injury and trachea-oesophageal fistula. Although these complications are rare their probability will increase over time and so operative reduction and stabilisation may perhaps be of more consideration the younger the patient. Closed reduction is only generally considered if the injury is less than 48 h old. Closed reduction manoeuvers after 48 h are discouraged, as they may result in tearing of posterior structures, owing to the formation of adhesions. Closed reduction is undertaken using a general anaesthetic and a radio-translucent table allowing access for fluoroscopy. A bolster is placed posteriorly between the scapulae with the patient supine. Abduction, traction and extension are applied to the affected arm and a towel clip is used to grasp the medial clavicle and to pull it anteriorly [20].

Closed reduction of an acute posterior dislocation is difficult, with a reported success rate of approximately 50% in those cases attempted within 48 h and of 31% between the second and fifth day [15]. In a multicentre series of 30 acute posterior dislocations, of the 16 cases that were treated within 48 h, 7 required an open reduction and 2 of the 7 cases that could be reduced re-dislocated within 7 days and required a subsequent open stabilisation [21]. If a closed reduction is successful, due to soft-tissue swelling and difficulties in interpreting fluoroscopy images around the SCJ, a repeat CT scan to confirm the reduction has been maintained should be undertaken the next day.

Considering the high potential failure rate for a closed reduction it is important to consider, pre-operatively, the potential need to proceed to an open reduction and stabilisation. This may mean that a patient requires transfer to an appropriate facility where cardiothoracic cover is available.

Open reduction in the acute phase is usually technically easier due to the lack of adhesions, and the consequent diminished risk to the posterior mediastinal structures. In the chronic situation preoperative planning with a CT arteriogram with discussion and collaboration with a cardiothoracic surgeon are essential. Any likely adhesions to the posterior mediastinal vascular structures, with the brachiocephalic veins in particular, can then be anticipated. A transverse incision is made over the SCJ and, after freeing any adhesions, the clavicle is reduced by anterior and laterally directed traction applied through a towel clip or bone holding forceps. The normal capsular and ligamentous stabilisers are usually only partially repairable and are not biomechanically sufficient to maintain the reduction and, as a result, an open reduction will usually require some form of additional reconstruction [22].

Various types of wires and pins have been used to stabilise the joint, however, due to reported lethal complications, these techniques have, in the most part, been abandoned [23]. Reconstruction using sutures alone through osseous drill holes or suture anchors have been reported but with only marginal biomechanical results. The most recent trend has been towards reconstruction techniques using autograft (palmaris longus, semitendinosis, gracilis or sternocleidomastoid) or allograft. Several techniques have been described and although satisfactory outcomes have been reported for most techniques, a figure-of-eight reconstruction appears to be biomechanically superior and may lead to better longer term outcomes [22]. In this technique the graft is shuttled through 3.2 mm drill holes in the strenum and medial end of the clavicle. Synthetic ultra-strong synthetic braided sutures, such as Orthocord (DePuy Mitek, Raynham, Massachussetts) and Fibrewire (Arthrex, Naples, Florida) may be useful in augmenting the graft. The ends of the graft are then tensioned and sutured together, any surrounding remnants of the capsule may be incorporated into the repair (Fig. 1.7).

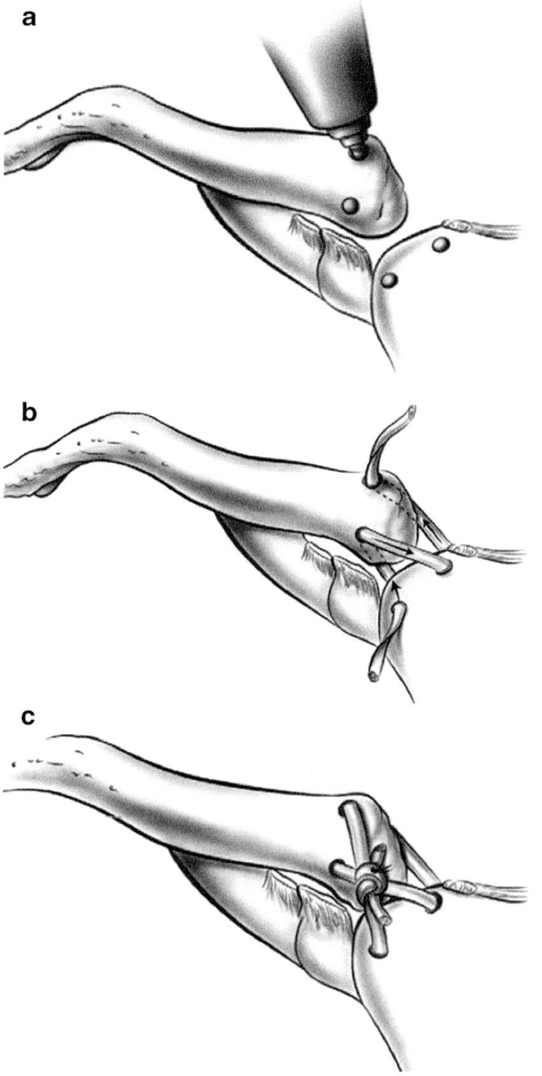

Fig. 1.7 SCJ reconstruction using a figure-of-eight hamstring tendon graft. (**a**) 3.2 mm drill holes are made in the medial end of the clavicle and the sternum. (**b**) Tendon graft is passed through the holes in a figure of eight. (**c**) The tendon ends are tensioned and sutured/tied together

Medial Physeal Clavicle Fractures

The medial clavicular epiphysis does not ossify until between 18 and 25 years of age. As a result, injury to the SCJ in patients younger than twenty five may actually lead to a displaced medial physeal fracture rather than a straightforward dislocation. A CT scan is the investigation of choice (Fig. 1.8). Fortunately, most physeal injuries are either un- or minimally displaced and rarely extend into the SCJ [24]. These injuries can be treated non-operatively with immobilisation in a sling.

More than 50% of patients with significantly displaced fractures that are treated non-operatively end up with persistent discomfort [14]. Some authors recommend an attempt at closed reduction for posteriorly displaced fractures within 7 days of injury. Open reduction should be

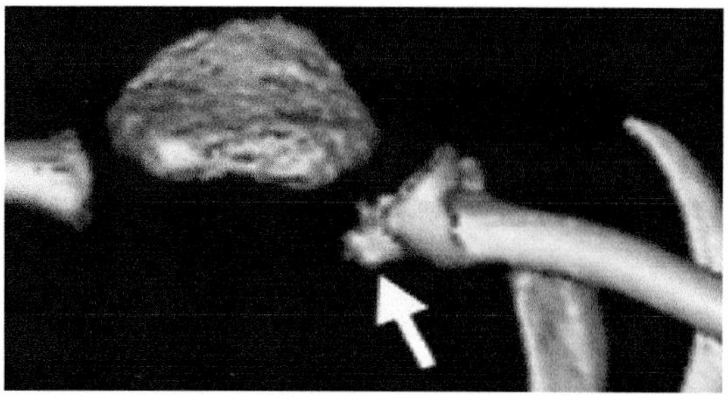

Fig. 1.8 CT 3D reconstruction of a right clavicular medial physeal fracture in a 19 year old man

reserved for injuries associated with mediastinal compressive symptoms [14]. Medial clavicle physeal injuries are stable once reduced and usually do not require fixation [25]. Anterior physeal injuries and posterior injuries presenting after 7 days may be treated symptomatically, with a degree of remodelling possible depending on the age of the patient.

Miscellaneous Causes of Type I Instability

Clavicular malunion resulting in relative anterior angulation of the medial end of the clavicle can give the appearance and sensation of anterior subluxation. This is particularly accentuated during retraction of the scapula and over time can lead to type II instability due to stretching out the anterior SCJ capsule. Other conditions which place the scapula in persistently abnormal positions, such as occurs with scoliosis, also predispose to atraumatic SCJ instability [11]. If the clavicular malunion induced SCJ symptoms are significant a corrective clavicular corrective osteotomy with a simultaneous SCJ stabilisation procedure may be necessary.

Type II Atraumatic Structural

Type II SCJ instability occurs as the result of either increased laxity or stretching out of the joint stabilising ligaments. It can be caused by a variety of pathologies including conditions that lead to ligamentous laxity (Marfan's, Ehlers Danlos) or those that can weaken or stretch the ligaments such as degenerative and inflammatory arthritis, infection and clavicular shortening, secondary to fracture malunion. Correct diagnosis therefore requires an accurate history and careful local and systemic examination.

In cases of capsular laxity clinical evidence of a generalised ligamentous laxity secondary to conditions such as Ehlers-Danlos and Marfan's may be present. Typically patients present in their teens with no specific history of trauma, with a prominence and subluxation of the medial clavicle and associated pain with overhead activities. The majority of patients can be managed successfully with physiotherapy and corticosteroid injections. In the largest reported series twenty nine of thirty seven patients (78%) returned to full activity when treated non operatively [26]. Eight of the patients (21%) had ongoing discomfort with evidence of persistent subluxation remaining in nearly all cases. The authors cautioned against surgical treatment of these cases as all of the patients that were managed surgically reported unsatisfactory results.

Owing to the much stronger posterior capsular restraints posterior atraumatic type II instability secondary to ligamentous laxity is much rarer than anterior [22, 27]. However, in a similar way to the traumatic posterior dislocations, if at any point a patient's symptoms should become suggestive of retrosternal compression an open operative reduction is indicated.

Type III Muscle Patterning

Type III instability is characterised by poorly co-ordinated afferent and efferent neuromuscular biofeedback loops in the presence of otherwise normal musculature and a structurally normal joint. The pectoralis major is the most commonly affected muscle and can be confirmed with EMG studies. Management focuses on re-learning the correct patterns of muscle contraction with proprioceptive feedback playing an important role [28]. Occasionally Botulinum toxin is can be used to suppress hypertonicity in pectoralis major, if slow progress is being made with physiotherapy treatment.

Muscle patterning can also arise secondary to type I or II instabilities, making the diagnosis lie on the I/III or II/III axis. In this situation, it is important that the biofeedback loops are addressed prior to any stabilisation surgery. Botulinum toxin should be considered routinely pre-operatively in order to protect the ligamentous stabilisation in the first 3 months post operatively.

Clinical Pearl

Acute dislocation of the SCJ is usually the result of a high-energy injury and should be treated expectantly. Plain radiographs are insufficient and a CT or MRI should be undertaken. Mediastinal symptoms occur in 30% of patients with a posterior dislocation and discussion and referral on to a specialist unit should be considered.

Sternoclavicular Joint Ostoearthritis

Osteoarthritis of the SCJ is relatively common in patients over the age of 50 and particularly in women. Evidence of osteoarthritic changes at the sternoclavicular joint (SCJ) have been shown to be present on computed tomography scans in over 90% of patients over the age of 60 years [29]. However, it is usually asymptomatic and may present as a painless lump secondary to effusion and osteophytes. When symptomatic patients complain of pain, crepitus and clicking. This is particularly on cross body adduction and related to overhead sports such as tennis and golf.

Non-operative treatment including physiotherapy, NSAID medications and ultrasound guided intra-articular steroid injection are adequate in the majority of cases. Occasionally, in patients with unremitting symptoms, resection of the degenerate disc and the medial end of the clavicle are indicated. When undertaken as an open procedure the patient requires a period of immobilisation to protect the repaired anterior SCJ ligament [30]. It is now possible to do this arthroscopically as a day case without immobilisation [31] (Fig. 1.9). The results of an excision arthroplasty of the medial end of the clavicle for SCJ osteoarthritis, whether undertaken as an open or arthroscopic procedure, are good, with over 80% of patients scoring their SCJ as good or excellent after a minimum follow-up of 2 years [30, 31].

Arthritic involvement of the SCJ has been reported in over 30% of patients with rheumatoid arthritis and in 90% of patients with severe psoriatic arthritis. The management of these conditions usually involves systemic pharmacological suppression and local intra-articular steroid injections. However, in severely affected cases debridement of the SCJ and stabilisation maybe considered.

Clinical Pearl

Excision arthroplasty of the medial end of the clavicle is usually a very successful treatment for patients with symptomatic SCJ osteoarthritis that have failed non-operative treatment.

Sternoclavicular Joint Disc Injuries

The SCJ is divided into medial and lateral halves by a complete fibrocartilaginous disc which resembles a discoid meniscus in the lateral compartment of the knee. Although rare, damage to the disc can cause symptoms of pain and clicking of the joint on movement. Sometimes this clicking can be mistaken for minor anterior subluxation. In younger patients a shearing injury results in a complex tear in the middle part of an otherwise normal disc. This can occur when the joint is both loaded and twisting, such as in serving in tennis. In older patients there is usually pre-existing degenerative change present and the disc usually has torn from the superior periphery

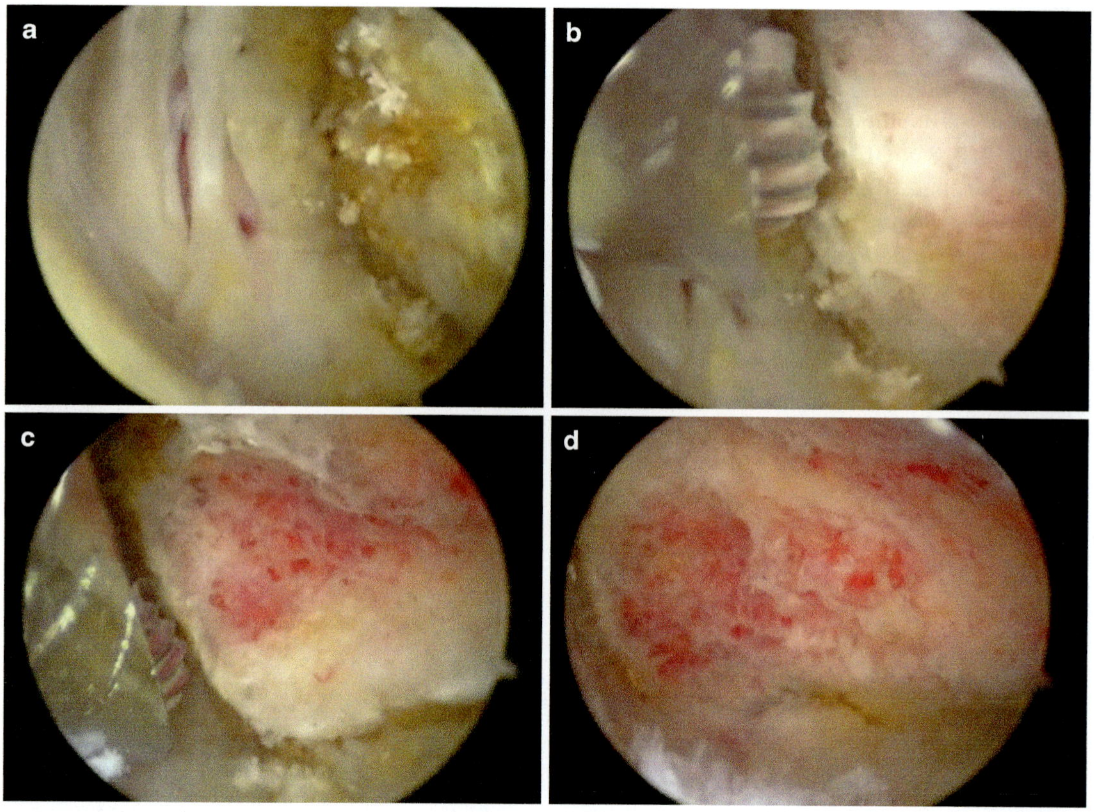

Fig. 1.9 Intra-operative arthroscopic pictures of a left SCJ arthroscopic excision. (**a**) The residual articular cartilage and soft-tissue has been resected off of the medial end of the clavicle (C). The intact posterior joint capsule (P) can be seen with the relatively well preserved sternal articular surface on the left (S). (**b**) A 4 mm acromioniser burr has been introduced through the superior portal and is beginning to resect the superior part of the medial end of the clavicle. (**c**) Boney resection has progressed inferiorly and medially to the inferior recess of the joint with the tip of the inferior osteophyte about to be resected. (**d**) Resection has been completed with the intact inferior capsule clearly visible

of the joint. There are often associated degenerative articular changes present within the joint.

An MRI scan can usually demonstrate a disc tear which has a characteristic wavy appearance when compared to the normal ipsilateral side (Fig. 1.10). A CT scan is not able to demonstrate the disc.

An ultrasound guided cortisone injection can be tried as the first line of treatment. If this is unsuccessful resection of the torn disc is indicated. This has previously been done as an open procedure but can now be undertaken arthroscopically [32, 33]. At surgery the whole of the disc is resected back to a stable rim. In the presence of a degenerative tear, resection of the medial end of the clavicle may also be undertaken if there are significant associated osteoarthritic symptoms.

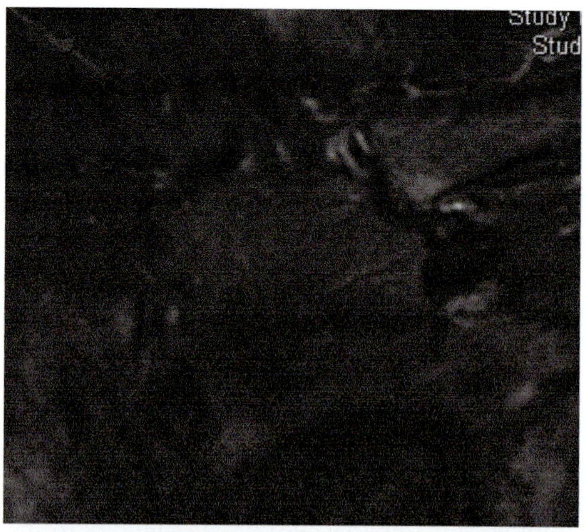

Fig. 1.10 MRI scan (T2) demonstrating a wavy appearance of the superior disc with a small joint effusion. This represent a tear/detatchment of the superior part of the discleft from the capsule. SCJ disc

Miscellaneous Sternoclavicular Pathologies

The SCJ can be the focus of a disparate group of other pathologies including inflammatory arthropathies, crystal-deposition arthropathies (gout and pseudogout), SAPHO syndrome (synovitis, acne, pustulosis hyperostosis and osteitis) and CRMO (chronic relapsing multifocal osteomyelitis). These conditions are all rare but the surgeon should be mindful of them as a potential differential diagnosis for a painful swollen SCJ. Initial investigations would be screening inflammatory markers (CRP, ESR) and either an MRI or CT scan.

Conclusion

Injury around the Sternoclavicular joint is relatively unusual. Injuries are usually high energy and result in instability and/or fracture of the medial end of the clavicle. An understanding of the complex arrangement of the ligaments, tendons and muscles that stabilise the joint and an appreciation of the posterior mediastinal structures is an essential requirement to treat these injuries successfully.

Osteoarthritis of the sternoclavicular joint is very common with increasing age and usually asymptomatic. Symptomatic osteoarthritis can usually be adequately treated with non-operative measures. In the unusual situation where symptoms persist, excision arthroplasty of the medial end of the clavicle, either as an open or arthroscopic procedure, is usually successful.

References

1. Warth RJ, Lee JT, Millett PJ. Anatomy and biomechanics of the sternoclavicular joint. Oper Tech Sports Med. 2014;22:248–52.
2. Lee JT, Campbell KJ, Mischalski MP, et al. Surgical anatomy of the sternoclavicular joint. J Bone Joint Surg Am. 2014;96(e166):1–10.
3. Emura K, Arakawa T, Terashima T, Miki A. Macroscopic and histological observations on the human sternoclavicular joint disc. Anat Sci Int. 2009;84(3):182–8.
4. Renfree KJ, Wright TW. Anatomy and biomechanics of the acromioclavicular and sternoclavicular joints. Clin Sports Med. 2003;22(2):219–37.
5. Spencer EE, Kuhn JE, Huston LJ, et al. Ligamentous restraints to anterior and posterior translation of the sternoclavicular joint. J Shoulder Elb Surg. 2002;11:43–7.
6. Tubbs RS, Loukas M, Slappey JB, et al. Surgical and clinical anatomy of the interclavicular ligament. Surg Radiol Anat. 2007;29:357–60.
7. Tubbs RS, Shah NA, Sullivan BP, et al. The costoclavicular ligament revisited: a functional and anatomical study. Romanian J Morphol Embryol. 2009;50(3):475–9.
8. Koch MJ, Wells L. Proximal clavicle physeal fracture with posterior displacement: diagnosis, treatment, and prevention. Orthopaedics. 2012;35(1):e108–11.
9. Webb PA, Schuey JM. Epiphyseal union of the anterior iliac crest and medial clavicle in a modern multiracal sample of American males and females. Am J Phys Anthropol. 1985;68:4567–466.
10. Ludewig PM, Behrens SA, Meyer SM, et al. Three-dimensional clavicular motion during arm elevation: reliability and descriptive data. J Orthop Sports Phys Ther. 2004;34:140–9.
11. Sewell MD, Al-Hadithy N, Le Leu A, Lambert SM. Instability of the sternoclavicular joint. Current concepts in classification, treatment and outcomes. Bone Joint J. 2013;95-B(6):721–31.
12. Mehta JC, Sachdev A, Collins JJ. Retrosternal dislocation of the clavicle. Injury. 1973;5:79–83.
13. Wirth MA, Rockwood CA Jr. Acute and chronic traumatic injuries of the sternoclavicular joint. J Am Acad Orthop Surg. 1996;4:268–78.
14. Thut D, Hergan D, Dukas A, et al. Sternoclavicular joint reconstruction: a systematic review. Bull NYU Hosp Jt Dis. 2011;69:128–35.
15. Tepolt F, Carry PM, Heyn PC. Posterior sternoclavicular joint injuries in the adolescent population: a meta-analysis. Am J Sports Med. 2014;42(10):2517–24.
16. Deutsch AL, Resnick D, Mink JH. Computed tomography of the glenohumeral and sternoclavicular joints. Orthop Clin North Am. 1985;16:497–511.
17. Yeh GL, Williams GR Jr. Conservative management of sternoclavicular injuries. Orthop Clin North Am. 2000;31:189–203.
18. Tytherleigh-Strong G, Pecheva M, Titchener A. Treatment of first-time traumatic anterior dislocation of the sternoclavicular joint with surgical repair of the anterior capsule augmented with internal bracing. Orthop J Sports Med. 2018;6(7):1–7.
19. Bak K, Fogh K. Reconstruction of the chronic anterior unstable sternoclavicular joint using a tendon autograft: medium-term to long-term follow-up result. J Shoulder Elb Surg. 2014;23:245–50.
20. Rockwood CA. Dislocations of the sternoclavicular joint. In: Evans EB, editor. American Academy of Orthopaedic Surgeons Instructional Course Lectures: Volume XXIV. CV Mosby: St Louis; 1975. p. 144–59.

21. Lafosse JM, Espie A, Bonnevialle N, Mansat P, Tricoire JL. Posterior dislocation of the sternoclavicular joint and epiphyseal disruption of the medial clavisle with posterior displacement in sports participants. J Bone Joint Surg Br. 2010;92:103–9.
22. Spencer EE, Kuhn JE. Biomechanical analysis of reconstructions for sternoclavicular joint instability. J Bone Joint Surg Am. 2014;86(1):98–105.
23. Morell DJ, Thyagarajan DS. Sternoclavicular joint dislocation and its management. A review of the literature. World J Orthop. 2016;7:244–50.
24. Nordqvist A, Petersson C. The incidence of fractures of the clavicle. Clin Orthop Relat Res. 1994;300:127–32.
25. Lyons FA, Rockwood CA Jr. Migration of pins used in operations on the shoulder. J Bone Joint Surg Am. 1990;72-A:1262–7.
26. Rockwood CA Jr, Odor JM. Spontaneous atraumatic anterior subluxation of the sternoclavicular joint. J Bone Joint Surg Am. 1989;71-A:1280–8.
27. Martin SD, Altcheck D, Erlanger S. Atraumatic posterior dislocation of the sternoclavicular joint: a case report and literature review. Clin Orthop Relat Res. 1993;292:159–64.
28. Sonazaki H, Mitsui H, Miyanaga Y, et al. Clinical features of 53 cases with pustulotic arthro-osteitis. Annals Rheum Dis. 1981;40:547–53.
29. Lawrence CR, East B, Rashid A, Tytherleigh-Strong GM. The prevalance of osteoarthritis of the sternoclavicular joint on computed tomography. J Shoulder Elbow. 2017;26:e18–22.
30. Kattahagen CJ, Tahal DS, Menge TJ, Horan MP, Millett PJ. Minimum-2-year outcomes and return to sport following resection arthroplasty for the treatment of sternoclavicular joint osteoarthritis. J Shoulder Elb Surg. 2017;26:e37–43.
31. Tytherleigh-Strong G, Griffiths D. Arthroscopic excision of the sternoclavicluar joint for the treatment of strenoclavicular osteoarthritis. Arthroscopy. 2013;29:1487–91.
32. Delos D, Shindle MK, Mintz DN, Warren RF. Menisectomy of the sternoclavicular joint: a report of two cases. J Shoulder Elb Surg. 2010;19(4):e9–e12.
33. Tytherleigh-Strong G, Rashid A, Lawrence C, Morrissey D. Arthroscopic intra-articular disk excision of the sternoclavicular joint. Arthrosco Tech. 2017;6:e599–605.

Clavice Fracture

2

Rajesh Nanda and Amar Rangan

Introduction

'Clavicle' is derived from the early seventeenth century Latin word clavicula that means 'small key'. It is named so, because of its shape and the fact that it rotates 'like a key' on shoulder abduction. Clavicle is the only long bone that lies horizontally connecting the scapula to the sternum and is entirely subcutaneous thus easily accessible to inspection and palpation.

Codman (1934) mentions in his book the functional importance of clavicle in development of humans- "We are proud that our brains are more developed than the animals: we might also boast of our clavicles. It seems to me that the clavicle is one of man's greatest skeletal inheritances, for he depends to a greater extent than most animals, except the apes and monkeys, on the use of his hands and arms" [1].

As far back as 400BC Hippocrates is said to have noted the displacement pattern of the fractured clavicle; the distal fragment sagging with the arm and the proximal fragment point upwards. He stated that the fractures were difficult to reduce and maintain reduction but usually unites with a prominent callus and deformity [2].

The traditionally held belief that these fractures could generally be treated non-operatively has been brought into question in recent years, and the controversy over the optimal treatment has continued. Recent studies have shown a high prevalence of symptomatic malunion and non-union after non-operative treatment of displaced midshaft clavicular fractures while some studies have shown that the shortening in a malunion may be well tolerated.

Embryology

The clavicle is the first bone to ossify in the developing embryo and the only long bone to ossify by intramembranous ossification. It is formed by two membranous primary ossification centres appearing by 5–6 weeks and fusing approximately 1 week later. Cartilage at both ends of the clavicle then develops. In time, the medial cartilaginous mass contributes more (80%) to the growth in length of the clavicle than the lateral cartilaginous mass [3, 4].

The sternal ossification centre appears between 12 and 19 years and fuses relatively late in life, by 22 to 25 years of age [5, 6].

McGraw et al. (2009) [7] have shown at 18 years of age the mean clavicle length +/-SD

R. Nanda (✉)
Department of Trauma & Orthopaedic Surgery, University Hospital of North Tees & Hartlepool, Hardwick Stockton on Tees, UK

A. Rangan
Department of Trauma & Orthopaedic Surgery, James Cook University Hospital, Middlesbrough, UK

University of Oxford, Oxford, UK

University of York, York, UK

I. A. Trail et al. (eds.), *Textbook of Shoulder Surgery*, https://doi.org/10.1007/978-3-319-70099-1_2

for females was 149+/−12 mm and for males it was 161+/−11 mm. They noted a statistically significant difference (P = 0.049) between the length of right and left clavicles though it was not clinically significant (0.036 mm). A steady growth rate was noted for both genders from birth to the age of 12 years (8.4 mm/y). Above the age of 12 years there were significant differences in the growth of the clavicles of girls (2.6 mm/y) versus boys (5.4 mm/y) (P < 0.001).

Girls achieve 80% of their clavicle length by 9 years of age and boys by 12 years of age. This could be useful in planning management of a displaced clavicular fracture in adolescent age.

Anatomy [8]

Clavicle has a double curve, the convexity being directed forward at the sternal end and the concavity at the scapular end. It articulates medially with the manubrium sterni, and laterally with the acromion of the scapula. Its lateral third is flattened from above downward, while its medial two-thirds is rounded to prismatic form.

The **lateral third of the clavicle** (Figs. 2.1 and 2.2) has 2 surfaces and 2 borders – **upper surface** with attachments of deltoid anteriorly and trapezius posteriorly. The **under surface** has 2 ridges named after the attachments of conoid and trapezoid ligaments; **anterior border** (deltoid attachment) and **posterior border** (trapezius attachment).

The **medial two-thirds** (Figs. 2.1 and 2.2) of the clavicle has 3 surfaces and 3 borders – **anterior surface** is continuous with the superior surface of the flattened portion. It is smooth, convex, and nearly subcutaneous, being covered only by the platysma. Pectoralis major and sternocleidomastoid is attached medially. The **posterior or cervical surface** is smooth, and looks backward toward the root of the neck. It gives attachment,

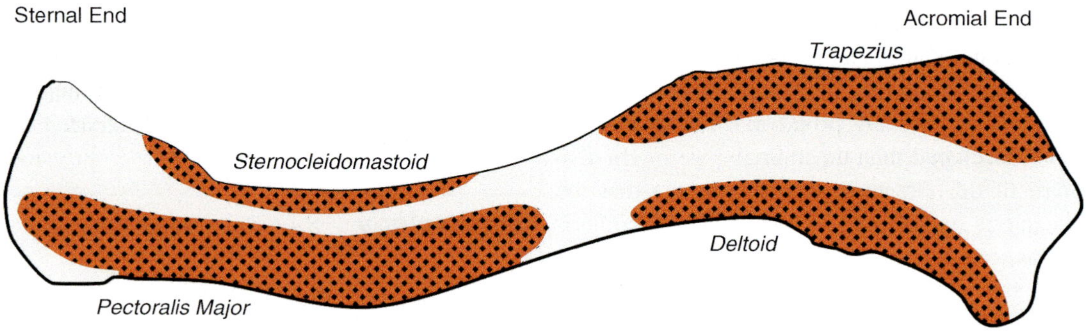

Fig. 2.1 Left clavicle –superior view and attachments

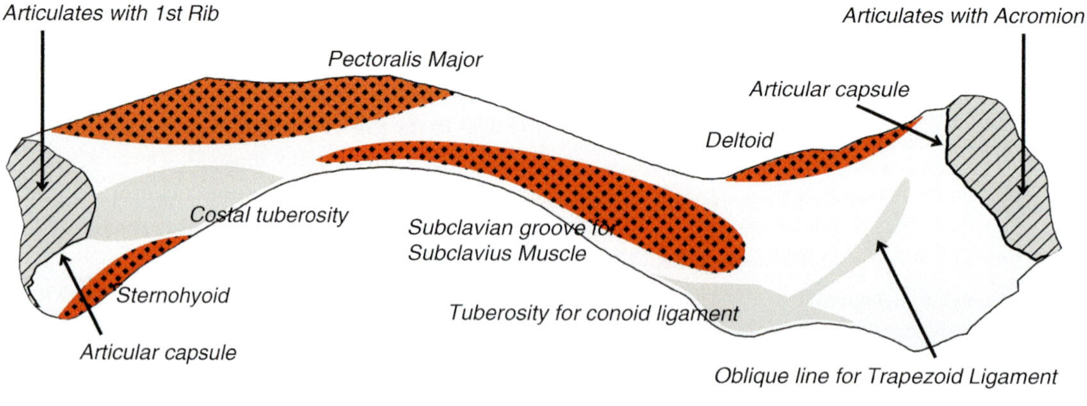

Fig. 2.2 Left clavicle – inferior view and attachments

near the sternal extremity, to part of the sternohyoid. Nutrient artery foramen is present on this surface. The **inferior or subclavian surface** is narrowed medially, but gradually increases in width laterally, and is continuous with the under surface of the flat portion. On its medial part is the attachment of the costoclavicular ligament. The rest of this surface is occupied by a groove, which gives attachment to the subclavius; The **anterior border** provides attachments of the pectoralis major. The **superior border** provides attachment to sternocleidomastoid. The **posterior or subclavian border** gives attachment to a layer of cervical fascia which envelops the omohyoid.

The Sternal End – the clavicle is prismatic (triangular). It presents an articular facet which articulates with the manubrium sterni with an articular disk. The lower part of the facet for articulation with the cartilage of the first rib.

The Acromial End is small, flattened, oval surface directed obliquely downward, for articulation with the acromion of the scapula. The circumference of the articular facet is rough for the attachment of the acromioclavicular ligaments. The scapula and clavicle are bound securely by both the acromioclavicular and coracoclavicular (conoid & trapezoid) ligaments.

Harrington et al. (1993) [9] studied the peculiar lazy 'S' shape of the clavicle and found varying porosity and bone density along its length. They found the most porosity and moments of inertia are located in the variably shaped sternal and acromial thirds of the bone as opposed to the denser, smaller, and more circular central third of the bone found to be weakest part of the bone. This attributed to the clavicle's biomechanical behavior and concur with the fracture location most commonly reported clinically.

Function

The clavicle provides attachment to various muscles of the shoulder girdle. It connects the axial skeleton (thorax) to the appendicular skeleton (shoulder girdle and arm) thus provides a stable linkage of the arm–trunk mechanism and contributes significantly to the power and stability of the arm and shoulder girdle, especially in movement above shoulder level [10, 11].

The clavicle provides skeletal protection for adjacent neurovascular structures and the superior aspect of the lung. The subclavian artery and vein and the brachial plexus (Fig. 2.3), pass from a posterosuperior to anteroinferior direction,

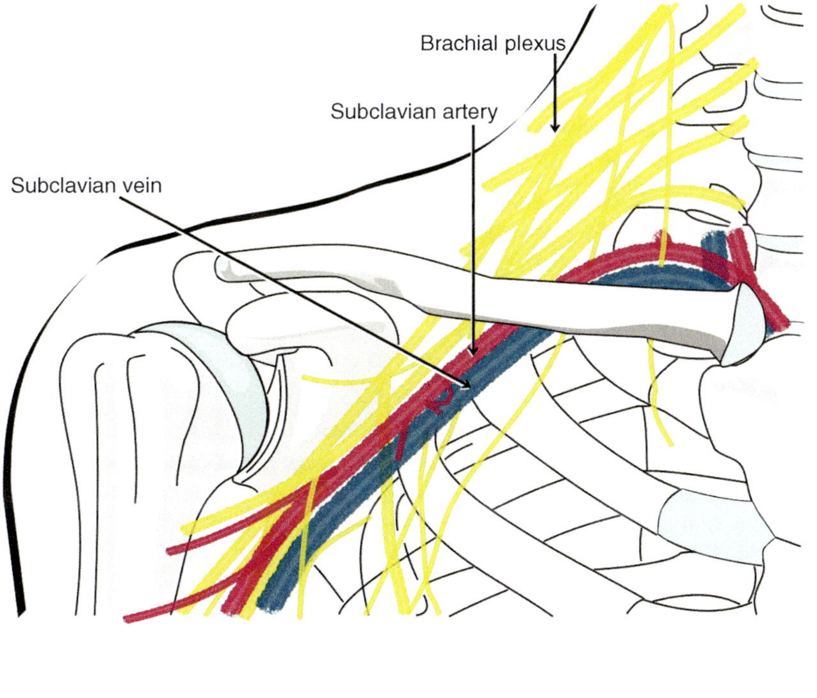

Fig. 2.3 Relationship of neurovascular structures to right clavicle – the subclavian artery and vein and the brachial plexus

between the first rib and the clavicle at the junction of its medial and middle thirds and are thus vulnerable during surgery and instrumentation. CT arteriogram have shown that at the medial end of the clavicle the subclavian vessels are situated behind it, with the vein intimately related to it. In some scans the vein was opposed to the posterior cortex of the clavicle. At the middle one-third of the clavicle the artery and vein are a mean of 17.02mm (5.4–26.8) and 12.45mm (5–26.1) from the clavicle, respectively, and at a mean angle of 50° [12–80] and 70° [38–100], respectively, to the horizontal. In the middle third or the tubular portion, the subclavius muscle and fascia protect the neurovascular structures from the fracture. At the lateral end of the clavicle the artery and vein are at mean distances of 63.4mm (46.8–96.5) and 75.67mm [50–109], respectively [12].

Epidemiology

Fractures of the clavicle are common, accounting for 2.6–4% of adult fractures and account for about a third of injuries to the shoulder girdle [13–15].

The annual incidence of clavicular fractures is estimated to be between 29 and 64 per 100,000 population per year [13, 14, 16].

Fractures of the shaft account for between 69% and 82%, the lateral-end account for 21–28%, and of the medial-end account for 2–3% of all clavicle fractures [13, 15, 17].

A study by Nowak in 2000 showed that the incidence of clavicle fractures in Uppsala, Sweden, was 50 per 100,000 population; however, the incidence in male patients was 71 per 100,000, and the incidence in female patients was 30 per 100,000 [16].

Another Swedish study showed 68% of the clavicle fractures occurred in males and 32% in females (male: female ratio of 2.2:1). Mean age was 48 years (SD 23 years). Mean age was higher in females (mean 59 years, SD 23 years) than in males (mean 43 years, SD 21 years). The fractures occurred more often in younger than in older individuals, with 15–24-year-olds representing 21% of the study population. Males in this age group represented 17% of the total fracture burden. As many as 45% of the females but only 17% of the males were 65 years or older [18].

Incidence of clavicle fractures is commonest in males less than 30 years. This is attributed to direct force trauma sustained during sporting activities. A second, smaller peak of incidence occurs in elderly patients (over 80 years of age), with a slight female predominance. These fractures tend to be related to osteoporosis, sustained during low-energy domestic falls [13].

Shaft fractures occur most commonly in young adults, whereas lateral and medial-end fractures are more common in older individuals [17].

Classifications of Fractures of the Clavicle

Allman classified fractures of the clavicle into 3 groups [19].

Group 1: fractures of the middle third – when there is displacement, the proximal fragment of the clavicle is usually elevated and the shoulder with the distal fragment is displaced downwards and inwards.

Group 2: fractures distal to the coraco-clavicular ligament.

Group 3: fractures of the proximal end of the clavicle – are infrequent and if the costo-clavicular ligament remains intact and attached to the outer fragment, there is little or no displacement.

Neer also classified clavicular fractures in 3 groups [20, 21]

1. Mid-clavicular fracture middle third (80%).
2. Fracture of the distal clavicle; or inter-ligamentous fracture (15%).
3. Fracture of the inner clavicle; inner third (5%).

Neer sub-divided the **fractures of the distal clavicle** into 3 different types

Type 1: minimal displacement with intact ligaments.

Type 2: displaced with detachment of the ligaments from the proximal fragment.

Type 3: fractures of the articular surface.

Neer suggested there were 4 displacing forces leading to distraction of distal clavicle fractures and leading to a higher risk of delayed / nonunion.

Trapezius muscle – This attaches upon the entire outer third of the clavicle and draws the large medial fragment posteriorly within its substance. Inter-position of this muscle is common. The skin may be tented posteriorly over the end of the shaft.

Weight of the arm – As the scapula and arm descend, the outer fragment, retaining its attachment to trapezoid ligament and the acromion, is pulled downwards and forwards.

Trunk muscles attaching the humerus and scapula. These displaced the outer fragment medially towards the apex of the thorax.

Rotary displacement – The scapular ligaments may rotate the outer fragment as much as 40° with movement of the arm. No similar rotation of the medial fragment occurs because it is detached.

Classification of Clavicular Fractures According to Craig [22, 23] (Table 2.1)

On the basis of Allman's classification, in 1990 Craig introduced a more detailed classification of clavicular fractures that was based on the variable fracture pattern seen within the 3 broad groups of Allman's clavicle fracture classification. See Table 2.1.

Group I fractures or fractures of the middle third are the most common fractures and accounts for 80% of clavicular fractures. They occur at the point at which the clavicle changes to a flattened cross-section from a prismatic cross-section. The force of the traumatic impact follows the curve of the clavicle and disperses on reaching the lateral curve. In addition, the proximal and distal fragments of the clavicle are mechanically secure by ligamentous structures and muscular attachments, whereas the central segment is relatively free.

Table 2.1 Classification of Clavicle Fractures according to Craig

Group I: fracture of the middle third
Group II: fracture of the distal third
Type I: minimal displacement (inter-ligamentous)
Type II: displaced secondary to a fracture medial to the coraco-clavicular ligaments
A – Conoid and trapezoid attached
B – Conoid torn, trapezoid attached
Type III: fractures of the articular surface
Type IV: ligaments intact to the periosteum (children) with displacement of the proximal fragment
Type V: comminuted with ligaments attached neither proximally or distally, but to an inferior, comminuted fragment
Group III: fracture of the proximal third
Type I: minimal displacement
Type II: displaced (ligaments ruptured)
Type III: intra-articular
Type IV: epiphyseal separation (children and young adults)
Type V: comminuted

Group II fractures account for 12–15% of all clavicle fractures and are sub-classified according to the location of the coraco-clavicular ligaments relative to the fracture fragments.

Type I fractures are the most common by a ratio of 4:1. In this fracture, the ligaments remain intact or hold the fragments together and prevent rotation, tilting or significant displacement. This fracture is an inter-ligamentous fracture that occurs between the conoid and trapezoid or between the coraco-clavicular and acromio-clavicular ligaments.

In ***type II*** distal clavicle fractures, the coraco-clavicular ligaments are detached from the medial segment. Both the conoid and trapezoid may be on the distal fragment, or the conoid ligament may be ruptured while the trapezoid ligament remains attached to the distal fragment. There is really no functional difference between these 2 fractures. The high rate of non-union in these fractures may be secondary to excessive motion at the fracture site. These fractures are equivalent to a serious acromio-clavicular separation in which the normal constraints to the antero-medial rotation of the scapula relative to the clavicle are lost. Craig (similar to Neer) described four forces that may impair healing and may be contributing factors to the reported high incidence of non-union act on this fracture. When the patient is erect, the outer fragment which retains the attachment of the trapezoid ligament to the scapula through the intact acromio-clavicular ligaments is pulled downwards and forward by the weight of the arm; The pectoralis major, pectoralis minor and latissimus dorsi draw the distal segment downwards and medially, thereby causing overriding; The scapula may rotate the distal fragment as the arm is moved; The trapezius muscle attaches upon the outer two-thirds of the clavicle, whereas the sternocleidomastoid muscle attaches to the middle third and these muscles act to draw the clavicular segment superiorly and posteriorly, often into the substance of the trapezius muscle.

Type III distal clavicle fractures involve the articular surface of the acromio-clavicular joint alone. Although type II fractures may have intra-articular extension, type III fractures are characterised by a break in the articular surface between a ligamentous injury. A type III injury may be subtle or may be confused with a first degree acromio-clavicular separation, and may require special views to visualise. It may, in fact, be manifested as late degenerative joint arthrosis of the acromio-clavicular joint. In addition, it has been suggested that in 'weightlifters' clavicle, resorption of the distal end of the clavicle may occur from increased vascularity secondary to the micro-trauma or of micro-fractures that lead to such resorption.

Type IV fractures occur in children and may be confused with complete acromio-clavicular separation. Called pseudo-dislocation of the acromio-clavicular joint, they typically occur in children younger than 16 years. The distal end of the clavicle is fractured, and the acromio-clavicular joint remains intact. In children and young adults, the attachment between bone and the periosteum is relatively loose. The proximal fragment ruptures through the thin periosteum and may be displaced upwards by muscular forces. The coraco-clavicular ligament remains attached to the periosteum or may be avulsed with a small piece of bone. Clinically and radiologically, it may be impossible to distinguish between grade III acromio-clavicular separations, type II fractures of the distal end of clavicle and type IV fractures involving rupture of the periosteum.

Group III fractures or fractures of the inner third of the clavicle, constitute 5–6% of clavicle fractures. As with distal clavicle fractures, they can be subdivided according to the integrity of the ligamentous structures. If the costoclavicular ligaments remain intact and attached to the outer fragment, little or no displacement develops. When these lesions occur in children, they are usually epiphyseal fractures. In adults, articular surface injuries can also lead to degenerative changes.

Classification of Fracture of the Clavicle in Adults According to Robinson – Edinburgh Classification [13] (Table 2.2)

Three different areas of fracture are identified: the diaphysis and the medial and lateral ends. Fractures are divided into sub-groups A and B depending on displacement (> or <100% translation) of the major fragment. This is often difficult because of the sigmoid shape of the clavicle, particularly at the end of the bone, but weight bearing, oblique 30° cephalic or caudal tilted or modified axial view X-rays are helpful in cases in which uncertainty existed

In their series of a 1000 clavicle fractures, Robinson found, Type-1 fractures were uncommon, at 2.8% of the fracture population; most were undisplaced and extraarticular (type 1A1). Type-2 injuries were the most common (69.2%) and most were displaced (type 2B); the most

Table 2.2 Classification of Fracture of the Clavicle in Adults According to Robinson – Edinburgh Classification

Type 1 – Fractures of the medial 5th – fifth of the bone lying medial to a vertical line drawn upwards from the center of the 1st rib.
Type 1A – Undisplaced or <100% translation of fracture fragments
Type 1A1 – Extra-articular
Type 1A2– Intra-articular
Type 1B – Displaced fracture (>100% translation of fracture fragments)
Type 1B1 – Extra-articular
Type 1B2– Intra-articular
Type 2 – Diaphyseal Fractures (Middle 3/5th)
Type 2A – Undisplaced diaphyseal fractures or <100% translation of fracture fragments
Type 2A1 – Undisplaced
Type 2A2 – Angulated
Type 2B – Displaced diaphyseal Fracture (>100% translation of fracture fragments)
Type 2B1 – Simple or wedge comminuted fractures
Type 2B2 – Isolated or Comminuted segmental fractures
Type 3 – fractures of the outer 5th – fifth of the bone lateral to a vertical line drawn upwards from the centre of the base of the coracoid process
Type 3A – Undisplaced fracture or <100% translation of fracture fragments
Type 3A1 – Extra-articular
Type 3A2– Intra-articular
Type 3B – Displaced fracture (>100% translation of fracture fragments)
Type 3B1 – Extra-articular
Type 3B2– Intra-articular

common was type 2B1. Of the type-2B1 fractures, 28.9% had wedge comminution and the remainder were simple. Type-2B2 fractures had an incidence of 25.5%. Of the type- 2B2 injuries 21.1% were the isolated segmental type and the remainder were comminuted segmental. Type-3 fractures, 28% of all, were predominantly undisplaced (type 3A). Type-1 and type-2 fractures were seen in a younger population and with a greater M:F ratio than type-3 fractures. Type-2A2 fractures occurred in a younger population than the other fractures; all but two were in patients aged 13 to 25 years. Type-2 fractures were mainly caused by sport or RTAs whereas simple falls were the commonest cause of type-1 and type-3 fractures [13].

Presentation

Birth Fractures – Fracture of the clavicle is one of the commonest birth injuries with an incidence of 0.5 to 7.2 per 1000 births [24].

Breech presentation has an increased risk of 160 per 1000. Other risk factors are increased birth weight of more than 3800 grams or larger babies that measure 52 cm or longer; increased maternal age; delivered by less experienced residents; instrument deliveries [25, 26].

Clavicle fractures in the new born are often missed and only recognised after a swelling (callus) is noticed about 7–11 days after birth. Sometimes, a crack may be heard / felt at the time of delivery as a clue of fracture [27].

Fractures in Children – Fractures of the clavicle are particularly common in childhood, and almost half occur in children younger than 7 years. Usually are a result of a fall on the point of the shoulder or on an outstretched hand. Sometimes the fracture may be a result of a direct blow front of the clavicle; like other fractures of long bones, fractures of the clavicle may be one of several signs of trauma in a physically abused child [28].

Commonly the diagnosis is obvious with a history of trauma, child complains of pain localized to the clavicle. At times a deformity due to displacement or angulation of the fracture may be obvious. The child is protective of the upper limb on the affected side. Fractures may only become apparent when a lump (of the healing callus) is noticed.

Fractures in Adults – Allman proposed different mechanisms of injury for each of the 3 types of fractures as per his classification. He suggested that in group I (fractures of the middle third), the most common mechanism of injury is a fall onto an outstretched hand, with the force being transmitted up the arm and across the glenohumeral joint and into the clavicle. Group II fractures occurred from a fall on the lateral aspect of the shoulder that drives the shoulder and scapula downward. Group III fractures, or proximal clavicle fractures, are usually due to direct violence caused by a force applied from the lateral side [19, 28].

Stanley et al. (1988) in a series of 150 fractures found 94% patients had fractured the clavicle due to a direct blow while only 6% of patients gave a history of fall on an outstretched hand [29]. Fowler (1962) and Sankarankutty and Turner (1975) reported that >90% fractures were caused by a fall or a blow on the point of the shoulder [30, 31].

A review of the Swedish fracture register in 2014 showed the most common cause of injury was either a fall, generally on the same level, or a transport accident. Bicycle accidents were by far the most common cause among the transport accidents, followed by motorcycle accidents. Males and younger patients most commonly sustained their clavicle fractures from transport accidents in comparison to females and older patients who more often sustained their clavicle fractures from a fall [18].

The patient will present with pain at the fracture site, be protective of the affected upper limb and have restricted shoulder movement. There is usually swelling, bruising, and ecchymosis at the fracture site. In displaced fractures, clinical deformity may be obvious with apparent shortening of the clavicle as compared to opposite side. The fracture may have a striking deformity, particularly if it is a displaced mid-shaft fracture, as the weight of the shoulder/arm pulls the lateral fragment caudally, whilst the sternocleidomastoid muscle pulls the medial end in a cephalad direction. The shoulder translates and rotates forward. Due to this malposition of the shoulder girdle, inspection of the patient from behind may reveal a subtle prominence of the inferior aspect of the scapula from scapular protraction as it moves with the distal fragment.

Shortening of the clavicle should be measured clinically (preferably with a tape measure). Measuring this length gives the difference between the involved and normal shoulder girdle. The degree of shortening at the fracture site is said to be important in the decision making of operative versus non-operative care, as it has been reported in multiple studies to be of prognostic significance (greater shortening, especially more than 1.5–2 cm, is associated with a worse prognosis) [32].

There may be bruising in the surrounding areas that might give a clue to mechanism of injury or associated injuries.

Polytrauma patients with fractures of the clavicular shaft have been found to have a mortality rate of up to 32%, mainly due to associated head and chest injuries. This high incidence of associated head/chest injuries mandates careful clinical and radiographic investigation [33].

Despite its subcutaneous nature open fractures of the clavicle are relatively uncommon. Most open fractures are associated with high-energy vehicular trauma. There is a high incidence of associated injuries – pulmonary injuries, head injuries, scapular fractures and facial trauma [34, 35].

Associated skeletal injuries can include sternoclavicular or acromioclavicular separations or fracture-dislocations through these joints. Fractures of the first rib are not infrequent and are easily overlooked. The floating shoulder consists of fractures of both the clavicle and the scapula and is associated with an extremely unstable shoulder girdle. Fractures of the clavicle may also be associated with disruption of the scapulothoracic articulation manifested as swelling of the shoulder, lateral displacement of the clavicle, severe neurovascular injury, and fracture of the clavicle or the acromioclavicular or sternoclavicular joint [36].

Associated pneumothorax or haemothorax with fractures of the clavicle because the apical pleura and upper lung lobes lie adjacent to this bone, have been reported. Patients with fractures of the clavicle may have decreased breath sounds or other physical findings that suggest pneumothorax. A thorough assessment is especially necessary in the polytrauma patient or unconscious patients [37, 38].

A careful neurological examination of the affected upper limb should be performed to rule out nerve injuries. Though uncommon, associated Brachial plexus injuries do occur. A clavicle fracture when presenting with an injury to the brachial plexus, a subclavian vascular injury often occurs concomitantly. Acute vascular injuries are uncommon but laceration, spasm or acute compression of the subclavian vessels associated with a clavicle fracture have been reported [28].

Though medial end clavicle fractures are uncommon injuries they have a high association with incidence of pneumothorax, haemothorax and facial or cervical injuries [39].

Investigations

It is essential to obtain at least 2 radiographic views to determine displacement and/or angulation of a clavicle fracture that may be difficult to assess on a single AP radiograph. For mid shaft fractures an AP and a cephalic tilt view (30–45°) is useful.

For distal third fractures, an AP view of the shoulder along with a cephalic tilt view and a scapular Y lateral view (of the trauma series) may be useful. Neer suggested an anterior and posterior 45° oblique view [21]. A weight bearing AP view or a Zanca view with a 15-degree tilt and soft tissue technique is said to detect intra articular fractures better than standard radiographs. Often, rupture of the conoid ligament is obvious on radiographs because the fracture is lateral to the conoid tubercle, the coracoclavicular interval is markedly increased and the fracture is markedly displaced. When both coracoclavicular ligaments are attached to the distal fragment, the fracture line is usually oblique, and the coracoclavicular interval is maintained with the lateral fragment [28].

A CT scan with 3D reconstruction may help to delineate the fracture anatomy better especially in intra articular extension though often not necessary as it does not alter treatment plan. MRI scan may also demonstrate the coracoclavicular ligament integrity or attachment.

Fractures of the medial third of clavicle are better seen on cephalic tilt views (30–45°) or the serendipity view. CT scan may be more useful to delineate the medial end fracture especially intra articular extensions or epiphyseal nature of the injury [28].

If clinically a vascular injury is suspected, an angiogram should be arranged.

Treatment Options and Evidence

Mid Shaft Clavicle Fractures

Non-operative Treatment

In a new-born with a birth injury, little treatment is needed as usually the fracture is noticed with the onset of callus formation, apart from keeping the baby comfortable. The fracture is well healed by 2 weeks usually with no sequelae.

Clavicle fractures in children are well known for their high potential for remodelling and healing despite their degree of displacement or angulation [40].

Therefore, they are traditionally treated non-operatively and seem to do well with time. In children with the undisplaced greenstick type of injury, the arm on the fractured side may be rested in a sling till symptoms ease. Displaced fractures may be treated similarly till comfortable followed by shoulder movements. Recent studies have noted that growth and remodelling potential of displaced clavicle fractures in the adolescent age group is not as predictable and may resemble that of an adult rather than that of a child [41, 42].

They believe that as most of the clavicle length is reached at a relatively early age (girls achieve 80% of their clavicle length by 9 years of age and boys by 12 years of age). In consideration of the age group, high functional demand, thinner periosteal tube, limited potential for complete remodelling, and a need to return to athletic activities as quickly as possible, the authors (Mehlman et al. and Namdari et al.) [41, 42] state that adolescent clavicle fractures represent a unique injury. They have reported excellent results with minimal complications of operative treatment of completely displaced clavicle shaft fractures in the adolescent age group.

Herzog et al. (2017) looked at functional outcomes following non-operative versus operative treatment of clavicle fractures in adolescents and found an increased variability in functional measures for the non-operative group suggests some patients may have dysfunction due to clavicle shortening [43].

Undisplaced mid-shaft fractures as well as majority of displaced or angulated fractures, which are closed injuries, are usually managed by conservative means with good outcomes [37, 44–46].

The use of a simple arm sling or the figure of eight bandage [47] is the most widely reported method of conservative management for a mid-shaft fracture of the clavicle. Andersen et al. following an RCT reported less discomfort and a trend towards fewer complications with a sling as compared to a figure of eight bandage. Both groups had similar clinical and functional results with either a sling or a figure of 8 bandage. However, 24% of those treated in a figure of eight bandage were dissatisfied of the treatment method [48].

An earlier study concluded that the functional and cosmetic sequelae of the two methods of treatment were identical and that alignment of the healed fracture was unchanged from the initial displacement with less complications in treatment with a sling [49].

Meta-analysis by Zlowdzki et al. showed that in sling versus figure-of-eight for non-operative treatment of acute midshaft clavicle fractures, patients treated with a sling were more satisfied (93% vs. 74%) [50].

A recent Cochrane Database Systematic Review that compared the figure-of-eight bandage with an arm sling for treating acute middle third clavicle fractures found no clear difference between the two groups in the time to return to school or work activities [51].

There is however no consensus on the optimal duration of immobilisation or on the rehabilitation protocol for these fractures. Recommended periods of immobilisation vary from 2 to 6 weeks, individualised to the patient's comfort level. Most authors recommend avoiding contact sports or heavy lifting for 4–6 months from the initial injury [44, 48, 52, 53].

Operative Treatment

Although good clinical outcomes can be achieved following non-operative treatment, even after significant radiographic malunion especially of displaced fractures several recent studies have reported unsatisfactory results and dissatisfied patient outcomes [32, 54–59]. Hill et al. were one of the first to use a patient-oriented outcome measure, and found 31% of patients described unsatisfactory outcome after non-operative care of displaced clavicle fracture [52]. They reported that shortening of >15mm is associated with shoulder discomfort and dysfunction.

The Canadian Orthopaedic Trauma Society (COTS) Study has been pivotal in changing opinions on management of completely displaced mid shaft clavicle fractures (no cortical contact between the main proximal and distal fragments). The study concluded that 'Operative fixation of a displaced fracture of the clavicular shaft results in improved functional outcome and a lower rate of malunion and non-union compared with non-operative treatment at 1 year of follow-up. This study supports primary plate fixation of completely displaced midshaft clavicular fractures in active adult patients' [32].

A meta-analysis of 13 recent publications has revealed that primary operative fixation could effectively reduce the rates of non-union, symptomatic malunion, neurological symptoms and overall complications [60].

The Clavicle Trial (2017) concluded that ORIF is a safe and reliable intervention with superior early functional outcomes and should be considered for patients who sustain this common injury [61].

Based on the available data from these recent studies there is growing consensus that a certain subset of individuals would benefit from surgical intervention. The aim of surgical intervention would be to restore normal alignment and stable fixation of the displaced (>2 cm or shortening of more than 2 cm) in the active, medically fit individual. A recent study by Goudie et al. suggests that there is no difference in outcome for patients with healed fractures with less than or equal to 2 cm of shortening compared with those with more than 2 cm of shortening. It is therefore likely that many patients can adapt and function well despite this degree of deformity. However, it should be noted that their study had only 5 patients with more than 2 cm shortening [62].

Table 2.3 Relative indications for Operative Treatment of Clavicle Fractures

Displacement >2 cm
Shortening >2 cm
Grossly comminuted Displaced Fracture
Open Fractures / Impending Soft Tissue Compromise
Floating Shoulder
Polytrauma especially with associated rib fractures
Vascular or Neurological Injury requiring repair

Table 2.3 shows relative indications for operative treatment of clavicle fractures. A range of implants are available for internal fixation of diaphyseal fractures but primarily there are two widely accepted methods – plate fixation or intramedullary devices. Any decision to treat fractures of the middle third of the clavicle operatively rather than non-operatively must carefully consider the risk factors for non-union and symptomatic malunion of non-operative treatment versus the possible complications inherent in operative treatment. These complications include deep or superficial wound infection, risk of neurovascular injury, hardware failure, hardware related irritation and poor cosmesis of a surgical scar. Recent publications have shown a decline in post-surgical complications probably resulting from improved surgical technique and implant technology [63–65].

Potter et al. concluded from their study that 'Late reconstruction of non-union and malunion after displaced midshaft fractures of the clavicle is a reliable and reproducible procedure that results in restoration of objective muscle strength similar to that seen with immediate fixation; however, there are subtle decreases in endurance strength and outcome compared with acute fracture repair.' They suggested that this should not be the sole reason to justify surgery but could be useful in decision making [66].

Plate Fixation

Plate fixation provides stability of the fracture, pain relief and facilitates early mobilisation of the shoulder. Dynamic compression plates, pre-contoured locking plates, semi-tubular and reconstruction plates have all been used though reconstruction plates and semi tubular plates have largely fallen out of favour due to their weakness and potential to deform at the site of the fracture leading to mal-union. Plating provides immediate rigid stabilisation of the fracture as it allows compression across the main fracture line and, if required, can be combined with the use of interfragmentary lag screws. Plate fixation also offers excellent rotational stability and maintains length control. Golish et al. demonstrated that plate fixation provides a superior construct, demonstrating decreased displacement at fixed loads, as well as greater loads at fixed levels of displacement during a wider range of movements. This allows for early mobilisation and early/ accelerated rehabilitation protocols [67] (Fig. 2.4).

Ianotti et al. compared biomechanical strength of plates and intramedullary devices for diaphyseal clavicle fractures and concluded that in the presence of comminution, which is usually inferior, locking plates are advantageous as their position on the superior aspect of the clavicle bestows greater stability than an intramedullary device [68].

Anatomic pre-contoured locking plates have gained prominence in recent times. They are increasingly used in displaced comminuted fractures to compress the fracture or where the fracture is bridged across using the plate as the degree of comminution does not allow for a compression plate. They may be less prominent after healing and may lead to less incidence of hardware removal [32, 69].

Surgeons should be aware of risk of injury to the underlying neurovascular structures from manipulation of the fracture, drilling of the screw holes, retracting the tissues and placing longer length screws. Some have suggested an antero-inferior placement of the plate that allows instrumentation directed away from potentially dangerous infraclavicular structures and a minimal incidence of implant prominence problems [65].

Formani et al. in their retrospective review found that both superior and anteroinferior techniques resulted in a similar time to radiographic union and identical union rates. They found that implant removal occurred more frequently after superior plating but was not significant [70].

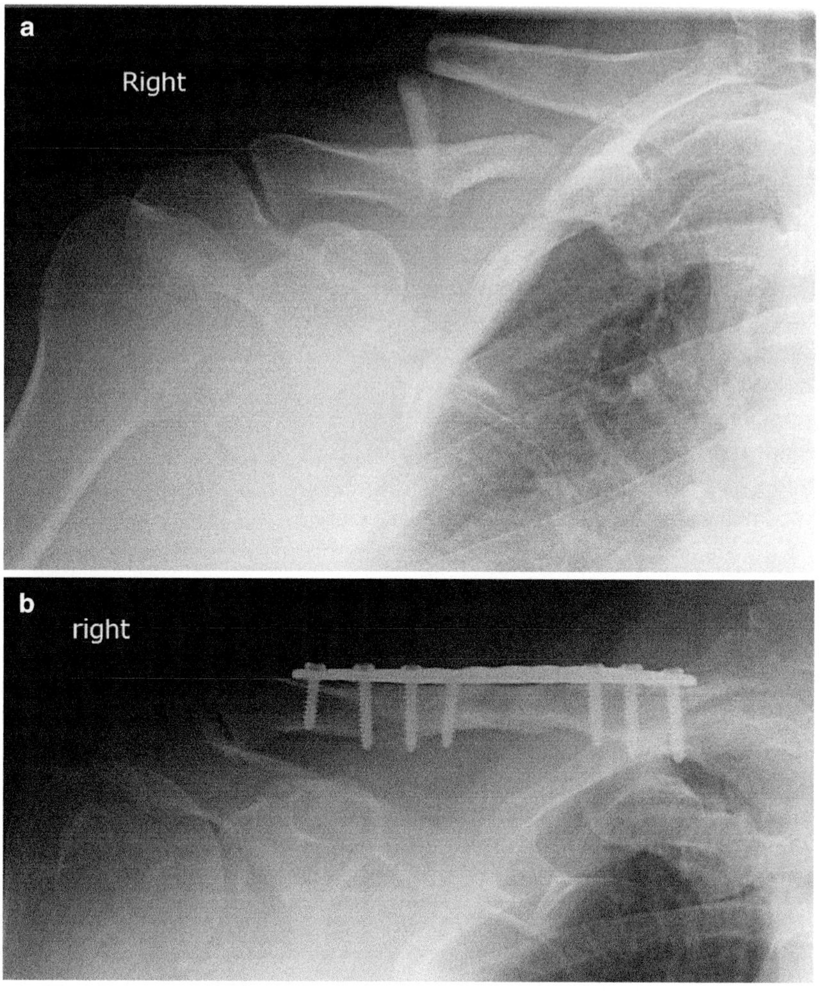

Fig. 2.4 (**a**) Displaced midshaft clavicle fracture. (**b**) Plate fixation

Intramedullary Fixation

Due to the sigmoid shape of the clavicle, intramedullary fixation of fractures has traditionally been difficult. There has a been a range of intramedullary fixation methods for the clavicle including; Knowles pins [71, 72], Rockwood pins [73], Hagie pins [45, 74] or titanium elastic nails [75, 76].

There are two methods for insertion of an intramedullary device – antegrade *via* an anteromedial entry point, and retrograde *via* a posterolateral entry point. Intramedullary fixation offers the advantages of being a soft tissue friendly and a minimally invasive or percutaneous procedure leading to less disruption to the periosteal blood supply and soft tissue stripping with the potential for improved cosmesis.

The main disadvantages intramedullary fixation is poor axial and rotational stability in non-transverse and comminuted fractures. In the absence of static locking, there may be shortening of the clavicle over time, more likely in comminuted fractures. Also, there have been reports of catastrophic migration of these implants -specifically smooth pins – elsewhere in the body [77–79].

A recent meta-analysis concluded that Intramedullary fixation may be superior to plate fixation in the treatment of mid-shaft clavicle fractures, with similar performance in terms of the union rate and shoulder function, better operative parameters and fewer complications [80].

Ferran et al. in their RCT found that both locked intramedullary fixation and plating produce good functional results, however, metalwork may need to be removed as a second procedure in 100% of intramedullary fixation and 53% of plate fixation cases [81].

Clinical results with intramedullary fixation or plate fixation are similar but many surgeons prefer plate fixation for primary operative treatment of clavicle fractures or non-union because of the superior rotational and axial stability of the plate construct, especially in comminuted fractures and not all plates need to be removed.

Lateral End Clavicle Fractures

Undisplaced fractures of the lateral end of the clavicle (Edinburgh type 3A) are generally treated conservatively as they have an intact periosteal sleeve and are relatively stable, due to the intact conoid and trapezoid CC ligaments. Good results have been reported with conservative measures using analgesia and an arm sling [82].

Displaced lateral clavicle fractures (Edinburgh type 3B) are often treated operatively as conservative measures are usually associated with increased incidence of non-union [13, 82].

A systematic review of lateral clavicle fractures, published in 2010, reported a 33.3% non-union rate in conservatively managed injuries and a 6% non-union rate in those treated operatively [83].

Robinson et al. who examined a cohort of 127 non-operatively treated patients concluded that 'non-operative treatment achieved good results in middle-aged and elderly patients, with only a small percentage (14%) requiring delayed surgery. Low demand, elderly and frail patients are usually treated non-operatively' [13].

For the majority of younger patients with these fractures, operative treatment is more appropriate. A range of techniques are described for fixation of these injuries including; plating (hook-plate, locking plates), coraco-clavicular screw, Kirschner wires and coracoclavicular ligament augmentation/reconstruction.

The difficulties faced during operative treatment of distal clavicle fractures is the fixation of the distal fragment. The distal fragment may have unexpected comminution or poor screw purchase when using anatomic plates (pre-contoured plates). This may necessitate a coracoclavicular fixation or use of a hook plate.

Plate Fixation

The hook-plate was specifically engineered for acromioclavicular injuries, such as dislocations, as well as to provide operative treatment for fractures with a small distal fragment where other plating techniques would be inappropriate. Good et al. prospectively reviewed 36 cases of distal clavicle fracture that underwent hook plate fixation as a primary procedure. Mean time to union was 3 months with a union rate of 95% [84]. There are concerns that the plate may induce shoulder stiffness and osteoarthritis of the acromioclavicular joint [85].

Improper positioning of the hook may lead a high incidence of incidence of subacromial impingement (32%) and of acromial osteolysis (25%) was noted. In all cases, symptoms resolved following removal of the plate allows early mobilisation and good subjective and objective functional outcome [86].

A high percentage of patients treated with hook plate fixation will require plate removal (recommended by most surgeons) to regain full range of shoulder motion. It is recommended to remove the hook plates 4 to 6 months after initial insertion to avoid said complications.

Pre-contoured locking plates designed for distal end clavicle fractures do overcome these acromial problems as well as the need for routine removal of the implant (Fig. 2.5). The new plating systems have multiple options of screw fixation in the broadened lateral end of the plate allowing for better screw purchase in the small distal fragment.

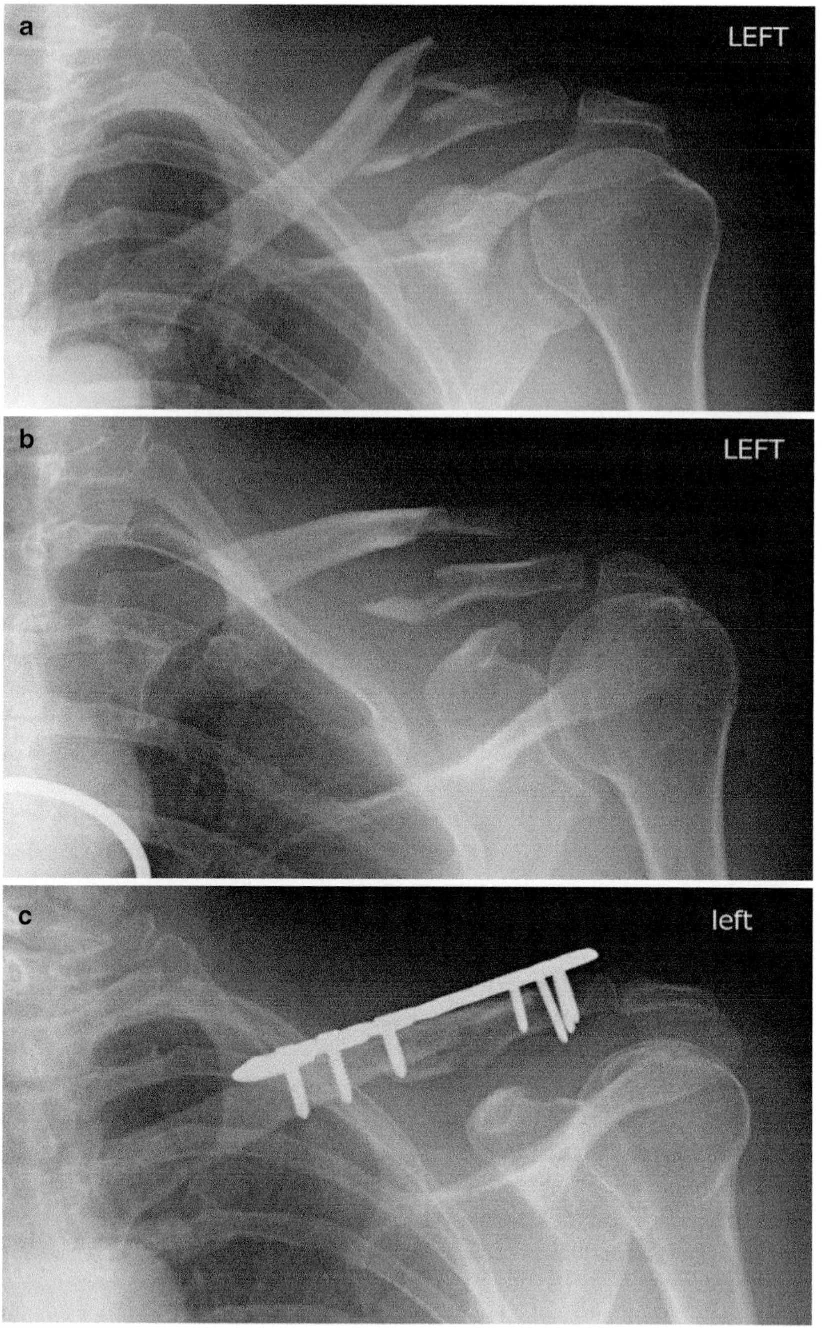

Fig. 2.5 (**a**) Displaced lateral end clavicle fracture- AP view. (**b**) 30° cephalad view. (**c**) Plate fixation

Suture and Sling Techniques

Surgical techniques, involving sutures and or ligament grafts, have been used either alone or alongside primary fixation to good effect [87, 88].

This is implemented by looping sutures around the coracoid process and the distal clavicle, or by drilling holes within the clavicle (Fig. 2.6). The 'tightrope technique,' which involves two EndoButtons in the clavicle and coracoid, and a loop of suture material through these, has been described as also demonstrating good early results for use in both fractures and dislocations. This method is useful in fractures

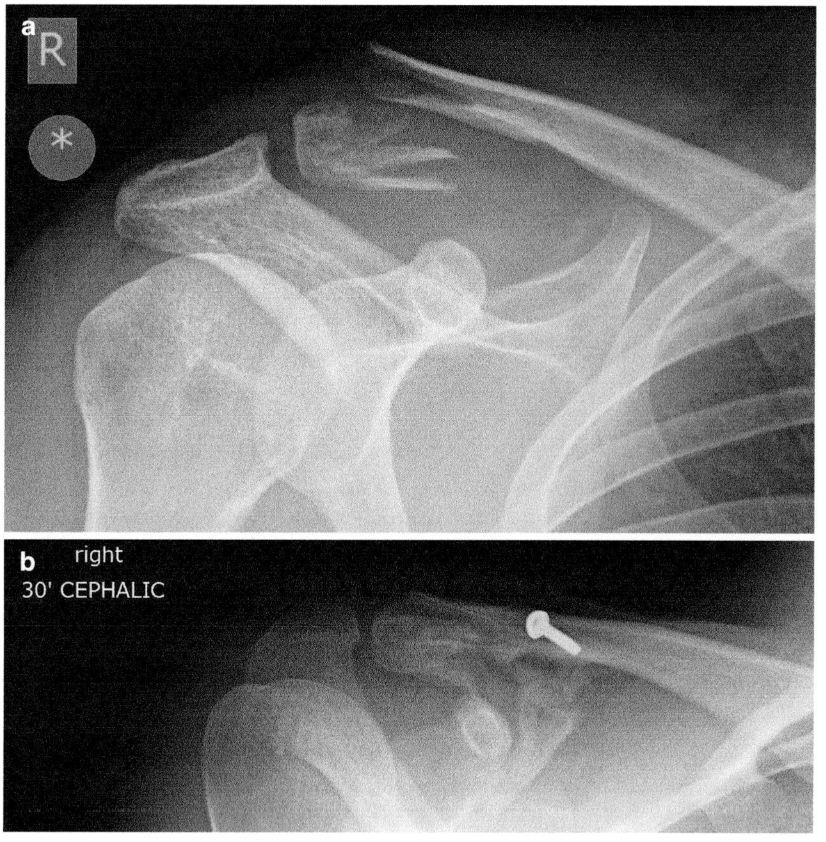

Fig. 2.6 (**a**) Displaced lateral end clavicle fracture (**b**) Fixation with reconstruction of coraco-clavicular ligaments

that have a small distal end fragment or a highly comminuted fracture. Also has the added advantage of there being no need for implant removal.

Coracoclavicular Screw

Coraco-clavicular screws have been described, as far back as 1941 by Bosworth, as a method of treatment for acromio-clavicular separation. It is worth noting that this procedure can be technically demanding because of the small area of coracoid that is available for screw insertion, which is associated with a higher rate of fixation failure.

Kirschner Wire Fixation

Kirschner wiring or K-wire tension banding has been used in the past but, as with mid-clavicular fractures, there are problems with pin migration as well as non-union and infection [89].

Oh et al. [83] described the outcome following various surgical interventions in 365 patients, and recommended that coracoclavicular fixation was preferred due to its low complication rate (4.8%) compared to hook plate fixation (40.7%) or K-wire tension banding (20.0%).

Medial End Clavicle Fractures

Medial end clavicle fractures are uncommon and account for less than 3% of all clavicular fractures. The medial clavicular epiphysis is the last long bone epiphysis to fuse in the body, and may persist in patients until 25 to 30 years of age. Therefore, medial clavicular fractures are often epiphyseal fracture- subluxations or fracture-dislocations. Even in cases in which the medial physis has already fused, these fractures heal well and majority of these fractures are managed non-operatively [90].

Fractures with anteriorly displaced fragments are nearly always managed non-operatively in a sling and heal well. A medial clavicle fracture with posterior displacement of fragments may impinge on the vital structures at the root of the neck. Patients may present with difficulty in swallowing or breathing or with any neurovascular compromise. This requires operative reduction of the fracture. Reduction manoeuvres should not be performed in the clinic or the emergency department unless the posterior position of the fragment is causing an airway or hemodynamic emergency. This reduction must be performed in the operating room under general anaesthesia with a thoracic surgeon present, in case a vascular problem occurs. A towel clip can be used to grasp the distal fragment and pull it forward to the proximal fragment. Simultaneous traction on the upper extremity helps in unlocking the fragments and allowing reduction. The reduction is generally stable [23].

The main difficulty with these injuries is the fixation in the medial fragment. The surgical approach is similar to that for a shaft fracture extended medially. It is important to remember that the subclavian vessels are in close proximity to the bone medially. Following reduction of the fracture, it can be temporarily held reduced with K-wires. If the medial fragment is large enough, then standard plate and screw fixation can be performed; a lateral end clavicle plate (with an expanded end section) may used to get a purchase with multiple screws at the expansion of the medial clavicle. Rarely the plate can be extended across the joint onto the sternum [28].

Fixation of the fracture using smooth wires or pins alone is contraindicated, due to the potential for migration and visceral injury.

Floating Shoulder

Ipsilateral Clavicle and scapular fractures are commonly referred by the term 'Floating Shoulder' was first described by Ganz and Noesberger [91, 92].

The term was first coined by Herscovici et al. [93], was considered an unstable injury that requires fixation. This injury is actually a double disruption of the superior shoulder suspensory complex (SSSC), a concept introduced by Goss [92] that describes a bone and soft tissue ring formed by the glenoid, coracoid process, coracoclavicular ligaments, clavicle (especially its distal part), AC joint, and acromion. This complex maintains the anatomic relationship between the upper extremity and the axial skeleton. The clavicle is the only bony connection between the two with the scapula suspended from it by the coracoclavicular and AC ligaments. Thus any injury that disrupts this ring at two or more locations is considered inherently unstable.

Concomitant fracture of scapular glenoid neck and clavicle is the commonest type of double disruptions of the SSSC. These injuries are extremely rare that result from high energy trauma. Associated ipsilateral upper extremity and thoracic injuries are common. There remains considerable controversy over optimal treatment. Owens et al. [94] and Rikli et al. [95] described excellent results in patients who had their floating shoulder treated with reduction and fixation of the clavicular fracture only. While Leung and Lam [96] described good or excellent results in 14 of 15 patients with this injury pattern following fixation of both the clavicle and glenoid fractures. There are cases series that have reported the results of non-operative treatment in patients with ipsilateral fractures of the clavicle and glenoid who had a good results and recovery to near-normal status [97].

Mckee [98] has suggested that an operative approach may be indicated in a young healthy individual who works overhead for a living whereas the same fracture pattern may be treated non-operatively in an elderly, low-demand patient with multiple medical comorbidities. Currently, standard operative indications include a clavicle fracture that warrants, in isolation, fixation, glenoid displacement of greater than 2.5 to 3 cm; displaced intra-articular glenoid fracture extension; Patient-associated indications (i.e., polytrauma with a requirement for early upper extremity weight bearing); severe glenoid angulation, retroversion, or anteversion 40° (Goss Type II);. Documented ipsilateral coracoacromial and/or AC ligament disruption or its equivalent (coracoid fracture, i.e., AC joint disruption).

Most surgeons now agree that the if operative treatment is planned then the clavicle fracture is fixed first and the shoulder then reimaged. If there is indirect reduction of the glenoid such that its alignment is within acceptable parameters, then no further intervention is required apart from close follow-up. If the glenoid remains in an "unacceptable" position, then fixation of the glenoid neck is performed, typically through a posterior approach [98].

Authors' Preferred Method

Indications for surgery are listed in Table 2.3. This list by no means is exhaustive or absolute indications for intervention. Figure 2.7 represents the authors' treatment rationale. Each case is decided on its merit and is an informed decision by the patient.

Use an anatomic pre-contoured plate to fit the 'S' shape of the clavicle. These plates also tend to have a low profile and help decrease soft tissue irritation. Our preference is to use a plate positioned on the superior surface of the clavicle.

Careful patient positioning improves access, particularly to the medial end. We use the 'reclining beach chair' position on a shoulder operating table in which the back of the table is about 30° angled from the plane of the floor. Unless cervical spinal problems preclude, the head is tilted to the opposite side of the fracture (with the anaesthetist's approval) and placed on a small head ring to ensure there is good access to the medial half of the clavicle to allow easy instrumentation and screw placement. The C-arm is adjusted to capture the field from either the opposite side or the head end of the patient to allow unhindered X-rays of the clavicle in AP view, 30–45° cephalad and caudad views. The operative area may be square draped, or the arm may be draped in a stockinette.

A superior approach plating is our preferred method. We use a transverse incision with the lateral part of the incision following Langer's lines and placed just inferior to the subcutaneous border of the clavicle. Incision is deepened, and care taken to isolate and protect the larger branches of the supraclavicular nerves. It is good practice to warn the patients prior to surgery that they may experience an area of numbness distal to the incision in the pectoral area. The myofascial layer (with platysma) is then divided to reach fracture site. The fracture ends are then exposed taking care not to denude the bone circumferentially away from the fracture ends. The major fragments are clearly identified and

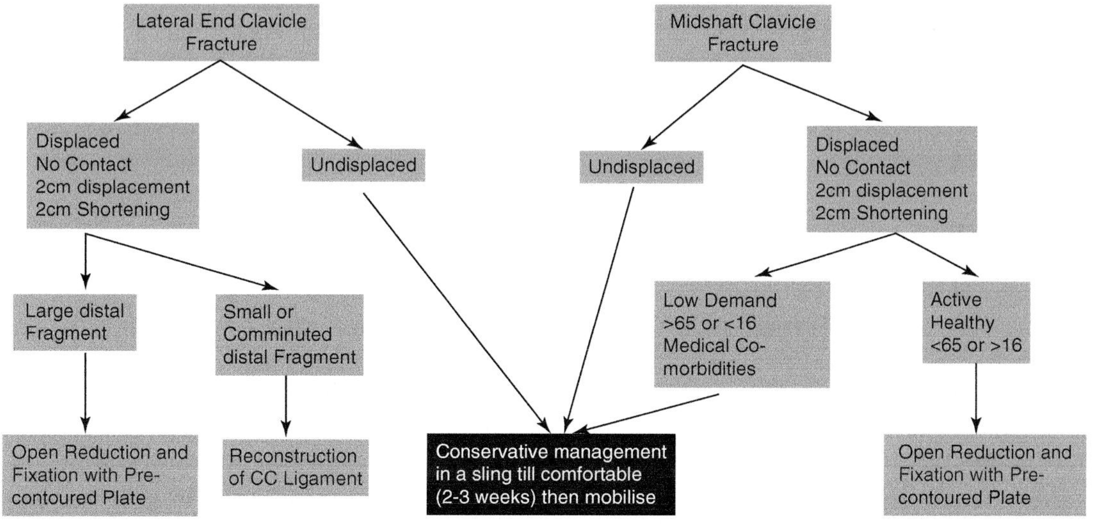

Fig. 2.7 Flowchart of Authors' preferred treatment rationale (these are not absolute indications for treatment choice)

cleaned of debris and hematoma, and a fixation strategy is formulated. Any 'butterfly' fragment should be gently eased in place without stripping soft tissue attachment and where possible, fixed with a lag screw. The aim should be to restore alignment and length, not necessarily perfect reduction at the cost of compromising local biology and soft tissue attachments. A pre-contoured plate of sufficient length is then applied to the superior surface. It is usually sufficient to secure the fracture with three bicortical screws (six cortices) on either side of the fracture. If the fracture configuration is stable, then the plate can be applied in a compression manner. If the fracture is comminuted or of an unstable pattern, then the plate should be applied in a bridging mode. Locking screws are an option for osteopenic bone, but we seldom use them as most patients who undergo fixation are younger and have good cortical bone.

Care should be taken when handling soft tissues and closure of the wound should be done in at least 2 layers – Deltoid Trapezial fascia; superficial fascia & skin.

Post-operatively the arm is placed in a sling for up to 2 weeks. Initially gentle pendular movements are allowed, followed by range of motion exercises from third week on removal of sling. Strengthening exercises, sporting activities and manual work are not allowed until after the 6th post-op week, and depends on progress with range of motion and progress with radiological union.

Complications

Non-union

Nonunion of the clavicle (Fig. 2.8b) is defined as the lack of radiographic healing at 6 months post injury. Initially thought to be an uncommon complication (less than 1%) [37, 46].

Non-union of clavicle fractures are said to be more common. Studies [99–102] suggesting up to 15% rate of non-union for all clavicle fractures and an even higher rate for fractures of the lateral end of clavicle (18% and 40%) [13, 103, 104].

According to Robinson et al. [99] who looked at 868 patients and found a non-union rate of 6.2%, but increased if fracture was displaced or comminuted the rate was higher (21%). Risk factors for nonunion include increasing age, female sex, fracture displacement, comminution and smoking [102].

Non-union of the lateral end of clavicle fractures may be asymptomatic, especially in the elderly but the majority of midshaft non-union occur in young active individuals, will be symptomatic enough to require treatment. Along with some discomfort or pain, the patient may have a clicking sensation on movement with restriction of shoulder movement, weakness and a cosmetic deformity. Clinical and radiographic signs of non-union include mobility or pain on stressing of the fracture and an absence of bridging callus on radiographs.

Wijdicks et al. [105] following a systematic review of 11 studies concluded that non-union rates were less than 10% following Plate fixation of Clavicle fractures. The COTS study [32] found a significant difference in rates of non-union with 2 out of 62 in the operative group versus 7 out of 49 in the conservatively managed patients.

A meta-analysis of 13 studies reported the pooled results of non-union incidence. They presented a significant difference favouring operative over non-operative treatment. Subgroup analysis concerning fixation methods showed that plate fixation, but not intramedullary nailing fixation, was associated with a reduced risk compared with non-operative treatment [60].

Surgical treatment for a midshaft non-union of the clavicle is open reduction and internal fixation with a pre-contoured anatomic clavicular plate (Fig. 2.8c) with the addition of an iliac crest bone graft or an osteoinductive bone graft substitute. If the non-union is hypertrophic (uncommon) then the morcellised autograft from the local bone is applied to the non-union site.

More commonly it is an atrophic non-union with loss of bone length. A structural or intercalary graft (tricortical iliac crest autograft) may be required in such cases where there has been excessive loss of length or failed previous surgery.

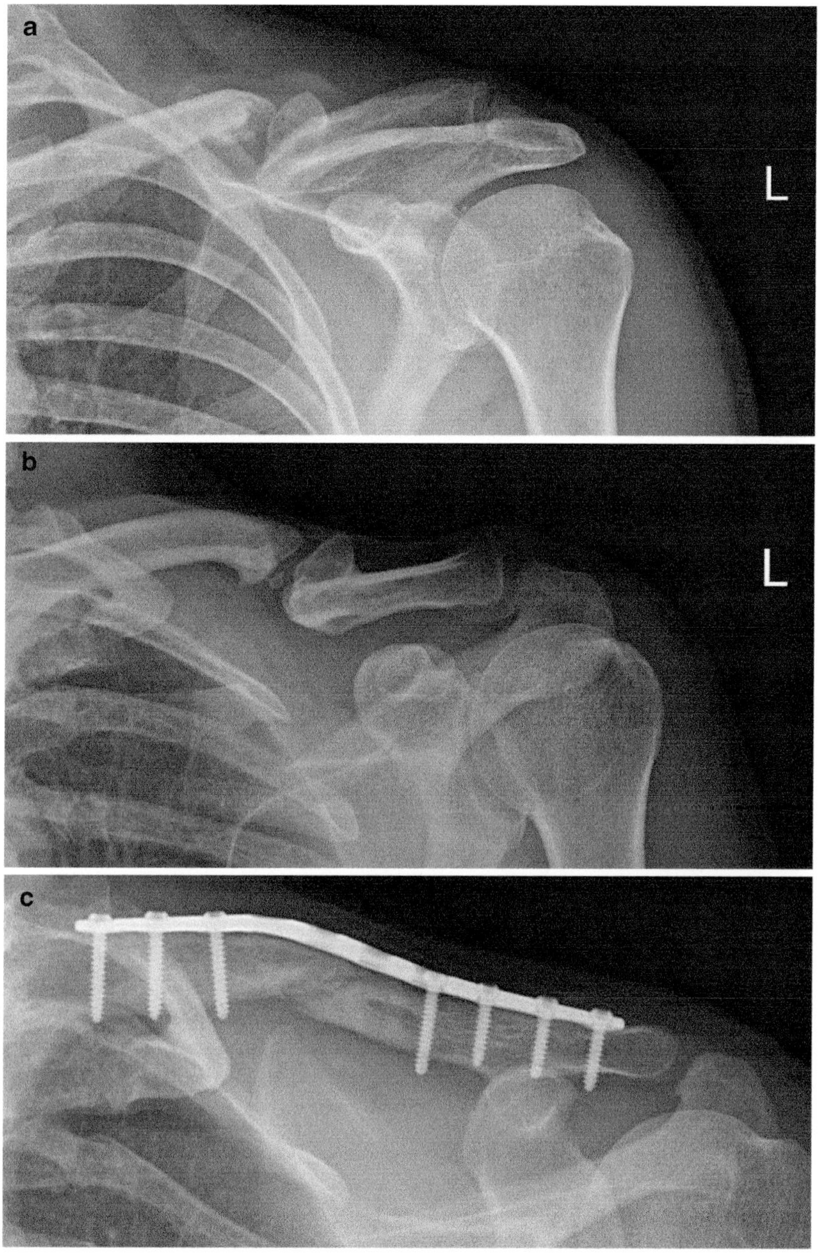

Fig. 2.8 (**a**) Displaced midshaft clavicle fracture – managed conservatively (**b**) Non-union of fracture (**c**) Plate Fixation for non-union

Malunion

All displaced fractures that are treated non-operatively heal with some degree of malunion due to angulation or shortening but often asymptomatic [106].

It was believed that malunion of the clavicle (Fig. 2.9b) was of radiographic interest only and clinically the fractures were deemed to have healed. However, more recently, several investigators have described a fairly consistent pattern of patient symptomatology following malunion of displaced midshaft fractures of the clavicle [52, 107].

Hill et al. were the first to use a patient-oriented outcome measure, and found 31% of patients

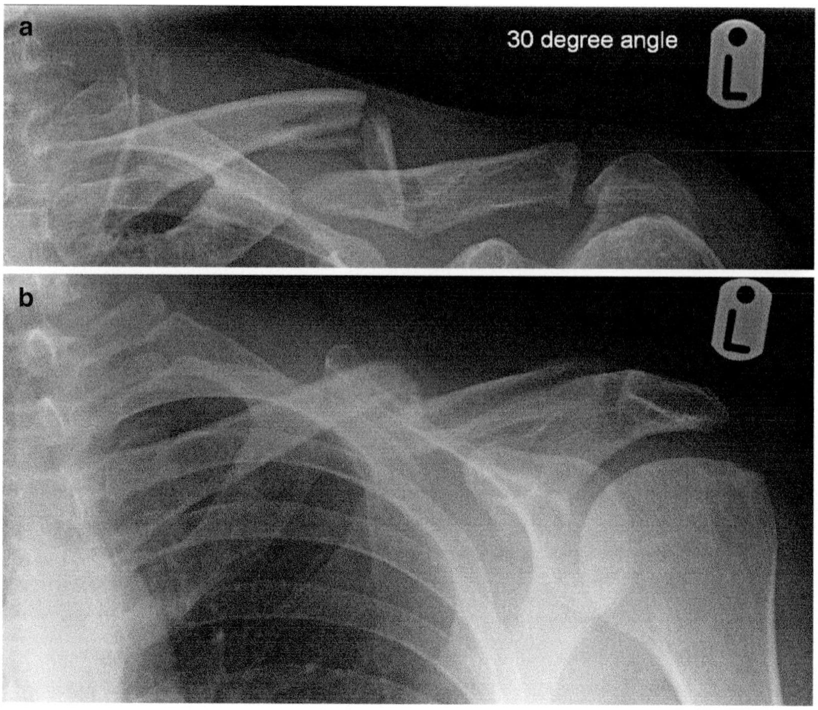

Fig. 2.9 (**a**) Displaced midshaft clavicle fracture – managed conservatively (**b**) Malunited and shortened clavicle

described unsatisfactory outcome after non-operative care of displaced clavicle fracture [52].

They reported that shortening of >15 mm is associated with shoulder discomfort and dysfunction. It has been suggested that the angular deformity and shortening change the orientation of the glenoid, altering the shoulder dynamics [107].

Malunion of the clavicle may cause pain, symptomatic parasthesia of the arm and hand with loss of strength and numbness, problems with sleeping on the back, as well as cosmetic complaints.

It is suggested that a shortened lever arm of the shoulder girdle changes the orientation of the glenoid with winging of the scapula, which leads to functional problems of the shoulder in overhead movements [106, 108].

Shortening of the clavicle has a negative effect on muscle-tendon tension and muscle balance, which may result in loss of strength and endurability; this can be measured in patients with a short malunion [106, 108].

The malunion results in a changed load of the acromioclavicular (AC Joint) and sternoclavicular joints. reported AC joint arthrosis in patients after follow-up of malunited clavicular fractures [52, 108].

Chan et al. suggested that malunited clavicle fracture that has united with deformity or shortening may have an adverse effect on normal shoulder girdle function. They reported that a malunited fracture of the clavicle was believed to be a contributing factor to shoulder girdle dysfunction. In each patient, the functional status of the involved limb was improved after corrective osteotomy at the site of deformity, realignment, and plate fixation [107].

Treatment can either be prevention in the acute phase, by means of primary fixation of displaced clavicle fracture or later when the symptomatic malunion is established, a correction osteotomy with or without an iliac crest autograft can be performed. Several reports on the operative treatment of malunited clavicular fractures have been published with all of them reporting good results and satisfied patients [106, 107, 109].

Major complications like bone healing problems and deep infections requiring implant removal were reported at a rate no higher than 7%. Reported rates for minor complications, such as wound infection and implant irritation that could be resolved without further surgery, were as high as 31% [60].

Neurovascular Injuries in Clavicle Fractures

Neurovascular injuries associated with clavicle fractures are relatively uncommon, despite the proximity of brachial plexus and subclavian vessels. These injuries / complications can be acute presentation, delayed presentation or iatrogenic [98].

Acute Neurovascular Injuries

Direct injury to the vessels and brachial plexus can occur at the time of the fracture [110, 111].

A thorough neurological and vascular examination should be carried out suspected cases especially clavicle fractures associated with high energy trauma or polytrauma patients.

If there is suspicion of a vascular injury then an urgent angiogram needs to be arranged. This may be done in the form of a CT angiogram. A vascular surgeon may need to be informed when the index of suspicion is high.

There have also been case reports of direct neurologic injury from clavicular fracture fragments. In this situation operative decompression of the brachial plexus by reduction and fixation of the clavicle fracture is indicated [112, 113].

Delayed Neurovascular Injuries

A number of synonyms have been applied to this condition, including 'thoracic outlet syndrome' [114], 'costoclavicular syndrome', and 'fractured clavicle-rib syndrome'. This is said to occur when there is entrapment of the medial cord of the brachial plexus by callus superiorly and by the first rib inferiorly producing predominantly ulnar nerve symptoms. This situation is more likely in the presence of a hypertrophic non-union or malunion. Rowe reported late neurovascular sequelae two out of 690 fractures (0.3%) [37], although higher rates have been reported in more recent studies [32, 52, 115].

A diagnosis is made when a patient has a suggestive clinical history with supportive evidence on electrophysiological testing. The treatment should be directed toward correction of the malunion or non-union. McKee et al. reported resolution of thoracic outlet syndrome symptoms in 16 patients who underwent corrective clavicular osteotomy to treat a malunion [106].

Iatrogenic Injuries

Brachial Plexus Injury

Iatrogenic neurovascular complications are rare. The incidence of brachial plexus injury is reported to be 0–1.5% [105, 116].

It is postulated that distraction of the fracture site and the delayed surgery (several weeks after their injury) can lead to a traction injury of the brachial plexus [117].

Patients with a significant brachial plexus injury following clavicle fracture surgery have a characteristic presentation of unremitting radicular pain, profound weakness and sensory loss in the immediate postoperative period. The lesion is usually incomplete, with the upper trunk and suprascapular nerve most commonly involved [118–120].

Recovery from postoperative brachial plexus injury occurs over many months and the final outcome is variable. All three cases following intramedullary fixation reported by Ring and Holovacs [117] were managed non-operatively and had complete resolution of symptoms within 6 months.

Jeyaseelan et al. [118] explored the plexus and performed a neurolysis in all their 21 cases. Four patients had nerve ruptures that were treated with nerve transfers or grafts. By 12 months, 71% of the 21 patients had recovered their MRC (Medical Research Council) power grade 4, and a further 14% to 3.

Significant postoperative plexopathy has severe symptoms and a variable outcome. Therefore, urgent revision surgery, including the support of a brachial plexus surgeon as neurolysis, repair, transfer or grafting may be required.

Vascular Injury

In a meta-analysis of 582 cases of clavicle fixation, all 11 studies did not report a single vascular complication [105]. Arterial injuries are rare and are usually pseudoaneurysms associated with prominent screws. These may be clinically silent for several years before presenting as subcritical upper limb ischaemia. They usually present as late upper limb claudication between 2 years and 10 years following surgery or may present as an acute deterioration to limb threatening ischaemia as a result of emboli to the upper limb [121].

The pseudoaneurysm can be diagnosed by an angiogram. Treatment usually involves removal of implant and a vascular stent or graft procedure by the vascular surgeon.

Venous injuries are a result of tearing of the vessel wall by fracture manipulation, drills or implants.

Once the injury is diagnosed, the two main goals are to gain rapid control of the bleeding and prevent air entering the circulation. An urgent vascular review should be sought for surgical repair of the subclavian vein that may require grafting.

Clavicle fractures with a higher risk for iatrogenic injury include a medial fracture, a grossly comminuted fracture, a fracture with over 2-week delay from the time of injury, or non-union, malunion and revision cases. To avoid significant iatrogenic neurovascular injuries, the surgeon must have a detailed understanding of the neurovascular anatomy of the region. All dissection around the medial and inferior clavicle should be performed in the subperiosteal plane. Screws should be placed along a safe trajectory and screw length should be accurately measured [98, 122].

Refracture

Refracture after non-operative treatment is uncommon. With increasing popularity of operative fixation of clavicle fractures and subsequent implant removal, there is a trend towards a reinjury following a new episode. Re-injury shortly after operative treatment may cause breakage or bending of the fixation device, or fracture around the implants non-union is relatively common after refracture, and internal fixation is often required.

Post Traumatic Osteoarthritis of the Acromioclavicular Joint

This complication occurs most frequently following an intraarticular fracture of lateral end of clavicle and may be seen after an extraarticular fracture that is treated with a hook plate fracture. In a medium-term study of 101 lateral-end clavicular fractures, three of eleven intra-articular (Edinburgh Type-3B2) fractures and six of ninety extra-articular (Edinburgh Type-3B1) fractures were associated with radiographic signs of osteoarthritis [123]. The major symptom is activity-related pain, which characteristically is worsened by cross-arm adduction.

Symptomatic osteoarthritis of the acromioclavicular joint may be treated with excision of the lateral end or fragment.

Infection Following Fixation of Clavicle Fractures

Infection following fixation of clavicle fractures has shown reduced rates in recent times following improvements in surgical techniques with better soft tissue handling, two-layered closure of the wound, biomechanically superior and more stable fixation methods and use of peri-operative antibiotic prophylaxis. Zlowodzki et al. reported a superficial infection rate of 4.4%, and a deep infection rate of only 2.2%; these figures are significantly improved compared to earlier studies [50].

Superficial infections are often treated with oral antibiotics with good results and seldom require implant removal. Deep infections should be treated initially with intravenous antibiotics for a certain period (following discussion with microbiologist) followed by oral antibiotics. The implant is removed in cases where the fixation is unstable, implant has loosened or there are few/no signs of the healing process. The implant is removed along with a thorough debridement of all infected and dead tissue including bone. Antibiotic impregnated cement may be placed in the residual space. A delayed surgery is then performed with or without a bone graft to replace the bone loss. Plastic surgery support may be required to provide soft tissue closure in form of local rotational flaps or free flaps [98].

Complications of Plate Fixation

Complications following the plate fixation of clavicular fractures may require another surgery to remove or revise the plate. Such major complications include non-union, symptomatic malunion, deep infection, mechanical failure, irritation due to the implant (that requires plate removal), breakage of the implant, angulation and refracture after plate removal. Iatrogenic neurovascular complications are rare. Minor complications may occur that do not need another surgery like wound infection (that require oral antibiotics), scar dysesthesia, implant irritation (not requiring plate removal) and transient neurological problems.

Due to subcutaneous nature of the clavicle local irritation from hardware prominence is relatively common. The incidence of hardware removal ranges from 5% to 100% [98]. A meta-analysis of plate fixation of clavicle fractures [105] reported that a vast majority of complications seem to be implant related, with irritation or failure of the plate being consistently reported on in almost every study, on average ranging from 9% to 64%. The same meta-analysis reported non-union and malunion rates of less than 10%. Wound and deep infection rates of less than 10% with the vast majority of these were wound infections requiring oral antibiotics. Neurovascular complications included brachial plexus symptoms and regional pain syndromes and ranged in prevalence from 0% to 23%, all reportedly were transient. They did not report a single vascular complication.

Complications of Intramedullary Fixation

Wijdicks et al. in their systematic review [105] reported rates for major complications like bone healing problems and deep infections requiring implant removal were no higher than 7%. Rates for minor complications, such as wound infection and implant irritation that could be resolved without further surgery, were as high as 31%. There were only 4 refractures after pin removal reported in a total of 3 studies. Overall, the rate of major complications requiring additional surgical treatment was low. Most complications were implant failures, breakages, irritations or implant migrations. Irritation is one of the main effects of migration, telescoping or protrusion of the intramedullary device. Migrating, telescoping or protruding devices may often remain asymptomatic not requiring additional treatment. Yet most intramedullary fixation techniques require routine surgical device removal once fracture healing has occurred [55, 59, 81, 124].

Owing to (routine) implant removal, treatment with intramedullary fixation often requires an additional surgical procedure.

Conclusion

Clavicle fractures are common upper extremity skeletal injuries. Most patients with clavicular fractures can be effectively treated conservatively in a sling for a period of immobilisation to allow initial healing, followed by structured rehabilitation. There is now good evidence that a subset of patients – the young, active, healthy patient with a completely displaced clavicle fracture with over 2 cm overlap – are likely to benefit from primary operative management. Use of an anatomic, pre-contoured compression plate placed on the superior aspect of the bone is the authors' preferred method of operative treatment.

References

1. Codman E, editor. The shoulder: rupture of the supraspinatus tendon and other lesions in or about the subacromial bursa. Boston: Thomas Todd; 1934.
2. Adams C. The genuine works of hippocrates. Baltimore: Williams & Wilkins; 1939.
3. Gardner E. The embryology of the clavicle. Clin Orthop Relat Res. United States. 1968;58:9–16.
4. Ogata S, Uhthoff HK. The early development and ossification of the human clavicle – an embryologic study. Acta Orthop Scand. England. 1990;61(4):330–4.
5. Jit I, Kulkarni M. Times of appearance and fusion of epiphysis at the medial end of the clavicle. Indian J Med Res. India. 1976;64(5):773–82.
6. Tyrnin A. The Bohler clavicular splint in the treatment of clavicular injuries. J Bone Joint Surg. 1937;19:417–24.
7. McGraw MA, Mehlman CT, Lindsell CJ, Kirby CL. Postnatal growth of the clavicle: birth to 18 years of age. J Pediatr Orthop. United States. 2009;29(8):937–43.

8. Gray H. Anatomy of the human body. Philadelphia: Lea & Febiger; 1918.
9. Harrington MAJ, Keller TS, Seiler JG 3rd, Weikert DR, Moeljanto E, Schwartz HS. Geometric properties and the predicted mechanical behavior of adult human clavicles. J Biomech. United States. 1993;26(4–5):417–26.
10. Moseley HF. The clavicle: its anatomy and function. Clin Orthop Relat Res. United States. 1968;58:17–27.
11. Abbott LC, Lucas DB. The function of the clavicle; its surgical significance. Ann Surg. United States. 1954;140(4):583–99.
12. Sinha A, Edwin J, Sreeharsha B, Bhalaik V, Brownson P. A radiological study to define safe zones for drilling during plating of clavicle fractures. J Bone Joint Surg Br. England. 2011;93(9):1247–52.
13. Robinson CM. Fractures of the clavicle in the adult. Epidemiology and classification. J Bone Joint Surg Br. England. 1998;80(3):476–84.
14. Nordqvist A, Petersson C. The incidence of fractures of the clavicle. Clin Orthop Relat Res. United States. 1994;300:127–32.
15. Postacchini F, Gumina S, De Santis P, Albo F. Epidemiology of clavicle fractures. J shoulder Elb Surg. United States. 2002;11(5):452–6.
16. Nowak J, Mallmin H, Larsson S. The aetiology and epidemiology of clavicular fractures. A prospective study during a two-year period in Uppsala, Sweden. Injury. Netherlands. 2000;31(5):353–8.
17. Khan LAK, Bradnock TJ, Scott C, Robinson CM. Fractures of the clavicle. J Bone Joint Surg Am. United States. 2009;91(2):447–60.
18. Kihlstrom C, Moller M, Lonn K, Wolf O. Clavicle fractures: epidemiology, classification and treatment of 2 422 fractures in the Swedish fracture register; an observational study. BMC Musculoskelet Disord. England. 2017;18(1):82.
19. FLJ A. Fractures and ligamentous injuries of the clavicle and its articulation. J Bone Joint Surg Am. United States. 1967;49(4):774–84.
20. Neer CS 2nd. Fractures of the clavicle. In: Rockwood CA, Green D, editors. Fractures in adults. Philadelphia: JB Lippincott; 1984. p. 707–13.
21. Neer CS 2nd. Fractures of the distal third of the clavicle. Clin Orthop Relat Res. United States. 1968;58:43–50.
22. Rockwood C Jr, Matsen F III. Fractures of the clavicle. In: The shoulder. Philadelphia: WB Saunders; 1990. p. 367–412.
23. Rockwood C Jr, Buckholz R, Heckman DG. Fractures of the clavicle. In: Fractures in adults. 4th ed. Philadelphia: Lippincott Raven; 1996. p. 1109–93.
24. Rubin A. Bith injuries: incidence, mechanism and incidents, mechanisms and end result. Obstet Gynecol. United States. 1964;23:218–21.
25. Beall MH, Ross MG. Clavicle fracture in labor: risk factors and associated morbidities. J Perinatol. United States. 2001;21(8):513–5.
26. Cohen AW, Otto SR. Obstetric clavicular fractures. A three-year analysis. J Reprod Med. United States. 1980;25(3):119–22.
27. Cumming WA. Neonatal skeletal fractures. Birth trauma or child abuse? J Can Assoc Radiol. Canada. 1979;30(1):30–3.
28. Basamania CJ, Rockwood CA. Rockwood and Matsen's the shoulder. Philadelphia: Elsevier – Health Sciences Division; 2016.
29. Stanley D, Trowbridge EA, Norris SH. The mechanism of clavicular fracture. A clinical and biomechanical analysis. J Bone Joint Surg Br. England. 1988;70(3):461–4.
30. Fowler AW. Fractures of the clavicle. J Bone Joint Surg. 1962;44:440.
31. Sankarankutty M, Turner BW. Fractures of the clavicle. Injury. Netherlands. 1975;7(2):101–6.
32. Canadian Orthopaedic Trauma Society. Nonoperative treatment compared with plate fixation of displaced midshaft clavicular fractures. A multicenter, randomized clinical trial. J Bone Joint Surg Am. United States. 2007;89(1):1–10.
33. McKee MD, Schemitsch EH, Stephen DJG, Kreder HJ, Yoo D, Harrington J. Functional outcome following clavicle fractures in polytrauma patients. J Trauma Acute Care Surg [Internet]. 1999;47(3):616.
34. Taitsman LA, Nork SE, Coles CP, Barei DP, Agel J. Open clavicle fractures and associated injuries. J Orthop Trauma. United States. 2006;20(6):396–9.
35. Gottschalk HP, Dumont G, Khanani S, Browne RH, Starr AJ. Open clavicle fractures: patterns of trauma and associated injuries. J Orthop Trauma. United States. 2012;26(2):107–9.
36. Ebraheim NA, An HS, Jackson WT, Pearlstein SR, Burgess A, Tscherne H, et al. Scapulothoracic dissociation. J Bone Joint Surg Am. United States. 1988;70(3):428–32.
37. Rowe CR. An atlas of anatomy and treatment of midclavicular fractures. Clin Orthop Relat Res. United States. 1968;58:29–42.
38. Dugdale T, Fulkerson J. Pneumothorax complicating a closed fracture of the clavicle: a case report. Clin Orthop Relat Res. 1987;221:212–4.
39. Throckmorton T, Kuhn JE. Fractures of the medial end of the clavicle. J shoulder Elb Surg. United States. 2007;16(1):49–54.
40. Calder JDF, Solan M, Gidwani S, Allen S, Ricketts DM. Management of paediatric clavicle fractures – is follow-up necessary? An audit of 346 cases. Ann R Coll Surg Engl. England. 2002;84(5):331–3.
41. Mehlman C, Yihua G, Bochang C, Zhingang W. Operative treatment of completely displaced clavicle shaft fractures inchildren. J Pediatr Orthop. 2009;29:81–5.
42. Namdari S, Ganley TJ, Baldwin K, Rendon Sampson N, Hosalkar H, Nikci V, et al. Fixation of displaced midshaft clavicle fractures in skeletally immature patients. J Pediatr Orthop. United States. 2011;31(5):507–11.
43. Herzog MM, Whitesell RC, Mac LM, Jackson ML, Culotta BA, Axelrod JR, et al. Functional outcomes following non-operative versus operative treatment of clavicle fractures in adolescents. J Child Orthop. England. 2017;11(4):310–7.

44. Nordqvist A, Petersson CJ, Redlund-Johnell I. Mid-clavicle fractures in adults: end result study after conservative treatment. J Orthop Trauma. United States. 1998;12(8):572–6.
45. Grassi FA, Tajana MS, D'Angelo F. Management of midclavicular fractures: comparison between nonoperative treatment and open intramedullary fixation in 80 patients. J Trauma. United States. 2001;50(6):1096–100.
46. Neer CS 2nd. Nonunion of the clavicle. J Am Med Assoc. United States. 1960;172:1006–11.
47. Quigley T. The management of simple fracture of the clavicle in adults. N Engl J Med. 1950;243:286–90.
48. Andersen K, Jensen P, Lauritzen J. Treatment of clavicular fractures: figure-of-eight versus a simple sling. Acta Orthop Scand. 1987;58:71–4.
49. McCandless D, Mowbray M. Treatment of displaced fractures of the clavicle: Sling vs. figure-of-eight bandage. Practitioner. 1979;223:266–7.
50. Zlowodzki M, Zelle BA, Cole PA, Jeray K, McKee MD. Treatment of acute midshaft clavicle fractures: systematic review of 2144 fractures: on behalf of the Evidence-Based Orthopaedic Trauma Working Group. J Orthop Trauma. United States. 2005;19(7):504–7.
51. Lenza M, Belloti JC, Andriolo RB, Faloppa F. Conservative interventions for treating middle third clavicle fractures in adolescents and adults. Cochrane database Syst Rev. England. 2014;(5):CD007121.
52. Hill JM, McGuire MH, Crosby LA. Closed treatment of displaced middle-third fractures of the clavicle gives poor results. J Bone Joint Surg Br. England. 1997;79(4):537–9.
53. Eskola A, Vainionpaa S, Myllynen P, Patiala H, Rokkanen P. Outcome of clavicular fracture in 89 patients. Arch Orthop Trauma Surg. Germany. 1986;105(6):337–8.
54. Judd DB, Pallis MP, Smith E, Bottoni CR. Acute operative stabilization versus nonoperative management of clavicle fractures. Am J Orthop (Belle Mead NJ). United States. 2009;38(7):341–5.
55. Smekal V, Irenberger A, Struve P, Wambacher M, Krappinger D, Kralinger FS. Elastic stable intramedullary nailing versus nonoperative treatment of displaced midshaft clavicular fractures-a randomized, controlled, clinical trial. J Orthop Trauma. United States. 2009;23(2):106–12.
56. Mirzatolooei F. Comparison between operative and nonoperative treatment methods in the management of comminuted fractures of the clavicle. Acta Orthop Traumatol Turc. Turkey. 2011;45(1):34–40.
57. Virtanen KJ, Remes V, Pajarinen J, Savolainen V, Bjorkenheim J-M, Paavola M. Sling compared with plate osteosynthesis for treatment of displaced midshaft clavicular fractures: a randomized clinical trial. J Bone Joint Surg Am. United States. 2012;94(17):1546–53.
58. Robinson CM, Goudie EB, Murray IR, Jenkins PJ, Ahktar MA, Read EO, et al. Open reduction and plate fixation versus nonoperative treatment for displaced midshaft clavicular fractures: a multicenter, randomized, controlled trial. J Bone Joint Surg Am. United States. 2013;95(17):1576–84.
59. Kulshrestha V, Roy T, Audige L. Operative versus nonoperative management of displaced midshaft clavicle fractures: a prospective cohort study. J Orthop Trauma. United States. 2011;25(1):31–8.
60. Wang X-H, Guo W-J, Li A-B, Cheng G-J, Lei T, Zhao Y-M. Operative versus nonoperative treatment for displaced midshaft clavicle fractures: a meta-analysis based on current evidence. Clinics (Sao Paulo). Brazil. 2015;70(8):584–92.
61. Ahrens PM, Garlick NI, Barber J, Tims EM. The clavicle trial: a multicenter randomized controlled trial comparing operative with nonoperative treatment of displaced midshaft clavicle fractures. J Bone Joint Surg Am. United States. 2017;99(16):1345–54.
62. Goudie EB, Clement ND, Murray IR, Lawrence CR, Wilson M, Brooksbank AJ, et al. The influence of shortening on clinical outcome in healed displaced midshaft clavicular fractures after nonoperative treatment. J Bone Joint Surg Am. United States. 2017;99(14):1166–72.
63. McKee MD, Seiler JG, Jupiter JB. The application of the limited contact dynamic compression plate in the upper extremity: an analysis of 114 consecutive cases. Injury. Netherlands. 1995;26(10):661–6.
64. Russo R, Visconti V, Lorini S, Lombardi LV. Displaced comminuted midshaft clavicle fractures: use of Mennen plate fixation system. J Trauma. United States. 2007;63(4):951–4.
65. Collinge C, Devinney S, Herscovici D, DiPasquale T, Sanders R. Anterior-inferior plate fixation of middle-third fractures and nonunions of the clavicle. J Orthop Trauma. United States. 2006;20(10):680–6.
66. Potter J, Jones C, Wild L, Schemitsch E, McKee M. The restoration of objectively measured shoulder strength and patient-oriented outcome after immediate fixation versus delayed reconstruction of displaced midshaft fractures of the clavicle. J Shoulder Elb Surg. 2007;5(16):514–8.
67. Golish SR, Oliviero JA, Francke EI, Miller MD. A biomechanical study of plate versus intramedullary devices for midshaft clavicle fixation. J Orthop Surg Res. England. 2008;3:28.
68. Iannotti MR, Crosby LA, Stafford P, Grayson G, Goulet R. Effects of plate location and selection on the stability of midshaft clavicle osteotomies: a biomechanical study. J shoulder Elb Surg. United States. 2002;11(5):457–62.
69. Huang JI, Toogood P, Chen MR, Wilber JH, Cooperman DR. Clavicular anatomy and the applicability of precontoured plates. J Bone Joint Surg Am. United States. 2007;89(10):2260–5.
70. Formaini N, Taylor BC, Backes J, Bramwell TJ. Superior versus anteroinferior plating of clavicle fractures. Orthopedics. United States. 2013;36(7):e898–904.
71. Lee Y, Lin C, Huang C, Chen C, Liao W. Operative treatment of midclavicular fractures in 62 elderly

patients: knowles pin versus plate. Orthopedics. 2007;30(11):959–64.
72. Chu C-M, Wang S-J, Lin L-C. Fixation of mid-third clavicular fractures with knowles pins: 78 patients followed for 2–7 years. Acta Orthop Scand. England. 2002;73(2):134–9.
73. Mudd CD, Quigley KJ, Gross LB. Excessive complications of open intramedullary nailing of midshaft clavicle fractures with the Rockwood clavicle pin. Clin Orthop Relat Res. United States. 2011;469(12):3364–70.
74. Strauss EJ, Egol KA, France MA, Koval KJ, Zuckerman JD. Complications of intramedullary Hagie pin fixation for acute midshaft clavicle fractures. J shoulder Elb Surg. United States. 2007;16(3):280–4.
75. Liu P-C, Chien S-H, Chen J-C, Hsieh C-H, Chou P-H, Lu C-C. Minimally invasive fixation of displaced midclavicular fractures with titanium elastic nails. J Orthop Trauma. United States. 2010;24(4):217–23.
76. Jubel A, Andermahr J, Schiffer G, Tsironis K, Rehm KE. Elastic stable intramedullary nailing of midclavicular fractures with a titanium nail. Clin Orthop Relat Res. United States. 2003;408:279–85.
77. Maget RJ. Migration of a Kirschner wire from the shoulder region into the lung: report of two cases. J Bone Joint Surg Am. 1943;25:477–83.
78. Lyons FA, Rockwood CAJ. Migration of pins used in operations on the shoulder. J Bone Joint Surg Am. United States. 1990;72(8):1262–7.
79. Sethi GK, Scott SM. Subclavian artery laceration due to migration of a Hagie pin. Surgery. United States. 1976;80(5):644–6.
80. Gao Y, Chen W, Liu Y-J, Li X, Wang H-L, Chen Z-Y. Plating versus intramedullary fixation for midshaft clavicle fractures: a systemic review and meta-analysis. PeerJ. United States. 2016;4:e1540.
81. Ferran NA, Hodgson P, Vannet N, Williams R, Evans RO. Locked intramedullary fixation vs plating for displaced and shortened mid-shaft clavicle fractures: a randomized clinical trial. J shoulder Elb Surg. United States. 2010;19(6):783–9.
82. Nordqvist A, Petersson C, Redlund-Johnell I. The natural course of lateral clavicle fracture. 15 (11–21) year follow-up of 110 cases. Acta Orthop Scand. England. 1993;64(1):87–91.
83. Oh JH, Kim SH, Lee JH, Shin SH, Gong HS. Treatment of distal clavicle fracture: a systematic review of treatment modalities in 425 fractures. Arch Orthop Trauma Surg. Germany. 2011;131(4):525–33.
84. Good DW, Lui DF, Leonard M, Morris S, JP ME. Clavicle hook plate fixation for displaced lateral-third clavicle fractures (Neer type II): a functional outcome study. J shoulder Elb Surg. United States. 2012;21(8):1045–8.
85. Flinkkilä T, Ristiniemi J, Lakovaara M, Hyvönen P, Leppilahti J. Hook-plate fixation of unstable lateral clavicle fractures: a report on 63 patients. Acta Orthop [Internet]. Taylor & Francis. 2006;77(4):644–9. Available from: https://doi.org/10.1080/17453670610012737.
86. Muramatsu K, Shigetomi M, Matsunaga T, Murata Y, Taguchi T. Use of the AO hook-plate for treatment of unstable fractures of the distal clavicle. Arch Orthop Trauma Surg. Germany. 2007;127(3):191–4.
87. Yang S-W, Lin LC, Chang SJ, Kuo SM, Hwang L-C. Treatment of acute unstable distal clavicle fractures with single coracoclavicular suture fixation. Orthopedics. United States. 2011;34(6):172.
88. Han L, Hu Y, Quan R, Fang W, Jin B, Huang L. Treatment of Neer IIb distal clavicle fractures using anatomical locked plate fixation with coracoclavicular ligament augmentation. J Hand Surg Am. United States. 2017;42(12):1036.e1–6.
89. Flinkkila T, Ristiniemi J, Hyvonen P, Hamalainen M. Surgical treatment of unstable fractures of the distal clavicle: a comparative study of Kirschner wire and clavicular hook plate fixation. Acta Orthop Scand. England. 2002;73(1):50–3.
90. Salipas A, Kimmel LA, Edwards ER, Rakhra S, Moaveni AK. Natural history of medial clavicle fractures. Injury. Netherlands. 2016;47(10):2235–9.
91. Ganz R, Noseberger B. Treatment of scapular fractures. Hefte Unfallheilkd. 1975;126:59–62.
92. Goss TP. Double disruptions of the superior shoulder suspensory complex. J Orthop Trauma. United States. 1993;7(2):99–106.
93. Herscovici DJ, Fiennes AG, Allgower M, Ruedi TP. The floating shoulder: ipsilateral clavicle and scapular neck fractures. J Bone Joint Surg Br England. 1992;74(3):362–4.
94. Owens BD, Goss TP. The floating shoulder. J Bone Joint Surg Br England. 2006;88(11):1419–24.
95. Rikli D, Regazzoni P, Renner N. The unstable shoulder girdle: early functional treatment utilizing open reduction and internal fixation. J Orthop Trauma. United States. 1995;9(2):93–7.
96. Leung KS, Lam TP. Open reduction and internal fixation of ipsilateral fractures of the scapular neck and clavicle. J Bone Joint Surg Am. United States. 1993;75(7):1015–8.
97. Ramos L, Mencia R, Alonso A, Ferrandez L. Conservative treatment of ipsilateral fractures of the scapula and clavicle. J Trauma. United States. 1997;42(2):239–42.
98. McKee M, Rockwood C, Green D. Clavicle fractures. In: Fracture in adults. Philadelphia: Lippincott; 2015. p. 1427–74.
99. Robinson CM, Court-Brown CM, McQueen MM, Wakefield AE. Estimating the risk of nonunion following nonoperative treatment of a clavicular fracture. J Bone Joint Surg Am. United States. 2004;86-A(7):1359–65.
100. Wilkins RM, Johnston RM. Ununited fractures of the clavicle. J Bone Joint Surg Am. United States. 1983;65(6):773–8.
101. Wick M, Muller EJ, Kollig E, Muhr G. Midshaft fractures of the clavicle with a shortening of more

than 2 cm predispose to nonunion. Arch Orthop Trauma Surg. Germany. 2001;121(4):207–11.
102. Murray IR, Foster CJ, Eros A, Robinson CM. Risk factors for nonunion after nonoperative treatment of displaced midshaft fractures of the clavicle. J Bone Joint Surg Am. United States. 2013;95(13):1153–8.
103. Edwards D, Kavanagh T, Flannery M. Fractures of the distal clavicle: a case for fixation. Injury. 1992;23:44–6.
104. Kavanagh T, Sarkar S. Complications of displaced fractures (Type II Neer) of the outer end of the clavicle. J Bone Jt Surg Br. 1985;67:492–3.
105. Wijdicks F-J, Van der Meijden O, Millett P, Verleisdonk E, Houwert R. Systematic review of the complications of plate fixation of clavicle fractures. Arch Orthop Trauma Sur. 2012;132(5):617–25.
106. McKee MD, Wild LM, Schemitsch EH. Midshaft malunions of the clavicle. J Bone Joint Surg Am. United States. 2003;85-A(5):790–7.
107. Chan KY, Jupiter JB, Leffert RD, Marti R. Clavicle malunion. J shoulder Elb Surg. United States. 1999;8(4):287–90.
108. Ledger M, Leeks N, Ackland T, Wang A. Short malunions of the clavicle: an anatomic and functional study. J shoulder Elb Surg. United States. 2005;14(4):349–54.
109. Bosch U, Skutek M, Peters G, Tscherne H. Extension osteotomy in malunited clavicular fractures. J shoulder Elb Surg. United States. 1998;7(4):402–5.
110. Tse DH, Slabaugh PB, Carlson PA. Injury to the axillary artery by a closed fracture of the clavicle. A case report. J Bone Joint Surg Am. United States. 1980;62(8):1372–4.
111. Kendall KM, Burton JH, Cushing B. Fatal subclavian artery transection from isolated clavicle fracture. J Trauma. United States. 2000;48(2):316–8.
112. Barbier O, Malghem J, Delaere O, Vande Berg B, Rombouts JJ. Injury to the brachial plexus by a fragment of bone after fracture of the clavicle. J Bone Joint Surg Br. England. 1997;79(4):534–6.
113. Howard FM, Shafer SJ. Injuries to the clavicle with neurovascular complications. A study of fourteen cases. J Bone Joint Surg Am. United States. 1965;47(7):1335–46.
114. Chen D, Chuang D, Wei F. Unusual thoracic outlet syndrome secondary to fractured clavicle. J Trauma. 2002;52:393–9.
115. Connolly JF, Dehne R. Nonunion of the clavicle and thoracic outlet syndrome. J Trauma. United States. 1989;29(8):1123–7.
116. Thyagarajan DS, Day M, Dent C, Williams R, Evans R. Treatment of mid-shaft clavicle fractures: A comparative study. Int J Shoulder Surg. South Africa. 2009;3(2):23–7.
117. Ring D, Holovacs T. Brachial plexus palsy after intramedullary fixation of a clavicular fracture. A report of three cases. J Bone Joint Surg Am. 2005;87(8):1834–7.
118. Jeyaseelan L, Singh VK, Ghosh S, Sinisi M, Fox M. Iatropathic brachial plexus injury: a complication of delayed fixation of clavicle fractures. Bone Joint J Engl. 2013;95-B(1):106–10.
119. Namdari S, Voleti P, Huffman G. Compressive brachial plexopathy after fixation of a clavicular fracture nonuniona case report. J Bone Joint Surg. 2012;2:261–4.
120. Thavarajah D, Scadden J. Iatrogenic postoperative brachial plexus compression secondary to hypertrophic non-union of a clavicle fracture. Ann R Coll Surg Engl [Internet]. Royal College of Surgeons. 2013;95(3):e55–7.
121. Bain GI, Galley IJ, Keogh ARE, Durrant AW. Axillary artery pseudoaneurysm after plate osteosynthesis for a clavicle nonunion: a case report and literature review. Int J Shoulder Surg. South Africa. 2010;4(3):79–82.
122. Clitherow HDS, Bain GI. Major neurovascular complications of clavicle fracture surgery. Shoul Elb [Internet]. Sage UK: London, England: SAGE Publications. 2015;7(1):3–12.
123. Robinson CM, Cairns DA. Primary nonoperative treatment of displaced lateral fractures of the clavicle. J Bone Joint Surg Am. United States. 2004;86-A(4):778–82.
124. Zenni EJJ, Krieg JK, Rosen MJ. Open reduction and internal fixation of clavicular fractures. J Bone Joint Surg Am. United States. 1981;63(1):147–51.

Acromioclavicular Joint Injuries

3

Simone Cerciello, Felix Dyrna, Leo Pauzenberger, Jeremiah D. Johnson, Knut Beitzel, and Augustus D. Mazzocca

Introduction

The AC joint is a diarthrodial joint; in association with the sterno-clavicular joint it connects the arm with the axial skeleton. Injuries of the (AC) joint were initially described by Hippocrates in the fourth century BC [1]. They are common in contact athletes and represent 40–50% of all sport injuries of the shoulder [2].

Proper treatment is important as failure may result in aesthetically unpleasant deformities of the clavicle, pain, fatigue, and muscle weakness especially with overhead activities. Dysfunction of scapulothoracic dynamics might result and this has been associated with inferior clinical outcomes. Unfortunately, controversies still exist on the classification and further treatment of these injuries.

S. Cerciello
Casa di Cura Villa Betania, Rome, Italy

Marrelli hospital, Crotone, Italy

F. Dyrna · K. Beitzel
Department of Orthopaedic Sportsmedicine, Technical University, Munich, Germany

L. Pauzenberger · J. D. Johnson · A. D. Mazzocca (✉)
Department of Orthopaedic Surgery, University of Connecticut, Farmington, CT, USA
e-mail: mazzocca@uchc.edu

Anatomy and Biomechanics

The AC joint is formed by the medial facet of the acromion and the lateral aspect of the clavicle. It has variable angles of inclination in both the sagittal and coronal planes ranging from a vertical orientation to 50° of obliquity [3]. The articular surface of the acromial end of the clavicle has hyaline cartilage until 17 years of age when it transitions to fibrocartilage. A similar evolution occurs at the clavicular side of the acromion around the age of 23 [4]. An AC joint meniscus has been described but its biomechanical role is poorly understood and it undergoes an involution process with aging and completely disintegrates by age 40 [5]. This may explain why degenerative changes affect this joint more frequently than the sterno-clavicular joint. Although the AC joint is particularly stable, it can undergo up to 6 mm of translation in anterior, posterior, and superior directions under a load [6]. In addition, the joint rotates 5–8° with scapulothoracic motion and 40–45° with shoulder abduction and elevation [7]. Stability of the joint is provided by passive (ligaments) and active restraints (muscles). Ligaments have been divided into intrinsic (acromioclavicular ligaments and capsule) and extrinsic (coraco-clavicular ligaments). Anterior-posterior plane stability is provided by the acromio-clavicular ligaments, which are thickenings of the joint capsule. Normal acromio-clavicular ligaments are about 2.5 mm in thickness [8]. The superior part is the strongest [9]

I. A. Trail et al. (eds.), *Textbook of Shoulder Surgery*, https://doi.org/10.1007/978-3-319-70099-1_3

and is further augmented by merging fibers of the deltoid-trapezial fascia [10]. The acromio-clavicular ligaments also act in the horizontal plane providing 50% and 90% restraint to anterior and posterior displacement respectively. The anterior-superior portion of the capsule may also play a role in preventing posterior displacement of the clavicle and the anterior and posterior area likely acts as a restraint to posterior rotation. The AC capsule attachments extend approximately 5–8 mm from the joint onto the adjacent bone. Therefore, excessive distal clavicle resection may result in increased posterior translation and rotation of the clavicle and should be avoided [11].

The superior-inferior stability is mainly provided by the coraco-clavicular (CC) ligaments. The trapezoid ligament is the most lateral. It originates on the lateral aspect of the undersurface of the clavicle (25.4 mm in males and 22.9 mm in females) and provides resistance to acromio-clavicular joint compression [12]. The conoid ligament insertion is more medial (47.2 mm in men and 42.8 mm in females from the lateral edge of the clavicle). It is responsible for about 60% of the restraint to anterior and superior clavicular displacement and rotation [9]. In addition, CC ligaments have a major role in stabilizing the joint against greater forces whereas AC ligaments are more effective against smaller loads [9]. Deltoid and trapezius muscles contribute to joint stability through their insertions on the superior aspect of the clavicle and the acromion process [13].

Epidemiology and Classification

AC joint injuries are common in contact sports; however, the real prevalence is likely underestimated as the diagnosis is missed in several patients [14]. Webb and Bannister reported a 45% incidence of AC injuries in first-class rugby players [15]. The spectrum of acromio-clavicular joint injury can range from minor sprains and subluxations to complete dislocations. The injury is often caused by a direct trauma to the shoulder with the arm in adduction. The acromion is then pushed inferiorly while the clavicle holds its anatomic position by resisting downward displacement through an interlocking of the sterno-clavicular and coraco-clavicular ligaments, and anteroposterior displacement through the acromio-clavicular ligaments [6, 16]. The endpoint of this mechanism is variable damage to the intrinsic and extrinsic ligaments. In the worst-case scenario, high-energy trauma can result in avulsion of deltoid and trapezius muscle attachments from the clavicle. Less frequently the injury is caused by indirect force. A fall onto the elbow can drive the humerus proximally involving the AC joint; however, in these circumstances the strain only affects intrinsic ligaments and not the coraco-clavicular ligaments. The extent of clavicle displacement varies based on the severity of the injury. Rockwood in 1984 developed a six stage radiographic classification of AC joint injuries (Table 3.1) [17]. Type I is a sprain of the joint with no involvement of intrinsic and extrinsic ligaments. In type II injuries AC ligaments are usually torn, while CC ligaments are sprained; CC displacement is usually <25%. A disruption of CC ligaments, AC ligaments, and a sprain of the deltopectoral fascia define type III injuries; 25–100% CC displacement is usually found. In type IV sprains the clavicle is dislocated posteriorly into the trapezial fascia; CC ligaments, AC ligaments, and deltopectoral fascia are generally torn. In type V injuries the AC, CC ligaments, and deltopectoral fascia are completely torn

Table 3.1 Rockwood's classification of AC joint injuries by soft tissue injury and radiographic findings [17]

Rockwood classification	Soft tissue injury	Radiographs
Type I	AC joint sprain	Normal
Type II	AC ligament disruption, CC ligaments sprain	CC displacement <25% contralateral
Type III	AC, CC ligament disruption	CC displacement is 25-100% contralateral
Type IV	AC, CC, and trapezial fascia disruption	Clavicle is displaced posteriorly on axillary view
Type V	AC, CC, and deltopectoral fascia disruption	CC displacement is >100% contralateral
Type VI	AC, CC ligament disruption	Clavicle is displaced inferiorly in a subcoracoid or subacromial position

leading to a CC displacement >100% compared with the contralateral side. Type VI injuries are rare and result from hyperabduction and external rotation of the shoulder girdle causing an inferior dislocation of the distal clavicle into a subcoracoid position. This classification system is useful in choosing the correct treatment protocol, but precise X-rays must be performed.

Clinical Presentation and Imaging

The majority of patients with an acute acromioclavicular injury will present with localized pain, swelling and tenderness over the joint. The injured upper extremity is typically held in an adducted and supported position to reduce the pain. Pain can be accentuated with abduction and cross-body adduction of the arm, which loads the acromioclavicular joint [18]. Standing examination may increase the extent of AC joint displacement. In type II and III injuries reduction of the AC joint is possible when a downward pressure is applied on the lateral aspect of the clavicle. Sternoclavicular pain may also be present in type IV injuries, when posterior displacement of the distal portion of the clavicle is associated with anterior dislocation of the sternoclavicular joint. Patients with type V and VI injuries may claim of pain in the neck or trapezius muscle as a result of soft-tissue injury and stripping of the deltotrapezial fascia. Transient paresthesia of the arm have been reported in type VI dislocations [19]. Clinical diagnosis is confirmed with imaging analysis. Standard X-rays should reduce the exposure of a standard shoulder radiograph by one-half to maximize the visualization of the AC joint. Standard radiographs include true anterior-posterior and axillary views. These views are generally sufficient to confirm the diagnosis and but not precise enough stage the injury especially when comparison with the unaffected side is missing. Therefore, a single film, bilateral Zanca view is recommended to increase visualization of the joint by directing the X-ray beam to 10–15° cephalic tilt and allows for contralateral comparison of the CC distance (Fig. 3.1) [20]. Additionally an axillary view or lateral stress X-ray like the

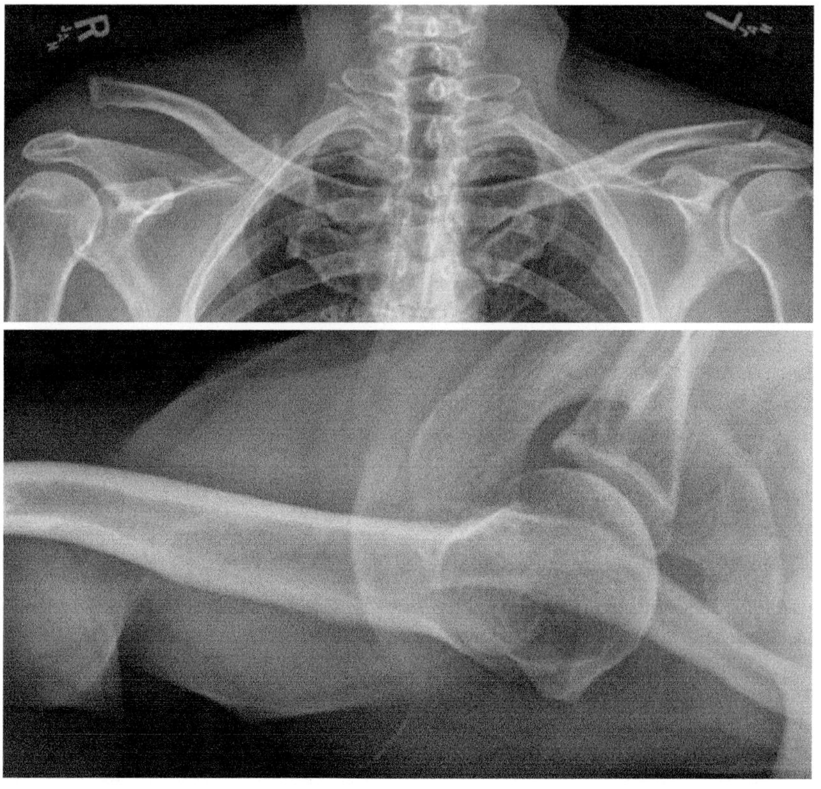

Fig. 3.1 Bilateral zanca view (top) and axillary view (below) of a high grade AC separation (Type V) in a patient following a dirt bike accident. The bilateral zanca view provides a good comparison of the CC distances. Note the increased CC distance on the right side

Alexander view [21] are essential to diagnose posterior displacement of the clavicle in type-IV and V acromioclavicular joint separations. The CC distance should be measured on the anterior-posterior view. In healthy subjects the AC joint is congruent and the CC distance is between 1.1 and 1.3 cm [22]. A 40–50% difference in CC distance between the normal and affected shoulders is predictive for complete disruption of the CC ligaments [22]. Rockwood et al. found a side-to-side CC difference of 25% in cases of complete AC joint disruption [13]. Additional imaging including MRI are helpful in assessing acromioclavicular and coracoclavicular ligamentous disruption. Moreover, MRI can be helpful in detecting associated injuries requiring surgical treatment. Approximately 18.2% of patients with grade III to V AC dislocations show an additional injury requiring surgery [23].

Management

Correct management depends on the grade of AC joint injury and timing. Conservative treatment with a sling has been shown to be successful in type I and II sprains [24]. Additional options include simple analgesia, anti-inflammatory medications, ice therapy, activity modification, and complete rest. Immobilization is usually shorter in type I injuries than in type II sprains as reported by Park et al. [25]. The sling should be discontinued once the patient is asymptomatic. Contact sports and heavy lifting should be avoided until the patient is free of pain and has symmetric shoulder range of motion and strength. Despite patient satisfaction rates of 80–90% [26], persistent pain at the AC joint with limitation of activities have been described. However, the rate of patients with persistent pain decreases with time [27] and is lower in type II than in type I injuries [26].

The treatment of type III dislocations is still debated. Both conservative treatment and surgery have been proposed with satisfactory outcomes and no statistically significant benefit from surgery has emerged [28]. Schlegel et al. compared the range of motion and rotational strength of conservatively treated shoulders with the contralateral side and found no differences [29]. Gumina et al. reported scapular dyskinesis at a rate of 70.6% and SICK scapula syndrome at 58.3% after conservative treatment of type III injuries. Although similar outcomes have been reported, surgical treatment is still preferred in young and active patients [30].

The goal of surgery is to restore anatomy and prevent hypermobility in horizontal, vertical, and rotational planes without limiting the physiologic AC joint function with regard to scapulothoracic motion. Multiple surgical options have been described to address AC injuries and include: primary fixation of the AC joint, fixation of the clavicle to the coracoid, ligament reconstruction, coracoid process transfer, and distal clavicle resection.

Primary fixation of the AC joint has been the treatment of choice for several decades. However severe complications have been reported with fixation devices such as K wires migrating to the thorax [31]. Hook plates were proposed with satisfactory results in combination with or without soft tissue augmentation. However, plate failure or dislocation, persistent pain, and infections have been reported [32]. Coraco-clavicular fixation with screws was initially popularised by Bosworth [33]. This technique was usually associated with CC ligament reconstruction in acute cases. Recent advancements in synthetic loops and arthroscopic techniques has renewed interest in this surgical option. There are several advantages of loops over screws. Most importantly, loops do not need to be removed, they are a less rigid construct, and their position can be adjusted to achieve a more anatomic reduction and reduced fracture risk. Major drawbacks of loops include clavicle osteolysis, suture cutout, and foreign body reaction [34, 35]. This technique is effective in acute cases when the healing potential of soft tissues such as the CC ligaments is maintained. In chronic cases the loop must be reinforced with ligament transfers (such as CA ligament) or ligament reconstruction. AC ligament transfer, that increase the stability of the AC joint was initially described by Cadenat in 1913 [36]. However, the technique was modified and popularized by Weaver and Dunn who described a transposition of the coracoacromial (CA) ligament in association with a distal clavicle resection to prevent the risk of late joint degeneration [37]. The CA ligament was detached from the acromion and fixed to the lateral end of the clavicle. Primary fixation could be increased by preserving some bone at the end of the CA ligament. Primary stability was also increased with a CC loop. Recently a similar procedure has been described with an all-arthroscopic approach [38]. Different autografts and allografts including semitendinosus and tibialis anterior and different looping configurations have been described to increase the stability of the joint in different planes. One potential drawback of techniques involving different tunnels through the lateral clavicle and coracoid is their potential osseous weakening and increased risk of fractures. Coracoid transfer was introduced by Dewar and Barrington for acute and chronic dislocations [39]. However, persistent AC joint pain and poor long-term outcomes have limited its use.

Distal clavicle resections have been proposed in symptomatic AC joints resulting from previous dislocations. However excessive resections may result in additional AC instability. Unfortunately, patients' outcomes have been generally poor with increased horizontal and vertical instability [40]. The conservative treatment of high-grade dislocations (stage IV, V and VI) with involvement of coraco-clavicular ligaments or the trapezius fascia often yelds unsatisfactory outcomes (20–40%) [41, 42]. Therefore these injuries are treated surgically with the previously outlined surgical options. Acute injuries may be stabilized with constructs such as hook plates or suture buttons. Both techniques reduce the joint and act as an internal brace while the ligaments are allowed to heal in an adequate position. Good outcomes have been reported with both hook plates and double suture buttons [43, 44]. Complications with these techniques include hardware migration, loss of reduction, wound problems, and osteolysis. It is important to act promptly in acute repairs to take full advantage of the biological healing window.

Author's Preferred Method

In high grade dislocations, senior author prefers an open, anatomic repair of the AC and CC ligaments with allograft tendon passed through bone tunnels and secured with interference screws [45]. Accurate repair of the deltoid and trapezoidal fascia is a crucial step since they are often damaged in severe cases. The technique involves an incision over the AC joint and curving inferiorly to better expose the coracoid. After elevating the deltotrapezial fascia of the clavicle and proper exposure of the ligaments, anatomic clavicular bone tunnels are prepared using a 5 mm reamer spaced 20 mm apart for the conoid and trapezoid ligament reconstruction. The trapezoid ligament tunnel should be medialized at least 15 mm from the lateral clavicle to prevent blow out (Fig. 3.2). Allograft tendon is wrapped around the coracoid (Fig. 3.3) with each end secured by a 5.5 mm bioabsorbable tenodesis screw (Fig. 3.4). The posterior and superior AC ligaments are reconstructed with excess graft exiting the lateral tunnel and sutured with strong nonabsorable suture ensuring a stable construct [46]. The deltotrapezial fascia is meticulously closed to provide adequate soft tissue coverage and further support the reconstruction (Fig. 3.5). Postoperative bilateral zanca views are useful in evaluating the reduction and CC distance (Fig. 3.6).

Postoperative management is crucial to protect the repaired AC joint. However several factors affect the protocol. In case of isolated distal clavicle resection, a short (1–3 days) period of immobilisation is indicated. It is then followed by range of motion activities. Strengthening begins at 4–6 weeks; heavy weight training starts at 3 months. After a coracoclavicular ligament reconstruction, the arm is supported with a sling or immobiliser. Gentle passive motion in the supine position is usually initiated at 7–10 days. Standing range of motion should be delayed to ensure early biologic stability. For an acute repair, this typically takes 4–6 weeks and may take up to 6–12 weeks for a chronic reconstruction. In the same manner, strengthening exercises start at 6–12 weeks after an acute repair and 4–5 months after a chronic repair.

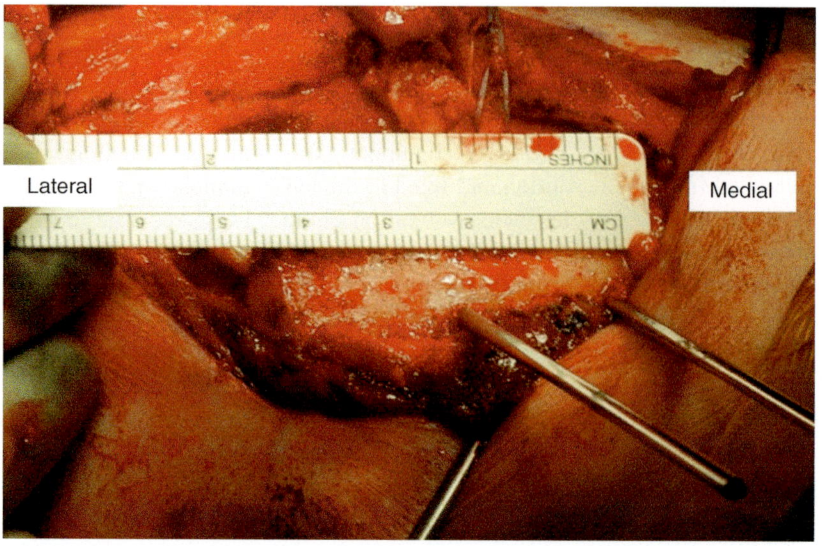

Fig. 3.2 The medial and lateral clavicle tunnels are medialised at least 15 mm from the lateral clavicle and the two tunnels are approximately 20 mm apart

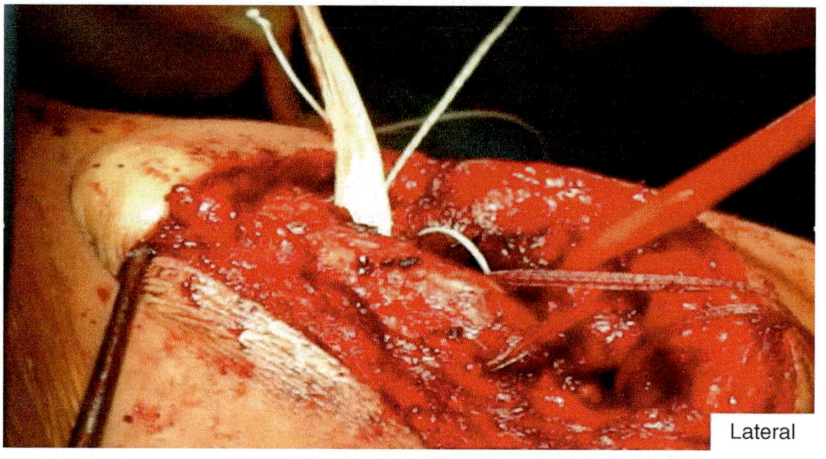

Fig. 3.3 The allograft is passed around the coracoid via suture

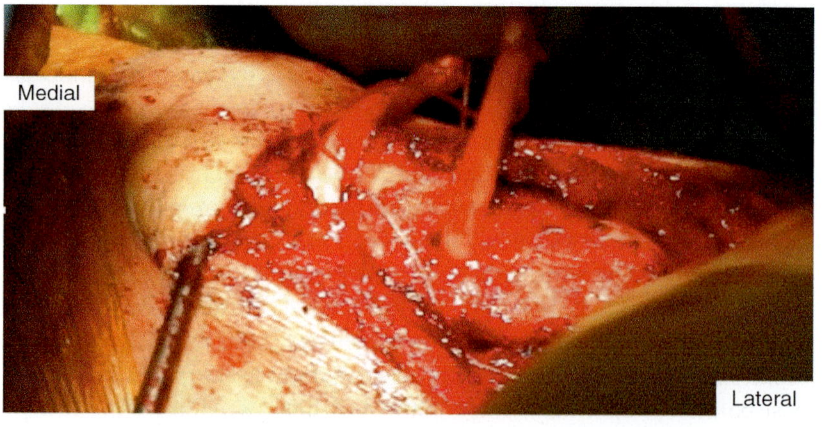

Fig. 3.4 Both ends of the allograft are passed through the bone tunnels via sutures. The AC ligament will then be reconstructed utilising the excess lateral limb of the allograft

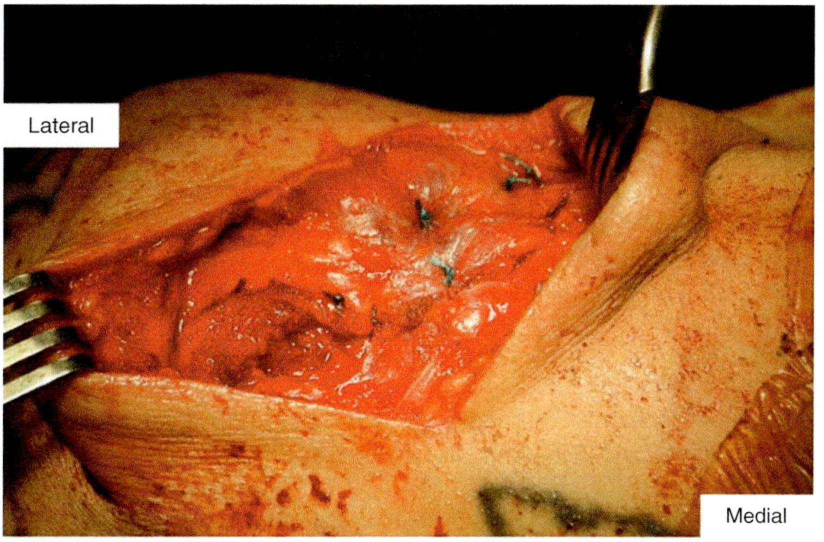

Fig. 3.5 The deltotrapezial fascia is thoroughly closed to provide good soft tissue coverage and further support the repair

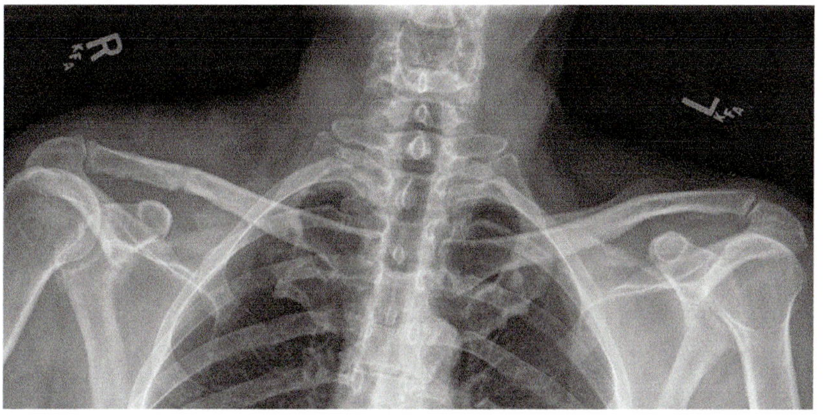

Fig. 3.6 Post-operative bilateral zanca view following a right anatomical reconstruction of the AC and CC ligaments utilizing allograft and interference screws. Note the interval improvement in the CC distance on the right

Results and Complications

Some key principles must be taken into account to achieve good functional outcomes. Anatomic and accurate reduction of the joint is mandatory to prevent recurrent superior displacement and anterior-posterior instability. Biologic aspects enhance late stability; therefore, direct repair in acute injuries and ligament reconstruction in chronic cases is highly recommended. Soft tissue repair or reconstruction must be initially protected with loops of synthetic materials (suture or tape) or rigid implants. Repair of the deltoid and trapezial fascia must be performed in high-grade injuries. Distal clavicle resection may increase postoperative instability and should be considered with caution. However, resection may be an option in chronic cases with radiographic or clinical evidence of AC joint osteoarthritis. The complexity of the local anatomy and biomechanics makes the AC joint susceptible to several complications. General complications include: residual pain or instability, infection, and soft tissue ossification. Chronic pain after surgery may be a disabling condition. Possible causes of chronic pain include horizontal instability (anterior to posterior) of the clavicle, subacromial disease, or neurologic injury. Loss of reduction has been reported in up to 28% of cases with poor clinical outcomes [47]. Loss of reduction maybe due to poor surgical technique or compliance with postoperative protocol. If the arm is not protected in a sling or immobilizer for an appropriate period the reconstructed joint is placed under high static forces affecting the stability. Postoperative infection rate ranges from 0% to 9% [48, 49]. Coracoclavicular ossification has also been reported with an incidence of 50–85% [50]. Specific complications have variable rates according to the different surgical techniques. Ghoring et al. reported an early postoperative complication rate of 43% with a tension band cerclage, 58% with hook plates, and 17% with PDS cord [51]. At 35 months, the residual instability rate was 32% with a tension band, 50% with plate fixation, and 24% with PDS cord treatment.

Complications after distal clavicle resection include excessive resection with violation of ligamentous structures and residual instability or insufficient resection (when less than 5 mm is removed) with persistent pain. Failure of fixation devices leads to loss of reduction and possible hardware migration. Osteolysis around screws has been reported with variable rates and may lead to late fractures. In a series by Fauci et al. osteolysis was 20% at 1 year and 65% at 4 years [52]. Arthroscopic techniques in the treatment of AC joint dislocations have been popularised for their advantages over open approaches such as reduced soft-tissue dissection, decreased skin and wound complication rates, easier rehabilitation, and earlier return to work or sport. However, drawbacks to arthroscopic techniques include: higher cost, longer operative times, and more difficult visualisation of anatomic landmarks. Poor visualisation may have a dramatic impact on tunnel positioning with additional complications such as loss of reduction, osteolysis, fractures, and hardware migration.

Conclusions

AC joint injuries are common in current practice. They often result from direct trauma. Disruption of the AC ligaments leads to anterior-to-posterior instability while failure of the CC ligaments results in superior instability. Recognising concomitant injuries is helpful in decreasing complications and poor outcomes. The bilateral Zanca view is essential for the diagnosing and staging of AC joint injuries by allowing for more accurate comparison of the CC distance. Appropriate treatment depends on the severity of clavicle displacement. A conservative approach is indicated in less severe injuries (type I and II) while surgery is recommended for high-grade dislocations (type IV, V and VI). The treatment of type III injuries is still debated. Surgical approach is generally indicated in young and high demand patients. Surgeons should be aware of complications including: infection, loss of graft or fixation failure, fractures, osteolysis, and hardware migration. However, poor outcomes can be minimised by a meticulous exposure and closure of the deltotrapezial fascia, reaming 5 mm or less for clavicle tunnels, spacing the lateral tunnel 20 mm from the AC joint, tapping tunnels, avoiding a distal clavicle excision, and protecting the repair for 6 weeks in a brace. Good patient outcomes following an AC joint injury can be achieved when these clinical principles are followed.

References

1. Adams FL. The genuine works of Hippocrates. Vols 1 and 2. New York: William Wood; 1886.
2. Kaplan LD, Flanigan DC, Norwig J, Jost P, Bradley J. Prevalence and variance of shoulder injuries in elite collegiate football players. Am J Sports Med. 2005;33(8):1142–6.
3. Bosworth BBM. Complete acromioclavicular dislocation. N Engl J Med. 1949;241:221–5.
4. Beim GM, Werner JJ. Clinical and radiographic evolution of the acromioclavicular joint. Oper Tech Sports Med. 1997;5:65–71.
5. DePalma AF. The role of the discs of the sternoclavicular and acromioclavicular joints. Clin Orthop Relat Res. 1959;13:7–12.
6. Debski RE, Parsons IM 4th, Woo SL, Fu FH. Effect of capsular injury on acromioclavicular joint mechanics. J Bone Joint Surg Am. 2001;83(9):1344–51.
7. Warth RJ, Martetschlager F, Gaskill TR, Millett PJ. Acromioclavicular joint separations. Curr Rev Muscoskelet Med. 2013;6:71–8.
8. Stine IA, Vangsness CT. Analysis of the capsule and ligament insertions about the acromioclavicular joint: a cadaveric study. J Arthrosc Relat Surg. 2009;25:968–74.
9. Fukuda K, Craig EV, An KN, Cofield RH, Chao EY. Biomechanical study of the ligamentous system

of the acromioclavicular joint. J Bone Joint Surg Am. 1986;68:434–40.
10. Epstein D, Day M, Rokito A. Current concepts in the surgical management of acromioclavicular joint injuries. Bull NYU Hosp Jt Dis. 2012;70:11–24.
11. Klimkiewicz JJ, Williams GR, Sher JS, Karduna A, Des Jardins J, Iannotti JP. The acromioclavicular capsule as a restraint to posterior translation of the clavicle: a biomechanical analysis. J Shoulder Elb Surg. 1999;8(2):119–24.
12. Rios CG, Arciero RA, Mazzocca AD. Anatomy of the clavicle and coracoid process for reconstruction of the coracoclavicular ligaments. Am J Sports Med. 2007;35(5):811–7.
13. Rockwood CA Jr, Young DC. Disorders of the acromioclavicular joint. In: Rockwood Jr CA, Hi MFA, editors. The shoulder. Philadelphia: WB Saunders; 1990. p. 413–76.
14. Copeland S. Shoulder surgery. London: WB Saunders; 1997.
15. Webb J, Bannister G. Acromioclavicular disruption in first class rugby players. Br J Sports Med. 1992;26:247–8.
16. Lee KW, Debski RE, Chen CH, Woo SL, Fu FH. Functional evaluation of the ligaments at the acromioclavicular joint during anteroposterior and superoinferior translation. Am J Sports Med. 1997;25(6):858–62.
17. Rockwood CA Jr. Injuries to the acromioclavicular joint. In: Rockwood Jr CA, Green DP, editors. Fractures in adults, vol. 1. 2nd ed. Philadelphia: JB Lippincott; 1984. p. 860–910.
18. Chronopoulos E, Kim TK, Park HB, Ashenbrenner D, McFarland EG. Diagnostic value of physical tests for isolated chronic acromioclavicular lesions. Am J Sports Med. 2004;32(3):655–61.
19. Gerber C, Rockwood CA Jr. Subcoracoid dislocation of the lateral end of the clavicle. A report of three cases. J Bone Joint Surg Am. 1987;69(6):924–7.
20. Zanca P. Shoulder pain: involvement of the acromioclavicular joint. (analysis of 1,000 cases). Am J Roentgenol Radium Therapy, Nucl Med. 1971;112(3):493–506.
21. Alexander OM. Radiography of the acromioclavicular articulation. Med Radiogr Photogr. 1954;30(2):34–9.
22. Bearden JM, Hughston JC, Whatley GS. Acromioclavicular dislocation: method of treatment. J Sports Med. 1973;1(4):5–17.
23. Tischer T, Salzmann GM, El-Azab H, Vogt S, Imhoff AB. Incidence of associated injuries with acute acromioclavicular joint dislocations types III through V. Am J Sports Med. 2009;37(1):136–9; Epub 2008 Aug 25.
24. Mouhsine E, Garofalo R, Crevoisier X, Farron A. Grade I and II acromioclavicular dislocations: results of conservative treatment. J Shoulder Elb Surg. 2003;12(6):599–602.
25. Park JP, Arnold JA, Coker TP, Harris WD, Becker DA. Treatment of acromioclavicular separations. A retrospective study. Am J Sports Med. 1980;8(4):251–6.
26. Bjerneld H, Hovelius L, Thorling J. Acromioclavicular separations treated conservatively. A 5-year follow-up study. Acta Orthop Scand. 1983;54(5):743–5.
27. Shaw MB, McInerney JJ, Dias JJ, Evans PA. Acromioclavicular joint sprains: the post-injury recovery interval. Injury. 2003;34(6):438–42.
28. Smith TO, Chester R, Pearse EO, Hing CB. Operative versus non-operative management following Rockwood grade III acromioclavicular separation: a metaanalysis of the current evidence base. J Orthop Traumatol. 2011;12(1):19–27.
29. Schlegel TF, Burks RT, Marcus RL, Dunn HK. A prospective evaluation of untreated acute grade III acromioclavicular separations. Am J Sports Med. 2001;29(6):699–703.
30. Gumina S, Carbone S, Postacchini F. Scapular dyskinesis and SICK scapula syndrome in patients with chronic type III acromioclavicular dislocation. Arthroscopy. 2009;25(1):40–5; Epub 2008 Oct 10.
31. Norrel H Jr, Lewellyn RC. Migration of a threaded Steinmann pin from an acromioclavicular joint into the spinal canal. A case report. J Bone Joint Surg Am. 1965;47:1024–6.
32. Faraj AA, Ketzer B. The use of a hook-plate in the management of acromioclavicular injuries. Report of ten cases. Acta Orthop Belg. 2001;67(5):448–51.
33. Bosworth BM. Acromioclavicullar separations. New method of repair. Surg Gynecol Obstet. 1941;73:866–71.
34. Stewart AM, Ahmad CS. Failure of acromioclavicular reconstruction using Gore-Tex graft due to aseptic foreign-body reaction and clavicle osteolysis: a case report. J Shoulder Elb Surg. 2004;13(5):558–61.
35. Boldin C, Fankhauser F, Ratschek M, Haller-Schober EM. Foreign-body reaction after reconstruction of complete acromioclavicular dislocation using PDS augmentation. J Shoulder Elb Surg. 2004;13(1):99–100.
36. Cadenat FM. Traitment des luxations et fractures externes de la clavicule. Thése médecine. Paris n° 195. 1913.
37. Weaver JK, Dunn HK. Treatment of acromioclavicular injuries, especially complete acromioclavicular separation. J Bone Joint Surg Am. 1972;5:1187–94.
38. Lafosse L, Baier GP, Leuzinger J. Arthroscopic treatment of acute and chronic acromioclavicular joint dislocation. Arthroscopy. 2005;21(8):1017.
39. Dewar FP, Barrington TW. The treatment of chronic acromio-clavicular dislocation. J Bone Joint Surg Br. 1965;47:32–5; PubMed PMID: 14296242.
40. Corteen DP, Teitge RA. Stabilization of the clavicle after distal resection: a biomechanical study. Am J Sports Med. 2005;33(1):61–7.
41. Bargren JH, Erlanger S, Dick HM. Biomechanics and comparison of two operative methods of treatment of complete acromioclavicular separation. Clin Orthop Relat Res. 1978;130:267–72.
42. Stam L, Dawson I. Complete acromioclavicular dislocations: treatment with a Dacron ligament. Injury. 1991;22(3):173–6. [PubMed].

43. Venjakob AJ, Salzmann GM, Gabel F, et al. Arthroscopically assisted 2-bundle anatomic reduction of acute acromioclavicular joint separations. Am J Sports Med. 2013;41(3):615–21. https://doi.org/10.2214/ajr.112.3.493.
44. Di Francesco A, Zoccali C, Colafarina O, Pizzoferrato R, Flamini S. The use of hook plate in type III and V acromio-clavicular Rockwood dislocations: clinical and radiological midterm results and MRI evaluation in 42 patients. Injury. 2012;43(2):147–52. https://doi.org/10.1016/j.injury.2011.04.002.
45. Carofino BC, Mazzocca AD. The anatomic coracoclavicular ligament reconstruction: surgical technique and indications. J Shoulder Elb Surg. 2010;19(2 Suppl):37–46. https://doi.org/10.1016/j.jse.2010.01.004.
46. Beitzel K, Obopilwe E, Apostolakos J, Cote MP, Russell RP, Charette R, Singh H, Arciero RA, Imhoff AB, Mazzocca AD. Rotational and translational stability of different methods for direct acromioclavicular ligament repair in anatomic acromioclavicular joint reconstruction. Am J Sports Med. 2014;42(9):2141–8. https://doi.org/10.1177/0363546514538947; Epub 2014 Jul 2.
47. Mayr E, Braun W, Eber W, Rüter A. Treatment of acromioclavicular joint separations. Central Kirschner wire and PDS augmentation. Unfallchirurg. 1999;102:278–86.
48. Winkler H, Schlamp D, Wentzensen A. Treatment of acromioclavicular joint dislocation by tension band and ligament suture. Aktuelle Traumatol. 1994;24(4):133–9.
49. Hessmann M, Gotzen L, Gehling H. Acromioclavicular reconstruction augmented with polydioxanonsulphate bands. Surgical technique and results. Am J Sports Med. 1995;23:552–6.
50. Lemos M, Tolo E. Complications of the treatment of the acromioclavicular and sternoclavicular joint injuries, including instability. Clin Sports Med. 2003;22(2):371–85.
51. Gohring H, Matusewicz A, Friedl W, Ruf W. Results of treatment after different surgical procedures for management of acromioclavicular joint dislocation. Chirurg. 1993;64:565–71.
52. Fauci F, Merolla G, Paladini P, Campi F, Porcellini G. Surgical treatment of chronic acromioclavicular dislocation with biologic graft vs synthetic ligament: a prospective randomized comparative study. J Orthop Traumatol. 2013;14(4):283–90. https://doi.org/10.1007/s10195-013-0242-2.

4 Scapular fractures

Jan Bartoníček, Michal Tuček, and Ondřej Naňka

Introduction

Until recently, scapular fractures were among the less common injuries, and of marginal interest. However, the situation has considerably changed lately. The incidence of scapular fractures is increasing, both in absolute terms due to the increase in number of injuries from traffic accidents and polytrauma; and in relative terms, as a result of improved diagnostic procedures. In addition, critical studies have appeared that question adequacy of the outcomes of non-operative treatment in displaced extraarticular scapular fractures, and an increasing number of authors recommend to fix these injuries surgically [1].

The growing interest in the scapula has been reflected also in the amount of published studies, largely debating fractures of the scapular body and neck, and the so-called floating shoulder. Opinions in the studies vary and are often contradictory [2–4]. Improving our understanding of scapular fractures requires revision of the traditional opinions on the anatomy of the scapula, diagnostic procedures, classification and treatment of scapular fractures.

Our experience in the treatment of scapular fractures is based on a cohort of 375 patients from January 2002 to December 2016, including 315 fractures documented by 3D CT reconstructions, and 128 treated surgically. Based on our findings and results we have developed our strategy for treatment of these injuries [5–15].

Anatomy

Scapula is part of the shoulder girdle. It is attached to the axial skeleton by the clavicle, functioning as a strut, and the acromioclavicular (AC) and sternoclavicular (SC) joints. This articulation chain keeps the scapula at a constant distance from the sternum. The scapula overlies the posterior chest wall between 2nd and 7th ribs and is held in its position by muscles, the trapezius in particular. It is inclined with the frontal plane at an angle of about 30°. Its main role is to provide an efficient support to the humeral head in all positions of the arm. The scapula is free to slide on the chest wall thanks to the thin gliding fibres

J. Bartoníček (✉)
Department of Orthopaedics, Charles University and Central Military Hospital Prague, Prague, Czech Republic

Department of Anatomy, Charles University, Prague, Czech Republic

M. Tuček
Department of Orthopaedics, Charles University and Central Military Hospital Prague, Prague, Czech Republic
e-mail: tucekmic@uvn.cz

O. Naňka
Department of Anatomy, Charles University, Prague, Czech Republic
e-mail: ondrej.nanka@lf1.cuni.cz

I. A. Trail et al. (eds.), *Textbook of Shoulder Surgery*, https://doi.org/10.1007/978-3-319-70099-1_4

that fill in the space between the muscles covering the anterior surface of the scapula and the chest.

Bone Anatomy Scapula is a flat, triangular bone bounded by the superior, medial and lateral borders including three angles. Two of them, the superior and inferior angles, are flat, while the lateral angle is a three-dimensional structure formed by the scapular neck and the glenoid fossa. On the posterior surface of the scapula, the scapular body and neck are separated by the *spinoglenoid notch*. The coracoid process curves forward from the anterosuperior surface of the scapular neck, with its base separated from the glenoid fossa by a variably defined *coracoglenoidal notch*. The pear-shaped glenoid surface is augmented by a robust fibrous ring, the glenoid labrum. A circle can be drawn in the inferior two thirds of the articular surface, which defines the *circular area*, the part of the glenoid exposed to the highest load. The anterior, concave surface of the scapula forms the subscapular fossa. The posterior surface is divided by a prominent triangular plate of bone, the scapular spine, into the smaller supraspinous fossa and the greater infraspinous fossa. Gradually the scapular spine becomes more elevated lateralward and ends in a flattened bony process curving forward, the acromion. The border between the scapular spine and the acromion is formed by a well palpable acromial angle.

Internal Architecture Distribution of bony mass of the scapula is highly uneven (Fig. 4.1). When held up to the light, the scapula shows its highest concentration in the glenoid, the scapular neck, including the base of the coracoid process, and the lateral border of the scapular spine. Cancellous bone can be found in the scapula only in the area of the lateral angle.

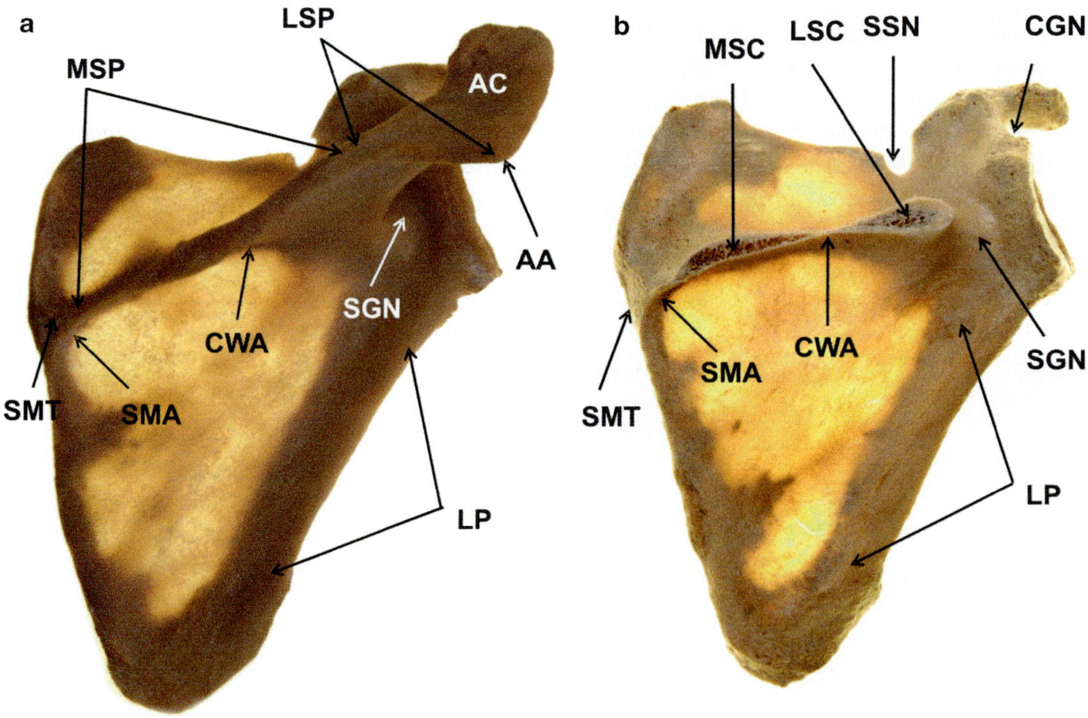

Fig. 4.1 Anatomy of scapula. (**a**) transluminated scapula – posterior view; (**b**) scapular spine removed: AA acromial angle, AC acromion, CGN coracoglenoidal notch, CWA central weakening of scapular spine, LSC lateral column of scapular spine, LSP lateral part of scapular spine, MSC medial column of scapular spine, MSP medial part of scapular spine, LP lateral pillar, SGN spinoglenoid notch, SMA spinomedial angle, SMT spinomedial triangle, SP spinous pillar, SSN suprascapular notch

Extending from the glenoid are two bony pillars that transmit compression forces from the glenoid fossa to the scapular body. *The lateral pillar* is identical with the lateral border of the scapular body, which connects the inferior border of the glenoid with the inferior angle. *The spinal pillar* arises from the central part of the glenoid and continues medially to become part of the base of the scapular spine. Its course can be seen better by viewing the scapula from the front against the light. The spinal pillar and the medial border of the scapular body include an obtuse *spinomedial angle*. From the posterior view it is evident that the two pillars connected by a markedly thinner medial border of the scapular body are its basic load-bearing structure. This triangle constitutes the *biomechanical body* of the scapula, as the superior angle and the superior border of the scapular body form merely an appendage, which serves as a surface of insertion or origin of muscles, but is not involved in transmission of compression forces from the glenoid. Therefore, it is necessary to distinguish between the *anatomical* and *biomechanical bodies* of the scapula [5].

The weakened area can be found primarily in the central parts of the supra- and infraspinous fossae, with the bone only several millimetres thick. The weakest area of the circumference of the biomechanical body of the scapula is the spinomedial angle, which is confirmed by the fact that in the majority of scapular body fractures one of the main fracture lines passes through this region. Another area of weak bone is in the central part of the scapular spine and is bound by its medial and lateral columns [5].

Muscles In total, 18 muscles are attached to the scapula. Only three of them, namely the subscapularis, the supraspinatus and the infraspinatus, that are part of the rotator cuff, originate from the broad surface of the scapula in their respective fossae. Other muscles reinforce with their attachments individual borders and angles of the scapula or its processes. The muscles of the scapula may be divided into two systems.

The first, the *scapuloaxial* system connects the scapula with the axial skeleton, particularly the vertebral column and the chest wall. This system stabilizes the position of the scapula relative to the spine and controls movement of the scapula over the chest wall.

The second, the *scapulobrachial* system is formed by the muscles originating from the scapula and attaching to the bones of arm, i.e. the humerus, proximal radius and proximal ulna. Its task is to control movements between the scapula and the humeral head, i.e. to control the glenohumeral joint.

Nerves and Blood Vessels The most significant of all the nerves and blood vessels in the region of the scapula are two structures. The *suprascapular nerve* passing under, but often also above the superior transverse scapular ligament continues across the supraspinous fossa together with the artery and vein of the same name. This neurovascular bundle travels below the inferior transverse scapular ligament (spinoglenoid ligament) to enter the spinoglenoid notch on the posterior surface of the scapular neck. The suprascapular nerve gradually sends motor branches to the supraspinatus, and to the infraspinatus. The terminal part of the *suprascapular artery* anastomoses in the spinoglenoid notch with one of the branches of the *circumflex scapular artery*. This branch, occasionally double, curves around the lateral border of the scapula, leaving an impression here, the *sulcus circumflexus*, when passing through the teres minor mostly 3 cm distal to the inferior pole of the glenoid fossa.

Epidemiology

According to the data in the literature, scapular fractures account for about 3–5% of all fractures of the shoulder girdle and approximately for 0.4% of all fractures [16, 17]. However, this data is either old [16], or obtained from small cohorts [17]. The only available recent epidemiological study, published by Zhang [18], based on a group of 595 scapular fractures, unfortunately misses a number of important details. Analysis of our own group of 250 patients documented by CT scans covering the period of 2008–2014 has provided the following data [8].

The cohort included 199 men (80%) and 51 women (20%). The mean age of the whole cohort was 45 years (range, 15–92), the mean age of men was 43.5 years and that of women 52.4 years. Patients older than 60 years comprised 17% of the whole group. The peak incidence of these fractures in men was in 4th to 6th age decade, in women in 5th to 7th age decade. As concerns the share of individual types of fractures, fractures of the scapular body accounted for 52%, fractures of the glenoid for 29%, fractures of processes and borders for 11% and fractures of the scapular neck for 8%.

Injury Mechanism

The scapula is well protected against injury by a robust muscular envelope, its mobility and location on the elastic chest wall. The statement that scapular fractures result mostly from high-energy trauma is not quite true. In terms of energy of the injury mechanism, we have identified in the literature and in our cohort three groups of patients [1–4, 15].

Energy of the Injury Mechanism The first group included patients with high-energy injuries caused most often during a traffic accident, or a fall from a great height, or by the fall of a heavy object on the patient. A majority of these patients were polytraumatised, with a wide range of injuries of individual organ systems. It is no surprise that up to 90% of these fractures were associated with other severe injuries, particularly to the chest (ribs, lungs), head, spine and abdomen. Prior to introduction of standard spiral CT examination scapular fractures were often diagnosed only coincidentally in polytrauma patients. Due to polytrauma, injury to the scapula is not the main focus of the treatment in these patients and its management depends on the patient's general condition.

The second largest group comprised patients with medium-energy trauma caused usually by a fall from the bicycle, or a slowly travelling motorcycle. The injury to the scapula and the shoulder girdle usually dominated, associated sometimes with cerebral contusion, or another injury (e.g., tibial fracture).

The third group comprised mostly elderly patients who sustained a scapular fracture in a simple fall onto flat ground, down stairs, or even as a result of fall of a smaller object onto the scapula. In the majority of these patients it was an isolated injury to the shoulder girdle.

In the second and third groups of patients, the scapular fracture can be treated quite early following the trauma, taking into account the local finding.

Injury Mechanism In terms of the type of violence, scapular fractures are caused by two mechanism patterns, namely the exogenous and endogenous ones.

With the exogenous mechanism, which is more frequent, the impact acts directly on the scapula, or is transmitted through the humeral head.

In cases of direct exogenous impact, the scapula hits surrounding objects, e.g., when the chest hits the car body, or vice versa, when for instance a heavy object hits the scapula. The result is most often a fracture of the scapular body or scapular processes.

With the endogenous mechanism, the forces are transmitted from the arm through the humeral head to the glenoid, the acromion or the coracoid. Thus the impactor is the humeral head. The fracture pattern depends on the position of the arm at the time of injury. With the arm in adduction, a blow on the elbow along the axis of the humeral shaft proximally dislocates the humeral head, which hits the acromion, or the coracoid, causing a fracture of these processes. With the arm in abduction, the humeral head is driven against the central part of the glenoid and, according to the degree of abduction, a smaller or greater inferior part of the articular surface separates off, rarely the entire glenoid is split. Anterior, or posterior, dislocation of the humeral head may result in a fracture of the respective rim of the glenoid.

The endogenous cause of scapular fractures is most frequently a violent muscle contracture, as the result of an electrical injury, or an epileptic seizure.

Quite rarely do scapular fractures occur in pathologically changed bone (e.g., bone cyst, bone ganglion, osteodystrophy, tumour metastasis). Fatigue fractures of the scapular spine and the acromion have been reported in cases of insufficiency of the rotator cuff. Exceptionally there occur gun shot and cut/stab injuries. A specific group are periprosthetic scapular fractures in patients following shoulder arthroplasty.

Clinical Examination

The diagnostic procedure in patients with scapular injuries depends on their general condition. In polytrauma patients, the priority is to save life. In a number of polytrauma patients, scapular fractures are often found coincidentally, e.g., on a radiograph of lungs. Introduction of the whole body spiral CT scans has considerably improved the diagnostic process. Patients in a less severe general condition, who are able to communicate, may undergo standard clinical examination.

Scapular fractures are often associated with other injuries and, therefore, it is essential first to conduct a thorough and comprehensive examination of the patient, before focusing on the shoulder. Where one fracture of a shoulder girdle is found, e.g., that of the clavicle, it is necessary to exclude other potential injuries!

Patient's Medical History Knowledge of the exact mechanism of the injury and the patient's subjective complaints are essential to a proper diagnosis. Elderly patients are asked about any past problems with the shoulder (rotator cuff lesion, osteoarthritis), or other systemic diseases (tumours, rheumatoid arthritis, metabolic disease).

Visual Assessment Careful examination of the shoulder and the entire chest, including the axilla, is performed. The shoulder may be deformed by a clavicular fracture, acromioclavicular dislocation, humeral head dislocation, by a markedly displaced scapular fracture, or significant swelling. Of great importance is examination of the integrity of the skin cover. A skin abrasion may indicate a site of impact.

Palpation A large part of the skeleton of the shoulder girdle may be examined by palpation, i.e. the clavicle, sternoclavicular joint, acromioclavicular joint, the scapular spine and acromion, the coracoid and the humeral head. In less muscular individuals, the inferior angle and medial border of the scapula are also accessible. Palpation may reveal crepitus, or pathological mobility. It is also important to palpate the axilla and the adjacent chest wall, and to identify the pulse of the axillary artery. As the fracture may be combined with a lesion of the brachial plexus, skin sensation in the area of the shoulder has to be examined.

Range of Motion Examination of the range of motion, mainly the active motion, in scapular fractures is significantly limited by pain. If possible, passive motion in the glenohumeral joint is carefully examined.

Periphery Of great importance is a thorough assessment also of other parts of the ipsilateral extremity in order to exclude associated injuries, and examination of its peripheral innervation and vascularity.

Imaging Methods

Radiological examination is essential to the diagnosis of scapular fractures, the determination of the fracture pattern and the treatment procedure. Other imaging methods may include MRI and ultrasound scanning, although they are indicated only exceptionally and their contribution is limited. The radiodiagnostic algorithm described below has to be adjusted to the patient's general condition.

Radiology Part of the basic examination is a general radiograph of the entire shoulder girdle covering the whole scapula, the proximal humerus and the whole clavicle, including the acromioclavicular and the sternoclavicular joints [15]. Scapular fractures are often associated with a clavicular fracture, and less frequently with a proximal humeral fracture or acromioclavicular dislocation. In cases of a detected, or suspected, scapular fracture, it should be combined with both Neer projections, if permitted by the patient's general condition.

Neer I projection or the true anteroposterior radiograph of the scapula, is used to assess the glenohumeral joint space, displacement of the glenoid in relation to the lateral border of the scapula and to measure the glenopolar angle (GPA). In this projection, the scapular plane is parallel to the x-ray cassette. A correctly performed projection visualises the glenohumeral joint line.

Neer II projection, also called Y-view, is a true lateral scapular projection. In this projection the scapular plane is perpendicular to the x-ray cassette. The Y-view projection allows assessment of scapular body fractures in terms of translation, angulation and overlap of fragments of the lateral border. In addition, it displays clearly the relationships between the coracoid, the acromion and the lateral clavicle, as well as the acromioclavicular joint. It can also help identify a fracture of the glenoid.

General radiograph of the chest, indicated to examine the lungs, heart and chest wall, is, in polytrauma patients, often the first clue leading to a diagnosis of a scapular fracture. It is important mostly for assessment of the position of both scapulae in relation to the spine (scapulothoracic dissociation).

Other special projections, axillary in particular, are recommended by some authors as complementary views, to diagnose fractures of the glenoid fossa, the acromion and the coracoid [19]. However, axillary projection is, for most patients with a scapular, or rib, fracture, highly unpleasant and should not substitute CT examination.

The complicated shape of the scapula and its position on the chest make very difficult, or even impossible, an unambiguous interpretation of findings and determination of the fracture pattern with the use of radiographic projections alone [20].

CT Examination This examination has fundamentally changed the radiodiagnostics of scapular fractures. It is always indicated when radiographic examination cannot reveal the exact fracture pattern, involvement of the articular surface, or displacements of fragments, which is the case in a majority of patients [6, 11, 21].

CT transverse sections are valuable in the assessment of the condition of the glenoid fossa. They also help to detect undisplaced fractures of the scapular processes, especially those of the coracoid and the acromion. However, they do not provide a three-dimensional image of the fracture anatomy.

Two-dimensional CT reconstructions (2D CT), mainly in the sagittal plane, are used to assess the articular surface, especially in fractures of the base of the coracoid process involving the glenoid fossa.

Three-dimensional CT reconstructions (3D CT) are the only way to determine reliably the exact fracture pattern, particularly in fractures of the scapular body and neck (Fig. 4.2), although they do not show fine fracture lines, especially in minimally displaced fractures. Reconstructions should be made in three basic views, namely with subtraction of ribs, clavicle and proximal humerus [6].

The anterior view is essential in fractures of the scapular neck (Fig. 4.2a). This view helps to identify different courses of fracture lines in fractures of the anatomical and surgical necks of the scapula.

The posterior view allows assessment of the course of fracture lines with regard to the scapular spine (Fig. 4.2b). It is important to visualize adequately the entire infraspinous and partially also the supraspinous fossae.

Glenoid fractures require a lateral view, always with subtraction of the humeral head (Fig. 4.2c). This is the only way how to get exact information about the number of fragments and course of the fracture lines in the glenoid. In fractures of the lateral border of the scapular body, this view helps to assess its shortening, angulation and translation, or the shape and displacement of small intermediate fragments.

In certain fracture patterns, also other complementary views may be valuable in the assessment

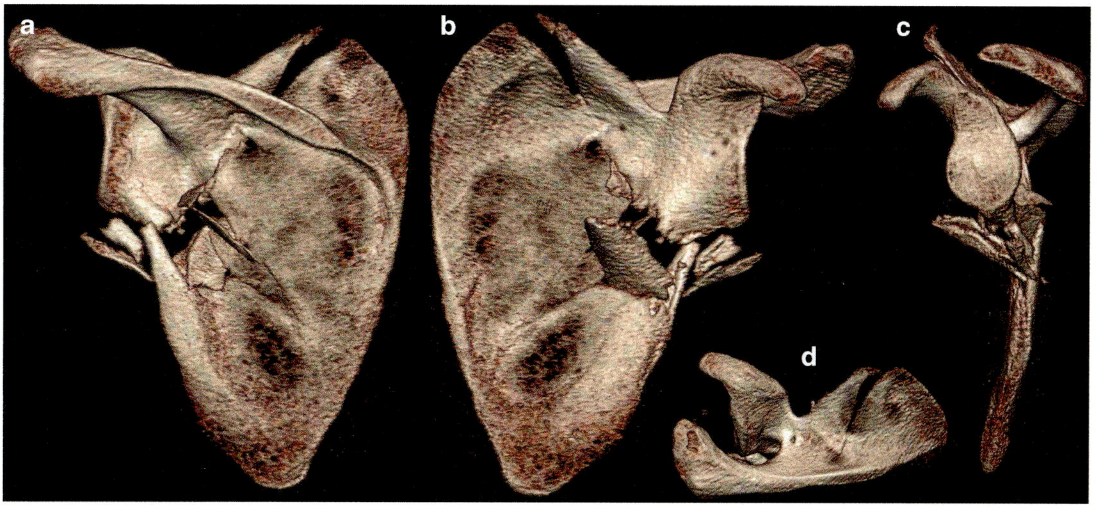

Fig. 4.2 Importance of 3D CT reconstructions for determination of fracture type (in this case trans-spinous fracture of scapular neck. (**a**) anterior view; (**b**) posterior view; (**c**) lateral view; (**d**) view into supraspinous fossa

of the course of the fracture line, e.g. a view of the supraspinous fossa (Fig. 4.2d), the spinoglenoid notch or a medial view. In some cases (fractures of the anatomical and surgical necks of the scapula), subtraction of the acromion may be helpful.

Radiometric Assessment of Fragment Displacement These measurements quantify different types of displacement of fragments, particularly of the lateral border of the scapula, and serve as supporting criteria for indication of operative treatment [15, 22]. Measurements may be made using both the Neer projections and 3D CT reconstructions. In decision-making about the method of treatment, it is important to assess primarily the degree of displacement of fragments of the lateral border of the scapula and displacement of the glenoid relative to the scapular body, preferably on 3D CT reconstructions.

Angulation of the main fragments of the lateral border of the scapula may be evaluated in the Neer II projection, or in the lateral view, based on 3D CT reconstructions. Operative treatment should be considered with an angulation angle of more than 30–45° [22].

Translation of the main fragments of the lateral border of the scapula in the anteroposterior direction is measured by means of the same views that are used to measure angulation. An indication for operative treatment is considered to be translation of fragments by 100% [22].

Medio-lateral displacement of the main fragments of the lateral border of the scapula, previously termed as medialisation of the glenoid, is measured in the Neer I projection on the anterior view or in 3D CT reconstructions. The term medialisation is not correct. In most cases there occurs lateral displacement of the infraglenoid part of the scapular body by pull of muscles as the intact clavicle maintains a constant distance between the glenoid and the sternum. Translation by 10–20 mm is considered to be an indication for operation [22].

Glenopolar Angle (GPA) This angle was defined by Bestard et al. [21] as an acute angle included by a line connecting the superior and inferior poles of the glenoid and a line connecting the superior pole of the glenoid and the inferior angle of the scapular body. Standard GPA values range according to Bestard between 30° and 45°. A detailed analysis has shown that neither GPA measurement, nor its normal and critical values have been standardized [7]. Individual authors measured GPA on ap radiographs of the shoulder, ap radiographs of the scapula (Neer I projection) and radiographs of the chest. Our study has proved that GPA is best measured with the use of the Neer I projection or 3D CT reconstructions [7]. Its mean value ranges around 43° (30–54°). Due to its variability, it is necessary to assess not only the absolute GPA value but also GPA on the intact side, as the side-to-side variability is minimal (1.4°).

A problem is also the critical value of GPA. Clinically relevant is considered a value of less than 20° [22, 23]. However, it has not been mentioned in the literature, yet, that in fractures of the anatomical neck of scapula the GPA values on the contrary increase and may reach up to 70° [7, 10].

Despite these reservations, measuring of the GPA, unlike that of medialisation, angulation and translation, is the only metric method where correlation between its value and the functional outcome has been found [23].

Classifications of Scapular Fractures

The common drawback of almost all current classifications is the fact that they are based on plain radiographs, often taken in a non-standard way [24–27]. As a result, a number of fracture patterns presented there do not correspond to reality. In spite of this, we may find them often in the newly developed classifications. Especially the AO classification is questionable, as its practical applicability is problematic [28, 29]. In addition, there is no exact definition of individual fracture patterns, the fractures of the scapular body and neck in particular.

Based on an analysis of the biomechanical architecture of the scapula [5], analysis of 315 scapular fractures documented by 3D CT reconstructions and experience gained in 132 operations, we have divided scapular fractures into four basic groups respecting the scapula anatomy [15], that may be combined:

- glenoid fractures
- scapular neck fractures
- scapular body fractures
- fractures of the processes and borders of scapula.

Glenoid fractures are intraarticular fractures of the articular surface that are distinguished according to the part of the glenoid involved (Fig. 4.3) [11].

Fractures of the superior glenoid are actually intraarticular fractures of the coracoid base and glenoidal fragment often carries also a part of the superior border of the scapular body. It is caused most probably by the humeral head hitting the coracoid base, with the arm in adduction. It is commonly associated with avulsion of the upper third, sometimes a half, of the articular surface (Fig. 4.3b).

Fractures of the anterior glenoid rim are in most cases caused by anterior dislocation of the shoulder. Involvement of the anteroinferior rim of the glenoid varies. With a larger fragment, the shoulder is unstable after reduction (Fig. 4.3c).

Fractures of the posterior glenoid rim are very rare, occurring in association with the posterior dislocation of the shoulder and usually affects only a part of the rim of the glenoid fossa (Fig. 4.3d).

Fractures of the inferior glenoid are the most common and highly severe glenoid fractures. They are caused by the humeral head hitting the glenoid fossa, with the arm in abduction. The humeral head is driven against the inferior glenoid and, consequently, also against the lateral border of the scapular body. The size of the avulsed part of the glenoid varies, ranging as a rule between one to two thirds of the articular surface. The fracture line extends as far as the lateral border of the scapula, at a variable distance. A majority of fractures of the inferior glenoid are combined with fractures of the scapular body that may be involved to a variable extent (Fig. 4.3e).

Fractures of the entire glenoid are the most severe intraarticular fractures of the scapula, when the articular surface is split into two or more parts, each of which is separated from the scapular neck or body. Anatomy of these fractures varies (Fig. 4.3f) [12].

Scapular neck fractures are extraarticular fractures of the lateral angle of the scapula, separating the glenoid from the scapular body. These fractures are infrequent. Three basic patterns may

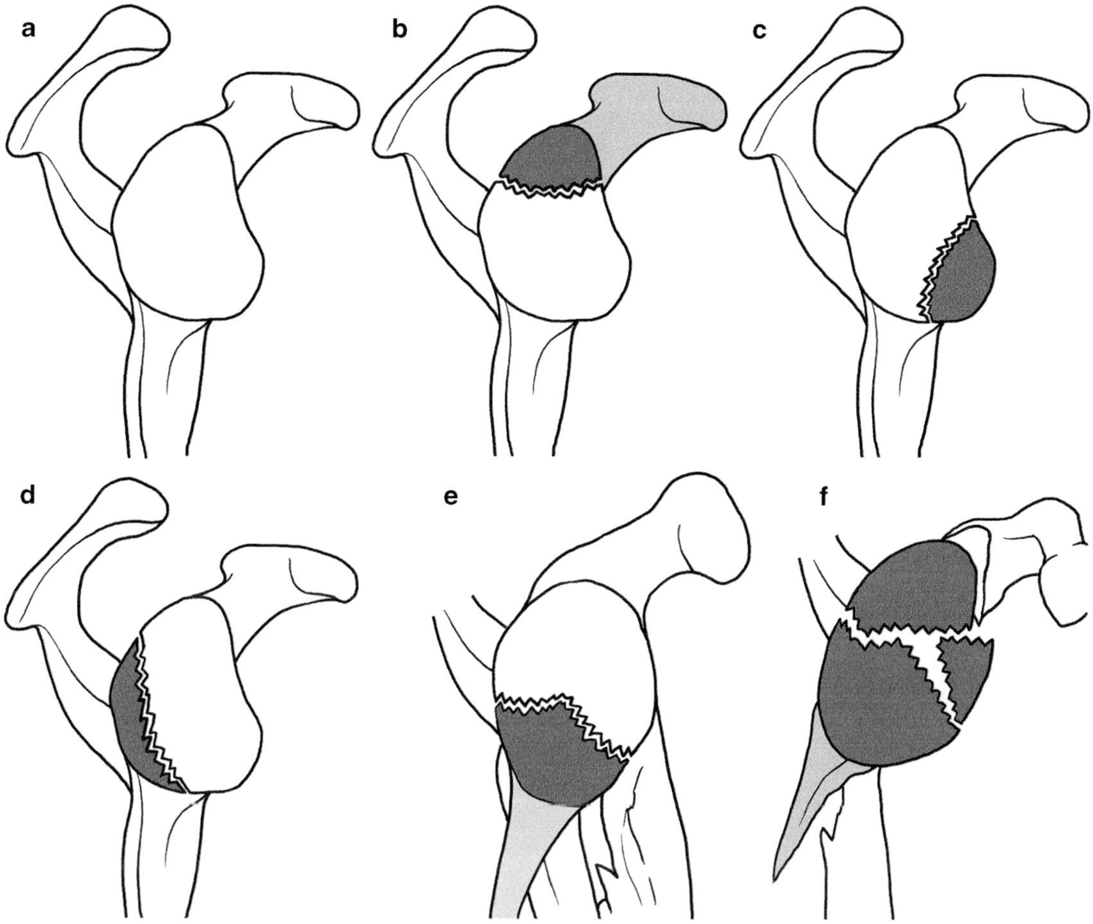

Fig. 4.3 Basic types of glenoid fractures: (**a**) anatomy of glenoid fossa; (**b**) superior glenoid fracture; (**c**) anterior glenoid fracture; (**d**) posterior glenoid fracture; (**e**) inferior glenoid fracture; (**f**) entire glenoid fracture. (From Bartoníček et al. [11])

be distinguished based on the course of the fracture line and the shape of the glenoid fragment (Fig. 4.4) [10].

Anatomical neck fractures separate only the glenoid fossa from the scapular body. The fracture line passes proximally between the upper rim of the glenoid and the coracoid base. This rare fracture is unstable, often associated with valgus displacement [10] (Fig. 4.4a).

Surgical neck fractures are the most frequently discussed of all three scapular neck fractures. Part of the glenoid fragment is the coracoid (Fig. 4.4b). Pull of muscles attached to this process (short head of the bicipitis brachii, the coracobrachialis and the pectoralis minor) may displace the glenoid fragment medially and distally. Displacement depends on the integrity of the coracoacromial and coracoclavicular ligaments. With intact ligaments, the fracture is *stable* relative to the acromion and clavicle. Rupture of the coracoacromial ligament has a negative impact on the relationship of the glenoid fragment to the acromion, but not to the clavicle. The fracture is *rotationally unstable*. Rupture of the coracoclavicular ligament results in a *completely unstable* fracture, with a typically greater distance between the coracoid and the clavicle [10]. A specific type of surgical neck fractures are *fractures with avulsion of the coracoid base*. This fracture type gets displaced in the same way as fractures of the anatomical neck, i.e., into valgus [10, 19].

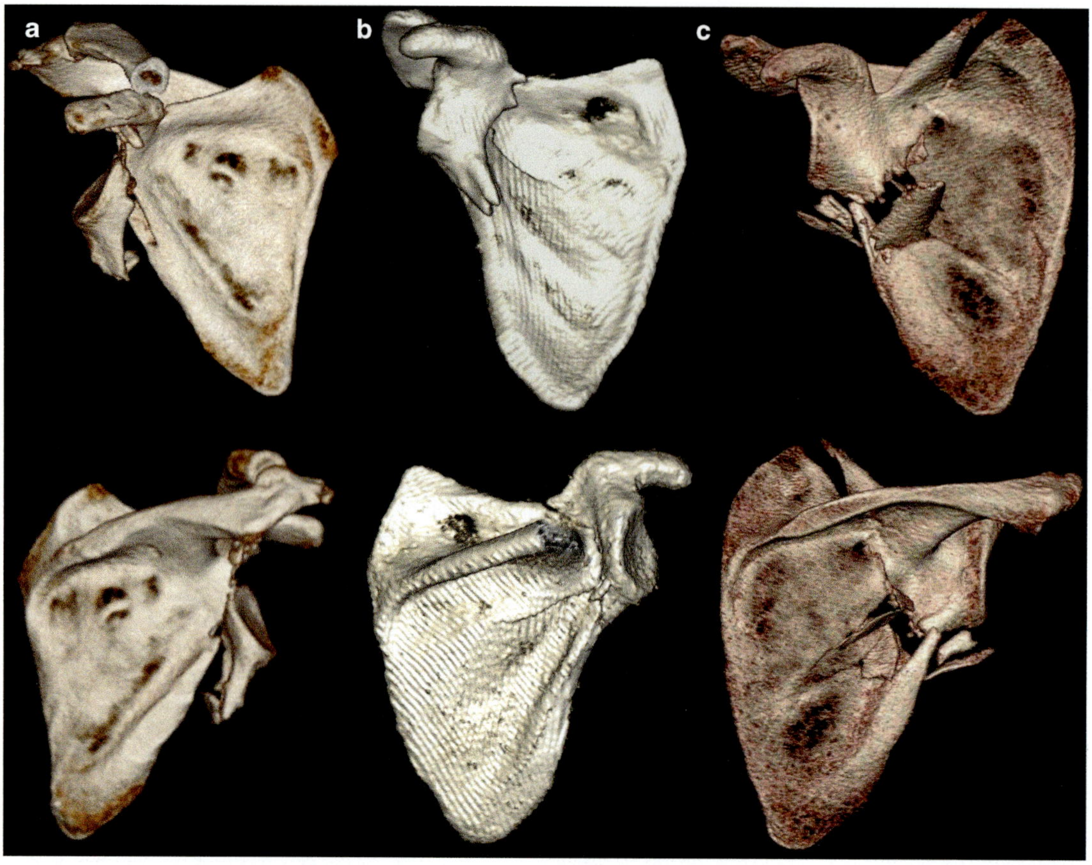

Fig. 4.4 Scapular neck fractures. (**a**) fracture of anatomic neck; (**b**) fracture of surgical neck, (**c**) trans-spinous scapular neck fracture

Trans-spinous neck fractures are little known and are similar to fractures of the anatomical body. Fracture line passes through the weakened central part of the scapular spine and the glenoid fragment is formed by the glenoid fossa, the coracoid and the acromion and the adjacent lateral part of the scapular spine and the acromion (Fig. 4.4c) [10, 15].

Scapular body fractures involve the biomechanical triangle, i.e., the main fracture line(s) run through one (spinal or lateral) of both pillars of the scapula (Fig. 4.5). Therefore they do not include isolated fractures of the superior border of the body, the superior or inferior angle of the scapula. The scapular fractures may be assessed also in view of their involving either only the infraspinous part of the scapula (the area of the infraspinous fossa) or the entire scapular body (both supra- and infraspinous part). Another important aspect is the number of fragments. Assessment covers only those fragments that carry part of the circumference of the biomechanical triangle. Intercalary fragments separated from the centre of the biomechanical triangle, i.e., from the central part of the infraspinous fossa, are excluded. Intercalary fragments are formed only by a thin bone and therefore are irrelevant from the viewpoint of reconstruction.

Spinal pillar fractures involve both posterior fossae. The fracture line runs through the centre of the scapular spine (spinal pillar) to the medial border of the infraspinous fossa. Less frequently, the base of the scapular spine is separated from the scapular body. The lateral pillar remains always intact and displacement of fragments is in most cases minimal (Fig. 4.5a).

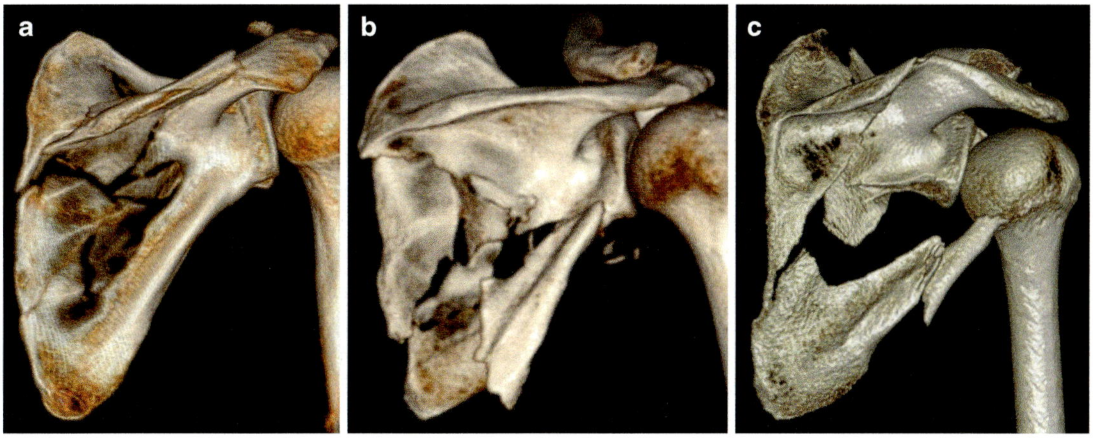

Fig. 4.5 Scapular body fractures. (**a**) fracture of spinal pillar; (**b**) fracture of lateral pillar, (**c**) fracture of both pillars

Lateral pillar fractures are the most common injuries. They involve only the infraspinous part of the scapula and are divided according to the number of circumferential fragments into 2-part, 3-part and comminuted. The most frequent are 2-part fractures with the fracture line passing transversely from the upper half of the lateral border to the spinomedial angle. Sometimes they are incorrectly referred to as infraglenoid fractures of the scapular neck. Approximately 30% of 2-part fractures are associated with a clavicle fracture. As a result, certain authors mistakenly classify these injuries as the floating shoulder. A significant part of the lateral pillar fractures is markedly displaced, primarily by pull of the infraspinatus, the subscapularis and the teres major (Fig. 4.5b).

Fractures of both pillars are caused mostly by high-energy violence and are often comminuted. These fractures have two patterns. In the first group the fracture line runs through the spinal pillar close to the spinomedial angle to the superior angle of the scapula. In the second group, the main fracture line passes through the central weakened part of the scapular spine (Fig. 4.5c).

Spinal pillar fractures are as a rule less frequently displaced than lateral pillar fractures. Of great importance in this respect is the shape of the glenoid fragment. It may be separated along the line of the anatomical, surgical or transspinous neck, which is decisive both for its displacement and the subsequent fixation.

Fractures of processes and peripheral fractures of the scapula include fractures of the coracoid, the acromion and the scapular spine, as well as fractures of the superior and inferior angle of the scapula. Except for the inferior angle, these fractures are caused by direct blow to the upper part of the scapula or by the displaced humeral head hitting the coracoacromial arch. Fractures are often reported to be caused by pull of muscles and ligaments. In case of the coracoid process this mechanism is highly questionable due to the distribution of the muscle and ligament attachments.

Coracoid process fractures may be divided into three types, primarily according to the relation of the fracture line to the attachment of the coracoclavicular ligament (CCL). The *first type* is an extraarticular fracture of the coracoid base (proximal to the CCL attachment), the *second type* is a fracture of the distal "finger-like" part of the coracoid (distal to the CCL attachment) and the *third type* is an impaction fracture of the apex. Almost all fractures of the coracoid in our cohort were only minimally displaced, mostly angulated, not distracted.

Fractures of the acromion and the lateral part of the scapular spine are sometimes classified separately, although in terms of anatomy it is the same structure. The separated fragment gets larger with the fracture line moving from the apex of the acromion as far as the base of the scapular spine. The conventional border between the acromion and the lateral part of the scapular spine is considered to be the acromial angle.

Acromion fractures are divided according to the size of fragments into peripheral fractures of the acromion and avulsion of the entire acromion when the fracture line passes close to the acromial angle. The latter fractures should be distinguished from the *os acromiale*. Exceptionally, both entities occur simultaneously.

Fractures of the lateral part of the scapular spine may be divided according to the course of the fracture line into fractures in the area of the acromial angle, fractures in the middle part of the lateral scapular spine and fractures at the base of the lateral part.

Fractures of the superior angle of the scapula involve in most cases only the superior angle, less frequently a part of the fragment is also the spinomedial triangle, i.e., the medial portion of the scapular spine. Fractures of the superior angle are usually slightly angulated, with minimal distraction. The distraction effect of the levator scapulae insertion is neutralised by insertions of the subscapularis and the supraspinatus.

Fractures of the inferior angle of the scapula result mostly from the combination of direct local violence and muscle pull (serratus anterior, teres maior). The avulsed inferior angle is typically angulated anteriorly. The size of the fragment varies but never exceeds the distal third of the infraspinous fossa.

Combined fractures of the scapula include two subgroups of injuries. The *first subgroup* comprises a combination of two or more basic scapular fracture patterns, e.g. a fracture of the glenoid and a fracture of processes. The *second* subgroup includes a combination of a scapular fracture with a fracture of the clavicle or injury of the AC joint. The most common is a combination of a scapular body fracture with a fracture of the shaft of the clavicle.

Treatment

The aim of treatment of scapular fractures is to restore normal function of the shoulder, i.e. a full, pain-free range of motion, and to prevent the development of late complications [2–4, 15, 19, 22], including pain, limited range of motion due to maluninon, nonunion, osteoarthritis of the glenohumeral joint or lesion of the rotator cuff. Specifically, it implies restoration of the congruence and stability of the glenohumeral joint in glenoid fractures; restoration of the anatomical form of the scapula, the biomechanical body in particular, and alignment of the scapular body and the glenoid in fractures of the scapular neck and body; and prevention of painful nonunion, or impingement of the humeral head, resulting from malunion of fractures of the acromion or the coracoid.

Treatment of scapular fractures depends on the fracture pattern; its displacement; the patient's general and local condition; and age [15, 19, 22].

Indication Undisplaced intra- and extraarticular scapular fractures are treated non-operatively, similarly as displaced intra- and extraarticular scapular fractures in patients when the patient's general or local condition does not allow operation.

Displaced intraarticular fractures involving more than 20–30% of the articular surface of the glenoid with a displacement, i.e. gap/step-off of more than 2–3 mm, are indicated for operative treatment and restoration of the congruence and stability of the glenohumeral joint [15, 19, 22, 30].

Treatment of *displaced extraarticular fractures* is currently the subject of an intense debate. The reported outcomes show that grossly displaced fractures of the scapular body and neck in active individuals can be better stabilised operatively, if permitted by their general and local condition. Operative treatment should be considered in fractures associated with [15, 19, 22]:

- 100% translation of fragments of the lateral border of the scapular body,
- angular displacement of fragments of the lateral border of the scapular body of more than 30–40°,
- mediolateral displacement of fragments of the lateral border of the scapular body of more than 1–2 cm,
- glenopolar angle (GPA) of less than 20° or more than 60°.

Nevertheless, these are only supporting criteria and it is always necessary to assess not only the local condition but also the personality of the patient.

In displaced fractures of the processes, particularly the coracoid, acromion and spine, which give attachments to prominent muscles and ligaments, the aim is to achieve healing in an anatomical position.

Non-operative Treatment Non-operative management consists of pain relief and about 2 weeks of sling immobilisation. It is then possible to start passive range of motion exercises with the aim of achieving a full passive range of motion within 1 month of the injury. Full active range of motion should be restored during the second month. Beginning from the third month, strengthening of the rotator cuff muscles and peri-scapular muscles may be started and during the fourth month all restrictions can be lifted [15, 22].

Operative Treatment Except for an open fracture, operation of scapular fractures is never acute and should be performed only after it is permitted by the patient's general, or local, condition. Therefore most patients are operated on at the interval of several days to weeks after the injury.

Surgical Approaches One of the following surgical approaches is chosen according to the fracture pattern:

Deltopectoral approach is indicated in isolated fractures of the anterior glenoid and in fractures of the coracoid.

Judet posterior approach provides an excellent exposure of the entire infraspinous fossa, lateral and medial borders of the scapula, the anatomical and surgical necks and the posterior and inferior rims of the glenoid [15]. It is used as a universal exposure in fractures of the scapular body, neck, the inferior or entire glenoid.

The skin incision curves from the acromial angle along the scapular spine and the medial border of the scapula. The spinal portion of the deltoid is released from the scapular spine and the infraspinatus is mobilised and carefully retracted proximally. It is not necessary to perform always the complete approach. It depends on the fracture pattern, the surgeon's experience and the injury-to-surgery interval, as the quickly progressing healing process and shortening of muscles make fragment reduction difficult. In certain cases it is possible to make after retraction of the deltoid only a medial and a lateral windows (in the interval between the infraspinatus and the teres minor) without mobilising the whole infraspinatus. The patients without full mobilisation of the infraspinatus have less pain and the range of motion is restored much more quickly.

Posterosuperior approach uses the horizontal part of the Judet incision. It extends along the posterior border of the acromion and the lateral part of the scapular spine. When necessary, this approach may be extended to the Judet approach. It is indicated in fractures of the acromion and the scapular spine, where appropriate also in fractures of the posterior rim of the glenoid.

Implants No special implants are required for scapular fractures, not even in elderly patients. The fractures can be usually fixed by 3.5 mm implants. Currently, we prefer 2.7 mm plates with standard 2.7 mm cortical screws. These implants are more gracile, but at the same time provide adequate stability. Locking plates and screws we use only exceptionally [15].

Internal Fixation In view of the distribution of the bony mass, implants can be firmly fixed mainly in the lateral pillar, in the scapular spine, neck and in the glenoid. Supplementary fixation is sometimes necessary in the spinomedial and inferior angles of the scapula.

Glenoid fractures are a heterogeneous group of injuries from the viewpoint of operative treatment [15, 30–33]. Fractures of the anterior rim of the glenoid are treated from the deltopectoral approach and the avulsed fragment is fixed with lag screws, and/or a buttress plate. Where appropriate, arthroscopically-assisted closed reduction and internal fixation with a lag screw may be performed as an alternative. Reduction and stabilisation of fractures of the superior pole of the glenoid are more difficult. Also in these fractures, the deltopectoral approach is indicated. Reduction is not always easy due to pull of the muscles attached to the coracoid. These fractures may be fixed using lag (cannulated) screws with washers, inserted through the coracoid into the glenoid, or the scapular neck.

Fractures of the inferior or entire glenoid are the biggest challenge. In case of multiple joint fragments it is important to reconstruct the circular area of the glenoid (Fig. 4.6). Fractures of the inferior glenoid are usually associated with a scapular body fracture and therefore it is necessary to restore the biomechanical triangle. Glenoid reconstruction should always be the first step. Reduction and fixation depend on the number and shape of joint fragments. Reconstruction of the articular surface of the glenoid often restores also integrity of the lateral border of the scapula. This is followed by reconstruction of the biomechanical triangle (Fig. 4.7). Fragments may be fixed using various techniques, usually by a combination of different plates, mostly 2.7 mm L- or T-shaped plates and lag screws.

Fractures of the scapular neck are operated on from the Judet approach [10, 34, 35]. Reduction and fixation of trans-spinous neck fractures are quite easy. Fractures of the surgical neck should be checked for a potential entrapment of the suprascapular nerve in the fracture line in the spinoglenoid notch. Reduction of unstable fractures of the surgical neck is difficult due to pull of the muscles attached to the coracoid. Fractures of the anatomical neck are difficult to stabilise due to the size of the glenoid fragment. Caution should be used to insert properly the screws into the glenoid fragment, to avoid their penetration into the joint cavity.

Fractures of the scapular body require restoration of continuity of so called biomechanical triangle, i.e., the circumference of the infraspinous fossa [9, 15, 34, 35]. Operative treatment is indicated mainly in fractures of the lateral pillar and of both pillars.

In fractures of the lateral pillar, the first step is restoration of its integrity. Majority of these fractures are associated with translation and overlap of the main fragments of the lateral pillar and, consequently, its significant shortening. The lateral pillar may be reduced using various techniques [9, 13, 15, 35]. Careful reduction by periosteal elevator inserted between the two fragments of the lateral pillar has proved to be a simple and efficient method. Another option is to drive a 3.5 mm cortical screw into each of the main fragments of the lateral border to facilitate manipulation of bone hooks. The fracture is reduced by pulling on the hooks. In unstable fractures of the lateral border, reduction may be maintained by the technique of the lost K-wire [13]. Final fixation may be completed with a 2.7 DCP or reconstruction plate fixed to each of the main fragments of the lateral border by two or three screws. In muscular individuals or in cases where it is necessary to eliminate shear or bending forces, we prefer 3.5 mm plates. Stabilisation of the medial border of the scapular body in the area of the spinomedial angle is a supplementary fixation to the fixation of the lateral border. It is used only in case when the stability of fragments is not adequate following internal fixation of the lateral border of the scapular body. Larger, thin, central, so called intercalary fragments are reduced only in case of gross displacement and are almost always left without fixation.

Treatment of fractures of both pillars starts usually with reduction and fixation of the spinal pillar which is less displaced than the lateral pillar. The lateral pillar is treated as the second. Fixation is performed preferably with the use of 2.7 mm, plates.

Processes fractures may be fixed by cerclage wiring, lag screws, or a plate. Displaced small fragments of the acromion or the coracoid apex should be excised and the muscle reinserted. Fractures of the distal finger-like part of the coracoid can be well fixed by a lag screw with a washer [36].

Clavicular fractures requiring internal fixation are treated only after completion of internal fixation of the scapula, similarly as injuries to the AC joint [15].

Postoperative Treatment Postoperatively, the arm is immobilised in a sling. Drainage, if used,

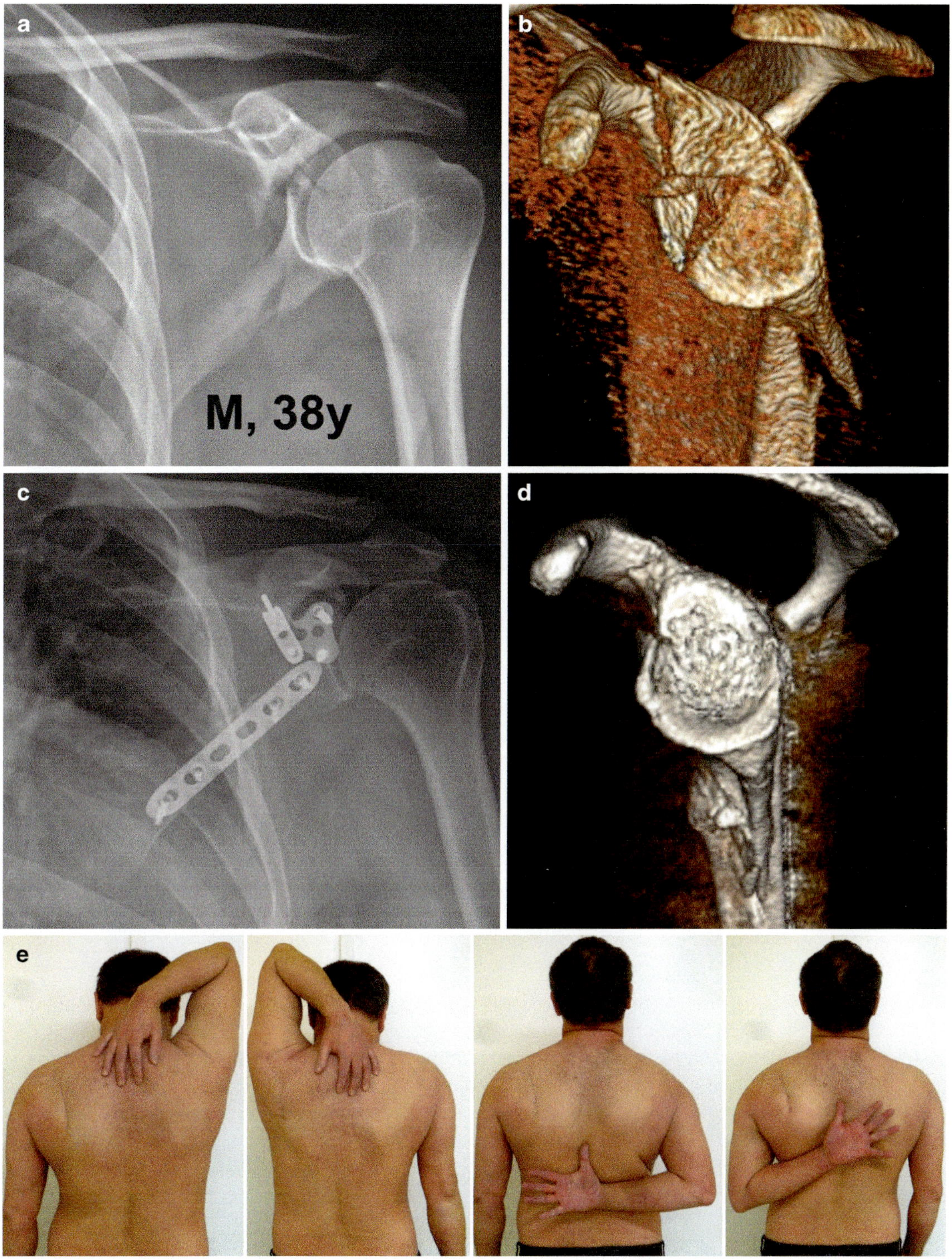

Fig. 4.6 Reconstruction of total glenoid fracture – three-part glenoid fossa fracture with fragment separation in anatomical neck. (**a**) post-injury radiograph, man 38 years old; (**b**) CT 3D reconstruction in lateral view demonstrating fragments separated in anatomical neck; (**c**) postoperative radiograph; (**d**) postoperative CT 3D reconstruction in lateral view demonstrating anatomical reconstruction of glenoid fossa, (**e**) functional result 3 years after surgery. (From Bartoníček et al. [12] with permission)

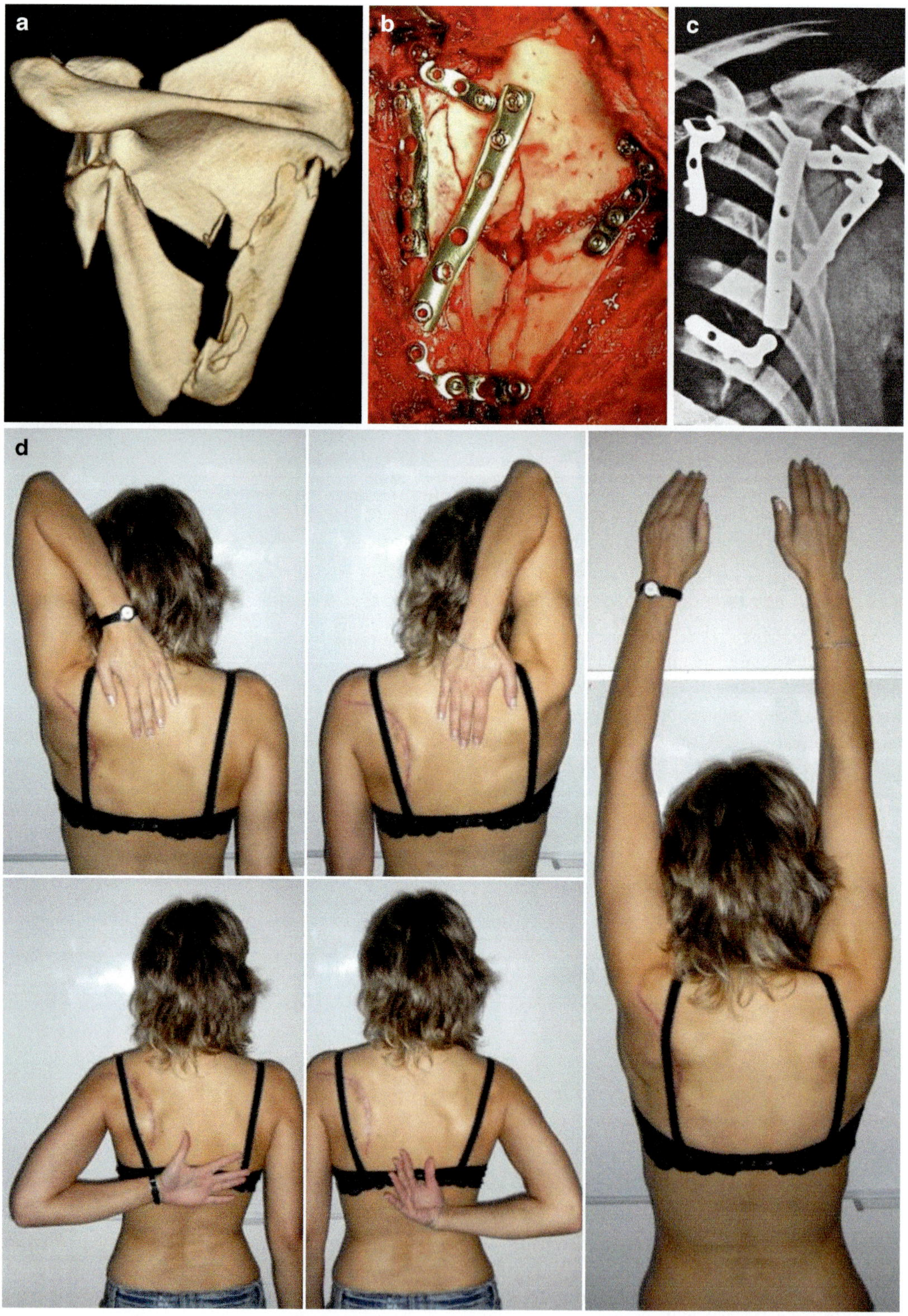

Fig. 4.7 Reconstruction of inferior glenoid fracture and three-part fracture of scapular body (lateral pillar), woman 19 years old. (**a**) 3D CT reconstruction – posterior view; (**b**) intraoperative view, (**c**) postoperative radiograph; (**d**) functional result 3 months after surgery. (From Bartoníček et al. [14] with permission)

is removed within 48 h after operation. Radiographs of the shoulder are obtained using the Neer I and II views. After discharge, the patient is checked for the first time 2 weeks after operation (wound healing, suture removal). Radiographs are taken at 6 weeks, 3 months, 6 months and 1 year after operation. Scapular fractures heal as a rule in 6–8 weeks.

Of great importance for the final outcome is proper rehabilitation. Passive range of motion exercises of the shoulder begin on the first postoperative day and continue for about 6 weeks. Continuous Passive Motion (CPM) machine may be helpful in this phase of rehabilitation. Active range of motion exercises start at approximately 4–5 weeks postoperatively, depending on the extent of the surgical approach and presence of other injuries (clavicular fracture, AC dislocation). The range of motion is assessed at 6 weeks and, if unsatisfactory, the motion is examined under general anesthesia and careful manipulation performed, as necessary. Active resistance exercises may be started approximately 8 weeks after operation. All restrictions of the shoulder range of motion are lifted, as a rule, 3 months postoperatively. The final subjective, objective and radiological outcomes of the operation cannot be assessed before 1 year after the operation, at the earliest.

Complications

Both non-operative and operative treatments of scapular fractures have a number of early and late complications, leading ultimately to pain and limitation of the range of motion of the shoulder [1–4, 15, 19, 22, 30–38].

Complications of Non-operative Treatment One of the most common complications is healing in a non-anatomical position, non-union and injury to the suprascapular nerve [1–4, 15, 19, 22].

Healing in a non-anatomical position is a typical complication of non-operative treatment. In extra-articular fractures, it changes the relation between the glenoid and the scapular body, and, consequently, the course of muscles of the rotator cuff. This has an impact on their function and may lead also to impingement syndrome. Fractures of the glenoid that have healed in displacement result in joint incongruity, instability, or both, and subsequently in post-traumatic osteoarthritis. Prominence of the bone fragment healed in displacement may be painful. Uneven surface of the costal scapular surface limits its smooth gliding over the chest wall.

Nonunions of the scapular body are rare. Reported also were nonunions of the acromion and the scapular spine. The solution is internal fixation of larger fragments and excision of small fragments.

Injury to the suprascapular nerve occurs most often in scapular neck fractures, when the nerve may become entrapped in the fracture line. This injury is manifested by atrophy of the infraspinatus.

Complications of Operative Treatment These complications may be divided into intraoperative, early postoperative and late postoperative ones. Their number reported by individual authors varies [2–4, 30–36].

Intraoperative complications include injuries to the suprascapular nerve, malreduction, intraarticular perforation by screws. In an analysis of 212 cases, Lantry [4] found injury to the suprascapular nerve in 2.4% of cases. It is difficult to distinguish whether the injury was caused by the initial trauma, or during surgery. In any case it is necessary to prevent overstretching of the suprascapular nerve during mobilisation of the infraspinatus. Reduction of the fragments may be hard to achieve in comminuted fractures of the scapular body, or in significantly displaced fractures of the scapular neck, particularly if operation is performed after a longer delay following the trauma. An infrequent complication is intraarticular perforation by the screws, which may happen especially during internal fixation of the glenoid, the scapular neck, or rarely of the lateral border of the scapula.

Early postoperative complications include first of all haematoma, and infection, either superficial or deep. According to Lantry [4], the infection rate is quite high – 4.2%, but our experience differs. Of 132 surgically treated cases we recorded deep infection only in two patients, one of whom was an alcoholic [12]. Haematoma has to be evacuated, most cases of superficial infection may be treated with antibiotics and local care. Deep infection requires débridement of the surgical wound. An early complication is also a limited range of motion of the shoulder, requiring manipulation, preferably within 6 weeks after surgery [15, 19].

Late complications are reported quite frequently. Failure of internal fixation [2–4, 9, 10, 12, 30–36], or non-union require reoperation [37, 38]. Malreduction of glenoid fractures results in incongruity. Hardegger [30] had to reoperate for joint instability. Schandelmeier [32] addressed acromial impingement after internal fixation of the glenoid by acromioplasty. Prominence of implants, requiring their removal, is a problem mainly in fractures of the acromion, scapular spine, or associated clavicular fractures. One report also described late infection 11 months after operation, requiring hardware removal [32].

Posttraumatic degenerative joint disease after scapular fractures occurs in 1.9%. Currently, the treatment of choice for such arthritis is shoulder arthroplasty.

Conclusion

Understanding of scapular fractures is impossible without a profound anatomical and clinical knowledge. Radiographic examination, first of all both Neer views and 3D CT reconstructions are essential for clear diagnosis and for planning treatment. In displaced fractures, it is necessary to consider operative treatment, which is not urgent and may be performed within up to 3 weeks after the injury. As these fractures are severe but rare injuries, it is better to refer the patients to specialist centres for definitive management.

References

1. Bartoníček J, Cronier P. History of the treatment of scapular fractures. Arch Orthop Trauma Surg. 2010;130:83–92.
2. Hersovici D, Roberts CS. Scapula fractures: to fix or not to fix? J Orthop Trauma. 2006;20:227–9.
3. Zlowodski M, Bhandari M, Zelle BA, Kregor PJ, Cole PA. Treatment of scapula fractures: systematic review of 520 fractures in 22 case series. J Orthop Trauma. 2006;20:230–3.
4. Lantry JM, Roberts CS, Giannoudis PV. Operative treatment of scapular fractures: a systematic review. Injury. 2008;39:271–83.
5. Tuček M, Bartoníček J, Frič V. Osseous anatomy of scapula: its importance for classification of scapular body. Ortopedie (Czech Orthopaedics). 2011;5:104–9.
6. Chochola A, Tuček M, Bartoníček J, Klika D. CT-diagnostic of scapular fractures. Rozhl Chir. 2013;92:385–8.
7. Tuček M, Naňka O, Malík J, Bartoníček J. Scapular glenopolar angle: standard values and side differences. Skelet Radiol. 2014;43:1583–7.
8. Tuček M, Bartoníček J, Klika D, Chochola A. Epidemiology of scapular fractures. Acta Orthop Belg. 2017;83:8–15.
9. Bartoníček J, Frič V. Scapular body fractures: results of the operative treatment. Int Orthop. 2011;35:747–53.
10. Bartoníček J, Tuček M, Frič V, Obruba P. Fractures of the scapular neck. Diagnosis-classifications-treatment. Int Orthop. 2014;38:2163–73.
11. Bartoníček J, Tuček M, Klika D, Chochola A. Pathoanatomy and computed tomography classification of glenoid fossa fractures based on 90 patients. Int Orthop (SICOT). 2016;40:2383–92.
12. Bartoníček J, Tuček M, Klika D, Obruba P. Total glenoid fractures. Rozhl Chir. 2016;95:386–93.
13. Bartoníček J, Frič V, Tuček M. Intra-operative reduction of the scapular body – a technical trick. J Orthop Trauma. 2009;23:294–8.
14. Bartoníček J, Tuček M, Frič V. Operative treatment of scapula fractures. Ortopedie (Czech Orthopaedics). 2010;4:204–10.
15. Bartoníček J. Scapular fractures. In: Court-Brown CH, Heckman AD, McMqQueen, Ricci WM, Tornetta P, editors. Rockwood and Green's fractures in adults. 8th ed. Philadelphia: Wolters Kluwer; 2015. p. 1475–501.
16. Reggio AW. Fracture of the shoulder girdle. In: Wilson PD, editor. Experience in the management of fractures and dislocations, based on an analysis of 4,390 cases. Philadelphia: Lippincott; 1938. p. 370–4.
17. Court-Brown CM, McQueen MM, Tornetta P. Trauma. Philadelphia: JB Lippincot, Williams and Wilkins; 2006. p. 76–81.
18. Zhang Y. Scapular fractures. In: Clinical epidemiology of orthopedic trauma. Stuttgart: Thieme; 2012. p. 580–617.

19. Goss TP. Scapula fractures and dislocations: diagnosis and treatment. J Am Acad Orthop Surg. 1995;3:22–33.
20. McAdams TR, Blevins FT, Martin TP, DeCoster TA. The role of plain films and computed tomography in the evaluation of scapula neck fractures. J Orthop Trauma. 2002;16:7–11.
21. Bestard EA, Schvene HR, Bestard EH. Glenoplasty inmanagement of recurrent shoulder dislocation. Contemp Orthop. 1986;12:47–55.
22. Cole PA, Gauger EM, Schroder LK. Management of scapular fractures. J Am Acad Orthop Surg. 2012;20:130–41.
23. Pace AM, Stuart R, Brownlow H. Outcome of glenoid neck fractures. J Shoulder Elb Surg. 2005;14:585–90.
24. Ada JR, Miller ME. Scapula fractures. Analysis of 113 cases. Clin Orthop Relat Res. 1991;269:174–80.
25. Euler E, Habermeyer P, Kohler W, et al. Skapulafrakturen – Klassifikation und Differentialtherapie. Orthopade. 1992;21:158–62.
26. Ideberg R, Grevsten S, Larsson S. Epidemiology of scapular fractures. Acta Orthop Scand. 1995;66:395–7.
27. Orthopaedic Trauma Association Fracture and dislocation compendium. Scapular fractures. J Orthop Trauma. 2007;21(Suppl 1):S68–71.
28. ter Meulen DP, Janssen SJ, Hageman MGJS, Ring DC. Quantitative htree-dimensional computed tomography analysis of glenoid fracture patterns according to the AO/OTA classification. J Shoulder Elb Surg. 2016;25:269–75.
29. Audigé L, Kellam JF, Lambert S, Madesn JE, Babst R, Andermahr LW, Jaeger M. The AO Foundation and Orthopaedic Trauma Association (AO/OTA) scapula fracture classification system focus on body involvement. J Shoulder Elb Surg. 2014;23:189–96.
30. Hardegger F, Simpson LA, Weber BG. The operative treatment of scapular fractures. J Bone Joint Surg (Br). 1984;66-B:725–31.
31. Bauer G, Fleuschmann W, Dussler E. Displaced scapular fractures: indication and long-term results of open reduction and internal fixation. Arch Orthop Trauma Surg. 1995;114:215–9.
32. Schandelmaier P, Blauth M, Schneider C, Krettek C. Fractures of the glenoid treated by operation. J Bone Joint Surg (Br). 2002;84-B:173–7.
33. Anavian J, Gauger EM, Schroder LK, Wijdicks CA, Cole PA. Surgical and functional outcomes after operative management of complex and displaced intra-articular glenoid fractures. J Bone Joint Surg Am. 2012;94:645–53.
34. Cole PA, Gauger EM, Herrera DA, Anavian J, Tarkin IS. Radiographic follow-up of 84 operatively treated scapula neck and body fractures. Injury. 2012;43:327–33.
35. Schroder LK, Gauger EM, Gilbertson JA, Cole PA. Functional outcomes after operative management of extra-articular glenoid neck and scapular body fractures. J Bone Joint Surg Am. 2016;98:1623–30.
36. Anavian J, Wijdicks CA, Schroder LK, Vang S, Cole PA. Surgery for scapula process fractures: good outcome in 26 patients. Acta Orthop. 2009;80:344–50.
37. Marek DJ, Sechriest VF, Swiontkowski MF, Cole P. Case report: reconstruction of a recalcitrant scapular neck nonunion and literature review. Clin Orthop Relat Res. 2009;467:1370–6.
38. Cole PA, Talbot M, Schroder LK, Anavian J. Extra-articular malunions of the scapula: a comparison of functional outcome before and after reconstruction. J Orthop Trauma. 2011;25:649–56.

Proximal Humeral Fractures

5

C. Spross and B. Jost

Introduction

There is no doubt that the number of proximal humeral fractures is high although will undoubtedly increase with an expanding elderly population. As such management of these fractures will become an increasing burden, not only on patients and clinicians but society generally. As such it is important that we develop good and clear evidence for treatment of the various fracture patterns and patient sub-groups. At the beginning of the twentieth century, conservative treatment was the mainstay as there were no viable alternatives. With the foundation of the AO (Association for the Study of Internal Fixation) in 1958 new treatment options were sought and devices for open reduction and internal fixation (ORIF) developed. In 1970 Charles Neer presented his results of hemiprosthetic replacements [1]. Subsequently, more fractures were treated operatively and with the development of anatomically pre-shaped angular stable implants at the beginning of the twenty first century, Open Reduction and Internal Fixation (ORIF) became the mainstay for the surgical treatment of proximal humeral fractures. The success of this, however, does not just depend on the implants themselves but also appropriate patient selection and surgical expertise. More recently there have been some reports of high complication and revision rates [2–7]. As such a number of authors have recommended a return to conservative treatment in many of these cases [8]. At one end of the spectrum in an elderly unfit patient with an undisplaced fracture, few would dispute the role of conservative treatment. Whilst at the other end with a comminuted fracture dislocation there is obviously a role for operative intervention. In between, however, there is a number of complex and perhaps only partially displaced fractures the management of which currently remains controversial. In this group the advantage of ORIF over conservative treatment would be weighed against the potential for significant complications.

More recently new and emerging technologies particularly Reverse Total Shoulder Arthroplasty (RTSA) has become a valuable option for treating severe fracture dislocation of the proximal humerus particularly in elderly patients [9, 10]. While reports of improved function with low revision rates are promising, long term follow up studies have yet to be reported. At this time, however, this implant does appear to be providing a satisfactory outcome for patients over 70.

Having considered the above it is our opinion that the aim of any fracture treatment should be to bring patients back as near as possible to their pre-injury function and quality of life. We do not believe there is one solution for all

C. Spross · B. Jost (✉)
Department of Orthopaedics and Traumatology, Kantonsspital St. Gallen, St. Gallen, Switzerland
e-mail: bernhard.jost@kssg.ch

I. A. Trail et al. (eds.), *Textbook of Shoulder Surgery*, https://doi.org/10.1007/978-3-319-70099-1_5

patients and that the whole range of treatment options should be considered for each individual. In this chapter we discuss the most recent literature on the treatment of proximal humerus fractures and will try to elucidate what is known and what is still controversial. Furthermore, we would like to share our first experiences and results with an evidence based treatment algorithm, accounting for patient-specific factors with the aim of finding the right treatment for each patient [11].

Aetiology

Epidemiology

Proximal humeral fractures account for nearly 6% of all fractures [12]. Although they can occur in any age group, over 80% of patients afflicted are older than 50 years and over 70% are female with the most common cause being a low-energy fall [13, 14]. The high percentage of postmenopausal women reflects the important role of osteoporosis with regard to these fractures [15].

Mechanism of Injury

The exact mechanism of injury leading to a proximal humeral fracture is often difficult to ascertain. The type of fracture depends on the position of the arm in relation to the torso at the moment of impact, when the humeral head is pushed against the glenoid or the acromion. For example, straight lateral impact from a fall or direct trauma to the adducted upper arm can result in a typical surgical neck fracture or a head split fracture as described in Neer's group VI [16]. Having the arm in a more abducted position results in more valgus impaction. Posterior fracture dislocation can result from direct trauma to the adducted and internally rotated extremity [17], whereas external rotation and abduction can lead to anterior dislocation with avulsion fracture of the greater tuberosity, especially in older patients [18, 19].

Presentations/Investigations/ Treatment Options

Clinical Examination

The first examination of the patient in the emergency department should include a full history particularly regarding to the mechanism of injury as to whether it was a high velocity injury or a low impact domestic fall. Whereas patients sustaining high velocity trauma are prone to associated injuries of the thoracic wall, cervical spine or other extremities as well as neurovascular damage [20], patients with severe osteoporosis or only secondary's a fracture may occur after minimal or indeed no trauma. It is also important to ascertain the patients pre-injury functional status eg dependence, activity level as well as any comorbidities. In our opinion this information is very important for later decision-making.

On physical examination, soft tissue swelling, ecchymosis and deformity may be present. The examiner should also look for concomitant injuries including the neurovascular status of the injured limb. Sensorimotor functions should be assessed and documented before further treatment. Special attention should be paid to the examination of axillary nerve function, which is the most commonly affected nerve in fractures or fracture-dislocations of the proximal humerus. By examining only the sensory function of the axillary nerve a lesion cannot be reliably excluded [21, 22]. Even in the presence of acute pain the motor function can be clinically assessed by feeling for isometric contraction of the deltoid muscle. This is done by putting one hand on the patient's elbow and the other one on the deltoid muscle. The patient is then told to attempt abduction of the elbow against the examiner's hand who can feel contractions of the deltoid muscle with the other hand. Any perceived contraction, even a weak one, of the deltoid, means that the axillary nerve is functioning.

Radiographic Examinations

Radiographic examination of suspected proximal humeral fractures or fracture-dislocations traditionally consists of a trauma series [antero-posterior (AP), scapular lateral and axillary view]. However, the axillary view can be painful for the patient and a recent study showed that it had no influence on further therapeutic decisions [23]. Furthermore, the classification of proximal humerus fractures based on radiographs is notoriously difficult and unreliable [24, 25]. As a consequence we obtain an AP and lateral view first and if we need further information, we have a low threshold for a CT scan with 3D reconstructions undoubtedly gives more accurate information with regard to fracture pattern and certainly allow better planning if surgery is contemplated [26, 27].

Bone Quality

After the first examination and the radiographic diagnosis, it is crucial to obtain more information for decision-making. Low bone mineral density (BMD) has been shown to be a risk factor for complications in the treatment of proximal humeral fractures [28–30].

The DEXA method is still the gold standard to diagnose osteoporosis but there are no defined threshold values for the proximal humerus yet and the examination is often not available at the time of fracture. The quantitative CT (pQCT) is an alternative method, but its availability is also limited and the analysis rather complicated [27]. Thus, several radiographic tools have been suggested to ascertain bone density [31–34]. We defined and validated the deltoid tuberosity index (DTI), which is a simple method to measure local bone quality directly proximal to the deltoid tuberosity on the AP fracture X-ray (Fig. 5.1). This structure is usually not affected by the fracture and well outlined on the AP radiograph due to the internally rotated relieving posture of the arm. The outer cortical diameter is divided by the inner endosteal diameter and does not need to be corrected for the magnification error. In a first study, we found a strong correlation between the DTI and the BMD of the humeral head (measured with pQCT). Furthermore, we were able to define a cut-off value (DTI < 1.4) for low BMD of the proximal humerus. Finally, we validated this index for its use on proximal humerus fractures and found that the DTI has a high intra- and interobserver reliability [35]. In a recent study, we were able to confirm the clinical relevance of this threshold value and its influence on complications after ORIF of proximal humerus fractures [30].

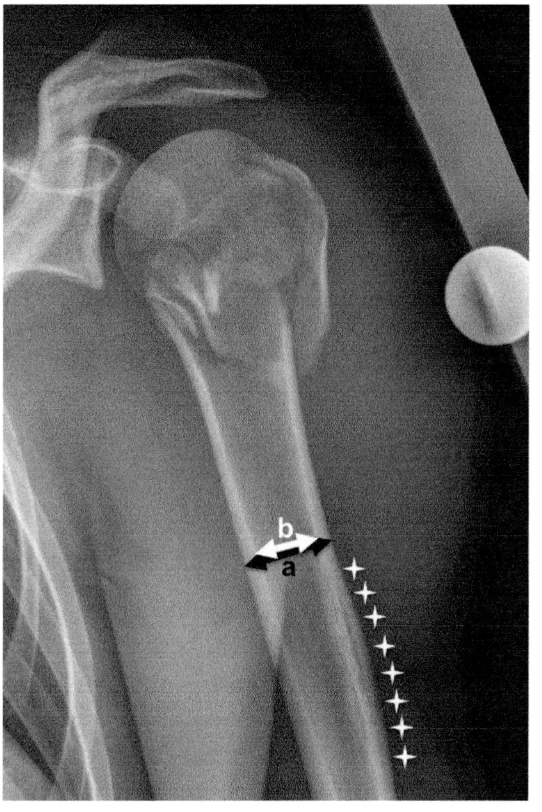

Fig. 5.1 The deltoid tuberositiy index (DTI) is measured directly proximal to the deltoid tuberosity (asterisks). At the level, where the outer cortical borders become parallel, the outer cortical diameter (**a**) is divided by the inner endosteal diameter (**b**)

Fracture Classification

In the past, a variety of classifications have been used to describe proximal humeral fractures and fracture-dislocations. Consequently, it has been difficult to compare the results of the early but also of current literature. Despite ample experience with these fractures, their treatment based on classifications remains controversial.

Codman/Neer Classification

Codman [36] noted that most proximal humeral fractures occur along the lines of the physeal scars at the proximal end of the humerus and described four possible fracture fragments: greater tuberosity, lesser tuberosity, anatomical head and shaft. Based on these four fragments, Neer [16] proposed the four-segment classification system. A segment (greater, lesser tuberosity, anatomical, surgical neck) is defined as a 'part' if its displacement is more than 1 cm or >45°. If none of the fragments meets these criteria, the fracture is called a 1-part fracture, even if all segments are fractured [37].

The AO/ASIF Classification System

The AO/ASIF (Arbeitsgemeinschaft für Osteosynthesefragen/Association for the Study of Internal Fixation) proposed a new classification, which was an expansion on and modification of the Neer classification [38]. Basically, the AO/ASIF system differentiates three types of fractures: extra articular unifocal (11-A), extra articular bifocal (11-B) and intra articular (11-C). Each of these groups is divided into further subgroups depending on impaction and dislocation.

Hertel's Classification and Predictors of Humeral Head Ischemia

Based on the original drawings of Codman, Hertel and colleagues [39, 40] proposed a "LEGO" classification system with 12 basic fracture patterns (+2 additional head split patterns). Furthermore, they found that a dorsomedial metaphyseal head extension of less than 8 mm, a more than 2 mm displaced medial hinge and fractures with isolated articular segments were good predictors for intraoperative head ischemia. However, these findings did not correlate with postoperative AVN in later follow-up studies [41, 42].

Authors' Opinion: Fracture Classification

The reproducibility of the Neer and the AO/ASIF classifications is difficult and has thus been subject to many studies with advantages for the Neer classification, especially with the help of 3D CT reconstructions [24, 26, 43–46]. However, more and more prospective randomised studies on conservative versus operative fracture treatment in elderly patients with three- or four-part fractures showed no functional benefits of surgery [8, 47–50]. Therefore, the discussion of fracture classification is becoming increasingly secondary, at least for elderly patients. However, in high energy injuries or head splitting fractures, particularly in younger patients where surgery is clearly indicated, interpretation of the fracture pattern remains eminently important for preoperative planning [42]. Therefore, in our institution CT scans are used for better imaging of fractures with subtle but potentially relevant displacement and for fractures where surgery is being considered. Based on that, we use the Neer classification and pay special attention to the displacement of the tuberosities in relation to the head and to certain fracture types and configurations, such as varus or valgus impaction of the head fragment [39, 51–60].

> **Clinical Pearl**
> Neer classification of fractures is still in widespread use. Special attention, however, should be paid to displacement of the tuberosity as any varus or valgus impactionof the humeral head.

Treatment Options

The literature regarding the treatment of fracture of the proximal humerus is indeed enormous. Most of the papers, however, are essentially cohort studies and could be used to justify literally every treatment strategy. When it comes to higher level evidence, however (Level 1 and 2 studies) the number shrinks to only a few prospective studies and even fewer prospective randomised studies. As such the evidence-based recommendations for the management of these fractures remains limited [61, 62]. A recent multicentre prospective randomised clinical trial (the PROFHER trial) performed in the UK involving over 30 centres [8]. Randomised patients older than 16 years with a proximal humerus fracture with sufficient displacement (for the treating surgeon to consider surgery) to either conservative or operative treatment. The authors concluded that there is no statistically significant benefit of surgery versus conservative treatment after 2 years. Not surprisingly this study has been criticised by way of its selection bias, inappropriate scoring and the involvement of too many surgeons and too many surgical techniques [63, 64]. There is no doubt, however, this study has stimulated discussion and has paved the way for further studies perhaps looking at individual sub-groups.

Personalising treatment for an individual patient however remains a challenge, particularly in the face of changing interventions. In the following sections, the authors present examples of published literature on individual interventions; and supplement this with the authors' preferred treatment algorithm.

Conservative Treatment

In the Elderly Patient

Since Neer [16] suggested conservative treatment for one-part fractures, they have been the subject of only a few studies of which most reported good functional results in the majority of patients treated [65–67]. Maybe it is due to the high complication rates after ORIF [2, 4, 7, 68, 69] or the restricted functional results after hemiarthroplasty [70–72] that also more extensively displaced fractures are being treated conservatively again. Several studies have been looking for patient and fracture characteristics amenable to conservative treatment. Court-Brown [73] found 80% of good or excellent results after conservative treatment of valgus impacted fractures (Fig. 5.2). The degree of displacement had a negative, and increasing age a positive influence on the final functional outcome after 1 year. The authors recommended conservative treatment for valgus impacted three-part fractures in elderly patients.

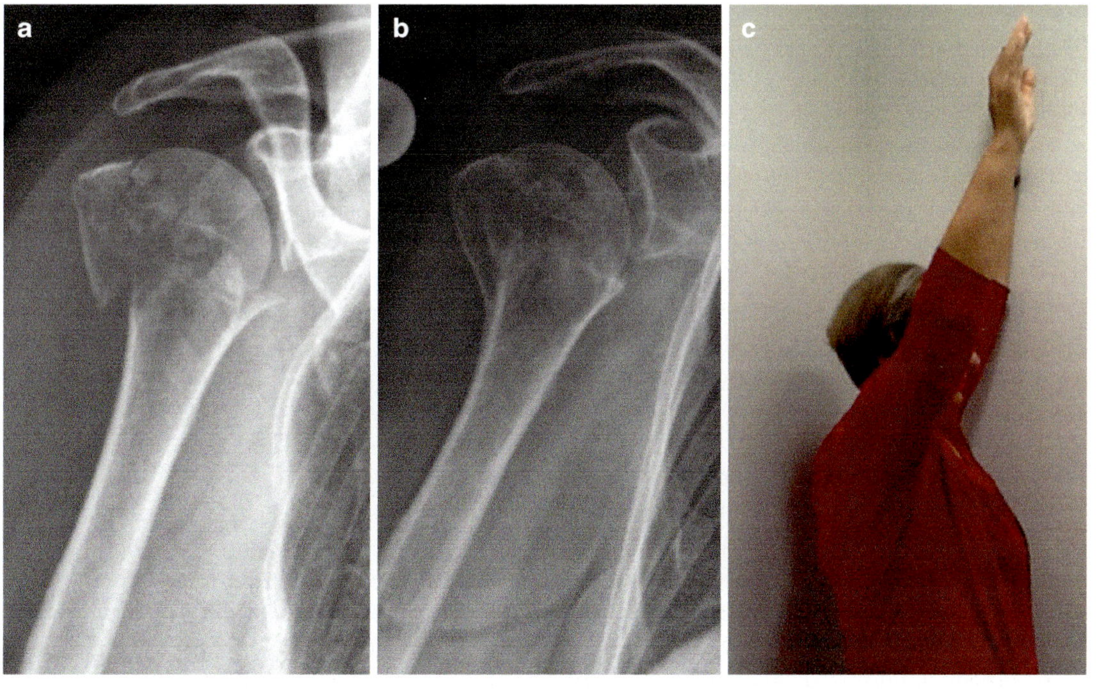

Fig. 5.2 (**a**) AP radiograph of a valgus impacted 2-part fracture of a 69 y.o. female. (**b**) AP radiographic follow-up after 1 year. (**c**) Clinical result (forward flexion) after 1 year

Scandinavian studies were then the first to prospectively randomise conservative versus surgical treatment for all three- and four-part fractures in the elderly (>60 years) [47, 48, 50]. None of these studies found a significant functional benefit of any operative treatment but they might have been underpowered to find such a difference. However, the authors concluded that the tendency of better functional results or quality of life after a surgical procedure has to be balanced against the higher risk of revision rates. They found that the overall acceptable outcome and limited need for surgical intervention might justify conservative treatment of elderly, low-demand patients with three- or four-part fractures.

Also the most recent Cochrane analysis found no difference between conservative and operative treatment in elderly patients with displaced proximal humerus fractures involving the surgical neck. However literature is not sufficient for strong treatment recommendations [62].

In Younger Patients

Now the question arises whether young(er) and active patients, who need maximal shoulder function to go back to work or sports as soon as possible, may tolerate less fracture displacement and malunion than elderly patients. Literature is scarce on this specific question, however a small number of studies had focused on conservative treatment and age groups. Koval et al. [66] found that conservative treatment in younger patients with one-part fractures showed a mainly successful outcome.

Hanson et al. also paid special attention to the conservative treatment of younger patients who are still working. They concluded that conservative treatment is safe and effective in AO 11-A and -B fractures (mainly one- and two-part surgical neck fractures).

This is in accordance to Court-Brown et al. [74] who looked at conservatively treated patients with varus impacted surgical neck fractures. All fractures healed and 79% showed good or excellent functional results independently from the final varus angle and age.

Therefore, it seems that even for young and active patients, conservative treatment of one-part fractures and some two-part fractures may be justified with acceptably satisfying results.

Conservative Treatment Protocol

Lefevre-Colau et al. [75] showed that physiotherapy with early mobilisation is safe for the conservative treatment of patients with stable impacted proximal humeral fractures. Patients in the early mobilisation group wore a sling for 4–6 weeks and started physiotherapy after 3 days with pendulum and passive ROM exercises. After 6 weeks, they started with active ROM exercises.

In case of unstable fractures, the arm can be immobilised in a sling for 2 weeks. Then physiotherapy may be started with pendulum exercises and passive elevation/abduction up to 90°. After 4–6 weeks, patients can be allowed a free active ROM [47, 48, 50].

Surgical Treatment

Despite the abundance of literature on surgical treatment of proximal humerus fractures, there is still no standard of care, and the main question of which patient and fracture is suitable for which surgical treatment remains unanswered. Surgeon's preference, patient's individuality, the high variety of fracture configurations, the difficulty in classification and the high number of different implants are the main reasons for these disagreements. Also, prospective studies comparing different treatment options for specific fracture types are relatively rare and the management and especially the surgical technique are mainly based on the surgeon's experience and preferences. However, with the large choice of different implants, there may not be a gold standard and it may be reasonable that each surgeon chooses the implant, which works best in their hands for the cases that need surgery. In the following, the most common implants for proximal humerus fractures are described including their range of indications according to the most recent literature.

Conventional (Non-locking) Plate

Before the appearance of anatomically preshaped, angular stable plates for the proximal humerus, one third tubular plates or T-plates were used for open reduction and internal fixation of all types of fractures of the proximal humerus [76–79]. Nowadays, some surgeons still use them mainly for more stable valgus impacted fractures.

However, newer and specifically preshaped plates have widely replaced the conventional ones.

Locking Plate

In biomechanical studies angular stable locking plates have shown some advantage compared to conventional plates [80]. These implants are currently the ones most widely used for proximal humeral fractures. Reports in the literature vary in terms of complications and revision rates but it seems that along with their broad use their indications have been expanded to all types of fractures. This might explain why reports about complication rates up to 49% can be found [2, 4–6, 69]. As a shoulder referral centre, we have seen several devastating situations after locking plate ORIF of proximal humerus fractures with often limited options for revision surgery [7]. Thus, it has been our priority to find predictors for complications and to consequently lower the complication rate after such operations. Further analysis of complications showed the following fracture characteristics to be at risk for later failure: a markedly displaced anatomical neck fragment, fracture-dislocations and head-splits [2, 3, 69]. Predictors for failure or impaired outcome were found to be: low BMD, increasing age, non-anatomical reduction of the medial hinge and smoking [2, 28–30, 81].

Percutaneous Fixation

The general advantage of closed reduction and fixation is minimal impairment of the vascular supply to the fragments. This technique has been modified from sole pin fixation to a "humerus block" fixation with pins and screws [82] or to a hybrid external fixation [83]. The indications for this technique are mainly based on the surgeon's experience with it. Good indications are described to be: surgical neck fractures with avulsion of the greater tuberosity and displaced articular segment fractures with valgus impaction or little medial displacement. Severely displaced articular segment fractures and fracture-dislocations [82] as well as comminution of the surgical neck, the medial calcar or the greater tuberosity are relative contraindications for this technique, as primary stability is much more difficult to achieve and maintain [28].

Intramedullary Nail

Some surgeons prefer the use of antegrade locked nails for the treatment of proximal humerus fractures, either minimally invasive [84] or through an open approach [85]. The results seem to be comparable to locking plate ORIF [84, 86]. However, a recent systematic review revealed that the indications for nailing may be limited to two-part surgical neck and three-part fractures as the complication rate of four-part fractures was found to be up to 63% [87].

The Da Vinci System

An interesting new device has been introduced by Russo et al. [88, 89]. The so-called "Da Vinci System" is a triangularly shaped, hollow cage, which can be put into the bone void after the reduction of the head fragment. This intraosseous device gives further support and stability to the head fragment and prevents secondary dislocation. This cage may be combined with screws, plates and screws or pins and according to the results of the inventor, even three- and four-part fractures may be treated successfully [89].

Hemiarthroplasty

Before reversed total shoulder arthroplasty (RTSA) was introduced, hemiarthroplasty was the mainstay of treatment for fractures that could not be reconstructed. Originally, Neer proposed primary hemiarthroplasty for four-part fractures, four-part fracture-dislocations and fractures with more than 50% of cartilage-covered articular defect [1]. The clinical results have consistently been reported as unpredictable mainly because of malunion of the tuberosities [90]. However, hemiarthroplasty may result in good functionality if the fragments heal in place and anatomical relations can be restored [70, 71, 91–94].

Reverse Total Shoulder Arthroplasty (RTSA)

Primary RTSA is becoming an increasingly popular option for the treatment of proximal humerus fractures, especially in the elderly patient. Compared to primary hemiarthroplasty, it has been shown that clinical results are better and more predictable with an even lower revision rate [95–99]. Looking at these results, one might be tempted to use this treatment option also in younger patients if the fracture is not reconstructable. However, long-term results on primary RTSA for fractures are only available from small case series [100, 101]. Considering the invasiveness of this implant and possible problems like infection or long-term deterioration of the deltoid muscle as well as glenoid loosening [102], stronger long-term data should first be available to guide its use. Therefore, primary RTSA should mainly be considered for patients over 70 years of age [103] with fractures that cannot be treated conservatively, either due to high functional demands or persistent pain.

One current dilemma is that, on one hand we have the RTSA promoted as an intervention with more predictable results but mainly reserved for elderly patients and on the other hand, a hemiprosthesis which results in less predictable results, recommended for younger patients with non-reconstructable fractures and higher functional demands. A possible solution may be to lower the age cut-off for RTSA with all its concomitant risks. In any case, more scientific efforts are needed to find better solutions for young patients to spare the glenoid, a structure not usually affected by the initial injury [104].

Authors' Preferred Treatment Algorithm

In our opinion, a 16-year-old patient with a three-part fracture needs different treatment than a 90-year-old patient with the same fracture who lives in a high level of care nursing home. If both had a displaced fractured neck of femur and were unable to walk, everybody would agree that both needed surgery. However, for proximal humerus fractures, the crucial question seems to be: "how much shoulder function does a patient need to reach his/her maximum quality of life after treatment?" Young patients have high expectations and need maximal shoulder function for their work and their lives at home, whereas some elderly patients may only desire to be free of pain and are content with limited shoulder function as long as they don't need surgery. In our opinion, treatment should be adapted to the patient's needs and expectations first and second to the biological conditions and then to the fracture pattern itself. As it is difficult to draw a clear line at a certain age, bone quality is helpful to assess at least the biological age of the patient's proximal humerus. Therefore, we developed and published a first suggestion of an evidence based treatment algorithm, which includes conservative and operative treatment for patients of different ages and with different demands [11]. In this section, we present and discuss the evidence the algorithm is based on, as well as our preliminary clinical results with the use of an adjusted version (Figs. 5.3 and 5.4).

The Young and Active Patient

These patients usually have good bone quality and need to return to work as soon as possible. Thus, the aim is to regain maximal shoulder function and our treatment pathway is depicted in Fig. 5.3. The range of non-surgical treatment in these patients is limited to one-part fractures except for isolated fractures of the tuberosities. We use CT scans to assess the exact degree of displacement and prefer operative treatment in the case of more than 5 mm of superior displacement of the greater or more than 5 mm of medial displacement of the lesser tuberosity [52, 53]. Small avulsions are usually treated arthroscopically with a double row or a suture bridge technique. For large fractures of the greater tuberosity we use a lateral one-third tubular buttress plate.

Two-, three- or four-part fractures as well as fracture-dislocations and head-split fractures are usually treated with ORIF in young patients.

We prefer the deltopectoral approach and use an angular stable implant. In case of unstable and severely displaced three- or four-part fractures ORIF is attempted whenever possible. However, if the head fragment shows no borehole bleeding and no stable reduction is possible, we change to primary hemiarthroplasty with modularity, which allows a later conversion to a RTSA without the need of changing the stem.

The Elderly Patient

We generally differentiate between elderly patients with high or low demands. Patients who exercise regularly (e.g.: walking, swimming, ski-

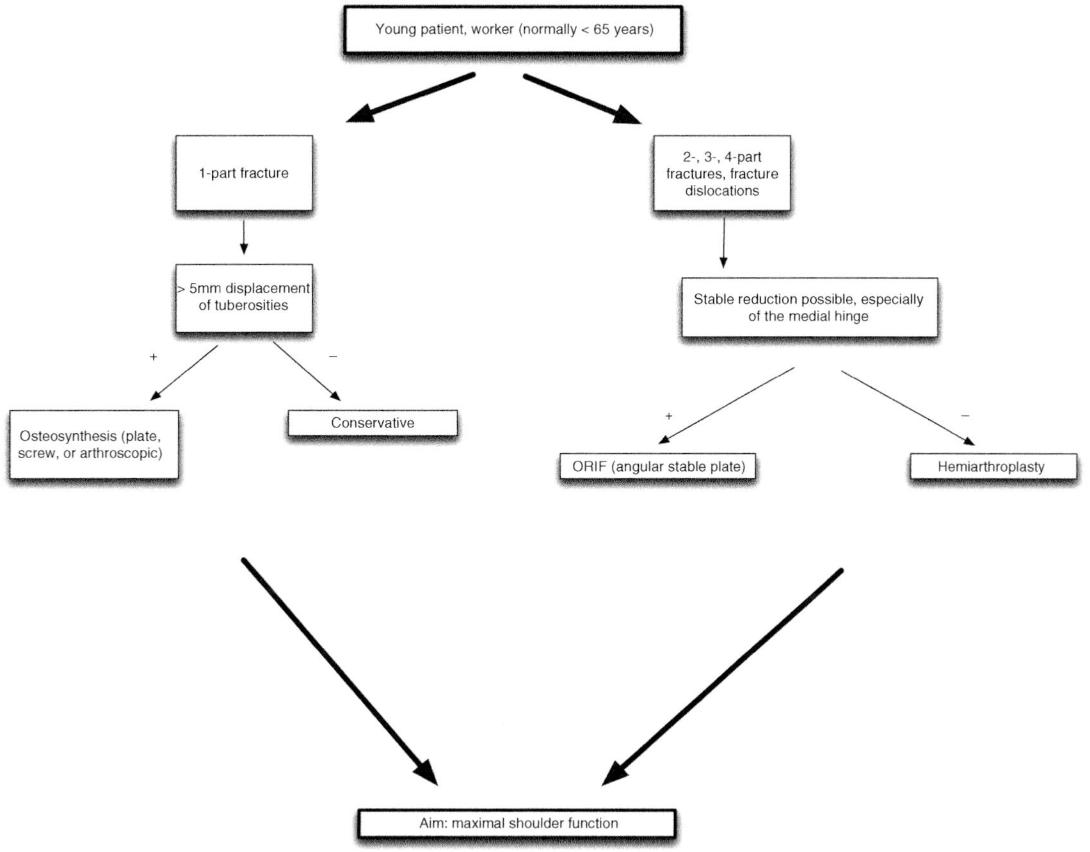

Fig. 5.3 Authors' preferred treatment strategy for younger and active patients with the aim of maximal shoulder function after treatment. (ORIF open reduction and internal fixation)

ing, golf, tennis) and live independently are classified as high-demand requiring maximal shoulder function. On the other hand, patients who can hardly fend for themselves and need regular help for daily living are classified as low-demand and do not require full shoulder function. We treat these patients conservatively whenever possible [47, 48, 50]. Only persistent pain would be an indication for surgery, which would then be a hemiprothesis.

Elderly patients with high needs are further assessed for osteoporosis using the Deltoid tuberosity index (DTI) (Fig. 5.1). If the bone quality is good (DTI > 1.4), we treat them in the same manner as young patients (Fig. 5.3) with the exception of using primary RTSA rather than hemiarthroplasty in patients older than 70 years. The algorithm for treatment of patients with osteoporosis is shown in Fig. 5.4. The indication for non-operative treatment is broader and includes all one-part fractures, even 1 cm displacement of the tuberosities. Also varus or valgus impacted two-part surgical neck and valgus impacted three-part fractures are treated conservatively (Fig. 5.2) [74, 105]. Valgus impacted four-part fractures with less than 1 cm displacement of the tuberosities in relation to the head fragment (centre of rotation) are not treated surgically either. Thus, in this population with limited bone quality our indications for angular stable ORIF are narrowed down to severely displaced fractures, which can be fixed in a stable manner, in patients <70 years (Fig. 5.5). Otherwise, we prefer prosthetic replacement for

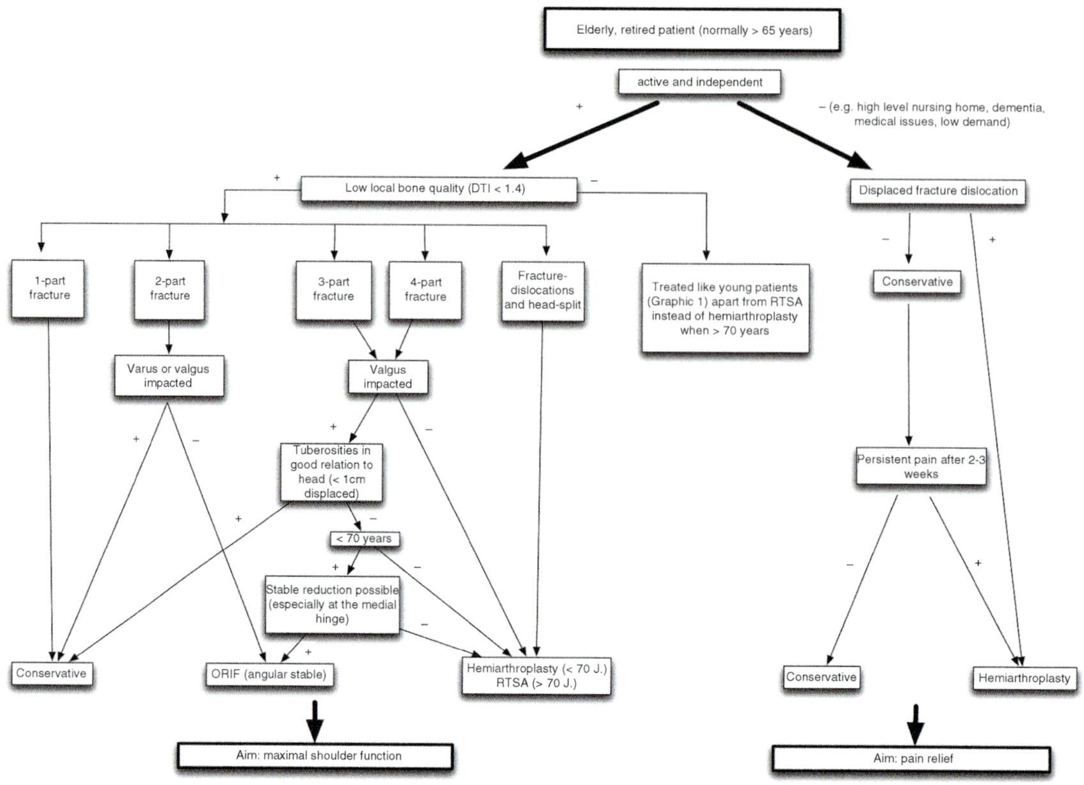

Fig. 5.4 Authors' preferred treatment strategy for elderly patients (>65 years) with either aim of maximal shoulder function or pain relief after treatment. (ORIF open reduction and internal fixation, RTSA reverse total shoulder arthroplasty)

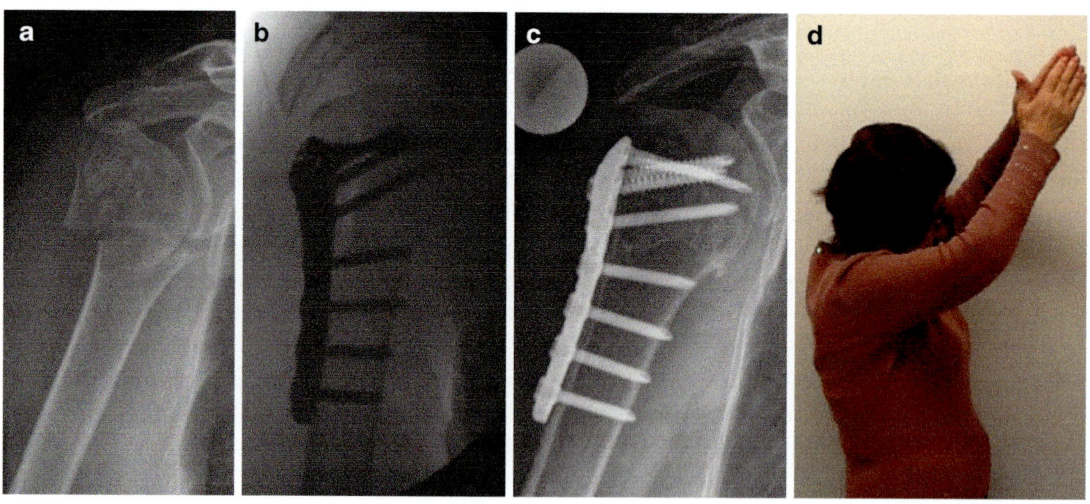

Fig. 5.5 (**a**) AP radiograph of a not impacted 2-part surgical neck fracture of a 65 y.o. female with limited bone quality (DTI < 1.4). The indication to ORIF was made according to the algorithm. (**b**) direct postoperative radiograph after angular stable ORIF. (**c**) AP radiographic follow-up after 1 year. (**d**) Clinical result (forward flexion) after 1 year

severely displaced three- and four-part fractures and fracture-dislocations (RTSA when patients are older than 70 years).

> **Clinical Pearl**
> There is significant debate and disagreement between the roles of conservative and operative intervention for proximal humeral fractures. Many factors have to be considered including the nature of the injury, the status or age of the patient, the bone quality and finally patient expectations.

Surgical Technique/Rehabilitation

Authors' Preferred Technique for Locking Plate ORIF

Positioning Techniques and Surgical Approach

The patient is positioned in a beach chair position, the arm draped free and positioned in a hydraulic device (e.g. Spider Limb Positioner; Smith & Nephew, London, U.K.). The image intensifier is placed over the shoulder from the top end of the table and covered with sterile drapes for free manipulation and independent use by the surgeon [106]. For open shoulder surgery we mainly use the deltopectoral approach, which has an internervous plane with minimal risk of nerve injury, can be safely extended distally and used for further revisions in the future. An approximately 8 cm long incision is made from the tip of the coracoid aiming to the middle of the upper arm. After identifying the cephalic vein, it is retracted laterally and the deltopectoral interval is sharply opened down to the conjoining tendon, which is retracted medially with a Langenbeck retractor. An 8 mm Hohman retractor is then placed on the top of the coracoid and the aperture is opened distally up to the insertion of the deltoid muscle. A blunt Eva retractor is placed laterally around the humerus directly proximal to the deltoid insertion. The plane between the deltoid and the rotator cuff is dissected in order to put a Browne Deltoid Retractor (Arthrex, Naples, Florida) around the proximal humerus. During this manoeuvre, special attention must be paid not to further displace the greater tuberosity fragment. As a next step, the tendon of the long head of the biceps is identified. If it is unstable and/or damaged, either the rotator interval or the cuff tear resulting from the fracture is extended slightly lateral to the bicipital groove towards the coracoid for tenotomy or tenodesis. We use heavy non-absorbable stay sutures (No 2 FiberWire; Arthrex, Naples, Florida), at least one for each tendon (subscapularis, supraspinatus, infraspinatus, teres minor). These stay sutures are kept during the surgery for better control of the reduction and later fixation to the plate as a tension band construct (even for two-part surgical neck fractures with intact tuberosities).

Reduction and Fixation Techniques

Generally, dissection and soft tissue damage should be kept minimal during the operation. The joint may be seen through the above-mentioned opening of the interval. The rest of the reduction depends on the type of fracture.

In case of valgus impacted fractures, the plate may be preliminarily fixed to the shaft with a conventional screw for indirect reduction using ligamentotaxis. The tuberosities can be pulled towards their anatomical position while the head is disimpacted and laterally lifted into normal angulation through the fracture gap between the tuberosities. Once the tuberosities can be brought together laterally, the plate can be slowly pressed against them by tightening the conventional screw. This results in an indirect reduction of the humeral head fragment with stable fixation of the fracture parts. If necessary, the space created behind the humeral head can be filled with bone substitute before this manoeuvre [78, 107], but we rarely use this option. Finally, further head and shaft screws may be applied and the tuberosities fixed to the plate using the stay sutures.

For unstable surgical neck fractures, we preposition two intramedullary K-wires (2 mm) (Fig. 5.6). To avoid later conflict with the plate, they are introduced percutaneously about 5 cm distal to the approach. The reduction may then be achieved with indirect manipulation of the arm (flexion and ab- or adduction) using the hydraulic positioner and the K-wires protruded to fix the head preliminary (Fig. 5.6b). In case of an unstable reduction at the calcar, we aim for impaction of the head on the shaft to prevent later varus collapse and secondary screw cut outs (Fig. 5.6c, d).

For severely displaced 3- and 4-part fractures, we try to proceed in the same way. Firstly, prepare the intramedullary K-wires, then we reduce the head fragment into a valgus position with as minimal soft tissue dissection as possible. Then the steps are the same as for the above-mentioned valgus fracture (Fig. 5.7).

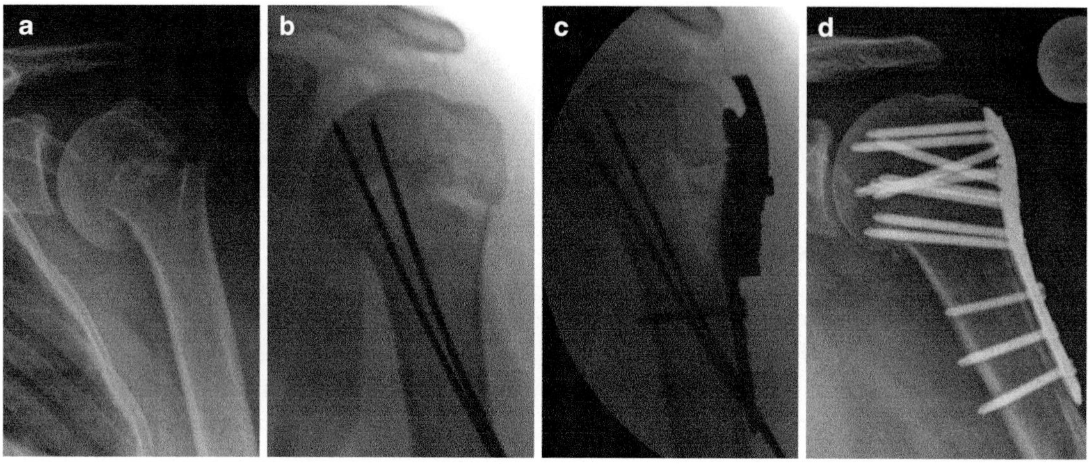

Fig. 5.6 (**a**) Radiograph of a varus displaced 2-part surgical neck fracture of a 35 y.o. female. (**b**) Reduction of the head fragment and preliminary fixation to the shaft with two previously introduced intramedullary K-wires (2 mm). (**c**) Final reduction by tightening the conventional screw of the plate first. (**d**) AP radiographic follow-up after 3 months

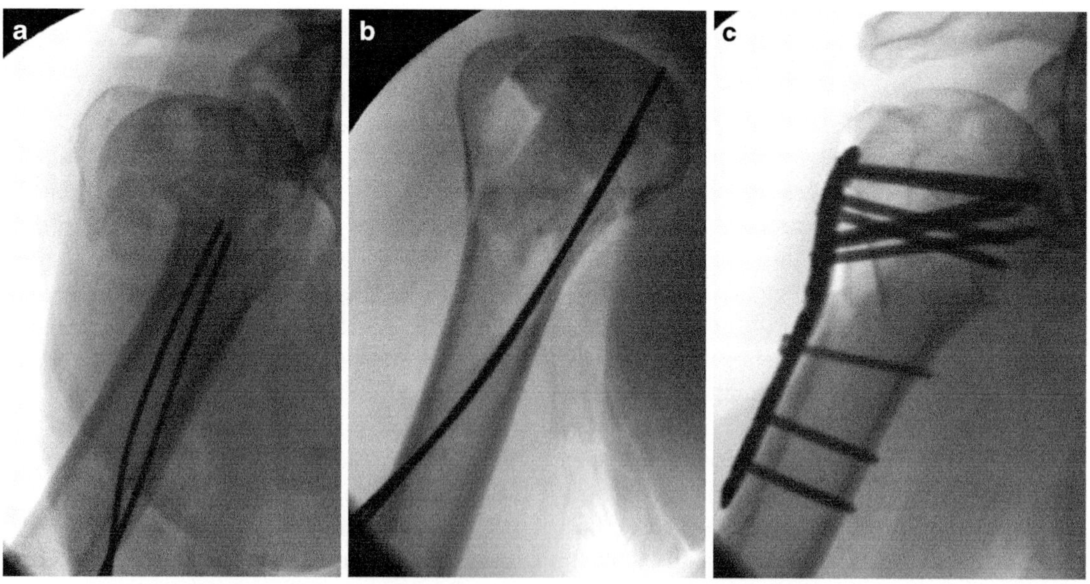

Fig. 5.7 (**a**) Intraoperative radiograph of a 4-part fracture of a 45 y.o. male. The head fragment has been put into a valgus position after the placement of two intramedullary K-wires. (**b**) From the valgus position, the head has been reduced to the shaft and preliminarily fixed with the K-wires. (**c**) Definitive fixation with plate and screws after the reduction of the tuberosities

The Minimal Invasive Plate Osteosynthesis (MIPO) Technique for Locking Plates

A minimally invasive technique has also been described for the use of locking plates [108–110]. The axillary nerve should be marked approximately 5–6 cm distal to the edge of the acromion. After the deltoid-split approach, sutures are placed in the rotator cuff tendons and preliminarily fixed to the plate. The plate is inserted underneath the deltoid muscle, always in contact to cortical bone, with a Langenbeck retractor securing the axillary nerve. Under fluoroscopic control, a stab incision is made for the most distal hole. Also, plate-specific aiming devices are available and useful for this technique. The plate is fixed to the head proximally with K-wires. The most distal hole of the plate must be placed in the middle of the shaft and can therefore be temporarily secured by drilling and leaving the bur in situ. A conventional screw is placed in the hole distal to the surgical neck fracture and tightened to the shaft. This results in indirect repositioning of the head in case of valgus displacement. At the end, the proximal locking screws and the already drilled distal locking shaft screw are inserted and the prepared rotator cuff sutures are fixed to the plate [108].

Percutaneous Fixation Techniques

Resch et al. described their detailed reduction technique [82, 111]. For reduction an elevator or a pointed hood retractor can be inserted through a small incision, the fragments can be fixed internally with 2–2.5 mm threaded K-wires. Depending on the displacement of the fragments they may be reduced with separate manoeuvres. First, axial traction to the adducted and internally rotated arm is needed to reduce the surgical neck fracture. The reduction is then secured with two or three K-wires drilled from inferior to superior, starting at the deltoid tuberosity. Then, the arm can be carefully returned to neutral position. In a second step, the greater tuberosity can be grasped with the help of a pointed hook retractor, which is inserted through the subacromial space. The greater tuberosity fragment is pulled in anterior and lateral direction until it reaches its anatomical position. It can be fixed with K-wires and its correct reduction is checked with internal and external rotation of the arm under fluoroscopy. Also, cannulated screws can be inserted over the K-wires for definitive fixation of the greater tuberosity. The pins can either be buried under the skin or left to protrude through the skin. They may be removed after 4–6 weeks under local anaesthesia.

Authors' Preferred Technique for Hemiarthroplasty

As a first step, all rotator cuff tendons are secured with at least one stay suture to secure the tuberosities. The articular segment is retrieved and saved as a potential bone graft.

The glenoid is examined for evidence of cartilage defects.

Together with preoperative CT planning, the medial calcar area is used as a bony landmark for proper positioning of the implant's humeral component. If the calcar is fractured as well, the insertion of pectoralis major may be used as a consistent reference to measure the height of the prosthesis with a specific measuring device. We aim for 20° of retroversion of the shaft to recreate anatomical conditions and perform a tenotomy (or tenodesis) of the long biceps tendon, as this has been shown to be beneficial for the functional outcome [112].

Before cementing the humeral implant, the shaft is prepared for the refixation of the tuberosities. Holes are drilled in the shaft so vertically oriented sutures can be used to repair each tuberosity. A preliminary reduction is then performed so that the tuberosities can be held together with a towel clip while determining proper head height.

We use a cemented implant in most of the cases as the fractured metaphysis may not allow enough press fit for the round shaft. We pay a lot of attention to the fixation of the tuberosities (No 2 FiberWire; Arthrex, Naples, Florida). We fix them to the humerus shaft and to the prosthetic stem with four sutures which go through the medial part of the prosthesis. Two of them are put around both tuberosities, the other two around each tuberosity separately. Then two further vertical sutures are used to fix each tuberosity to the stem through the pre-drilled shaft holes. Finally the stay suture of the greater is fixed to the stay sutures of the lesser tuberosity.

Authors' Preferred Technique for Reverse Total Shoulder Arthroplasty

We use a CT scan to assess the glenoid bone quality (e.g. cysts) and version, which should be corrected to 0° during surgery, but this is rarely necessary in fracture cases. The tuberosities are grasped with sutures as described above and retracted to remove the head fragment. The most anterior part of the supraspinatus tendon and the long biceps tendon are cut for better exposure of the glenoid. In our opinion it is important that the tuberosities are reduced and fixed to the shaft and prosthesis to restore at least some external and internal rotation [9, 10, 113]. Fixation of the greater tuberosity is of higher priority compared to fixation of the lesser tuberosity.

The anteroinferior capsule is only partially removed for good access to the glenoid; the labrum is completely removed circumferentially; the triceps is slightly released to identify the lateral border of the scapula. After reaming off the cartilage and correcting the glenoid version to 0° (if necessary), the baseplate should be orientated flush to its inferior border and centred in the anterior-posterior direction with a slight inclination of maximally 10°. After fixation of the baseplate and the insertion of the glenosphere, the shaft is prepared aiming to achieve 20° of retroversion. The correct height of the prosthesis is crucial; if the calcar is intact it can be used as reference together with preoperative CT planning. If the calcar is fractured, the correct height can be planned with additional full length X-rays of both upper arms [114]. A preliminary reduction can be made to test the laxity and stability of the joint before the definitive stem is inserted (cemented or uncemented) to the planned height. The sutures for fixation of the tuberosities are prepared the same way as described for hemiarthroplasty (see description above). After a careful trial reduction, soft tissue tension and distraction of the components is assessed and can be corrected with the use of different inlays. The goal is to achieve stability in all directions with no gapping when pulling on the arm. Finally, the tuberosities are fixed back to the stem and the humerus shaft as described above (Fig. 5.8).

Postoperative Rehabilitation

Independently from the type of technique for osteosynthesis, postoperative treatment mainly depends on the stability achieved. Stable reductions and fixations may be passively mobilised immediately after surgery and a sling used for 6 weeks. Active ROM exercises are usually started after 6 weeks and muscle strengthening exercises after 3 months. However, the relatively high rate of reduction failures even with the use of rigid angular stable implants has called early mobilisation after this procedure into question [115].

In our opinion, follow up care of three- or four-part ORIF, primary hemiarthroplasty or RTSA is limited by the healing of the tuberosities to the stem and to each other. As a stiff shoulder or prosthesis is still better to treat than displaced tuberosities, we use a more restrictive mobilisation algorithm. Patients wear a sling for 6 weeks and pendulum exercises are started 2 weeks postoperatively. Passive and active assisted mobilisation with the arm in neutral rotation is allowed up to an elevation and flexion of 90° in the fifth and sixth postoperative weeks. After the first clinical and radiographic control at 6 weeks, free active and passive ROM are permitted. Muscle strengthening is usually started after 3 months.

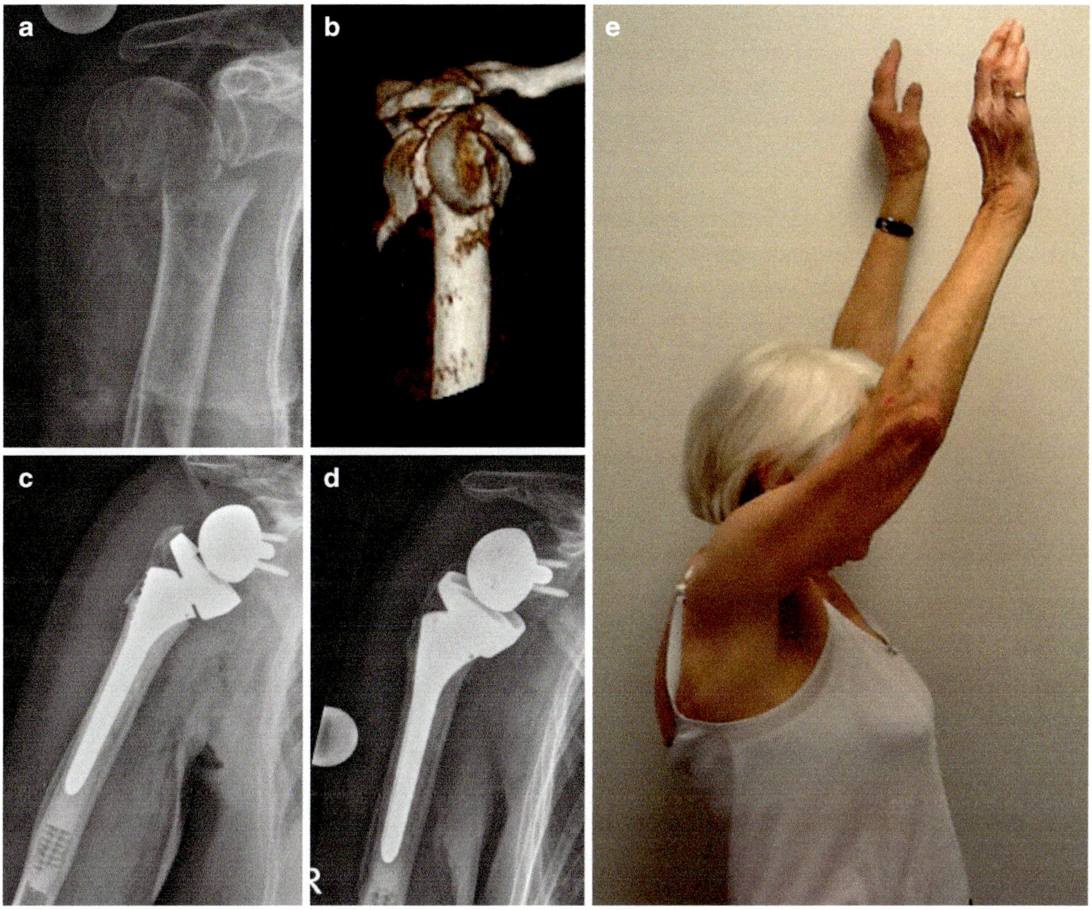

Fig. 5.8 (**a**) AP radiograph of a proximal humerus fracture of a 78 y.o. female. (**b**) 3D CT-reconstruction of the fracture shows severe displacement and involvement of the tuberosities. The indication for primary RTSA was made according to the algorithm. (**c**) Directly postoperative after implantation of a RTSA. (**d**) AP radiographic follow-up after 1 year. (**e**) Clinical result (forward flexion) after 1 year

Results

Outcome After Open and Minimally Invasive Osteosynthesis

The fragile blood supply and the often limited bone quality of the humeral head may be the two main reasons for failure after any kind of osteosynthesis. However, if a stable construct can be achieved with any kind of fixation, it appears that the fracture will heal without limiting sequelae resulting in good function. As it seems, any kind of technique has its pros and cons and is dependent on the surgeon's experience with it.

Conventional ORIF

Wanner et al. [76] reported their results after the use of double-plates in mainly three- and four-part fractures. The mean Constant score was 61 points (75% of the contralateral side) at a mean follow-up of 17 months. The functional results were rated to be good or excellent in 63% of patients. The authors concluded that the use of double-plates achieved good stability that allowed early mobilisation.

Bastian and Hertel [41] reported their results with mainly three- and four-part fractures, they found a mean Constant score of 77 points and a mean SSV of 92% after a mean follow-up of

5 years. They concluded that conventional osteosynthesis is worth considering in displaced fractures when adequate and stable reduction can be achieved intraoperatively.

Angular Stable ORIF

Südkamp et al. [6] first reported on a relatively large collective retrospectively. All types of fractures were included. After a mean follow-up of 12 months, the mean Constant score was 70 points (85% of the contralateral side) and 34% of complications were found, of which most were due to incorrect surgery. They concluded that angular stable ORIF provides good functional results as long as used with correct surgical technique.

Sproul et al. [5] did a systematic review. They found a complication rate of 33%. The mean Constant score was 74 points and the reoperation rate 16%. They concluded that the complication and reoperation rate is high with the use of these implants.

Acklin and colleagues [109] conducted a prospective study on patients treated with the MIPO technique. The mean Constant score at the latest follow-up was 75 points and the complication rate 19%, of which 4% of axillary nerve lesions were observed without clinical consequences. They concluded that the MIPO technique resulted in a relatively low complication rate with good functional results.

Percutaneous Fixation Techniques

Resch et al. [82, 111] found good reduction and healing results for almost all treated fracture types in their initial study with Constant scores around 90% compared to the uninjured side.

Also Brunner et al. [116] found mainly good functional results after the use of "humerus block". The overall mean Constant score was 73 points, 88% compared to the uninjured side. However, the 40% rate of unplanned surgery with either change or removal of the implant was relatively high.

Outcome After Hemiarthroplasty

The results after hemiprosthesis are very inconsistent and it still seems difficult to achieve a predictable and reliable clinical outcome. The main reason for this is the unsolved problem of the tuberosities. If they heal in anatomical position, the clinical result is usually good, but if they don't, the outcome will usually be a pain free shoulder without function. As long as there is no better solution to improve the healing of the tuberosities, hemiarthroplasty will mainly remain a good treatment for pain with low revision rates.

Boileau and colleagues [70] retrospectively reviewed their patients after a mean of 27 months after hemiarthroplasty and found Constant scores of 56 points with 58% of satisfied or very satisfied subjective results and a mean forward flexion of 101°. Final malposition of the tuberosities correlated with unsatisfactory results.

Fucentese et al. [93] reported their series with the use of a large metaphyseal volume prosthesis and found a mean Constant score of 59 points after at least 2 years of follow-up. However, White et al. [90] were not able to reproduce these results with the same prosthesis and found only a mean Constant score of 34 points after at least 2 years. They reported resorption of the tuberosities in more than 50% of their patients.

Park et al. [94] published their retrospective series of a low volume metaphysis prosthesis with bone block autograft. After a mean follow-up of 54 months, they found mainly good clinical results with a mean forward flexion of 125° and only two patients where the tuberosities did not heal.

Outcome After Reverse Total Shoulder Arthroplasty

Throughout recent literature, it seems that very consistent clinical results may be achieved with the use of RTSA for proximal humerus fractures. The tuberosities should be fixed, at least the greater tuberosity, to restore some external rotation. The complication and revision rate is still low. However, the longest follow-ups are small case series with a mean of 5–8 years.

Cazeneuve et al. [100] have so far the longest follow-up period with a mean of 86 months. They resected the tuberosities in nearly 2/3 of the patients. In their analysis, they found a mean Constant score of 60 points, with better results in terms of internal and external rotation in patients with fixed tuberosities.

Russo et al. [101] reported their results with a mean of 5 years of experience. They paid special attention to attaching the tuberosities with the help of a bone graft retrieved from the head. They found mean Constant scores of 73 points.

Grubhofer et al. [10] published their results after a mean of 35 months. In their retrospective case series, they found a mean Constant score of 62 points (86% compared to the uninjured side) and a mean subjective shoulder value of 83% with significantly better function in patients with healed tuberosities.

Chun et al. [9] did a recent study on their outcome after RTSA for proximal humerus fractures. Their mean follow-up was 36 months and they analysed their patients with special focus on the healing of the tuberosities. The Constant score was not different between patients with and without healing of the tuberosities (68 and 64 points). However, in terms of external rotation, patients with healed tuberosities had significantly better results.

Authors' Opinion: Preliminary Results of the Treatment Algorithm

In 2014, we started to treat our patients with proximal humerus fractures according to an evidence-based treatment algorithm and followed them prospectively (Figs. 5.3 and 5.4). In the emergency department, patients are first evaluated in terms of their needs and dependency and the pre-injury quality of life is assessed with the EQ-5D score. Clinical and radiographic examinations take place at first presentation, after 3 months, after 1 and 2 years. With this study, it is our aim to assess the clinical feasibility of such an algorithm in a teaching hospital like ours (level-1 trauma centre in Switzerland) and to follow all the patients closely with special focus on their quality of life 1 and 2 years after the injury. This prospective non-randomised study is still on going but we are able to present preliminary 1-year results of the first 60 patients included.

The mean age of the patients was 69 years (SD: 17.4) with 75% females and 25% males included. A total of 84% of the patients have been treated according to the algorithm, whereas unclear fracture criteria and intraoperative decisions were the main reason for deviation from the algorithm. In total, 36 patients (60%) have been treated conservatively, 14 (23%) with locking plate ORIF and 10 (17%) with hemiarthroplasty (n = 2) or RTSA (n = 8). Whereas the collective is too small to perform subgroup analyses of each treatment option, we are able to draw a first conclusion on the overall results and it looks promising so far. On one hand, the spectrum of treatment seems to be well balanced with nearly equal distribution of ORIF and arthroplasty and conservative treatment as the mainstay. On the other hand, the mean objective and subjective functional results are satisfying for each group (Table 5.1). Especially good quality of life 1 year after trauma supports our theory of tailored indications for the treatment of proximal humerus fractures (Table 5.2).

Overall, 7 patients (12%) had further surgery. Five of them were from the ORIF group including one conversion to RTSA due to secondary fracture displacement; the plate was removed four times due to patient's wish, stiffness and/or impingement. One infection occurred in a patient treated

Table 5.1 Preliminary clinical 1-year results

Mean	CS (pts)	Percentage of uninjured side (%)	SSV (%)
Conservative (n = 36)	76	95	87
ORIF (n = 14)	62	76	73
Prosthesis (n = 10)	70	87	83

CS constant score, *SSV* subjective shoulder value

Table 5.2 Preliminary 1-year quality of life

Mean	EQ-5D (1 = max.)		
	Pre Fx	3mt	1y
Conservative (n = 36)	0.9	0.8	0.9
ORIF (n = 14)	0.87	0.75	0.85
Prosthesis (n = 10)	0.9	0.75	0.9

with hemiarthroplasty that needed revision and finally implantation of RTSA. Of the conservatively treated patients, only one secondary ORIF was needed due to further fracture displacement.

Complications

Complications After Nonoperative Treatment

In our experience with a specifically selected collective of patients for conservative treatment (Figs. 5.3 and 5.4), we found mainly satisfying objective and subjective results 1 year later (Fig. 5.2). Impingement or limited ROM may be a sequelae of the not anatomically healed fracture. However, most of the patients don't wish further treatment, as they are not significantly bothered by these symptoms. In the above-mentioned collective, only 1 patient with conservative treatment needed secondary surgery due to severe early displacement of the fracture.

Looking at the literature, conservatively treated one-part fractures may result in limited ROM, especially internal and external rotation [67]. Markedly limited shoulder function, mainly due to stiffness, occurred in up to 10% of the patients [66]. However, nonunion and avascular necrosis (AVN) are very rare and have not been described for such fractures [66, 67]. Conservatively treated two- and three-part fractures can result in impingement, nonunion, and also AVN has been described. But the rate of these complications depends on the primary stability of the fracture type [58, 74, 105].

Complications After Open and Minimally Invasive Osteosynthesis

Looking at our preliminary results of specifically chosen patients for locking plate ORIF (Figs. 5.3 and 5.4), we still see a relatively high complication rate with need for secondary surgery. About one-third of our patients required at least a second operation to remove the plate either due to patient's wish or some kind of impingement or stiffness. Furthermore, we performed one secondary RTSA for a patient with early failure after ORIF. However, as bone quality is a high selection criterion in our treatment algorithm, we have not seen any secondary head screw cut out so far, which used to be the most common complication of these implants. As a consequence of these results, we changed our implant to a less prominent one. Further analysis of our results will show whether the selection criteria for ORIF, especially in elderly patients with limited bone quality, should be even stricter to not put them at risk for a second operation.

Complications After Conventional ORIF

The most frequently reported complication after open reduction with conventional plate fixation is partial or total AVN with a large range from 0% to 50%, [42, 76, 78, 79] occurring less often in valgus impacted fractures [78]. Total head collapse was reported in about 15% of patients treated [42, 79]. Further complications which led to revisions were: impingement, loss of reduction, loosening of screws and failure of the implant. The revision rate is reported to be between 0% and 40%, whereas most revisions included removal of screws or the implant [42, 76, 78, 79]. The rate of conversion to arthroplasty was about 1–5% [76, 79].

Complications After Angular Stable ORIF

Generally, the complication rate after angular stable implants varies between 10% and 49% with revision rates up to 25% [2, 4–6, 109, 117]. The rigid fixation of multiple head screws in the plate led to new, implant-specific complications such as screw cut outs into the joint involving the glenoid as a further devastating complication [7]. Thus, it is crucial to check the screws first intraoperatively to preclude primary screw cut outs [6, 7, 117]. We published a series of intraoperative fluoroscopic projections including AP views in internal, neutral and 30° external rotation as well as an axial view with 30° abduction to detect primary screw cut outs [118].

In larger series or systematic reviews, the rate of partial or total avascular necrosis (AVN) is reported to be between 4% and 54%, depending on type of fracture (highest for fracture-dislocations and head-splits) [2, 3, 5, 6, 117, 119]. The rate of secondary varus displacement is reported to be up to 25% [4, 5]. The occurrence of secondary screw cut out, after AVN or secondary varus displacement, is consistently reported to be between 6% and 11% and thus the most common complication of these implants needing revision surgery [2, 5, 6, 109, 117]. A further complication, which is primarily related to the MIPO technique, is axillary nerve injury. This reported to be between 0% and 4% [109, 110].

Complications After Percutaneous Fixation Techniques

Low BMD and comminuted medial hinge are relative contraindications for this technique because of increased risk of reduction failure or pin migration [28].

If the pins are left outside the skin, pin track infection can require early removal of the pins and additional treatment with systemic antibiotics. The rate of this complication is reported to be 8% [120]. Pin migration however, is a frequent complication related to this technique. It was mainly found in patients with osteoporotic bone [28, 82, 83, 111]. To solve this problem, angular stability of the pins with either a "humerus block" [82] or a hybrid external fixation [83] has been invented. However, even with this more rigid fixation technique the pin cut out rate has been reported to be up to 22%. The 40% rate of unplanned surgery including early change or implant removal was also afound to be relatively high [116]. The rate of partial or total AVN has been reported to occur in 4–21% of patients treated [82, 83, 120].

Complications After Hemiarthroplasty

In our above-mentioned collective, we implanted only two hemiprostheses in younger patients with not reconstructable fractures. One of these patients contracted an infection and later required revision to RTSA. This number is too small to draw conclusions on complication and revision rates, but it shows that we hardly use this implant any longer. In younger patients with good bone quality, we encourage osteosynthesis and in the elderly, we prefer primary RTSA.

Generally, the main reason for limited function after hemiarthroplasty is malpositioning or secondary displacement of the greater tuberosity, which is reported to occur in up to 50% of the patients treated [70, 71, 90]. Increasing age, osteoporosis and female gender are risk factors for this type of complication [70, 71, 121]. Also proximal migration of the prosthesis with decrease of the acromio humeral distance is a relatively frequently observed complication with an incidence of up to 30%, correlated to impaired shoulder function [70, 72, 122]. Radiographic signs of heterotopic ossification are reported in up to 25% of the patients treated but its clinical relevance is debatable [70, 72]. The dislocation and infection rate of primary hemiarthroplasty is about 1% [70, 122, 123]. The general revision rate is low and the overall rate of prosthetic survival was found to be 97% at 1 year, 95% at 5 years and 94% at 10 years [99, 121].

Complications After Reversed Total Shoulder Arthroplasty

In our experience, primary RTSA leads to more predictable and satisfying results. So far, none of our patients with primary RTSA needed any kind of revision surgery. But we need to keep in mind, that, generally, the threshold to revise RTSA may be much higher than to revise hemiarthroplasty.

As no strong long-term data on RTSA for fracture treatment is available, we have to look up these results for RTSA in general. Bacle and Walch recently published their experience with a mean follow-up of 150 months. They report a general decrease in function between midterm and long-term follow-up. An explanation for this finding may be the general ageing of the patients as well as deterioration of deltoid function. In their series, the complication rate was 29% and revision rate 12%. In the first 2 years of follow-up, the main reasons for revision were dislocation and infection, whereas implant loosening was the main reason for revision in the long-term. However, the 10-year over-all survival of the prosthesis was 93%.

A recent review on RTSA after fracture treatment included 256 patients with a mean follow-up of around 2 years. The most common complication was found to be scapular notching (38%) which might be rather a radiographic problem than a real complication followed by malunion, nonunion or resorption of the tuberosities in 21%. The revision rate was 3% mainly due to instability or infection [124].

In terms of limited function, it seems that mal-, nonunion or resection of the tuberosities is at least associated with decreased external rotation [9, 10].

Conclusions

Despite the relatively high incidence of fractures of the proximal humerus and an abundance of literature there is still not enough good evidence to give clear treatment recommendations. There is moderately good evidence in elderly patients that surgical management does not necessarily result in better clinical function when compared to conservative treatment [62]. These studies, however, do not take into account the individual needs of patients. For younger patients, at least most one-part fractures may be treated conservatively with early mobilisation. However, there is still controversy as to how much displacement of the greater tuberosity may be accepted to achieve maximal shoulder function in these patients. What is also important to remember is that the results of rigid fixation in good quality bone may not necessarily apply for older patients with severe osteoporosis [28, 30] and as such any extrapolation should be viewed with caution.

Primary hemiarthroplasty has been shown to result in good pain relief with a relatively low rate of revision surgery. However, the consistently high failure rate of the tuberosities to heal makes the functional outcome unpredictable [90, 94]. As a consequence reverse total shoulder arthroplasty is now becoming the mainstay of arthroplasty management of difficult fractures particularly in elderly patients. With this implant the functional results appear more satisfying and predictable and again has a low revision rate [95, 99]. However, there is currently not yet enough long-term evidence for its widespread use in fracture treatment and as such it is still restricted to patients over 70 years of age. Going forward, however, it may well be that this cut-off age for primary RTSA may be lowered as further long-term data becomes available.

Finally with the help of our evidence-based treatment algorithm, we are trying to find the best solution for each patient using the currently available treatment methods. The highest priority is given to the patients needs, then to their biological condition (local bone quality) and finally to the fracture pattern. We believe this algorithm is a helpful tool for decision making, for which we have achieved good overall clinical results with high satisfaction and low revision rates. However, we do accept that there will be deviations from these guidelines and exceptions need to be made with even more tailored solutions. We will further continue to analyse, improve and adjust our algorithm to meet these patients needs.

References

1. Neer CS. Displaced proximal humeral fractures. II. Treatment of three-part and four-part displacement. J Bone Joint Surg Am. 1970;52:1090–103.
2. Spross C, Platz A, Rufibach K, et al. The PHILOS plate for proximal humeral fractures – risk factors for complications at one year. J Trauma Acute Care Surg. 2012;72:783–92. https://doi.org/10.1097/TA.0b013e31822c1b5b.
3. Spross C, Platz A, Erschbamer M, et al. Surgical treatment of Neer group VI proximal humeral fractures: retrospective comparison of PHILOS® and hemiarthroplasty. Clin Orthop Relat Res. 2012;470:2035–42. https://doi.org/10.1007/s11999-011-2207-1.
4. Owsley KC, Gorczyca JT. Fracture displacement and screw cutout after open reduction and locked plate fixation of proximal humeral fractures [corrected]. J Bone Joint Surg Am. 2008;90:233–40. https://doi.org/10.2106/JBJS.F.01351.
5. Sproul RC, Iyengar JJ, Devcic Z, Feeley BT. A systematic review of locking plate fixation of proximal

humerus fractures. Injury. 2011;42:408–13. https://doi.org/10.1016/j.injury.2010.11.058.
6. Südkamp NP, Bayer J, Hepp P, et al. Open reduction and internal fixation of proximal humeral fractures with use of the locking proximal humerus plate. Results of a prospective, multicenter, observational study. J Bone Joint Surg. 2009;91:1320–8. https://doi.org/10.2106/JBJS.H.00006.
7. Jost B, Spross C, Grehn H, Gerber C. Locking plate fixation of fractures of the proximal humerus: analysis of complications, revision strategies and outcome. J Shoulder Elb Surg. 2012:1–8. https://doi.org/10.1016/j.jse.2012.06.008.
8. Rangan A, Handoll HHG, Brealey S, et al. Surgical vs nonsurgical treatment of adults with displaced fractures of the proximal humerus. JAMA. 2015;313:1037. https://doi.org/10.1001/jama.2015.1629.
9. Chun Y-M, Kim D-S, Lee D-H, Shin S-J. Reverse shoulder arthroplasty for four-part proximal humerus fracture in elderly patients: can a healed tuberosity improve the functional outcomes? J Shoulder Elb Surg. 2017:1–6. https://doi.org/10.1016/j.jse.2016.11.034.
10. Grubhofer F, Wieser K, Meyer DC, et al. Reverse total shoulder arthroplasty for acute head-splitting, 3- and 4-part fractures of the proximal humerus in the elderly. J Shoulder Elb Surg. 2016;25:1690–8. https://doi.org/10.1016/j.jse.2016.02.024.
11. Spross C, Jost B. Chapter 48B proximal humeral fractures and fracture-dislocation. In: Browner BD, Jupiter JB, Krettek C, Anderson PA, editors. Skeletal trauma: basic science, management, and reconstruction. 5th ed. Philadelphia: Elsevier Science; 2014. p. 1423–53. released 09 Dec 2014.
12. Court-Brown CM, Caesar B. Epidemiology of adult fractures: a review. Injury. 2006;37:691–7. https://doi.org/10.1016/j.injury.2006.04.130.
13. Rose SH, Melton LJ, Morrey BF, et al. Epidemiologic features of humeral fractures. Clin Orthop Relat Res. 1982;168:24–30.
14. Bergdahl C, Ekholm C, Wennergren D, et al. Epidemiology and patho-anatomical pattern of 2,011 humeral fractures: data from the Swedish Fracture Register. BMC Musculoskelet Disord. 2016;17:1–10. https://doi.org/10.1186/s12891-016-1009-8.
15. Wilson J, Bonner TJ, Head M, et al. Variation in bone mineral density by anatomical site in patients with proximal humeral fractures. J Bone Joint Surg Br. 2009;91:772–5. https://doi.org/10.1302/0301-620X.91B6.22346.
16. Neer CS. Displaced proximal humeral fractures. I. Classification and evaluation. J Bone Joint Surg Am. 1970;52:1077–89.
17. McLaughling HL. Posterior dislocation of the shoulder. J Bone Joint Surg Am. 1952;24-A(3):584–90.
18. McLaughling H. Dislocation of the shoulder with tuberosity fracture. Surg Clin North Am. 1963;43:1615–20.
19. Robinson CM. Injuries associated with traumatic anterior glenohumeral dislocations. J Bone Joint Surg Am. 2012;94:18. https://doi.org/10.2106/JBJS.J.01795.
20. Pierce RO, Hodurski DF. Fractures of the humerus, radius, and ulna in the same extremity. J Trauma. 1979;19:182–5.
21. Visser CP, Tavy DL, Coene LN, Brand R. Electromyographic findings in shoulder dislocations and fractures of the proximal humerus: comparison with clinical neurological examination. Clin Neurol Neurosurg. 1999;101:86–91.
22. de Laat EA, Visser CP, Coene LN, et al. Nerve lesions in primary shoulder dislocations and humeral neck fractures. A prospective clinical and EMG study. J Bone Joint Surg Br. 1994;76:381–3.
23. Berkes MB, Dines JS, Birnbaum JF, et al. The axillary view typically does not contribute to decision making in care for proximal humeral fractures. HSS J. 2015;11:192–7. https://doi.org/10.1007/s11420-015-9445-9.
24. Siebenrock KA, Gerber C. The reproducibility of classification of fractures of the proximal end of the humerus. J Bone Joint Surg Am. 1993;75:1751–5.
25. Gracitelli MEC, Dotta TAG, Assunção JH, et al. Intraobserver and interobserver agreement in the classification and treatment of proximal humeral fractures. J Shoulder Elb Surg. 2017:1–6. https://doi.org/10.1016/j.jse.2016.11.047.
26. Brunner A, Honigmann P, Treumann T, Babst R. The impact of stereo-visualisation of three-dimensional CT datasets on the inter- and intraobserver reliability of the AO/OTA and Neer classifications in the assessment of fractures of the proximal humerus. J Bone Joint Surg Br. 2009;91:766–71. https://doi.org/10.1302/0301-620X.91B6.22109.
27. Krappinger D, Roth T, Gschwentner M, et al. Preoperative assessment of the cancellous bone mineral density of the proximal humerus using CT data. Skelet Radiol. 2012;41:299–304. https://doi.org/10.1007/s00256-011-1174-7.
28. Krappinger D, Bizzotto N, Riedmann S, et al. Predicting failure after surgical fixation of proximal humerus fractures. Injury. 2011;42:1283–8. https://doi.org/10.1016/j.injury.2011.01.017.
29. Jung S-W, Shim S-B, Kim H-M, et al. Factors that influence reduction loss in proximal humerus fracture surgery. J Orthop Trauma. 2015;29:276–82. https://doi.org/10.1097/BOT.0000000000000252.
30. Spross C, Zeledon R, Zdravkovic V, Jost B. How bone quality may influence intraoperative and early postoperative problems after angular stable open reduction–internal fixation of proximal humeral fractures. J Shoulder Elb Surg. 2017:1–7. https://doi.org/10.1016/j.jse.2017.02.026.
31. Giannotti S, Bottai V, Dell'osso G, et al. Indices of risk assessment of fracture of the proximal humerus. Clin Cases Miner Bone Metab. 2012;9:37–9.
32. Hepp P, Theopold J, Osterhoff G, et al. Bone quality measured by the radiogrammetric parameter "cortical index" and reoperations after locking plate osteosynthesis in patients sustaining

proximal humerus fractures. Arch Orthop Trauma Surg. 2009;129:1251–9. https://doi.org/10.1007/s00402-009-0889-6.
33. Tingart MJ, Apreleva M, Stechow v D, et al. The cortical thickness of the proximal humeral diaphysis predicts bone mineral density of the proximal humerus. J Bone Joint Surg Br. 2003;85:611–7.
34. Newton AW, Selvaratnam V, Pydah SK, Nixon MF. Simple radiographic assessment of bone quality is associated with loss of surgical fixation in patients with proximal humeral fractures. Injury. 2016;47:904–8. https://doi.org/10.1016/j.injury.2015.12.029.
35. Spross C, Kaestle N, Benninger E, et al. Deltoid tuberosity index: a simple radiographic tool to assess local bone quality in proximal humerus fractures. Clin Orthop Relat Res. 2015;473:3038–45. https://doi.org/10.1007/s11999-015-4322-x.
36. Codman EA. The shoulder. Kreiger Publishing; 1934. p. 313–31. ISBN 0898747317, 9780898747317.
37. Neer CS. Four-segment classification of proximal humeral fractures: purpose and reliable use. J Shoulder Elb Surg. 2002;11:389–400. https://doi.org/10.1067/mse.2002.124346.
38. Müller ME. The comprehensive classification of fractures of long bones. Berlin/Heidelberg/New York: Springer; 1990.
39. Hertel RW, Hempfing A, Stiehler M, Leunig M. Predictors of humeral head ischemia after intracapsular fracture of the proximal humerus. J Shoulder Elb Surg. 2004;13:427–33. https://doi.org/10.1016/S1058274604000795.
40. Sukthankar A, Leonello DT, Hertel RW, et al. A comprehensive classification of proximal humeral fractures: HGLS system. J Shoulder Elb Surg. 2013:1–6. https://doi.org/10.1016/j.jse.2012.09.018.
41. Bastian JD, Hertel RW. Initial post-fracture humeral head ischemia does not predict development of necrosis. J Shoulder Elb Surg. 2008;17:2–8. https://doi.org/10.1016/j.jse.2007.03.026.
42. Bastian JD, Hertel RW. Osteosynthesis and hemiarthroplasty of fractures of the proximal humerus: outcomes in a consecutive case series. J Shoulder Elb Surg. 2009;18:216–9. https://doi.org/10.1016/j.jse.2008.09.015.
43. Kristiansen B, Andersen UL, Olsen CA, Varmarken JE. The Neer classification of fractures of the proximal humerus. An assessment of interobserver variation. Skelet Radiol. 1988;17:420–2.
44. Brien H, Noftall F, MacMaster S, et al. Neer's classification system: a critical appraisal. J Trauma. 1995;38:257–60.
45. Sjödén GO, Movin T, Güntner P, et al. Poor reproducibility of classification of proximal humeral fractures. Additional CT of minor value. Acta Orthop Scand. 1997;68:239–42.
46. Sidor ML, Zuckerman JD, Lyon T, et al. The Neer classification system for proximal humeral fractures. An assessment of interobserver reliability and intraobserver reproducibility. J Bone Joint Surg Am. 1993;75:1745–50.
47. Olerud P, Ahrengart L, Ponzer S, et al. Hemiarthroplasty versus nonoperative treatment of displaced 4-part proximal humeral fractures in elderly patients: a randomized controlled trial. J Shoulder Elb Surg. 2011;20:1025–33. https://doi.org/10.1016/j.jse.2011.04.016.
48. Olerud P, Ahrengart L, Ponzer S, et al. Internal fixation versus nonoperative treatment of displaced 3-part proximal humeral fractures in elderly patients: a randomized controlled trial. J Shoulder Elb Surg. 2011;20:747–55. https://doi.org/10.1016/j.jse.2010.12.018.
49. Boons HW, Goosen JH, Grinsven S, et al. Hemiarthroplasty for humeral four-part fractures for patients 65 years and older: a randomized controlled trial. Clin Orthop Relat Res. 2012;470:3483–91. https://doi.org/10.1007/s11999-012-2531-0.
50. Fjalestad T, Hole MO, Hovden IAH, et al. Surgical treatment with an angular stable plate for complex displaced proximal humeral fractures in elderly patients: a randomized controlled trial. J Orthop Trauma. 2012;26:98–106. https://doi.org/10.1097/BOT.0b013e31821c2e15.
51. Court-Brown CM, Garg A, McQueen MM. The epidemiology of proximal humeral fractures. Acta Orthop Scand. 2001;72:365–71. https://doi.org/10.1080/000164701753542023.
52. Park TS, Choi IY, Kim YH, et al. A new suggestion for the treatment of minimally displaced fractures of the greater tuberosity of the proximal humerus. Bull Hosp Jt Dis. 1997;56:171–6.
53. Bono CM, Renard R, Levine RG, Levy AS. Effect of displacement of fractures of the greater tuberosity on the mechanics of the shoulder. J Bone Joint Surg Br. 2001;83:1056–62.
54. Platzer P, Thalhammer G, Oberleitner G, et al. Displaced fractures of the greater tuberosity: a comparison of operative and nonoperative treatment. J Trauma. 2008;65:843–8. https://doi.org/10.1097/01.ta.0000233710.42698.3f.
55. Gruson KI, Ruchelsman DE, Tejwani NC. Isolated tuberosity fractures of the proximal humeral: current concepts. Injury. 2008;39:284–98. https://doi.org/10.1016/j.injury.2007.09.022.
56. Parsons BO, Klepps SJ, Miller S, et al. Reliability and reproducibility of radiographs of greater tuberosity displacement. A cadaveric study. J Bone Joint Surg Am. 2005;87:58–65. https://doi.org/10.2106/JBJS.C.01576.
57. Jakob RP, Miniaci A, Anson PS, et al. Four-part valgus impacted fractures of the proximal humerus. J Bone Joint Surg Br. 1991;73:295–8.
58. Court-Brown CM, Cattermole H, McQueen MM. Impacted valgus fractures (B1.1) of the proximal humerus. The results of non-operative treatment. J Bone Joint Surg Br. 2002;84:504–8.
59. Robinson CM. Complex posterior fracture-dislocation of the shoulder – epidemiology, injury patterns, and results of operative treatment. J Bone Joint Surg Am. 2007;89:1454. https://doi.org/10.2106/JBJS.F.01214.

60. Hersche O, Gerber C. Iatrogenic displacement of fracture-dislocations of the shoulder. A report of seven cases. J Bone Joint Surg Br. 1994;76:30–3.
61. Handoll HHG, Ollivere BJ, Rollins KE. Interventions for treating proximal humeral fractures in adults. Cochrane Database Syst Rev. 2012;12:CD000434. https://doi.org/10.1002/14651858.CD000434.pub3.
62. Handoll HHG, Brorson S. Interventions for treating proximal humeral fractures in adults. Cochrane Database Syst Rev. 2015:CD000434. https://doi.org/10.1002/14651858.CD000434.pub4.
63. Krieg JC. Surgical and nonsurgical treatment produced similar outcomes for proximal humeral fractures. J Bone Joint Surg Am. 2015;97:1890. https://doi.org/10.2106/JBJS.9722.ebo102.
64. Steinhaus ME, Dare DM, Gulotta LV. HSS J. 2016:1–4. https://doi.org/10.1007/s11420-015-9479-z.
65. Clifford PC. Fractures of the neck of the humerus: a review of the late results. Injury. 1980;12:91–5.
66. Koval KJ, Gallagher MA, Marsicano JG, et al. Functional outcome after minimally displaced fractures of the proximal part of the humerus. J Bone Joint Surg Am. 1997;79:203–7.
67. Tejwani NC, Liporace F, Walsh M, et al. Functional outcome following one-part proximal humeral fractures: a prospective study. J Shoulder Elb Surg. 2008;17:216–9. https://doi.org/10.1016/j.jse.2007.07.016.
68. Agudelo J, Schürmann M, Stahel P, et al. Analysis of efficacy and failure in proximal humerus fractures treated with locking plates. J Orthop Trauma. 2007;21:676–81. https://doi.org/10.1097/BOT.0b013e31815bb09d.
69. Solberg BD, Moon CN, Franco DP, Paiement GD. Locked plating of 3- and 4-part proximal humerus fractures in older patients: the effect of initial fracture pattern on outcome. J Orthop Trauma. 2009;23:113–9. https://doi.org/10.1097/BOT.0b013e31819344bf.
70. Boileau P, Krishnan SG, Tinsi L, et al. Tuberosity malposition and migration: reasons for poor outcomes after hemiarthroplasty for displaced fractures of the proximal humerus. J Shoulder Elb Surg. 2002;11:401–12.
71. Kralinger FS, Schwaiger R, Wambacher M, et al. Outcome after primary hemiarthroplasty for fracture of the head of the humerus. A retrospective multicentre study of 167 patients. J Bone Joint Surg Br. 2004;86:217–9.
72. Mighell MA, Kolm GP, Collinge CA, Frankle MA. Outcomes of hemiarthroplasty for fractures of the proximal humerus. J Shoulder Elb Surg. 2003;12:569–77. https://doi.org/10.1016/S1058274603002131.
73. Court-Brown CM, Garg A, McQueen MM. The translated two-part fracture of the proximal humerus. Epidemiology and outcome in the older patient. J Bone Joint Surg Br. 2001;83:799–804.
74. Court-Brown CM, McQueen MM. The impacted varus (A2.2) proximal humeral fracture: prediction of outcome and results of nonoperative treatment in 99 patients. Acta Orthop Scand. 2004;75:736–40.
75. Lefevre-Colau MM. Immediate mobilization compared with conventional immobilization for the impacted nonoperatively treated proximal humeral fracture: a randomized controlled trial. J Bone Joint Surg Am. 2007;89:2582–90. https://doi.org/10.2106/JBJS.F.01419.
76. Wanner GA, Wanner-Schmid E, Romero J, et al. Internal fixation of displaced proximal humeral fractures with two one-third tubular plates. J Trauma. 2003;54:536–44. https://doi.org/10.1097/01.TA.0000052365.96538.42.
77. Hertel RW. Fractures of the proximal humerus in osteoporotic bone. Osteoporos Int. 2005;16(Suppl 2):S65–72. https://doi.org/10.1007/s00198-004-1714-2.
78. Robinson CM, Page RS. Severely impacted valgus proximal humeral fractures. Results of operative treatment. J Bone Joint Surg Am. 2003;85-A:1647–55.
79. Gerber C, Werner CML, Vienne P. Internal fixation of complex fractures of the proximal humerus. J Bone Joint Surg Br. 2004;86:848–55.
80. Hessmann MH, Hansen WSM, Krummenauer F, et al. Locked plate fixation and intramedullary nailing for proximal humerus fractures: a biomechanical evaluation. J Trauma. 2005;58:1194–201. https://doi.org/10.1097/01.TA.0000170400.68994.AB.
81. Osterhoff G, Hoch A, Wanner GA, et al. Calcar comminution as prognostic factor of clinical outcome after locking plate fixation of proximal humeral fractures. Injury. 2012;43:1651–6. https://doi.org/10.1016/j.injury.2012.04.015.
82. Resch H, Hübner C, Schwaiger R. Minimally invasive reduction and osteosynthesis of articular fractures of the humeral head. Injury. 2001;32(Suppl 1):SA25–32.
83. Blonna D, Castoldi F, Scelsi M, et al. The hybrid technique: potential reduction in complications related to pins mobilization in the treatment of proximal humeral fractures. J Shoulder Elb Surg. 2010;19:1218–29. https://doi.org/10.1016/j.jse.2010.01.025.
84. Gradl G, Dietze A, Kääb M, et al. Is locking nailing of humeral head fractures superior to locking plate fixation? Clin Orthop Relat Res. 2009;467:2986–93. https://doi.org/10.1007/s11999-009-0916-5.
85. Park J-Y, An J-W, Oh J-H. Open intramedullary nailing with tension band and locking sutures for proximal humeral fracture: hot air balloon technique. J Shoulder Elb Surg. 2006;15:594–601. https://doi.org/10.1016/j.jse.2006.01.001.
86. Konrad G, Audigé L, Lambert S, et al. Similar outcomes for nail versus plate fixation of three-part proximal humeral fractures. Clin Orthop Relat Res. 2011;470:602–9. https://doi.org/10.1007/s11999-011-2056-y.
87. Wong J, Newman JM, Gruson KI. Outcomes of intramedullary nailing for acute proximal humerus fractures: a systematic review. J Orthop Traumatol. 2015;17:113–22.https://doi.org/10.1007/s10195-015-0384-5.

88. Russo R, Visconti V, Lombardi LV, et al. Da Vinci System: clinical experience with complex proximal humerus fractures. Musculoskelet Surg. 2010;94(Suppl 1):S57–64. https://doi.org/10.1007/s12306-010-0066-7.
89. Russo R, Cautiero F, Ciccarelli M, Lombardi LV. Reconstruction of unstable, complex proximal humeral fractures with the da Vinci cage: surgical technique and outcome at 2 to 6 years. J Shoulder Elb Surg. 2013;22:422–31. https://doi.org/10.1016/j.jse.2012.04.010.
90. White JJE, Soothill JR, Morgan M, et al. Outcomes for a large metaphyseal volume hemiarthroplasty in complex fractures of the proximal humerus. J Shoulder Elb Surg. 2017;26:478–83. https://doi.org/10.1016/j.jse.2016.08.004.
91. Reuther F, Mühlhäusler B, Wahl D, Nijs S. Functional outcome of shoulder hemiarthroplasty for fractures: a multicentre analysis. Injury. 2010;41:606–12. https://doi.org/10.1016/j.injury.2009.11.019.
92. Greiner SH, Diederichs G, Kröning I, et al. Tuberosity position correlates with fatty infiltration of the rotator cuff after hemiarthroplasty for proximal humeral fractures. J Shoulder Elb Surg. 2009;18:431–6. https://doi.org/10.1016/j.jse.2008.10.007.
93. Fucentese SF, Sutter R, Wolfensperger F, et al. Large metaphyseal volume hemiprostheses for complex fractures of the proximal humerus. J Shoulder Elb Surg. 2014;23:427–33. https://doi.org/10.1016/j.jse.2013.06.010.
94. Park YK, Kim SH, Oh JH. Intermediate-term outcome of hemiarthroplasty for comminuted proximal humerus fractures. J Shoulder Elb Surg. 2017;26:85–91. https://doi.org/10.1016/j.jse.2016.05.008.
95. Wang J, Zhu Y, Zhang F, et al. Meta-analysis suggests that reverse shoulder arthroplasty in proximal humerus fractures is a better option than hemiarthroplasty in the elderly. Int Orthop. 2016;40:531–9. https://doi.org/10.1007/s00264-015-2811-x.
96. Ferrel JR, Trinh TQ, Fischer RA. Reverse total shoulder arthroplasty versus hemiarthroplasty for proximal humeral fractures: a systematic review. J Orthop Trauma. 2015;29:60–8. https://doi.org/10.1097/BOT.0000000000000224.
97. Sebastiá-Forcada E, Cebrián-Gómez R, Lizaur-Utrilla A, Gil-Guillén V. Reverse shoulder arthroplasty versus hemiarthroplasty for acute proximal humeral fractures. A blinded, randomized, controlled, prospective study. J Shoulder Elb Surg. 2014;23:1419–26. https://doi.org/10.1016/j.jse.2014.06.035.
98. Cuff DJ, Pupello DR. Comparison of hemiarthroplasty and reverse shoulder arthroplasty for the treatment of proximal humeral fractures in elderly patients. J Bone Joint Surg. 2013;95:2050–5. https://doi.org/10.2106/JBJS.L.01637.
99. Boyle MJ, Youn S-M, Frampton CMA, Ball CM. Functional outcomes of reverse shoulder arthroplasty compared with hemiarthroplasty for acute proximal humeral fractures. J Shoulder Elb Surg. 2012;22:32–7. https://doi.org/10.1016/j.jse.2012.03.006.
100. Cazeneuve JF, Cristofari D-J. Grammont reversed prosthesis for acute complex fracture of the proximal humerus in an elderly population with 5 to 12 years follow-up. Orthop Traumatol Surg Res. 2014;100:93–7. https://doi.org/10.1016/j.otsr.2013.12.005.
101. Russo R, Rotonda Della G, Cautiero F, Ciccarelli M. Reverse shoulder prosthesis to treat complex proximal humeral fractures in the elderly patients: results after 10-year experience. Musculoskelet Surg. 2015;99:1–7. https://doi.org/10.1007/s12306-015-0367-y.
102. Bacle G, Nové-Josserand L, Garaud P, Walch G. Long-term outcomes of reverse total shoulder arthroplasty. J Bone Joint Surg Am. 2017;99:454–61. https://doi.org/10.2106/JBJS.16.00223.
103. Jobin CM, Galdi B, Anakwenze OA, et al. Reverse shoulder arthroplasty for the management of proximal humerus fractures. J Am Acad Orthop Surg. 2015;23:190–201. https://doi.org/10.5435/JAAOS-D-13-00190.
104. Li F, Zhu Y, Lu Y, et al. Hemiarthroplasty for the treatment of complex proximal humeral fractures: does a trabecular metal prosthesis make a difference? A prospective, comparative study with a minimum 3-year follow-up. J Shoulder Elb Surg. 2014;23:1437–43. https://doi.org/10.1016/j.jse.2014.04.017.
105. Hanson B, Neidenbach P, de Boer P, Stengel D. Functional outcomes after nonoperative management of fractures of the proximal humerus. J Shoulder Elb Surg. 2009;18:612–21. https://doi.org/10.1016/j.jse.2009.03.024.
106. Spross C, Grueninger P, Gohil S, Dietrich M. Open reduction and internal fixation of fractures of the proximal part of the humerus. J Bone Joint Surg Am Surg Tech. 2015;5:e15. https://doi.org/10.2106/JBJS.ST.N.00106.
107. Resch H, Beck E, Bayley I. Reconstruction of the valgus-impacted humeral head fracture. J Shoulder Elb Surg. 1995;4:73–80.
108. Acklin YP, Sommer C. Plate fixation of proximal humerus fractures using the minimally invasive anterolateral delta split approach. Orthop Traumatol. 2012;24:61–73. https://doi.org/10.1007/s00064-011-0051-9.
109. Acklin YP, Stoffel K, Sommer C. A prospective analysis of the functional and radiological outcomes of minimally invasive plating in proximal humerus fractures. Injury. 2013;44:456–60. https://doi.org/10.1016/j.injury.2012.09.010.
110. Röderer G, Erhardt JB, Graf M, et al. Clinical results for minimally invasive locked plating of proximal humerus fractures. J Orthop Trauma. 2010;24:400–6. https://doi.org/10.1097/BOT.0b013e3181ccafb3.
111. Resch H, Povacz P, Fröhlich R, Wambacher M. Percutaneous fixation of three- and four-part fractures of the proximal humerus. J Bone Joint Surg Br. 1997;79:295–300.

112. Soliman OA, Koptan WMT. Proximal humeral fractures treated with hemiarthroplasty: does tenodesis of the long head of the biceps improve results? Injury. 2013;44:461–4. https://doi.org/10.1016/j.injury.2012.09.012.
113. Anakwenze OA, Zoller S, Ahmad CS, Levine WN. Reverse shoulder arthroplasty for acute proximal humerus fractures: a systematic review. J Shoulder Elb Surg. 2014;23:e73–80. https://doi.org/10.1016/j.jse.2013.09.012.
114. Spross C, Ebneter L, Benninger E, et al. Short- or long-stem prosthesis for intramedullary bypass of proximal humeral fractures with severe metaphyseal bone loss: evaluation of primary stability in a biomechanical model. J Shoulder Elb Surg. 2013:1–7. https://doi.org/10.1016/j.jse.2013.02.012.
115. Schulte LM, Matteini LE, Neviaser RJ. Proximal periarticular locking plates in proximal humeral fractures: functional outcomes. J Shoulder Elb Surg. 2011;20:1234–40. https://doi.org/10.1016/j.jse.2010.12.015.
116. Brunner A, Weller K, Thormann S, et al. Closed reduction and minimally invasive percutaneous fixation of proximal humerus fractures using the Humerusblock. J Orthop Trauma. 2010;24:407–13. https://doi.org/10.1097/BOT.0b013e3181c81b1c.
117. Brunner F, Sommer C, Bahrs C, et al. Open reduction and internal fixation of proximal humerus fractures using a proximal humeral locked plate: a prospective multicenter analysis. J Orthop Trauma. 2009;23:163–72. https://doi.org/10.1097/BOT.0b013e3181920e5b.
118. Spross C, Jost B, Rahm S, Winklhofer S, Erhardt JB, Benninger E. How many radiographs are needed to detect angular stable head screw cut outs of the proximal humerus – A cadaver study. Injury. 2014;45(10):1557–63. https://doi.org/10.1016/j.injury.2014.05.025.
119. Thanasas C, Kontakis G, Angoules A, et al. Treatment of proximal humerus fractures with locking plates: a systematic review. J Shoulder Elb Surg. 2009;18:837–44. https://doi.org/10.1016/j.jse.2009.06.004.
120. Jaberg H, Warner JJ, Jakob RP. Percutaneous stabilization of unstable fractures of the humerus. J Bone Joint Surg Am. 1992;74:508–15.
121. Robinson CM, Page RS, Hill RMF, et al. Primary hemiarthroplasty for treatment of proximal humeral fractures. J Bone Joint Surg Am. 2003;85-A:1215–23.
122. Grönhagen CM, Abbaszadegan H, Révay SA, Adolphson PY. Medium-term results after primary hemiarthroplasty for comminute proximal humerus fractures: a study of 46 patients followed up for an average of 4.4 years. J Shoulder Elb Surg. 2007;16:766–73. https://doi.org/10.1016/j.jse.2007.03.017.
123. Kontakis G, Koutras C, Tosounidis T, Giannoudis P. Early management of proximal humeral fractures with hemiarthroplasty: a systematic review. J Bone Joint Surg Br. 2008;90:1407–13. https://doi.org/10.1302/0301-620X.90B11.21070.
124. Longo UG, Petrillo S, Berton A, Denaro V. Reverse total shoulder arthroplasty for the management of fractures of the proximal humerus: a systematic review. Musculoskelet Surg. 2016;100:83–91. https://doi.org/10.1007/s12306-016-0409-0.

Outcome Measures Following Upper Limb Trauma

6

Ramsay Refaie and Amar Rangan

Not everything that can be counted counts and not everything that counts can be counted

– Albert Einstein

Introduction

The impact of trauma to the upper limb is significant with the presence of pain or associated symptoms affecting quality of life; and functional impairment following such an injury often having a direct impact on activities of daily living including tasks such as basic dressing, eating and personal hygiene. Structured assessment of outcomes following shoulder trauma becomes important when evaluating the effectiveness of individual treatments or philosophies of care; the impact of such trauma on quality of life of affected individuals; and in informing service organisation and healthcare policy. The impact of such injuries can typically be evaluated using an outcome measurement tool specific to the injured part of the body and a more general quality of life outcome score.

Outcome measurement has become a key component of orthopaedic research and audit alike. Several general, region specific and pathology specific outcome scores have evolved over the past 30 or so years. Early outcome scoring systems tended to be clinician or caregiver reported with a focus on the objective measurement of clinical parameters e.g., radiographic union, range of motion and strength. Whilst some of these outcomes, particularly fracture healing is still considered important, increasingly a greater importance is now placed on patient reported outcome measurement systems (PROMS) as a way of reporting the impact of particular injuries and their treatments in clinical research. PROMS tend to focus not only on biomedical parameters but also incorporate an assessment of psychosocial factors [1].

There is an increasing body of evidence showing that disability following orthopaedic trauma better correlates with measures of the subjective experience of illness rather than objective measureable criteria [2, 3]. As such it has become established best practice in orthopaedic research to assess both a region specific PROM as well as a more general quality of life measure [4] e.g. Euro-Qol-5D questionnaire (EQ-5D) or short form 36 (SF-36).

R. Refaie (✉)
Department of Trauma & Orthopaedic Surgery, James Cook University Hospital, Middlesbrough, UK

A. Rangan
Department of Trauma & Orthopaedic Surgery, James Cook University Hospital, Middlesbrough, UK

University of Oxford, Oxford, UK

University of York, York, UK

I. A. Trail et al. (eds.), *Textbook of Shoulder Surgery*, https://doi.org/10.1007/978-3-319-70099-1_6

Recent work comparing the impact of upper extremity injuries with all other injuries has demonstrated that in fact upper extremity trauma has a greater impact on quality of life and that this effect becomes more pronounced with more proximal injuries [5] thus highlighting the particular value of evaluating more general quality of life parameters particularly in upper limb research. Furthermore research focusing specifically on proximal humeral fractures has shown that in fact strength and range of movement correlate poorly with patient reported measures of impairment [6] providing further evidence of the need for more patient reported outcome measures.

The process of developing and validating an outcome score is complex and lengthy [7], when selecting an outcome score for a particular study investigators should utilise available guidance like the COSMIN checklist [8]. The COSMIN checklist was developed as a framework to ensure the most appropriate scoring systems are used by assessing their reliability, validity, responsiveness and interpretability. It can however be difficult to establish how PROMS have been derived [1] which can lead to their inappropriate use.

Whilst the use of PROMS can provide useful reliable information about the impact of a particular injury and / or its treatment these are not a panacea and investigators should be mindful of the potential impact of response burden on study participants leading to so called 'response fatigue'. It has been suggested that excessively burdening study participants with questionnaires can negatively impact the quality of their responses [9, 10]. This has led to many commonly used PROMS and general quality of life measures adopting abbreviated formats such as the quick DASH and short form 12 (SF12).

Current Trends in Outcome Measurement

As healthcare has moved to becoming more patient centred in its ethos we have seen a move away from outcome measures based on caregivers' priorities towards measuring outcomes based on function and wellbeing i.e., more patient centred and led criteria.

Patient Reported Outcome (PRO) has been defined as any report of the status of a patient's health condition that comes directly from the patient, without interpretation of the patient's response by a clinician or anyone else [11]. PRO measures take account of the fact that patients focus on different areas following intervention, that their views may differ from those of an observer scoring their outcome for them and they give a better overall assessment of the patient's experience of disease. PRO also overcomes the inherent inaccuracy or bias in assessment within and between observers when more clinimetric outcomes are used. An important advantage of PROMS is that they can be collected remotely without the patient having to return to clinic for assessment. Postal, telephonic, electronic or online collection of PROMS has made this the outcome assessment of choice for longer term follow up, and also in other areas such as joint arthroplasty registries.

PROMS can best capture the nature of symptoms; nature and severity of any disability; impact of the injury on the daily life of the patient; patient's perception of the effects of the injury and the treatment provided. Selecting which PROM to use can itself be a challenge and in an attempt to address this the COMET (Core Outcome Measures in Effectiveness Trials) [12, 13] intiative aims to define core outcome sets representing agreed minimum standards for use in reporting clinical trials for particular areas of interest. Another tool The Patient Reported Outcome and Quality of Life Instruments Database (PROQOLID) [14] is another useful source of information particularly with regards to selecting appropriate and relevant outcome measures.

Despite this many PROMS are used beyond the conditions that were used in their development. This is in part because the process of developing and validating PROMS is arduous.

The importance of using the right PROMS cannot be overstated. Criteria from the COSMIN framework and other important considerations as set out by Fitzpatrick et al. [15] are summarised in Table 6.1.

Table 6.1 Criteria for selecting an appropriate outcome measure

Criteria	Assessment
Appropriateness	Is the content of the instrument appropriate to the questions of the clinical trial?
Reliability	Does the instrument produce results that are reliable and internally consistent? Are the results from an instrument reproducible?
Validity	Does the instrument measure what it claims to measure? Consider face, content and construct validity. Has the instrument been validated for particular purposes?
Responsiveness	Does the instrument measure changes over time that matter to patients? How sensitive and specific to change is the score?
Precision	How precise are the scores of the instrument? Can small changes be detected?
Interpretability	How interpretable are the scores of an instrument? Has the Minimal clinically important difference (MCID) been defined?
Acceptability	Is the instrument acceptable to patients? Take into account for example time to complete and any cultural issues

In addition to PROMS there is also emerging evidence of at least an association between patient reported experience and patient reported outcome and it may be that measuring patient experience as well as outcome becomes the norm. Tools such as the Picker Patient Experience Questionnaire [16] have been used for this purpose.

Whilst PROMS measurement is widely used for research purposes it is also important to consider the wider societal impact of treatments. Quality Adjusted Life Years (QALY) [17] is a combined measure of the benefits afforded by a treatment in terms of both duration and magnitude of improvement. QALYs are not however considered in isolation and healthcare providers will look at these in relation to costs and typically evaluate treatments in terms of their cost per QALY gain. Therefore, whilst a treatment may provide a large improvement in QALYs it may be prohibitively expensive and therefore deemed a treatment that is not good 'value for money' in a health economic analysis. Commissioning decisions and national guidance (for example NICE guidance in England) tends to be based on both health economic analysis and clinical outcome, as opposed to the latter in isolation. Commonly used outcome measures in shoulder trauma are summarised in Table 6.2 and examples of frequently

Table 6.2 Commonly used outcome scores in shoulder trauma research

Scoring systems – shoulder		
Score	**Parameters**	**Scoring**
OSS [18] (Oxford Shoulder Score)	PRO 12 items assessing both pain and function	Range 12 (Best) – 60 (worst)
DASH [19] (Disability of Arm, Shoulder & Hand)	PRO 30 item disability/symptom scale	Range 30 (Best) – 150 (worst)
Quick DASH [20]	PRO Abbreviated version of original DASH, containing 11 items assessing disability and symptoms	Range 11 (Best) – 55 (worst)
Constant [21]	Combination of PRO and objective parameters. Pain and ADLs are patient reported and range of motion and strength are objective measures	Total 100 points Pain (15 points) ADLs (20 points) Strength (25 points) ROM (40 points)
SST [22] (Simple Shoulder Test)	PRO 12 item Yes/No	N/A

(continued)

Table 6.2 (continued)

ASES [23] (American Shoulder & Elbow Surgeons Score)	PRO 11 items pain (VAS) function/disability (10 items)	Range 10 (worst) – 100 (Best)
Scoring systems – ACJ and clavicle		
Score	**Parameters**	
Nottingham clavicle Score [24]	PRO. 10 item score assessing both pain and function	Range 20 (worst) – 100 (Best
Imatani score [25]	PRO 3 domains, pain, function and range of movement	Range 0 (worst) – 100 (Best)
General quality of life scores		
Score	**Parameters**	
SF-36 [26] (Short Form-36)	36 item score across 3 domains of health (functional status, well-being and health perception)	Transformed to range of 0 (Worst) – 100 (Best)
SF-12 [27] (Short Form – 12)	Shorter version of SF36, using only 12 of the original 36 items	SF-36 condensed to Physical component & Mental component scores (PCS 12 & MCS 12)
EQ5D (3 L) [28] (EuroQOL 5 Dimensions – 3 Levels)	Generic measure of health across 5 domains (Mobility, Self-Care, Usual Activities, Pain/ Discomfort, and Anxiety/ Depression) All domains scored on 3 point scale	3 Levels of scores for each domain Scores for individual domains is the norm, may be converted to a single index value
EQ5D (5 L) [29]	Similar to EQ5D (3 L) but 5 point scale	5 Levels of scores for each domain Scores for individual domains is the norm, may be converted to a single index value

used scoring systems are provided in the Appendix at the end of this chapter.

Summary

The choice of type of outcome measurement used depends on the purpose of the evaluation. The current trend is to move towards PROMS, with a combination of region or disease specific score and a general health score used for assessing clinical effectiveness of interventions. Health economic evaluation of treatments or philosophies of care is becoming increasingly important in order to inform healthcare policy. Patient experience measures tend to help engineer quality and service improvement for healthcare providers. When evaluating outcomes from shoulder trauma, as with outcome assessment in other areas, attention should be paid to the criteria within the COSMIN checklist to choose a validated assessment tool that would be most appropriate for specific injuries and their treatment.

Appendix

Examples of frequently used scores for outcome evaluation following shoulder trauma

OXFORD SHOULDER SCORE

Tick(✓) one box for every question.

1. During the past 4 weeks...

How would you describe the **worst** pain you had from your shoulder ?

None	Mild	Moderate	Severe	Unbearable
☐	☐	☐	☐	☐

2. During the past 4 weeks...

Have you had any trouble dressing yourself because of your shoulder?

No trouble at all	A little bit of trouble	Moderate trouble	Extreme difficulty	Impossible to do
☐	☐	☐	☐	☐

3. During the past 4 weeks...

Have you had any trouble getting in and out of a car or using public transport because of your shoulder?

No trouble at all	A little bit of trouble	Moderate trouble	Extreme difficulty	Impossible to do
☐	☐	☐	☐	☐

4. During the past 4 weeks...

Have you been able to use a knife and fork - at the same time?

Yes, easily	With little difficulty	With moderate difficulty	With extreme difficulty	No, impossible
☐	☐	☐	☐	☐

5. During the past 4 weeks...

Could you do the household shopping on your own?

Yes, easily	With little difficulty	With moderate difficulty	With extreme difficulty	No, impossible
☐	☐	☐	☐	☐

6. During the past 4 weeks...

Could you carry a tray containing a plate of food a cross a room?

Yes, easily	With little difficulty	With moderate difficulty	With extreme difficulty	No, impossible
☐	☐	☐	☐	☐

7. During the past 4 weeks...

Could you brush/comb your hair with the affected arm?

Yes, easily	With little difficulty	With moderate difficulty	With extreme difficulty	No, impossible
☐	☐	☐	☐	☐

8. During the past 4 weeks...

How would you describe the pain you usually had from your shoulder?

None	Very mild	Mild	Moderate	Severe
☐	☐	☐	☐	☐

9. During the past 4 weeks...

Could you hang your clothes up in a wardrobe, using the affected arm?

Yes, easily	With little difficulty	With moderate difficulty	With great difficulty	No, impossible
☐	☐	☐	☐	☐

10. During the past 4 weeks...

Have you been able to wash and dry yourself under both arms?

Yes, easily	With little difficulty	With moderate difficulty	With extreme difficulty	No, impossible
☐	☐	☐	☐	☐

11. During the past 4 weeks...

How much has pain from your shoulder interfered with your usual work (including housework)?

Not at all	A little bit	Moderately	Greatly	Totally
☐	☐	☐	☐	☐

12. During the past 4 weeks...

Have you been troubled by pain from your shoulder in bed at night?

No nights	Only 1 or 2 nights	Some nights	Most nights	Every night
☐	☐	☐	☐	☐

Finally, please check back that you have answered each question.
Thank you very much.

Constant Shoulder Score

Clinician's Name: ______________________ Patient's Name: ______________________

Answer all questions, selecting just one unless otherwise stated

During the past 4 weeks......

1. Pain

- ☐ Severe
- ☐ Moderate
- ☐ Mild
- ☐ None

2. Activity Level (check all that apply)

- ☐ Unaffected Sleep
- ☐ Full Recreation/Sport
- ☐ Full Work

3. Arm Positioning

- ☐ Up to Waist
- ☐ Up to Xiphoid
- ☐ Up to Neck
- ☐ Up to Top of Head
- ☐ Above Head

4. Strength of Abduction [Pounds]

- ☐ 0
- ☐ 1-3
- ☐ 4-6
- ☐ 7-9
- ☐ 10-12
- ☐ 13-15
- ☐ 15-18
- ☐ 19-21
- ☐ 22-24
- ☐ >24

RANGE OF MOTION

5. Forward Flexion

- ☐ 31-60 degrees
- ☐ 61-90 degrees
- ☐ 91-120 degrees
- ☐ 121-150 degrees
- ☐ 151-180 degrees

6. Lateral Elevation

- ☐ 31-60 degrees
- ☐ 61-90 degrees
- ☐ 91-120 degrees
- ☐ 121-150 degrees
- ☐ 151-180 degrees

7. External Rotation

- ☐ Hand behind Head, Elbow forward
- ☐ Hand behind Head, Elbow back
- ☐ Hand to top of Head, Elbow forward
- ☐ Hand to top of Head, Elbow back -
- ☐ Full Elevation

8. Internal Rotation

- ☐ Lateral Thigh
- ☐ Buttock
- ☐ Lumbosacral Junction
- ☐ Waist (L3)
- ☐ T12 Vertebra
- ☐ Interscapular (T7)

The Constant Shoulder Score is: 0 ______________________

Grading the Constant Shoulder Score

>30 Poor	21-30 Fair	11-20 Good	<11 Excellent

1. Name of instrument	***American Shoulder and Elbow Surgeons (ASES) Assessment Form***
2. What it is designed to assess (specific anatomic area)	***Shoulder and elbow***
3. Method of administration (patient, clinician, or combined)	***Combined***
4. How to obtain the instrument	***ASES office*** ***6300 N. River Road, Suite 727*** ***Rosemont, IL 60018***
5. Cost involved in obtaining instrument	***None***
6. Method of design	***Physician-designed***
7. Statistical validation	Michener LA, McClure PW, Sennett BJ. American Shoulder and Elbow Surgeons Standardized Shoulder Assessment Form, patient self-report section: reliability, validity, and responsiveness. *J Shoulder Elbow Surg.* 2002;11:587–594.
8. Normative data available	***None***
9. Disease-specific data available	***None***
10. References for scientific basis and reference data	Richards RR, An K-N, Bigliani LU, et al. A standardized method for the assessment of shoulder function. *J Shoulder Elbow Surg. 1994;3:347–352.* Kirkley A, Griffin S, Dainty K. ISAKOS Scientific Committee Report: scoring systems for the functional assessment of the shoulder. *Arthroscopy.* 2003;19:1109–1120. Placzek JD, Lukens SC, Badalanmenti S, et al. Shoulder outcome measures: a comparison of 6 functional tests. *Am J Sports Med.* 2004;32:1270–1277. King GJW, Richards RR, Zuckerman JD, et al. A standardized method for assessment of elbow function. *J Shoulder Elbow Surg.*1999;8:351–354.
11. Scoring module	*Yes*
12. What kind of total and subscales do you get	***Shoulder Score Index Pain, Instability, ADL, ROM, Signs, Strength***
13. Format and number of questions	***Combination of VAS,Yes/No, scaled questions***
14. Time for administration	***Patient subjective = 3 minutes*** ***Physician objective: not documented***
15. Additional notes	***0 to100 (best)***
16. The questionnaire	***See page S115***

PATIENT SELF-EVALUATION		
Are you having pain in shoulder? (circle correct answer)	Yes	No
Mark where your pain is on this diagram: 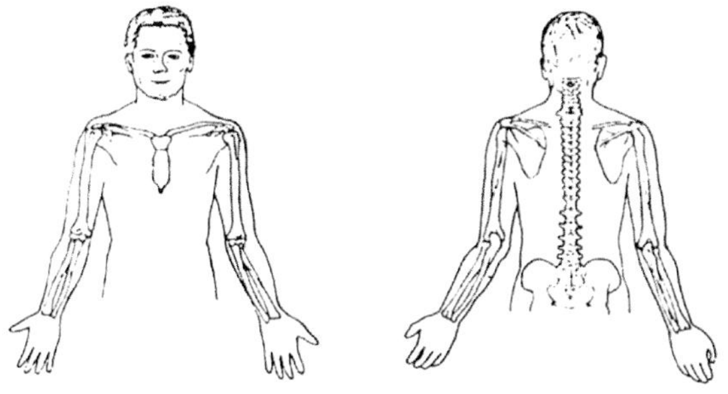		
Do you have pain in your shoulder at night?	Yes	No
Do you take pain medication (aspirin, Advil, Tylenol etc.)?	Yes	No
Do you take narcotic pain medication (codeine or stronger)?	Yes	No
How many pills do you take each day (average)?	pills	
How bad is your pain today (mark line)? 0 ____ 10 No pain at all — Pain as bad as it can be		
Does your shoulder feel unstable (as if it is going to dislocate?)	Yes	No
How unstable is your shoulder (mark line)? 0 ____ 10 Very stable — Very unstable		
Circle the number in the box that indicates your ability to do the following activities: 0 = **Unable** to do; 1 = **Very** difficult to do; 2 = **Somewhat** difficult; 3 = **Not** difficult		

ACTIVITY	RIGHT ARM	LEFT ARM
1. Put on a coat	0 1 2 3	0 1 2 3
2. Sleep on your painful or affected side	0 1 2 3	0 1 2 3
3. Wash back/do up bra in back	0 1 2 3	0 1 2 3
4. Manage toiletting	0 1 2 3	0 1 2 3
5. Comb hair	0 1 2 3	0 1 2 3
6. Reach a high shelf	0 1 2 3	0 1 2 3
7. Lift 10 lbs. above shoulder	0 1 2 3	0 1 2 3
8. Throw a ball overhand	0 1 2 3	0 1 2 3
9. Do usual work - List:	0 1 2 3	0 1 2 3
10. Do usual sport - List:	0 1 2 3	0 1 2 3

STRENGTH
(record MRC grade)

0 = no contraction; 1 = flicker; 2 = movement with gravity eliminated
3 = movement against gravity; 4 = movement against some resistance; 5 = normal power.

	Right	Left
Testing affected by pain?	Y N	Y N
Forward elevation	0 1 2 3 4 5	0 1 2 3 4 5
Abduction	0 1 2 3 4 5	0 1 2 3 4 5
External rotation (Arm comfortably at side)	0 1 2 3 4 5	0 1 2 3 4 5
Internal rotation (Arm comfortably at side)	0 1 2 3 4 5	0 1 2 3 4 5

INSTABILITY

0 = none; 1 = mild (0-1 cm translation)
2 = moderate (1-2 cm translation or translated to glenoid rim)
3 = severe (> 2 cm translation or over rim of glenoid)

Anterior translation	0 1 2 3	0 1 2 3
Posterior translation	0 1 2 3	0 1 2 3
Inferior translation (sulcus sign)	0 1 2 3	0 1 2 3
Anterior apprehension	0 1 2 3	0 1 2 3
Reproduces symptoms?	Y N	Y N
Voluntary instability?	Y N	Y N
Relocation test positive?	Y N	Y N
Generalized ligamentous laxity?	Y N	

Other physical findings:

Examiner's name:

____________________ ____________Date

SHOULDER ASSESSMENT FORM
AMERICAN SHOULDER AND ELBOW SURGEONS

Name:		Date
Age:	Hand dominance: R L Ambi	Sex: M F
Diagnosis:		Initial Assess? Y N
Procedure/Date:		Follow-up: M; Y

PHYSICIAN ASSESSMENT

RANGE OF MOTION Total shoulder motion Goniometer preferred	RIGHT		LEFT	
	Active	Passive	Active	Passive
Forward elevation (Maximum arm-trunk angle)				
External elevation (Arm comfortably at side)				
External rotation (Arm at 90° abduction)				
Internal rotation (Highest posterior anatomy reached with thumb)				
Cross-body adduction (Antecubital fossa to opposite acromion)				

SIGNS

0 = none; 1 = mild; 2 = moderate; 3 = severe

SIGN		Right	Left
Supraspinatus/greater tuberosity tenderness		0 1 2 3	0 1 2 3
AC joint tenderness		0 1 2 3	0 1 2 3
Biceps tendon tenderness (or rupture)		0 1 2 3	0 1 2 3
Other tenderness - List:		0 1 2 3	0 1 2 3
Impingement I (Passive forward elevation in slight internal rotation)		Y N	Y N
Impingement II (Passive internal rotation with 90° flexion)		Y N	Y N
Impingement III (90° active abduction - classic painful arc)		Y N	Y N
Subacromial crepitus		Y N	Y N
Scars - location		Y N	Y N
Atrophy - location:		Y N	Y N
Deformity : describe		Y N	Y N

THE *Quick*DASH OUTCOME MEASURE

INSTRUCTIONS

This questionnaire asks about your symptoms as well as your ability to perform certain activities.

Please answer *every question*, based on your condition in the last week, by circling the appropriate number.

If you did not have the opportunity to perform an activity in the past week, please make your *best estimate* of which response would be the most accurate.

It doesn't matter which hand or arm you use to perform the activity; please answer based on your ability regardless of how you perform the task.

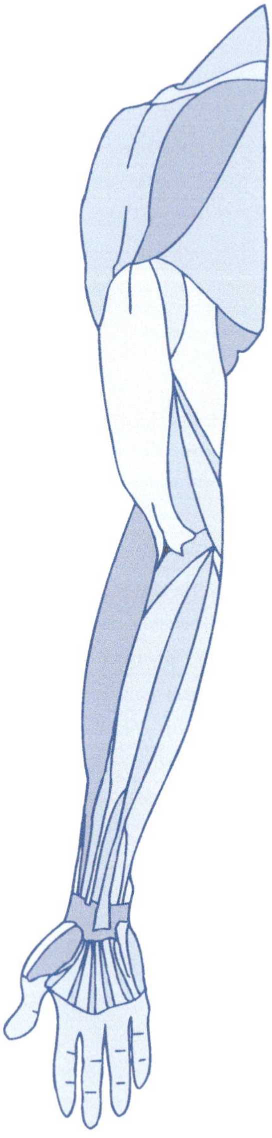

*Quick*DASH

Please rate your ability to do the following activities in the last week by circling the number below the appropriate response.

	NO DIFFICULTY	MILD DIFFICULTY	MODERATE DIFFICULTY	SEVERE DIFFICULTY	UNABLE
1. Open a tight or new jar.	1	2	3	4	5
2. Do heavy household chores (e.g., wash walls, floors).	1	2	3	4	5
3. Carry a shopping bag or briefcase.	1	2	3	4	5
4. Wash your back.	1	2	3	4	5
5. Use a knife to cut food.	1	2	3	4	5
6. Recreational activities in which you take some force or impact through your arm, shoulder or hand (e.g., golf, hammering, tennis, etc.).	1	2	3	4	5

	NOT AT ALL	SLIGHTLY	MODERATELY	QUITE A BIT	EXTREMELY
7. During the past week, *to what extent* has your arm, shoulder or hand problem interfered with your normal social activities with family, friends, neighbours or groups?	1	2	3	4	5

	NOT LIMITED AT ALL	SLIGHTLY LIMITED	MODERATELY LIMITED	VERY LIMITED	UNABLE
8. During the past week, were you limited in your work or other regular daily activities as a result of your arm, shoulder or hand problem?	1	2	3	4	5

Please rate the severity of the following symptoms in the last week. *(circle number)*	NONE	MILD	MODERATE	SEVERE	EXTREME
9. Arm, shoulder or hand pain.	1	2	3	4	5
10. Tingling (pins and needles) in your arm, shoulder or hand.	1	2	3	4	5

	NO DIFFICULTY	MILD DIFFICULTY	MODERATE DIFFICULTY	SEVERE DIFFICULTY	SO MUCH DIFFICULTY THAT I CAN'T SLEEP
11. During the past week, how much difficulty have you had sleeping because of the pain in your arm, shoulder or hand? *(circle number)*	1	2	3	4	5

*Quick***DASH DISABILITY/SYMPTOM SCORE** = $\left(\left[\frac{\text{(sum of n responses)}}{\text{n}}\right] - 1\right) \times 25$, where n is equal to the number of completed responses.

A *Quick*DASH score may <u>not</u> be calculated if there is greater than 1 missing item.

*Quick*DASH

WORK MODULE (OPTIONAL)

The following questions ask about the impact of your arm, shoulder or hand problem on your ability to work (including homemaking if that is your main work role).

Please indicate what your job/work is:____

❐ I do not work. (You may skip this section.)

Please circle the number that best describes your physical ability in the past week.

Did you have any difficulty:	NO DIFFICULTY	MILD DIFFICULTY	MODERATE DIFFICULTY	SEVERE DIFFICULTY	UNABLE
1. using your usual technique for your work?	1	2	3	4	5
2. doing your usual work because of arm, shoulder or hand pain?	1	2	3	4	5
3. doing your work as well as you would like?	1	2	3	4	5
4. spending your usual amount of time doing your work?	1	2	3	4	5

SPORTS/PERFORMING ARTS MODULE (OPTIONAL)

The following questions relate to the impact of your arm, shoulder or hand problem on playing *your musical instrument or sport or both*. If you play more than one sport or instrument (or play both), please answer with respect to that activity which is most important to you.

Please indicate the sport or instrument which is most important to you:______________________________

❐ I do not play a sport or an instrument. (You may skip this section.)

Please circle the number that best describes your physical ability in the past week.

Did you have any difficulty:	NO DIFFICULTY	MILD DIFFICULTY	MODERATE DIFFICULTY	SEVERE DIFFICULTY	UNABLE
1. using your usual technique for playing your instrument or sport?	1	2	3	4	5
2. playing your musical instrument or sport because of arm, shoulder or hand pain?	1	2	3	4	5
3. playing your musical instrument or sport as well as you would like?	1	2	3	4	5
4. spending your usual amount of time practising or playing your instrument or sport?	1	2	3	4	5

SCORING THE OPTIONAL MODULES: Add up assigned values for each response; divide by 4 (number of items); subtract 1; multiply by 25.
An optional module score may <u>not</u> be calculated if there are any missing items.

Institute for Work & Health | Research Excellence Advancing Employee Health

EQ-5D Health Questionnaire

Client ID ☐ New User ☐ Existing User ☐

Date ☐

By placing a tick in one box in each group below, please indicate which statements best describe your own health state today.

Mobility

I have no problems in walking about ☐

I have some problems in walking about ☐

I am confined to bed ☐

Self-Care

I have no problems with self-care ☐

I have some problems with washing or dressing myself ☐

I am unable to wash or dress myself ☐

Usual Activities (*e.g. work, study, housework, family or leisure activities*)

I have no problems with performing my usual activities ☐

I have some problems with performing my usual activities ☐

I am unable to perform my usual activities ☐

Pain / Discomfort

I have no pain or discomfort ☐

I have moderate pain or discomfort ☐

I have extreme pain or discomfort ☐

Anxiety / Depression

I am not anxious or depressed ☐

I am moderately anxious or depressed ☐

I am extremely anxious or depressed ☐

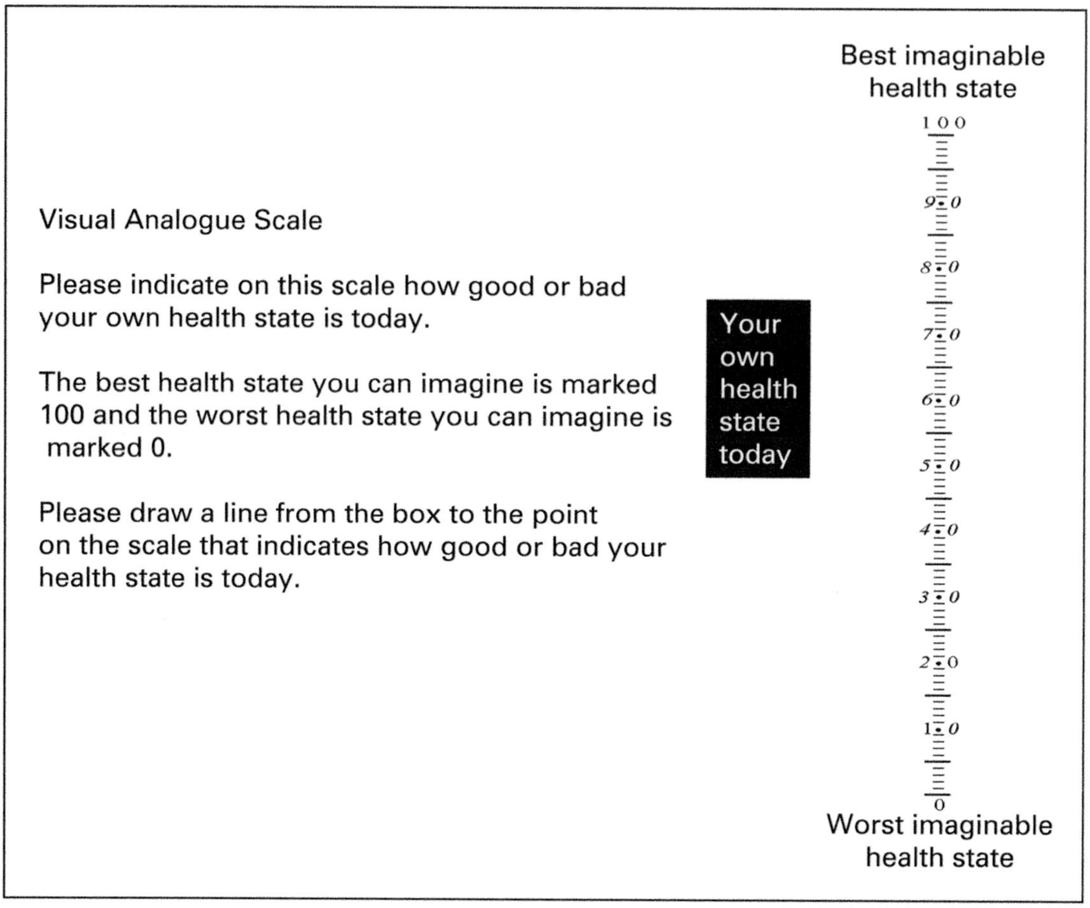

Now, please write the number you marked on the scale in the box below.

YOUR HEALTH TODAY = ☐

References

1. Jayakumar P, Williams M, Ring D, Lamb S, Gwilym S. A systematic review of outcome measures assessing disability following upper extremity trauma. JAAOS Global Res Rev. 2017;1(4):e021.
2. Nota SPFT, Bot AGJ, Ring D, Kloen P. Disability and depression after orthopaedic trauma. Injury. 2015;46(2):207–12.
3. Levin PE, MacKenzie EJ, Bosse MJ, Greenhouse PK. Improving outcomes: understanding the psychosocial aspects of the orthopaedic trauma patient. Instr Course Lect. 2014;63:39–48.
4. Van Beeck EF, Larsen CF, Lyons RA, Meerding W-J, Mulder S, Essink-Bot M-L. Guidelines for the conduction of follow-up studies measuring injury-related disability. J Trauma Acute Care Surg. 2007;62(2):534–50.
5. de Putter CE, Selles RW, Haagsma JA, Polinder S, Panneman MJM, Hovius SER, et al. Health-related quality of life after upper extremity injuries and predictors for suboptimal outcome. Injury. 2014;45(11):1752–8.
6. Slobogean GP, Noonan VK, Famuyide A, O'Brien PJ. Does objective shoulder impairment explain patient-reported functional outcome? A study of proximal humerus fractures. J Shoulder Elb Surg. 2011;20(2):267–72.

7. Rothrock NE, Kaiser KA, Cella D. Developing a valid patient-reported outcome measure. Clin Pharmacol Ther. 2011;90(5):737–42.
8. Mokkink LB, Terwee CB, Patrick DL, Alonso J, Stratford PW, Knol DL, Bouter LM, de Vet HCW. The COSMIN checklist for assessing the methodological quality of studies on measurement properties of health status measurement instruments: an international Delphi study. Qual Life Res. 2010;19:539–49. http://www.cosmin.nl/images/upload/files/COSMIN%20checklist%20manual%20v9.pdf. Accessed 26 Jan 2018.
9. Diehr P, Chen L, Patrick D, Feng Z, Yasui Y. Reliability, effect size, and responsiveness of health status measures in the design of randomized and cluster-randomized trials. Contemp Clin Trials. 2005;26(1):45–58.
10. Snyder CF, Watson ME, Jackson JD, Cella D, Halyard MY, Mayo FDAP-ROCMG. Patient-reported outcome instrument selection: designing a measurement strategy. Value Health. 2007;10:S76–85.
11. McLeod LD, Coon CD, Martin SA, Fehnel SE, Hays RD. Interpreting patient-reported outcome results: US FDA guidance and emerging methods. Expert Rev Pharmacoecon Outcomes Res. 2011;11(2):163–9.
12. Williamson PR, Altman DG, Bagley H, Barnes KL, Blazeby JM, Brookes ST, et al. The COMET handbook: version 1.0. Trials. 2017;18(Suppl 3):280.
13. The COMET initiative website: http://www.comet-initiative.org/. Accessed 26 Jan 2018.
14. Emery M-P, Perrier L-L, Acquadro C. Patient-reported outcome and quality of life instruments database (PROQOLID): frequently asked questions. Health Qual Life Outcomes. 2005;3:12.
15. Fitzpatrick R, Davey C, Buxton MJ, Jones DR. Evaluating patient-based outcome measures for use in clinical trials. Health Technol Assess. 1998;2(14):i-iv, 1–74.
16. Jenkinson C, Coulter A, Bruster S. The picker patient experience questionnaire: development and validation using data from in-patient surveys in five countries. Int J Qual Health Care. 2002;14(5):353–8.
17. Nord E. Cost-value analysis in health care: making sense out of QALYs. Cambridge: Cambridge University Press; 1999.
18. Dawson J, Fitzpatrick R, Carr A. Questionnaire on the perceptions of patients about shoulder surgery. J Bone Joint Surg Br. 1996;78(4):593–600.
19. Hudak PL, Amadio PC, Bombardier C, Beaton D, Cole D, Davis A, et al. Development of an upper extremity outcome measure: the DASH (disabilities of the arm, shoulder, and hand). Am J Ind Med. 1996;29(6):602–8.
20. Beaton DE, Wright JG, Katz JN; Upper Extremity Collaborative G. Development of the QuickDASH: comparison of three item-reduction approaches. JBJS. 2005;87(5):1038–46.
21. Constant CR, Murley AG. A clinical method of functional assessment of the shoulder. Clin Orthop Relat Res. 1987;214:160–4.
22. Lippitt SB, Harryman DT, Matsen FA, Fu FH, Hawkins RJ. A practical tool for evaluating function: the simple shoulder test. In: The shoulder: a balance of mobility and stability. Rosemont: American Academy of Orthopaedic Surgeons; 1993. p. 501–18.
23. Michener LA, McClure PW, Sennett BJ. American shoulder and elbow surgeons standardized shoulder assessment form, patient self-report section: reliability, validity, and responsiveness. J Shoulder Elb Surg. 2002;11(6):587–94.
24. Charles ER, Kumar V, Blacknall J, Edwards K, Geoghegan JM, Manning PA, et al. A validation of the Nottingham Clavicle Score: a clavicle, acromioclavicular joint and sternoclavicular joint-specific patient-reported outcome measure. J Shoulder Elb Surg. 2017;26(10):1732–9.
25. Imatani RJ, Hanlon JJ, Cady GW. Acute, complete acromioclavicular separation. JBJS. 1975;57(3):328–32.
26. Ware JE Jr, Sherbourne CD. The MOS 36-item short-form health survey (SF-36). I. Conceptual framework and item selection. Med Care. 1992;30(6):473–83.
27. Jenkinson C, Layte R, Jenkinson D, Lawrence K, Petersen S, Paice C, et al. A shorter form health survey: can the SF-12 replicate results from the SF-36 in longitudinal studies? J Public Health. 1997;19(2):179–86.
28. Group TE. EuroQol-a new facility for the measurement of health-related quality of life. Health Policy. 1990;16(3):199–208.
29. Herdman M, Gudex C, Lloyd A, Janssen M, Kind P, Parkin D, et al. Development and preliminary testing of the new five-level version of EQ-5D (EQ-5D-5L). Qual Life Res. 2011;20(10):1727–36.

Part II

Soft Tissue Disorders of the Shoulder

Glenohumeral Joint Instability

7

Paolo Paladini, Giovanni Merolla,
and Giuseppe Porcellini

Clinical Pearls

1) Always evaluate scapula dyskinesia in MDI
2) Never operate on a patient with MDI without six months of prior tailored rehabilitation
3) Arthroscopic and Open Bankart procedure have the same indications and outcomes. If an arthroscopic approach is not indicated, then consider a Latarjet procedure.
4) Do not consider Latarjet purely on glenoid bone loss alone. Time from first dislocation to surgery, number of dislocations and numerous episode of subluxation are sufficient to justify a Latarjet procedure.
5) If glenoid bone loss is greater than 30% of the entire glenoid surface, the coracoid transfer Latarjet procedure, may not be enough to cover the defect. In these cases consider an Eden-Hybinette operation with bone graft from iliac crest.

Introduction

Shoulder instability is characterized by a symptomatic loss of contact between the glenohumeral joint components [1]. Trauma is the most common cause, with an incidence of about 24 cases in 100,000 population. In some patients it is difficult to identify a clear mechanism of injury, because the onset of instability can be the result of very mild trauma or of repeated microtrauma [2]. The first traumatic dislocation may result in glenoid and humeral bony lesions or in soft tissue injuries, which can then lead to multiple episodes of instability [3]. A number of factors, such as age, level of sport activity practiced, ligamentous laxity, and scapular dyskinesis, can influence the evolution to chronic instability [1]. Matsen et al. [4] have divided recurrent instability into two major groups: TUBS (Traumatic Unidirectional Bankart lesion Surgery) and AMBRI (Atraumatic Multidirectional Bilateral Rehabilitation). In 2002 Gerber and Nyffeler [5] proposed a new classification of instability into dynamic, static, and voluntary dislocation. Dynamic instability is characterized by an initial trauma that leads to secondary capsular or labral tears or hyperlaxity. This classification emphasizes the distinction between unidirectional and multidirectional instability and between instability with and without hyperlaxity.

P. Paladini (✉) · G. Merolla
Unit of Shoulder and Elbow Surgery,
Cervesi Hospital, Cattolica, Italy

G. Porcellini
Università di Modena - Clinica Ortopedica,
Modena, MO, Italy

I. A. Trail et al. (eds.), *Textbook of Shoulder Surgery*, https://doi.org/10.1007/978-3-319-70099-1_7

Biomechanics

Shoulder instability can be associated with a wide range of lesions, whose extent determines clinical evolution. Most injuries are sustained during the initial episode of dislocation and involve capsuloligamentous or bony structures [6]. Provencher et al. [7] have demonstrated that glenohumeral joint stability rests on the health and integrity of its static (bony architecture, compression concavity mechanism, capsulolabral structures) and dynamic stabilizers (coordinated muscle contraction).

Unidirectional Traumatic Instability

The direction of traumatic instability is anterior in 95% of cases, posterior in 4%, and inferior in the remaining 1% [1–7]. The lesion that is typically associated with acute anterior traumatic dislocation is anterior-inferior capsulolabral detachment (Bankart lesion), found in 97% of cases [8]. A Bankart lesion is sufficient per se to induce instability. However, the glenoid provides a considerable contribution to joint stability, and its fracture in the acute episode or its gradual wear with each successive dislocation can result in a bony Bankart lesion [9]. These progressive morphological changes ultimately result an "inverse pear" shape when the anterior-inferior glenoid bone deficiency exceeds 20% [10]. Numerous biomechanical studies have described the progressive loss of joint stability that occurs as the glenoid defect grows [11]. In posterior dislocations, detachment of the labrum involves the posterior portion of the capsulolabral complex and in rare cases also the bone (posterior bony Bankart lesion). Hill-Sachs fractures are the result of the forceful impaction of the posterior-superior portion of the humeral head against the anterior glenoid rim – are also common. [12]. In anterior dislocations these injuries involve the posterior-lateral side of the humeral head, whereas in posterior dislocations they involve the anterior-medial side (McLaughlin fracture). The morphology of these lesions varies according to several factors that include dislocation number and chronicity and the energy of the trauma. Their combination determines the depth and width of the Hill-Sachs fracture. A bone deficiency involving less than 20% of the humeral head has little clinical relevance, whereas one ranging between 20 and 40% and especially exceeding 40% increases the likelihood of further dislocations [13]. Burkhart and De Beer [14] defined the injury where the head fracture is combined with glenoid bone loss as engaging Hill-Sachs lesion. In these patients, when the arm is abducted (90°) and externally rotated (0°–135°), the humeral head is pushed forward towards the edge of the glenoid until it dislocates. In 2007 Yamamoto et al. [15] introduced the concept of "glenoid track" (GT) to measure the risk of engagement and to illustrate the glenohumeral instability dynamics in case of combined glenoid and humeral bone defects. GT represents the contact area between the humeral head and the glenoid in a position that is conducive to anterior dislocation, and shrinks in presence of glenoid bone deficiency, increasing the risk of engagement. The same risk is involved in presence of a Hill-Sachs fracture extending medially into the GT [15].

Multidirectional Instability

Multidirectional instability (MDI) is characterized by symptomatic inferior instability associated with instability in at least another direction, anterior and/or posterior [16]. The main characteristic of this condition is capsular redundancy, which results in increased joint volume. Generalized joint laxity is a predisposing factor for MDI [17]. Dewing et al. [18] have demonstrated that MDI patients have a wider transverse capsular area compared with both healthy subjects and patients with anterior or posterior traumatic unidirectional instability. Although this finding is often related to constitutional ligamentous laxity, repeated traumatic dislocation can promote its development [19]. Some authors believe that capsular redundancy is an evolutionary anatomical variant rather than the consequence of trauma, since it has been described in

23% of foetal and embryonic shoulders [20]. Other researchers have related it to a connective tissue abnormality based on the finding that MDI often affects individuals with connective tissue diseases [21]. In particular Rodeo et al. [22], in a study of the distribution of collagen and elastin fibrils in subjects with unidirectional anterior instability, MDI, or no clinical history of shoulder instability described similar capsular biological properties in the two patient groups. Since the average diameter of the skin collagen fibrils differed significantly in the two groups of patients, the authors suggested a possible positive correlation with an underlying connective tissue abnormality [22]. Another factor that is believed to predispose to MDI is the position of the scapula in relation to the chest, since the scapula is directly responsible for the orientation of the glenoid both at rest and during movement [23]. An increase in frontal scapular tilt prevents the inferior dislocation of the humeral head, both because the upper capsular structures are tensioned and because the slope of the glenoid fossa is increased [24]; in contrast, a reduced frontal tilt compounds the inferior instability. These findings have been confirmed by Warner et al. [25], who demonstrated a direct correlation between reduced scapular tilt and shoulder instability. Dynamic scapular alterations are important predisposing factors for MDI. These patients show an increased scapulothoracic movement starting from 90 ° of elevation until the end of the movement that is associated with an abnormal upward rotation and with an anterior tilt and excessive scapular internal rotation [26]. Proprioception contributes to the maintenance of functional integrity and joint stability through a neuromuscular control system that serves as a sort of "anti-injury mechanism" [27]. It has been suggested that altered proprioception may play a role in MDI development [28]. A recent study of movement analysis data obtained with a 3D video system has demonstrated a significantly greater positioning error in subjects with MDI compared with healthy controls [27].

MDI may also be voluntary. These patients can dislocate their shoulder through muscle activation [29] and tend to hold the shoulder in internal rotation, which results in a typical scapular protraction that affects the inferior-medial angle (type I dyskinesis) or the entire medial border of the scapula (type II dyskinesia). In an electromyographic study combined with kinematic analysis with a motion capture system (Vicon, Oxford, UK), De Santis et al. [30] showed that the abnormal scapular movement of these patients is due to altered muscle coordination, where hyperactivation of the internal rotation muscles of the shoulder and of the anterior deltoid, pectoralis major, and latissimus dorsi is associated with a reduced activity of the external rotation muscles and of the posterior deltoid [29]. Induction of posterior shoulder subluxation occurs when the arm is actively placed in internal rotation. Patients who can dislocate the humeral head either anteriorly or anteriorly and posteriorly are less common.

Clinical Evaluation

An accurate history is critical to classify shoulder instability. Indeed, whereas in trauma patients the cause of instability is clear, in MDI it is more difficult to establish. History can highlight repeated micro-trauma, especially in subjects who participate in sports or overhead activities. In some there is no history of any trauma or micr-trauma (atraumatic). Patients with MDI often have generalized ligamentous laxity, either familial or acquired. Symptom onset is often subtle. Patients report non-specific pain elicited by a number of activities; often the pain prompts changes in lifestyle and patients learn to avoid painful positions and develop compensatory movements. Among the clinical tests employed to evaluate shoulder instability, the Apprehension-Relocation test is the one used most frequently to assess traumatic instability [31], whereas suspected MDI is assessed with an apprehensive Sulcus sign [1], the Load-and-Shift test [31], and Gagey's hyperabduction test [32]. A rotational imbalance is a common finding in MDI patients and overhead athletes, who exhibit a significantly increased external rotation range when the limb is in abduction and external rotation (ABER) and reduced mobility in internal rotation (glenohumeral internal rotation deficit, GIRD) due to tightness of posterior structures [23]. In atraumatic MDI the glenohumeral ROM can be normal or limited by apprehension [32]. In case of MDI, the clinician should seek signs of generalized hyperlaxity like joint hyperextension at the level of the elbow or the metacarpophalangeal joints, thumb hyperabduction, knee hyperextension, and patellar instability [33]. The Sulcus sign is often positive and associated with posterior subluxation when the limb is actively held in internal rotation; the Drawer test and the Load-and-Shift tests are also usually positive [29].

Imaging

Plain radiographs obtained in anteroposterior and axillary view are useful to establish the static relationship between the humeral head and the glenoid and to depict any bone abnormalities such as humeral head defects, glenoid dysplasia or hypoplasia, and bone loss. However, the best imaging modality to depict bone loss is CT, which clearly identifies and quantifies the humeral bone defect (Hill-Sachs) and the glenoid lesion. Glenoid bone deficiency can be measured with CT using the PICO method, i.e. by comparing the eroded glenoid surface with the healthy contralateral glenoid and quantifying the defect as a percentage of the lost glenoid surface [10]. This preoperative assessment is essential for treatment planning, because when the glenoid deficit exceeds 15–20% an augmentation intervention should be considered. MRI Arthrogram is the gold standard for the diagnosis of instability, since it provides excellent soft-tissue detail, especially of capsule and ligaments. MR arthrography, by extending the capsule, allows visualization of the glenoid labrum, the rotator interval, and the glenohumeral ligaments [34]. Bankart lesions are the most common MRI findings in patients with traumatic instability, whereas a pathological distension of the joint capsule and increased glenohumeral joint volume are typical of MDI. Recently, diagnostic signs and parameters have been measured on MRI scans taken both in neutral rotation and in ABER position, to identify the capsular redundancy [35]. Provencher et al. [36] have evaluated by MR arthrography the relationships between increased rotator interval dimension and shoulder instability; they concluded that the interval is almost identical in patients with unidirectional instability and MDI and not significantly different from that of controls.

Treatment

The treatment of shoulder instability has undergone considerable evolution in recent years, due to both a greater knowledge of the aetiology of shoulder conditions and to advances in surgical techniques. To select the correct therapeutic approach several factors need to be considered, chiefly the cause of the instability, patient age, the number of episodes of dislocation, the interval between the first and the latest episode, the demands from sport/work activities, and the presence of glenoid and/or humeral bone fractures [10].

Conservative Treatment

The treatment of choice after a first episode of dislocation is conservative with limb immobilization in a brace for about 3 weeks in most cases [37]. Some studies have reported that the disease course is not influenced by the duration of immobilization, whereas according to others immobilization of the humerus in external rotation reduces the risk of recurrence [37]. The subsequent phase is a rehabilitation programme which aims at full ROM restoration and at strengthening the scapulohumeral muscles, especially the scapular stabilizers [37]. Surgery after the first episode of instability is indicated in young patients, especially professional athletes whose high functional demands on the shoulder increase the risk of recurrence. Recent studies have demonstrated that athletes under the age of 20 conservative treatment is associated with a higher rate of recurrence (96%) compared with arthroscopic surgery [38].

The first approach in MDI patients is, non-operative and involves a tailored rehabilitation programme [39] to restore the neuromotor mechanisms that contribute to the dynamic stability of the shoulder, strengthen the scapular stabilizers and glenohumeral protectors, and restore the scapulo-thoraco-humeral rhythm. The rationale of this approach is that muscle strengthening should compensate for the lack of passive stability, assisting in the active control of the shoulder [40]. Several researchers have described an improvement after rehabilitation. According to Rowe [41] and to Burkhead and Rockwood [39], most patients with non-traumatic instability respond well to a targeted rehabilitation programme, whereas Misamore et al. [42] concluded that non-surgical treatment is associated with relatively poor outcomes in young athletes. When this fails to restore shoulder stability, surgical treatment offers a satisfactory rate of good outcomes.

Arthroscopy

Arthroscopic capsuloplasty is the treatment of choice for patients with capsulolabral lesions, either isolated or associated, and moderate glenoid bone deficiency (<15–20%). Its objective is to restore normal anatomy by reinserting the avulsed capsulolabral complex into the glenoid and correcting the capsular elongation generated by the first episode of dislocation [7]. Joint stability is always tested under anaesthesia with an interscalene block and compared with the contralateral side, to assess its severity and direction. The patient is placed in lateral or beach-chair decubitus. We prefer the lateral decubitus position with the shoulder in about 30° of abduction and 15° of anterior flexion and a tractions of 5 kg applied to the arm. The camera is inserted through the posterior portal (2 cm below the posterior acromial angle) [43] and an anterosuperior and an anteroinferior portal are created [44, 45] above the subscapularis and lateral to the coracoid. After inspection of the joint cavity and of the lesions through the posterior portal, the arthroscope is switched to the anterosuperior portal and

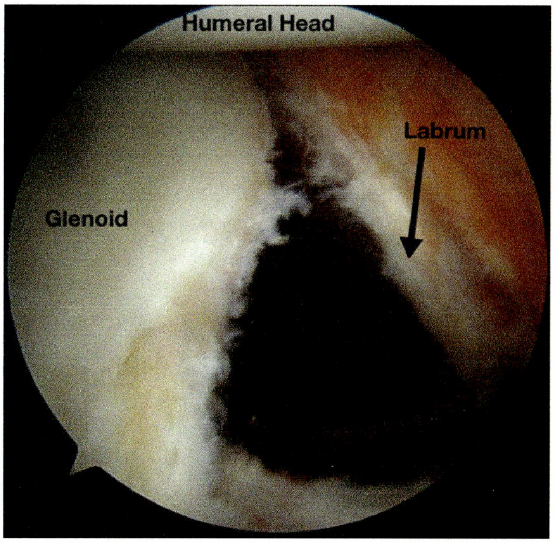

Fig. 7.1 Bankart lesion: arthroscopic view from the anterior-superior portal. Arrow: detached labrum. The humeral head is shifted anteriorly due to the slack ligament

a 8.5 mm cannula is passed through the anteroinferior portal. The posterior portal is kept as a secondary portal with a 6 mm cannula. The Bankart lesion is mobilized (Fig. 7.1), absorbable or soft non-metal anchors are placed on the glenoid edge with an inclination of 45° with respect to the glenoid surface and more proximal with respect to the capsule, to tension the capsule. The anchors should be placed on the glenoid surface, on the border between cartilage and bone, not on the glenoid neck [46]. The sutures from the anchors are then passed through the capsule and under the labrum using a sharp suture relay or shuttle system and knotted [46] (Fig. 7.2). Both the number of anchors and their configuration are chosen by the surgeon based on the type of instability to be treated and on the quality of the capsular and ligamentous tissue. In MDI patients the labrum can be folded on the anterior and posterior side using free wires (simple plication) or anchors (anchor plication).

Large unrecognized glenoid bone deficits and a hyperlax shoulder are the main risk factors for recurrence after arthroscopic stabilization [47]. An open capsuloplasty can also be performed using a deltopectoral approach with subscapularis split [48]. Since the recurrence rates associ-

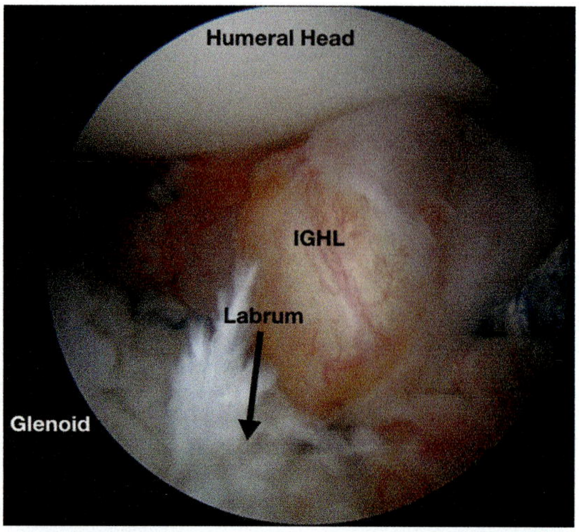

Fig. 7.2 Bankart lesion: arthroscopic view from the anterior-superior portal. The labrum is attached to the glenoid rim with two screws. The inferior glenohumeral ligament is tensioned and the humeral head seems centred on the glenoid surface

ated with open and arthroscopic procedures have become very similar (8% vs. 8.5%, respectively) [49], the minimally invasive arthroscopic approach is preferable. Among the researchers who have assessed the risk factors for recurrence after arthroscopic repair, Porcellini et al. [50] analysed the results of arthroscopic capsuloplasty performed in patients without bone defects. They reported that male gender, age less than 22 years, and interval from the first episode of dislocation to surgery >6 months are predisposing factors for recurrence.

As regards humeral bone deficiency, there is no consensus on the lesions to be treated by surgery. According to Sekiya et al. [51], surgical treatment is required to treat defects exceeding 12.5%. Wolf and Pollack [52] described arthroscopic "remplissage", a posterior capsular tenodesis, to manage medium-large Hill-Sachs lesions showing the classic "engaging" mechanism in patients without large glenoid bone defects. The procedure is performed with the standard arthroscopic technique described above. The extent of the lesion is dynamically evaluated by arthroscopy with the arm in abduction, flexion and external rotation [14]. After debridement of the surface of the humeral defect with a bur, to identify its borders, an anchor is passed through the posterior cannula in the Hill-Sachs fracture. The suture threads from the anchor are passed through the capsule and the lower portion of the infraspinatus tendon using a grasper [53]. To avoid postoperative joint stiffness, the anchor is placed directly on the bottom of the bone defect, not too close to the edge of the humeral head, and the suture threads are carefully woven through the soft tissues close to the bone defect [54]. A mattress suture is performed and knotted through the posterior portal. Therefore, all the knots are outside the joint, in the subdeltoid space, while in the joint the humeral bone defect is completely filled by the capsule and the infraspinatus tendon [53]. A study by Merolla et al. [13] has confirmed the effectiveness of remplissage in unstable shoulders with extensive Hill-Sachs lesions; the authors reported that the strength of the infraspinatus was not impaired, and that although the procedure induced a reduction of external rotation with the arm in adduction, it did not affect limb function.

The surgical approach to symptomatic MDI involves stabilization by open or arthroscopic surgery, although the arthroscopic approach has become the reference method. A recent systematic review has demonstrated that the results of arthroscopic plication are comparable to those obtained with open surgery in terms of recurrence, return to sports, loss of external rotation, and rate of general complications [55]. The procedure involves the execution of multiple capsular plications (anterior, posterior, and inferior) in distal-proximal direction, to retension the anterior and posterior band of the inferior glenohumeral ligament and to augment the height and consistence of the labrum, thus enhancing its "bumper" effect. Using the standard arthroscopic technique described above, the joint cavity is inspected through the posterior portal and the decision regarding the number, size, and thickness of the plicae is based on the identification of a positive "drive-through sign" and on the degree of capsule laxity [56]. The plication is performed with a pinch-tuck technique, each plica folding a centimetre of capsule tissue. Viewing the glenoid surface as a clock face, an absorbable thread is passed through the anterior capsule and placed in 5:30–4:30 o'clock position using a dedicated 45° left- or right-angled instrument, pulling the capsule in superior-medial direction, and then knotting the suture [57]. The posterior plication is performed through the posterior portal with the camera passed through the anterosuperior portal. The procedure begins at 6:30 o'clock and usually involves three plicae, pulling the capsule in superior direction [57]. Follow-up studies have described good or excellent short- and medium-term outcomes in 80–94% of cases [56]. In particular, Fleega and Shewy [58] reported complete recovery of movement and a recurrence rate of 4% in patients managed by arthroscopy. Other researchers have stressed the limited rate of return to the same level of sport performance [56, 57, 59]. Notably, the outcomes of arthroscopic management for MDI are less satisfactory than those of unidirectional instability.

Open Surgery

Biomechanical and clinical studies [10, 60] have demonstrated that an anterior-inferior glenoid bone defect of 20–25% significantly affects the outcome of arthroscopic capsuloplasty and should be treated by a bone-block procedure. The most widely used technique is the Bristow-Latarjet technique, which involves transposition of the coracoid on the glenoid neck [61]. The procedure is performed through a deltopectoral approach. After identification of the coracoid, the pectoralis minor is detached from the medial side of the bone. The coracoacromial ligament is cut from the lateral side leaving a stump on the coracoid. The coracoid is detached from the scapula using a 90°-angled saw. The insertion of the conjoined tendon is spared and the tendon is transferred with the coracoid. The coracoid is released from the underlying soft tissues, carefully avoiding injury to the musculocutaneous nerve. After dissection, two holes are drilled in the coracoid graft for two 4.0 mm partially threaded bicortical screws. The glenohumeral space is accessed through a split in the subscapularis and the joint capsule is incised to expose and refresh the glenoid neck. After the holes for the screws have been drilled the coracoid graft is fixed on the glenoid [62] (Figs. 7.3, 7.4, and 7.5). The effectiveness of the technique is based on biomechanical criteria: (a) the increase in glenoid surface provided by the coracoid transfer increases glenoid congruence; (b) the dynamic 'hammock' effect produced by the conjoint tendon prevents excessive frontal translation of the humeral head; and (c) the anterior capsular repair and retensioning of the inferior subscapularis contributes to stability [61]. The grafting site on the anterior glenoid neck should carefully be selected, because too lateral a position would involve exposure on the glenoid rim and impingement with the humeral head, whereas too medial a position is associated with a high failure rate [63]. Cerciello et al. [64] reported excellent functional recovery and a recurrence rate of 3.5% in professional athletes

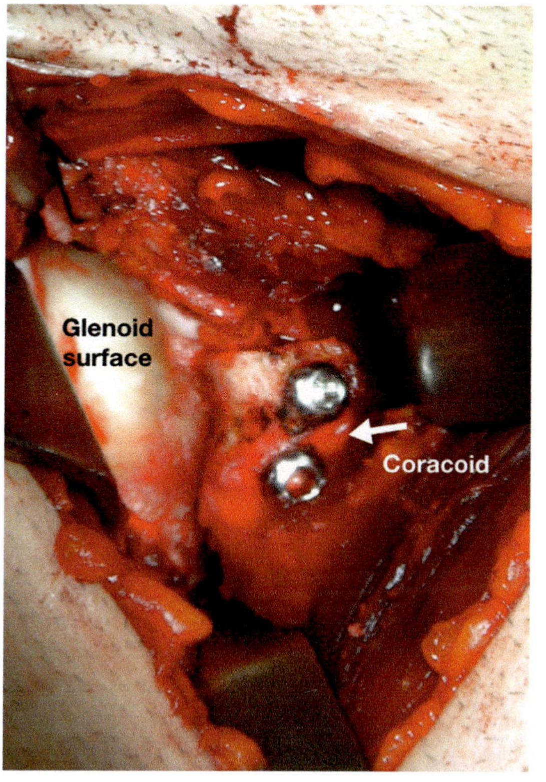

Fig. 7.3 Intraoperative view of an open Latarjet procedure. Arrow: transposed coracoid, flush with the glenoid surface. The coracoid is fixed with two 4.0 partially treaded screws

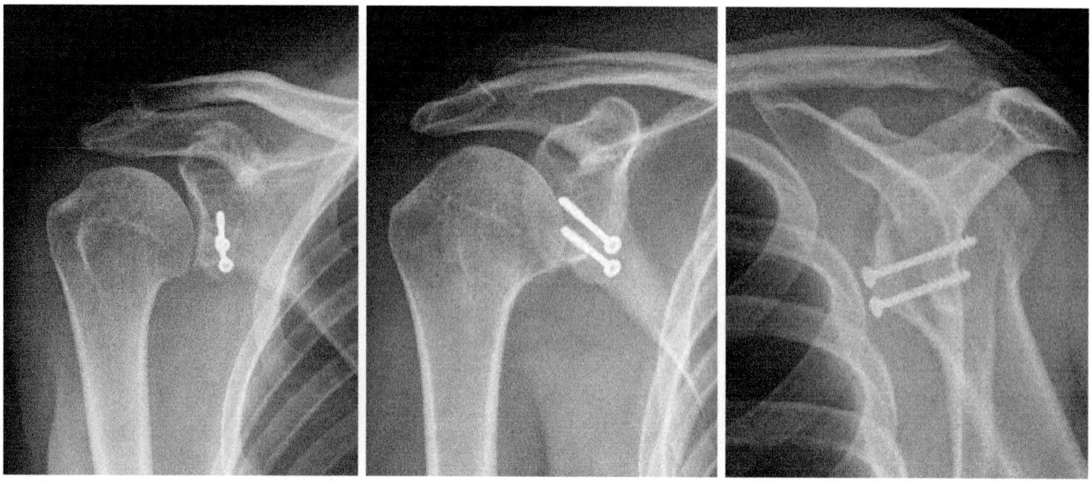

Fig. 7.4 Follow-up radiographs at 2 years (same patient as in Fig. 7.3)

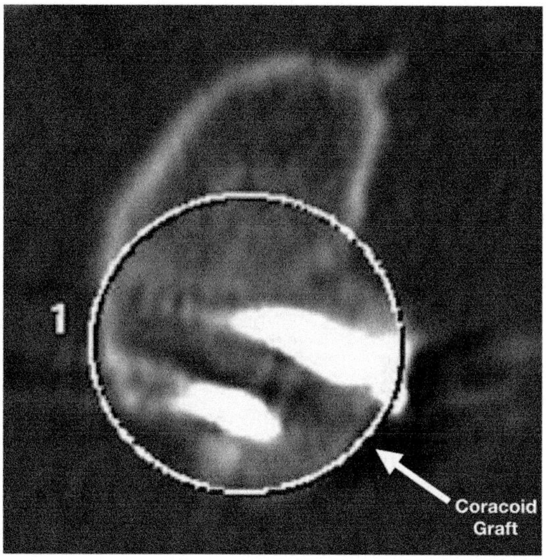

Fig. 7.5 Follow-up CT scan at 2 years (same patient as in Figs. 7.3 and 7.4). The coracoid graft (arrow) is still clearly visible and the glenoid surface is surrounded by a white circle

with a glenoid bone defect managed by Latarjet stabilization. The procedure can be performed arthroscopically, as originally described by Lafosse et al. in 2007 [65] and subsequently perfected by the author and his team [66]. Although the arthroscopic Latarjet procedure is highly complex, it combines the advantages of arthroscopic surgery and the low recurrence rate ensured by the Latarjet method [67].

Conclusions

Several issues, either diagnostic and therapeutic, remain outstanding in shoulder instability Accurate clinical examination allows identifying the underlying cause of the instability and selecting the most appropriate imaging approaches. Recent advances in imaging and surgical techniques have changed the therapeutic approach to traumatic unidirectional instability, leading to the recommendation of an early surgical approach to manage the first episode of dislocation. MDI instability requires careful evaluation and prolonged conservative treatment before surgery, preferably by arthroscopy.

References

1. Matsen FA, Harryman DT, Sidles JA. Mechanics of glenohumeral instability. Clin Sports Med. 1991;10:783–8.
2. Leroux T, Wasserstein D, Veillette C, et al. Epidemiology of primary anterior shoulder dislocation requiring closed reduction in Ontario, Canada. Am J Sports Med. 2014;42:442–50.
3. Te Slaa RL, Wijffels MP, Brand R, et al. The prognosis following acute primary glenohumeral dislocation. J Bone Joint Surg Br. 2004;86(1):58–64.
4. Matsen FA, Thomas SC, Rockwood CA Jr. Anterior G lenohumeral instability. In: Rockwood Jr CA, Matsen FA, editors. The shoulder. Philadelphia: Saunders; 1990. p. 611–754.

5. Gerber C, Nyffeler RW. Classification of glenohumeral joint instability. Clin Orthop Relat Res. 2002;400:65–76.
6. Atef A, El-Tantawy A, Gad H, Hefeda M. Prevalence of associated injuries after anterior shoulder dislocation: a prospective study. Int Orthop. 2016;40(3):519–24. https://doi.org/10.1007/s00264-015-2862-z. Epub 2015 Jul 2.
7. Provencher MT, Ghodadra N, Romeo AA. Arthroscopic management of anterior instability: pearls, pitfalls, and lessons learned. Orthop Clin North Am. 2010;41(3):325–37.
8. Owens BD, Nelson BJ, Duffey ML, et al. Pathoanatomy of first-time, traumatic, anterior glenohumeral subluxation events. J Bone Joint Surg Am. 2010;92(7):1605–11.
9. Patel RM, Amin NH, Lynch TS. Management of Bone Loss in Glenohumeral Instability. Orthop Clin N Am. 2014;45:523–39.
10. Provencher MT, Bhatia S, Ghodadra NS, et al. Recurrent shoulder instability: current concepts for evaluation and management of glenoid bone loss. J Bone Joint Surg Am. 2010;92(2):133–51.
11. Itoi E, Lee SB, Amrami KK, et al. Quantitative assessment of classic anteroinferior bony Bankart lesions by radiography and computed tomography. Am J Sports Med. 2003;31(1):112–8.
12. Hill HA, Sachs MD. The grooved defect of the humeral head. A frequently unrecognized complication of dislocations of the shoulder joint. Radiology. 1940;35:690–700.
13. Merolla G, Paladini P, Di Napoli G, et al. Outcomes of arthroscopic Hill-Sachs remplissage and anterior Bankart repair: a retrospective controlled study including ultrasound evaluation of posterior capsulotenodesis and infraspinatus strength assessment. Am J Sports Med. 2015;43(2):407–14.
14. Burkhart SS, De Beer JF. Traumatic glenohumeral bone defects and their relationship to failure of arthroscopic Bankart repairs: significance of the inverted-pear glenoid and the humeral engaging Hill-Sachs lesion. Arthroscopy. 2000;16(7):677–94.
15. Yamamoto N, Itoi E, Abe H, et al. Contact between the glenoid and the humeral head in abduction, external rotation, and horizontal extension: a new concept of glenoid track. J Shoulder Elb Surg. 2007;16(5):649–56.
16. Pollock RG, Owens JM, Flatow EL, et al. Operative results of the inferior capsular shift procedure for multidirectional instability of the shoulder. J Bone Joint Surg Am. 2000;82:919–28.
17. Johnson SM, Robinson CM. Shoulder instability in patients with joint hyperlaxity. J Bone Joint Surg Am. 2010;92(6):1545–57.
18. An analysis of capsular area in patients with anterior, posterior, and multidirectional shoulder instability. Am J Sports Med 2008; 36(3):515–22. https://doi.org/10.1177/0363546507311603.
19. Ahmad CS, Freehill MQ, Blaine TA, Levine WN, Bigliani LU. Anteromedial capsular redundancy and labral deficiency in shoulder instability. Am J Sports Med. 2003;31(2):247–52.
20. Uhthoff HK, Piscopo M. Anterior capsular redundancy of the shoulder: congenital or traumatic? An embryological study. J Bone Joint Surg Br. 1985;67:363–6.
21. Jerosch J, Castro WH. Shoulder instability in Ehlers-Danlos syndrome: an indication for surgical treatment? Acta Orthop Belg. 1990;56:451–3.
22. Rodeo SA, Suzuki K, Yamauchi M, et al. Analysis of collagen and elastic fibers in shoulder capsule in patients with shoulder instability. Am J Sports Med. 1998;26:634–43.
23. Oyama S, Myers JB, Wassinger CA, et al. Asymmetric resting scapular posture in healthy overhead athletes. J Athl Train. 2008;43:565–70.
24. Ludewig PM, Phadke V, Braman JP, et al. Motion of the shoulder complex during multiplanar humeral elevation. J Bone Joint Surg. 2009;91:378–89.
25. Warner JJ, Deng XH, Warren RF, et al. Static capsuloligamentous restraints to superior-inferior translation of the glenohumeral joint. Am J Sports Med. 1992;20:675–85.
26. Illye's A, Kiss RM. Kinematic and muscle activity characteristics of multidirectional shoulder joint instability during elevation. Knee Surg Sports Traumatol Arthrosc. 2006;14:673–85.
27. Barden JM, Balyk R, Raso VJ, et al. Dynamic upper limb proprioception in multidirectional shoulder instability. Clin Orthop Relat Res. 2004;420:181–9.
28. Beard DJ, Dodd CAF, Simpson HARW. Sensorimotor changes after anterior cruciate ligament reconstruction. Clin Orthop. 2000;372:205–16.
29. Merolla G, De Santis E, Cools AMJ, et al. Functional outcomes and quality of life after rehabilitation for voluntary posterior shoulder instability: a prospective blinded cohort study. Eur J Orthop Surg Traumatol. 2014;25(2):263–72.
30. De Santis E, Parel I, Paladini P, Porcellini G, Merolla G. Kinematics and electromyographic findings in subjects with symptomatic voluntary posterior shoulder instability: a prospective laboratory study. Abstract Book SECEC Congress 2015; p. 159.
31. Gerber C, Ganz R. Clinical assessment of instability of the shoulder: with special reference to anterior and posterior drawer tests. J Bone Joint Surg Br. 1984;66:551–6.
32. Gagey OJ, Gagey N. The hyperbaduction test. J Bone Joint Surg Br. 2001;83:69–74.
33. Gaskill TR, Taylor DC, Millett PJ. Management of multidirectional instability of the shoulder. J Am Acad Orthop Surg. 2011;19:758–67.
34. Dewing CB, McCormick F, Bell SJ, Solomon DJ, et al. An analysis of capsular area in patients with anterior, posterior, and multidirectional shoulder instability. Am J Sports Med. 2008;36:515–22.
35. Schaeffeler C, Waldt S, Bauer JS, et al. MR arthrography including abduction and external rotation images in the assessment of traumatic multidirectional instability of the shoulder. Eur Radiol. 2014;24:1376–85.

36. Provencher MT, Dewing CB, Bell SJ, et al. An analysis of the rotator interval in patients with anterior, posterior, and multidirectional shoulder instability. Arthroscopy. 2008;24:921–9.
37. Dodson CC, Cordasco FA. Anterior glenohumeral joint dislocations. Orthop Clin North Am. 2008;39(4):507–18.
38. Crall TS, Bishop JA, Guttman D, et al. Cost-effectiveness analysis of primary arthroscopic stabilization versus nonoperative treatment for first-time anterior glenohumeral dislocations. Arthroscopy. 2012;28(12):1755–65.
39. Burkhead WZ, Rockwood CA Jr. Treatment of instability of the shoulder with an exercise program. J Bone Joint Surg Am. 1992;74:890–6.
40. Magarey ME, Jones MA. Dynamic evaluation and early management of altered motor control around the shoulder complex. Man Ther. 2003;8:195–206.
41. Rowe CR. Prognosis in dislocations of the shoulder. J Bone Joint Surg Am. 1956;38:957–77.
42. Misamore GW, Sallay PI, Didelot W. A longitudinal study of patients with multidirectional instability of the shoulder with seven- to ten-year follow-up. J Shoulder Elb Surg. 2005;14:466–70.
43. Snyder SJ. Shoulder arthroscopy. New York: Lippincott Williams and Wilkins; 2003. p. 22–8.
44. Matthews LS, Zarins B, Michael RH, et al. Anterior portal selection for shoulder arthroscopy. Arthroscopy. 1985;1:33–9.
45. Wolf EM. Anterior portals in shoulder arthroscopy. Arthroscopy. 1989;5:201–8.
46. Snyder SJ, Strafford BB. Arthroscopic management of instability of the shoulder. Orthopedics. 1993;16(9):993–1002.
47. Boileau P, Villalba M, Héry JY, et al. Risk factors for recurrence of shoulder instability after arthroscopic Bankart repair. J Bone Joint Surg Am. 2006;88(8):1755–63.
48. Rhee YG, Ha JH, Cho NS. Anterior shoulder stabilization in collision athletes: arthroscopic versus open Bankart repair. Am J Sports Med. 2006;34(6):979–85.
49. Harris JD, Gupta AK, Mall NA, et al. Long term outcomes after Bankart shoulder stabilization. Arthroscopy. 2013;29(5):920–33.
50. Porcellini G, Campi F, Pegreffi F, et al. Predisposing factors for recurrent shoulder dislocation after arthroscopic treatment. J Bone Joint Surg Am. 2009;91(11):2537–42.
51. Sekiya JK, Wickwire AC, Stehle JH, et al. Hill-Sachs defects and repair using osteoarticular allograft transplantation: biomechanical analysis using a joint compression model. Am J Sports Med. 2009;37(12):2459–66.
52. Wolf EM, Pollack ME. Hill-Sachs "remplissage": an arthroscopic solution for the engaging Hill-Sachs lesion. Arthroscopy. 2004;20(Suppl 1):e14–5.
53. Purchase RJ, Wolf EM, Hobgood ER, et al. Hill-sachs "remplissage": an arthroscopic solution for the engaging hill-sachs lesion. Arthroscopy. 2008;24(6): 723–6.
54. Elkinson I, Giles JW, Boons HW, et al. The shoulder remplissage procedure for Hill-Sachs defects: does technique matter? J Shoulder Elb Surg. 2013;22(6):835–41.
55. Jacobson ME, Riggenbach M, Wooldridge AN, et al. Open capsular shift and arthroscopic capsular plication for treatment of multidirectional instability. Arthroscopy. 2012;28:1010–7.
56. Cicak N, Klobucar H, Bicanic G, et al. Arthroscopic extracapsular plication to treat multidirectional instability of the shoulder. Arthroscopy. 2005;21:1278.
57. Merolla G, Cerciello S, Chillemi C, et al. Multidirectional instability of the shoulder: biomechanics, clinical presentation, and treatment strategies. Eur J Orthop Surg Traumatol. 2015;25(6): 975–85.
58. Fleega BA, El Shewy MT. Arthroscopic inferior capsular shift: long-term follow-up. Am J Sports Med. 2012;40:1126–32.
59. Lubiatowski P, Ogrodowicz P, Wojtaszek M, et al. Arthroscopic capsular shift technique and volume reduction. Eur J Orthop Surg Traumatol. 2012;22:437–41.
60. Yamamoto N, Itoi E, Abe H, et al. Effect of an anterior glenoid defect on anterior shoulder stability: a cadaveric study. Am J Sports Med. 2009;37(5):949–54.
61. Latarjet M. Treatment of recurrent dislocation of the shoulder. Lyon Chir. 1954;49(8):994–7.
62. Mizuno N, Denard PJ, Raiss P, et al. Long-term results of the Latarjet procedure for anterior instability of the shoulder. J Should Elbow Surg Am Should Elbow Surg. 2014;23(11):1691–9.
63. Gupta A, Delaney R, Petkin K, et al. Complications of the Latarjet procedure. Curr Rev Musculoskelet Med. 2015;8(1):59–66.
64. Cerciello S, Edwards TB, Walch G. Chronic anterior glenohumeral instability in soccer players: results for a series of 28 shoulders treated with the Latarjet procedure. J Orthop Traumatol. 2012;13(4):197–202.
65. Lafosse L, Lejeune E, Bouchard A, et al. The arthroscopic Latarjet procedure for the treatment of anterior shoulder instability. Arthroscopy. 2007;23(11):1242.e1–5.
66. Lafosse L, Boyle S, Gutierrez-Aramberri M, et al. Arthroscopic Latarjet procedure. Orthop Clin North Am. 2010;41(3):393–405.
67. Dumont GD, Fogerty S, Rosso C, et al. The arthroscopic Latarjet procedure for anterior shoulder instability: 5-year minimum follow-up. Am J Sports Med. 2014;42(11):2560–6.

8 Rotator Cuff Pathology

Teruhisa Mihata

Introduction

The most common signs of rotator cuff tears are pain from subacromial impingement, muscle weakness in the shoulder joint, and, consequently, functional impairment, including limited range of motion [11, 19]. These signs result mainly from loss of the superior stability of the glenohumeral joint because of dysfunction of the rotator cuff muscles. The various treatment options for rotator cuff tears include conservative treatment, anatomic repair, and alternative surgical techniques. The current research on the treatment and management of rotator cuff tears are summarized.

Etiology

The cause of rotator cuff tears is thought to include both intrinsic factors within the rotator cuff itself and extrinsic factors. In 1934, Codman [12] reported that degenerative changes within the rotator cuff promote tearing of the tendon. In 1972, Neer [66] suggested that most rotator cuff tears are caused by impingement of proliferative acromial spurs upon the rotator cuff tendons. Recent studies have shown that both intrinsic and extrinsic factors should be evaluated to determine the most suitable treatment for rotator cuff tears [13, 29, 62, 77, 84].

Radiographic studies showed that rotator cuff tears increase superior glenohumeral translation, causing subacromial impingement [16, 17]. The altered kinematics causes pathological osseous changes in the shoulder joint. The most common signs of rotator cuff tears are pain from subacromial impingement [17, 24], muscle weakness in the shoulder joint, 11,19 and as a result, limitation of arm elevation [17, 24]. These signs result mainly from a loss of the superior stability of the glenohumeral joint because of dysfunction of the rotator cuff muscles.

Epidemiologic study showed the prevalence of rotator cuff tear in the general population was 22.1%, which increased with age, and more than half of the rotator cuff tears were asymptomatic [60]. In the symptomatic tears, which were treated by conservative management, or the asymptomatic tears, the severity of torn tendon may become worse with time. Once the tear become chronic and large size, complete repair is challenging because of the development of tendon retraction with inelasticity [3, 69], muscle atrophy [3, 27, 49, 50, 67], and fatty infiltration [3, 27, 49, 50, 67, 69].

T. Mihata (✉)
Department of Orthopedic Surgery, Osaka Medical College, Takatsuki, Osaka, Japan

Orthopaedic Biomechanics Laboratory, Congress Medical Foundation, Pasadena, CA, USA

First Towakai Hospital, Takatsuki, Osaka, Japan

Katsuragi Hospital, Kishiwada, Osaka, Japan
e-mail: tmihata@osaka-med.ac.jp

I. A. Trail et al. (eds.), *Textbook of Shoulder Surgery*, https://doi.org/10.1007/978-3-319-70099-1_8

Treatment Options

Conservative Treatment

Natural History

Investigations of the anatomic and clinical progression of rotator cuff tears have revealed that whereas 36% (18 of 50) of patients with initially asymptomatic rotator cuff tears developed symptoms during the follow-up period (18 ± 9.6 months) [64], 29% (7 of 24) patients with symptomatic isolated tears of the supraspinatus tendon became asymptomatic without surgical treatment at a median duration of follow-up of 42 months (range, 27–87 months) after diagnosis [21]. In addition, asymptomatic rotator cuff tears were smaller than they had been at initial diagnosis in 9 of 24 patients (38%) but had progressed in size in 6 patients (25%) [17], whereas only 5 of 61 (8%) symptomatic rotator cuff tears had decreased in size, and 30 (50%) had increased in size [80]. The increase in tear size in the anteroposterior direction in newly symptomatic patients (10.6 mm) was significantly larger than that in the still-asymptomatic group (3.3 mm) [64]. Furthermore, the presence of considerable pain was significantly correlated with an increase in tear size [80]. Progression of the Goutallier grade (fatty degeneration) occurred in 6 of the 16 cases (35%) in the newly symptomatic group but in only 1 of the 25 cases (4%) in the still-asymptomatic group [64]. Therefore, the progression of tear size and of fatty degeneration was severe in symptomatic tears, although the pattern of the natural history of rotator cuff tears varied. Given the likelihood of an increase in the size of the tear and of progressive fatty degeneration, which may cause shoulder disability and render the tear irreparable, rotator cuff repair should be considered early during management and therapy, especially in symptomatic patients.

Subacromial Injection

Subacromial injection of a corticosteroid or sodium hyaluronate is one nonsurgical treatment for rotator cuff disease. Corticosteroid injection reportedly is highly effective in decreasing the clinical symptoms of rotator cuff tendinopathy or full-thickness rotator cuff tears for at least 3 months after injection [20, 65]. Two injections, 21 days apart, did not prolong or potentiate pain relief [25]. For patients with rotator cuff tendinopathy without any tears, a series of three or four subacromial injections of sodium hyaluronate may provide pain relief for approximately 3 months after injection [51, 61]. However, corticosteroid injection may induce the progression of rotator cuff tears: in one report, 66.6% of partial-thickness rotator cuff tears had become full-thickness tears by 12 weeks after the injection of a corticosteroid [75].

Physical Therapy

Physical therapy of rotator cuff tears includes stretching, passive and active range-of-motion exercises, and muscle strengthening exercises. Both the patient's complaint and physical status must be assessed carefully and are the most important factors in treating rotator cuff tears with physical therapy [32, 53]. According to recent reports, physical therapy yields excellent short-term results. For example, a non-operative protocol using physical therapy was effective for treating atraumatic, full-thickness rotator cuff tears in approximately 75% of patients followed for 2 years [44]. In another study, 70 of 93 (75%) patients were classified as having a successful outcome after 3 months of physical therapy, in that both surgeon and patient agreed that surgery was no longer necessary [6]. Even home-based exercise achieved results comparable to those of traditional occupational therapy for conservative treatment of rotator cuff tears when patients were thoroughly educated by using an exercise guide booklet with detailed instructions and demonstrations [43]. An investigation to identify modifiable factors that could be addressed nonoperatively to improve or possibly eliminate symptoms in patients willing to undergo an initial trial of physical therapy for an atraumatic, full-thickness rotator cuff tear found that scapulothoracic dyskinesis, decreased range of motion in active abduction and forward elevation, and reduced strength in abduction and forward elevation contributed significantly to pain and loss of function [28]. Another group assessed the physical and MRI findings on initial examination that were characteristic of responders by comparing patients who responded well to conservative treatment (including physical therapy) with those who responded poorly [83]. The following parameters showed significant differences between patient groups: [1] impingement sign; [2] active external rotation angle on physical examination; [3] integrity of the intramuscular tendon of the supraspinatus on MRI; and [4] presence of supraspinatus muscle atrophy on MRI. However, while physical therapy is performed, the quality of the torn rotator cuff and of clinical outcome may become worse [72]. Among 103 patients with rotator cuff tears no longer than 3 cm who were randomized to receive primary tendon repair ($n = 52$) or physical therapy ($n = 51$) [63], 75% (38 patients among the 51 treated with physiotherapy) experienced ultrasonography-diagnosed increases of >5 mm in tear size within 5 years; this condition was associated with an inferior outcome. In addition, 12 patients in whom physiotherapy failed to ameliorate clinical symptoms underwent secondary surgery within the first 2 years. The clinical results after physiotherapy plus secondary repair were inferior to those after primary tendon repair, with between-group mean differences of 5.3 points on the Constant score, 9.0 points on the American Shoulder and Elbow Surgeons score, 1.1 cm on a 10-cm visual analog scale for pain, and 1.0 cm on a 10-cm visual analog scale for patient satisfaction [55].

Surgical Treatment

Reparable Tears

Factors Affecting Outcome

Key factors prognostic of re-tearing after rotator cuff repair include primary tear size, tendon quality, repair tension, cuff retraction, footprint coverage, and poor patient compliance with postoperative rehabilitation [1]. Among 80 patients treated with arthroscopic rotator cuff repair [65], tendon healing was greater for those younger than 50 years ($n = 40$), but functional gain was at least equivalent in patients younger than 50 years and those older than 70 years ($n = 40$). In addition, post-operative scores according to the Short Western Ontario Rotator Cuff, American Shoulder and Elbow Surgeons, or American College of Sports Medicine scales did not differ between patients younger than 55 years of age ($n = 84$) and those 55 years and older ($n = 260$) [18].

Retear Rate and Clinical Outcome

According to recent literature, recurrent rotator cuff tears typically are associated with inferior clinical outcomes. In addition, a long-term follow-up study showed that 93% (13 of 14) of patients with postoperative recurrent tears also experienced proximal humeral migration or cuff tear arthropathy [73]. Therefore, surgeons need to consider how to increase healing rate.

On the other hand, some literatures reported controversial results [22, 39, 47, 52]. Several studies [32, 42, 47] showed no significant correlation between the clinical and anatomic outcomes after arthroscopic single-row rotator cuff repair. In contrast, another group [18] concluded that arthroscopic rotator cuff repair with defect recurrence achieved excellent pain relief and improvement in the ability to perform activities of daily living despite an average postoperative American Shoulder and Elbow Surgeons score of only 79.9 points, which is lower than that of healed repairs in other studies [34, 42, 47]. However, all of the cited studies had inherent limitations of small sample size (18 [22], 24 [39], 62 [47], and 17 [52] shoulders) and high retear rates (94% [22], 88% [39], 48% [47], and 48% [52], respectively), suggesting the influence of technical problems, such as inexperienced surgical technique, and excessively aggressive postoperative protocols.

Surgical Options to Increase Healing Rates

To improve the healing rate after surgical repair of rotator cuff tears, several new techniques have been developed recently. The following sections review published studies that have investigated the effects of various new surgical options on healing rate, clinical outcome, and shoulder biomechanics.

Arthroscopic Versus Open Repair

Most studies show that both arthroscopic and mini-open rotator cuff repair techniques improve functional outcome and range of motion and decrease the Visual Analog Scale for Pain score of treated patients [33, 86, 88]. However, reported advantages specific to arthroscopic surgery compared with open repair techniques include more rapid treatment benefit [86], less severe night pain at 6 months postoperatively, less extreme pain, a lower retear rate, and greater patient satisfaction with the overall shoulder condition [88].

Single-Row Versus Double-Row Repair

Although both single-row and double-row repairs significantly improve clinical outcomes relative to preoperative status [9, 15, 42, 46, 48, 59], double-row repair is associated with unique advantages. In one study [15], the percentage of patients reporting that their shoulders felt close to normal was greater in those that received double-row repair than in those receiving single-row repair; a double-row repair was 4.9 times more likely to lead to a good or excellent outcome. In addition, arthroscopic rotator cuff repair with double-row compared with single-row fixation gave better shoulder strength in patients with large tears (minimum, 3 cm) [48]. A multicenter randomized controlled trial showed that use of a double-row fixation technique was associated with higher healing rates, as assessed with ultrasonography or MRI [46].

Double-Row Repair Versus Suture-Bridge (Transosseous-Equivalent) Repair

Both double-row and suture-bridge (transosseous-equivalent) repairs are associated with substantial improvements in pain and function [40, 59, 71]. Two groups [40, 71] reported no significant difference in clinical outcome between double-row and suture-bridge repair at final follow-up. However, when medial mattress sutures, such as rip-stop fixation, were added to suture-bridge repair, the retear rate associated with large and massive rotator cuff tears decreased [59].

Biomechanical Considerations for Rotator Cuff Repair

Cyclic loading of transosseous-equivalent suture-bridge repairs causes loosening of the bridging suture and medial tendon movement [45]. Adding medial mattress sutures significantly increases the failure load compared with that of suture-bridge repair only [36, 55]. In addition, the knots of medial mattress sutures decrease the gap between the edge of the supraspinatus tendon and the greater tuberosity [8]. These studies suggest that adding medial-row fixation to a knotless construct enhances the stability of rotator cuff repairs, ultimately improving patient outcomes.

In some studies, medial-row fixation has been associated with an increased retear rate at the musculotendinous junction, especially in cases of severe degeneration of the rotator cuff tendon [30, 76]. However, these findings do not necessarily support the conclusion that medial-row fixation worsens clinical outcome and the biomechanical properties of the repaired tendon, because many previous studies have shown the efficacy of double-row repair or suture-bridge repair with medial-row fixation [8, 9, 36, 46, 55, 74]. Rather, in some chronic rotator cuff tears, the medial-row fixation has to be placed in a severely degenerated and atrophied tendon or at the musculotendinous junction because of excessive shortening of the tendon portion, thus increasing the likelihood of retearing. In these cases, retear at the musculotendinous junction can be minimized by modifying the suturing technique. Increasing the bite size of the mattress stitches increases the strength of the repaired tendon with slightly mobile medial knots, which can be tightened by lateral fixation [82]. Another group reported that the sliding of sutures through tissue weakens the suture–tendon interface in mattress stitch constructs, suggesting that medial mattress stitches using "non-sliding" knots may decrease the rate of retear at the musculotendinous junction [81]. Moreover, increasing the number of sutures reportedly decreases cyclic gap formation and increases load to failure [35].

Other Surgical Options

The margin-convergence and interval-slide techniques have been introduced to obtain acceptable mobility of the torn tendon, especially in large and massive rotator cuff tears. However, in some studies, neither technique has yielded better clinical or structural outcomes than does a partial-repair strategy [39, 41].

Early suture-bridge repairs [72] paired a couple of medial mattress-suture configurations using 0.5-mm-diameter suture material (FiberWire, Arthrex, Naples, FL) with lateral fixation using knotless or suture anchors [55, 59, 72]. Recently, the suture-bridge procedure has shifted to a 4-strand, knotless, double-row construct using 2-mm-wide suture tapes [19, 85, 87]. In a comparison of an arthroscopic, tied, suture-bridging technique with knot-less bridging using suture tape [7], mean pain relief, range of motion, strength, and Constant score improved significantly in both groups. In addition, the two groups did not differ significantly during the post-operative period.

Multiple channeling in the greater tuberosity of the proximal humerus has been reported to improve the healing environment at the repair site of the rotator cuff tendon. Healing elements, including mesenchymal stem cells, are thought to migrate from the bone marrow cavity to the repair site through these multiple channels [34, 70]. In one study, multiple channeling significantly decreased the retear rate after arthroscopic rotator cuff repair [34].

A marginal dog-ear deformity is defined as a noncompression site at the tendon-to-bone interface that develops at the anterior and posterior aspects of the bridging suture limbs after repair with the suture-bridge technique. The dog-ear deformity is thought to interfere with rotator cuff healing and to cause retear initiating at the gap between the unhealed rotator cuff tendon and the greater tuberosity footprint [37, 38]. Compared with the conventional technique, a suture-bridge technique that was modified to prevent marginal dog-ear deformity significantly decreased the tendon retear rate after arthroscopic rotator cuff repair of full-thickness medium-sized to massive tears [78].

Irreparable Tears

Despite the many surgical options developed to increase the healing rate after the repair of rotator cuff tears, it never reaches 100%. Specifically, in chronic tears involving severely atrophied [3, 27, 49, 50, 68], fatty-infiltrated [3, 27, 49, 50, 68, 69], and retracted [3, 69] tendons, the retear rate after rotator cuff repair is relatively high [4, 39, 41]. Therefore, irreparable rotator cuff tears are those that affect severely degenerated tendons as well as those with a lateral edge that fails to reach the original footprint. The following section presents the published literature regarding alternative treatments for irreparable rotator cuff tears.

Superior Capsule Reconstruction

The most recently developed alternative surgery for irreparable rotator cuff tears is superior capsule reconstruction (Fig. 8.1) [57, 58]. The correct graft size is the most important point regarding this surgery: clinical outcome invariably is poor after complete re-tears and most partial re-tears. The optimal graft thickness is 6–8 mm; we achieved this thickness by folding the fascia lata. Typically we folded the fascia lata twice, but when the fascia lata was particularly thin, we folded the tissue three or four times. Also, the fascia lata includes an intermuscular septum that consists of the tissues of two tendons and connects the fascia lata to the femur. To make a thicker graft, this intermuscular septum should be included in the graft. We removed all fatty tissue and muscles from the graft. The medial side of the fascia lata was then attached to the superior glenoid by using two suture anchors. The lateral side of the graft was attached to the rotator cuff footprint on the greater tuberosity in 30° of shoulder abduction by using the compression double-row technique, which is a combination of the conventional double-row technique and the suture-bridge technique [56, 59], or SpeedBridge, and uses SwiveLock and FiberTape (Arthrex). Finally, side-to-side sutures were added between the graft and the infraspinatus – teres minor tendon and between the graft and the residual anterior supraspinatus – subscapularis tendon to improve force coupling in the shoulder joint [54].

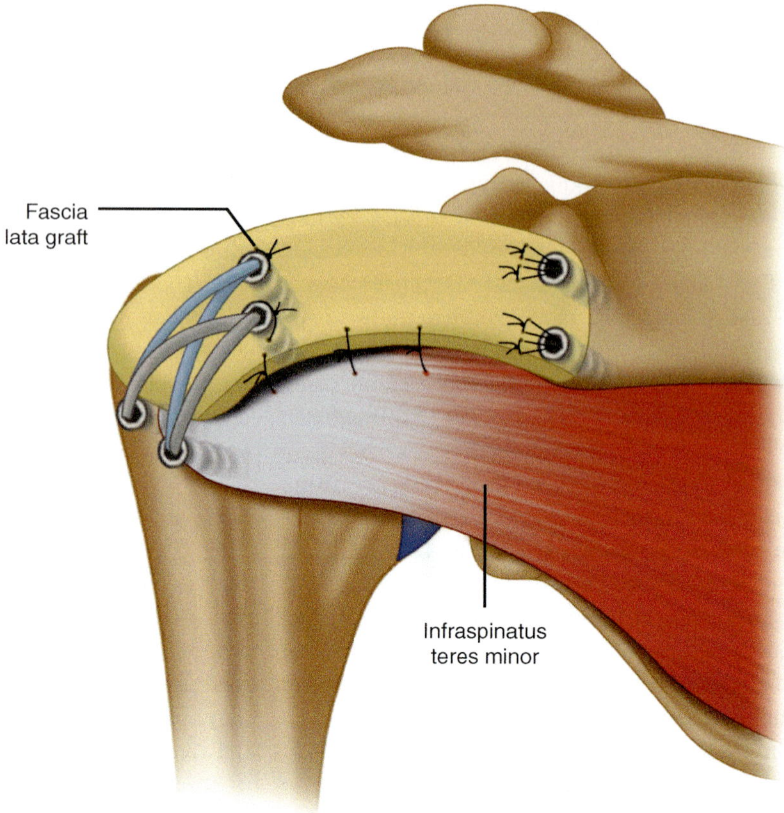

Fig. 8.1 Superior capsule reconstruction

In a biomechanical cadaveric study, superior capsule reconstruction using a fascia lata patch graft completely restored the superior stability of the glenohumeral joint, whereas patch grafting to the supraspinatus tendon only partially restored superior translation [58]. After arthroscopic superior capsule reconstruction, the mean active elevation increased from 91° to 147°, external rotation increased from 26° to 41°, and the American Shoulder and Elbow Surgeons score improved from 36 to 92 points. In addition, 95 of the 100 patients (95%) had no graft tear or tendon retear during follow-up (24–88 months) [56].

Reverse Total Shoulder Arthroplasty

Reverse total shoulder arthroplasty was developed to treat patients with pseudoparalysis due to cuff tear arthropathy. In a 5-year follow-up study [2], mean abduction improved from 64° to 100°, and forward flexion increased from 55° to 110°. In addition, the high rate of scapular notching did not affect overall functional outcomes. Another study assessed the clinical outcomes of 68 shoulders among patients with a mean age of 66 years (range, 53–84 years) and a minimum of 2 years of follow-up [79]. In this population, active anterior elevation significantly increased from 34° to 125°, and active external rotation decreased from 14.1° to 13.9°. These clinical results proved beneficial in terms of increased range of motion and improved pain relief [68]. However, the high rates of complications associated with reverse total shoulder arthroplasty remain a matter of concern. In previous studies, 13.3–32.8% of patients have required revision surgery owing to complications of reverse total shoulder arthroplasty [20, 90]. The most common complications of reverse total shoulder arthroplasty are hematoma [90], dislocation of the prosthesis [11, 90], acromial or spinal fracture [11, 14, 90], loosening of the glenoid component [11, 20, 79, 90], loosening of the prosthesis stem [11, 79, 90], infection [5, 11, 20, 79, 90], and nerve lesions [5, 79, 90].

Tendon Transfer

Tendon transfer protocols have been described as salvage procedures for irreparable posterosuperior rotator cuff tears. Specifically, transfer of the latissimus dorsi tendon was introduced to compensate for loss of function of the supraspinatus and infraspinatus tendons and to restore external rotation [23]. In another method, the tendon of the teres major is transferred to the insertion of the supraspinatus tendon on the greater tuberosity of the humerus. Among 28 consecutive patients (average age, 60 years) who underwent teres major tendon transfer to correct an irreparable posterosuperior rotator cuff tear after failed conservative or surgical treatment, the mean active abduction improved from 79° (range, 0°–150°) preoperatively to 105° (range, 20°–180°) postoperatively, and the mean active external rotation in 90° abduction improved from 25° (range, 0°–70°) to 55° (0°–90°) [10]. Developed to treat irreparable tears of the subscapularis, trapezius tendon transfer led to clinical improvements in pain, daily activity, and Constant scores, although active shoulder range of motion and strength remained unchanged [26].

Partial Rotator Cuff Repair

Partial rotator cuff repair, in which the torn tendons are repaired as much as possible, was developed as a means to improve shoulder function after irreparable rotator cuff tears. Among patients who underwent partial repair to treat large, retracted rotator cuff tears, the active range of motion improved from 133° of forward flexion before surgery to 163° afterward and from 111° of abduction preoperatively to 156° postoperatively [89]. However, among these same patients, the active range of external rotation decreased from 44° preoperatively to 36° postoperatively, and the mean acromiohumeral distance decreased from 7.0 mm before surgery to 5.6 mm after surgery [89]. In another study, partial repair for massive rotator cuff tears yielded clinical outcomes comparable to those after complete repair of tears [31].

My Treatment Strategy for Rotator Cuff Tears

Our surgical indication for the treatment of rotator cuff tears has been determined by using preoperative MRI to assess [1] muscle degeneration (MILD degeneration: fat area in the supraspinatus fossa is less than muscle area; SEVERE degeneration: fat area in the supraspinatus fossa is equal to or larger than muscle area); [2] tendon degeneration (MILD degeneration: slightly thinned, or slight fatty degeneration in the tendon part; SEVERE degeneration: markedly thinned, with fatty degeneration in the tendon part, or no tendon); and [3] tendon retraction (MILD retraction: the torn tendon edge is on the greater tuberosity or the lateral half of the humeral head; SEVERE retraction: the torn tendon edge lies in the medial half of the humeral head or on the glenoid) (Fig. 8.2). Patients with SEVERE degeneration or retraction in only one category or in none receives ARCR only; the patients with SEVERE degeneration or retraction in two or three of the supraspinatus assessment categories undergo arthroscopic SCR (Fig. 8.3). Reducibility of the torn rotator cuff tendons is assessed during diagnostic arthroscopy. For patients with SEVERE degeneration or retraction of the supraspinatus in two or three categories on the basis of the preoperative MRI and who are judged as having irreducible tears during diagnostic arthroscopy, SCR only is performed (Figs. 8.3, 8.4). When the torn tendon reaches the original footprint in patients with SEVERE degeneration or retraction in two or three categories according to preoperative MRI, arthroscopic SCR is performed for reinforcement, after which the torn tendon is repaired over a fascia lata graft (ARCR with SCR) (Figs. 8.3, 8.5).

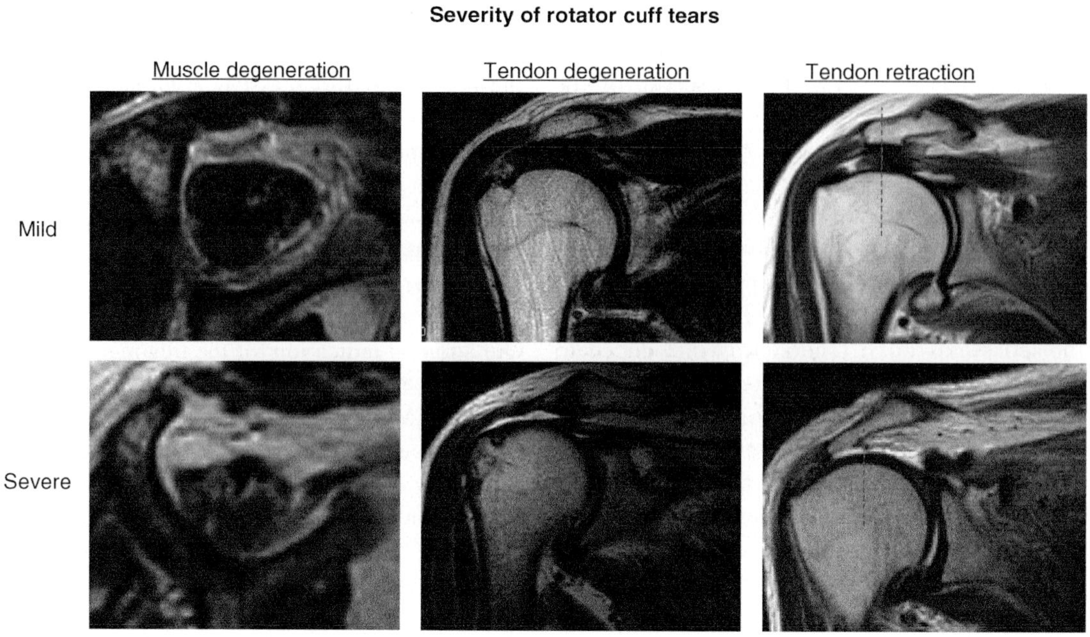

Fig. 8.2 Severity of degeneration in the torn supraspinatus tendon was evaluated by using preoperative MRI. (**a**) Muscle degeneration (MILD degeneration: fat area in the supraspinatus fossa is equal to or smaller than that in muscle, SEVERE degeneration: fat area in the supraspinatus fossa is larger than in muscle). (**b**) Tendon degeneration (MILD degeneration: slightly thinned, or slight fatty degeneration in the tendon part, SEVERE degeneration: severely thinned, with fatty degeneration in the tendon part, or no tendon). (**c**) Tendon retraction (MILD retraction: the torn tendon edge is located on the greater tuberosity or on the lateral half of the humeral head, SEVERE retraction: the torn tendon edge is located on the medial half of the humeral head or on the glenoid)

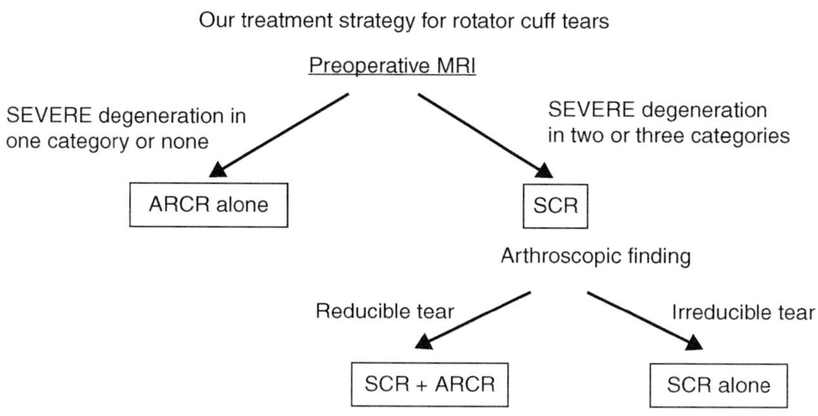

Fig. 8.3 Our treatment strategy for rotator cuff tears

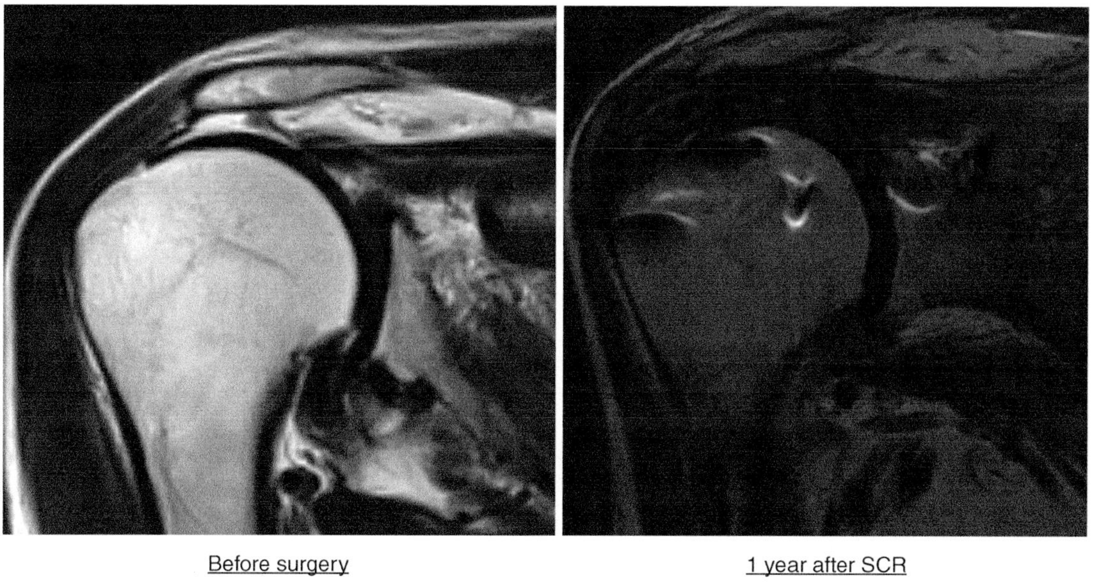

Fig. 8.4 Magnetic resonance imaging. (**a**) Coronal image before surgery. (**b**) Coronal image at 1 year after SCR

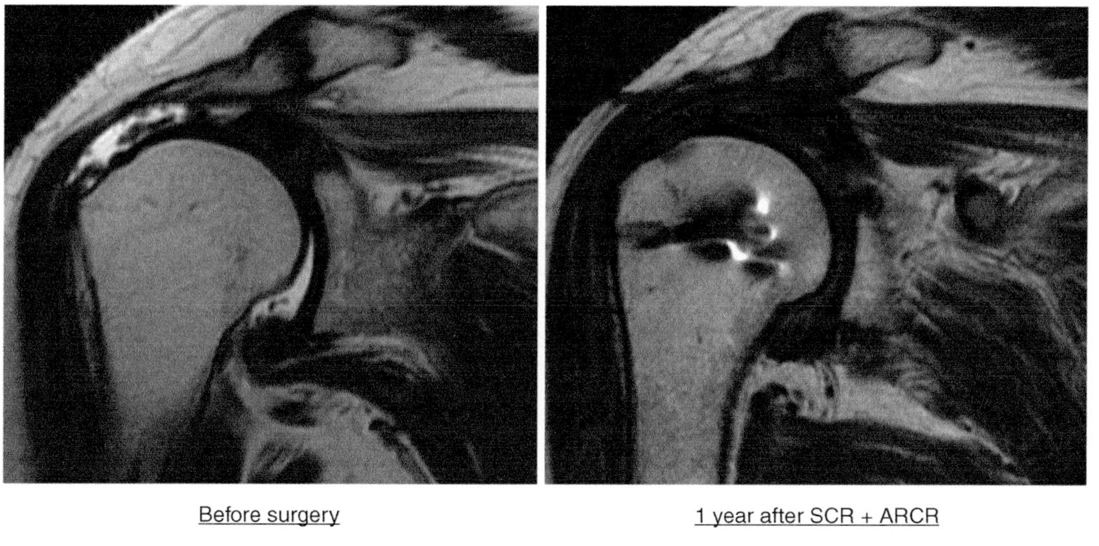

Fig. 8.5 Magnetic resonance imaging. (**a**) Coronal image before surgery. (**b**) Coronal image at 1 year after ARCR with SCR

Conclusions

Management of both reparable and irreparable rotator cuff tears is developing rapidly. Biomechanical studies are useful to improve surgical technique and provide better clinical outcome. Both clinical and biomechanical researches are expected to greatly contribute to the further development of management of rotator cuff tears.

Clinical Pearls

1. Patient's complaint and physical status must be assessed carefully to decide the most appropriate treatment for rotator cuff tears.
2. When surgical treatment is performed, the severity of the rotator cuff tears (muscle degeneration, tendon degeneration, and tendon retraction) should be evaluated by using preoperative MRI.
3. Superior capsule reconstruction is a reliable and useful alternative treatment for irreparable rotator cuff tears.
4. Superior capsule reconstruction for reinforcement prevents postoperative re-tear after arthroscopic rotator cuff repair and improved the quality of the repaired tendon on MRI.

References

1. Ahmad S, Haber M, Bokor DJ. The influence of intraoperative factors and postoperative rehabilitation compliance on the integrity of the rotator cuff after arthroscopic repair. J Shoulder Elb Surg. 2015;24:229–35.
2. Al-Hadithy N, Domos P, Sewell MD, Pandit R. Reverse shoulder arthroplasty in 41 patients with cuff tear arthropathy with a mean follow-up period of 5 years. J Shoulder Elb Surg. 2014;23:1662–8.
3. Bedi A, Dines J, Warren RF, Dines DM. Massive tears of the rotator cuff. J Bone Joint Surg Am. 2010;92:1894–908.
4. Berdusco R, Trantalis JN, Nelson AA, Sohmer S, More KD, Wong B, Boorman RS, Lo IK. Arthroscopic repair of massive, contracted, immobile tears using interval slides: clinical and MRI structural follow-up. Knee Surg Sports Traumatol Arthrosc. 2015;23:502–7.
5. Boileau P, Chuinard C, Roussanne Y, Bicknell RT, Rochet N, Trojani C. Reverse shoulder arthroplasty combined with a modified latissimus dorsi and teres major tendon transfer for shoulder pseudoparalysis associated with dropping arm. Clin Orthop Relat Res. 2008;466:584–93.
6. Boorman RS, More KD, Hollinshead RM, Wiley JP, Brett K, Mohtadi NG, Nelson AA, Lo IK, Bryant D. The rotator cuff quality-of-life index predicts the outcome of nonoperative treatment of patients with a chronic rotator cuff tear. J Bone Joint Surg Am. 2014;96:1883–8.
7. Boyer P, Bouthors C, Delcourt T, Stewart O, Hamida F, Mylle G, Massin P. Arthroscopic double-row cuff repair with suture-bridging: a structural and functional comparison of two techniques. Knee Surg Sports Traumatol Arthrosc. 2015;23:478–86.
8. Busfield BT, Glousman RE, McGarry MH, Tibone JE, Lee TQ. A biomechanical comparison of 2 technical variations of double-row rotator cuff fixation: the importance of medial row knots. Am J Sports Med. 2008;36:901–6.
9. Carbonel I, Martinez AA, Calvo A, Ripalda J, Herrera A. Single-row versus double-row arthroscopic repair in the treatment of rotator cuff tears: a prospective randomized clinical study. Int Orthop. 2012;36:1877–83.
10. Celli A, Marongiu MC, Rovesta C, Celli L. Transplant of the teres major in the treatment of irreparable injuries of the rotator cuff (long-term analysis of results). Chir Organi Mov. 2005;90:121–32.
11. Clark JC, Ritchie J, Song FS, Kissenberth MJ, Tolan SJ, Hart ND, Hawkins RJ. Complication rates, dislocation, pain, and postoperative range of motion after reverse shoulder arthroplasty in patients with and without repair of the subscapularis. J Shoulder Elb Surg. 2012;21:36–41.
12. Codman EA. The shoulder: rupture of the supraspinatus tendon and other lesions in or about the subacromial bursa. Boston: Thomas Todd; 1934. p. 65–107.
13. Cofield RH, Parvizi J, Hoffmeyer PJ, Lanzer WL, Ilstrup DM, Rowland CM. Surgical repair of chronic rotator cuff tears. A prospective long-term study. J Bone Joint Surg Am. 2001;83-A:71–7.
14. Crosby LA, Hamilton A, Twiss T. Scapula fractures after reverse total shoulder arthroplasty: classification and treatment. Clin Orthop Relat Res. 2011;469:2544–9.
15. Denard PJ, Jiwani AZ, Ladermann A, Burkhart SS. Long-term outcome of arthroscopic massive rotator cuff repair: the importance of double-row fixation. Arthroscopy. 2012;28:909–15.
16. Deutsch A, Altchek DW, Schwartz E, Otis JC, Warren RF. Radiologic measurement of superior displacement of the humeral head in the impingement syndrome. J Shoulder Elb Surg. 1996;5:186–93.
17. Duralde XA, Bair B. Massive rotator cuff tears: the result of partial rotator cuff repair. J Shoulder Elb Surg. 2005;14:121–7.
18. Dwyer T, Razmjou H, Holtby R. Full-thickness rotator cuff tears in patients younger than 55 years: clinical outcome of arthroscopic repair in comparison with older patients. Knee Surg Sports Traumatol Arthrosc. 2015;23:508–13.

19. El-Azab H, Buchmann S, Beitzel K, Waldt S, Imhoff AB. Clinical and structural evaluation of arthroscopic double-row suture-bridge rotator cuff repair: early results of a novel technique. Knee Surg Sports Traumatol Arthrosc. 2010;18:1730–7.
20. Frankle M, Siegal S, Pupello D, Saleem A, Mighell M, Vasey M. The reverse shoulder prosthesis for glenohumeral arthritis associated with severe rotator cuff deficiency. A minimum two-year follow-up study of sixty patients. J Bone Joint Surg Am. 2005;87:1697–705.
21. Fucentese SF, von Roll AL, Pfirrmann CW, Gerber C, Jost B. Evolution of nonoperatively treated symptomatic isolated full-thickness supraspinatus tears. J Bone Joint Surg Am. 2012;94:801–8.
22. Galatz LM, Ball CM, Teefey SA, Middleton WD, Yamaguchi K. The outcome and repair integrity of completely arthroscopically repaired large and massive rotator cuff tears. J Bone Joint Surg Am. 2004;86-A:219–24.
23. Gerber C. Latissimus dorsi transfer for the treatment of irreparable tears of the rotator cuff. Clin Orthop Relat Res. 1992:152–60.
24. Gerber C, Maquieira G, Espinosa N. Latissimus dorsi transfer for the treatment of irreparable rotator cuff tears. J Bone Joint Surg Am. 2006;88:113–20.
25. Gialanella B, Prometti P. Effects of corticosteroids injection in rotator cuff tears. Pain Med. 2011;12:1559–65.
26. Goutallier D, De Abreu L, Postel JM, Le Guilloux P, Radier C, Zilber S. Is the trapezius transfer a useful treatment option for irreparable tears of the subscapularis? Orthop Traumatol Surg Res. 2011;97:719–25.
27. Goutallier D, Postel JM, Bernageau J, Lavau L, Voisin MC. Fatty muscle degeneration in cuff ruptures. Pre- and postoperative evaluation by CT scan. Clin Orthop Relat Res. 1994;304:78–83.
28. Harris JD, Pedroza A, Jones GL. Predictors of pain and function in patients with symptomatic, atraumatic full-thickness rotator cuff tears: a time-zero analysis of a prospective patient cohort enrolled in a structured physical therapy program. Am J Sports Med. 2012;40:359–66.
29. Hartzler RU, Sperling JW, Schleck CD, Cofield RH. Clinical and radiographic factors influencing the results of revision rotator cuff repair. Int J Shoulder Surg. 2013;7:41–5.
30. Hayashida K, Tanaka M, Koizumi K, Kakiuchi M. Characteristic retear patterns assessed by magnetic resonance imaging after arthroscopic double-row rotator cuff repair. Arthroscopy. 2012;28:458–64.
31. Iagulli ND, Field LD, Hobgood ER, Ramsey JR, Savoie FH 3rd. Comparison of partial versus complete arthroscopic repair of massive rotator cuff tears. Am J Sports Med. 2012;40:1022–6.
32. Itoi E. Rotator cuff tear: physical examination and conservative treatment. J Orthop Sci. 2013;18:197–204.
33. Ji X, Bi C, Wang F, Wang Q. Arthroscopic versus mini-open rotator cuff repair: an up-to-date meta-analysis of randomized controlled trials. Arthroscopy. 2015;31:118–24.
34. Jo CH, Shin JS, Park IW, Kim H, Lee SY. Multiple channeling improves the structural integrity of rotator cuff repair. Am J Sports Med. 2013;41:2650–7.
35. Jost PW, Khair MM, Chen DX, Wright TM, Kelly AM, Rodeo SA. Suture number determines strength of rotator cuff repair. J Bone Joint Surg Am. 2012;94:e100, e1–7.
36. Kaplan K, Elattrache NS, Vazquez O, Chen YJ, Lee T. Knotless rotator cuff repair in an external rotation model: the importance of medial-row horizontal mattress sutures. Arthroscopy. 2011;27:471–8.
37. Kim KC, Rhee KJ, Shin HD. Deformities associated with the suture-bridge technique for full-thickness rotator cuff tears. Arthroscopy. 2008;24:1251–7.
38. Kim KC, Rhee KJ, Shin HD, Kim YM. A modified suture-bridge technique for a marginal dog-ear deformity caused during rotator cuff repair. Arthroscopy. 2007;23:562 e1–4.
39. Kim KC, Shin HD, Cha SM, Kim JH. Repair integrity and functional outcomes for arthroscopic margin convergence of rotator cuff tears. J Bone Joint Surg Am. 2013;95:536–41.
40. Kim KC, Shin HD, Lee WY, Han SC. Repair integrity and functional outcome after arthroscopic rotator cuff repair: double-row versus suture-bridge technique. Am J Sports Med. 2012;40:294–9.
41. Kim SJ, Kim SH, Lee SK, Seo JW, Chun YM. Arthroscopic repair of massive contracted rotator cuff tears: aggressive release with anterior and posterior interval slides do not improve cuff healing and integrity. J Bone Joint Surg Am. 2013;95:1482–8.
42. Koh KH, Kang KC, Lim TK, Shon MS, Yoo JC. Prospective randomized clinical trial of single- versus double-row suture anchor repair in 2- to 4-cm rotator cuff tears: clinical and magnetic resonance imaging results. Arthroscopy. 2011;27:453–62.
43. Krischak G, Gebhard F, Reichel H, Friemert B, Schneider F, Fisser C, Kaluscha R, Kraus M. A prospective randomized controlled trial comparing occupational therapy with home-based exercises in conservative treatment of rotator cuff tears. J Shoulder Elb Surg. 2013;22:1173–9.
44. Kuhn JE, Dunn WR, Sanders R, An Q, Baumgarten KM, Bishop JY, Brophy RH, Carey JL, Holloway BG, Jones GL, Ma CB, Marx RG, McCarty EC, Poddar SK, Smith MV, Spencer EE, Vidal AF, Wolf BR, Wright RW. Effectiveness of physical therapy in treating atraumatic full-thickness rotator cuff tears: a multicenter prospective cohort study. J Shoulder Elb Surg. 2013;22:1371–9.
45. Kummer F, Hergan DJ, Thut DC, Pahk B, Jazrawi LM. Suture loosening and its effect on tendon fixation in knotless double-row rotator cuff repairs. Arthroscopy. 2011;27:1478–84.
46. Lapner PL, Sabri E, Rakhra K, McRae S, Leiter J, Bell K, Macdonald P. A multicenter randomized controlled trial comparing single-row with double-row fixation in arthroscopic rotator cuff repair. J Bone Joint Surg Am. 2012;94:1249–57.
47. Lee KW, Seo DW, Bae KW, Choy WS. Clinical and radiological evaluation after arthroscopic rotator cuff

repair using suture bridge technique. Clin Orthop Surg. 2013;5:306–13.
48. Ma HL, Chiang ER, Wu HT, Hung SC, Wang ST, Liu CL, Chen TH. Clinical outcome and imaging of arthroscopic single-row and double-row rotator cuff repair: a prospective randomized trial. Arthroscopy. 2012;28:16–24.
49. Melis B, Nemoz C, Walch G. Muscle fatty infiltration in rotator cuff tears: descriptive analysis of 1688 cases. Orthop Traumatol Surg Res. 2009;95:319–24.
50. Melis B, Wall B, Walch G. Natural history of infraspinatus fatty infiltration in rotator cuff tears. J Shoulder Elb Surg. 2010;19:757–63.
51. Merolla G, Bianchi P, Porcellini G. Ultrasound-guided subacromial injections of sodium hyaluronate for the management of rotator cuff tendinopathy: a prospective comparative study with rehabilitation therapy. Musculoskelet Surg. 2013;97(Suppl 1):49–56.
52. Meyer M, Klouche S, Rousselin B, Boru B, Bauer T, Hardy P. Does arthroscopic rotator cuff repair actually heal? Anatomic evaluation with magnetic resonance arthrography at minimum 2 years follow-up. J Shoulder Elb Surg. 2012;21:531–6.
53. Mihata T. Current concepts: arthroscopic treatment of articular-sided partial-thickness rotator cuff tears. In: Park JY, editor. Sports injuries to the shoulder and elbow. Heidelberg: Springer; 2015. p. 85–97.
54. Mihata T. Superior capsule reconstruction for irreparable rotator cuff tears. In: Tamai K, editor. Advances in shoulder surgery. Tokyo: Springer JP; 2015.
55. Mihata T, Fukuhara T, Jun BJ, Watanabe C, Kinoshita M. Effect of shoulder abduction angle on biomechanical properties of the repaired rotator cuff tendons with 3 types of double-row technique. Am J Sports Med. 2011;39:551–6.
56. Mihata T, Lee TQ, Fukunishi K, Itami Y, Fujisawa Y, Kawakami T, Ohue M, Neo M. Return to sports and physical work after arthroscopic superior capsule reconstruction in patients with irreparable rotator cuff tears. Am J Sports Med. 2018;46:1077–83.
57. Mihata T, Lee TQ, Watanabe C, Fukunishi K, Ohue M, Tsujimura T, Kinoshita M. Clinical results of arthroscopic superior capsule reconstruction for irreparable rotator cuff tears. Arthroscopy. 2013;29:459–70.
58. Mihata T, McGarry MH, Pirolo JM, Kinoshita M, Lee TQ. Superior capsule reconstruction to restore superior stability in irreparable rotator cuff tears: a biomechanical cadaveric study. Am J Sports Med. 2012;40:2248–55.
59. Mihata T, Watanabe C, Fukunishi K, Ohue M, Tsujimura T, Fujiwara K, Kinoshita M. Functional and structural outcomes of single-row versus double-row versus combined double-row and suture-bridge repair for rotator cuff tears. Am J Sports Med. 2011;39:2091–8.
60. Minagawa H, Yamamoto N, Abe H, Fukuda M, Seki N, Kikuchi K, Kijima H, Itoi E. Prevalence of symptomatic and asymptomatic rotator cuff tears in the general population: from mass-screening in one village. J Orthop. 2013;10:8–12.
61. Moghtaderi A, Sajadiyeh S, Khosrawi S, Dehghan F, Bateni V. Effect of subacromial sodium hyaluronate injection on rotator cuff disease: a double-blind placebo-controlled clinical trial. Adv Biomed Res. 2013;2:89.
62. Moor BK, Wieser K, Slankamenac K, Gerber C, Bouaicha S. Relationship of individual scapular anatomy and degenerative rotator cuff tears. J Shoulder Elb Surg. 2014;23:536–41.
63. Moosmayer S, Lund G, Seljom US, Haldorsen B, Svege IC, Hennig T, Pripp AH, Smith HJ. Tendon repair compared with physiotherapy in the treatment of rotator cuff tears: a randomized controlled study in 103 cases with a five-year follow-up. J Bone Joint Surg Am. 2014;96:1504–14.
64. Moosmayer S, Tariq R, Stiris M, Smith HJ. The natural history of asymptomatic rotator cuff tears: a three-year follow-up of fifty cases. J Bone Joint Surg Am. 2013;95:1249–55.
65. Moraiti C, Valle P, Maqdes A, Boughebri O, Dib C, Giakas G, Kany J, Elkholti K, Garret J, Katz D, Leclere FM, Valenti P. Comparison of functional gains after arthroscopic rotator cuff repair in patients over 70 years of age versus patients under 50 years of age: a prospective multicenter study. Arthroscopy. 2015;31:184–90.
66. Neer CS 2nd. Anterior acromioplasty for the chronic impingement syndrome in the shoulder: a preliminary report. J Bone Joint Surg Am. 1972;54:41–50.
67. Oh JH, Kim SH, Choi JA, Kim Y, Oh CH. Reliability of the grading system for fatty degeneration of rotator cuff muscles. Clin Orthop Relat Res. 2010;468:1558–64.
68. Oh JH, Kim SH, Choi JA, Kim Y, Oh CH. Reliability of the grading system for fatty degeneration of rotator cuff muscles. Clin Orthop Relat Res. 2009;468:1558–64.
69. Oh JH, Kim SH, Kang JY, Oh CH, Gong HS. Effect of age on functional and structural outcome after rotator cuff repair. Am J Sports Med. 2010;38:672–8.
70. Osti L, Del Buono A, Maffulli N. Microfractures at the rotator cuff footprint: a randomised controlled study. Int Orthop. 2013;37:2165–71.
71. Park JY, Lee SY, Chung SW, Zulkifli H, Cho JH, Oh KS. Clinical comparison between double-row and transosseous-equivalent repairs for medium to large size rotator cuff tears. Arch Orthop Trauma Surg. 2013;133:1727–34.
72. Park MC, Elattrache NS, Ahmad CS, Tibone JE. "Transosseous-equivalent" rotator cuff repair technique. Arthroscopy. 2006;22:1360 e1–5.
73. Paxton ES, Teefey SA, Dahiya N, Keener JD, Yamaguchi K, Galatz LM. Clinical and radiographic outcomes of failed repairs of large or massive rotator cuff tears: minimum ten-year follow-up. J Bone Joint Surg Am. 2013;95:627–32.
74. Prasathaporn N, Kuptniratsaikul S, Kongrukgreatiyos K. Single-row repair versus double-row repair of full-thickness rotator cuff tears. Arthroscopy. 2011;27:978–85.
75. Ramirez J, Pomes I, Cabrera S, Pomes J, Sanmarti R, Canete JD. Incidence of full-thickness rotator cuff tear

after subacromial corticosteroid injection: a 12-week prospective study. Mod Rheumatol. 2014;24:667–70.
76. Rhee YG, Cho NS, Parke CS. Arthroscopic rotator cuff repair using modified Mason-Allen medial row stitch: knotless versus knot-tying suture bridge technique. Am J Sports Med. 2012;40:2440–7.
77. Rockwood CA Jr, Williams GR Jr, Burkhead WZ Jr. Debridement of degenerative, irreparable lesions of the rotator cuff. J Bone Joint Surg Am. 1995;77:857–66.
78. Ryu KJ, Kim BH, Lee Y, Lee YS, Kim JH. Modified suture-bridge technique to prevent a marginal dog-ear deformity improves structural integrity after rotator cuff repair. Am J Sports Med. 2015;43:597–605.
79. Sadoghi P, Vavken P, Leithner A, Hochreiter J, Weber G, Pietschmann MF, Muller PE. Impact of previous rotator cuff repair on the outcome of reverse shoulder arthroplasty. J Shoulder Elb Surg. 2011;20:1138–46.
80. Safran O, Schroeder J, Bloom R, Weil Y, Milgrom C. Natural history of nonoperatively treated symptomatic rotator cuff tears in patients 60 years old or younger. Am J Sports Med. 2011;39:710–4.
81. Savage AJ, Spruiell MD, Schwertz JM, McGwin G, Eberhardt A, Ponce BA. The effect of sliding knots on the suture-tendon interface strength: a biomechanical analysis comparing sliding and static arthroscopic knots. Am J Sports Med. 2013;41:296–301.
82. Tamboli M, Mihata T, Hwang J, McGarry MH, Kang Y, Lee TQ. Biomechanical characteristics of the horizontal mattress stitch: implication for double-row and suture-bridge rotator cuff repair. J Orthop Sci. 2014;19:235–41.
83. Tanaka M, Itoi E, Sato K, Hamada J, Hitachi S, Tojo Y, Honda M, Tabata S. Factors related to successful outcome of conservative treatment for rotator cuff tears. Ups J Med Sci. 2010;115:193–200.
84. Umans HR, Pavlov H, Berkowitz M, Warren RF. Correlation of radiographic and arthroscopic findings with rotator cuff tears and degenerative joint disease. J Shoulder Elb Surg. 2001;10:428–33.
85. Vaishnav S, Millett PJ. Arthroscopic rotator cuff repair: scientific rationale, surgical technique, and early clinical and functional results of a knotless self-reinforcing double-row rotator cuff repair system. J Shoulder Elb Surg. 2010;19:83–90.
86. van der Zwaal P, Thomassen BJ, Nieuwenhuijse MJ, Lindenburg R, Swen JW, van Arkel ER. Clinical outcome in all-arthroscopic versus mini-open rotator cuff repair in small to medium-sized tears: a randomized controlled trial in 100 patients with 1-year follow-up. Arthroscopy. 2013;29:266–73.
87. Voigt C, Bosse C, Vosshenrich R, Schulz AP, Lill H. Arthroscopic supraspinatus tendon repair with suture-bridging technique: functional outcome and magnetic resonance imaging. Am J Sports Med. 2010;38:983–91.
88. Walton JR, Murrell GA. A two-year clinical outcomes study of 400 patients, comparing open surgery and arthroscopy for rotator cuff repair. Bone Joint Res. 2012;1:210–7.
89. Wellmann M, Lichtenberg S, da Silva G, Magosch P, Habermeyer P. Results of arthroscopic partial repair of large retracted rotator cuff tears. Arthroscopy. 2013;29:1275–82.
90. Werner CM, Steinmann PA, Gilbart M, Gerber C. Treatment of painful pseudoparesis due to irreparable rotator cuff dysfunction with the Delta III reverse-ball-and-socket total shoulder prosthesis. J Bone Joint Surg Am. 2005;87:1476–86.

Calcific Tendinitis

9

Simon Boyle and Geoffrey C. S. Smith

Introduction

Intra-tendinous calcific deposition has been referred to as calcifying tendinitis, calcific tendinitis, calcified tendinitis, calcareous tendinitis, tendinosis calcarea, calcific periarthritis and periarticular apatite deposition. Whilst any tendinous insertion may be affected, the shoulder and the hip are the most commonly involved sites in clinical practice. The variable nomenclature of this condition reflects the lack of understanding of the pathogenesis and that different pathological processes may be involved at different sites.

Intra-tendinous calcific deposition in the rotator cuff may be due to calcific tendinitis or dystrophic calcification. Calcific tendinitis is characterized by the deposition of calcium hydroxyapatite within a viable healthy tendon [1, 2]. The area of calcification in calcific tendinitis typically occurs in the mid-substance of the tendon, approximately 1–2 cm proximal to its insertion. In contrast, dystrophic calcification occurs within a degenerate tendon close to its insertion or around the edge of a rotator cuff tear. Calcium may be deposited as a variety of crystals in dystrophic calcification (calcium pyrophosphate, hydroxyapatite, tri-calcium phosphate) [3]. Dystrophic calcification is sometimes referred to as insertional calcific tendinitis, however this terminology implies a common pathogenesis and pathology which is most likely to be inaccurate.

Background

Epidemiology

Bosworth first reported an incidence of 2.7% of calcification within the subacromial space with 35% of shoulders being symptomatic [4].

Louwerens et al. later identified calcification in the rotator cuff in 7.8% of asymptomatic patients and calcification was found to be present in 42.5% of patients with subacromial pain syndrome [5]. Calcific tendinitis tends to affect patients between 30 and 60 years of age and is slightly more common in women [6, 7]. Most patients have sedentary or low demand occupations [8].

Aetiology & Pathogenesis

The aetiology and pathogenesis of calcific tendinitis in the shoulder has been controversial with two predominant theories:

Multiphasic theory/Reactive calcification – Uhthoff postulated that the condition is predominantly cell-mediated in which chondrocytes appear within the tendon and as a result calcifica-

S. Boyle (✉)
York Teaching Hospital, York, UK

G. C. S. Smith
St George Hospital, Sydney, NSW, Australia

I. A. Trail et al. (eds.), *Textbook of Shoulder Surgery*, https://doi.org/10.1007/978-3-319-70099-1_9

tion occurs. The area of calcification is phagocytosed after a period of time and is replaced by normal tendon [9]. This process is considered to be different from that which leads to calcific tendinitis at other sites [10].

Degenerative theory – Codman originally proposed a degenerative process that is identical to that which results in rotator cuff tears, with calcification developing secondarily in areas of degenerate tissue [11, 12].

The natural history of eventual resolution of calcific tendinitis, its epidemiology (relatively young age, increased incidence in sedentary occupations and females) and pathology (occurrence in viable tissue, different composition of calcium compounds) support the multiphasic theory, whilst the degenerative theory supports the formation of dystrophic calcification.

Uhthoff and Loehr [9] described calcific tendinitis occurring as a three-phase process: pre-calcific, calcific and post-calcific. All phases may occur simultaneously in the same tendon.

Pre-calcific Phase

This is characterized by a fibrocartilaginous metaplasia. This period is usually asymptomatic.

Calcification Phase

Characterized by formation of the calcium deposit. This is divided into three subphases:

(a) Formative: calcium crystals are deposited primarily in matrix vesicles that coalesce to form large foci of calcification separated by chondrocytes, fibrocartilaginous and fibrocollagenous septae. The calcific deposit appears chalky during this phase.
(b) Resting: The formative phase ends when fibrocollagenous tissue borders the areas of calcification. This period is variable in length.
(c) Resorptive: Neoangiogenesis, beginning at the periphery of the deposit develops. Infiltration of macrophages and multinucleated giant cells is evident. These surround the deposit and phagocytose the calcium. This is the most painful period. The calcium deposit is liquefied and has a toothpaste-like consistency.

Post-calcific Phase

The calcific deposit disappears and is replaced by normal appearing rotator cuff tendon.

It is widely accepted that the chondrocytes are linked to the formation of the calcific deposits. The origin of the chondrocytes may be the metaplastic transformation of tenocytes into chondrocytes [9] or the differentiation of tendon derived stem cells [13]. The molecular pathways involved in the pathogenesis of calcific tendinitis remain largely unresolved and are an area of ongoing research but there is evidence for the involvement of extracellular matrix proteins such as osteopontin, cathepsin K, and BMP's [10].

Pathology

Loew et al. demonstrated that the supraspinatus tendon was most commonly affected either alone (63%) or combined with a deposit in the subscapularis (20%). Isolated deposits in the infraspinatus (7%) and subscapularis (3%) are uncommon [14].

Associated Conditions

Ischemic heart disease, hypertension, diabetes and endocrine diseases (in particular hypothyroidism) are known associated medical conditions that seem to predispose patients to the development of calcific tendinitis. Patients with endocrine diseases have an earlier age of onset of symptoms, a longer disease course, and more recalcitrant symptoms that require surgery more frequently [15].

Presentation

The presentation of calcific tendinitis depends on the stage of the disease process. Symptoms may be absent in the precalcification stage and in the formative and resting phase. However large deposits may cause impingement symptoms. During the resorptive phase, the pain can so severe and relatively acute in onset that it may mimic a septic arthritis. There may be concomitant stiffness giving rise to a picture of adhesive capsulitis. Because of the prevalence of asymptomatic intra-tendinous calcification consideration must be given to other causes of shoulder pain.

Investigations

Usually the diagnosis is made based on the clinical features and radiographic findings. Occasionally inflammatory markers and an glenohumeral aspiration may be required if there is a clinical suggestion of septic arthritis.

Imaging

A standard shoulder radiographic series, including anteroposterior (AP), Grashey, outlet, and axillary views are recommended. Plain films are useful for monitoring progression and/or resorption. In calcific tendinitis the typical location of calcification is within 1.5 to 2 cm from the tendon insertion on the greater tuberosity. Deposits within the supraspinatus can best be seen in neutral rotation, whilst those in the infraspinatus and teres minor may be seen in internal rotation. The axillary view is useful to diagnose deposits in the subscapularis. Deposits are usually well-visualized during the formative phase as homogenous masses with clearly-defined borders. During the resorptive phase, some fragmentation of the calcific deposit can be seen.

In dystrophic calcification the area of calcification is localised more towards the tendon insertion and tend to have a more stippled appearance.

Ultrasound or MRI may be useful if additional pathology is suspected. Areas of calcification are of low signal intensity on all MRI sequences. On T2 weighted images there may be an area of surrounding oedema which should not be confused with a rotator cuff tear. Calcific regions appear as hyperechoic foci on USS often with acoustic shadowing.

Radiographic Classification

Multiple radiographic classifications have been proposed based on size and morphology, each with significant inter-observer variability. In general, the lesion appears dense, homogenous and well-defined during the formative phase whereas during the resorptive phase, the lesion is irregularly dense and not clearly delineated, with a fluffy or cloud-like appearance [16, 17].

Radiographic Classification of Calcific Tendinitis		
Gartner and Heyer [16]	I	Well circumscribed, dense (Fig. 9.1)
	II	Soft contour/dense or sharp/transparent
	III	Translucent and cloudy appearance without clear circumscription
Mole [17]	A	Dense, homogeneous, sharp contours
	B	Dense, segmented, sharp contours (Fig. 9.2)
	C	Heterogeneous, soft contours
	D	Dystrophic calcifications at cuff insertions

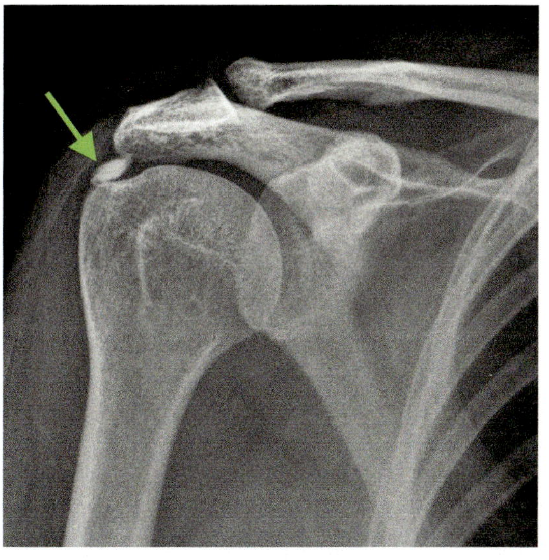

Fig. 9.1 Well circumscribed dense deposit - Gartland and Heyer grade I

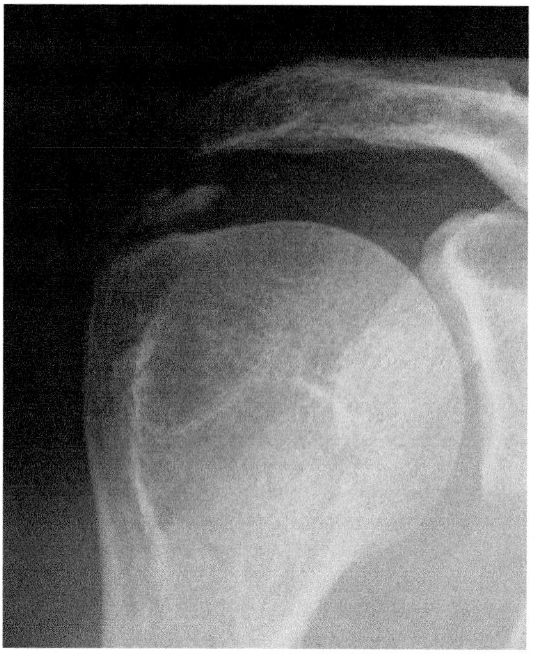

Fig. 9.2 Dense segmented deposit - Mole Type B

Treatment

Conservative Management

Calcific tendinitis is generally a self-limiting condition and as such, the first line of treatment should be non-surgical. In the first instance, activity modification, non-steroidal anti-inflammatory drugs (NSAID's) and gentle physiotherapy should be considered. Noel [18] reported good to excellent results in 50% of 125 patients managed non-operatively by 6 months. Ogon et al. [19] examined the prognostic factors related to the success or failure of conservative management in their study of 488 shoulders. They found that analgesia and corticosteroid injections were successful in treating 73% of cases of chronic symptomatic calcific tendinitis. Failure of this treatment approach was more likely when the disease was bilateral, when the deposits were found in the superior aspect of the cuff, where deposits extended medial to the undersurface of the acromion and with large volume deposits.

Cho et al. [20] found in their study of 92 shoulders that 60% of deposits decreased in size during the study period (12–42 months) with the use of NSAID's and physiotherapy. Overall, they achieved 72% good to excellent results with conservative management.

Sub-Acromial Injections

Infiltration of local anaesthetic and corticosteroid into the subacromial space is an easily performed intervention for pain arising from calcific tendinitis. This can be performed in the office/clinic environment and usually leads to a rapid improvement in painful symptoms.

A recent RCT suggests that there is no discernible clinical difference for the effectiveness of injections performed blind or under ultrasound guidance when used to manage the pain of impingement syndrome [21]. It is worth noting that animal studies suggest that repeated use of steroid injections can be harmful to rotator cuff tendons and has a negative effect on bone mineral density in the tuberosity [22].

Ultrasound Guided Needle Aspiration and Barbotage (UGNB)

Where these initial conservative measures have failed, further treatments can be employed to both improve the pain from calcific tendinitis and to encourage deposit resorption and resolution. Needle aspiration and barbotage is one such option to achieve both these goals. This is best performed under ultrasound guidance to allow accurate visualisation and localisation of the deposit. Aspiration can be performed using a one or two needle technique [23]. In the one needle technique, the needle is inserted into the deposit and an attempt at aspiration made. Should this fail to yield any calcium then 2–3 mls of saline can be introduced and re-aspirated. This will often result in a cloudy aspirate within the syringe (Fig. 9.3). An alternative is to use two needles in an inflow/outflow system. Both techniques are continued until the cloudy aspirate becomes clear.

If it is not possible to aspirate any calcium, then multiple perforations/punctures can be per-

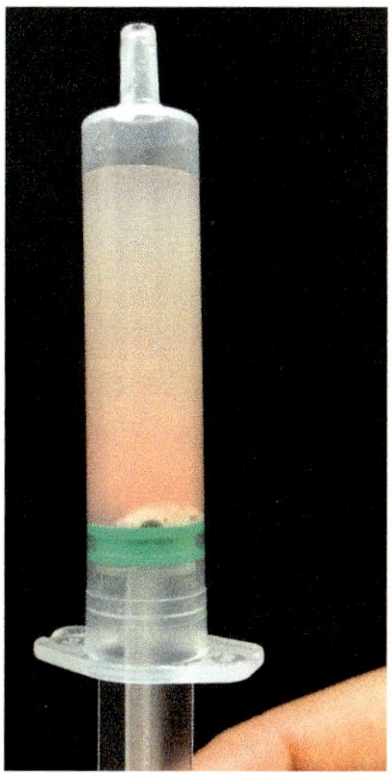

Fig. 9.3 Aspirate of calcific deposit - calcific sediment can be seen at the base of the syringe

formed to decompress the deposit. It is thought that this decompression promotes the subsequent resorption of the deposit. This procedure can be supplemented with a subacromial injection of local anaesthetic and corticosteroid to improve post procedural pain. Yoo et al. [24] report in their cohort of 35 shoulders that deposit aspiration was possible in only 20% of cases with the remaining shoulders requiring barbotage decompression. Overall, they found 71.4% of patients experienced almost complete resolution of pain by 6 months. Painful symptoms were more likely to persist in those patients whose deposit size had failed to reduce by 6 months post treatment. Furthermore, needle barbotage had a higher failure rate in SFA type A [17] deposits (sharply delineated, dense and homogeneous) as compared to type B deposits (sharply delineated, dense and multilobulated). Deposit morphology was found to influence the outcome of UGNB in a further study by Oodelar et al. [25]. They reported that the need for multiple procedures was more likely in Gartner and Heyer type I deposits and that smoking was an independent risk factor for overall treatment failure.

Needle decompression can be uncomfortable and as such, patients are advised to rest and take NSAID's for the first 48 h post procedure. Occasionally sedation may be used for the duration of the procedure where a patient is particularly anxious.

When UGNB alone is compared with UGNB combined with subacromial injections of corticosteroids for calcific tendinitis, clinically and radiologically superior results are seen at 1-year post intervention in those cases where steroids have been infiltrated [26]. However these outcomes appear to be equal by 5 years [27].

Complications are uncommon from this form of treatment but can include syncope [28], bursitis [29] and adhesive capsulitis.

Extracorporeal Shockwave Therapy (ESWT)

ESWT is a non-invasive procedure that is used to encourage the breakdown and resorption of calcific deposits and is easy to perform in a clinic setting. ESWT utilises acoustic shock waves which are generated by either electrohydraulic, piezoelectric or electromagnetic devices. The amount of energy released is quantified by area and is known as the Energy Flux Density (EFD – mJ/mm^2). Arbitrarily, the energy values have been stratified into low energy ESWT (energy flux density below 0.08 mJ/mm^2), medium energy (0.08 to 0.28 mJ/mm^2) and high energy ESWT (0.28–0.60 mJ/mm^2) [30]. Ultrasound scanning or fluoroscopy can be used in conjunction to enable the shock waves to be focussed on the cuff areas containing the deposits. Alternatively, some operators elect to focus the shock waves on the area of maximal tenderness in the cuff. The shock waves are then delivered by a probe. The delivery frequency (no. of shocks per minute), total no. of shocks and total energy (mJ/mm^2) varies between operators. As this can be a painful procedure, analgesia and local anaesthetic patches can be used to reduce discomfort.

The mechanisms through which ESWT exerts its effects are thought to be both mechanical and cellular. The mechanical effect occurs due to the increase in pressure inside the deposit leading to fragmentation. The cellular/molecular effect arises as a result of an inflammatory response, neovascularisation and leucocyte chemotaxis.

This eventually leads to phagocytosis of the deposit. Daeke et al. [31] performed a 4 year follow up study with regard to the effects of ESWT for calcific tendinitis. They reported 78–87% patient reported successful outcome but conceded that by 4 years 20% of their original 115 patients had undergone surgical intervention. Patients who had complete radiographic resorption of the deposit reported superior subjective success rates compared to those with partial resorption (80% vs 52%).

Several studies have been undertaken to determine the most effective energy dose of ESWT to be applied. Overall, high energy therapy seems to result in better clinical outcomes than low energy treatment although there is no consensus as to the most effective energy flux density, number of pulses or the number of sessions required [32–35]. Gerdesmeyer et al. [34] compared the effectiveness of high energy therapy vs low energy vs sham treatment in 144 patients. They found significantly greater improvements in the Constant scores in the high energy treatment group over both the low energy and sham groups.

Greater effectiveness can also be seen for both pain and function scores at up to 1 year where the therapy is focused on the calcific deposit rather than the tender areas of the greater tuberosity [36].

A large variation exists as to the radiological response to ESWT. Albert et al. [32] reported just 15% complete resorption of the deposits at 3 months in their trial using high energy ESWT whereas Gerdesmeyer et al. report 86% resorption by 1 year [34]. Despite these differing results, both studies demonstrated good functional and pain improvements.

Kim et al. [37] compared UGNB (with subacromial steroid infiltration but without deposit aspiration) and ESWT in an RCT including 54 patients. They reported a significant improvement in pain and outcome scores in both groups, however the greater effects were seen in the group who underwent needling. A similar significant difference was seen between the two groups when reduction in deposit size was compared (72.2% complete resolution in the needling group vs 42.6% in the ESWT group).

Krasny et al. [38] performed an RCT comparing one group treated with UGNB alone with a further group who were treated with ESWT combined with UGNB. They reported improved results in both groups but with significantly better pain and outcome scores as well as better deposit resorption in the combined treatment group (60% vs 32.5%). Despite this evidence for combination treatment, most clinicians tend to opt for single therapy.

Complications of ESWT include pain, erythema, subcutaneous haematomas and very rarely cases of avascular necrosis have been reported [39].

Other Non-operative Therapies

Further treatment modalities have been used in the treatment of calcific tendinitis in the shoulder including therapeutic ultrasound [40], laser therapy and platelet rich plasma [41]. Unfortunately these tend to be small studies and case series and as such there is insufficient evidence to be able to recommend these in the routine treatment of calcific tendinitis

Surgery

Despite the relative success of non-operative treatments, some patients will continue to struggle with pain that affects their activities of daily living. In these patients, surgery offers a viable option to improve their symptoms. Historically this procedure was performed through an open approach [42] using a deltoid split, however the increased familiarity of shoulder arthroscopy now makes these open approaches less common. Early case series comparing both open and arthroscopic techniques showed good outcomes. This was confirmed in a small RCT by Rubenthaler et al. in 2003 [43] who showed no difference between open and arthroscopically decompressed groups.

Ark and colleagues in 1992 published their series of 23 cases of arthroscopically decompressed shoulders with calcific tendinitis resulting in 91% good or satisfactory results [44].

Complete removal of the deposit was not possible in 14 of these patients but significant pain relief was achieved in 12 of these 14 patients. Seil et al. [45] reported 90% successful outcome at final follow up (24 months) in their study of 54 patients undergoing arthroscopic deposit excision. They found that the pattern and severity of post op pain was irregular but 78% of patients returned to work at 6 weeks regardless of profession.

Few studies have compared surgery to non-operative techniques. Castagna et al. [46] compared arthroscopic needling of the deposit vs arthroscopic excision and cuff repair after failure of non-operative management (all of whom had tried ESWT). Both groups demonstrated significant improvements in their clinical scores (Constant, ASES, SST, UCLA, VAS) but there was no statistically relevant difference between either group. Interestingly, the presence of residual calcification was not associated with persistent symptoms.

Surgical Technique

The patient can be positioned in the beach chair or lateral decubitus position. DVT prophylaxis is managed using compression stockings and intermittent pneumatic calf compression pumps. A brachial plexus block may be undertaken to reduce post-operative pain.

A standard posterior portal is made and anarthroscopic glenohumeral joint examination performed. If the deposit can be seen on the articular side of the rotator cuff tendon, then some surgeons opt to pass a percutaneous needle through the deposit, traversing the subacromial space, and a monofilament marker suture may be shuttled through. The suture will be visible within the subacromial space to allow easier localisation of the deposit. One potential downside to this technique is that it can theoretically introduce inflammatory calcium into the glenohumeral joint.

We prefer to decompress the deposit through the subacromial space. This is entered via the posterior portal. It is common to find the bursa to be thickened and hypertrophic and for the cuff to be injected and hypervascular.

The pre-operative imaging is used to assist in localising the deposit. If available, skin markings can be made pre-operatively using ultrasound [47]. The exact site of the deposit is found intraoperatively using a needle in a systematic probing fashion. The hub end of the needle is occluded with the surgeons finger tip to prevent washout of the deposit which plugs up the bevel end of the needle. Once localised, a partial thickness incision is made on the bursal side of the cuff in the line of the fibres of the tendon.

In cases where the deposit is soft, this may extrude in a toothpaste like fashion (Fig. 9.4). This can be assisted or "milked" with pressure from a probe over the surrounding deposit. The extruded material is then aspirated using the suction on the arthroscopic shaver. When the deposit exists in a more solid state it requires removal using a combination of a probe, curette and the arthroscopic shaver, taking care not to remove or damage any surrounding healthy tendon. We feel it is important to aspirate all the liberated calcium to minimise any post-operative inflammatory response.

Subscapularis deposits are much less frequently encountered than deposits in the superior cuff. These can be approached using a midlateral or anterolateral subacromial viewing portal after clearance of the anterior subdeltoid bursa. The deposit can then be localised using spinal needle and an accessory anterior portal created. A radial horizontal incision is made in line with the sub-

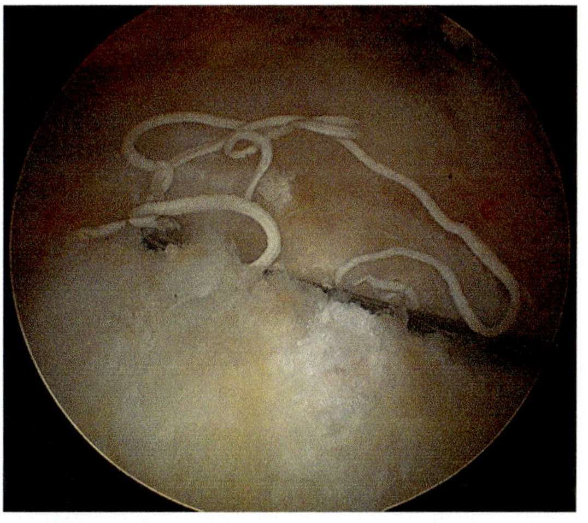

Fig. 9.4 Soft toothpaste like calcific being "milked" from the rotator cuff during arthroscopy

scapularis fibres and the deposit excised using the probe, curette and arthroscopic shaver.

The Role of Tendon Repair

The role of rotator cuff tendon repair after excision of the deposit remains contentious. Balke et al. [48] re-evaluated the rotator cuff tendons in 48 shoulders who had previously undergone excision of a calcific deposit after a mean of 6 years follow up (no tendon repair had been performed). They reported ultrasound evidence of partial thickness cuff tears in 11 of their 48 operated shoulders as compared to the 3 shoulders on the asymptomatic opposite side. There were no significant differences in the clinical scores when comparing the partial thickness tears with the intact tendons. Similar findings were reported by Seil et al. [45] who found 60% of their post-operative patients had ultrasound evidence of tendon change at 2 years post deposit excision but this did not lead to any clinical issues or major tendon structural changes. Conversely, Porcellini et al. [49] reported their 2 year ultrasound follow up of arthroscopic deposit excision in 63 shoulders. Within their cohort they had repaired any tendon defect >1 cm (49%) and any full thickness defect (13%). Those tendons with a radial incision that was partial thickness and 1 cm < were left unrepaired (38%). Their 2 year post-operative ultrasound surveillance did not reveal any tendon tears.

The Role of Acromioplasty

Acromial morphology in patients with calcific tendinitis has been demonstrated to be most similar to the morphology in patents experiencing subacromial impingement and different to controls in comparative studies [48]. This may lend some support to the addition of an acromioplasty as part of calcific deposition removal surgery where a type II or II acromion is present. Balke et al. reported their series of decompressions of calcific deposits where they undertook an additional acromioplasty when there were signs of impingement (fraying of the CAL or abrasions on the underside of the acromion). In these cases, the patients were found to have a Bigliani type II or III acromion. They further reported that in the patients who had undergone an subacromial decompression in addition to the deposit excision, there was a significant improvement in the pain component of the Constant-Murley score [50].

Seil et al. [45] and Porcellini et al. [49] both reported their outcomes when combining a subacromial decompression with deposit excision. The subacromial decompression was only undertaken when there were signs of impingement. Both studies showed no clinical difference in the subacromial decompression group. This was further confirmed in an RCT by Clement et al. [51] where patients were randomised to deposit removal alone or deposit removal and acromioplasty. They did not demonstrate any clinically significant difference between their two groups at 1 year post operatively and concluded that a routine acromioplasty is not necessary with calcific deposit removal. Finally, Marder et al. [52] found in their comparison of arthroscopic deposit excision vs deposit excision plus subacromial decompression that both groups experienced good improvements in their symptoms but the subacromial decompression group had a significantly longer return to normal activities.

Complications

Adhesive Capsulitis – calcific tendinitis is considered to be an intrinsic cause of a secondary frozen shoulder or adhesive capsulitis [53, 54]. The inflammatory nature of the calcific deposit may well be the stimulus for the development of the capsular contracture although the mechanism remains unclear [55]. Adhesive capsulitis is also more frequently seen in post-surgical patients where calcific tendinitis has been a component of their pathology [56, 57].

Rotator Cuff Tears – calcific tendinitis has long been associated with rotator cuff tears with studies showing a 28–90% probability of having a cuff tear in the presence of a calcific deposit [57–60]. The surgical approach to removing a deposit requires and incision in the cuff and therefore the creation of a cuff defect. Current opinion is mixed in its support for leaving or repairing these tears (see above).

Greater Tuberosity Osteolysis – this is an uncommon complication of calcific tendinitis and can lead to prolonged symptoms and impairment of function [45, 61]. This tends to occur when the deposit lies close to the tendon insertion and has bony involvement or extension [62]. Porcellini reported that tuberosity osteolysis was more likely where the deposit came in to contact with the bone of the tuberosity resulting in a cortical lesion [63]. Porcellini also reported more severe symptoms and longer recoveries in this subgroup of patients with cortical involvement. They advocated consideration of arthroscopic management and cleaning of the bone in cases resistant to non-operative management.

Ossifying Tendinitis – this exceptionally rare complication [64] represents a form of heterotopic ossification. In these cases there is hydroxyapatite deposition occuring with a histological pattern similar to lamellar bone [65].

Conclusion

Calcific tendinitis is a commonly encountered and frequently painful disorder presenting to general practitioners, musculoskeletal specialists and orthopaedic surgeons. Many patients may be managed symptomatically with NSAID's and gentle physiotherapy as the natural history of a calcific deposit can be one of resolution and resorption over time. It is the author's preference to supplement this early painful phase with a subacromial injection of local anaesthetic and steroid.

When symptoms fail to resolve then ultrasound guided needle aspiration and barbotage or extracorporeal shock wave therapy offer safe and effective treatment options.

A final option is of arthroscopic excision which can result in up to 90% successful outcomes. We do not routinely repair the rotator cuff post excision of the calcific deposit but would do so in the presence of a large or full thickness defect. We reserve a subacromial decompression for those cases where there have been clear signs of impingement.

Clinical Pearls

1. Pain presents most commonly during the painful resorptive phase.
2. Clinical history, examination and plain x-rays lead to the diagnosis of this condition.
3. Non-operative management can lead to the symptom improvement and resorption of calcific deposits. This includes the administration of subacromial injections of local anaesthetic and steroid, ultrasound guided needle aspiration and barbotage (UGNB) or extra-corporeal shock wave therapy (ESWT).
4. Surgical excision can offer good results. The addition of an acromioplasty or cuff repair remains contentious.

References

1. Gärtner J, Simons B. Analysis of calcific deposits in calcifying tendinitis. Clin Orthop Relat Res. 1990;254:111–20.
2. Hernandez-Santana A, Yavorskyy A, Loughran ST, McCarthy GM, McMahon GP. New approaches in the detection of calcium-containing microcrystals in synovial fluid. Bioanalysis. 2011;3(10):1085–91.
3. Riley GP, Harrall RL, Constant CR, Cawston TE, Hazleman BL. Prevalence and possible pathological significance of calcium phosphate salt accumulation in tendon matrix degeneration. Ann Rheum Dis. 1996;55(2):109–15.
4. Bosworth B. Calcium deposits in the shoulder and subacromial bursitis. A survey of 12,122 shoulders. JAMA. 1941;116:2477–82.
5. Louwerens JK, Sierevelt IN, van Hove RP, van den Bekerom MP, van Noort A. Prevalence of calcific deposits within the rotator cuff tendons in adults with and without subacromial pain syndrome: clinical and radiologic analysis of 1219 patients. J Shoulder Elb Surg. 2015;24(10):1588–93.
6. Speed CA, Hazleman BL. Calcific tendinitis of the shoulder. N Engl J Med. 1999;340(20):1582–4.
7. Uhthoff HK. Calcifying tendinitis. Ann Chir Gynaecol. 1996;85(2):111–5.
8. Depalma AF, Kruper JS. Long-term study of shoulder joints afflicted with and treated for calcific tendinitis. Clin Orthop. 1961;20:61–72.
9. Uhthoff HK, Loehr JW. Calcific tendinopathy of the rotator cuff: pathogenesis, diagnosis, and management. J Am Acad Orthop Surg. 1997;5(4):183–91.

10. Oliva F, Via AG, Maffulli N. Physiopathology of intratendinous calcific deposition. BMC Med. 2012;10:95.
11. Codman EA, Akerson IB. The pathology associated with rupture of the supraspinatus tendon. Ann Surg. 1931;93(1):348–59.
12. Refior HJ, Krödel A, Melzer C. Examinations of the pathology of the rotator cuff. Arch Orthop Trauma Surg. 1987;106(5):301–8.
13. Rui YF, Lui PP, Chan LS, Chan KM, Fu SC, Li G. Does erroneous differentiation of tendon-derived stem cells contribute to the pathogenesis of calcifying tendinopathy? Chin Med J. 2011;124(4):606–10.
14. Loew M, Jurgowski W, Mau HC, Thomsen M. Treatment of calcifying tendinitis of rotator cuff by extracorporeal shock waves: a preliminary report. J Shoulder Elb Surg. 1995;4(2):101–6.
15. Harvie P, Pollard TC, Carr AJ. Calcific tendinitis: natural history and association with endocrine disorders. J Shoulder Elb Surg. 2007;16(2):169–73.
16. Gärtner J, Heyer A. Calcific tendinitis of the shoulder. Orthopade. 1995;24(3):284–302.
17. Molé D, Kempf JF, Gleyze P, Rio B, Bonnomet F, Walch G. Results of endoscopic treatment of non-broken tendinopathies of the rotator cuff. 2. Calcifications of the rotator cuff. Rev Chir Orthop Reparatrice Appar Mot. 1993;79(7):532–41.
18. Noël E. Treatment of calcific tendinitis and adhesive capsulitis of the shoulder. Rev Rhum Engl Ed. 1997;64(11):619–28.
19. Ogon P, Suedkamp NP, Jaeger M, Izadpanah K, Koestler W, Maier D. Prognostic factors in nonoperative therapy for chronic symptomatic calcific tendinitis of the shoulder. Arthritis Rheum. 2009;60(10):2978–84.
20. Cho NS, Lee BG, Rhee YG. Radiologic course of the calcific deposits in calcific tendinitis of the shoulder: does the initial radiologic aspect affect the final results? J Shoulder Elb Surg. 2010;19(2):267–72.
21. Cole BF, Peters KS, Hackett L, Murrell GA. Ultrasound-guided versus blind subacromial corticosteroid injections for subacromial impingement syndrome: a randomized, double-blind clinical trial. Am J Sports Med. 2016;44(3):702–7.
22. Maman E, Yehuda C, Pritsch T, Morag G, Brosh T, Sharfman Z, et al. Detrimental effect of repeated and single subacromial corticosteroid injections on the intact and injured rotator cuff: a biomechanical and imaging study in rats. Am J Sports Med. 2016;44(1):177–82.
23. Sconfienza LM, Viganò S, Martini C, Aliprandi A, Randelli P, Serafini G, et al. Double-needle ultrasound-guided percutaneous treatment of rotator cuff calcific tendinitis: tips & tricks. Skelet Radiol. 2013;42(1):19–24.
24. Yoo JC, Koh KH, Park WH, Park JC, Kim SM, Yoon YC. The outcome of ultrasound-guided needle decompression and steroid injection in calcific tendinitis. J Shoulder Elb Surg. 2010;19(4):596–600.
25. Oudelaar BW, Ooms EM, Huis In 't Veld R, Schepers-Bok R, Vochteloo AJ. Smoking and morphology of calcific deposits affect the outcome of needle aspiration of calcific deposits (NACD) for calcific tendinitis of the rotator cuff. Eur J Radiol. 2015;84(11):2255–60.
26. de Witte PB, Selten JW, Navas A, Nagels J, Visser CP, Nelissen RG, et al. Calcific tendinitis of the rotator cuff: a randomized controlled trial of ultrasound-guided needling and lavage versus subacromial corticosteroids. Am J Sports Med. 2013;41(7):1665–73.
27. de Witte PB, Kolk A, Overes F, Nelissen RGHH, Reijnierse M. Rotator cuff calcific tendinitis: ultrasound-guided needling and lavage versus subacromial corticosteroids: five-year outcomes of a randomized controlled trial. Am J Sports Med. 2017;45(14):3305–14.
28. del Cura JL, Torre I, Zabala R, Legórburu A. Sonographically guided percutaneous needle lavage in calcific tendinitis of the shoulder: short- and long-term results. AJR Am J Roentgenol. 2007;189(3):W128–34.
29. Serafini G, Sconfienza LM, Lacelli F, Silvestri E, Aliprandi A, Sardanelli F. Rotator cuff calcific tendonitis: short-term and 10-year outcomes after two-needle us-guided percutaneous treatment – nonrandomized controlled trial. Radiology. 2009;252(1):157–64.
30. Rompe JD, Kirkpatrick CJ, Küllmer K, Schwitalle M, Krischek O. Dose-related effects of shock waves on rabbit tendo Achillis. A sonographic and histological study. J Bone Joint Surg Br. 1998;80(3):546–52.
31. Daecke W, Kusnierczak D, Loew M. Long-term effects of extracorporeal shockwave therapy in chronic calcific tendinitis of the shoulder. J Shoulder Elb Surg. 2002;11(5):476–80.
32. Albert JD, Meadeb J, Guggenbuhl P, Marin F, Benkalfate T, Thomazeau H, et al. High-energy extracorporeal shock-wave therapy for calcifying tendinitis of the rotator cuff: a randomised trial. J Bone Joint Surg Br. 2007;89(3):335–41.
33. Louwerens JK, Veltman ES, van Noort A, van den Bekerom MP. The effectiveness of high-energy extracorporeal shockwave therapy versus ultrasound-guided needling versus arthroscopic surgery in the management of chronic calcific rotator cuff tendinopathy: a systematic review. Arthroscopy. 2016;32(1):165–75.
34. Gerdesmeyer L, Wagenpfeil S, Haake M, Maier M, Loew M, Wörtler K, et al. Extracorporeal shock wave therapy for the treatment of chronic calcifying tendonitis of the rotator cuff: a randomized controlled trial. JAMA. 2003;290(19):2573–80.
35. Lee SY, Cheng B, Grimmer-Somers K. The midterm effectiveness of extracorporeal shockwave therapy in the management of chronic calcific shoulder tendinitis. J Shoulder Elb Surg. 2011;20(5):845–54.
36. Haake M, Deike B, Thon A, Schmitt J. Exact focusing of extracorporeal shock wave therapy for calcifying tendinopathy. Clin Orthop Relat Res. 2002;397:323–31.
37. Kim YS, Lee HJ, Kim YV, Kong CG. Which method is more effective in treatment of calcific tendinitis in the shoulder? Prospective randomized compari-

son between ultrasound-guided needling and extracorporeal shock wave therapy. J Shoulder Elb Surg. 2014;23(11):1640–6.
38. Krasny C, Enenkel M, Aigner N, Wlk M, Landsiedl F. Ultrasound-guided needling combined with shock-wave therapy for the treatment of calcifying tendonitis of the shoulder. J Bone Joint Surg Br. 2005;87(4):501–7.
39. Liu HM, Chao CM, Hsieh JY, Jiang CC. Humeral head osteonecrosis after extracorporeal shock-wave treatment for rotator cuff tendinopathy. A case report. J Bone Joint Surg Am. 2006;88(6):1353–6.
40. Ebenbichler GR, Erdogmus CB, Resch KL, Funovics MA, Kainberger F, Barisani G, et al. Ultrasound therapy for calcific tendinitis of the shoulder. N Engl J Med. 1999;340(20):1533–8.
41. Louwerens JK, Sierevelt IN, van Noort A, van den Bekerom MP. Evidence for minimally invasive therapies in the management of chronic calcific tendinopathy of the rotator cuff: a systematic review and meta-analysis. J Shoulder Elb Surg. 2014;23(8):1240–9.
42. Bosworth B. Examination of the shoulder for calcium deposits. Technique of fluoroscopy and spot film roentgenography. J Bone Joint Surg. 1942;23:567–77.
43. Rubenthaler F, Ludwig J, Wiese M, Wittenberg RH. Prospective randomized surgical treatments for calcifying tendinopathy. Clin Orthop Relat Res. 2003;410:278–84.
44. Ark JW, Flock TJ, Flatow EL, Bigliani LU. Arthroscopic treatment of calcific tendinitis of the shoulder. Arthroscopy. 1992;8(2):183–8.
45. Seil R, Litzenburger H, Kohn D, Rupp S. Arthroscopic treatment of chronically painful calcifying tendinitis of the supraspinatus tendon. Arthroscopy. 2006;22(5):521–7.
46. Castagna A, DE Giorgi S, Garofalo R, Conti M, Tafuri S, Moretti B. Calcifying tendinitis of the shoulder: arthroscopic needling versus complete calcium removal and rotator cuff repair. A prospective comparative study. Joints. 2015;3(4):166–72.
47. Ambacher T, Kirschniak A, Holz U. Intraoperative localization of calcification in the supraspinatus via a percutaneous marking suture after preoperative ultrasound. J Shoulder Elb Surg. 2007;16(2):146–9.
48. Balke M, Banerjee M, Vogler T, Akoto R, Bouillon B, Liem D. Acromial morphology in patients with calcific tendinitis of the shoulder. Knee Surg Sports Traumatol Arthrosc. 2014;22(2):415–21.
49. Porcellini G, Paladini P, Campi F, Paganelli M. Arthroscopic treatment of calcifying tendinitis of the shoulder: clinical and ultrasonographic follow-up findings at two to five years. J Shoulder Elb Surg. 2004;13(5):503–8.
50. Balke M, Bielefeld R, Schmidt C, Dedy N, Liem D. Calcifying tendinitis of the shoulder: midterm results after arthroscopic treatment. Am J Sports Med. 2012;40(3):657–61.
51. Clement ND, Watts AC, Phillips C, McBirnie JM. Short-term outcome after arthroscopic bursectomy debridement of rotator cuff calcific tendonopathy with and without subacromial decompression: a prospective randomized controlled trial. Arthroscopy. 2015;31(9):1680–7.
52. Marder RA, Heiden EA, Kim S. Calcific tendonitis of the shoulder: is subacromial decompression in combination with removal of the calcific deposit beneficial? J Shoulder Elb Surg. 2011;20(6):955–60.
53. Rokito A, Loebenberg M. Frozen shoulder and calcific tendonitis. Curr Opin Orthop. 1999;10:294–304.
54. Neviaser RJ. Painful conditions affecting the shoulder. Clin Orthop Relat Res. 1983;173:63–9.
55. Chen SK, Chou PH, Lue YJ, Lu YM. Treatment for frozen shoulder combined with calcific tendinitis of the supraspinatus. Kaohsiung J Med Sci. 2008;24(2):78–84.
56. Jacobs R, Debeer P. Calcifying tendinitis of the rotator cuff: functional outcome after arthroscopic treatment. Acta Orthop Belg. 2006;72(3):276–81.
57. Huberty DP, Schoolfield JD, Brady PC, Vadala AP, Arrigoni P, Burkhart SS. Incidence and treatment of postoperative stiffness following arthroscopic rotator cuff repair. Arthroscopy. 2009;25(8):880–90.
58. Wolfgang GL. Surgical repair of tears of the rotator cuff of the shoulder. Factors influencing the result. J Bone Joint Surg Am. 1974;56(1):14–26.
59. Hsu HC, Wu JJ, Jim YF, Chang CY, Lo WH, Yang DJ. Calcific tendinitis and rotator cuff tearing: a clinical and radiographic study. J Shoulder Elb Surg. 1994;3(3):159–64.
60. Gotoh M, Higuchi F, Suzuki R, Yamanaka K. Progression from calcifying tendinitis to rotator cuff tear. Skelet Radiol. 2003;32(2):86–9.
61. Chan R, Kim DH, Millett PJ, Weissman BN. Calcifying tendinitis of the rotator cuff with cortical bone erosion. Skelet Radiol. 2004;33(10):596–9.
62. Flemming DJ, Murphey MD, Shekitka KM, Temple HT, Jelinek JJ, Kransdorf MJ. Osseous involvement in calcific tendinitis: a retrospective review of 50 cases. AJR Am J Roentgenol. 2003;181(4):965–72.
63. Porcellini G, Paladini P, Campi F, Pegreffi F. Osteolytic lesion of greater tuberosity in calcific tendinitis of the shoulder. J Shoulder Elb Surg. 2009;18(2):210–5.
64. Merolla G, Dave AC, Paladini P, Campi F, Porcellini G. Ossifying tendinitis of the rotator cuff after arthroscopic excision of calcium deposits: report of two cases and literature review. J Orthop Traumatol. 2015;16(1):67–73.
65. Ozaki J, Kugai A, Tomita Y, Tamai S. Tear of an ossified rotator cuff of the shoulder. A case report. Acta Orthop Scand. 1992;63(3):339–40.

10 Long Head of the Biceps Tendon Complex: Pathology and Treatment Approach

Brian B. Gilmer, Sarah D. Lang, and Dan Guttmann

Background

Lesions of the biceps tendon had been documented since the middle ages mostly in response to spontaneous dislocation or rupture and based upon anatomic studies. Codman [1], in his seminal text *The Shoulder*, felt the biceps were more likely a recipient of the collateral damage from associated shoulder pathologies than a primary source of shoulder pain. Shortly thereafter however, a series of authors began to express their disagreement Lippmann [2], Tarsy [3], Hitchcock et al. [4] , DePalma [5]; and a series of procedures for tenodesis of the LHBT were introduced.

The significance of the intraarticular biceps tendon was introduced when Andrews described lesions of the superior labrum and Snyder et al. [7], coined the term *SLAP tear (superior labrum anterior to posterior)* and described the relationship of the superior labrum to the LHBT [6].

B. B. Gilmer (✉) · S. D. Lang
Mammoth Orthopedic Institute, Mammoth Lakes, CA, USA
e-mail: brian.gilmer@mammothhospital.com; sarah.lang@mammothhospital.com

D. Guttmann
Taos Orthopaedic Institute Sports Medicine Fellowship and Research Foundation, Taos, NM, USA
e-mail: drg@taosortho.com

Anatomy

Many aspects of the anatomy of the biceps tendon are variable. It is generally agreed the tendon is approximately 9 cm [8, 9]; in length, 5–6 mm in diameter, and can generally be divided into an intraarticular portion, a portion within the biceps groove just lateral to the insertion of the subscapularis tendon, and a subpectoral portion.

Because the tendon has been shown to glide in the groove, it is important to understand these relationships as dynamic rather than static as the same portion of the tendon can be located in a different zone based upon arm position [10].

The LHBT is most commonly described as originating from the supraglenoid tubercle, but this origin too, is variable. In fact, Habermeyer et al. [11] described origin from the supraglenoid tubercle in only 20% of specimens versus an origin from the posterosuperior labrum in most cases (48%), or a shared origin. Additional studies have confirmed a predominant relationship with the posterior labrum and little to no microscopic origin occurring from the more anterior labrum (Fig. 10.1).

The tendon begins as a relatively flat structure until it reaches the intratubercular groove around 20 mm from its origin, at which point it becomes more tubular in the middle and distal portions [12, 13]. It is important to understand flattening as a normal feature as it is often one of the reported pathologic changes of the tendon noted at arthroscopy.

I. A. Trail et al. (eds.), *Textbook of Shoulder Surgery*, https://doi.org/10.1007/978-3-319-70099-1_10

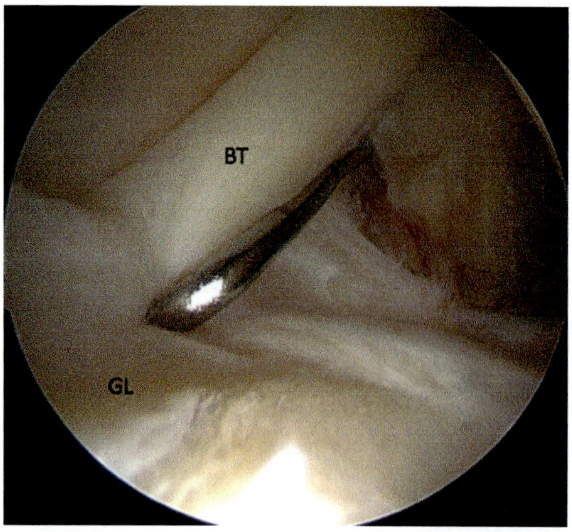

Fig. 10.1 Right shoulder, lateral decubitus position view through a standard posterior viewing portal with a 30 degree arthroscope. Probe is entering through an anterior rotator interval portal and demonstrates the normal relationship of the biceps tendon (BT) to the superior glenoid labrum (GL). Note the lack of displacement of the superior labrum and biceps anchor on the superior glenoid despite probe

Blood supply to the tendon is chiefly from the brachial artery by means of the anterior humeral circumflex artery. The portion of the tendon within the groove is supplied by a branch of the anterior humeral circumflex artery. This vessel provides perfusion to the most proximal part of the tendon in a retrograde fashion [14].

Notably, the arterial supply to the underlying supraglenoid tubercle is largely absent, particularly in the anterior superior quadrant, and no vessel from the proximal end supplies the superior labrum or biceps tendon [14, 15]. This vascular anatomy has significant biologic implications in SLAP repair where the relatively avascular tissue is secured to the poorly perfused quadrant of the glenoid bone with suture anchors (Fig. 10.2).

Neurologically, Alpantaki et al. [16] demonstrated a rich plexus of sympathetic fibers supplying the biceps anchor and a relatively less innervated pattern more distally. The presence of sympathetic fibers in pathologic conditions was confirmed with immunohistochemical studies [17]. These findings

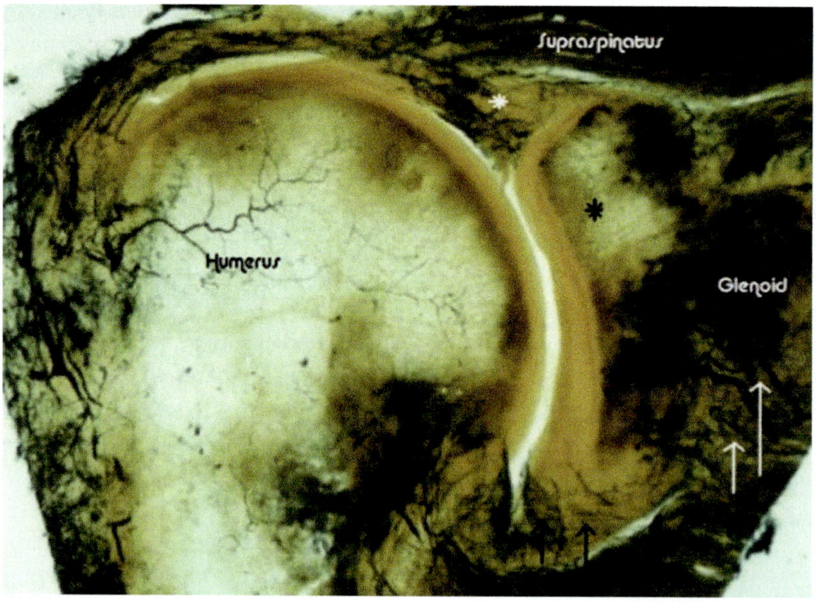

Fig. 10.2 Mid coronal section of the glenohumeral joint demonstrating the avascular area of superior glenoid bone (black asterisk) and superior glenoid labrum (white asterisk) compared to the inferior glenoid bone and labrum (white and black arrows respectively). Note that the cartilage extends superiorly beyond the articulating glenoid surface preventing communication of vessels in this region and contributing to the generally poor vascularity. (Photo courtesy of Dr. S. Arnoczky, DVM)

support the role of the biceps tendon as a potential pain generator in the shoulder.

Surprisingly, the presence of proprioceptive fibers has not been confirmed [18]. The presence of pain fibers in the absence of proprioception may explain the vague nature of the pain often described by patients with LHBT pathology and their difficulty in localizing the source of discomfort accurately.

Soft tissue restraint of the LHBT in the glenohumeral joint is provided by the biceps sling, or pulley, which is composed of tissue surrounding the rotator interval. This structure is relevant to surgical treatment of the LHBT as it is the primary restraint to medial dislocation of the tendon [19]. This pulley structure is composed of fibers of the superior glenohumeral ligament (SGHL), the coracohumeral ligament (CHL), and parts of the subscapularis tendon. It is intimately related to both the subscapularis and supraspinatus tendons as well as the superior capsule [20] (Fig. 10.3).

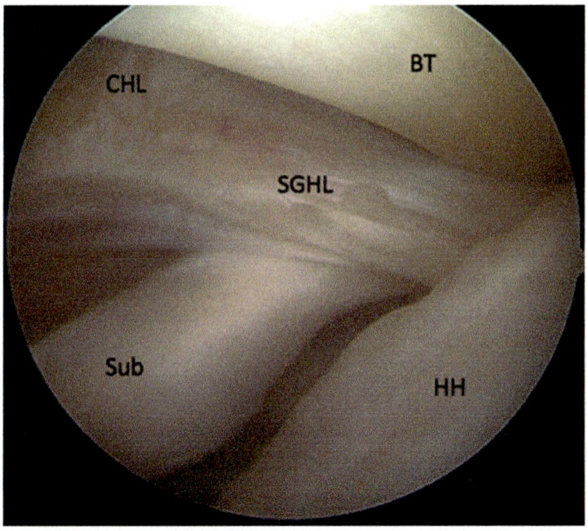

Fig. 10.3 Right shoulder, beach chair position view through a standard posterior viewing portal with a 30 degree arthroscope. The anatomy of the biceps pulley sling is demonstrated. The coracohumeral ligament (CHL) and the (SGHL) ligament provide resistance to displacement of the intraarticular biceps tendon (BT). The subscapularis tendon (Sub) is seen inserting on the lesser tuberosity. The humeral head (HH) is visualized. More laterally the supraspinatus tendon (not illustrated in this image) prevents posterior and lateral displacement of the tendon

More distally the biceps groove is covered by a transverse ligament which provides a secondary role in stabilization of the tendon; however, dislocation of the biceps tendon has been noted in specimens where the transverse ligament is intact. Conversely, complete transection of the transverse ligament does not lead to biceps dislocation in the setting of an intact rotator cuff.

Relevant osseous anatomy includes the bony groove itself which has a higher medial ridge formed by the lesser tuberosity and a lower lateral ridge formed by the anterior border of the greater tuberosity. The relationship of the groove to the humeral epicondylar axis is a consistent 45° and can be used as a landmark in establishing version in the setting of a proximal humerus fracture treated with arthroplasty. The groove has an opening angle of 30–40° into the glenohumeral joint which is consistent with reports regarding the course of the biceps tendon in the setting of an intact biceps pulley [21]. The medial wall angle (meaning the angle formed by the bottom of the groove and the top of the medial wall) is constant in apes but varies in a human which probably represents a varying degree of physiologic adaptation to throwing [4]. This angle has been inversely correlated to likelihood of biceps dislocation.

Function

The shoulder joint is one of the most morphologically labile structures in the fossil record following the evolution of our species. In a clear case of form following function the steady shift from brachiating hominids to bipedal hominids to modern homosapiens is marked by a steady change in shoulder anatomy [22].

In quadruped species the biceps tendon is still attached at the labrum and supraglenoid tubercle but takes a direct course into the groove and down the axis of the forelimb such that it is an effective elevator of the arm in the forward plane. In primates, the course of the tendon is progressively more oblique with humans developing the most oblique course [4]. This angle has been inversely correlated to likelihood of biceps dislocation. This adaptive position subjects the tendon to stress and creates potential for impingement and degenerative change of the tendon as it changes course before entering the intertubercular groove.

The biceps tendon is theorized to have been a source of storage of potential energy in the shoulder. This adaptation allowed forceful throwing motion which in turn allowed hunting and incorporation of animal proteins into the hominid diet. This expanded the range of early hominids and may have facilitated the diaspora from Africa – or so the theory goes [23].

Multiple older biomechanical studies have suggested a role of the long head of the biceps tendon as a depressor of the humeral head, and this has long been propagated as fact [24, 25]. However, in vivo studies using radiographs have failed to reproduce these findings [26, 27]. Electromyography studies by Sakurai et al. [28] have shown no activation of the biceps tendon when the elbow is immobilized. Thus, the direct function of the biceps tendon in humans remains uncertain. As discussed later, the loss of biceps tendon function due to either traumatic rupture or through iatrogenic means seems to leave little functional impairment in most patients calling further into question the purpose of the LHBT in the native anatomic state.

Clinical Presentation and Diagnosis of LHBT Lesions

History

Biceps tendon pain most commonly presents as exertional anterior shoulder pain. There is often no specific history of trauma. Because the pain can radiate to the deltoid origin it can be difficult to distinguish from rotator cuff tendonitis or glenohumeral pain from an intraarticular source such as a labral tear, subtle glenohumeral instability, or degenerative joint disease. In cases of biceps tendon subluxation or rupture there may be a history of a discrete pop which is heard or felt. Both subluxation and rupture are commonly associated with traumatic or degenerative changes of the rotator cuff, particularly the anterior aspect of the supraspinatus and the upper portion of the subscapularis.

In the case of SLAP lesions, a history of repetitive overhead activities is common and may be associated with vague posterior shoulder pain over the area of the posterior deltoid and rotator cuff which is exacerbated with activity and improved with rest. Patients often complain of being unable to sleep on that shoulder, unable to reach behind i.e. into the backseat of a car, unable to perform military press during weight-lifting.

Physical Examination

As is the case with the history, the examination of the biceps is confounded by the associated structures in close proximity.

Direct palpation of the biceps tendon is best performed with the arm in slight internal rotation and by placing the examiners fingers just lateral to the coracoid process and the palpable divot formed by the glenohumeral joint. Because of the relationship of the biceps tendon to the humeral shaft this same position should become less tender with larger angles of internal and external rotation. It is worth noting that tenderness to direct palpation is more specific to pathology of the extraarticular biceps tendon and may not be present in the setting of SLAP tear or lesions of the biceps anchor.

Provocative tests for biceps tendonitis have been shown to be of generally low sensitivity and specificity, Hegedus et al. [29]; and the same is true for SLAP tears [30]. Regardless, the most common tests for the distal biceps are Speed's test and Yergason's sign; for SLAP tears O'Brien's test is the most frequently described.

Speed's test can be performed with the patient seated with the arm in 90° of forward elevation, the elbow extended, and the arm fully supinated. The examiner provides downward pressure on the hand while the patient resists. The reported sensitivity for this test has been described as 90% but with a specificity of only 13% [31].

Yergason's sign is present when pain is reproduced in the anterior shoulder with resisted supination of the elbow with the arm at the side and the elbow at 90°.

These tests were reviewed by Holtby and Razmjou [32] in a level one diagnostic study who found while both had reasonable specificity, they did not generate a large change in the posttest probability and therefore were useful in preoperative diagnosis and decision making.

O'Brien's test is performed with the patient seated with the arm in slight adduction, forward elevation to 90°, and full pronation of the forearm with the elbow extended. Again, the examiner provides downward force while the patient resists. The arm is then fully supinated and the test is repeated. The test is positive when the pain is recreated in pronation and relieved in supination. Since the development of this classic test a variety of new tests have been described in an effort to improve diagnostic accuracy. Unfortunately, no single test has demonstrated a consistent diagnostic reliability [33] (Fig. 10.4).

Often a combination of tests, provide the most reliable method of diagnosis. It is helpful to first test the opposite arm for comparison. Do not allow the patient to torque their body or scapula to compensate or lean on something with their other arm during testing of the affected limb.

Imaging

In the absence of reliable history and physical exam findings, diagnostic imaging can play a significant role. Unfortunately, most studies have demonstrated limitations of common imaging modalities.

X-Ray Plain radiographs are normal in the setting of SLAP tears and biceps tendinopathy. Specialized views have been described to visualize the biceps groove, but the relevance of groove morphology to pathologic conditions of the tendon remains unclear [34, 35]. A standard screening series of plain radiographs including anteroposterior in external rotation (AP), Grashey AP (oblique with internal rotation), scapular Y, and axillary lateral are still useful as a screening tool to identify other sources of shoulder pain.

Ultrasound More recently, ultrasonography has emerged as a common tool for diagnosis of biceps tendon pathology. The advantages are the study can be performed in the office, performed dynamically with patient cooperation, is non-invasive, and is less expensive than MRI. Armstrong et al. [36] confirmed the utility of ultrasound for diagnosis of lesions of the LHBT in the groove including subluxation, rupture, or dislocation, but noted its inability to diagnose intraarticular partial thickness tears and SLAP tears.

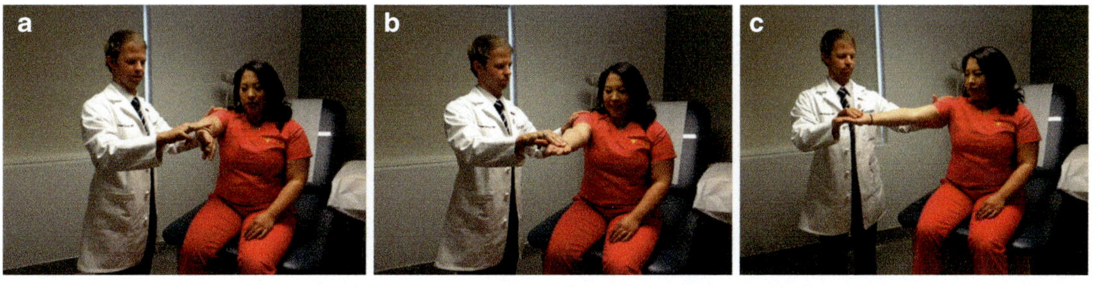

Fig. 10.4 Physical Examination for Biceps Tendon Pathology (**a**) O'Briens Test- arm is in 90 degrees of forward elevation and 10 degrees of adduction with the elbow extended and forearm pronated. Examiner applies downward pressure. (**b**) O'Briens Test continued-maintain position of the shoulder and supinate the forearm. Examiner again applies downward pressure. Improvement in pain with supination suggests SLAP tear or lesion of the biceps anchor. (**c**) 'Speed's' test – Arm is positioned in 90 degrees of forward elevation, 30 degrees of abduction, and full supination. Examiner applies downward pressure. Pain in the shoulder anteriorly suggests biceps tendon pathology without specificity towards the biceps anchor or groove

Ultrasound is highly user dependent and a learning curve exists for achieving competency. Studies on rotator cuff tears have suggested that with experience, surgeons can achieve a high degree of diagnostic accuracy comparable to magnetic resonance arthrography (MRA); however, studies specific to biceps tendon pathology are lacking [37, 38].

Magnetic Resonance Imaging (MRI) MRI has evolved to become the advanced imaging modality of choice for the diagnosis of a multitude of musculoskeletal pathologies. Advances in medical technology have improved the quality of imaging and specific sequences have been developed to increase diagnostic accuracy. The addition of contrast, MRA, has increased the clinician's ability to detect SLAP lesions [39].

Unfortunately, in multiple comparisons of MRI to arthroscopy, MRI has been shown to incompletely evaluate the LHBT for pathology. Malavolta et al. [40] demonstrated a sensitivity of MRI of only 67% for complete tears [41]. The ability to identify more subtle lesions such as fraying, partial tearing, or degeneration is probably even more limited. The correlation between LHBT lesions and rotator cuff tears has been well established, and MRI is very useful for diagnosis of associated pathology. Thus, MRI is a useful but incomplete screening tool for both SLAP lesions and lesions of the LHBT itself (Fig. 10.5).

It is not uncommon for an MRI and even an MRA report stating "Normal Labrum and Biceps" demonstrate clear pathologic changes during diagnostic arthroscopy. The shoulder surgeon needs to have an index of suspicion based on the history and physical exam and explain to the patient a dynamic arthroscopic examination is still the gold standard to diagnose lesions of the LHBT and SLAP tears. When preoperative diagnostic studies are unclear, it is encouraged to initiate non-surgical treatment with rest, modification of activity, physical therapy, medication etc. If pain persists, it can be useful to apply a Single Assessment Numeric Evaluation (SANE) rating. Even in the face of a normal MRI, if the patient states the affected shoulder is 50 or below out of 100, after reasonable non-operative treatment, surgery is a rational option.

Arthroscopy Direct arthroscopy is typically the gold standard used in studies comparing other

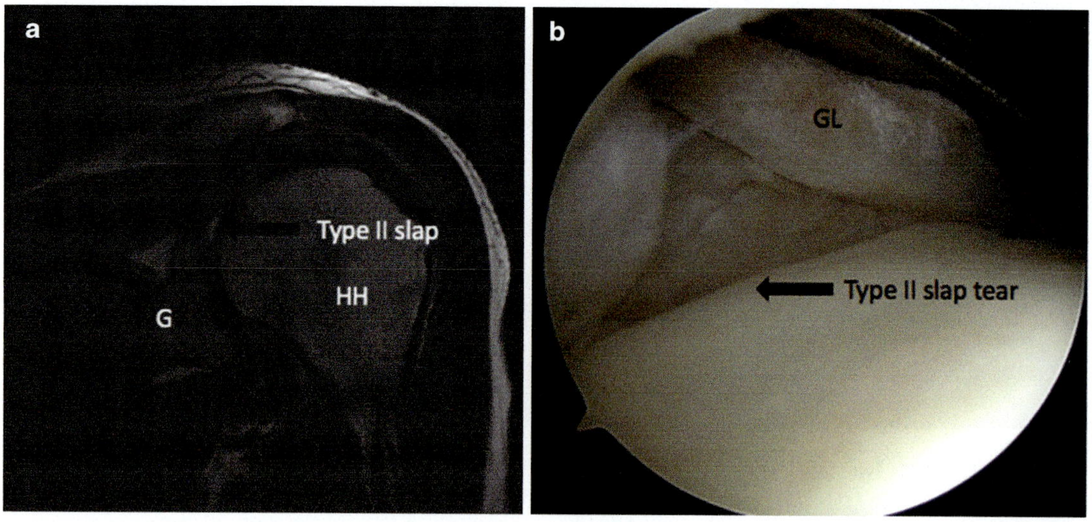

Fig. 10.5 (**a**) Coronal T2 MRI arthrogram image of a type II SLAP lesion (black arrow). Note the contrast medium extending between the superior aspect of the glenoid labrum and the superior labrum. Glenoid (G) and humeral head (HH). (**b**) Corresponding arthroscopic image of type II SLAP lesion in the same patient. Left shoulder, lateral decubitus position view with a 30 degree arthroscope in a standard posterior viewing portal demonstrates clear displacement of the superior glenoid labrum (GL) and biceps anchor by probe

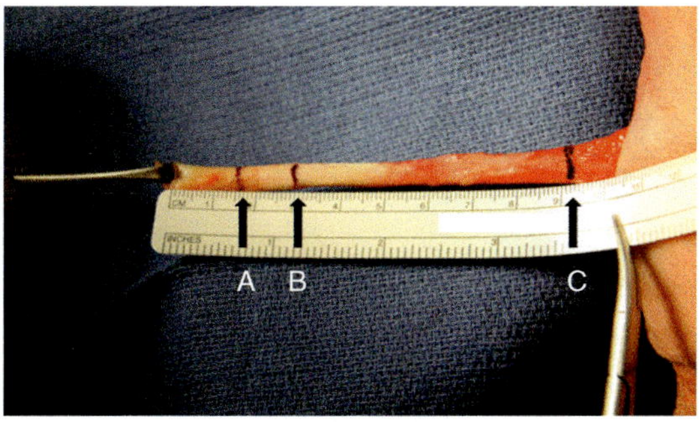

Fig. 10.6 In vivo gross examination of right shoulder biceps tendon after arthroscopic tenotomy in preparation for open subpectoral biceps tenodesis. The proximal tendon end is held in the Alice clamp in the lefthand portion of the image. (**a**) Indicates portion of tendon visualized arthroscopically. (**b**) Indicates portion of tendon visualized arthroscopically with assistance of arthroscopic grasper. (**c**) Myotendinous junction

modalities. Our group, Gilmer et al. [8], evaluated arthroscopy in evaluation of LHBT lesions in patients undergoing biceps tenodesis. We identified that only approximately only 32% of the biceps tendon is evaluated arthroscopically even with use of an arthroscopic probe. Furthermore, arthroscopy only identified 67% of pathology that was identified by open examination during tenodesis (Fig. 10.6).

In summary, no single diagnostic tool has clearly been identified for definitive diagnosis of all lesions of the LHBT. A combination of history, physical exam, advanced imaging, and even arthroscopy is necessary to fully evaluate the LHBT anchor and distal tendon.

Treatment of the LHBT Lesions

The treatment of LHBT pathology lies along a spectrum ranging from simple debridement to tenotomy, to one of the multitude of procedures developed for tenodesis. The decision to perform a tenodesis versus primary SLAP repair has evolved over recent years as the rate of SLAP repair has declined in response to disappointing outcomes in some patient populations. The location of tenodesis remains a topic of controversy as does the debate between arthroscopic versus open techniques.

Tenotomy One of the simplest techniques described for treatment of LHBT is simple arthroscopic tenotomy.

The patient is in the beachchair or lateral position. After the patient is prepped and draped, a standard posterior viewing portal is placed. As the arthroscope is placed into the glenohumeral joint, identification of a lesion of LHBT is confirmed. A spinal needle is used to identify the anterior portal and then an incision made in the skin. A switching stick is used to enter the glenohumeral joint in the superior anterior portion. Dilators are used and an arthroscopic scissor is introduced. The LHBT is then cut at the origin of the biceps anchor cutting the LHBT but leaving the labral attachment intact. This is a biceps tenotomy and can be done very quickly from an arthroscopic standpoint.

Some authors have advocated simple debridement of the LHBT. The procedure is performed as above but an arthroscopic shaver is introduced through the anterior portal and the lesion is debrided to a stable base (Fig. 10.7).

Arthroscopic SLAP Repair A SLAP repair can be done in the beachchair or lateral position. After the patient is prepped and draped in sterile fashion a posterior viewing portal is placed into the glenohumeral joint. The arthroscope visualizes the superior labrum and identifies a SLAP tear. This typically involves a lesion of the labrum including the biceps anchor, occurring more commonly posterior to the biceps anchor versus anterior. An anterior portal is made at the level of the biceps tendon. A cannula is placed with a minimum of a 7 mm diameter. A shaver is introduced and the labrum is debrided and the bone of the superior glenoid is also carefully debrided and prepared for repair.

The senior author's preference is to use a percutaneous technique for repair of the superior labrum. A percutaneous insertion kit will include a long spinal needle that allows an obturator to be placed and then a dilator followed by a cannula which has a minimum of 4.7 mm inner diameter, and a 5.4 mm outer diameter. This is placed at the anterior superior to posterior portion of the lateral aspect of the acromion (depending on the posterior extent of the lesion). Once the cannula

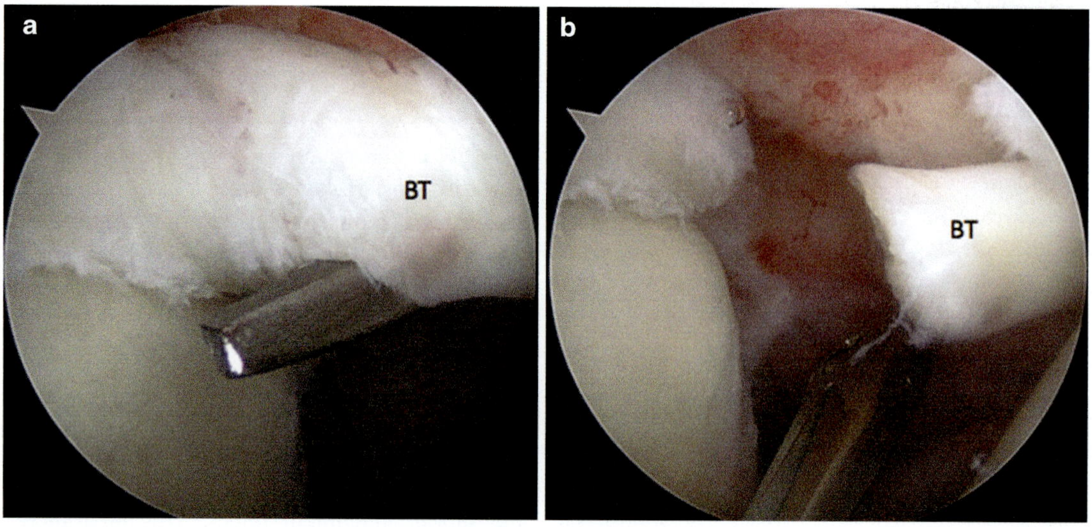

Fig. 10.7 Arthroscopic image demonstrating technique for biceps tenotomy. Right shoulder, beach chair position view through a posterior viewing portal with a 30 degree arthroscope. (**a**) An arthroscopic scissor is visualized entering through a standard anterior rotator interval portal. The biceps tendon (BT) is surrounded just distal to its origin from the superior labrum. (**b**) The biceps tendon (BT) has been truncated and released completely by the arthroscopic scissor

is placed using a percutaneous technique, a 45° curved lasso-type device is used through the anterior cannula, to pass suture around the posterior aspect of the labrum superiorly and posterior to the biceps anchor. In a right shoulder the 45° curved lasso suture passing instrument is curved to the left and vice versa. A suture can be passed that can be either cinched or a tape could be passed around the labrum either in a simple fashion or in a mattress fashion with a second pass using the lasso-type device. This suture having been passed through the labrum is then docked in the anterior portal. A drill is then used through the percutaneous cannula to drill into the glenoid superiorly at approximately the 11 o'clock position. The drill is then removed. The suture and/or tape is then brought out through the percutaneous placed cannula, it is loaded onto a 2.9 mm push lock anchor. In a knotless technique, the anchor is impacted into the previously drilled hole at approximately the 11 o'clock position and the first anchor/suture repair of the SLAP repair is completed. A second identical repair can be placed at approximately the 10 o'clock position and if needed, anterior to the biceps anchor. It is important to not strangulate the biceps anchor and tendon. The knotless technique is preferred because some surgeons have reported the knots from SLAP repairs can cause cartilage or rotator cuff damage (Fig. 10.8).

Sub-Pectoral Biceps Tenodesis For a sub-pectoral biceps tenodesis, the LHBT is first tenotomized arthroscopically. The correct location for the incision is identified by abducting the arm which makes the inferior border of the pectoralis major tendon easily palpable. The incision is made just lateral to the axilla extending from the inferior border of the pectoralis major distally approximately 2 cm. An incision is made through the skin then subcutaneous tissue. The pectoralis major is identified and retracted superiorly. The biceps groove is palpated and the fascia is carefully released. The LHBT is identified, having been previously released at its origin, is pulled carefully out of the incision. It is critical to protect the neurovascular structures and avoid dissection medially. Starting at the musculotendinous junction of the LHBT, a looped suture with a straight needle is used to whipstitch the tendon. Approximately

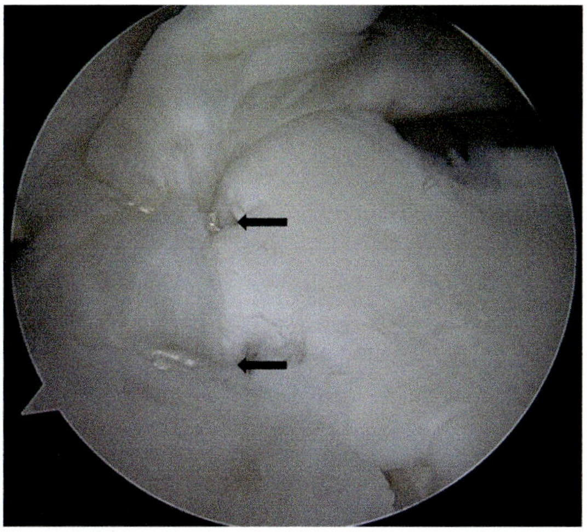

Fig. 10.8 Arthroscopic image demonstrating final construct after SLAP repair using a knotless technique. Right shoulder, lateral decubitus position view through a posterior viewing portal with a 30 degree arthroscope. Note placement of two anchors (black arrows) posterior to the biceps anchor. Note the absence of anchors or capsular imbrication anterior to the biceps tendon in the anterosuperior quadrant. Fixation in this location can lead to postoperative stiffness and pain

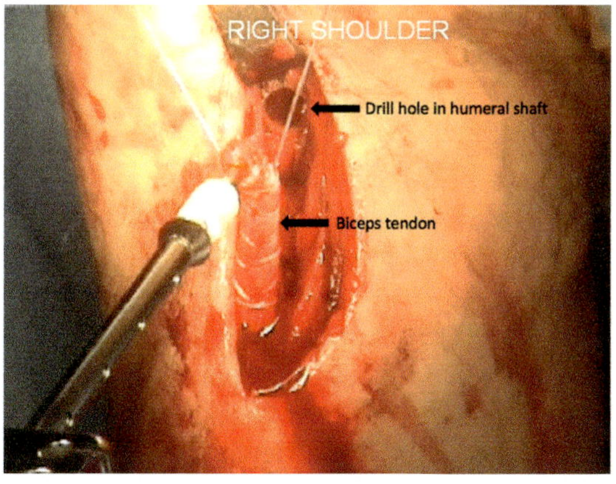

Fig. 10.9 Open view, right shoulder in preparation for subpectoral biceps tenodesis with interference screw. The biceps tendon has been whip-stitched along its course and a unicortical hole has been drilled in the humeral shaft in the subpectoral location corresponding to the anatomic location of the musculotendinous junction

five throws are placed with the second to last throw being a locking stitch. The remaining portion of the tendon may be excised. A method of fixation is then selected (Fig. 10.9).

Sub-Pectoral Biceps Tenodesis: Biotenodesis Screw Technique The screw technique involves cutting the wire from the straight needle and keeping the loop on the whip-stitched suture. Approximately 1.5–2 cm of the proximal portion of the long head of the biceps tendon is removed which allows return of the correct length tension relationship.

By marking the musculotendinous junction at the sub-pectoral region on the humerus prior to pulling the tendon from it's position in the groove allows the surgeon to plan where to cut the tendon after whip-stitching to restore the correct length tension relationship. Using a screw assumes approximately 1.5 cm of tendon will be placed into the humerus along with the screw in an interference technique.

Retractors are used to expose the bicipital groove just inferior to the pectoralis major. Once identifying the correct location, a drill is placed into the proximal humerus in the area of intertubercular groove at the sub-pectorally unicortically. Once a unicortical drill has engaged the humerus, a reamer is used to enlarge the hole depending on the size of the screw; commonly an 8 × 23 screw is used. Measurement of the length of the screw can be confirmed using another guide pin after the unicortical first pin has been placed. A wire is then used to place the looped suture through the cannulated tenodesis screw. Then using a biotenodesis screw technique with a screw handle and paddle, the screw with the tendon is placed into the proximal humerus to complete the tenodesis of the LHBT. If there is any laxity noted or if additional reinforcement is desired, a limb of one suture can be placed using a free needle back through the tendon to adjust for tension and strength. Arthroscopic knot tying technique is employed to complete the repair and then subcutaneous closure and skin closure are completed.

Sub-Pectoral Biceps Tenodesis: Unicortical Button Technique For the unicortical button technique, a tenodesis button 8.5 mm long is used which has angled edges to promote a toggle effect when the button contacts the humeral far cortex allowing it to flip unicortically.

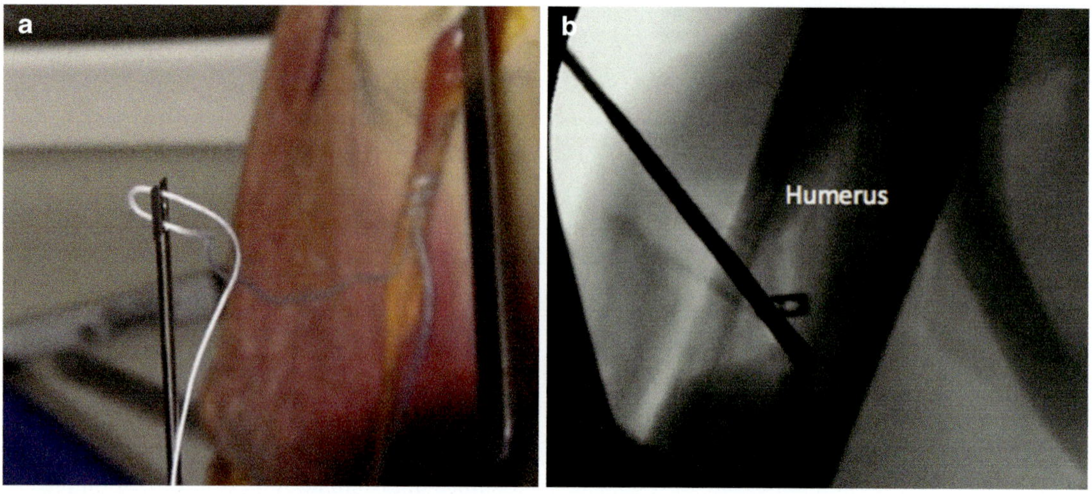

Fig. 10.10 Open view, right shoulder in preparation for subpectoral biceps tenodesis with unicortical button. (**a**) Suture from the previously prepared biceps tendon is passed through the button. (**b**) Intraoperative fluoroscopic image confirming intramedullary placement of the button

After whip-stitching the suture the proximal LHBT is then cut as described above. Using a button assumes the tendon will be placed onto the humerus, and therefore more tendon is excised in this technique than the interference screw technique. Having marked the humerus prior to displacing the tendon again allows for restoration of the correct length tension relationship.

The two ends of the suture are looped through the button. One limb is placed proximally and distally and then distally and proximally with the other limb. A drill is then used to make a unicortical hole in the humerus approximately 1 cm above the inferior border of the pectoralis tendon using a 3.2 mm drill pin. A drill guide can be used to protect the soft tissues. The button is then inserted with a special insertion device to allow the button to make contact with the far cortex. Then by unthreading the button from the inserter and turning counterclockwise and simultaneously pulling on the sutures gently, the button is flipped in the canal and the inserter is removed. Fluoroscopy can be used to confirm the button deployment. The suture limbs are then pulled to reduce the tendon onto the humerus and once the tendon is fully reduced a free needle can be used to pass one limb of the suture through the tendon and knots are tied to complete the repair. Similar soft tissue closure (Fig. 10.10).

Rehabilitation

Tenotomy The rehabilitation for a biceps tenotomy is immediate range of motion with no restrictions. Once pain free and full range of motion is regained, a gentle strengthening program may be initiated. A postoperative sling is not required.

SLAP Repair After SLAP repair a postoperative sling is utilized for approximately four weeks. For the first three weeks, active biceps exercises are prohibited. Gentle range of motion is allowed with table slides and passive motion to approximately 90° of forward flexion and internal/external rotation as tolerated. Over the next three to six weeks, passive range of motion progresses to full motion. Once passive motion has been restored, active biceps motion is then initiated with no resistance. At six weeks a strengthening program is initiated for the rotator cuff and biceps followed by a gradual return to throwing sports occurring over the next two to three months.

Tenodesis After a biceps tenodesis, whether it is using a screw or button the patient is placed in a sling for at least six weeks. The patient is encouraged to remove the sling at least three to five times a day and work on passive and active-assisted (without resistance) range of motion of the elbow and shoulder. Active biceps exercises begin at approximately three to four weeks. After six weeks biceps strengthening is initiated.

Importantly, rehabilitation will often be influenced by concomitant procedures such as rotator cuff repair. In those cases, the range of motion and strengthening may be advanced more carefully.

Outcomes

Tenotomy Most authors agree that tenotomy provides good pain control but cramping and weakness are common. Boileau et al. [42] described cramping in 62% of those treated with tenotomy but according to their report "none were bothered by it".

The other primary concern with tenotomy is the development of a clinical deformity caused be retraction of the biceps muscle belly distally, the so-called Popeye deformity. In one series 70% had a Popeye sign and 38% had fatigue discomfort with resisted elbow flexion but most had good pain control improvements [43].

SLAP Repair Results after SLAP repair, while initially encouraging, have been brought into question over time. Recently there has been a trend away from SLAP repair, especially in certain patient populations [44].

Most studies comparing SLAP repair to tenodesis are limited by a selection bias as younger patients and overhead athletes tend to receive SLAP repair over tenodesis. Despite this limitation results have been conflicting.

Gupta et al. [45] and Ek et al. [46] retrospectively compared the cases of 10 patients who underwent SLAP repair (mean age, 32 years) and compared them to 15 who underwent biceps tenodesis (mean age, 47 years). There was no significant difference in outcome scores.

By contrast, in another study of isolated type II SLAP lesions, 60% of patients were dissatisfied with the results of SLAP repair versus a 93% satisfaction rate among patients undergoing tenodesis. Dissatisfied patients after SLAP repair reported persistent pain and failure to return to previous level of sport. In total 13 patients (87%) were able to return to their previous levels of sports participation following biceps tenodesis, compared with only 20% after SLAP repair. Furthermore, four patients with a failed SLAP repair were revised to biceps tenodesis and reported successful return to previous level of sports activity [47].

Failure of SLAP Repairs Provencher et al. [48] found that 36.8% had problems postoperatively and were unable to return to work or sports successfully. Provencher also discovered that patients greater than 36 years of age had a high-risk for failure.

Using American Shoulder and Elbow Surgeons (ASES) scores (<75), return to full military duties and no need for revision procedures to mark successful cases, the investigators found that 66 patient (36.8%) had failures. Of these, 50 patients failures opted for corrective surgery including 42 patients who underwent biceps tenodesis, four patients had biceps tenotomy and four patients required debridement.

Age was a major factor in whether the repair was successful. The mean age in the failures was 39 years; successes were 29 years. There was no association with etiology, smoking history or preoperative outcome scores.

Waterman et al. [49] studied a similar population of 192 patients with two year follow up and found 37% of patients reported some level of activity-related shoulder pain and 16% were described as failures. Among the failures those revised to biceps tenodesis had a 76% return to activity versus 17% with revision SLAP repair.

Denard et al. [50] reviewed isolated type II SLAP lesions in patient's older than 35 years of age and found equivalent results for postoperative ASES, University of California, Los Angeles (UCLA) and SANE ratings. However, full range of motion recovery was delayed by approximately three months in the repair group compared with the tenodesis group and two patients in the repair group required a secondary capsular release. They concluded that individuals greater than 35 years of age with an isolated type II SLAP lesion had a shorter postoperative recovery, a more predictable functional outcome, a higher rate of satisfaction and return to activity with a biceps tenodesis compared to those who had a biceps repair.

Given the tenuous blood supply, the uncertain function of the intraarticular LHBT, the exponential difference in recovery time, and the marginal outcomes for some patient populations, it is not surprising that there is a trend towards SLAP repair only in younger and more active patients while expanding the relative prevalence of primary tenodesis.

The young, overhead throwing athlete remains the most compelling candidate for SLAP repair as it restores native anatomy while biceps tenodesis does not. Chalmers et al. [52] recently described motion analyses with simultaneous surface electromyography measurements in 18 baseball pitchers. Of these 18 players, seven were uninjured (controls), six were pitching after SLAP repair, and five were pitching after subpectoral biceps tenodesis. There were no significant differences between controls and postoperative patients with respect to pitching kinematics. Interestingly, compared with the controls and the patients who underwent open biceps tenodesis, the patients who underwent SLAP repair had altered patterns of thoracic rotation during pitching. However, the clinical significance of this finding and the impact of this finding on pitching efficacy are not currently known [45].

Werner et al. [51] confirmed that biceps tenodesis was a successful treatment after failed SLAP repair.

Considering the superior results, shorter rehabilitation, and uncertain functional changes in high level throwing athletes as well as the fact the tenodesis appears to be an effective treatment in the revision of the failed SLAP repair, it is reasonable to consider whether tenodesis should be the treatment of choice in the management of the primary SLAP tear in all populations. Unfortunately, high quality studies are not currently available to definitively answer this questions.

Tenodesis The high rates of deformity prompted development of techniques for restoring the length tension relationship of the biceps. Techniques using screws or buttons are the most common and have shown good outcomes ([53, 54], and [55]). Despite similar subjective reports, tenodesis has reported supination peak torque is better preserved with tenodesis over tenotomy [56].

Concern about proximal humerus fracture due to the large size of the drill hole required for some tenodesis screw fixation prompted development of unicortical and bicortical button techniques that required smaller drill holes [57]. Clinical results of this technique are still pending publication.

Location of Tenodesis More proximal tenodesis of the biceps lends itself to arthroscopic techniques; however, the primary argument against arthroscopic suprapectoral tenodesis is that lesions of the biceps groove may not be treated as effectively. Moon et al. [58] found that in approximately 80% of the intra-articular biceps tears evaluated in their study, a "hidden lesion" was observed going beyond the bicipital groove and extending to the distal extra-articular portion. Therefore, the subpectoral portion may be considered the optimal tenodesis site for the complete removal of all hidden biceps lesions.

Despite this, Millett et al. [55] showed that many patients complain of groove tenderness despite technically successful biceps tenodesis.

To date, most studies reviewing this question support equal clinical results for supraspinatus or subpectoral tenodesis and a systematic review has supported this finding, citing 98% good to excellent results for both techniques [59]. Others have confirmed arthroscopic biceps tenodesis performed at the articular margin results in a low surgical revision rate, a low rate of residual pain, and significant improvement in objective shoulder outcome scores [60].

Fixation Methods Golish et al. [61] found biceps tenodesis with interference screw fixation has been shown to be superior to placing a suture anchor and tying the tendon to the bone itself. However, other authors have demonstrated equivalent biomechanical properties for all fixation techniques except a simple bone tunnel technique [62].

Use of a unicortical button has been validated as a reasonable alternative to a screw and has the potential advantage of a smaller drill hole in the humerus [63]. Indeed, it may be superior to screw fixation as in one small cadaveric study intramedullary cortical button fixation showed no failure during cycling testing while interference screw fixation had a 30% failure rate [64].

Complications

Complications of biceps tenotomy as described above are cramping, strength deficits in elbow flexion and supination, and cosmetic deformity which can be common.

Complications after SLAP repair include recurrent SLAP tear, failure of SLAP repair, continued pain, stiffness, decreased throwing velocity, adhesive capsulitis, and inability to return to previous level of sport [65, 66].

Complications after subpectoral biceps tenodesis have been reported around 2% and can include deep infection, hardware failure, reflex sympathetic dystrophy, neurologic injury, and persistent bicipital pain [67].

While uncommon, proximal humerus fracture has been described after subpectoral tenodesis. Euler et al. [68] performed a biomechanical analysis and determined laterally eccentric malpositioned biceps tenodesis caused significant reduction in humeral strength and concluded that concentric screw placement and a smaller screw size would minimize this risk (Fig. 10.11).

The use of a bicortical button in a suprapectoral location results in instrumentation in close proximity to the axillary nerve where it lies posterior to the posterior cortex of the humerus. Therefore, an intramedullary button fixation is preferred in this area. In the subpectoral location, unicortical or bicortical fixations are safe as long as the direction of drilling is perpendicular to the axis of the humerus [69, 70].

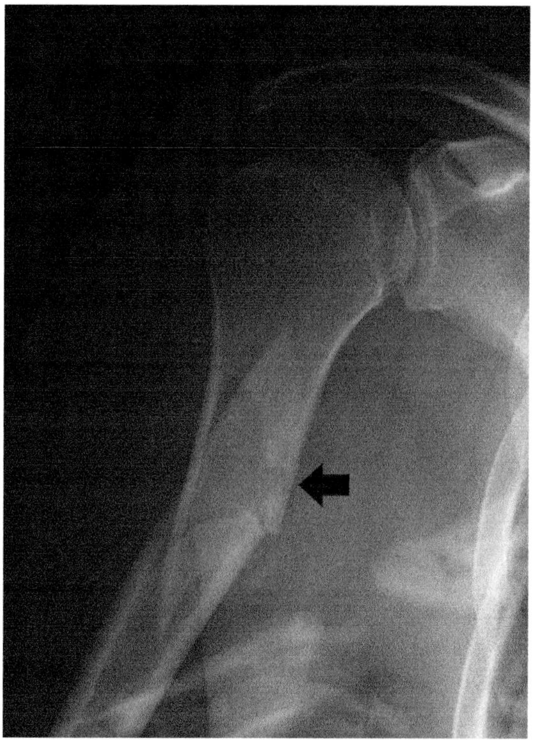

Fig. 10.11 X-ray image demonstrating proximal humerus fracture through prior subpectoral tenodesis drill hole (black arrow)

Summary

The role of the LHBT complex in shoulder pain is well established. However, anatomic and functional questions remain. Diagnosis of lesions of the LHBT requires a thorough history and combination of physical exam maneuvers. No single diagnostic test is confirmatory in all cases.

In the setting of continued or severe shoulder dysfunction surgical treatment of LHBT pathology should be considered. Treatment options include tenotomy, SLAP repair, and one of a myriad of forms of tenodesis.

Recovery after SLAP repair can be prolonged, complicated by postoperative stiffness, and may result in not returning to their previous level of sport. As such, the role and frequency of biceps tenodesis as a primary treatment for all LHBT complex disorder is expanding.

Further research is required to compare primary biceps tenodesis in a young active population of throwing athletes to primary SLAP repair.

Clinical Pearls

- Patients with SLAP tears often complain of being unable to sleep on that shoulder, unable to reach behind i.e. into the back-seat of a car, unable to perform military press during weight-lifting.
- Often a combination of physical exam tests provides the most reliable method of diagnosis. It is helpful to first test the opposite arm for comparison. Do not allow the patient to torque their body or scapula to compensate or lean on something with their other arm during testing of the affected limb.
- It is not uncommon an MRI and even an MRA report stating "Normal Labrum and Biceps" demonstrate clear pathologic changes during diagnostic arthroscopy. The shoulder surgeon needs to have an index of suspicion based on the history and physical exam and explain to the patient that a dynamic arthroscopic examination is still the gold standard to diagnose lesions of the LHBT and SLAP tears. When preoperative diagnostic studies are unclear, it is encouraged to initiate non-surgical treatment with rest, modification of activity, physical therapy, medication etc. If pain persists, it can be useful to apply a SANE rating. Even in the face of a normal MRI, if the patient states the affected shoulder is 50 or below out of 100, after reasonable non-operative treatment, surgery is a rational option.
- By marking the musculotendinous junction at the sub-pectoral region on the humerus prior to pulling the tendon from it's position in the groove allows the surgeon to plan where to cut the tendon after whip-stitching to restore the correct length tension relationship. Using a screw assumes approximately 1.5 cm of tendon will be placed into the humerus along with the screw in an interference technique.
- SLAP repair results in lower return to previous level of activity, requires a longer recovery, and has inferior outcomes in patients over 35 years of age when compared to biceps tenodesis.
- Results of arthroscopic suprapectoral and open subpectoral biceps tenodesis appear to be equivalent.

References

1. Codman EA. The shoulder. Boston: Thomas Todd; 1934.
2. Lippmann RK. Bicipital tenosynovitis. N Y State J Med. 1944;90:2235–41.
3. Tarsy JM. Bicipital syndromes and their treatment. N Y State J Med. 1946;46:996–1001.
4. Hitchcock HH, Bechtol CO. Painful shoulder. Observations on the role of the tendon of the long head of the biceps brachii in its causation. J Bone Joint Surg Am. 1948;30:263–73.
5. Depalma AF. Surgery of the shoulder. Philadelphia: JB Lippincott; 1950.
6. Andrews J, Carson W, McLeod W. Glenoid labrum tears related to the long head of the biceps. Am J Sports Med. 1985;13:337–41.
7. Snyder SJ, Karzel RP, Del Pizzo W, et al. SLAP lesions of the shoulder. Arthroscopy. 1990;6:274–9.
8. Gilmer BB, DeMers AM, Guerrero D, Reid JB, Lubowitz JH, Guttmann D. Arthroscopic versus open comparison of long head of biceps tendon visualization and pathology in patients requiring Tenodesis. Arthroscopy. 2014;31:29–34.
9. Denard PJ, Dai X, Hanypsiak BT, Burkhart SS. Anatomy of the biceps tendon: implications for restoring physiological length-tension relation during biceps tenodesis with interference screw fixation. Arthroscopy. 2012;28:1352–8.
10. Braun S, Millett PJ, Yongpravat C, et al. Biomechanical evaluation of shear force vectors leading to injury of the biceps reflection pulley: a biplane fluoroscopy study on cadaveric shoulders. Am J Sports Med. 2010;38:1015–24.
11. Habermeyer P, Kaiser E, Knappe M, et al. Functional anatomy and biomechanics of the long biceps tendon. Unfallchirurg. 1987;90:319–29. 3659929
12. McGough R, Debski RE, Taskiran E, et al. Tensile properties of the long head of the biceps tendon. Knee Surg Sports Traumatol Arthrosc. 1996;3:226–9. 8739718
13. Ahrens PM, Boileau P. The long head of biceps and associated tendinopathy. J Bone Joint Surg Br. 2007;89:1001–9.
14. Boesmueller S, Fialka C, Pretterklieber ML. The arterial supply of the tendon of the long head of the

biceps brachii in the human: a combined anatomical and radiological study. Ann Anat. 2014;196:449–55.
15. Abrassart S, Stern R, Hoffmeyer P. Arterial supply of the glenoid: an anatomic study. J Shoulder Elb Surg. 2016;15:232–8.
16. Alpantaki K, McLaughlin D, Karagogeos D, Hadjipavlou A, Kontakis G. Sympathetic and sensory neural elements in the tendon of the long head of the biceps. J Bone Joint Surg Am. 2005;87:1580–3.
17. Tosounidis T, Hadjileontis C, Triantafyllou C, Sidiropoulou V, Kafanas A, Kontakis G. Evidence of sympathetic innervation and α1-adrenergic receptors of the long head of the biceps brachii tendon. J Orthop Sci. 2013;18:238–44.
18. Ryu JHJ, Pedowitz RA. Rehabilitation of biceps tendon disorders in athletes. Clin Sports Med. 2010;29(229–46):vii–viii.
19. Bennett WF. Subscapularis, medial and lateral head coracohumeral ligament insertion anatomy: arthroscopic appearance and incidence of "hidden" rotator interval lesions. Arthroscopy. 2001;17(2):173–80.
20. Clark J, Sidles JA, Matsen FA. The relationship of the glenohumeral joint capsule to the rotator cuff. Clin Orthop Relat Res. 1990;254:29–34.
21. Pfahler M, Branner S, Refior HJ. The role of the bicipital groove in tendopathy of the long biceps tendon. J Shoulder Elb Surg. 1999;8:419–24.
22. Young NM, Capellini TD, Roach NT, Alemseged Z. Fossil hominin shoulders support an African ape-like last common ancestor of humans and chimpanzees. Proc Natl Acad Sci U S A. 2015;112:11829–34.
23. Roach NT, Venkadesan M, Rainbow MJ, Lieberman DE. Elastic energy storage in the shoulder and the evolution of high-speed throwing in homo. Nature. 2013;498:483–6.
24. Pagnani MJ, Deng XH, Warren RF, Torzilli PA, O'Brien SJ. Role of the long head of the biceps brachii in glenohumeral stability: a biomechanical study in cadavera. J Shoulder Elb Surg. 1996;5:255–62.
25. Itoi E, Kuechle DK, Newman SR, Morrey BF, An KN. Stabilizing function of the biceps in stable and unstable shoulders. J Bone Joint Surg Br. 1993;75:546–50.
26. Warner JJ, McMahon PJ. The role of the long head of the biceps brachii in superior stability of the glenohumeral joint. J Bone Joint Surg Am. 1995;77:366–72.
27. Kido T, Itoi E, Konno N, Sano A, Urayama M, Sato K. The depressors function of biceps on the head of the humerus in shoulders with tears of the rotator cuff. J Bone Joint Surg Br. 2000;82:416–9.
28. Sakurai G, Ozaki J, Tomita Y, et al. Morphologic changes in the long head of biceps brachii in rotator cuff dysfunction. J Orthop Sci. 1998;3:137–42.
29. Hegedus EJ, Goode AP, Cook CE, Michener L, Myer CA, Myer DM, Wright AA. Which physical examination tests provide clinicians with the most value when examining the shoulder? Update of a systematic review with meta-analysis of individual tests. Br J Sports Med. 2012;46:964–78.
30. Karrlson J. Physical examination tests are not valid for diagnosing SLAP tears: a review. Clin J Sport Med. 2010;20:134–5.
31. Bennett WF. Specificity of the Speed's test: Arthroscopic technique. Arthroscopy. 1998;14:789–96. 9848587
32. Holtby R, Razmjou H. Accuracy of the Speed's and Yergason's tests in detecting biceps pathology and SLAP lesions: comparison with arthroscopic findings. Arthroscopy. 2004;20(3):231–6.
33. Cook C, Beaty S, Kissenberth MJ, Siffri P, Pill SG, Hawkins RJ. Diagnostic accuracy of five orthopedic clinical tests for diagnosis of superior labrum anterior posterior (SLAP) lesions. J Shoulder Elb Surg. 2012;21:13–22.
34. Cone RO, Danzig L, Resnick D, Goldman AB. The bicipital groove: Radiographic, anatomic, and pathologic study. AJR Am J Roentgenol. 1983;141:781–8. 6351569
35. Ahovuo J. The radiographic anatomy of the intratubercular groove of the humerus. Eur J Radiol. 1985;2:83–6.
36. Armstrong A, Teefey SA, Wu T, Clark AM, Middleton WD, Yamaguchi K, Galatz LM. The efficacy of ultrasound in the diagnosis of long head of the biceps tendon pathology. J Shoulder Elb Surg. 2006;15:7–11.
37. Ok J-H, Kim Y-S, Kim J-M, Yoo T-W. Learning curve of office-based ultrasonography for rotator cuff tendons tears. Knee Surg Sports Traumatol Arthrosc. 2013;21:1593–7.
38. Jeyam M, Funk L, Harris J. Are shoulder surgeons any good at diagnosing rotator cuff tears using ultrasound?: a comparative analysis of surgeon vs radiologist. Int J Shoulder Surg. 2008;2:4–6.
39. De Maeseneer M, Boulet C, Pouliart N. Assessment of the long head of the biceps tendon of the shoulder with 3T magnetic resonance arthrography and CT arthrography. Eur J Radiol. 2012;81(5):934–9.
40. Malavolta EA, Assunção JH, Guglielmetti CLB, de Souza FF, Gracitelli MEC, Ferreira Neto AA. Accuracy of preoperative MRI in the diagnosis of disorders of the long head of the biceps tendon. Eur J Radiol. 2015;84:2250–4.
41. Taylor SA, Newman AM, Nguyen J, Fabricant PD, Baret NJ, Shorey M, Ramkumar P, O'Brien SJ. Magnetic resonance imaging currently fails to fully evaluate the biceps-labrum complex and bicipital tunnel. Arthroscopy. 2016;32:238–44.
42. Boileau P, Baqué F, Valerio L, Ahrens P, Chuinard C, Trojani C. Isolated arthroscopic biceps tenotomy or tenodesis improves symptoms in patients with massive irreparable rotator cuff tears. J Bone Joint Surg Am. 2007;89:747–57.
43. Kelly AM, Drakos MC, Fealy S, Taylor SA, O'Brien SJ. Arthroscopic release of the long head of the biceps tendon: functional outcome and clinical results. Am J Sports Med. 2015;33:208–13.
44. Erickson BJ, Jain A, Abrams GD, Nicholson GP, Cole BJ, Romeo AA, Verma NN. (2016) SLAP lesions: trends in treatment. Arthroscopy. 2016;32:976–81.
45. Gupta AK, Chalmers PN, Klosterman EL, Harris JD, Bach BR, Verma NN, Cole BJ, Romeo AA. Subpectoral biceps tenodesis for bicipital tendonitis with SLAP tear. Orthopedics SLACK Incorporated. 2015;38:e48–53.

46. Ek ETH, Shi LL, Tompson JD, Freehill MT, Warner JJP. Surgical treatment of isolated type II superior labrum anterior-posterior (SLAP) lesions: repair versus biceps tenodesis. J Shoulder Elb Surg. 2014;23:1059–65.
47. Boileau P, Parratte S, Chuinard C, Roussanne Y, Shia D, Bicknell R. Arthroscopic treatment of isolated type II SLAP lesions: biceps tenodesis as an alternative to reinsertion. Am J Sports Med. 2009;37:929–36.
48. Provencher MT, McCormick F, Dewing CB, Solomon DJ. A prospective analysis of 179 type 2 superior labrum anterior and posterior repairs: Outcomes and factors associated with success and failure. Am J Sports Med. 2013; Apr;41(4):880–6.
49. Waterman BR, Arroyo W, Heida K, Burks R, Pallis M. SLAP repairs with combined procedures have lower failure rate than isolated repairs in a military population: surgical outcomes with minimum 2-year follow-up. Orthop J Sports Med. 2015; SAGE Publications.
50. Denard PJ, Ladermann A, Parsley BK, Burkhart SS. Arthroscopic biceps tenodesis compared with repair of isolated type II SLAP lesions in patients older than 35 years. Orthopedics. 2014;37:e292–7.
51. Werner BC, Pehlivan HC, Hart JM, Lyons ML, Gilmore CJ, Garrett CB, Carson EW, Diduch DR, Miller MD, Brockmeier SF. Biceps tenodesis is a viable option for salvage of failed SLAP repair. J Shoulder Elb Surg. 2014;23:e179–84.
52. Chalmers PN, Trombley R, Cip J, Monson B, Forsythe B, Nicholson GP, Bush-Joseph CA, Cole BJ, Wimmer MA, Romeo AA, Verma NN. Postoperative restoration of upper extremity motion and neuromuscular control during the overhand pitch: evaluation of tenodesis and repair for superior labral anterior-posterior tears. Am J Sports Med. 2014;42:2825–36.
53. Lo I, Burkhart S. Arthroscopic biceps tenodesis using a bioabsorbable interference screw. Arthroscopy. 2004;20:85–95.
54. Mazzocca A, Cote M, Arciero C, Romeo A, Arciero R. Clinical outcomes after subpectoral biceps tenodesis with an interference screw. Am J Sports Med. 2008;36:1922–9.
55. Millett P, Sanders B, Gobezie R, Braun S, Warner J. Interference screw vs. suture anchor fixation for open subpectoral biceps tenodesis: does it matter? BMC Musculoskelet Disord. 2008;9:121.
56. Wittstein JR, Queen R, Abbey A, Toth A, Moorman CT. Isokinetic strength, endurance, and subjective outcomes after biceps tenotomy versus tenodesis: a postoperative study. Am J Sports Med. 2011;39:857–65.
57. Snir N, Hamula M, Wolfson T, Laible C, Sherman O. Long head of the biceps tenodesis with cortical button technique. Arthrosc Tech. 2013;2:e95–7.
58. Moon SC, Cho NS, Rhee YG. Analysis of "hidden lesions" of the extra-articular biceps after subpectoral biceps tenodesis: the subpectoral portion as the optimal tenodesis site. Am J Sports Med. 2015;43:63–8.
59. Abraham VT, Tan BHM, Kumar VP. Systematic review of biceps Tenodesis: arthroscopic versus open. Arthroscopy. 2016;32:365–71.
60. Brady PC, Narbona P, Adams CR, Huberty D, Parten P, Hartzler RU, Arrigoni P, Burkhart SS. Arthroscopic proximal biceps tenodesis at the articular margin: evaluation of outcomes, complications, and revision rate. Arthroscopy. 2015; Mar;31(3):470–6.
61. Golish SR, Caldwell PE, Miller MD, Singanamala N, Ranawat AS, Treme G, Pearson SE, Costic R, Sekiya JK. Interference screw versus suture anchor fixation for subpectoral tenodesis of the proximal biceps tendon: a cadaveric study. Arthroscopy. 2008;24:1103–8.
62. Mazzocca AD, Bicos J, Santangelo S, Romeo AA, Arciero RA. The biomechanical evaluation of four fixation techniques for proximal biceps tenodesis. Arthroscopy. 2015;21:1296–306.
63. Arora AS, Singh A, Koonce RC. Biomechanical evaluation of a unicortical button versus interference screw for subpectoral biceps tenodesis. Arthroscopy. 2015;29:638–44.
64. Buchholz A, Martetschläger F, Siebenlist S, Sandmann GH, Hapfelmeier A, Lenich A, Millett PJ, Stöckle U, Elser F. Biomechanical comparison of intramedullary cortical button fixation and interference screw technique for subpectoral biceps tenodesis. Arthroscopy. 2013;29:845–53.
65. McDonald LLS, Dewing CCB, Shupe LPG, Provencher CMT. Disorders of the proximal and distal aspects of the biceps muscle. J Bone Joint Surg. 2013;95:1235–45.
66. Weber SC, Martin DF, Seiler JG. Superior labrum anterior and posterior lesions of the shoulder: incidence rates, complications, and outcomes as reported by American Board of Orthopedic Surgery Part II candidates. Am J Sports Med. 2012; Jul;40(7):1538–43.
67. Nho SJ, Reiff SN, Verma NN, Slabaugh MA, Mazzocca AD, Romeo AA. Complications associated with subpectoral biceps tenodesis: low rates of incidence following surgery. J Shoulder Elb Surg. 2010;19:764–8.
68. Euler SA, Smith SD, Williams BT, Dornan GJ, Millett PJ, Wijdicks CA. Biomechanical analysis of subpectoral biceps tenodesis: effect of screw malpositioning on proximal humeral strength. Am J Sports Med. 2015;43:69–74.
69. Saithna A, Longo A, Jordan RW, Leiter J, MacDonald P, Old J. A cadaveric assessment of the risk of nerve injury during open subpectoral biceps tenodesis using a bicortical guidewire. Knee Surg Sports Traumatol Arthrosc. 2017;25(9):2858–63.
70. Sethi PM, Vadasdi K, Greene RT, Vitale MA, Duong M, Miller SR. Safety of open suprapectoral and subpectoral biceps tenodesis: an anatomic assessment of risk for neurologic injury. J Shoulder Elb Surg. 2015;24:138–42.

The Stiff Shoulder

11

Richard S. Page and Goran Mitreski

Clinical Pearls

1. Adhesive capsulitis is mainly a clinical diagnosis, with the minimum of a plain x-ray is required to exclude other diagnoses.
2. The natural history and duration of AC may vary and the pain is often severe, so a detailed history of the onset of pain and reduced motion may aide in determining which patients are on a shorter verses a more prolonged trajectory.
3. Diabetics, particularly those on insulin, have a more resistant disease course.
4. Intra-articular local anaesthetic and corticosteroid +/− hydrodilatation are more effective in the early course of the disease (Stage I) with a supportive home based stretching programme.
5. Manipulation +/− intra-articular injection have a role in early (Stage II) disease, however, the risks of excessive trauma to the joint may increase with maturity of the fibrosis over time.
6. Arthroscopic capsular release is a safe and reliable treatment modality, particularly in more chronic and resistant disease (late resistant Stage II).
7. Adequate pain management is crucial in all treatment pathways to enable the patient to engage in their rehabilitation programme to restore function.

R. S. Page (✉)
Barwon – Centre of Orthopaedic Research and Education, University Hospital Geelong and St John of God Hospital, Geelong, VIC, Australia

School of Medicine, Deakin University, Geelong, VIC, Australia
e-mail: richard.page@deakin.edu.au

G. Mitreski
Barwon – Centre of Orthopaedic Research and Education, University Hospital Geelong and St John of God Hospital, Geelong, VIC, Australia

Introduction

The stiff shoulder covers a heterogeneous group of conditions resulting in reduced shoulder range of motion, usually associated with a variable element of pain. The key two elements covered in this chapter are adhesive capsulitis (AC, also known as frozen shoulder) and post-surgical/traumatic (PTS) stiffness. Osteoarthritis and inflammatory arthritis of the shoulder are important causes of loss of motion in which pain may not be a strong early feature, but predominates later. These latter conditions are important to exclude and are covered in other chapters.

I. A. Trail et al. (eds.), *Textbook of Shoulder Surgery*, https://doi.org/10.1007/978-3-319-70099-1_11

Adhesive capsulitis describes a condition of shoulder pain and stiffness of unknown aetiolgy. It is disabling, often severely painful and commonly managed in the primary care setting. The condition was originally attributed to Duplay in 1872 coining the term periarthritis [1]. Codman was the first to introduce the phrase of frozen shoulder in 1934, describing pain down to the deltoid insertion with a gradual progressive loss of motion [2]. The term 'Adhesive Capsulitis' was introduced by Nervaiser in 1945, in recognition of the inflammatory and fibrosis features as part of the pathogenesis [3].

Shoulder range of motion decreases over a period of month's until it becomes functionally limiting [4]. True AC has a protracted natural history that usually ends in resolution [5]. Yet patients with this disease face months to years of pain and disability [6]. Recent literature challenges the natural history of AC with persisting symptoms including pain and biomechanical deficits seen in up to 6% of patients followed long term [7].

Evidence suggests an underlying inflammatory process affecting the joint capsule and shoulder ligaments, but conjecture remains [8]. As such, optimal management and treatment for AC is unclear as its pathophysiology remains incompletely understood [9].

Post-surgical or post-traumatic stiffness (PTS) is a secondary cause of stiff shoulder, characterized by loss of motion from a prior injury or trauma, which may include surgery. The resultant fibrosis often involves both intra-articular and extra-articular structures around the shoulder including the capsule, bursa, rotator cuff and glenohumeral and coracohumeral ligaments. Consequently, the natural history may differ, with resultant chronic reduction in shoulder functional range. Shoulder surgery associated with stiffness includes subacromial decompression, rotator cuff repair, shoulder stabilization, joint replacement surgery and fracture fixation around the shoulder girdle. Classically in PST the subacromial bursa is fibrosed and with adhesions between the bursal surface of the rotator cuff and the deltoid. Non-shoulder surgery that has been associated with shoulder stiffness includes breast surgery +/− associated axillary lymph node sampling or clearance and open cardiac surgery.

Shoulder stiffness may also be linked to pathology affecting the neuromuscular structures driving the shoulder, the articular surface and adjacent connective tissues. Weakness leading to an inability achieve a normal range of motion, may over time may result in fixed, non-corrigible loss of motion. Peri-articular tissue pathology resulting in fibrosis and/or reduced tissue compliance such as heterotopic ossification is rare around the shoulder, but may also result in significant irreversible loss of motion.

Demographics/Epidemiology

Adhesive capsulitis occurs in 2–5% of the population [6] affecting females more than males, with as much as a 70% preponderance toward the female sex [8, 10]. Patients typically develop AC in the 40–60 year old age bracket [11, 12] with the non-dominant arm mostly involved [6]. In 6–17% of patients, the other shoulder becomes affected, usually within 5 years, and after the first has resolved [5]. Recurrence in the ipsilateral shoulder is rare [13]. A genetic link, using twin studies has found genetic associations [14] yet supporting data has not been published.

Further those with diabetes, prolonged shoulder immobility (trauma, overuse injuries or surgery) or systemic disease (hyperthyroidism, hypothyroidism, cardiovascular disease, autoimmune disease or Parkinson's disease) are at higher risk [15]. The incidence of adhesive capsulitis increases to 10% and 20% in patients with diabetes [16]. Further, bilateral involvement is more frequent in patients with diabetes than in non-diabetic patients (33–42% vs. 5–20%) [16–18]. AC also remains the most common musculoskeletal complaint in diabetic patients and is more resistant to treatment in this group [5, 19].

Protease inhibitors used for antiretroviral therapy have been also been implicated, as well as an association with Dupuytren's disease and the development of AC [20].

Despite epidemiological data establishing a relationship between diabetes mellitus and frozen shoulder, a pathophysiological association has yet been reported [21]. This is the subject of ongoing research by the senior author among others.

Table 11.1 Classification and Epidemiology of Adhesive capsulitis

Classification	Cause	Examples
Primary AC	Unknown	Idiopathic
	Predisposing conditions	Diabetes mellitus, Dupuytren contracture, thyroid disorders, myocardial infarction, Parkinsons disease
Secondary AC	Intra-articular	Chondral lesion, labral tear, loose bodies
	Capsular	Capsular injury, surgery, joint immobilization
	Extra-articular	Muscle tightness, heterotropic ossification, skin scarring following burns
	Neurological	Cervical spine, brachial plexus injuries or upper motor neuron lesions with spasticity

Adapted from Itoi et al. [21]

Definition

Adhesive capsulitis (AC), also known as frozen shoulder (FS) can be grouped into two categories: Primary and secondary adhesive capsulitis.

Primary Adhesive capsulitis is defined as an idiopathic condition of the shoulder, characterized by the spontaneous onset of shoulder pain accompanied by increasingly severe limitation of glenohumeral movement in all directions with restricted active and passive movement. AC is largely a clinical diagnosis and there is lack of consensus around the defined functional loss of motion. Most authors agree on the loss in range of motion of at least 25% in at least two directions, up to 50% reduction in external rotation [22–26]. The pain, persisting for more than 4 weeks, is often severe and characteristically disturbs the sleep [11].

This definition excludes: sub acromial bursitis, acute calcinosis of the rotator cuff, supraspinatus tendinitis and isolated bicipital tendinitis.

Secondary adhesive capsulitis develops when there is a known intrinsic, extrinsic or systemic cause. Possible causes of secondary adhesive capsulitis include macro trauma, micro trauma or postsurgical intervention [11, 12]. Postoperative stiff shoulder seen after open rotator cuff repair is a common complaint with resolution of symptoms in 6–12 months and good long-term results, in itself does not constitute true AC [27]. Adhesive capsulitis has also been linked to numerous medical conditions in the literature, including diabetes and thyroid dysfunction [5, 11, 13, 21, 28] (see Table. 11.1).

Pathogenesis

The pathological findings have been well documented by Neviaser (1945), who found a tight capsule, along with dense adhesions between the humeral head and the capsule. He further described an inflammatory reaction in the capsule and synovium that subsequently led to adhesions to the attachment of the capsule to the humeral head [29]. Watson et al. (2010) describe the pathological change as a fibrotic expansion of the synovium and joint capsule that results in painful loss of function [30]. Kabbabe et al. (2010) further found evidence of inflammatory changes in the synovium of all recorded patients with AC having capsular thickenings with higher degrees of proliferation than controls [4].

There is still disagreement whether the underlying pathology is inflammatory [29], fibrotic in nature [30] or a transitional process [4].

Pathology

Inflammatory Changes

Cytokines

Cytokines have been recently implicated in the inflammation and subsequent fibrosis seen in shoulder joints during arthroscopy. Cytokines are involved in the initiation and repair processes in multiple musculoskeletal tissues, with sustained activity attributable to increased tissue [13]. Rodeo et al. (1997) reported an increased in transforming growth factor-B (TGFb1), platelet derived growth factor (PDGF) and hepatocyte staining growth factor (HGF), IL-1beta and TNFα in patients with adhesive capsulitis. TGFb1 has been shown to induce arthrofibrosis and chondrometaplasia with delivery and over expression in rat models, as outlined in Fig. 11.1 [31]. Further Rodeo et al., found that the synovium contained few T-cells and no B-cells, predominating with synovial hyperplastic change and that the cytokines were more frequently localized to the synovial cells than the capsular fibroblasts.

As such, they postulate these cytokines and their role in cell proliferation, angiogenesis and matrix synthesis to produce the fibrotic changes seen in adhesive capsulitis. Kabbabe et al. had also shown in samples collected significant lower values of macrophage colony stimulating factor (M-CSF) in AC patients who had diabetes as compared to AC patients without diabetes [4]. New and novel modalities investigating the inflammatory mRNA pathways and subsequent protein synthesis have been proposed by Page et al. using NexGen sequencing technology. These techniques have the potential to shed new light on the diagnosis, mediating pathways and possible intervention points to treat AC [32].

Immunoglobulins

ICAM-1 (intercellular adhesion molecule 1) is a member of the immunoglobulin superfamily. It is typically expressed on endothelial cells and has been reported in association with inflammation, infection and malignancy. It plays a central role to the inflammatory response mediated by leukocytes and lymphocytic proliferation. Kim et al. 2013 found significantly elevated levels of ICAM-1 in glenohumeral capsular tissue, synovial fluid and serum in patients with adhesive capsulitis compared to controls. Further, elevated ICAM-1 levels were found in patients with diabetes mellitus. However, patients with diabetes mellitus who have high circulating ICAM-1 may not have symptoms of adhesive capsulitis nor are symptoms of adhesive capsulitis correlated to ICAM-1 levels in the serum. ICAM-1 levels are not specific to adhesive capsulitis; they only strengthen the idea that the key pathophysiological response is a multi-factorial inflammatory cascade [33].

Matrix Metalloproteases

Matrix metalloproteases (MMPs) and the inhibitors of MMP (TIMP's) regulate the remodeling of the extracellular matrix that fibroblasts produce [4]. The expression of MMP's are tightly controlled by cytokines and other growth factors, including TGFbeta1, TNFα, and IL-1, which either stimulate or repress their genetic transcription, and further can act on TIMP's [34, 35]. It is believed mismatches in these proteases and their inhibitors can trigger aggressive healing, scarring, contracture and failure of remodeling, accounting for the phases and clinical course of AC.

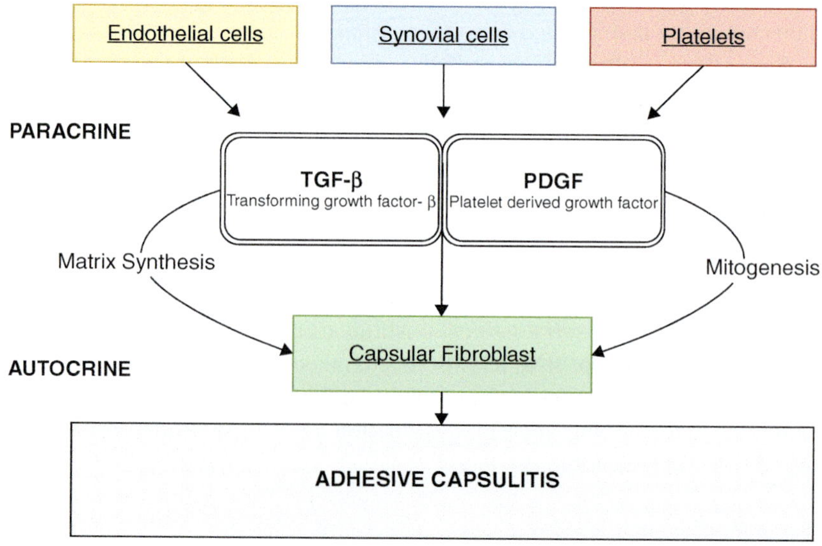

Fig. 11.1 Proposed cellular pathway for the activation of TGF-B and PDGF, which in turn stimulate the capsular fibroblasts with resultant capsular hypertrophy and restricted motion. (Modified from Rodeo et al. [31])

Along with higher levels of cytokines IL-1 and IL6 in arthroscopic samples, Kabbabe et al. also found changes in the levels of fibrogenic cytokines, with matrix metalloprotease 3 (MMP3) and a disintigrin and metalloprotease with thrombospondin motifs 4 (ADAMTS4) to be elevated in adhesive capsulitis patients compared to controls [4].

Richards et al. (1993) found increased levels of TIMPs to be increased in comparison to MMPs 1, 2 and 3 which were also elevated. The mRNA for MMP-14 was absent in all specimens ($n = 14$) of AC, with its action to secrete and activate MMP-2; essential for degradation of collagen in connective tissue [34, 35]. Hutchinson et al. (1998) further described the MMP: TIMP ratio, with changes influencing pathological change. They discussed the possible aetiolgy of AC being due to a decrease in the MMP: TIMP ratio [36].

The implications of TIMP's in AC was further implicated in the treatment of patients with inoperable gastric cancer, where their treatment with a broad spectrum MMP inhibitor (Marimastat) induced bilateral AC in 6 of the 12 treated, with 3 also exhibiting signs of Dupuytrens contracture [36]. De Ponti et al. (2006) also discussed the increased incidence of AC in HIV-1 affected patients receiving highly active antiretroviral therapy which included protease inhibitor (indinavir), where 6 out of 50 developed AC, with no other causes of secondary AC present [20].

Fibrotic Changes

Adhesive capsulitis has been regarded as an inflammatory response leading to fibrosis [29]. Killian et al. (2007) sought to investigate collagen synthesis during the fibrotic stages of AC. They found a significant increase in alpha1 mRNA in AC compared to control, with type I collagen representing the major extracellular matrix protein in capsule and tendon tissue [29, 37]. This secondary fibrotic change in the shoulder follows the initial inflammatory synovitis, induced by cytokines growth factors and matrix metalloproteases [34].

Pathoanatomy and Histology

Histology and Histochemical Studies

The underlying histology in AC patients has shown to be a process of fibroplasia and capsular contractures [38, 39]. Bunker et al. (2000) showed an increase in fibrogenic growth factors, MMP's and TIMPS, whilst Rodeo et al. demonstrated elevated levels of inflammatory cytokines within the capsule [31, 34].

Rodeo et al. established on histological examination, deposition of dense collagen fibres, with high degrees of staining for collagen type I and type III in the matrices of AC and control yet higher qualitative degrees of type I staining in AC group. Further, they noted definite matrix staining for TGF-B and PDGF in tissues of AC, whereas matrix did not stain for cytokines in controls, additionally, increased receptor staining in AC samples was seen compared with controls. Histologically, massive proliferation of synovial fibroblasts has been shown with high degrees of differentiation into myofibroblasts in rat models over expressing TGFbeta1 [30]. Further such differentiation and specific cellularity with predominating myofibroblasts and fibroblasts have also been reviewed by Bunker (2011) in AC [40]. Of note is the cross over association of fibroblastic proliferation in AC and Dupuytren's disease in the hand. Although an association between AC and Dupuytren's has been demonstrated, [17, 41, 42] the exact mechanisms are not well understood. A feature of the myofibroblast is the response to tension, whereby the cell shortens under tension which does not reverse with the load is removed. This and the production of extracellular collagen forming fibrosis, result in fixed contracture and therefore loss of capsular length and shoulder motion.

In a tissue study on arthroscopic samples, Hettrich [43] demonstrated a high prevalence of myofibroblasts in affected tissue, containing alpha smooth muscle actin in AC patients. The prior treatment with an intra-articular corticosteroid injection resulted in a decrease in the presence of fibromatosis, vascular hyperplasia and fibrosis, with a reduction in fibroblasts, the typical hallmarks of AC.

The staining of increased type III collagen in the capsule of AC samples indicates new deposition of connective tissue [31]. Nago et al. (2010) also demonstrated chronic non-specific inflammation with synovial hyperplasia, proliferation of blood vessels and fibroblasts, along with an increase in extracellular matrix in samples of AC, with such findings not evident in patients who had rotator cuff disease without AC [44].

Clinical Conditions Associated with Shoulder Stiffness

Conditions Associated with Adhesive Capsulitis

Varying conditions have been affiliated with adhesive capsulitis in the literature (see Table 11.2). These have been grouped as to those associated with trauma, endocrine, cardiac, neurological and other conditions.

Other Causes of Stiff Shoulder

Stiffness of the shoulder can result from a range of other conditions, secondary causes as opposed to associated conditions where the causal link is unclear. Secondary conditions relate to those where either direct capsular scaring and thickening occurs, or where there is immobility with resultant shortening of the joint capsular fibers with resultant restricted motion such and post-surgical or post-traumatic stiffness (PTS). The later associated conditions include endocrine, cardiac, pulmonary and Dupuytren's Disease where the causal link is unclear.

Neurological

Neurological conditions resulting in shoulder stiffness are uncommon, but important and often over-

Table 11.2 Conditions associated with adhesive capsulitis

Authors	Condition
	Trauma
Stam [45]	Upper limb trauma
Patten and Hillel [46]	Radical neck dissection
	Endocrine
Arkkila et al. [47]	Diabetes
Choy et al. [48]	ACTH deficiency
Wohlgethan [49]	Hyperthyroidism
Bowman et al. [50]	Hypothyroidism
Okamura and Ozaki [51]	Reduced bone mineral density
Lundberg and Nilsson [52]	Osteopenia
	Cardiac
Tuten et al. [53]	Cardiac surgery
Pineda et al. [54]	Cardiac catheterisation through the brachial artery
Boyle-walker et al. [55]	Cardiac disease
	Neuroligcal
Bruckner and Nye [56]	Neurosurgery
Tanishima and Yoshimasu [57]	Aneurysm surgery
Riley et al. [58]	Parkinson's disease
Jayson [59]	Stroke
	Other
Wadsworth [60]	Pulmonary disease
Smith et al. [42]	Dupuytren's disease
Bunker and Esler [61]	Hyperlipidemia
Hutchinson et al. [36]	Treatment with matrix metalloproteinase inhibitor
Saleh et al. [62]	Pneumococcal and influenza vaccine
Kim et al. [33]	Immunogenic

Adapted from Chambler and Carr [63]

looked. These can be divided into upper motor and lower motor lesions. Upper motor neuron lesions generally result in spasticity and chronic reduction in motion, such as in stroke or Parkinson's disease patients. The reduced range can initially be related to loss of length of the musculotendinous unit. This in turn leads to long-term loss of capsular stretch and adaptive shortening of the collagen matrix fibers with excess cross-linking of these fibers in the capsule. In time, these changes may become permanent if the joint is not regularly taken through a range of motion.

Lower motor neuron lesions cause muscle weakness and a flaccid paralysis, with associated loss of reflexes and later muscle wasting. This flaccid pattern is typically seen in complete brachial plexus injuries such as following high energy trauma, penetrating injuries or uncommonly Parsonage Turner syndrome. The changes in muscle volume may become fixed and irreversible after 12–24 months with fixed reduction in the length of the musculotendinous unit. Secondary posturing is more pronounced when there is partial brachial plexus involvement. The normal motor level supply to the shoulder is C5–6, and the when upper trunk is injured the loss of C5 results in an internal rotation/adduction contracture, with loss of external rotation at the shoulder. This is as a result of muscle imbalance and loss of motion due to weakness compared to normal, intact muscle groups. Joint capsule contracture may occur over time as an adaptive change, similar to upper motor neuron lesions.

Neuropathic osteoarthropathy also known as Charcot neuroarthropathy, is a chronic degenerative arthropathy associated with decreased sensory innervation and afferent signaling, largely proprioception, pain and temperature sensation [64]. Chronic peripheral neuropathy in diabetes tends to affect the lower limbs whereas patients with cervical syrinx and syringomyelia tend to have shoulder and elbow involvement [65, 66]. Clinically, there is marked joint swelling, pain and deformation along with restrictions in movement, both passive and active.

Heterotopic Ossification

Heterotopic ossification (HO) is the formation of lamellar bone in non-osseous tissues. This differs from calcific tendinosis affecting the rotator cuff, which involves the deposition of calcium hydroxyapatite crystals in the tendon but not the maturation into osseous tissue. HO is rare around the shoulder in the absence of trauma (including brain or local injury) or surgery. The formation of ossification differs from tendinosis in that other tissue layers may be involved, notably local muscles around the shoulder with associated myositis. The rotator cuff and capsule can also be involved, unlike calcific tendinopathy which is usually self-limiting with eventual resorption of the calcium crystals without permanent loss of shoulder motion. In contrast, HO tissue matures into lamellar bone that does not usually recede. This significant increase in tissue compliance results in the loss of motion, which in extreme cases may result in ankylosis of the joint (see Fig. 11.2).

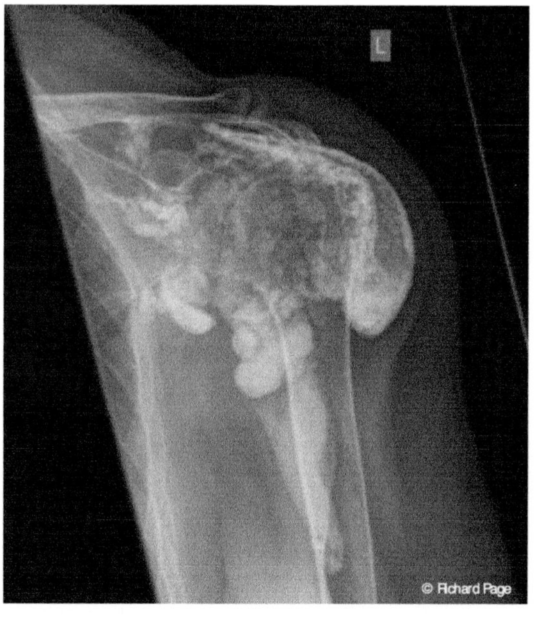

Fig. 11.2 Extensive heterotopic ossification of the shoulder affecting peri-bursal as well as capsular and muscular elements around the shoulder presenting as a progressive loss of motion, to a point of virtual ankylosis

Stages of Adhesive Capsulitis/Frozen Shoulder

Adhesive capsulitis progresses through 4 stages described by Neviaser in 1987. These 4 stages are based on the correlation of history, physical examination and arthroscopic examination (see Table. 11.3).

Clinical Assessment

There is lack of consensus as to the exact range of motion restriction required to diagnose adhesive capsulitis [9] yet criteria have been established: severe shoulder pain that interfered with successful performance of activities of daily living, night pain, painful restriction of both active and passive elevation to less than 100 degrees and 50% restriction of the external rotation, with normal radiological findings and no secondary cause [9, 11, 13, 67].

Signs and Symptoms

Patients suffering from adhesive capsulitis typically have had the condition for several weeks or months prior to presenting for physical therapy. Pain and gradually deteriorating shoulder function motivate the patient to seek help [10]. Pain is aggravated by motion, especially external rotation and alleviated by limiting use of the affected limb [5, 10]. The pain is generally worse at night and most often, the pain associated with adhesive capsulitis is located to the deltoid region, but may be felt in the anterior and posterior joint lines.

Functional impairment includes difficulty putting on a coat, reaching into the hip pocket or combing the hair, with difficulty in personal hygiene and toileting and in fastening bras in women. At rest the arm is usually held in a position of adduction and internal rotation. In gait, arm swing is limited or absent.

Physical signs include muscle spasm (pectoralis major and prei-scapular muscles) early on or muscle atrophy (deltoid and supraspinatus) in later cases [5, 10]. Early in the disease process, the only physical examination finding might be pain produced at end range of shoulder motion [12]. On palpation, there is diffuse tenderness over the glenohumeral joint, extending to the trapezius and interscapular area [5]. The tenderness may be increased along both the anterior and posterior joint lines and below the acromium, along

Table 11.3 The four stages of Adhesive capsulitis

Stages	Symptoms	Signs	Arthroscopic appearance	Biopsy
Stage 1	Pain referred to deltoid insertion Pain at night	Capsular pain on deep palpation Empty end feel at extreme of motion Full motion under anesthesia	Fibrous synovial inflammatory reaction No adhesions or capsular contracture	Rare inflammatory cell infiltrate Hypervascular hypertrophic synovitis Normal capsular tissue
Stage 2	Severe night pain Stiffness	Motion restricted in forward flexion, abduction, internal and external rotation Some motion loss under anesthesia	Christmas tree synovitis Some loss of axillary fold	Hypertrophic hypervascular synovitis Perivascular, sub synovial capsular scar
Stage 3	Profound stiffness Pain only at the end of range of motion	Significant loss of motion Tethering at ends of motion No improvement under anesthesia	Complete loss of axillary fold Minimal synovitis	Hyper cellular, collagenous tissue with a thin synovial layer Similar features to other fibrosis conditions
Stage 4	Profound stiffness Pain minimal	Significant motion loss Gradual improvement in motion	Full mature adhesions Identification of intra-articular structures difficult	Not reported

Adapted from Neviaser and Neviaser [29]

the coracohumeral ligament line in thinner patients. In those with significant pain, a local anesthetic can be used. Those with adhesive capsulitis will still have a decreased range of abduction and external rotation [15].

Natural History

Duration of Symptoms

Adhesive capsulitis is largely a self-limiting condition [11]. It is a disease that improves over an 18 to 36 month period, [7] with symptom's persisting up to 52 months in up to a half of patients [68]. Dominant arm involvement has been shown to have a good prognosis; associated intrinsic pathology or insulin dependent diabetes are poor prognostic indicators [7, 12]. However, during this time there may be significant limitation in shoulder and upper limb function, sleep and social activities, as well as severe pain and suffering. In younger patients, this can lead to limitations in the capacity to work, particularly in the early stages.

Phases of Recovery

Adhesive capsulitis passes through three phases, pain, stiffness and recovery [63]. The first stage is the 'freezing stage' in which there is insidious onset of pain. This stage ends with limited range of movement [12]. The second stage is the stiff or 'frozen stage', where range of motion remains compromised, but pain is less a feature. The third stage is the recovery or 'thawing' stage where range of movement recovers but over a period of months to years. Most patients regain near full function yet discussion remains for some have continual pain and disability [12, 69, 70].

Four phases of Adhesive capsulitis have also been described, [13, 29] where stage 1 shows pain with active and passive movement lasting up to 3 months. Stage 2 is classed as the 'freezing stage', where symptoms have been present 3–9 months with chronic pain and progressive loss of range of movement. Stage 3 is classed the 'frozen stage' similar to other published phases, this stage correlates with poor range of movement in the absence of pain. In this phase, symptoms have been present for 9–15 months. Stage 4, coinciding with the 'thawing stage' describes functional recovery with little to no pain (Fig. 11.3).

Prognostic Factors for Non-Operative Treatment and Recovery

Diabetes mellitus and severely reduced joint motion elicited at the initial clinical visit respond poorly to non-operative treatment [18]. Patients who do not improve with non-operative treatment, including those with diabetes, have shown to respond to manipulation and arthroscopic release [71]. Patients aged 60 years or over, conversely, have shown good response to non-operative treatment.

Resolution of Symptoms and Return of Function with Non-operative Treatment

Although some literature supports complete resolution of pain, [72] other studies have shown contrary results. Reeves (1975) [70] showed in a

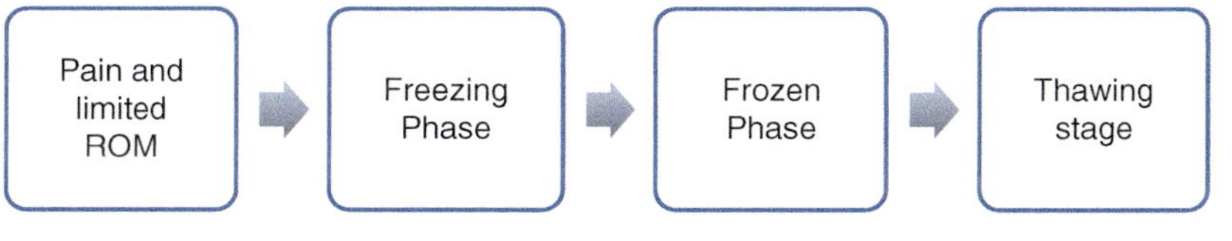

Fig. 11.3 The four phases of Adhesive Capsulitis. (Adapted from Sheriden and Hannafin [8], Neviaser and Neviaser [29])

5–10 year follow up, 54% of patients having clinical limitation without functional disability, with 7% having remaining disability whilst Shaffer et al. (1992) [69] showed in patients treated non-operatively, 50% had some degree of pain and stiffness seven years after onset of disease with 11% having functional limitation. More recent literature has strengthened the idea that condition does not fully resolve [7, 9, 73]. Vastamaiki et al. (2012) had found 94% of patients with spontaneous adhesive capsulitis recover to normal levels of function without treatment over a mean follow up period of 14 years. As such, the natural history of adhesive capsulitis remains variable and there remains discussion as to whether this disease runs a benign course or if its progression retains clinically significant disability, be it pain or mobility. This also points to there being a spectrum of disease involvement without clear markers or factors to point to which patients will fully recover and over what time course.

Diagnosis

Laboratory Studies

Laboratory data are relatively normal in adhesive capsulitis, however in patients with other medical issues, thyroid stimulating hormone (TSH), lipid levels and blood sugar levels (BSL) might be elevated. Human leukocyte antigen B27, C-reactive protein (CRP) and erythrocyte sedimentation rate (ESR) are normal [5].

Radiography

No diagnostic x-ray modality exists for AC. In chronic cases, there could be osteoporotic changes of the humeral head which are well visualised with plain film imaging. Radiography is better suited to differentiate AC from other shoulder conditions such as fractures, arthritis, malignancy, calcific tendinitis or chondocalcinosis. In the early stages of disease, AC may not be clinically distinguishable from glenohumeral arthritis, hence basic plain radiography is important for exclusion. The basic views required are true anteroposterior (AP), axillary and a lateral of the shoulder; external rotation and outlet views are also helpful to excluded other pathology.

Magnetic Resonance Imaging (MRI)

MRI enhanced with either, indirect (intravenous gadolinium) or direct (intraarticular contrast) can visualise thickening of the joint capsule and synovium along with hypervascularity when compared to controls, yet shows little difference when comparing rheumatoid to AC on MRI perfusion scans [74]. MRI can demonstrate the rotator interval and axillary recess, which are common sites affected by AC, with reduced joint volume. Imaging is best performed using T1-weighted and T2-weighted fat suppressed (T2-FS) sequences; intravenous contrast is much more commonly used over intraarticular [75]. Table 11.4 outlines imaging findings that can aid in the radiological diagnosis of AC.

Ultrasound (US)

Ultrasound can show thickening of the coracohumeral ligament and increased blood flow on Doppler scans. However, the efficacy of US is questionable as the worst pathological change occurs beneath the coracoid process and US cannot visualize past bone [40]. Ancillary features

Table 11.4 Signal characteristics on MRI in AC

Site	Process	Signal characteristics
Rotator interval	Thickening of the coracohumeral and superior glenohumeral ligament Thickened rotator interval capsule Biceps tendon anchor	T2-FS increased signaling obscuring adjacent fat planes Increased signal intensity on T2-FS in adjacent synovial structures
Axillary recess	Thickened inferior glenohumeral ligament	T2-FS increased signaling and inferior glenohumeral ligament >4 mm in thickness Axillary recess thickness ≥1.3 cm

on US that may assist the clinician in diagnosis include thickening of the coracohumeral ligament [76] and limited supraspinatus movement under the acromion [77]. A key function of US is to differentiate alternate sources of shoulder pain involving pathology of the rotator cuff or bursal impingement.

Arthrography

Arthrography was the investigation of choice for many years; with a joint volume less than 10 ml and a marked loss of normal axillary folds making the correct diagnosis [29]. However it is no longer routinely used, as it is invasive, technically challenging and has largely been replaced by MRI which provides a greater range of diagnostic and anatomical information [39, 78].

Arthroscopy

The early findings in arthroscopy are a low volume joint, neo-angiogenesis (Figs. 11.4 and 11.5) and loss of the inferior articular recess. Granulation tissue (neoangiogenesis) can be present, occurring in the rotator cuff area and extending onto biceps, subscapularis and supraspinatus tendons. In the late stage, the angiogenesis reduces in intensity, the joint is less inflamed but bands of scar tissue adhere to adjacent structures of the capsule. Further the joint volume can be reduced [40] with loss of the normal rotator interval space and overall joint volume. There is also the added benefit of high sensitivity to identifying other intra-articular pathology which may be treated. It is important to note that arthroscopy is not a means of establishing a diagnosis [29].

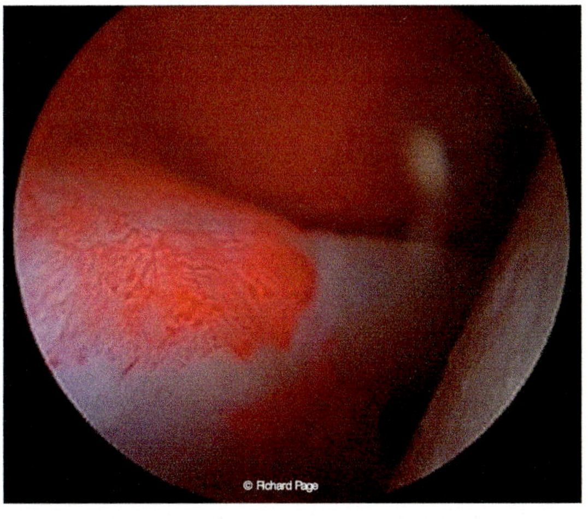

Fig. 11.4 Arthroscopic image showing inflammatory neo-angiogenesis at the biceps anchor insertion and superior rotator interval, enveloping those structures. Features similar to this may be seen in the retina associated with diabetic retinopathy

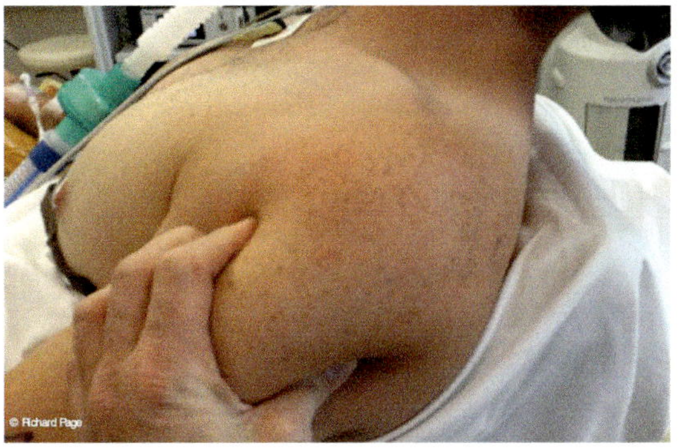

Fig. 11.5 Low beach chair position on a shoulder table, universally adaptable for examination under anaesthetic, manipulation and arthroscopic capsular release as required

Treatment

Prophylaxis

Prevention is ideally the best form of treatment. It is important to maintain shoulder movement, both active and passive in those over 50 years of age (especially diabetics) who have: shoulder pain, immobilization secondary to trauma, myocardial infarction, intracranial haemorrhage, brain injury or prolonged hospitalization [10].

Non-Surgical / Conservative Treatment

Anti-Inflammatories

Treatment of adhesive capsulitis often involves anti-inflammatories (NSAIDs) or corticosteroids. There is a paucity of data on the efficacy of NSAIDs in adhesive capsulitis within any phase as an attempt to relieve symptoms. The natural history of adhesive capsulitis has not been shown to change with NSAID use [79]. Despite no significant evidence, they are still widely used due to their analgesic effect. NSAIDs require cautious use as prolonged use can precipitate gastric bleeding or worsen renal function, particularly in older patients.

Oral Corticosteroids

A short course of oral steroid therapy (Prednisolone 30 mg Daily for 3 weeks) has been shown to improve pain, range of motion and disability. This treatment is a short-term option with benefits beyond 6 weeks' treatment nearing placebo [80]. Like anti-inflammatories, prolonged use of steroid therapy carries unfavorable side effects including weight gain, sleep and mood disturbance, myopathy and osteoporosis. These side effects become important with the understanding that adhesive capsulitis affects middle aged patients (40–60 years) with a female predilection.

Acupuncture

The role of acupuncture in adhesive capsulitis has not been thoroughly investigated. Improvement in flexion and abduction movements at the shoulder have been described 1.5 months after commencing treatment and after 3 months when compared to physiotherapy [81]. There is no consensus on timing for acupuncture or duration, yet with all non-operative treatment approaches, treatment should be early in the course of disease where pain and limited range of movement are apparent.

Low-Level Laser Therapy (LLLT)

LLLT is postulated to normalize cellular function through photo-biomodulation. The literature suggests favorable anti-inflammatory effects of LLLT, by reducing, in a dose-dependent manner, levels of prostaglandin, interleukin and tumour necrosis factor. A study by Ip and Fu (2015) had shown improvement in shoulder mobility and pain in patients whom were treated with LLLT after failing initial oral analgesic options to treat adhesive capsulitis. This improvement in function and pain was effective in the short-term through to the 2 year follow up [82].

Therapeutic Exercise

Increased range of movement with exercise regimes is associated with increased motion and decreased pain when treating AC. Gentle stretching and active movement are encouraged. Emphasis should be on external rotation whilst keeping as much range of motion in the shoulder [10].

Mobilization

Mobilisation aims to passively stretch the joint capsule to sufficiently restore normal glenohumeral motion and biomechanics [10]. Any assistance in elevation needs to avoid excessive pain that may lead to secondary inhibition of active motion and reduced use and function of the affected shoulder. Combined pharmacological and rehabilitative regimes are effective in 96% of patients with adhesive capsulitis with improved movement in the shoulder and decreased levels of pain. Specific programs for capsule and muscle stretching may mitigate the requirement for manipulation under anesthesia or surgery [83]. Counter traction exercises in conjunction with physiotherapy and muscle stretching may also improve shoulder function compared with physiotherapy alone [84].

Corticosteroid Injection

Injection of corticosteroids have been reported to alleviate the pain and fibrosis associated with AC, offering superior symptom relief and increased range of motion [85]. Concomitant physical therapy shows better results than injections alone [10, 86]. Treatment with injected corticosteroids are recommended in the early stages of disease and are not indicated in the freezing stage (Phase II) of adhesive capsulitis as the inflammatory stage has passed. The injections are usually directed to the joint, however bursal injections have also demonstrated a positive effect. Recent literature has shown no significant difference in the efficacy of high dose to low dose corticosteroid injection, suggesting a preference to low dose steroids in the initial stage of intra-articular treatment [87].

Hydrodilatation and Intra-Articular Corticosteroid Injection

First described by Andren and Lundberg in 1965, [88] hydrodilatation (HD) or distension arthrography aims to disrupt fibrous connections within the shoulder joint, using a large volume of irrigation solution, mainly sterile saline (0.9% NaCl) under ultrasound or fluoroscopy with an anterior approach favored. This procedure carries less risk than surgical interventions including manipulation and capsular release. The efficacy of hydrodilatation has been extensively investigated with randomized clinical trials, but conjecture remains. Utilising HD in combination with intra-articular corticosteroids (Kenacort A-40; triamcinolone acetonide; Methylprednisolone acetate) have shown no significant difference in functional outcome over corticosteroid injections alone [89]. With previous outcomes perhaps confounded by the concurrent use of intra-articular corticosteroids, Yoon et al. (2016) sought to randomize and assess the therapeutic use of HD over intra-articular steroid therapy or subacromial injection. They found that HD alone provided significantly improved return of function with decreased visual analog pain scores up to 6 months follow up with no significant differences between the three treatment groups at the final 6-month follow-up [90]. No significant difference was found between glenohumeral steroid injection compared to subacromial injection at 6 months, a finding consistent with previous randomized control studies [91].

Hydrodilatation has traditionally sought to rupture the joint capsule [88, 92, 93] in an attempt to disrupt developing intra-articular adhesions. Average volumes to rupture the joint capsule have been measured using 24.4 ± 8.9 mL of NaCl. Due to significant variation, both in volume and pressure distension required, no standardized approach has yet been accepted [94]. More recent literature suggests joint preservation as a means to distend the joint, preserve joint capsule integrity and encourage microdissection of adhesion bands [95]. Sites of rupture also tend to occur in in deficient areas of the capsule including the subscapularis bursa or the long head of biceps tendon sheath as opposed to focal areas of fibrosis [96, 97]. Rupture of the capsule also leads to loss of intra-articular steroid into the surrounding soft tissues. Hypertonic saline (3% NaCl) has also been trialed as a means to increase intra-articular fluid distension whilst reducing tissue oedema and prolonging the degree of intra-articular fluid in capsule preserving hydrodilatation [98].

As with any procedure involving a sterile joint, utmost care must be undertaken to prevent iatrogenic joint infection. Further, hydrodilatation can be painful and may not be tolerated by all patients due to the large volumes of fluid used to disrupt capsular fibrosis and multiple injections have not been shown to improve the efficacy.

Suprascapular Nerve Block +/– Corticosteroid Injection

The use of regional anaesthesia in AC is widely described as a treatment modality for the management of pain and as an adjunct to either physical therapy or manipulation. The use of long acting local anaesthesia has been augmented with the addition of corticosteroid in attempt to prolong the analgesic affect and in attempt to provide a local anti-inflammatory affect.

The utility of suprascapular nerve block (SSNB) in AC has been suggested in the outpatient setting for pain management either using topographical surface markings or under ultrasound guidance. In two level one studies improvements in short term pain relief were demonstrated, although differences in function compared to controls were not significant at one month [99, 100].

In a primary care setting a randomized control trial comparing SSNB to intra-articular injection demonstrated faster resolution of pain and improvement in motion at 12 weeks for SSNB

[101]. Most studies do not clarify the duration of precedent symptoms of include patients with short term presentations, diluting the evaluation of the treatment effect in the more chronic setting that normal presents for surgical intervention.

Surgical Interventions

Manipulation under Anesthesia

A more aggressive form of passive manipulation; intended to decrease the symptomatic course of the disease by severing adhesions in the joint capsule with passive movement whilst under anesthesia. It requires immediate post-operative therapy to maintain advances in physical mobility and prevent further scarring [5, 10]. Manipulation is often combined with intra-articular injection of local anesthetic and corticosteroid and or regional anaesthesia at the time of manipulation. The benefit of manipulation to improving range of movement appears to persist long term, along with decreased pain levels in studies following patients through up to 23 years after manipulation [102]. Manipulation may confer benefit in patients who have failed non-operative treatment without progressing to intra-articular surgical release.

Timing of manipulation may also contribute to effective treatment, patients manipulated between 6 and 9 months have shown significantly improved shoulder movement and decreased pain than those manipulated earlier or after 9 months [103]. Others have shown no significant differences in outcome in timing of manipulation, where improvement in function was independent of duration of symptoms or timing of manipulation [104].

Manipulation under anesthesia requires care and experience given the risk of iatrogenic damage to the shoulder complex. Such complications may range from expectant haemarthrosis to glenohumeral dislocation [105, 106] or humeral fracture [107]. Other injuries can include brachial plexus injuries [108] and glenoid fractures [109]. Rotator cuff integrity has been shown to be spared in small prospective studies [110] with limited data to confer otherwise.

Senior Author's Tips:
The patient is given a short general anaesthetic (+/− supra-scapular nerve block) and positioned supine, the shoulder range of motion is examined to determine and record the end points of passive motion, where the manipulation is to take effect from. Immediately prior to manipulation a short acting relaxant such as suxamethonuim is administered to eliminate muscle spasm that may result in undue force to joint and bony structures. The scapula and clavicle is stabilized with one hand and the shoulder taken through each plane with a careful steady force, holding the humerus proximally to reduce excessive rotational torque that may risk fracture. Manipulation is started in flexion, then abduction, external rotation by the side, external rotation and internal rotation in abduction and lastly cross body adduction in that order. This is continued until the capsular adhesions are no longer felt to be breaking down. This sequence almost invariably restores full passive motion under the anaesthetic, with an expected haemarthrosis.

The patient is then rolled onto their side, still under anaesthetic and the extension range manipulated. Finally, the glenohumeral joint is injected using a straight spinal needle via the posterior joint line with a mixture of corticosteroid and local anaesthetic (40 mg methyl prednisolone and 20 mL 1% ropivocaine).

Post-operatively the patient is given a sling for symptomatic support only and adequate regular oral analgesia. Active assisted and passive range of motion exercises are commenced the same day while the intra-articular local anaesthetic is still active. It is important to enable the patient to visualise the potential achievable motion range, whilst still free of pain and have a clear target range during the early rehabilitation phase. Early experienced physiotherapy follow-up is helpful to 'coach' patients through the recovery phase to restoration of active motion and finally a graded resistance programme.

Arthroscopic Capsular Release

Selective capsular release is considered effective for the treatment for resistant cases, especially in diabetics. It allows a more controlled release of the contracted capsule than manipulation under anesthesia, particularly in chronic cases exceeding 12 months [5]. Further manipulation is easier when adhesions are initially torn through arthroscopic release [13].

Capsular arthrotomy at the anteroinferior portion of the dependent axillary fold can be performed with release of the coracohumeral and coracoacromial ligaments. However, the use, timing and extent of surgery in AC remains unclear. Further, the safety profile for an invasive intervention must be considered; with the risk of axillary nerve damage if the release is extended too far inferiorly and the established risks of anesthesia, infection and bleeding.

Senior Author's Tips:

The patient is given a general anaesthetic and a regional block (brachial plexus or suprascapular nerve block). The set up can be the surgeons choice, although the author's preference is the beach chair position (Fig. 11.5). This allows examination of the shoulder range of motion and in the very tight shoulder (< 40% retained passive range) partial manipulation in flexion and external rotation, to increase the joint volume, make entry of the arthroscope easier and reduce the risk of chondral trauma. If manipulation is required it is best to limit this prior to arthroscopy, to minimize the haemarthrosis that may cause visualisation issues during a capsular release.

Intra-articular saline injection (10 mL) immediately prior to insertion of the arthroscope can also assist to allow safer insertion by distending the joint capsule. Standard anterior, posterior and lateral portals (for bursoscopy if required) are used to allow a full diagnostic arthroscopy and capsular release as needed to restore motion. Controlled release can be achieved using a combination of arthroscopic punches and heat protected radiofrequency probe. The authors recommended routine for release is as follows:

- Clearance of the rotator interval
- Exposure of the articular tendinous portion of subscapularis
- Release interval tissue and corocoid insertion of coracohumeral ligament
- Extend release vertically down in the mid capsular plane, preserving the capsulolabral insertion
- Repeat EUA once capsule is released to the 5.30 position to determine if further release required – avoid releasing more inferiorly to protect the axillary nerve.
- If further release required, address the posteroinferior capsule by switching visualisation to the anterior portal, allowing clear access to the posterior capsule. Usually this in only necessary in less than 20% of cases and release from 10 to 7 o'clock is adequate (Fig. 11.6).

Bursoscopy is not routinely required, however in the setting of acute or pre-existing bursitis, it may aid recovery to add a subacromial bursectomy. In this setting, the author would add a subacromial local anaesthetic wound infusion catheter is added to augment post-operative analgesia and aid early range of motion exercises.

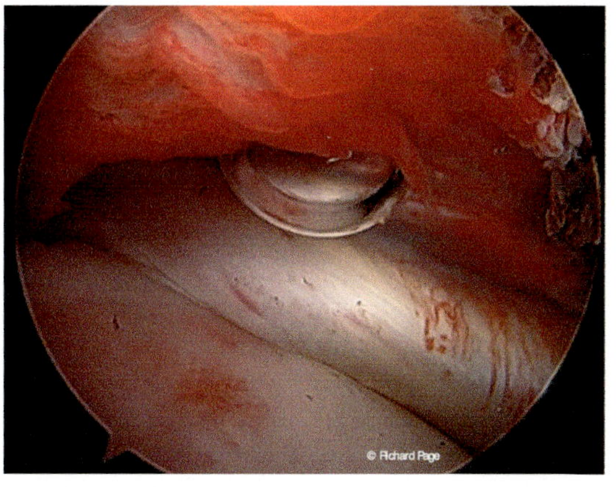

Fig. 11.6 Arthroscopic image of capsulitis with associated synovitis unresolved twelve months after the commencement of painful symptoms. Vascular proliferation with neo-vascularisation can be seen extending from the rotator interval, articular side of the supraspinatus and onto the biceps tendon

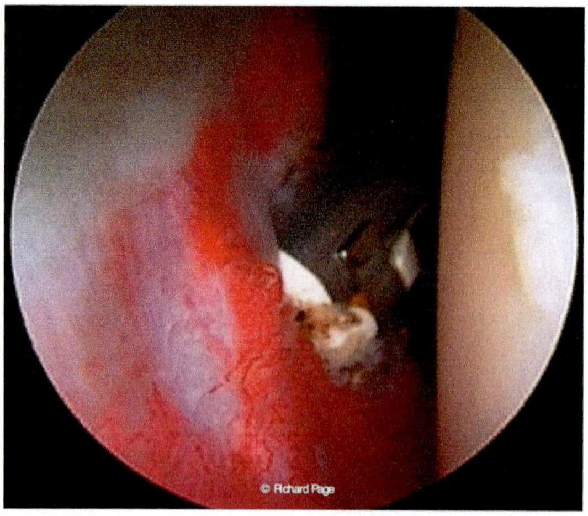

Fig. 11.7 Antero-inferior capsule being released with radiofrequency tissue ablation, seen down to the 5 o'clock position in a right shoulder. Prominent neo-angiogenesis is again evident affecting the surrounding tissue, but remains clear from the articular margins as opposed to the synovial panus encroaching on the articular surface seen in rheumatoid arthritis

Post-operatively the initial focus is good analgesia to allow active-assisted and passive range of motion exercises, aiming to obtain 80% of motion in the first 6–8 weeks. The next phase is terminal range stretching and the commencement of resistance exercises after 8–12 weeks as motion improves and pain subsides (Fig. 11.7).

Senior Author's Preferred Approach

In the majority of patients, the time of onset of symptoms can be reasonably determined from the presenting history. This gives some guidance to the trajectory an individual patient may be on and in particular whether there has been a shift in symptoms from predominantly pain to some reduction in pain but progressive loss of motion. That is from stage I to stage II disease. In the patient who has already progressed from painful stage I disease over a shorter period of time (3–4 months) and is functioning with adequate symptom control and early improvement in motion, a more conservative approach maybe appropriate – the 'ELM POPI' non-operative approach, with 'masterly observation'.

However, where pain and restriction persist or progress beyond 3 months and particularly in the presence of sleep disruption, intervention is warranted. In early disease, when capsular fibrosis is less mature, the theoretical efficacy for intra-articular injection and hydrodilatation should be greatest. In this setting image guided (ultrasound or CT) intra-articular local anaesthetic, saline +/− corticosteroid (methyl prednisolone) injected under pressure to the point of reduced resistance (mark breach of the capsule). This is usually well tolerated and with the dual benefit of shutting down the inflammatory response and increasing the capsular volume.

In the mid-term (3–6 months), with either a delayed presentation or failure of earlier hydrodilatation, then next modality of choice is a manipulation and injection under anaesthetic MUA + CSI –methyl prednisolone 80 mg + 20 mls ropivocaine local anaesthetic, either as a day case or overnight stay to enable early physiotherapy.

When symptoms, including restricted motion have persisted beyond 6 months, the capsular fibrosis is more mature warranting a more controlled release. In this setting, I prefer a formal arthroscopic capsular release to allow release of the rotator interval and anterior capsule in a controlled fashion. Therefore, reducing the complication risk of damage to the labrum, articular surface, rotator cuff or bony anatomy. This enables restoration of the joint volume and the range of motion can be assessed whilst the patient is still under general anaesthesia and if necessary completion with a gentle manipulation.

In all the above staged treatments, the reduction in pain is usually an early benefit. However, it is important to inform patients that improvement in range may take at least 6–12 weeks to show significant and sustained improvement. An ongoing supported home exercise programme with physiotherapy support is an important part of the treatment programme. This is supplemented with regular adequate simple analgesia in

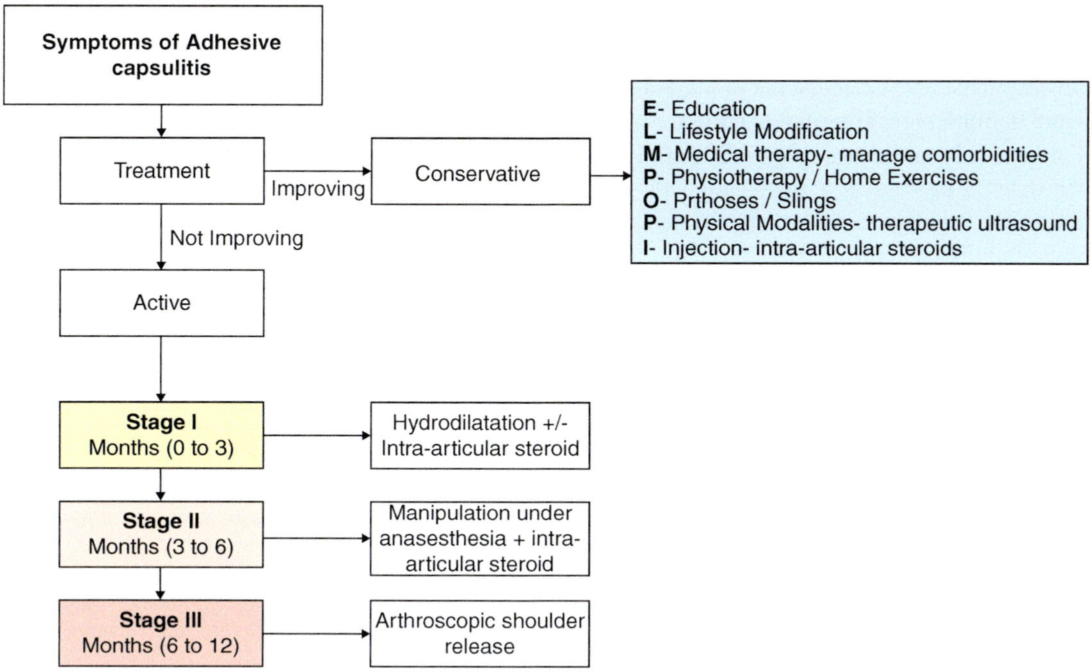

Fig. 11.8 Treatment flow chart as recommended by the authors

Table 11.5 Summary table of authors non-operative and operative treatment

Conservative – 'ELM POPI' approach	Active symptomatic disease
E – Education	*Stage I – Months* 0–3
L – Lifestyle modifications	Hydrodilatation +/−corticosteroid
M – Medical therapy / analgesia Manage co-morbidities e.g. diabetes / thyroid disease	*Stage II – Months* 3–6 Manipulation under anaesthetic + intra-articular corticosteroid injection with local anaesthetic
P – Physiotherapy and/or home exercise program	
O – Orthoses / slings	*Stage III – Months* 6–12+ Arthroscopic capsular release
P – Physical modalities – e.g. therapeutic ultrasound (limited role in this setting)	
I – Injection – Intra-articular corticosteroid	

the early post-operative period to allow patients to confidently undertake their exercises (see Fig. 11.8 and Table 11.5).

Summary

Shoulder stiffness is seldom an isolated complaint and is usually accompanied by pain. Clinical history, examination and radiology are important in determining the diagnosis and excluding associated causes such as osteoarthritis, rotator cuff disease and neurological weakness. Adhesive capsulitis is a common cause of pain and stiffness in the community and although the natural history is for improvement over time, the natural history can vary widely and cause significant morbidity and dysfunction during the recovery phase. This is particularly so in the setting of associated co-morbidities such as diabetes mellitus.

There is a knowledge gap on the triggers, mechanisms and genetic predispositions for the development, severity and patient specific natural history of AC. Consequently, there is lack of consensus on the best management of patients with a more debilitating and prolonged disease process. Further study and research on AC to understand the disease process at a molecular and genetic level and develop tools to better diagnose and stage the disease will improve targeting the correct treatment at the right time.

However, a pragmatic approach demands treatment options for patients with persistent symptoms after 3 months, escalating after 6 months, ranging from low invasive options in the first 3 to 6 months to more invasive and surgical options after 6 months. This generally provides predictable improvement in symptoms, function and a reduction in the disease timeline.

References

1. Duplay ES. De la péri-arthrite scapulo-humérale et des raideurs de l'épaule qui en sont la conséquenc. Archives générales de médecine. 1872;20:513–42.
2. Codman E. The shoulder: rupture of the supraspinatus tendon and other lesions in or about the subacromial Bursa. Thomas Todd Co: Boston; 1934.
3. Neviaser JS. Adhesive capsulitis of the shoulder. A Study of the Pathological Findings in Periarthritis of the Shoulder. J Bone Joint Surg. 1945;27(2):211–22.
4. Kabbabe B, Ramkumar S, Richardson M. Cytogenetic analysis of the pathology of frozen shoulder. Int J Shoulder Surg. 2010;4(3):75–8.
5. Dias R, Cutts S, Massoud S. Frozen shoulder. BMJ. 2005;331(7530):1453–6.
6. Neviaser AS, Hannafin JA. Adhesive capsulitis: a review of current treatment. Am J Sports Med. 2010;38(11):2346–56.
7. Vastamaki H, Kettunen J, Vastamaki M. The natural history of idiopathic frozen shoulder: a 2- to 27-year followup study. Clin Orthop Relat Res. 2012;470(4):1133–43.
8. Sheridan MA, Hannafin JA. Upper extremity: emphasis on frozen shoulder. Orthop Clin North Am. 2006;37(4):531–9.
9. Brue S, Valentin A, Forssblad M, Werner S, Mikkelsen C, Cerulli G. Idiopathic adhesive capsulitis of the shoulder: a review. Knee Surg Sports Traumatol Arthrosc. 2007;15(8):1048–54.
10. Grubbs N. Frozen shoulder syndrome: a review of literature. J Orthop Sports Phys Ther. 1993;18(3):479–87.
11. Baslund B, Thomsen BS, Jensen EM. Frozen shoulder: current concepts. Scand J Rheumatol. 1990;19(5):321–5.
12. Tasto JP, Elias DW. Adhesive capsulitis. Sports Med Arthrosc Rev. 2007;15(4):216–21.
13. Hannafin JA, Chiaia TA. Adhesive capsulitis. A treatment approach. Clin Orthop Relat Res. 2000;372:95–109.
14. Hakim AJ, Cherkas LF, Spector TD, MacGregor AJ. Genetic associations between frozen shoulder and tennis elbow: a female twin study. Rheumatology (Oxford, England). 2003;42(6):739–42.
15. Wong PL, Tan HC. A review on frozen shoulder. Singap Med J. 2010;51(9):694–7.
16. Crispin JC, Alcocer-Varela J. Rheumatologic manifestations of diabetes mellitus. Am J Med. 2003;114(9):753–7.
17. Bunker TD, Anthony PP. The pathology of frozen shoulder. A Dupuytren-like disease. J Bone Joint Surg. 1995;77(5):677–83.
18. Ando A, Sugaya H, Hagiwara Y, Takahashi N, Watanabe T, Kanazawa K, Itoi E. Identification of prognostic factors for the nonoperative treatment of stiff shoulder. Int Orthop. 2013;37(5):859–64.
19. Del Rosso A, Cerinic MM, De Giorgio F, Minari C, Rotella CM, Seghieri G. Rheumatological manifestations in diabetes mellitus. Curr Diabetes Rev. 2006;2(4):455–66.
20. De Ponti A, Vigano MG, Taverna E, Sansone V. Adhesive capsulitis of the shoulder in human immunodeficiency virus-positive patients during highly active antiretroviral therapy. J Shoulder Elb Surg. 2006;15(2):188–90.
21. Itoi E, Arce G, Bain GI, Diercks RL, Guttmann D, Imhoff AB, Mazzocca AD, Sugaya H, Yoo YS. Shoulder stiffness: current concepts and concerns. Arthroscopy. 2016;32(7):1402–14.
22. Carette S, Moffet H, Tardif J, Bessette L, Morin F, Fremont P, Bykerk V, Thorne C, Bell M, Bensen W, et al. Intraarticular corticosteroids, supervised physiotherapy, or a combination of the two in the treatment of adhesive capsulitis of the shoulder: a placebo-controlled trial. Arthritis Rheum. 2003;48(3):829–38.
23. Ryans I, Montgomery A, Galway R, Kernohan WG, McKane R. A randomized controlled trial of intra-articular triamcinolone and/or physiotherapy in shoulder capsulitis. Rheumatology (Oxford). 2005;44(4):529–35.
24. Sharad KS. A comparative study on the efficacy of end range mobilization techniques in treatment of adhesive capsulitis of shoulder. Indian J Physiother Occup Ther. 2011;5(3):28–31.
25. Yang JL, Chang CW, Chen SY, Wang SF, Lin JJ. Mobilization techniques in subjects with frozen shoulder syndrome: randomized multiple-treatment trial. Phys Ther. 2007;87(10):1307–15.
26. Vermeulen HM, Rozing PM, Obermann WR, le Cessie S, Vliet Vlieland TP. Comparison of high-grade and low-grade mobilization techniques in the management of adhesive capsulitis of the shoulder: randomized controlled trial. Phys Ther. 2006;86(3):355–68.

27. Vastamaki H, Vastamaki M. Postoperative stiff shoulder after open rotator cuff repair: a 3- to 20-year follow-up study. Scand J Surg. 2014;103(4):263–70.
28. Nathan DM. The pathophysiology of diabetic complications: how much does the glucose hypothesis explain? Ann Intern Med. 1996;124(1 Pt 2):86–9.
29. Neviaser RJ, Neviaser TJ. The frozen shoulder. Diagnosis and management. Clin Orthop Relat Res. 1987;223:59–64.
30. Watson RS, Gouze E, Levings PP, Bush ML, Kay JD, Jorgensen MS, Dacanay EA, Reith JW, Wright TW, Ghivizzani SC. Gene delivery of TGF-beta1 induces arthrofibrosis and chondrometaplasia of synovium in vivo. Lab Investig. 2010;90(11):1615–27.
31. Rodeo SA, Hannafin JA, Tom J, Warren RF, Wickiewicz TL. Immunolocalization of cytokines and their receptors in adhesive capsulitis of the shoulder. J Orthop Res. 1997;15(3):427–36.
32. Page RS, Gill S. Analysing genes, blood, urine and clinical outcomes in people with frozen shoulder. https://www.anzctr.org.au/Trial/Registration/TrialReview.aspx?ACTRN=12618000431224.
33. Kim YS, Kim JM, Lee YG, Hong OK, Kwon HS, Ji JH. Intercellular adhesion molecule-1 (ICAM-1, CD54) is increased in adhesive capsulitis. J Bone Joint Surg Am. 2013;95(4):e181–8.
34. Bunker TD, Reilly J, Baird KS, Hamblen DL. Expression of growth factors, cytokines and matrix metalloproteinases in frozen shoulder. J Bone Joint Surg. 2000;82(5):768–73.
35. Richards CD, Shoyab M, Brown TJ, Gauldie J: Selective regulation of metalloproteinase inhibitor (TIMP-1) by oncostatin M in fibroblasts in culture. J Immunol (Baltimore: 1950). 1993;150(12):5596–5603.
36. Hutchinson JW, Tierney GM, Parsons SL, Davis TR. Dupuytren's disease and frozen shoulder induced by treatment with a matrix metalloproteinase inhibitor. J Bone Joint Surg. 1998;80(5):907–8.
37. Kilian O, Pfeil U, Wenisch S, Heiss C, Kraus R, Schnettler R. Enhanced alpha 1(I) mRNA expression in frozen shoulder and dupuytren tissue. Eur J Med Res. 2007;12(12):585–90.
38. Thomas SJ, McDougall C, Brown ID, Jaberoo MC, Stearns A, Ashraf R, Fisher M, Kelly IG. Prevalence of symptoms and signs of shoulder problems in people with diabetes mellitus. J Shoulder Elb Surg. 2007;16(6):748–51.
39. Arkkila PE, Gautier JF. Musculoskeletal disorders in diabetes mellitus: an update. Best Pract Res Clin Rheumatol. 2003;17(6):945–70.
40. Bunker T. (ii) Frozen shoulder. J Orthop Trauma. 2011;25(1):11–8.
41. Degreef I, Steeno P, De Smet L. A survey of clinical manifestations and risk factors in women with Dupuytren's disease. Acta Orthop Belg. 2008;74(4):456–60.
42. Smith SP, Devaraj VS, Bunker TD. The association between frozen shoulder and Dupuytren's disease. J Shoulder Elb Surg. 2001;10(2):149–51.
43. Hettrich CM, DiCarlo EF, Faryniarz D, Vadasdi KB, Williams R, Hannafin JA. The effect of myofibroblasts and corticosteroid injections in adhesive capsulitis. J Shoulder Elb Surg 2016 Aug;25(8):1274–9. https://doi.org/10.1016/j.jse.2016.01.012. Epub 2016 Mar 31
44. Nago M, Mitsui Y, Gotoh M, Nakama K, Shirachi I, Higuchi F, Nagata K. Hyaluronan modulates cell proliferation and mRNA expression of adhesion-related procollagens and cytokines in glenohumeral synovial/capsular fibroblasts in adhesive capsulitis. J Orthop Res. 2010;28(6):726–31.
45. Stam HW. Frozen shoulder: a review of current concepts. Physiotherapy. 1994;80(9):588–98.
46. Patten C, Hillel AD. The 11th nerve syndrome. Accessory nerve palsy or adhesive capsulitis? Arch Otolaryngol Head Neck Surg. 1993;119(2):215–20.
47. Arkkila PE, Kantola IM, Viikari JS, Ronnemaa T. Shoulder capsulitis in type I and II diabetic patients: association with diabetic complications and related diseases. Ann Rheum Dis. 1996;55(12):907–14.
48. Choy EH, Corkill MM, Gibson T, Hicks BH. Isolated ACTH deficiency presenting with bilateral frozen shoulder. Br J Rheumatol. 1991;30(3):226–7.
49. Wohlgethan JR. Frozen shoulder in hyperthyroidism. Arthritis Rheum. 1987;30(8):936–9.
50. Bowman CA, Jeffcoate WJ, Pattrick M, Doherty M. Bilateral adhesive capsulitis, oligoarthritis and proximal myopathy as presentation of hypothyroidism. Br J Rheumatol. 1988;27(1):62–4.
51. Okamura K, Ozaki J. Bone mineral density of the shoulder joint in frozen shoulder. Arch Orthop Trauma Surg. 1999;119(7–8):363–7.
52. Lundberg BJ, Nilsson BE. Osteopenia in the frozen shoulder. Clin Orthop Relat Res. 1968;60:187–91.
53. Tuten HR, Young DC, Douoguih WA, Lenhardt KM, Wilkerson JP, Adelaar RS. Adhesive capsulitis of the shoulder in male cardiac surgery patients. Orthopedics. 2000;23(7):693–6.
54. Pineda C, Arana B, Martinez-Lavin M, Dabague J. Frozen shoulder triggered by cardiac catheterization via the brachial artery. Am J Med. 1994;96(1):90–1.
55. Boyle-Walker KL, Gabard DL, Bietsch E, Masek-Vanarsdale DM, Robinson BL. A profile of patients with adhesive capsulitis. Hand Ther. 1997;10(3):222–8.
56. Bruckner FE, Nye CJ. A prospective study of adhesive capsulitis of the shoulder ("frozen shoulder") in a high risk population. Q J Med. 1981;50(198):191–204.
57. Tanishima T, Yoshimasu N. Development and prevention of frozen shoulder after acute aneurysm surgery. Surg Neurol. 1997;48(1):19–22.
58. Riley D, Lang AE, Blair RD, Birnbaum A, Reid B. Frozen shoulder and other shoulder disturbances in Parkinson's disease. J Neurol Neurosurg Psychiatry. 1989;52(1):63–6.
59. Jayson MI. Frozen shoulder: adhesive capsulitis. Br Med J (Clin Res Ed). 1981;283(6298):1005–6.

60. Wadsworth CT. Frozen shoulder. Phys Ther. 1986;66(12):1878–83.
61. Bunker TD, Esler CN. Frozen shoulder and lipids. J Bone Joint Surg. 1995;77(5):684–6.
62. Saleh ZM, Faruqui S, Foad A. Onset of frozen shoulder following pneumococcal and influenza vaccinations. J Chiropr Med. 2015;14(4):285–9.
63. Chambler AFW, Carr AJ. The role of surgery in frozen shoulder. J Bone Joint Surg (Br). 2003;85-B(6):789–95.
64. Johnson JT. Neuropathic fractures and joint injuries. Pathogenesis and rationale of prevention and treatment. J Bone Joint Surg Am. 1967;49(1):1–30.
65. Browne RF, Murphy SM, Torreggiani WC, Munk PL: Musculoskeletal case 29. Neuropathic shoulder secondary to syringomyelia. Can J Surg. 2003;46(4):300, 309–310.
66. Nozawa S, Miyamoto K, Nishimoto H, Sakaguchi Y, Hosoe H, Shimizu K. Charcot joint in the elbow associated with syringomyelia. Orthopedics. 2003;26(7):731–2.
67. Fernando DJ, Vernidharan J. Limited joint mobility in Sri Lankan patients with non-insulin-dependent diabetes. Br J Rheumatol. 1997;36(3):374–6.
68. Hand C, Clipsham K, Rees JL, Carr AJ. Long-term outcome of frozen shoulder. J Shoulder Elb Surg. 2008;17(2):231–6.
69. Shaffer B, Tibone JE, Kerlan RK. Frozen shoulder. A long-term follow-up. J Bone Joint Surg Am. 1992;74(5):738–46.
70. Reeves B. The natural history of the frozen shoulder syndrome. Scand J Rheumatol. 1975;4(4):193–6.
71. Rill BK, Fleckenstein CM, Levy MS, Nagesh V, Hasan SS. Predictors of outcome after nonoperative and operative treatment of adhesive capsulitis. Am J Sports Med. 2011;39(3):567–74.
72. Grey RG. The natural history of "idiopathic" frozen shoulder. J Bone Joint Surg Am. 1978;60(4):564.
73. Wong CK, Levine WN, Deo K, Kesting RS, Mercer EA, Schram GA, Strang BL. Natural history of frozen shoulder: fact or fiction? A systematic review. Physiotherapy. 2017;103(1):40–7.
74. Tamai K, Yamato M. Abnormal synovium in the frozen shoulder: a preliminary report with dynamic magnetic resonance imaging. J Shoulder Elb Surg. 1997;6(6):534–43.
75. Connell D, Padmanabhan R, Buchbinder R. Adhesive capsulitis: role of MR imaging in differential diagnosis. Eur Radiol. 2002;12(8):2100–6.
76. Homsi C, Bordalo-Rodrigues M, da Silva JJ, Stump XM. Ultrasound in adhesive capsulitis of the shoulder: is assessment of the coracohumeral ligament a valuable diagnostic tool? Skelet Radiol. 2006;35(9):673–8.
77. Ryu KN, Lee SW, Rhee YG, Lim JH. Adhesive capsulitis of the shoulder joint: usefulness of dynamic sonography. J Ultrasound Med. 1993;12(8):445–9.
78. Sofka CM, Ciavarra GA, Hannafin JA, Cordasco FA, Potter HG. Magnetic resonance imaging of adhesive capsulitis: correlation with clinical staging. HSS J. 2008;4(2):164–9.
79. Manske RC, Prohaska D. Diagnosis and management of adhesive capsulitis. Curr Rev Muscoskelet Med. 2008;1(3–4):180–9.
80. Buchbinder R, Hoving J, Green S, Hall S, Forbes A, Nash P. Short course prednisolone for adhesive capsulitis (frozen shoulder or stiff painful shoulder): a randomised, double blind, placebo controlled trial. Ann Rheum Dis. 2004;63(11):1460–9.
81. Asheghan M, Aghda AK, Hashemi E, Hollisaz M. Investigation of the EFFECTIVENESS of acupuncture in the treatment of frozen shoulder. Mater Soc. 2016;28(4):253–7.
82. Ip D, Fu NY. Two-year follow-up of low-level laser therapy for elderly with painful adhesive capsulitis of the shoulder. J Pain Res. 2015;8:247–52.
83. Russo A, Arrighi A, Vignale L, Molfetta L. Conservative integrated treatment of adhesive capsulitis of the shoulder. Joints. 2014;2(1):15–9.
84. Paul A, Rajkumar JS, Peter S, Lambert L. Effectiveness of sustained stretching of the inferior capsule in the management of a frozen shoulder. Clin Orthop Relat Res. 2014;472(7):2262–8.
85. Lorbach O, Anagnostakos K, Scherf C, Seil R, Kohn D, Pape D. Nonoperative management of adhesive capsulitis of the shoulder: oral cortisone application versus intra-articular cortisone injections. J Shoulder Elb Surg. 2010;19(2):172–9.
86. Bal A, Eksioglu E, Gulec B, Aydog E, Gurcay E, Cakci A. Effectiveness of corticosteroid injection in adhesive capsulitis. Clin Rehabil. 2008;22(6):503–12.
87. Yoon S-H, Lee HY, Lee HJ, Kwack K-S. Optimal dose of intra-articular corticosteroids for adhesive capsulitis. Am J Sports Med. 2013;41(5):1133–9.
88. Andren L, Lundberg BJ. Treatment of rigid shoulder by joint distension during arthrography. Acta Orthop Scand. 1965;36:45–53.
89. Tveitå EK, Tariq R, Sesseng S, Juel NG, Bautz-Holter E. Hydrodilatation, corticosteroids and adhesive capsulitis: a randomized controlled trial. BMC Musculoskelet Disord. 2008;9(1):53.
90. Yoon JP, Chung SW, Kim JE, Kim HS, Lee HJ, Jeong WJ, Oh KS, Lee DO, Seo A, Kim Y. Intra-articular injection, subacromial injection, and hydrodilatation for primary frozen shoulder: a randomized clinical trial. J Shoulder Elb Surg. 2016;25(3):376–83.
91. Oh JH, Oh CH, Choi JA, Kim SH, Kim JH, Yoon JP. Comparison of glenohumeral and subacromial steroid injection in primary frozen shoulder: a prospective, randomized short-term comparison study. J Shoulder Elb Surg. 2011;20(7):1034–40.
92. Buchbinder R, Green S, Forbes A, Hall S, Lawler G. Arthrographic joint distension with saline and steroid improves function and reduces pain in patients with painful stiff shoulder: results of a randomised, double blind, placebo controlled trial. Ann Rheum Dis. 2004;63:302–9.

93. Mulcahy KA, Baxter AD, Oni OO, Finlay D. The value of shoulder distension arthrography with intraarticular injection of steroid and local anaesthetic: a follow-up study. Br J Radiol. 1994;67:263–6.
94. Chung SG, Lee KJ, Kim HC, Seo KS, Lee YT. Intra-articular pressure profiles of painful stiff shoulders compared with those of other conditions. PM R. 2009;1(4):297–307.
95. Kim K, Lee KJ, Kim HC, Lee KJ, Kim DK, Chung SG. Capsule preservation improves short-term outcome of hydraulic distension in painful stiff shoulder. J Orthop Res. 2011;29(11):1688–94.
96. Bell S, Coghlan J, Richardson M. Hydrodilatation in the management of shoulder capsulitis. Australas Radiol. 2003;47:247–51.
97. Amoretti N, Grimaud A, Brocq O, Roux C, Dausse F, Fournol M, Chevallier P, Bruneton JN. Shoulder distension arthrography in adhesive capsulitis. Clin Imaging. 2006;30(4):254–6.
98. Lee JH, Kim SB, Lee KW, Lee SJ, Lee JU. Effect of hypertonic saline in intra-articular hydraulic distension for adhesive capsulitis. PM R. 2015;7(7):721–6.
99. Klc Z, Filiz MB, Cakr T, Toraman NF. Addition of suprascapular nerve block to a physical therapy program produces an extra benefit to adhesive capsulitis: a randomized controlled trial. Am J Phys Med Rehabil. 2015;94(10 Suppl 1):912–20.
100. Dahan TH, Fortin L, Pelletier M, Petit M, Vadeboncoeur R, Suissa S. Double blind randomized clinical trial examining the efficacy of bupivacaine suprascapular nerve blocks in frozen shoulder. J Rheumatol. 2000;27(6):1464–9.
101. Jones DS, Chattopadhyay C. Suprascapular nerve block for the treatment of frozen shoulder in primary care: a randomized trial. Br J Gen Pract. 1999;49(438):39–41.
102. Vastamäki H, Vastamäki M. Motion and pain relief remain 23 years after manipulation under anesthesia for frozen shoulder. Clin Orthop Relat Res. 2013;471(4):1245–50.
103. Vastamaki H, Varjonen L, Vastamaki M. Optimal time for manipulation of frozen shoulder may be between 6 and 9 months. Scand J Surg. 2015;104(4):260–6.
104. Thomas WJC, Jenkins EF, Owen JM, Sangster MJ, Kirubanandan R, Beynon C, Woods DA. Treatment of frozen shoulder by manipulation under anaesthetic and injection. Does the timing of treatment affect the outcome? J Bone Joint Surg. 2011;93-B(10):1377–81.
105. Othman A, Taylor G. Manipulation under anaesthesia for frozen shoulder. Int Orthop. 2002;26(5):268–70.
106. Hamdan TA, Al-Essa KA. Manipulation under anaesthesia for the treatment of frozen shoulder. Int Orthop. 2003;27(2):107–9.
107. Amir-Us-Saqlain H, Zubairi A, Taufiq I. Functional outcome of frozen shoulder after manipulation under anaesthesia. J Pak Med Assoc. 2007;57(4):181–5.
108. Birch R, Jessop J, Scott G. Brachial plexus palsy after manipulation of the shoulder. J Bone Joint Surg. 1991;73(1):172.
109. Magnussen RA, Taylor DC. Glenoid fracture during manipulation under anesthesia for adhesive capsulitis: a case report. J Shoulder Elb Surg. 2011;20(3):e23–6.
110. Atoun E, Funk L, Copland SA, Even T, Levy O, Rath E. The effect of shoulder manipulation on rotator cuff integrity. Acta Orthop Belg. 2013;79(3):255–9.

Muscle Ruptures of the Shoulder Girdle

12

Ewan Bigsby and Alex A. Malone

Introduction

Muscle ruptures of the shoulder girdle are rare with the exception of the long head of biceps and the rotator cuff tendons, which are discussed in Chap. 30.

Muscle ruptures generally occur from contraction of the muscle against resistance but may occur from direct impact. Partial ruptures are more common than complete but tend to be managed non-operatively and are under-represented in the literature. In this chapter we discuss complete ruptures of the main muscles of the shoulder girdle; Pectoralis Major, Latissimus Dorsi, Teres Major, Deltoid, Coracobrachialis and Serratus Anterior.

Pectoralis Major

Anatomy

The Pectoralis Major (PM) muscle comprises a clavicular head (CH) arising from the medial half of the clavicle, and a sternal head (SH) arising from the second to sixth ribs, the costal margin of the sternum and the External Oblique aponeurosis. The tendons of the clavicular and sternal heads form a bilaminate tendon comprising anterior (Clavicular) and posterior (Sternal) layers, which insert in the lateral edge of the intertubercular groove (Fig. 12.1). In the anatomical position these tendons form a spiral configuration which untwists as the shoulder elevates to provide a more direct line of pull in both portions.

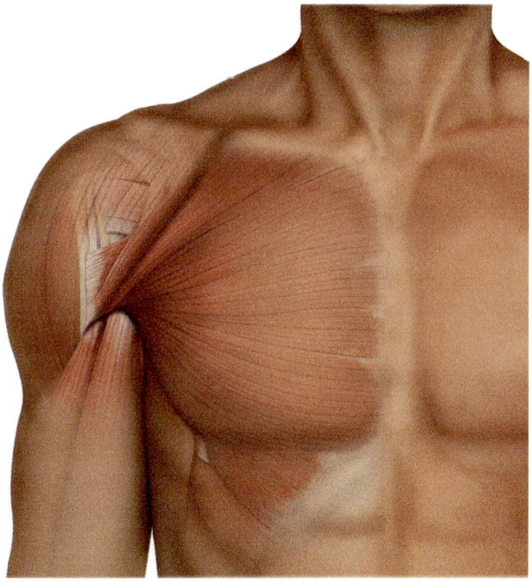

Fig. 12.1 Anatomy of pectoralis major. Note the clavicular tendinous insertion lies superficial and distal to the sternal head

E. Bigsby (✉) · A. A. Malone
University of Otago, Christchurch, New Zealand

I. A. Trail et al. (eds.), *Textbook of Shoulder Surgery*, https://doi.org/10.1007/978-3-319-70099-1_12

Background Literature

A pectoralis major (PM) rupture was first reported by Patissier in 1822 in a butcher boy who went on to have surgery but unfortunately died from an infected haematoma. Since then numerous case reports, case series and more recently a meta-analysis [1] and systematic review [2] have been published. Studies by [3] of 291 cases and Nute et al. [4] of 257 military personnel have added considerably to the literature. The only incidence reported is that for ruptures going on to have surgery, in the United States military, which was 60 episodes per 100,000 person years (0.6 per 1000) [3].

There are two main groups of patients presenting with a PM rupture, the first being the young active, usually male weightlifter and the second the elderly patient group. Balzas et al. [3] reported that most patients of their group of 291 military personnel sustained the injury whilst weight lifting (64%), or performing other physical training activities (12%). There were 19 cases of injury that occurred during airborne operations where the parachutist's arm became entangled in a static parachute line or riser which causes forced extension and abduction of the shoulder. Bak et al. [1] in a meta-analysis of 112 cases of rupture reported the mechanism as using weights (42%), sport (36%), and work (15%).

Site of Rupture

It has been suggested that the PM tears in a predictable sequence of steps, with the most inferior muscle segments rupturing first, followed by the remaining sternal head segments and finally the clavicular head [5], while this does not explain isolated clavicular head ruptures, it does explain why bench presses are a common mechanism of rupture with the abduction and extension position of a bench press placing more stretch on the shorter fibers of the inferior sternal head segments compared to the rest of the pectoralis major tendon [5]. Nute et al. [4] reported both heads ruptured in 47% of cases, while if only one head was ruptured it was usually the sternal head (97%) of cases.

Bak et al. [1] reported of the 86 cases where the rupture had been surgically verified, there were 7 incomplete and 79 complete ruptures. There have been few reports of either incomplete ruptures or those treated conservatively with regard to their rupture location, so the report by Bak et al. [1] is interesting in that of 7 cases of incomplete rupture, 4 were at the tendon insertion, 2 in the tendon substance and 1 in the muscle belly. Complete PM tears are usually at the myotendinous junction (33–50%) or the tendonous insertion (33–55%), but also occur in the midsubstance of the tendon (2–12%), the muscle belly (1–5%), and as a boney avulsion (8%) and even at multiple locations (3%) [1, 3, 4].

Clinical Features and Associated Injuries

PM rupture is usually associated with sudden onset pain in the upper chest and medial aspect of the brachium, with ecchymosis developing over the anterolateral chest wall and brachium. A loss of anterior axillary fold is seen with asymmetric muscle contours and a lump medially representing the retracted muscle (Fig. 12.2).

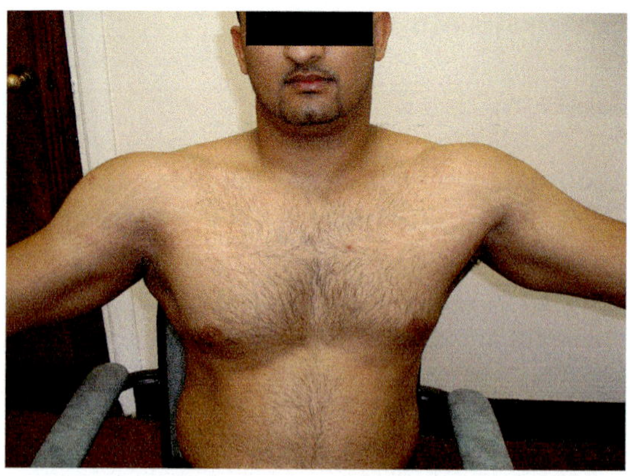

Fig. 12.2 Right pectoralis major tendon rupture. Note asymmetry of the axilla with loss of the prominent anterior axillary fold due to tendon rupture

While rupture of the PM is usually an isolated injury, Arciero et al. [6] reported a case of PM rupture associated with an anterior glenohumeral dislocation and Berghs et al. [7] report a case with a proximal humerus fracture. The tendon injury was only noted at the time of surgery. The humeral fracture was fixed with a proximal humeral plate and the avulsed PM tendon fixed to the plate at the level of its anatomical insertion.

Investigations

Radiographs may rarely show bony avulsions and can indicate a rupture by a change in the shadow of PM, although this may be subtle. Soft tissue imaging modalities such as ultrasound or magnetic resonance imaging (MRI) are the usual investigations. However, it is worth noting that ruptures are not always seen on MRI [8], and the scan needs to extend sufficiently to view the tendonous insertion, focusing on the PM and not the shoulder (Fig. 12.3).

Non-operative Treatment

While conservative treatment has been reported to be effective in some groups, particularly elderly low demand patients [9], others have reported a significant loss of torque [5, 10], reduced strength [11] and a lower satisfaction with cosmesis [11] when compared with surgical treatment. Bak et al. [1] analysed 72 patients (15 non-operative and 57 operative cases) and found the outcome of operative treatment to be substantially better than non-operative treatment, (although publishing bias may mean that non operatively treated PM ruptures with satisfactory outcomes may not be deemed worth of publication).

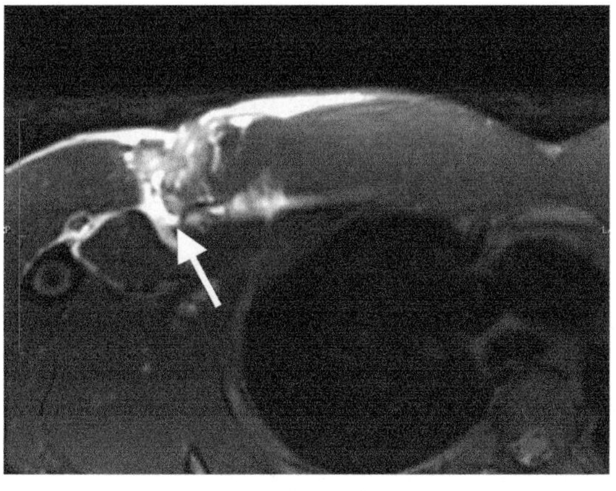

Fig. 12.3 MRI PM rupture TBA

Operative Treatment

The patient is positioned in a low angled beach chair with the arm supported. The incision is in line with the distal end of a standard deltopectoral incision, although a slightly more medially and inferiorly placed (Axillary) incision may be more cosmetic. Mobilisation is achieved with blunt division of adhesions to the subcutaneous and deep tissue. If the CH fibers remain intact, these can be used to help in identification of the PM. Once mobilised, the lateral edge of the bicipital groove is identified and cleared of any residual tendon tissue. Various methods exist to secure the tendon to the bone. These include sutures to secure the PM to the clavipectoral fascia [12], a screw and washer [13], staples [14], bone anchors [15], transosseous sutures, as well as those specific techniques such as the PM endobutton [16]. A variety of techniques of late surgical reconstruction of the PM have been described where direct repair is not possible. These include the use of autografts such as Hamstring, Fascia Lata, and bone-patellar tendon [17–21] as well as allograft options such as Achilles tendon [12, 22]. The authors preferred method consists of using two fibretape sutures which are individually whipstitched into the tendon up to the musculotendinous junction. The two lengths of suture can be engaged with each other to reinforce the purchase on the tendon. Two unicortical 3.5 mm tunnels are placed at the mid axis of the humerus with a bone bridge no less than 10 mm. The tapes are loaded onto endobuttons which are then inserted into the medullary canal and flipped. Pulling on the suture through the button advances the tendon end to the humeral shaft and this is then tied to the other suture end (Fig. 12.4).

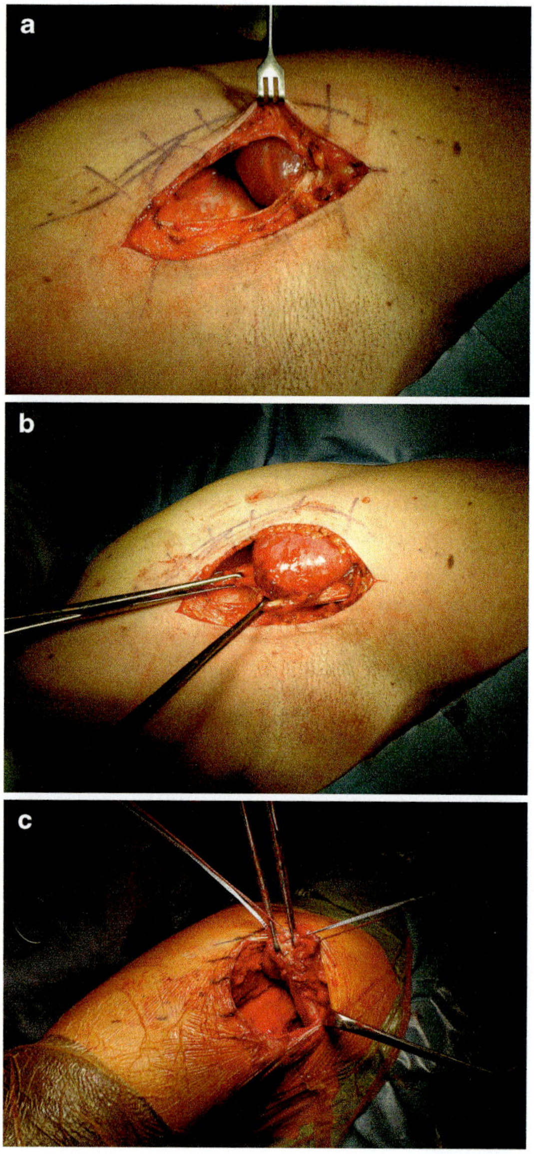

Fig. 12.4 (**a**) Identification of the ruptured right pectoralis major muscle within the sheath. Chest to the right humerus to left. (**b**) Retrieval of the tendon deep to the muscle belly. (**c**) Interlocking whip stitch suture with tape

In terms of the outcome of surgical repair of PM ruptures, Balzas et al. (2016) reported that of the 214 patients for which they had 1 year or more clinical follow-up, 10 (4.7%) were physically unable to return to military service, nine of these because of persistent weakness and one because of chronic regional pain syndrome. Nute et al. [4] reported that 94% of patients returned to full unrestricted duty within 7.1 (+/−4.4) months. Of the 8 patients who underwent revision repair 88% were able to return to full military duty. Overall there was 90% good to excellent results. In the meta-analysis by Bak et al. [1] there was outcome data on 72 of 112 patients. In the 57 of 72 treated surgically, 88% had excellent or good outcomes versus 27% of the 15 treated conservatively. Such a difference was even more statistically significant when the 9 surgical cases after failed conservative treatment were excluded (90% excellent or good versus 17%). Of the surgically treated patients the group treated within 8 weeks of injury had better outcomes than those treated later.

Balzas et al. [3] reported of the 291 patients, 7 patients (2%) required revision surgery and 29 patients (10%) experienced complications, with the commonest being infection (12 superficial and 6 deep requiring further surgery). There were 4 clinical repair failures (3 following trauma and 1 after a deep infection). Two patients experienced hardware failure (one button failed radiologically and one suture anchor pulled out) but neither went on to have further surgery. Two patients experienced a temporary neurological injury of the Musculocutaneous or Axillary nerves. Nute et al. [4] in a study of 257 military personnel reported complications in 23% of patients. Minor complications included persistent shoulder pain and residual weakness. Major complications occurred in 12% of patients including re-rupture in 5% and further surgery for wound complications in 5%. Eight patients (3%) underwent revision surgery for re-rupture and were reported to have "returned to function".

Less common complications include hypertrophic scarring, chronic regional pain syndrome, proximal humeral osteomyelitis, adhesive capsulitis humeral fracture through drill holes (and myositis ossificans.

Clinical Pearls

Asymmetry of the PM tendons at the anterior axillary fold can be demonstrated clinically by asking the patient to face the examiner, place both hands on his/her shoulders and press down with adduction of the arms. The thin residual empty tendon sheath can be compared with the normal side in which tension in the PM creates a prominent anterior axillary fold.

In an acute injury the ruptured tendon can usually be identified intra operatively within a fluid filled space from the haematoma. This sheath also directs the surgeon towards the location of detachment from the humerus.

Latisimus Dorsi

The Latissimus Dorsi (LD) is a large muscle in the back, which extends from the spinous processes of the lower thoracic vertebra, sacrum, posterior iliac crest, lower ribs and scapula. It forms the lower border of the posterior wall of the axilla and inserts on the humerus in the intertubercular groove in front of Pectoralis Major. It is closely associated with the Teres Major tendon proximally. Latissimus Dorsi acts to extend, internally rotate and adduct the arm.

Background

While numerous cases of LD rupture have been reported in the literature, they are all case reports or small case series. While the majority are complete tears, Martin et al. [23] report on a partial tear in the context of a Teres Major tear. Complete LD ruptures tend to be in young patients following sporting injuries: baseball (39%), waterskiing (16%), gym work (6%), golf (3%), cricket (3%), rock climbing (3%), tennis (3%), steer wrestling (6%), grabbing / holding an overhead bar 10%), fall onto arm (6%), and following a crush injury (3%).

Site of Rupture

The most common site of rupture is at the site of the tendon insertion on the humerus in 90% of cases, although bony avulsion from the humerus [24] rupture at the myotendonous junction [25–28] have been reported.

Clinical Features and Associated Injuries

In the majority of cases patients describe an immediate tearing or popping sensation at the time of injury, with pain localising to the back of the shoulder or axilla. Ecchymosis develops with a defect in the posterior axilla and asymmetry of the posterior axillary fold. On palpation, a tender lump representing the end of the ruptured tendon may be identified. In other cases, a tight band in the posterior axilla has been reported which can become painful on contraction of the LD and may represent either a remnant of the LD tendon or a pseudo sheath [24, 29]. While the patient usually has full passive range of movement there is often weakness and pain on resisted adduction, extension and internal rotation.

The commonest associated injury is that to the Teres Major [30–32]. In cases of higher energy injuries, multiple tendons and other neurovascular structures are at risk [25, 33].

Investigations

The initial investigation of a plain radiograph may identify a bony avulsion [32]. alert the clinician to the possible, but an MRI can define the tear location, degree of retraction and assess for other concomitant soft tissue injuries.

Non-operative Treatment

Non-operative treatment has been described with some patients having residual symptoms of pain, asymmetry of axillary contour and some weakness but others returning to full sporting activities, including throwing athletes. In the literature, of those patients treated non-operatively, 13 had returned to full activity by 18 months, while 1 professional baseball pitcher had been unable to return to full function and 1 army officer remained dissatisfied because of ongoing pain and activity limitation.

Operative Treatment

Surgical repair of the LD has been reported in a number of cases [26, 29, 33–41]. Patients tend to be positioned in a beach chair or semilateral position and a single anterior axillary or dual anterior and posterior approaches used, identifying the tendon, retrieving it, then securing it back to the humerus. In one case, ultrasound was used preoperatively to mark the ruptured site [26]. Authors have reported a number of methods of fixing the tendon back to bone, including bone anchors [34, 37, 39–41], bone tunnels [29], bone tunnels and interference screw [36], and the use of an anterior cruciate ligament reconstruction guide [41]. Repair is usually possible within the first 12 weeks of injury [26, 36, 37, 39–42], although Livsey et al. [29] repaired the tendon to bone using non-absorbable sutures through three drill holes in the humerus at over two and a half years from injury.

Outcomes for acute repair in the literature is generally good, with a full return to normal strength and sporting activities usually expected. Some patients describe a painful band in the posterior of the axilla following non-operative treatment of LD ruptures which may represent either a remnant of the tendon or a pseudosheath. In these cases, Turner and Stewart [24] suggested an alternative treatment to repair, was to simply divide the painful residual band of latissimus tendon or scar tissue to enable development of accessory muscles around the shoulder.

The authors preferred technique for surgical repair is to place the patient in the lateral position with an arm holder (Fig. 12.5). A single posterior axillary fold incision is made through which the tendon is retrieved, mobilized and repaired to the humerus with a dual unicortical endobutton technique with 2 tape whipstiches in a manner similar to the Pectoralis Major repair. Adduction and

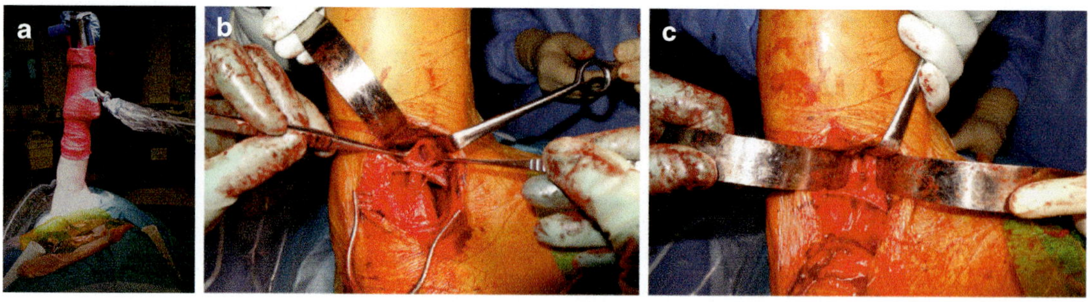

Fig. 12.5 (**a**) Lateral position with arm abducted and internally rotated by arm holder. (**b**) Identification of the latissimus dorsi sheath which leads to the point of humeral attachment. (**c**) Unicortical drill holes in preparation for docking the buttons

internal rotation of the humerus reduces the tension on the tendon to ensure full reduction to the humeral shaft.

> **Clinical Pearls**
> In order to enable adequate internal rotation of the humerus the arm holder attachment may need to be modified by placing the metal bar along the dorsal aspect of the pronated forearm (Fig. 12.5a). Ensure there is protective bandaging around the wrist to prevent irritation of the superficial radial nerve.
>
> During identification and dissection of the ruptured tendon preserve the residual sheath to protect adjacent neurovascular structures.

Teres Major

Anatomy

The Teres Major (TM) originates at the inferolateral aspect of the scapula and inserts at the medial lip of the intertubercular groove. The tendon is closely associated with the Latissimus Dorsi tendon at its insertion. The Teres Major internally rotates, extends, and adducts the arm [43].

Background

There have been 17 cases of complete Teres Major (TM) ruptures reported in the literature, with an additional 3 partial ruptures [30, 44] and 10 cases of TM strains [30, 45] in baseball pitchers. The commonest sporting activities in the 10 reported cases are baseball (throwing or pitching?) [30, 31, 46], followed by waterskiing. The specific mechanism during waterskiing included a traction injury when the tow rope suddenly became taught [47, 48], a fall to the side when the tow rope forcibly jerked the arm [49], and a traction injury from a fall [50]. Other sports leading to TM injuries include ice hockey, where a professional player sustained a partial rupture during the windup phase of a slapshot [44], while another player sustained a partial TM rupture with rapid resisted internal rotation of the shoulder during face off, involving an impact of the players stick against the opponents stick [44]. Teres major ruptures have also been reported when hitting an overhead shot in tennis [51], when throwing out a ball by a goal keeper in football [52], and when a professional boxer was readying an uppercut [23].

Site of Rupture

Tearing can occur within the muscle belly [51], at the myotendinous junction [23, 50] within the tendon [48, 52], and at the tendon bone interface [30, 31, 46, 47, 49], with the latter being the commonest site.

Clinical Features and Associated Injuries

Patients frequently report a pop in the shoulder with immediate onset of symptoms and ecchymosis. A change of contour in the posterior axilla is often noted with asymmetry of the posterior axillary fold and a tender mass. While full passive range of movement is often present, resisted extension, adduction and internal rotation may cause pain. The ruptured TM muscle belly mass is accentuated with extension, adduction and internal rotation.

Latissimus Dorsi ruptures have been identified in conjunction with injury to the TM [30, 31].

Investigations

The initial investigation of plain radiographs may show a boney avulsion. Fitzpatrick et al. [50] recommend coronal oblique and sagittal oblique MRI images of the TM to provide parallel and perpendicular views of the tendon and muscle fibers. It is also important that imaging is centered on the upper arm and chest since a standard shoulder MRI can miss a complete rupture [49].

Non-operative Treatment

The majority of cases in the literature describe non-operative treatment [23, 30, 31, 46, 47, 50–52]. One case of surgical treatment is described [49].

Takase [51] reported a 21 year old tennis player who was pain free and had made a full recovery back to tennis by 6 months. The 33 year old football goalkeeper reported by Maciel et al. [52] had returned to competitive football with no pain or functional limitation by 18 days and at 1 year review had no functional limitations or pain. A 28 year old boxer who sustained a TM rupture had resumed competitive boxing without symptoms at 2 months, although a 25% reduction in internal rotation strength was noted at a 3 months review [23]. Lester et al. [47] reported that the 30 year old waterskier was pain free at 16 weeks from injury with no limitations in sport, although there was a persistent bulge present. Fitzpatrick et al. [50], reporting on a 53 year old waterskier reported no pain and a full range of movement at 14 weeks from injury. The baseball pitcher reported by Malcolm et al. [46] was symptom free at 1 month from injury and had returned to pitching. Of the baseball pitchers reported by Schickendantz et al. [31], three returned to full speed pitching within 4 months, another within 6 months, and the last (a combined Latissimus Dorsi and Teres Major tear) returned at 10 months. The TM avulsions reported by Nagda et al. [30] generally lost a season of baseball in recovering from their injury although all returned to their prior level of play, including the patient that had combined LD and TM tendon avulsions.

Operative Treatment

Garrigues and Lazarus [49] report on a 33 year old right hand dominant executive who sustained a complete TM rupture whilst waterskiing. After 1 month of non-operative treatment, the patient reported continued pain and weakness. An MRI showed complete rupture of the TM tendon from bone with retraction. The patient was positioned in the lateral decubitus position and a low posterior axillary incision made. The TM was mobilised taking care to include the neurovascular pedicle. The roughened area of bone was identified adjacent to the LD tendon. The tendon was repaired with 2 bone anchors and a Krakow weave At 1 year post-operatively, there was normal symmetrical appearance. There was a full range of movement and the patient felt the shoulder was nearly back to normal but had some tightness in overhead throwing. Strength on dynamometer testing was 73% internal rotation and 76% extension after normalising for handedness. The authors concluded that operative repair does not provide complete recovery of strength and results in a similar outcome to the non-operatively treated patients.

Deltoid

Anatomy

The deltoid is a large multipennate muscle which originates on the clavicle, acromion and scapula spine and inserts on to the humeral shaft. It comprises three main portions: anterior, middle and posterior, however, seven smaller segments have been described which are separated by intramuscular tendons. The anterior most segment attaches to the clavicle, the middle four to the acromion and the posterior two to the scapula spine. The anterior three segments are considered the classic anterior deltoid, and the posterior three segments comprise the classic posterior deltoid. The deltoid acts to move the arm at the glenohumeral joint, with the specific movement being dependent on the component of the deltoid which is activated.

Background

Rupture of the deltoid is rare in the absence of previous surgery. Ilslan et al. [53] investigated 8562 shoulder MRI scans performed in patients with rotator cuff tears and identified partial or full thickness deltoid ruptures in only 0.3%. While there are numerous accounts of deltoid dehiscence following surgery [54–56], there are only case reports and small case series of acute deltoid rupture [57–63]. The first report of such was by Clemens in 1913 [57], who described a hernia of the deltoid muscle resulting from a sudden jerking movement when a co-worker dropped one end of a track that was being carried. The hernia became bigger and harder on contraction of the deltoid and was associated with pain. The patient declined surgery so no surgical confirmation of the diagnosis was possible.

In addition to acute traumatic muscle ruptures, spontaneous ruptures have also been reported, occurring in the elderly population and associated with massive rotator cuff tears, possibly resulting from attrition of the humeral head on the coracoacromial arch [64]. In addition to the two cases described by Panting and Hunter [64] they refer to two other cases in the literature, and of a discussion with R. J. A. Tregonning who had also observed a similar case. Blazar et al. [59] reported on three patients, with an average age of 73 years, with four affected shoulders. While one patient was involved in a motor vehicle accident with minor trauma to the shoulder the others presented with spontaneous onset of extreme weakness and a decrease in shoulder function, while passive movement was relatively preserved. MRI imaging performed for two of the shoulders confirmed the clinical diagnosis with rupture being from the acromion. All patients were treated non-operatively with outcomes not being presented.

The recorded mechanisms of acute ruptures have included: manual work [59], a motor vehicle accident [59], a seatbelt [61], a pull-up [62] and after massage therapy [63]. Allen and Drakos [60] report a case of partial detachment of the deltoid in a cricketer and while they attribute the rupture to bowling, they recognise there was no specific traumatic incident, rather a 4 months period of shoulder pain, making a direct causal link with bowling difficult.

Site of Rupture

In acute traumatic cases, rupture occurs in the muscle belly mid substance [58] and from the origin on the acromion and clavicle [61, 62]. In terms of which component of the deltoid is involved; anterior deltoid ruptures [61, 62], ruptures of the mid portion [53, 59], as well as posterior deltoid ruptures [60, 62] have all been recorded. One of the authors of this chapter (AM) has treated a patent with rupture of all components of Deltoid from the acromion. (Fig. 12.6a).

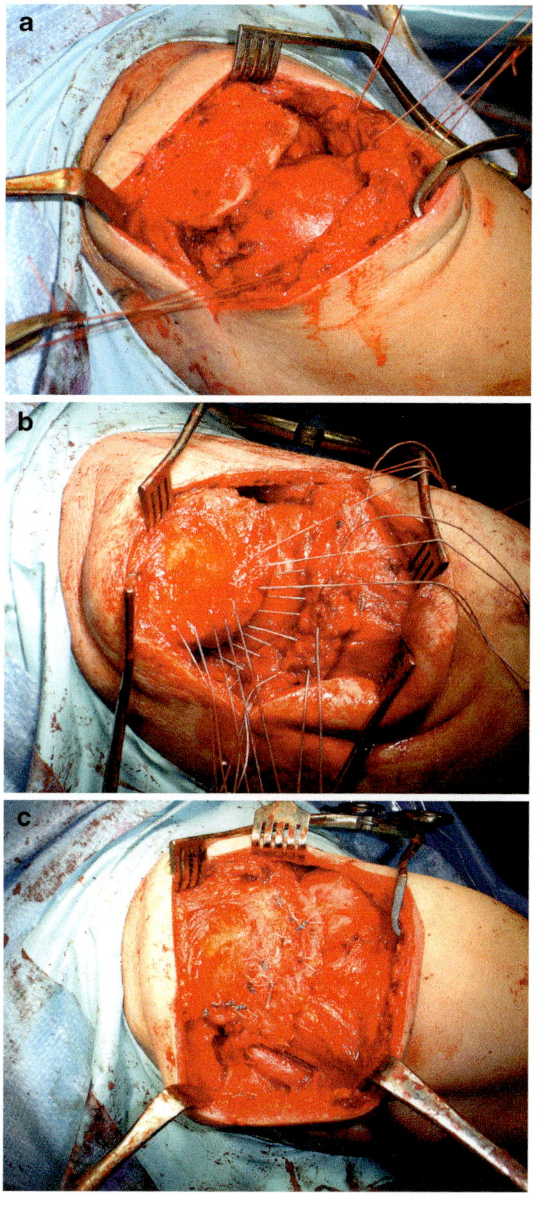

Fig. 12.6 (**a**) Complete avulsion of the deltoid from acromion. (**b**) Multiple transosseous sutures placed. (**c**) Bony attachment restored prior to repair of deltitrapezial fascia

Clinical Features and Associated Injuries

With acute tears, ecchymosis and swelling are common, with a loss of normal shoulder contour developing and becoming more prominent with activation of the deltoid. A palpable defect may be present, or a prominent bulge which is soft when the deltoid is relaxed but firm and immoveable when the deltoid is contracted. Pain may or may not be a feature but weakness is universal with the involvement of the particular component of the deltoid dictating whether the weakness is predominantly in resisted shoulder abduction, flexion or extension.

Tears in the cuff tendons have been associated with deltoid ruptures, either as a prelude [58, 59] or in conjunction with the deltoid injury itself [61].

Investigations

Radiographs are usually the initial imaging modality to exclude boney avulsions. MRI with or without arthrography has been usedto provide information on the site and size of the rupture and the quality of the muscle.

Non-operative Treatment

Non-operative management tends to be for partial ruptures or those in elderly low demand patients. The partial detachment of the deltoid in a 31 year old patient reported by Allen and Drakos [60] was treated with a supervised rehabilitation programme with the patient making a full recovery, with pain free bowling at 8 weeks. Lin and Nagler [65] report on a 75 year old patient with a partial tear in the posterior fibres of the deltoid which was also treated non-operatively. With a return to golf at 4 weeks and full strength at 6 weeks. The three patients reported by Blazar et al. [59] had a mean age of 73 years and were all treated non-operatively due to the chronic nature of the deltoid and the associated rotator cuff tear. One 80 year old patient, Morisawa [58] was treated non-operativelyand continued to have pain with motion and an impairment of active shoulder function.

Operative Treatment

Gilcreest [66] suggested that repair as soon as possible should be performed for deltoid muscle injuries, with splinting afterwards in an abducted forward elevated position and this remains the recommended treatment for complete ruptures in active patients. A 71 year old operatively treated patient reported by Morisawa [58] had an associated massive rotator cuff tear. Three months after surgery the patient could actively elevate the shoulder to more than 160°. In the case reported by Chiba et al. [61] of a 53 year old man who ruptured their deltoid from a seatbelt during a road traffic accident, surgical repair was performed 2 months after injury, with the Deltoid being reattached to the clavicle using a pull-out suture technique. At 12 months from surgery the patient had returned to work without any problems. The most recent case reported in the literature is that of a 21 year old army trainee whose Deltoid was repaired to the distal clavicle and anterior acromion using drill holes and non-absorbable sutures [62]. After 6 months, he had returned to work including upper limb training without any problems. There was no tenderness or palpable defect over the deltoid which had been present preoperatively. Both the range of motion and muscle strength had recovered completely. The Author's case of complete deltoid avulsion was repaired through multiple drill holes in the acromion and non absorbable suture and made a reasonable recovery but had some residual weakness (Fig. 12.6).

Pearls: Care should be taken to restore continuity of the deltotrapezial fascia in addition to the bony origins during repair of a deltoid avulsion from the acromion.

Serratus Anterior

Anatomy

The Serratus Anterior (SA) muscle is composed of three principle components (upper, middleand lower parts). Various authors have investigated the contribution of the various parts to movement. Hamada et al. [67], in their study of 35 cadavers (70 specimens), suggest that the upper part of the muscle stabilises rotational motion of the scapula on the thorax during shoulder elevation, while the middle part provides scapular abduction and the lower part contributes to upward rotation, abduction and posterior tilting.

Background

There have been nine cases of serratus anterior (SA) rupture reported in the literature, although only four have been proved on imaging or surgical exploration. All occurred in young active patients. Fitchet [68] reported 4 cases which he diagnosed on clinical examination as SA ruptures and an additional fifth case of a long thoracic nerve injury with possible SA rupture. Hayes et al. [69] reported a traumatic injury to a 25 year old man, while Gaffney [70] reported a case of a 21 year old who noticed a problem with his shoulder 3–4 h after a gym session, although there was not a specific injury event. Two patients sustained a SA rupture playing sports, the first was a 16 year old baseball pitcher [71] and the second a 19 year old rower [72]. An additional case of a 19 year old who sustained an injury lifting heavy goods from the ground was report by Singh and Vargaonkar [73] as a rupture of SA although an MRI only showed inflammatory change. Carr et al. [72] reported a 19 year old who sustained a rupture while rowing.

Site of Rupture

The site of rupture of serratus anterior was shown on MRI as being at the musculotendinous junction of the fourth and fifth interdigitations in the case of a 21 year old with the gym injury [70] and partial tearing of SA muscle along the seventh through ninth ribs in the case of a 19 year old rower [72]. A surgical assessment showed avulsion from the seventh rib in the case of the 16 year old baseball pitcher [71]. In the case of Hayes et al. [69], following surgical exploration it was apparent that the Rhomboid major and Serratus Anterior muscles had become detached from the vertebral border of the scapula, in addition, the inferior angle of scapula was avulsed and remained attached to small part of Serratus Anterior.

Clinical Features and Associated Injuries

There may be a history of sudden onset pain in the chest wall, some patients reported a grating sensation along posterior wall of chest and under the shoulder blade. Weakness and fatigue of shoulder with activities of arm elevated in front and above head has also been reported. Generally, there is no pain at rest. There may be winging of scapula which is more prominent with forward flexion of the arm and resistance against the outstretched hand. A soft tissue mass may be present in the mid lateral chest wall which is tender and becomes firmer when the muscle is activated. Ecchymosis on the chest wall where the Serratus Anterior muscles attach may develop.

Hayes et al. [69] reported an associated Rhomboid Major detachment following a traumatic injury in a 25 year old man.

Investigations

Plain radiographs are the first investigation of choice and may show a displaced fracture of the inferior angle of the scapula [69]. An MRI is the most common definitive investigation and may show the presence of haematoma, oedema, or a defect in the muscle or tendon. If winging of the scapula is present and an MRI is inconclusive of rupture, then, nerve conduction studies or electromyography may be helpful to rule out a long thoracic nerve injury [73, 74].

Non-operative Treatment

A 21 year old gym goer [70] and a 19 year old female rower [72] were treated non-operatively and reported no pain and full strength at 4 weeks. Meythaler et al. [74] treated a 64 year old man with rheumatoid arthritis conservatively and after 16 weeks he was independent of activities of daily living with a full range of movement, although strength was reduced and the scapula winging persisted [74].

Operative Treatment

In the case of a 25 year old man, Hayes et al. [69] initially employed a non-operative approach, but after 9 months although the patient had returned to work he continued to experience weakness and a grating sensation around the shoulder so went on to have surgery. The patient was positioned in the prone position and an incision made along the inferior medial border of the scapula. The Rhomboid Major and Serratus Anterior muscles were detached from the vertebral border of the scapula and there was an associated bone fragment that had avulsed from the inferior angle of the scapula. The bone fragment was excised and the Rhomboid Major and Serratus Anterior muscles were reattached to the freshened border of the scapula with silk sutures. At 1 year from surgery, the patient had regained full strength and normal range of motion and no winging [69].

Otoshi et al. [71] who reported on a 16 year old student who had severe pain, with an associated tender lump in the chest wall went on to have surgical exploration and SA repair. A longitudinal incision was made along the lateral edge of the scapula and the SA was noted to have avulsed from the seventh rib with the periosteum. The serratus anterior was repaired directly to the residual periosteum with non-absorbable sutures. The patient returned to competitive baseball 7 months after surgery [71].

Coracobrachialis

Anatomy

Coracobrachialis originates from the coracoid process and from the medial, lateral and posterior aspects of the short head of Biceps rachii and inserting into the medial surface of the humeral shaft. Anatomical variations exist with an additional muscle belly noted by El Naggar and Zahir [75] that inserts into the medial head of the Triceps Brachii. Coracobrachilais acts to assist with the flexion and adduction of the humerus and helps maintain the head of the humerus within the glenoid fossa.

Background

There have been four cases reported in the literature. The first was by Gilcreest [76] which 'occurred from direct violence'. The patient went on to have early surgery where a large complete rupture in the belly of the muscle was noted. Two years later, Tobin et al. [77] described a parachute injury where the static line became entangled in the jumper's axilla leading to the complete tear of the short head of biceps and the coracobrachialis. More recently Spiegl et al. [78] described a 41 year old oil rig worker who sustained a rupture of the Coracobrachialis muscle when their arm was forcefully elevating with flexion of the elbow) by a lifting machine. The most recent case, in a 57 year old, was that of a proximal Coracobrachialis tendon rupture from its origin after traumatic anterior shoulder dislocation after a fall from standing height [79].

Site of Rupture

Of the four cases in the literature, one was a rupture of the proximal tendon [79], one a rupture of the muscle belly [76], one a distal rupture at the distal musculotendinous junction [78], while the fourth doesn't specify an exact location of rupture.

Clinical Features and Associated Injuries

Because of the paucity of reported cases it is difficult to provide a comprehensive account of expected findings. However, a tearing sensation was reported following injury in one case, with ecchymosis developing down the arm. Irritation of the musculocutaneous nerve affecting sensation over the lateral forearm and weakness in elbow flexion and shoulder forward elevation have also been described.

A complete tear of the short head of Biceps was reported by Tobin et al. [77] in association with a complete Coracobrachialis tear. In the case of the 57 year old woman with a traumatic anterior shoulder dislocation, there were numerous additional pathologies noted. These included a Subscapularis tear, and dislocation of LHB (short head of biceps was intact), although it is difficult to be sure that these were as a direct result of the trauma [79].

Investigations

Of the two accounts that reported investigations, these were in the form of MRI scans [78, 79]. It is worth noting that in the case the oil rig worker, initial MRI scans of both his shoulder and elbow were normal and only when an MRI of the arm was performed, was the coracobrachialis rupture identified [78].

Non-operative Treatment

Non-operative treatment has not been reported in the literature.

Operative Treatment

Gilcreest and Albi [76] reported that an early operation resulted in complete recovery for their patient. In the case of Spiegl et al. [78], surgery 2 months after injury identified significant retraction of the Coracobrachilais and tenodesis to the adjacent Biceps muscle was performed. Four months later the neurological symptoms in the lateral cutaneous nerve had partially improved only. The patient had resumed full activities including work without pain or discomfort.

Saltzman et al. [79] performed surgery 2 weeks after injury in a patient with multiple injuries The coracobrachialis tendon was tenodesed to the lateral border of short head of biceps and at 6 months from surgery the patient was pain free, with a good range of movement and power.

References

1. Bak K, Cameron EA, Henderson IJP. Rupture of the pectoralis major: a meta-analysis of 112 cases. Knee Surg Sports Traumatol Arthrosc. 2000;8(2):113–9.
2. ElMaraghy AW, Devereaux MW. A systematic review and comprehensive classification of pectoralis major tears. J Shoulder Elb Surg. 2012;21(3):412–22.
3. Balazs GC, Brelin AM, Donohue MA, Dworak TC, Rue JPH, Giuliani JR, Dickens JF. Incidence rate and results of the surgical treatment of pectoralis major tendon ruptures in active-duty military personnel. Am J Sports Med. 2016;44(7):1837–43.
4. Nute DW, Kusnezov N, Dunn JC, Waterman BR. Return to function, complication, and reoperation rates following primary pectoralis major tendon repair in military service members. JBJS. 2017;99(1):25–32.
5. Wolfe SW, Wickiewicz TL, Cavanaugh JT. Ruptures of the pectoralis major muscle: an anatomic and clinical analysis. Am J Sports Med. 1992;20(5):587–93.
6. Arciero RA, Cruser DL. Pectoralis major rupture with simultaneous anterior dislocation of the shoulder. J Shoulder Elb Surg. 1997;6(3):318–20.
7. Berghs BM, Van Tongel A, De Bo T, De Wilde LF. Fracture of the proximal humerus with disruption of the tendon of the pectoralis major. Int J Shoulder Surg. 2016;10(1):44.
8. Alho A. Ruptured pectoralis major tendon: a case report on delayed repair with muscle advancement. Acta Orthop Scand. 1994;65(6):652–3.
9. Roi GS, Respizzi S, Dworzak F. Partial rupture of the pectoralis major muscle in athletes. Int J Sports Med. 1990;11(01):85–7.
10. McEntire JE, Hess WE, Coleman SS. Rupture of the pectoralis major muscle: a report of eleven injuries and review of fifty-six. JBJS. 1972;54(5):1040–6.
11. Schepsis AA, Grafe MW, Jones HP, Lemos MJ. Rupture of the pectoralis major muscle: outcome after repair of acute and chronic injuries. Am J Sports Med. 2000;28(1):9–15.

12. Butt U, Mehta S, Funk L, Monga P. Pectoralis major ruptures: a review of current management. J Shoulder Elb Surg. 2015;24(4):655–62.
13. Kehl T, Holzach P, Matter P. Rupture of the pectoralis major muscle. Unfallchirurg. 1987;90(8):363–6.
14. Egan TM, Hall H. Avulsion of the pectoralis major tendon in a weight lifter: repair using a barbed staple. Can J Surg. 1987;30(6):434–5.
15. Miller MD, Johnson DL, Fu FH, Thaete FL, Blanc RO. Rupture of the pectoralis major muscle in a collegiate football player: use of magnetic resonance imaging in early diagnosis. Am J Sports Med. 1993;21(3):475–7.
16. Metzger PD, Bailey JR, Filler RD, Waltz RA, Provencher MT, Dewing CB. Pectoralis major muscle rupture repair: technique using unicortical buttons. Arthrosc Tech. 2012;1(1):e119–25.
17. de Castro Pochini A, Ejnisman B, Andreoli CV, Monteiro GC, Silva AC, Cohen M, Albertoni WM. Pectoralis major muscle rupture in athletes: a prospective study. Am J Sports Med. 2010;38(1):92–8.
18. Joseph TA, DeFranco MJ, Weiker GG. Delayed repair of a pectoralis major tendon rupture with allograft: a case report. J Shoulder Elb Surg. 2003;12(1):101–4.
19. Schachter AK, White BJ, Namkoong S, Sherman O. Revision reconstruction of a pectoralis major tendon rupture using hamstring autograft: a case report. Am J Sports Med. 2006;34(2):295–8.
20. Sikka RS, Neault M, Guanche CA. Reconstruction of the pectoralis major tendon with fascia lata allograft. Orthopedics. 2005;28(10):1199–201.
21. Zafra M, Muñoz F, Carpintero P. Chronic rupture of the pectoralis major muscle: report of two cases. Acta Orthop Belg. 2005;71(1):107–10.
22. Zacchilli MA, Fowler JT, Owens BD. Allograft reconstruction of chronic pectoralis major tendon ruptures. J Surg Orthop Adv. 2013;22(1):95–102.
23. Martin E, Lotito G, Le Corroler T, Coudreuse JM, Bensoussan L, Delarque A, Viton JM. Teres major tendon tears in a professional boxer. Ann Phys Rehabil Med. 2014;57(9–10):727–33.
24. Turner J, Stewart MP. Latissimus dorsi tendon avulsion: 2 case reports. Inj Extra. 2005;9(36):386–8.
25. Butterwick DJ, Mohtadi NG, Meeuwisse WH, Frizzell JB. Rupture of latissimus dorsi in an athlete. Clin J Sport Med. 2003;13(3):189–91.
26. Park JY, Lhee SH, Keum JS. Rupture of latissimus dorsi muscle in a tennis player. Orthopedics. 2008;31(10).
27. Çelebi MM, Ergen E, Üstüner E. Acute traumatic tear of latissimus dorsi muscle in an elite track athlete. Clin Pract. 2013;3(2).
28. Friedman MV, Stensby JD, Hillen TJ, Demertzis JL, Keener JD. Traumatic tear of the latissimus dorsi myotendinous junction: case report of a CrossFit-related injury. Sports Health. 2015;7(6):548–52.
29. Livesey JP, Brownson P, Wallace WA. Traumatic latissimus dorsi tendon rupture. J Shoulder Elb Surg. 2002;11(6):642–4.
30. Nagda SH, Cohen SB, Noonan TJ, Raasch WG, Ciccotti MG, Yocum LA. Management and outcomes of latissimus dorsi and teres major injuries in professional baseball pitchers. Am J Sports Med. 2011;39(10):2181–6.
31. Schickendantz MS, Kaar SG, Meister K, Lund P, Beverley L. Latissimus dorsi and teres major tears in professional baseball pitchers: a case series. Am J Sports Med. 2009;37(10):2016–20.
32. Spinner RJ, Speer KP, Mallon WJ. Avulsion injury to the conjoined tendons of the latissimus dorsi and teres major muscles. Am J Sports Med. 1998;26(6):847–9.
33. Kawashima M, Sato M, Torisu T, Himeno R, Iwabuchi A. Rupture of the pectoralis major. Report of 2 cases. Clin Orthop Relat Res. 1975;(109):115–9.
34. Ellman MB, Yanke A, Juhan T, Verma NN, Nicholson GP, Bush-Joseph C, Bach BR, Romeo AA. Open repair of an acute latissimus tendon avulsion in a Major League Baseball pitcher. J Shoulder Elb Surg. 2013;22(7):e19–23.
35. Cox EM, McKay SD, Wolf BR. Subacute repair of latissimus dorsi tendon avulsion in the recreational athlete: two-year outcomes of 2 cases. J Shoulder Elb Surg. 2010;19(6):e16–9.
36. Levine JW, Savoie FH. Traumatic rupture of the latissimus dorsi. Orthopedics. 2008;31(8).
37. Burks R, Burke W, Stevanovic M. Rehabilitation following repair of a torn latissimus dorsi tendon. Phys Ther. 2006;86(3):411.
38. Barnes DA, Tullos HS. An analysis of 100 symptomatic baseball players. Am J Sports Med. 1978;6(2):62–7.
39. Lim JK, Tilford ME, Hamersly SF, Sallay PI. Surgical repair of an acute latissimus dorsi tendon avulsion using suture anchors through a single incision. Am J Sports Med. 2006;34(8):1351–5.
40. Hiemstra LA, Butterwick D, Cooke M, Walker RE. Surgical management of latissimus dorsi rupture in a steer wrestler. Clin J Sport Med. 2007;17(4):316–8.
41. Henry JC, Scerpella TA. Acute traumatic tear of the latissimus dorsi tendon from its insertion: a case report. Am J Sports Med. 2000;28(4):577–9.
42. Budoff JE, Gordon L. Surgical repair of a traumatic latissimus dorsi avulsion: a case report. Am J Orthop (Belle Mead NJ). 2000;29(8):638–9.
43. Broome HL, Basmajian JV. The function of the teres major muscle: an electromyographic study. Anat Rec. 1971;170(3):309–10.
44. Grosclaude M, Najihi N, Laedermann A, Menetrey J, Ziltener JL. Teres major muscle tear in two professional ice hockey players: cases study and literature review. Orthop Traumatol Surg Res. 2012;98(1):122–5.
45. Leland JM, Ciccotti MG, Cohen SB, Zoga AC, Frederick RJ. Teres major injuries in two professional baseball pitchers. J Shoulder Elb Surg. 2009;18(6):e1–5.

46. Malcolm PN, Reinus WR, London SL. Magnetic resonance imaging appearance of teres major tendon injury in a baseball pitcher. Am J Sports Med. 1999;27(1):98–100.
47. Lester JD, Boselli KJ, Kim PD, Ahmad CS. Isolated rupture of the teres major tendon. Orthopedics. 2010;33(11).
48. Maldjian C, Adam R, Oxberry B, Chew F, Kelly J. Isolated tear of the teres major: a waterskiing injury. J Comput Assist Tomogr. 2000;24(4):594–5.
49. Garrigues GE, Lazarus MD. Operative treatment of isolated teres major ruptures. J Shoulder Elb Surg. 2012;21(6):e6–e11.
50. Fitzpatrick D, Cagle P, Flatow E. Isolated Teres major rupture: a case report with a suggested dedicated imaging protocol and review of the literature. J Radiol Case Rep. 2016;10(4):31.
51. Takase K. Isolated rupture of the teres major muscle. J Orthop Sports Phys Ther. 2008;38(7):439.
52. Maciel RA, Zogaib RK, Pochini ADC, Ejnisman B. Case report: isolated rupture of teres major in a goalkeeper. BMJ Case Rep. 2015;2015.
53. Ilaslan H, Iannotti JP, Recht MP. Deltoid muscle and tendon tears in patients with chronic rotator cuff tears. Skelet Radiol. 2007;36(6):503–7.
54. Arntz CT, Matsen FA 3rd. Partial scapulectomy for disabling scapulo-thoracic snapping. Orthop Trans. 1990;14(2):252–3.
55. Gumina S, Di Giorgio G, Perugia D, Postacchini F. Deltoid detachment consequent to open surgical repair of massive rotator cuff tears. Int Orthop. 2008;32(1):81–4.
56. Akgün U, Kocaoglu B, Karahan M. Full recovery of muscle function after delayed primary repair of deltoid muscle detachment. Int J Shoulder Surg. 2008;2(4):79.
57. Clemens H. Traumatische hernie des M. deltoideus [in German]. Deutsch Med Wochenschr. 1913;39:2197.
58. Morisawa K, Yamashita K, Asami A, Nishikawa H, Watanabe H. Spontaneous rupture of the deltoid muscle associated with massive tearing of the rotator cuff. J Shoulder Elb Surg. 1997;6(6):556–8.
59. Blazar PE, Williams GR, Iannotti JP. Spontaneous detachment of the deltoid muscle origin. J Shoulder Elb Surg. 1998;7(4):389–92.
60. Allen AA, Drakos MC. Partial detachment of the deltoid muscle. Am J Sports Med. 2002;30(1):133–4.
61. Chiba D, Sano H, Nakajo S, Fujii G. Traumatic deltoid rupture caused by seatbelt during a traffic accident: a case report. J Orthop Surg. 2008;16(1):127–9.
62. Han F, Tan HMB, Tan CH, Kumar VP. Traumatic rupture of the deltoid muscle during a pull-up: a case report. J Shoulder Elb Surg. 2012;21(9):e8–e10.
63. Pointud P, Clerc D, Manigand G, Deparis M. Spontaneous rupture of the deltoid muscle. La Nouvelle presse medicale. 1976;5(35):2315.
64. Panting AL, Hunter MH. Spontaneous rupture of the deltoid [abstract]. J Bone Joint Surg. 1983;65B:518.
65. Lin JT, Nagler W. Use of surface scanning for creation of transparent facial orthoses: a report of two cases. Burns. 2003;29(6):599–602.
66. Gilcreest EL. Unusual lesions of muscles and tendons of the shoulder girdle and upper arm. Surg Gynecol Obstet. 1939;68:903–17.
67. Hamada J, Igarashi E, Akita K, Mochizuki T. A cadaveric study of the serratus anterior muscle and the long thoracic nerve. J Shoulder Elb Surg. 2008;17(5):790–4.
68. Fitchet SM. Injury of the serratus magnus (anterior) muscle. N Engl J Med. 1930;203(17):818–23.
69. Hayes JM, Zehr DJ. Traumatic muscle avulsion causing winging of the scapula. A case report. JBJS. 1981;63(3):495–7.
70. Gaffney KM. Avulsion injury of the serratus anterior: a case history. Clin J Sport Med. 1997;7(2):134–6.
71. Otoshi KI, Itoh Y, Tsujino A, Hasegawa M, Kikuchi SI. Avulsion injury of the serratus anterior muscle in a high-school underhand pitcher: a case report. J Shoulder Elb Surg. 2007;16(6):e45–7.
72. Carr JB, John QE, Rajadhyaksha E, Carson EW, Turney KL. Traumatic avulsion of the serratus anterior muscle in a collegiate rower: a case report. Sports Health. 2017;9(1):80–3.
73. Singh VK, Vargaonkar GS. Winging of scapula due to serratus anterior tear. Chin J Traumatol. 2014;17(5):305–6.
74. Meythaler JM, Reddy NM, Mitz M. Serratus anterior disruption: a complication of rheumatoid arthritis. Arch Phys Med Rehabil. 1986;67(10):770–2.
75. El-Naggar MM, Zahir FI. Two bellies of the coracobrachialis muscle associated with a third head of the biceps brachii muscle. Clin Anat. 2001;14(5):379–82.
76. Gilcreest EL, Albi P. Unusual lesions of muscles and tendons of the shoulder girdle and upper arm. Surg Gynecol Obstet. 1939;68:903–17.
77. Tobin WJ, Cohen LJ, Vandover JT. Parachute injuries. J Am Med Assoc. 1941;117(16):1318–21.
78. Spiegl UJ, Faucett SC, Millett PJ. Traumatic rupture of the coracobrachialis muscle: a case report. JBJS Case Connect. 2014;4(3):e54.
79. Saltzman BM, Harris JD, Forsythe B. Proximal coracobrachialis tendon rupture, subscapularis tendon rupture, and medial dislocation of the long head of the biceps tendon in an adult after traumatic anterior shoulder dislocation. Int J Shoulder Surg. 2015;9(2):52.

Part III

Arthritis of the Shoulder: I

Design of Polyethylene Glenoid Components

13

Ian A. Trail

Introduction

A range of factors, including general factors and those local to the shoulder, affect the long-term survival of the glenoid component in total shoulder arthroplasty (TSA) [1–3]. Unfortunately many of these factors are unknown and, of the ones that have been determined, it is often unclear how they affect glenoid survival.

Of those that are known, general factors include the quality and amount of bone, which is highly dependent on the disease process (many rheumatoid arthritis patients have very thin osteoporotic bone), and patient attitudes towards, and expectations of, their prosthesis. For example, a patient who subjects their joint replacement to high loads is likely to wear out or loosen the glenoid component more quickly than one who respects the joint. Surgeons can have little impact on these factors.

Local factors associated with the long-term survival of the glenoid component include: glenoid component design; glenoid preparation and cementing techniques; position and alignment of the glenoid component; position of the humeral head; and, finally, surgical technique.

I. A. Trail (✉)
Wrightington Hospital, Upper Limb Research Department, Hall Lane, Appley Bridge, Wigan, Lancashire, UK
e-mail: upperlimb@wrightington.org.uk

Glenoid Component Design

It is difficult to recreate normal shoulder biomechanics, as it is a very complex joint that is neither a ball-and-socket nor a hinge. What is of note, however, is that the movement of the shoulder does involve both translation and rotation. The articular surface geometry of the various glenoid components available can vary, with some conforming more to the humeral head than others. The non-conforming components, which have a mismatch or incongruity similar to the normal anatomy of the shoulder, have been shown to perform better than more rigidly conforming components [4–6], with the result that the articular surface geometry is now standard for the majority of implants, typically with a mismatch between the radius of curvature of the humeral and glenoid components of 6 mm. This allows translation, as well as angulation and rotation (Fig. 13.1). Nho et al. demonstrated in a retrieval study that closely conforming glenoid components suffered from greater abrasion and delamination, while the non-conforming, standard implant showed significantly greater burnishing of the articular surface [6]. Testing data for non-conforming glenoid and humeral components, at a 750 N load under 100,000 cycles, showed that there was less than 0.2 mm deformation [7].

I. A. Trail et al. (eds.), *Textbook of Shoulder Surgery*, https://doi.org/10.1007/978-3-319-70099-1_13

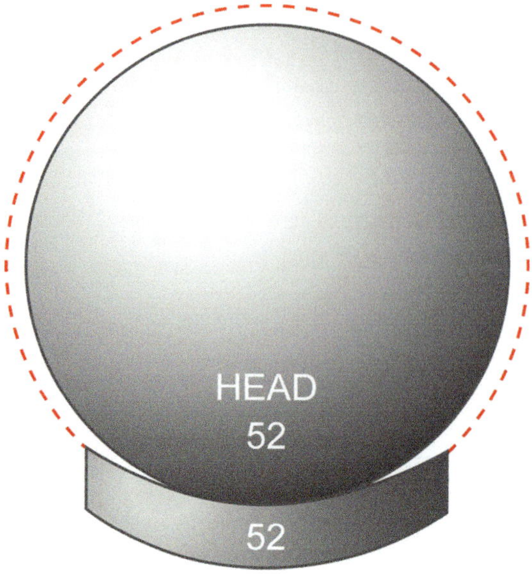

Fig. 13.1 Typical mismatch between the radius of curvatures of the humerus and glenoid component

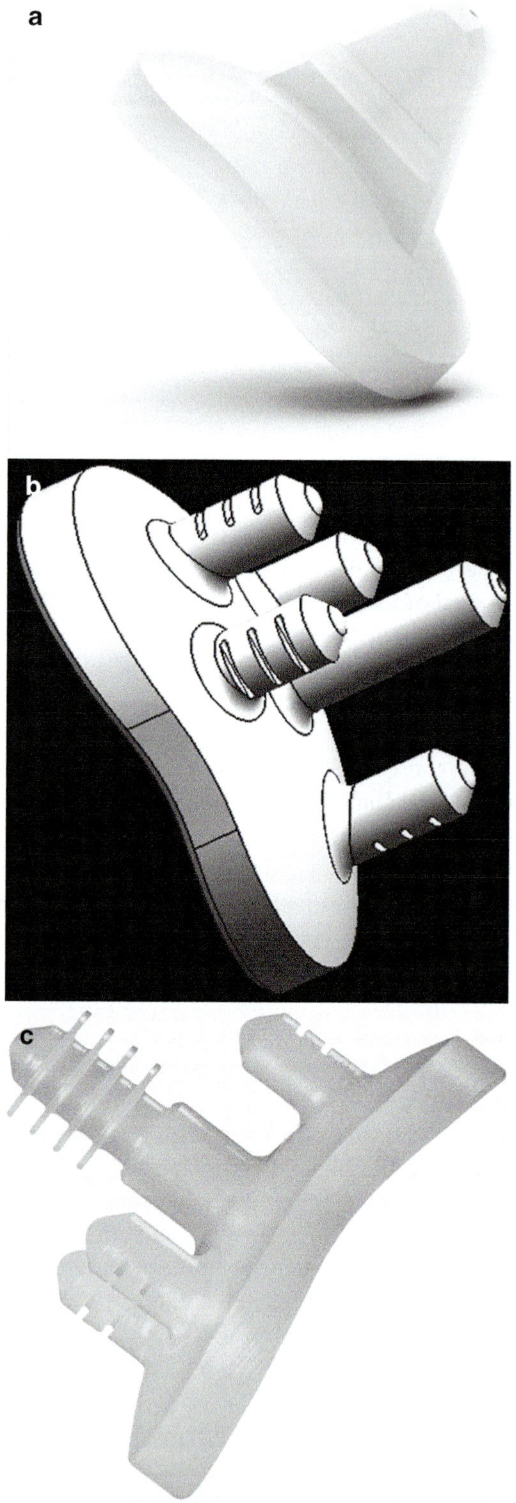

Fig. 13.2 Keeled, pegged and Anchor pegged glenoid components. (**a**) keeled glenoid implant, (**b**) pegged glenoid implant, (**c**) anchor peg component

The shape of the glenoid component is often an ellipse or oval in order to best mirror the normal articular surface.

The back of the glenoid component may be convex or flat. The convex-backed glenoid component has been shown to perform better than the flat-backed version on immediate postoperative radiographic analysis [8]. Longer term analysis, however, up to 10 years from the same centre revealed no difference, with no progression in the presence or progression of radiolucent lines [9].

Furthermore, a keel or pegs may be used to facilitate insertion into the glenoid. Since the introduction of the pegged components, designs have varied from three to five pegs. 'Anchor pegged' components, with a larger, finned, central peg to encourage bone ingrowth and three smaller pegs fixed with cement, have recently become popular (Fig. 13.2). Studies have suggested that, overall, pegged components appear to perform better than keeled components again on postoperative radiographic analysis [10–13], particularly in normal bone [14].

Studies from our institution revealed that on radiostereographic analysis both keeled and pegged components migrated after implantation and in the same anteroposterior direction.

However, the degree of rotation was significantly greater with the keeled component, at up to 6°. The maximum total point movement was also greater for the keeled compared with the pegged component, at up to 2 mm in 2 years [15].

Studies by Rahme et al. and Throckmorton et al. [16, 17] disputed these findings, specifically whether the new pegged components translated into better clinical and radiographical outcomes. However, a more detailed analysis indicated that these authors compared the keeled with an 'in-line' peg design, rather than a triangular or rectangular pattern, as used in other implants. It may be that this 'in-line' system of pegs is really little different to a keel.

Metal-backed glenoid components theoretically have the potential for improved fixation. However, the reduced thickness of the polyethylene layer on these prostheses can have an impact on outcomes, with this thin layer resulting in higher rates of wear, particularly if there is misalignment. This may also result in polyethylene dissociation from the metal tray [18]. To prevent this, previous designs were often too large, in that the combination of metal and polyethylene was too thick, leading to lateralisation of the humeral head. However, the metal backing of the glenoid can, with modern techniques, such as screw fixation and hydroxyapatite coating, lead to sound fixation. It may be that this type of glenoid component has a role in revision or where there is significant glenoid erosion.

More recently the 'Anchor peg' design has become popular. This combines a central fluted peg which is uncemented to allow bone ingrowth, combined with 3 shorter peripheral pegs which are cemented in situ. To date opinion amongst clinicians has been split in that some units have reported higher rates of migration and loosening compared to the standard cemented pegged component [19, 20].

Four other studies have described the clinical and radiographic analysis of this specific glenoid implant [21–23]. They have independently used modifications of the Lazurus method which was originally designed to assess the standard 5-pegged glenoid component [12]. One of these studies found evidence of osseointegration in 24 of 83 implants (29%) and reported no observed radiolucency; there was no mention of the presence or absence of focal lucency [23]. The second study of 20 implants observed that 15 had evidence of osseointegration, but 5 showed a decrease or absence of bone around the central peg [22]. It is well known that any misalignment from a perfect orthogonal view can lead to a gross underestimate of lucency [24]. The third study also reported radiolucencies using CT scans where 23 of 35 had complete osseointegration and 3 showed absence of bone around the central peg [21]. The final study was by Noyes et al. in 2015. Having analysed the x-rays of 42 consecutive total shoulder arthroplasties using this glenoid component identified complete incorporation with no lucent lines in 81% [25].

For polyethylene-only components, newer, cross-linked versions appear to have a lower osteolytic potential than conventional polyethylene components [26]. However, the problems that occurred with the introduction of the Hylamer ultra-high molecular weight polyethylene implant in 1990 should not be forgotten. Sterilisation with gamma radiation in an air environment, which was used between 1990 and 1993, increased rates of wear, osteolysis and loosening, thus increasing the need for revision. From 1995, the implants were sterilised using a gas plasma process, and the risk of degradation as a result of sterilisation was eliminated [27].

The use of non-standard glenoid components for bone deficiencies in shoulder arthroplasty were investigated by Cofield et al. [28]. They studied a group of patients who underwent a primary or revision anatomical shoulder replacement with one of three designs of non-standard glenoids. The first a polyethylene component with an angled keel for posterior glenoid wear without posterior subluxation. A second polyethylene component with 2 mm of extra thickness for central glenoid erosion and finally a posteriorly augmented metal-backed glenoid component for posterior glenoid wear and posterior subluxation. At the most recent follow-up, 3 glenoid components had loosened and 3 were at risk of loosening (14% at an average of 5.5 years). Of the group of 38, 7 patients had undergone revision surgery for various reasons. As a consequence they did not recommend non-standard glenoid components for addressing glenoid bone deficiency.

Finally, the use of a porous tantalum-backed glenoid component has been reported by Budge et al. who after an average follow-up of 38 months noted 4 of the components (21%) had failed by fracture at the keel-glenoid face junction [29]. As a consequence of this unacceptably high rate of glenoid component failure they cautioned against continued use.

Clinical Pearl
Pegged polyethylene components appear to migrate less and have a lower incidence of loosening when compared to keeled components.

Glenoid Preparation and Cementing Techniques

Just as important as the design of the glenoid components are glenoid preparation and cementing techniques, particularly as the majority of polyethylene implants are cemented. For example, preparation using a modern cannulated reaming system and an instrumented cement pressurisation technique for a three-pegged glenoid is, compared with results from the literature, associated with a lower incidence of early radiolucencies around the glenoid component [30]. The role of drying the glenoid prior to cementation was assessed by Edwards et al. in 2007, with three techniques investigated: thrombin-soaked gel foam; compressed gas lavage; and saline solution lavage with sponge drying. There were no significant radiological differences between the three preparation techniques, although the material costs were significantly higher in the first two groups [31].

The importance of cementing has been underlined by two studies. Cementless metal-backed components were shown by Boileau et al. to be inferior to cemented polyethylene implants in terms of fixation [32]. Furthermore, Pelletier et al. concluded that noncemented metal-back glenoids produce areas of higher cortical shear strains compared with cemented all-polyethylene implants [33].

The importance of a full back-side cementation rather than peg only was confirmed by Glennie et al. who in a cadaveric study showed that loading characteristics are more favourable when the cement is placed along the entire back of the implant contacting the subchondral bone [34].

At our institution, we conducted a study to evaluate the uniformity of the cement mantle under glenoid components inserted into cadaver shoulders using computed tomography [35]. The results were that keeled prostheses generally had a satisfactory cement mantle of 2 mm around the implant and no cortical encroachment. Despite pegged prostheses typically having a satisfactory cement mantle, the posterior peg of a pegged prosthesis often penetrated the posterior cortex (Fig. 13.3). In light of this, we felt that, while most glenoid prostheses were satisfactory with regard to the radius of curvature, shape and size, the margin of error for insertion of the pegged prosthesis was narrow due to the potential cortical perforation. The results of this study suggest that a smaller posterior peg size and side specific prostheses may prevent cortical perforations [35].

Whether a glenoid component needs to be 100% seated however, has been brought into recent focus in a paper by Dilisio et al. who con-

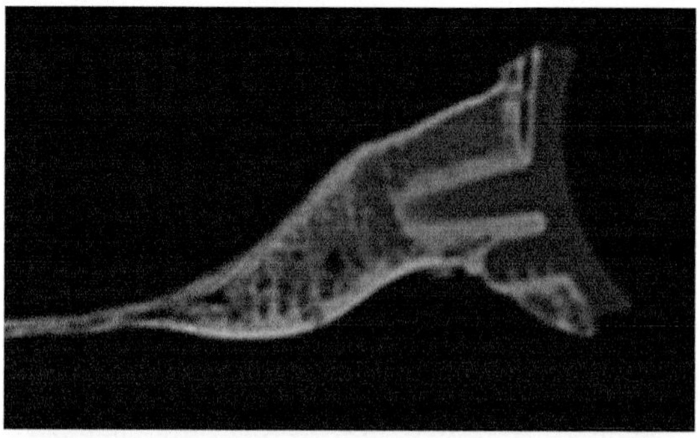

Fig. 13.3 Five pegged component cemented to glenoid showing perforation of the cortex by the posterior peg

cluded having undertaken a CT study on 36 total shoulder arthroplasties, at a minimum of two-year follow-up, which showed that radiolucencies around the cemented glenoid component were not related to the degree of component seating [36].

Finally, the use of cement at all has been brought into focus by De Wilde et al. in 2013, who reported on 34 shoulders in whom they had inserted a pegged polyethylene glenoid component without the use of cement. At a mean follow-up of 28 months they were able radiologically to demonstrate signs of loosening in only 4 shoulders. Clinically the outcome was satisfactory [37].

Position and Alignment

The position and alignment of both glenoid and humeral components is an obvious area in which the survival of an implant can be improved. Although there is no evidence to support this assumption, common sense suggests that, if the implant is in as near an anatomically perfect position as possible, it should survive longer than one that is mal-aligned. Wang et al. in a laboratory study were able to demonstrate that polyethylene implants inserted in neutral version after eccentric reaming had superiorly less subsequent loosening compared to an angle backed augmented glenoid component [38].

Several findings in the literature emphasise the importance of proper component positioning in glenoid survival. In 2007, Cheung et al. showed that displacement of the polyethylene was a primary reason for revision arthroplasty [18]. In addition, Nyffeler et al. demonstrated that even small variations in the degree of glenoid version influences the loading pattern of the glenoid component and may increase the risk of instability and glenoid loosening [39]. In a study of glenoid components removed for loosening and instability, many cases revealed asymmetric deformation, particularly located at the inferior quadrant of the glenoid, suggesting impingement with bone at the edge of the humeral component and/or edge deformation caused by eccentric loading from off the humeral head [40]. Finally, Favre et al. demonstrated that a superiorly placed humeral component can predispose to impingement and component failure [41].

What most surgeons, however, agree upon is that where possible as much subchondral bone should be preserved. This was confirmed in a study by Walch et al. [42].

Computer-aided surgery (Patient Specific Instrumentation, PSI) would be an ideal technique for placing a glenoid implant in the correct alignment and achieving a near-perfect anatomical position. Nguyen et al. showed in a cadaveric study that computer-aided surgery resulted in more accurate version during glenoid component implantation, as measured by post-implantation computed tomography [43]. However, there is little manual instrumentation available even today to aid the surgeon with alignment of the glenoid component. Consequently, this area of surgical technique would seem key to future development.

> **Clinical Pearl**
> Glenoid exposure, alignment of the prosthesis and good cement technique should lead to better survivalship, although this has never been scientifically proven.

The Position of the Humeral Head

Emphasis on humeral head positioning was much less 20 years ago than it is today. Research by Roberts et al. in 1991 showed in normal cadaveric humeri that, rather than purely retroverted, the humeral head has a median retroversion of 21.4° and a median posterior offset of 4.7 mm [44]. These findings were underscored by Walch and Boileau in 1999, who demonstrated that an adaptable prosthesis, with eight possible positions for the humeral head to allow the shoulder anatomy to be replicated, can achieve good functional and radiographic results [45].

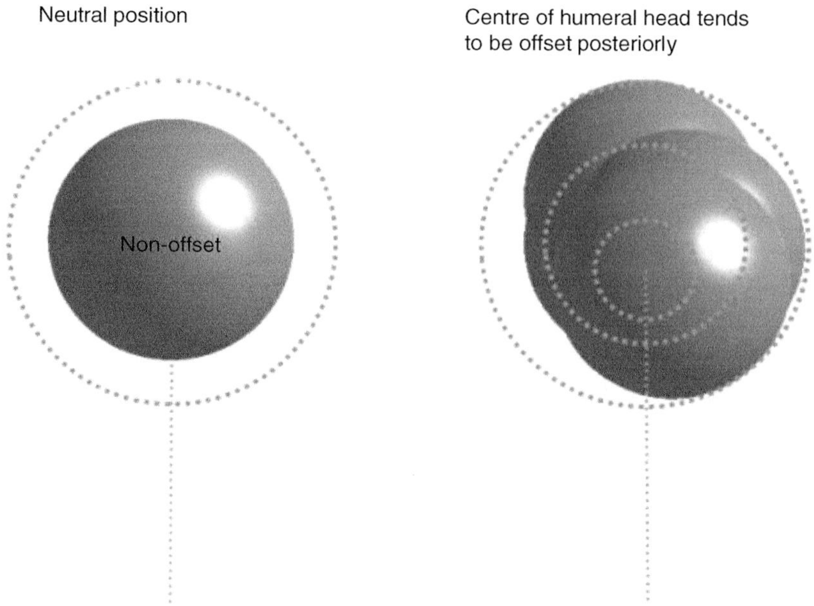

Fig. 13.4 Non-offset and offset humeral heads

At our institution, we used radiostereographic analysis to investigate the effect of offset versus non-offset humeral heads (Fig. 13.4) on the micromovement of glenoid components. While there was no significant difference in clinical outcomes between the offset and non-offset groups, there was significantly greater migration of the glenoid component around the anterior/posterior, ante/retroversion and varus/valgus axes with the non-offset humeral head. Furthermore, correction of glenoid erosion appeared to have a detrimental effect on glenoid migration [46].

With regard to the optimal degree of mismatch studies by Sabesan et al. using a laboratory model concluded that a radial mismatch of less than 10 mm may decrease the risk of glenoid micromotion [47].

Clinical Pearl

It would appear that the more anatomical the humeral head is replaced then this diminishes glenoid component migration.

Surgical Technique

While it is relatively easy to expose the humeral head in TSA, it is more difficult to fully expose the glenoid. A glenoid component can only be implanted in the appropriate position once the whole of the glenoid articular surface is clearly visible and accessible. In 2006, Chin et al. observed that surgical technique was a critical variable in component placement, with the overall complication rate of TSA decreasing dramatically with the advent of newer techniques [48]. An in vitro analysis also showed that the component can be stabilised against eccentric loads with careful preparation of the bone and reaming [49]. Again, improvements in instrumentation, such as the availability of smaller and/or two-headed reamers, would aid surgical technique, resulting in better congruity and conformity of the glenoid component.

Conclusion

If we are to improve the key outcome of TSA, which is survival of the glenoid component, the most important factor appears to be improved surgical technique, particularly exposure of the glenoid. Specifically, surgeons should be able to expose the posterior aspect of the glenoid easily. Secondly, the glenoid component should be inserted in the correct anatomical position, with instruments developed to allow alignment to the correct inclination, even in the presence of erosion. Thirdly, cementing techniques for fixation should continue to improve. Finally, further research is needed to determine the long-term survival of the anchor peg and the effect of more anatomical humeral head replacements (Fig. 13.5).

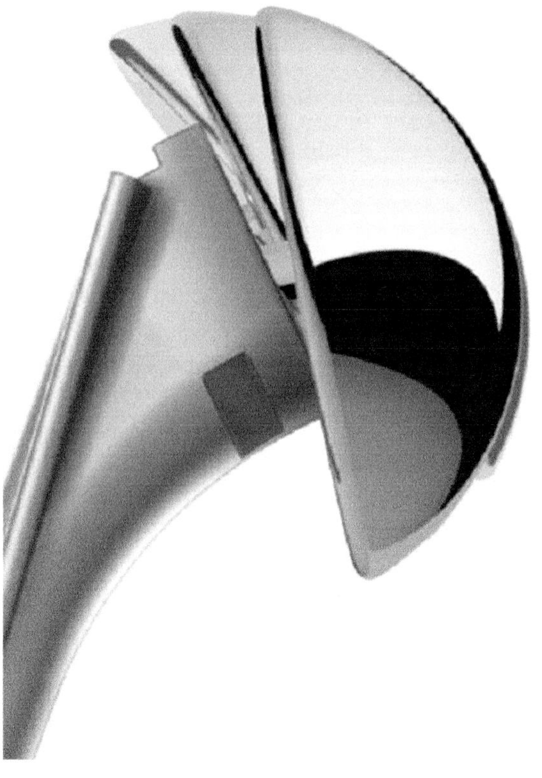

Fig. 13.5 Humeral head replacements to allow both offset and inclination

References

1. Trail IA, Nuttall D. The results of shoulder arthroplasty in patients with rheumatoid arthritis. J Bone Joint Surg Br. 2002;84(8):1121–5.
2. Fox TJ, Cil A, Sperling JW, Sanchez-Sotelo J, Schleck CD, Cofield RH. Survival of the glenoid component in shoulder arthroplasty. J Shoulder Elb Surg. 2009;18(6):859–63.
3. Greiner S, Berth A, Kääb M, Irlenbusch U. Glenoid morphology affects the incidence of radiolucent lines around cemented pegged polyethylene glenoid components. Arch Orthop Trauma Surg. 2013;133(10):1331–9.
4. Craig EV, Nho S, Warren RF, Owen A, Figgie MP, Wright T, Dodson C. Comparison of conforming and non-conforming retrieved glenoid components. J Bone Joint Surg. 2007;16(2):e58.
5. Walch G, Edwards TB, Boulahia A, Boileau P, Mole D, Adeleine P. The influence of glenohumeral prosthetic mismatch on glenoid radiolucent lines: results of a multicenter study. J Bone Joint Surg Am. 2002;84(12):2186–91.
6. Nho SJ, Ala OL, Dodson CC, Figgie MP, Wright TM, Craig EV, Warren RF. Comparison of conforming and nonconforming retrieved glenoid components. J Shoulder Elb Surg. 2008;17:914–20.
7. Anglin C, Wyss UP, Nyffeler RW, Gerber C. Loosening performance of cemented glenoid prosthesis design pairs. Clin Biomech (Bristol, Avon). 2001;16:144–50.
8. Szabo I, Buscayret F, Edwards TB, Nemoz C, Boileau P, Walch G. Radiographic comparison of flat-back and convex-back glenoid components in total shoulder arthroplasty. J Shoulder Elb Surg. 2005;14(6):636–42.
9. Collin P, Tay AK, Melis B, Boileau P, Walch G. A ten-year radiologic comparison of two-all polyethylene glenoid component designs: a prospective trial. J Shoulder Elb Surg. 2011;20(8):1217–23.
10. Edwards TB, Labriola JE, Stanley RJ, O'Connor DP, Elkousy HA, Gartsman GM. Radiographic comparison of pegged and keeled glenoid components using modern cementing techniques: a prospective randomized study. J Shoulder Elb Surg. 2010;19(2):251–7.
11. Gartsman GM, Elkousy HA, Warnock KM, Edwards TB, O'Connor DP. Radiographic comparison of pegged and keeled glenoid components. J Shoulder Elb Surg. 2005;14(3):252–7.
12. Lazarus MD, Jensen KL, Southworth C, Matsen FA 3rd. The radiographic evaluation of keeled and pegged glenoid component insertion. J Bone Joint Surg Am. 2002;84(7):1174–82.
13. Haines JF, Trail IA, Nuttall D, Birch A, Barrow A. The results of arthroplasty in osteoarthritis of the shoulder. J Bone Joint Surg Br. 2006;88:496–501.
14. Lacroix D, Murphy LA, Prendergast PJ. Three-dimensional finite element analysis of glenoid replacement prostheses: a comparison of keeled

and pegged anchorage systems. J Biomech Eng. 2000;122(4):430–6.
15. Nuttall D, Haines JF, Trail IA. A study of the micromovement of pegged and keeled glenoid components compared using radiostereometric analysis. J Shoulder Elb Surg. 2007;16(3):S65–70.
16. Rahme H, Mattsson P, Wikblad L, Nowak J, Larsson S. Stability of cemented in-line pegged glenoid compared with keeled glenoid components in total shoulder arthroplasty. J Bone Joint Surg Am. 2009;91:1965–72.
17. Throckmorton TW, Zarkadas PC, Sperling JW, Cofield RH. Pegged versus keeled glenoid components in total shoulder arthroplasty. J Shoulder Elb Surg. 2010;19(5):726–33.
18. Cheung EV, Sperling JW, Cofield RH. Polyethylene insert exchange for wear after total shoulder arthroplasty. J Shoulder Elb Surg. 2007;16(5):574–8.
19. Nuttall D, Haines JF, Trail IA. The early migration of a partially cemented fluted pegged glenoid component using radiostereometric analysis. J Shoulder Elb Surg. 2012;21:1191–6.
20. Nuttall D, Birch A, Haines JF, Watts AC, Trail IA. Migration of a partially cemented fluted glenoid component, inserted using a cannulated preparation system, as measured using radiostereometric analysis and it's relation to lucency as seen on CT scans. Bone Joint Surg. 2017;99B:674–9.
21. Arnold RM, High RR, Grosshans KT, Walker CW, Fehringer EV. Bone presence between the central peg's radial fins of a partially cemented pegged all poly glenoidcomponent suggest few radiolucencies. J Shoulder Elb Surg. 2011;20:315–21.
22. Churchill RS, Zellmer C, Zimmers HJ, Ruggero R. Clinical and radiographic analysis of a partially cemented glenoid implant: five-year minimum follow-up. J Shoulder Elb Surg. 2010;19: 1091–7.
23. Groh GI. Survival and radiographic analysis of a glenoid component with a cementless fluted central peg. J Shoulder Elb Surg. 2010;19:1265–8.
24. Nagels J, Valstar ER, Stokdijk M, Rozing PM. Patterns of loosening of the glenoid component. J Bone Joint Surg Br. 2002;84:83–7.
25. Noyes MP, Meccia B, Spencer EE. Five-to-ten-year follow-up with a partially cemented all-polyethylene bone-ingrowth glenoid component. J Shoulder Elb Surg. 2015;24:1458–62.
26. Wirth MA, Klotz C, Deffenbaugh DL, McNulty D, Richards L, Tipper JL. Cross-linked glenoid prosthesis: a wear comparison to conventional glenoid prosthesis with wear particulate analysis. J Shoulder Elb Surg. 2009;18(1):130–7.
27. Rockwood CA. Observation on retrieved Hylamer glenoids in shoulder arthroplasty: problems associated with sterilization by gamma irradiation in air. J Shoulder Elb Surg. 2002;11(2):191–7.
28. Cil A, Sperling JW, Cofield RH. Nonstandard glenoid components for bone deficiencies in shoulder arthroplasty. J Shoulder Elb Surg. 2014;23(7):e149–57.
29. Budge MD, Nolan EM, Heisey MH, Baker K, Wiater JM. Results of total shoulder arthroplasty with a monoblock porous tantalum glenoid component: a prospective minimum 2-year follow-up study. J Shoulder Elb Surg. 2013;22(4):535–41.
30. Barwood S, Setter KJ, Blaine TA, Bigliani LU. The incidence of early radiolucencies about a pegged glenoid component using cement pressurization. J Shoulder Elb Surg. 2008;17(5):703–8.
31. Edwards TB, Sabonghy EP, Elkousy H, Warnock KM, Hammerman SM, O'Connor DP, Gartsman GM. Glenoid component insertion in total shoulder arthroplasty: comparison of three techniques for drying the glenoid before cementation. J Shoulder Elb Surg. 2007;16(3 Suppl):S107–10.
32. Boileau P, Avidor C, Krishnan SG, Walch G, Kempf JF, Mole D. Cemented polyethylene versus uncemented metal-backed glenoid components in total shoulder arthroplasty: a prospective, double-blind, randomized study. J Shoulder Elb Surg. 2002;11(4):351–9.
33. Pelletier MH, Langdown A, Gillies RM, Sonnabend DH, Walsh WR. Photoelastic comparison of strains in the underlying glenoid with metal-backed and all-polyethylene implants. J Shoulder Elb Surg. 2008;17(5):779–83.
34. Glennie RA, Giles JW, Johnson JA, Athwal GS, Faber KJ. An in vitro study comparing limited to full cementation of polyethylene glenoid components. J Orthop Surg Res. 2015;17(10):142.
35. Kumar G, Page R, Trail IA. CTA analysis of glenoid fixation in a cadaveric model. J Bone Joint Surg Br. 2004;86(Suppl 1):100.
36. Dilisio MF, May NR, Vincent SA, High RR, Walker CW, Manzer MN, Apker KA, Fehringer EV. The association of incomplete glenoid component seating and periprosthetic glenoid radiolucencies after total shoulder arthroplasty. J Shoulder Elb Surg. 2015;8:S1058–2746.
37. De Wilde L, Dayerizadeh N, De Neve F, Basmania C, Van Tongel A. Fully uncemented glenoid component in total shoulder arthroplasty. J Shoulder Elb Surg. 2013;22(10):e1–7.
38. Wang T, Abrams GD, Behn AW, Lindsey D, Giori N, Cheung EV. Posterior glenoid wear in total shoulder arthroplasty: eccentric anterior reaming is superior to posterior augment. Clin Orthop Relat Res. 2015;473(12):3928–36.
39. Nyffeler RW, Sheikh R, Atkinson TS, Jacob HA, Favre P, Gerber C. Effects of glenoid component version on humeral head displacement and joint reaction forces: an experimental study. J Shoulder Elb Surg. 2006;15(5):625–9.
40. Nho SJ, Nam D, Ala OL, Craig EV, Warren RF, Wright TM. Observations on retrieved glenoid components from total shoulder arthroplasty. J Shoulder Elb Surg. 2009;18(3):371–8.
41. Favre P, Moor B, Snedeker JG, Gerber C. Influence of component positioning on impingement in conventional total shoulder arthroplasty. Clin Biomech (Bristol, Avon). 2008;23(2):175–83.

42. Walch G, Young AA, Boileau P, Loew M, Gazielly D, Molé D. Patterns of loosening of polyethylene keeled glenoid components after shoulder arthroplasty for primary osteoarthritis: results of a multicentre study with more than five years of follow-up. J Bone Joint Surg Am. 2012;94(2):145–50.
43. Nguyen D, Ferreira LM, Brownhill JR, King GJ, Drosdowech DS, Faber KJ, Johnson JA. Improved accuracy of computer assisted glenoid implantation in total shoulder arthroplasty: an in-vitro randomized controlled trial. J Shoulder Elb Surg. 2009;18(6):907–14.
44. Roberts SN, Foley AP, Swallow HM, Wallace WA, Coughlan DP. The geometry of the humeral head and the design of prostheses. J Bone Joint Surg Br. 1991;73(4):647–50.
45. Walch G, Boileau P. Prosthetic adaptability: a new concept for shoulder arthroplasty. J Shoulder Elb Surg. 1999;8(5):443–51.
46. Nuttall D, Haines JF, Trail IA. The effect of the offset humeral head on the micromovement of pegged glenoid components: a comparative study using radiostereometric analysis. J Bone Joint Surg Br. 2009;91(6):757–61.
47. Sabesan VJ, Ackerman J, Sharma V, Baker KC, Kurdziel MD, Wiater JM. Glenohumeral mismatch affects micromotion of cemented glenoid components in total shoulder arthroplasty. J Shoulder Elb Surg. 2015;24(5):814–22.
48. Chin PY, Sperling JW, Cofield RH, Schleck C. Complications of total shoulder arthroplasty: are they fewer or different? J Shoulder Elb Surg. 2006;15:19–22.
49. Collins D, Tencer A, Sidles J. Matsen Fr. Edge displacement and deformation of glenoid components in response to eccentric loading. The effect of preparation of the glenoid bone. J Bone Joint Surg Am. 1992;74(4):501–7.

Design of Humeral Stems

14

Emmet John Griffiths, Ian A. Trail, and Gilles Walch

Introduction

The first attempt at prosthetic replacement of the humeral head was performed in 1893 by Pean to treat a shoulder infected with tuberculosis. Modern total shoulder arthroplasty, however, really began in the 1950s with the cemented Neer prosthesis [1] (Fig. 14.1) which gave reasonable short and long term results in terms of pain relief, function and movement and a low

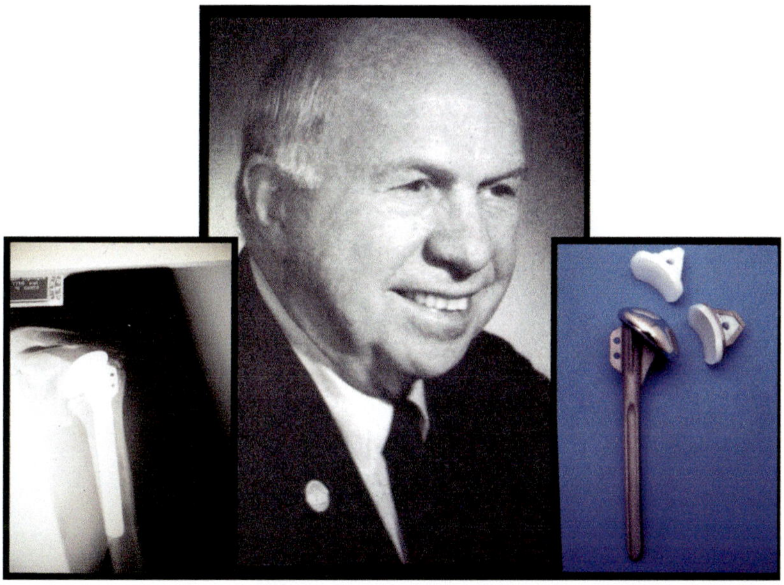

Fig. 14.1 Neer monoblock prosthesis

E. J. Griffiths
Norfolk & Norwich University Hospital, Norwich, UK

I. A. Trail
Wrightington Hospital, Wigan, Lancashire, UK
e-mail: upperlimb@wrightington.org.uk

G. Walch (✉)
Centre Orthopédique Santy-Ramsay Generale de Santé, Lyon, France

I. A. Trail et al. (eds.), *Textbook of Shoulder Surgery*, https://doi.org/10.1007/978-3-319-70099-1_14

incidence of humeral loosening [2]. Since then there has been significant evolution both in terms of materials but also in design of the humeral prostheses. Initially humeral components were monoblocks available in limited sizes. These evolved into second generation implants which allowed a degree of modularity in terms of variable head sizes to better match the resected head (Fig. 14.2). This purported to allow better soft tissue tensioning and hence a better outcome although clinical studies have not yet bourne this out [3, 4]. They also facilitated revision surgery by allowing separate head removal which exposes the bone-cement interface proximally as well as the glenoid. The third-generation implants added further modularity in terms of eccentricity of the head compared to the stem, head thickness and diameter as well as head-neck angulation (in some systems) (Fig. 14.3). These are commonly referred to as an anatomic replacement [5]. More recently the introduction of platform systems has added further complexity to the design of humeral stems as the ability to change from an anatomic stem to a reverse polarity stem requires further modularity of the body of the stem. Finally there has also been the development of both resurfacing systems (Fig. 14.4) and short stem, (or metaphyseal fit/stemless) prostheses (Fig. 14.5). At this time again there is little clinical evidence to support one over the other. However, there is no doubt that the use of resurfacing and stemless prosthesis again makes revision simpler.

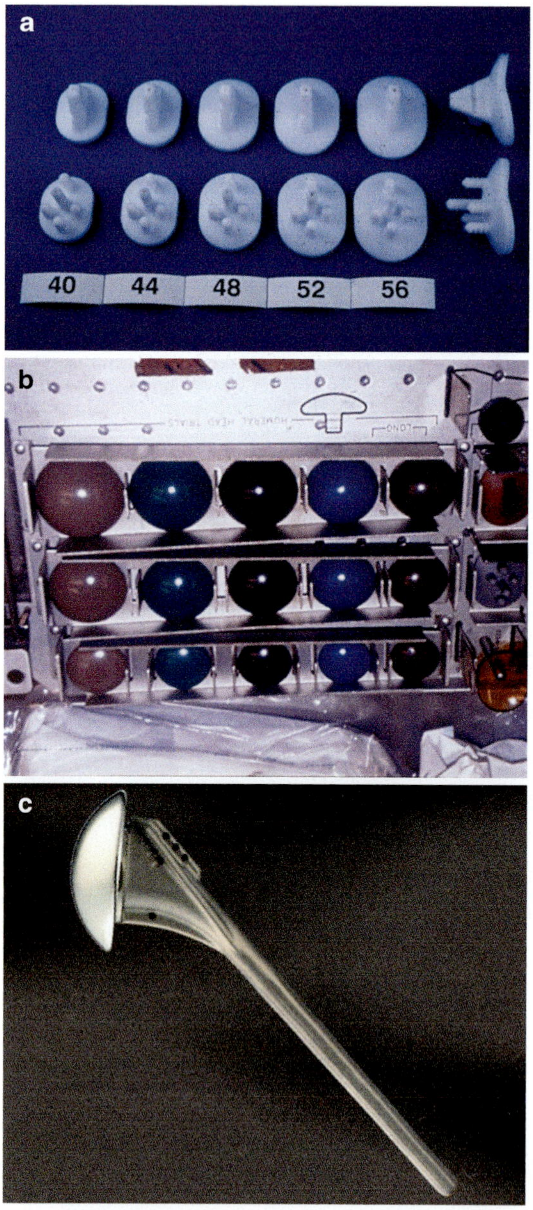

Fig. 14.2 Global advantage modular prosthesis

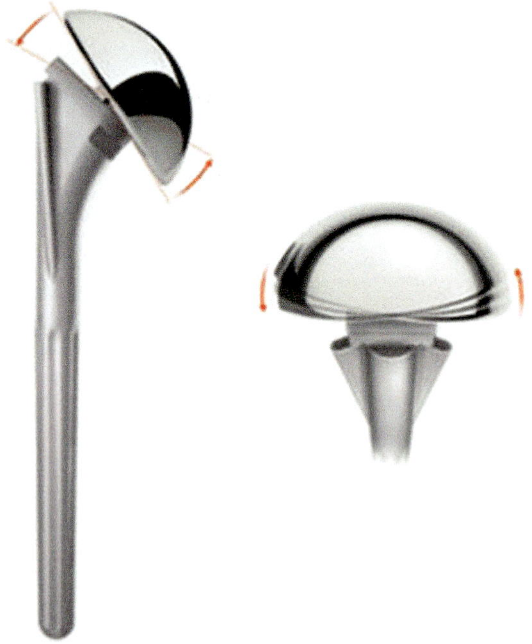

Fig. 14.3 Global AP with increased variability

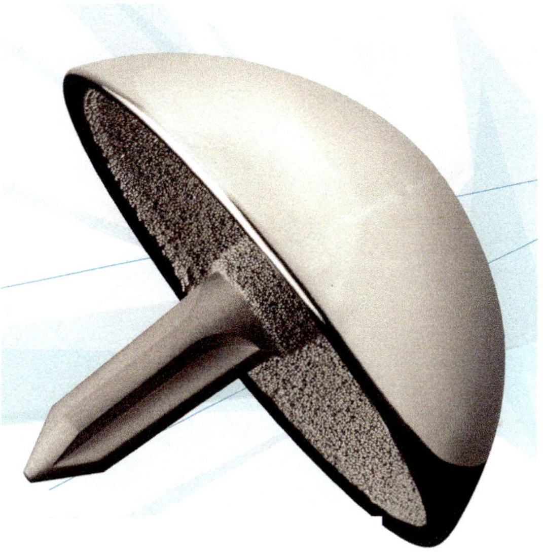

Fig. 14.4 Copeland resurfacing

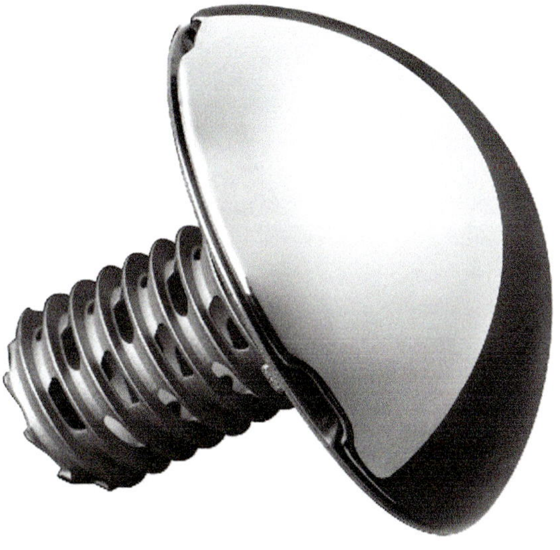

Fig. 14.5 Habermeyer stemless prosthesis

Anatomical Considerations

The aim of arthroplasty is to restore the anatomy of the joint that is replaced. The rationale follows that the more closely the anatomy is replicated the better the implant should be expected to perform. This is particularly pertinent when the joint that is replaced has a large soft tissue component for example the shoulder. The initial evolution of shoulder prostheses however was not based upon rigorous anatomic studies but rather on seeking to replicate or improve on the original Neer prosthesis. It wasn't until the 1990's that proximal humeral anatomy was examined more closely with reference to prosthetic design and the large variability in 'normal' anatomy was uncovered.

Version of the humeral head is very variable both between individuals and even between the 2 shoulders in a single individual (Fig. 14.6). There is also some variability in how it is measured. It equates to the difference in orientation between the proximal humeral articular surface and the trochlear of the distal humerus. The vast majority of individuals show retroversion of the proximal humeral articular surface with a mean retroversion of roughly 20° as shown in the largest cadaveric study [6].

The radius of curvature of the humeral head may be measured in both frontal and saggital planes and this again reveals significant variation. As expected the radius of curvature is smaller in women compared to men. The ratio of frontal to saggital size is relatively constant (roughly 10% mismatch) and shows that the humeral head is not circular in cross sectional area but rather elliptical (Fig. 14.7). The long axis of the ellipse is aligned with the version axis of the humerus. There is also striking correlation between the radius of curvature and the head thickness. The head thickness is approximately 70% of the frontal radius of curvature.

The offset (eccentricity) of the humeral head is the relationship between the head of the humerus and the longitudinal axis of the humeral shaft (Fig. 14.8). There are two dimensions to offset, antero-posterior and medio-lateral. Due to the conical shape of the proximal humeral medullary cavity it may be difficult to accurately define the shaft axis on standard AP radiographs. The mean offset is generally regarded as being 6 mm medially and between 2.6 ± 1.8 mm [5] or 1.4 ± 1.4 mm [6] posterior compared to the shaft axis.

Head-shaft angle or inclination (Fig. 14.9) may be measured off a frontal view of the humerus and is the angle created by a line drawn perpendicular to the midpoint of the humeral articular surface and the long axis of the humerus. It is less variable with a mean of 137°.

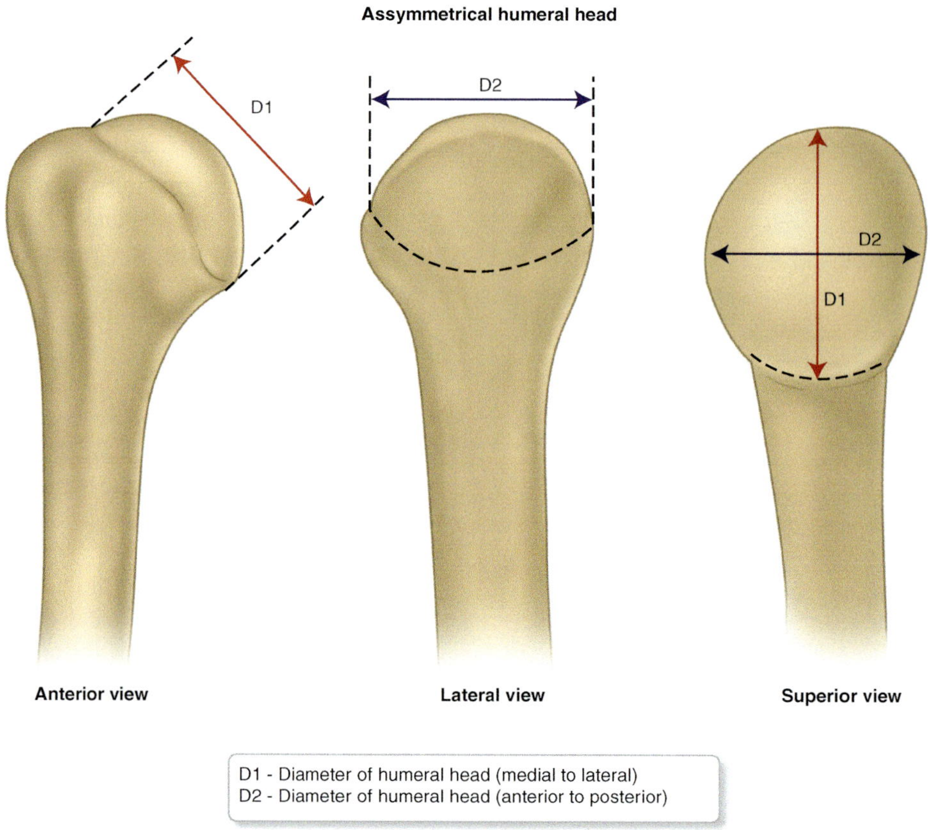

Fig. 14.6 Version of humeral head

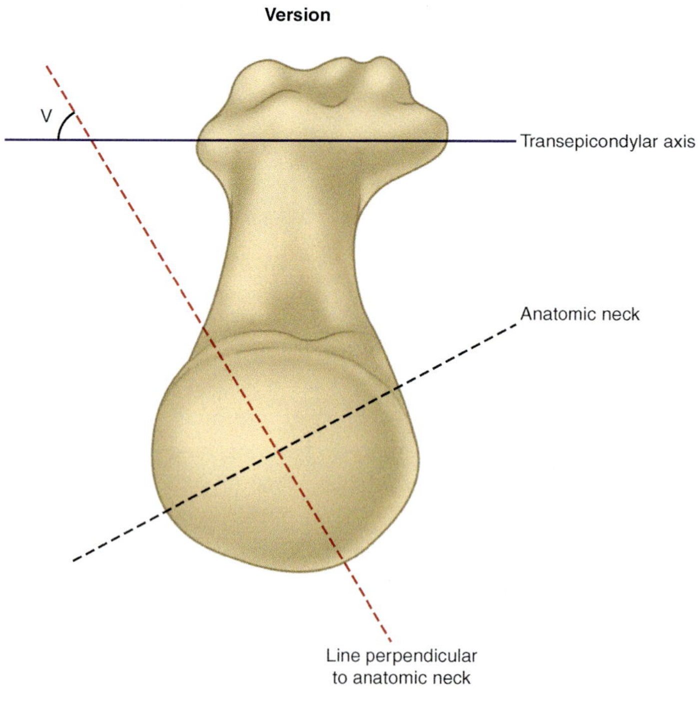

Fig. 14.7 Radius of curvature and shape of humeral head

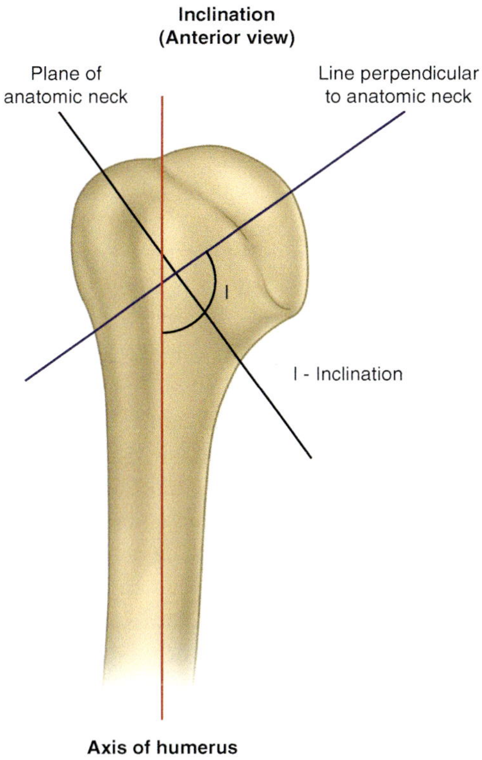

Fig. 14.8 Offset of humeral head

Surgical Considerations

The incorrect sizing of the humeral head component may have considerable detrimental effects. In vitro study would suggest that an increase in thickness of the head component of 5 mm reduces the range of movement at the glenohumeral joint of between 20° and 30° [7]. This also causes earlier obligate translation of the humeral component on the glenoid component. Whether this effect is seen in vivo where there is often slight medialisation of the joint line due to glenoid wear is unknown. Similarly undersizing the head may also reduce range of movement by a similar amount [8]. This is due to the reduction in the surface arc and hence the angular movement permitted before impingement occurs. There may also be concerns with the theoretical increased longitudinal wear of a smaller bearing surface. However it may be beneficial clinically to err on the side of a smaller component at least in the short term rather than potentially overstuffing the joint [8].

Due to the elliptical shape of the native head matching the circular prosthetic head in the frontal

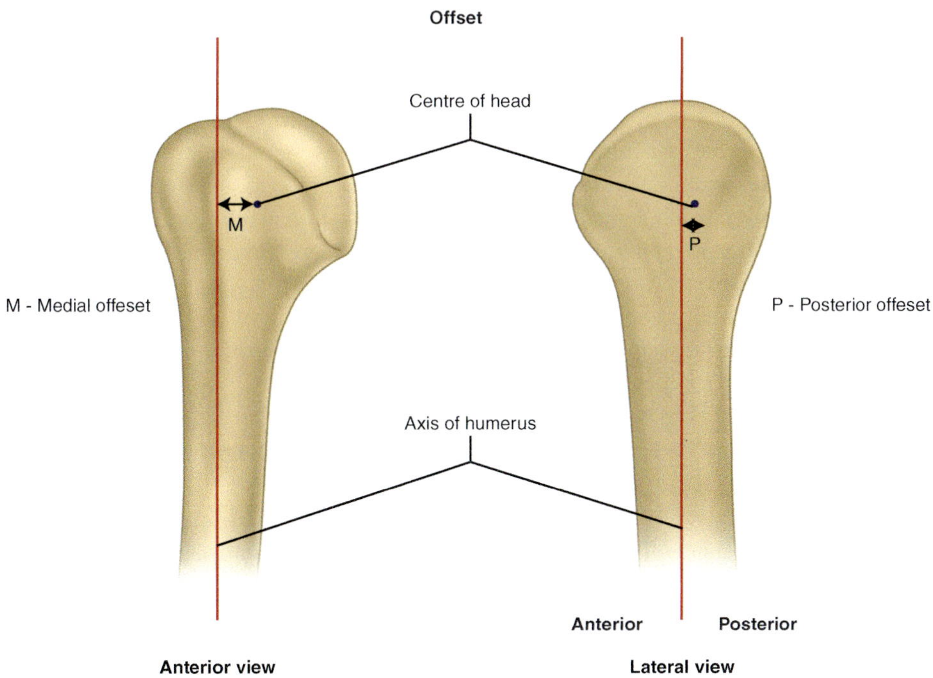

Fig. 14.9 Head shaft angle

plane results in an overlap of approximately 3 mm in the sagittal plane. The clinical effect of this is unknown. The key area to avoid overlap is laterally as any overlap here impinges on the rotator cuff insertion and increases cuff tension at the point of most vulnerability. This is one of the benefits of an eccentric humeral head component.

Similarly significant variability in proximal humeral anatomy means that a straight stem will disrupt the cuff insertion in a proportion of individuals (less than 10%). This is related to the critical distance and is measured as the distance between the lateral border of the greater tuberosity and the longitudinal axis of the humerus.

Clinical Pearl

It is important at surgery not to overstuff the joint as this can diminish range of motion and result in an increase in soft tissue tension.

Added to that it is also important that the metal head does not impinge on the rotator cuff insertion as this can lead to early rotator cuff failure.

The Effects of Modularity

The large variability in proximal humeral anatomy between individuals and a desire to closely replicate patient anatomy has led to increasingly modular designs. The aim of modularity is to allow maximum variability without increasing requirements for the manufacture and storage of a huge number of different monoblocks. Modularity allows the surgeon to control several aspects of the soft tissue and bony reconstruction. It also may allow revision procedures to be technically easier, allowing the removal of the head separate to the stem and hence easier access to revise the glenoid component. This ability to leave the humeral stem in situ is the basis of the argument for the current platform systems. This has recently been confirmed by Weber-Spickschen et al. [9] following a retrospective study of 15 shoulder replacements that were converted from an anatomic to a reverse implant using the convertible prosthetic system (SMR, Lima, Italy) concluded that this reduced the rate of complication and that mid-term clinical and radiological results were promising [9].

Varied modularity of humeral head size does allow for a more accurate matching of the prosthesis to the patient. Whilst the early implants really only allowed tension to be adjusted, the addition of offset heads allowed improved matching. More recently later designs have incorporated the option of tilt such that the inclination of the head can be adjusted. Again further improving anatomy. Whilst there is little or any evidence that this is translated into improved outcomes there is some evidence that a more anatomic humeral head replacement has a beneficial effect on the adjacent glenoid replacement [10].

There are however possible disadvantages of modularity. With each additional component the potential points of failure increase. There is also the creation of additional wear surfaces which may or may not prove clinically relevant. The incidence of backside wear in knee arthroplasty and trunnion wear in hip arthroplasty shows that these considerations are worth bearing in mind. To date there have been no reported failures causing clinical significance at the shoulder. Indeed Teeter et al. [11] whilst showing tribocorrosion on the heads and stems of some retrieved shoulder implants noted that this was significantly lower than in the cases of retrieved hip implants. The greatest changes were in the lower zone of the taper where the connections may be exposed to the surrounding joint fluid. Again, however, whether this was of any clinical significance is unclear [11].

Use of Cement and Stem Length

The role of cementation remains unclear. Whilst it undoubtedly has a role in trauma and revision for fixation of implants, it's role generally has diminished with time. In 2010 Throckmorton et al. analysed the radiological outcome of 76 patients who had a circumferential metaphyseal porous coated humeral stem inserted. They were not able to find any radiolucencies initially although subsequent x-rays did reveal small areas of radiolucency with a mean follow up of 4.6 years. These implants, however, were not felt to be at risk. As such, they concluded in treatment of osteoarthritis cement was not required [12]. More recently work by Raiss et al. [13] analysed the radiological outcome of both cemented and uncemented humeral stems in patients with primary osteoarthritis with a mean follow up of 8.2 years. They were able to demonstrate comparable results and no difference between humeral loosening. They were, however, able to identify stress shielding particularly in patients who had undergone an uncemented humeral stem [13].

The length of humeral stems has again diminished with time. For certain the original 10 cm humeral stems have become redundant. More recent work by Schnetzke et al. [14] evaluated a shorter cementless humeral stem made of titanium (Aequalis Ascend) in 52 patients with a minimum follow up of 2 years. They were not able to identify any loosening, (subsidence) or osteolysis in any of the cases, although they did see cortical thinning and osteopenia in a number of cases. They concluded that the results of the stem at least in the short term are comparable to that of standard stem design [14].

Finite element analysis undertaken by Razfar et al. [15] concluded that reducing the stem length produced humeral stresses that more closely matched the intact stress distribution in proximal cortico bone. Conversely stresses in a more proximal trabecular bone were significantly elevated particularly when stemless implants were used [15].

With the increased use of a reverse design prosthesis more attention has been given to the design but also the humeral position in this type of implant and its effect on range of motion, impingement and notching etc. Work by Lädermann et al. [16] using a 3 dimensional computer model compared the traditional inlay Grammont stem with a short curved onlay stem with different inclinations (155°, 145°, 135°) and offset (lateralised vs medialised). They concluded the shorter stem design lead to a nearly 7 mm change in humeral offset. Different inclinations of the stems, however, had little influence on humeral offset and a large influence on decreasing the acromiohumeral distance. There was also a 10° decrease in abduction and a 5° increase in adduction between an inlay Grammont design and an onlay design with the same inclination. Compared to the 155° model, the 135° model improved adduction by 28°, extension by 24° and external rotation by 15°. There was however a decrease in abduction of 9°. They concluded that with a varus inclination prostheses of 135° and 145° elevation remained unchanged, abduction slightly decreases but there was a dramatic improvement in adduction, extension and external rotation [16]. Similar work was undertaken by Berhouet et al. [17] using a 3 dimensional shoulder simulation model to investigate the biomechanical effect of humeral tray positioning in reverse shoulder arthroplasty. Conclusions were that if the humeral tray was positioned as an offset posteriorly this offered a biomechanical advantage by decreasing superior impingement and increasing the internal rotation moment arm of subscapularis without creating inferior impingement [17].

Clinical Pearl

Whilst one should accept in certain clinical circumstances, for example trauma, revision or essentially poor bone stock the need for cemented fixation of a humeral stem generally this has become much less common.

The Need for a Stem

One way to accurately replicate the anatomy of the proximal humerus would be to perform a resurfacing procedure and several designs of resurfacing have excellent medium and long term outcomes [18]. They are especially attractive in patients with associated proximal humeral deformity that would otherwise require an associated osteotomy or custom stem. They may also be useful in patients suffering with rheumatoid arthritis who also require an elbow arthroplasty. The stem of the humeral component of the elbow prosthesis may interfere with insertion of the shoulder component or leave a very narrow segment between the two stems, which may increase the risk of a periprosthetic fracture. However, resurfacing also has some disadvantages. It may be difficult to achieve adequate stability of the prosthesis if the local bone stock is compromised. In addition, the implantation of a glenoid component is more difficult, as the exposure is limited by preservation of the humeral head. Soft-tissue balance may also be difficult to achieve, as the size and position of humeral head cannot be altered much. Finally, it is difficult to assess the radiographic bone-implant interface.

The technical challenge of glenoid access to perform a glenoid replacement in association with a resurfacing has led to the development of short stem (or metaphyseal fit) prostheses. These maintain the advantage of essentially removing the effect of variable humeral axis on the position of the humeral head. This removes the need for eccentric heads and hence reduces the number of 'moving parts' and potential points of failure. As the diameter of head and thickness of head have a relatively stable relationship it minimises the need for a large inventory. If done properly it also deals with off-set and inclination. Added to that the improvement in uncemented technology has meant that a secure and long lasting hold between the implant and bone is achievable without the use of cement. This philosophy has now to have appeared to have borne fruit, in that recent publications have been able to demonstrate consistently good function and radiological outcome of this type of implant. Uschok et al. [19] compared the clinical and radiological outcome of 20 patients with a stemless shoulder prosthesis and 20 patients with a standard humeral stem. Clinical outcome showed no significant difference at a minimum of 2 and 5 year follow up. There was, however, a significant difference in the radiographic analysis of the zone adjacent to the humeral calcar, with a lower bone mineral density in the stem group compared to the stemless. There are also statistically more radiolucent lines around the stemmed implant. Hence a short stem anatomic with its ability to uncouple the humeral head anatomy from the humeral shaft anatomy combined with the theoretical advantage of bone preservation may be the future stem of choice for anatomic replacement [19].

With regard to stemless reverse humeral components, these are currently under design, and early results are promising. The medium term results are comparible to stemmed designs [20]. This is in keeping with the good results of this type of stem utilised in an anatomic shoulder replacement [21]. This may be surprising when one considers the different forces on the humeral stem in anatomic and reverse shoulder replacement.

Clinical Pearl

Stemless implants have a number of theoretical advantages. If the initial cut or removal of the humeral head is accurate, at a stroke this can address offset and inclination. This combined with the new bony ingrowth technology can offer a stable platform.

References

1. Neer CS, Watson KC, Stanton FJ. Recent experience in total shoulder replacement. J Bone Joint Surg [Am]. 1982;64(3):319–37.
2. Torchia ME, Cofield RH, Settergren CR. Total shoulder arthroplasty with the neer prosthesis: long term results. J Shoulder Elb Surg. 1997;6(6):495–505.
3. Trail IA, Nuttall D. The results of shoulder arthroplasty in patients with rheumatoid arthritis. J Bone Joint Surg (Br). 2002;84:1121–4.
4. Haines JF, Trail IA, Nuttall D, Birch A, Barrow A. Results of arthroplasty in osteoarthritis of the shoulder. J Bone Joint Surg (Br). 2006;88:496–501.
5. Walch G, Boileau P. Prosthetic adaptability: a new concept for shoulder arthroplasty. J Shoulder Elb Surg. 1999;8(5):443–51.
6. Hertel R, Knothe U, Ballmer FT. Geometry of the proximal humerus and implications for prosthetic design. J Shoulder Elb Surg. 2002;11(4):331–8.
7. Harryman DT, Sidles JA, Harris SL, Lippitt SB, Matsen FA. The effect of articular conformity and the size of the humeral head component on laxity and motion after glenohumeral arthroplasty. J Bone Joint Surg [Am]. 1995;77(4):555–63.
8. Jobe CM, Iannotti JP. Limits imposed on glenohumeral motion by joint geometry. J Shoulder Elb Surg. 1995;4(4):281–5.

9. Weber-Spickschen TS, Alfke D, Agneskirchner JD. The use of a modular system to convert an anatomical total shoulder arthroplasty to a reverse shoulder arthroplasty. Bone Joint J. 2015;97-B: 1662–7.
10. Nuttall D, Haines JF, Trail IA. The effect of the offset humeral head on the micromovement of pegged glenoid components; a comparative study using radiostereometric analysis. J Bone Joint Surg (Br). 2009;91(6):757–61.
11. Teeter MG, Carroll MJ, Walch G, Athwal GS. Tribocorrosion in shoulder arthroplasty humeral component retrievals. J Shoulder Elb Surg. 2016;25:311–5.
12. Throckmorton TW, Zarkadas PC, Sperling JW, Cofield RH. Radiographic stability of ingrowth humeral stems in total shoulder arthroplasty. Clin Orthop Relat Res. 2010;468:2122–8.
13. Raiss P, Bradley Edwards T, Deutsch A, Shah A, Bruckner T, Loew M, Boileau P, Walch G. Radiographic changes around humeral components in shoulder arthroplasty. J Bone Joint Surg Am. 2014;96(7):e54.
14. Schnetzke M, Coda S, Raiss P, Walch G, Loew M. Radiologic bone adaptations on a cementless short-stem shoulder prosthesis. J Shoulder Elb Surg. 2016;25:650–7.
15. Razfar N, Reeves JM, Langohr DG, Willing R, Athwal GS, Johnson JA. Comparison of proximal humeral bone stresses between stemless, short stem, and standard stem length: a finite element analysis. J Shoulder Elb Surg. 2016;25:1076–83.
16. Lädermann A, Denard PJ, Boileau P, Farron A, Deransart P, Terrier A, Ston J, Walch G. Effect of humeral stem design on humeral position and range of motion in reverse shoulder arthroplasty. Inter Orthop (SICOT). 2015;39:2205–13.
17. Berhouet J, Kontaxis A, Gulotta LW, Craig E, Warren R, Dines J, Dines D. Effects of the humeral tray component positioning for onlay reverse shoulder arthroplasty design: a biomechanical analysis. J Shoulder Elb Surg. 2015;24:569–77.
18. Nuttall D, Birch A, Haines JF, Trail IA. Radiostereographic analysis of a shoulder surface replacement: does hydroxyapatite have a place? Bone Joint J. 2014;96-B(8):1077–81.
19. Uschok S, Magosch P, Moe M, Lichtenberg S, Habermeyer P. Is the stemless humeral head replacement clinically and radiographically a secure equivalent to standard stem humeral head replacement in the long-term follow up? A prospective randomized trial. J Shoulder Elb Surg. 2017;26:225–32.
20. Ballas R, Béguin L. Results of a stemless reverse shoulder prosthesis at more than 58 months mean without loosening. J Shoulder Elb Surg. 2013;22(9):e1–6.
21. Huguet D, DeClercq G, Rio B, Teissier J, Zipoli B. Results of a new stemless shoulder prosthesis: radiologic proof of maintained fixation and stability after a minimum of three years' follow-up. J Shoulder Elb Surg. 2010;19(6):847–52.

Results of Anatomical Shoulder Arthroplasty

15

Clemens Abel and Frank Gohlke

Introduction

The modern era of shoulder replacement began with the first generation of anatomical shoulder arthroplasty as pioneered by Charles Neer in 1953 [59] firstly as fracture hemiarthroplasty and later [60] as total joint replacement for glenohumeral osteoarthritis. His simple monobloc design of a stemmed humeral component combined with a cemented polyethylene resurfacing of the glenoid has been modified over the course of 60 years. Excellent pain relief and gain of active elevation of 44° on average was confirmed by Cofield [15] who evaluated the results of 73 patients with mixed aetiology after a mid-term follow-up of 2–6.5 years. Although he noted that "postoperatively there was little or no pain even with vigorous activities in most shoulders" there was a revision rate of 6.8%, glenoid loosening in 11% and "some radiolucency" in 80% of the cases. In 1997 Torchia et al. published the long-term results of this series and described 44% glenoid loosening. They stated that "glenoid loosening was associated with pain" which seemingly did not influence the survival rate of 87% after 15 years. When compared to recently published data the rate of aseptic glenoid loosening has persisting as the "weak link" [7].

C. Abel, M.D. · F. Gohlke, M.D. (✉)
KLinik für Schulterchirurgie,
Rhön Kliniken, Campus Bad Neusrtadt,
Bad Neustadt an der Saale, Germany
e-mail: frank.gohlke@schulterchirurgie-bad-neustadt.de

The next step of development towards better anatomical reconstruction was the introduction of two piece modularity of the humeral component using variable head sizes [58]. This second generation of humeral components was later combined with a metal-backed glenoid resurfacing. Unfortunately, true anatomic fit was not always possible and good clinical results sometimes difficult to achieve.

In 1995 and 1997 Boileau and Walch showed that inclination, retroversion, diameter and thickness of the articular surface vary widely [4, 5]. They proposed eccentric modular heads and initiated the third generation of humeral implants. Although the new design restored the posterior and medial offset in relation to the shaft axis, studies have never proven superior clinical results [87].

Resurfacing of the humeral head was introduced by Zippel in Germany in 1976. Subsequently Jonsson, Kelly and later Copeland popularized its use in the 1990s. The hydroxyapatite coated Mark 3 implant aimed at cementless metaphyseal fixation and bone ingrowth. The preservation of bone stock was believed to be a significant advantage for any subsequent revision surgery.

After poor results with metal-backed glenoid components, resurfacing was often used as a hemiarthroplasty. Unfortunately, bone loss caused by glenoid erosion and humeral stress shielding were observed [94]. Reports of

I. A. Trail et al. (eds.), *Textbook of Shoulder Surgery*, https://doi.org/10.1007/978-3-319-70099-1_15

unexpectedly high failure rates related to technical errors and overstuffing [54, 93] led to newer designs with cementless metaphyseal fixation of a tray combined with modular humeral heads. Since 2004 a great variety of these stemless or short-stemmed implants have been developed. However, it was not the longevity of stemless anatomical implants but the ease of component removal during revisions turned out to be their strongest selling point.

The growing clinical use of Grammont-type reverse shoulder arthroplasty (RSA) in Europe in the mid-90s improved the results of patients with irreparable massive rotator cuff tears, the so called "limited goals" group. Within the following decade different aetiologies [42] were added to the spectrum of reverse arthroplasty. Gross instability, fracture sequelae and severe glenoid deformity currently show better results when treated with RSA than with anatomical joint replacement. This leads to a decreasing use of the anatomic design but on the other hand to improved success rates by proper patient selection.

Today's Main Issues

Still many questions remain unanswered due to a lack of comprehensive clinical studies with comparable cohorts regarding aetiology, sufficient follow-up and sufficient numbers of cases for each new design.

While improvements have been made on the humeral component side, the glenoid fixation still seems to be the most important limiting factor for implant survival in the mid- to long-term. Initial total shoulder arthroplasties designed by Neer followed the concept of Charnley's low friction arthroplasty used a polyethylene glenoid component with a keel that was cemented into the bone. Although considerable thought has been spent on size and form of the polyethylene articular surface and various types of pegs and keels have been tried, it does not seem to have influenced the long-term survival and revision rate. Moreover most of the metal-backed glenoid components revealed unacceptably high failure rates even at mid-term follow-up [62].

Gregory et al. [32] stated "TSA has a relatively short survival rate as compared to knee and hip replacement, of on average 10 years". Therefore the most important question is how to improve glenoid component survival rates, thereby moving towards the longevity of hip and knee replacements.

> **Clinical Pearl**
> Currently the biggest hurdle in anatomic total shoulder arthroplasty is to improve glenoid component survival rates, thereby moving towards the longevity of hip and knee replacements.

How to Get Reliable Data: From Original Studies, Reviews or Registries?

Clinical results deteriorate between mid- and long-term follow-up [73] due to aseptic loosening particularly of the glenoid component. The ideal investigation into joint replacement would be a long-term study involving a large number of centres and surgeons contributing to a registry with compulsory participation. The drop out of patients would be controlled by independent project managers. Aetiology should be listed separately, patient related co-factors identified, the functional outcome documented and all complications reported. Ideally the influence of commercial interests on data analysis should be minimized. This ideal type of study unfortunately does not exist (Fig. 15.1).

In the field of shoulder arthroplasty prospective randomized studies with a control group are extremely rare. Most of the data derives from retrospective studies with an evidence level of 3–4. Therefore most review articles rely on data provided by mid to long-term retrospective clinical outcome studies and national joint registries. Even long-term studies can provide outcome measures with bias [49]. The survival rates reported in clini-

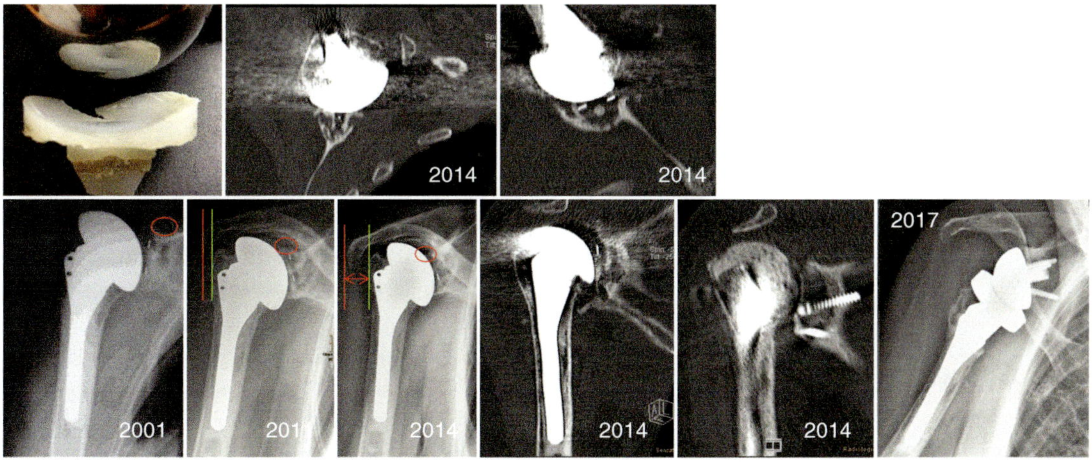

Fig. 15.1 Anatomical stemmed total shoulder arthroplasty (modular Aequalis stem and flat back cemented glenoid) for osteoarthritis: Aseptic loosening at least since 2011, which required a 2-stage revision using iliac crest autograft 13 years after primary implantation. Aseptic loosening caused over several years a "floating" glenoid with advanced bone loss 5°. Note the progressive amount of medialization of the glenoid and bone loss in the CT scan

cal follow-up studies depend on the decision to perform revision surgery. This may reflect the surgeon's motivation, level of experience and available resources and not necessarily the performance of the implant or complaints of the patient or indeed the patients fitness for surgery.

National joint registries mostly deliver survival rates with the endpoint "death" or "revision" rather than functional deterioration or radiological signs of loosening. Radiolucency lines (RLL) in standard radiographs are often underestimated and detection varies from one observer to the other. Yian et al. [99] have demonstrated that 40% of RLL on CT-scans were not diagnosed in plain radiographs. Moreover, in some national registries many clinical outcome measures are not provided, such as complication rate, active range of motion, muscle strength or pain relief. Shoulder specific outcome measures like the Constant score are rarely provided. On the positive side national joint registries are not influenced by developers' interests and represent the performance of an implant in the hands of multiple surgeons.

National shoulder arthroplasty registries have been running in Finland (since 1980), Norway (1994), Sweden (1999), Denmark (2004), New Zealand (2000), Australia (2004) [1], UK (2012). Some of them are government funded, some by a levy on orthopaedic implants. Reporting is voluntary except for Denmark and Finland where it is mandatory. Reporting rates in these countries are mostly higher than 90% of hospitals. Implant survival is mainly used as a primary outcome measure, with revision including partial exchange of the components as an indicator. Revision has to be seen as a surrogate endpoint where factors such as the patient's general condition, skill and experience of the surgeon, the implant's modularity and waiting lists will influence all revision rates.

Nevertheless, the Danish registry has confirmed high revision rates for resurfacing arthroplasty [85] and the Australian [1] and New Zealand registries showed high failure rates of metal backed glenoid components and identified two designs in particular with problems [14].

Labek et al. [48, 49] analysed the data from several national joint registries and reported a revision rate of 1.39 per 100 observed component years in shoulder replacements, 1.29 in hip replacements, 1.26 in knee replacements and 3.29 in ankle replacements. Hemiarthroplasties interestingly had lower revision rates in the Norwegian and New Zeeland joint registry than TSA. The Norwegian joint registry [25] documented 1531 hemiarthroplasties (as opposed to 69 TSA's) over the course of 12 years and showed a failure rate of 6% after five and 8% after

10 years. The risk of revision for patients older than 70 years was half of that of younger patients. The main reasons for revision were pain or dislocation. Different time periods within the Norwegian joint registry were compared [26]. TSA's improved their respective 5-year survival rate from 75% (1994–1999) to 95% (2006–2012), whereas hemiarthroplasties remained at around 95%.

Outcome Measures

Since the 90s it is generally accepted that anatomical shoulder arthroplasty leads to significant improvement in pain reduction and patient satisfaction. In osteoarthritis with intact rotator cuff good or excellent functional results can be expected. Unfortunately, there is little agreement as to how outcome is measured best in shoulder arthroplasty. Many scoring systems were introduced before appropriate methods to establish their validity were developed. Due to limited resources patient questionnaires have often been used for assessment. Despite the introduction of several validated scales in the 1990s, there is not a single generally accepted score for shoulder arthroplasty. How to compare the quality of shoulder replacements in regards to pain relief, active range of motion, strength and quality of life between different studies, is still a subject of research [69]. The European Shoulder and Elbow Society (SECEC) recommends the Constant and Murley score as the most appropriate and effective tool for outcome assessment [17]. English and German versions as patient questionnaires are available and widely used.

Carter et al. [8] evaluated twenty studies (1576 total shoulder replacements) with outcome measures after a mean follow-up of 3.7 years. On average there was an improvement of the VAS pain score from 7.2 to 1.4. The Constant score improved from 31.7 to 69.8 and ASES score from 34.8 to 82.5 was found. The Simple Shoulder Score revealed a gain from 3.1 to 9.6. The Short-form-36 demonstrated significant improvement only in physical component summary scores. Shoulder specific measures of function consistently showed the greatest degree of improvement with large effect sizes.

Bekerom et al. [83] analysed 18 studies published since 1990 dealing with clinical long-term results of both, TSA and HA. The search included a total of 1958 patients (HA: 316 and TSA: 1642) and 2111 shoulders. The weighted mean improvement in active anteflexion, external rotation and abduction were 33°, 15° and 31° respectively in the HA group and 56°, 21° and 48° in the TSA group. The mean decrease in pain (VAS) scores was 4.2 in the HA group and 5.5 in the TSA group. TSA resulted in less revision surgery, but had a trend to show more complications.

Amongst patient-reported outcome measures (PROMs), which are frequently used instead of objective shoulder-specific scores or as a supplement to registry data, the DASH, the Oxford shoulder score [65] and the Simple shoulder test enjoy popularity. Hsu et al. [40] proposed the Simple Shoulder Test (SST) as a brief, inexpensive patient-reported tool for shoulder arthroplasty outcome assessment. However Matsen et al. [55] recommended using both subjective and objective measures as they cover complementary aspects of shoulder function.

Factors Influencing Clinical Outcome

Patient Related Outcome Factors

Age, Morbidity and Gender

General medical condition and comorbidities are considered to be more important for complication rates than postoperative outcome and implant failure [23]. Previous surgery has to be taken into account especially when it has altered the anatomy and compromising the rotator cuff. The status of the rotator cuff; subscapularis, infraspinatus tendon tear and fatty muscle degeneration (exceeding Goutallier 2°), as well as eccentric glenoid deformity are crucial factors for clinical outcome and early implant failure.

Younger age seems to influence the survival rates of both, stemmed and stemless anatomical TSA.

The 2012 Australian Joint Registry Report showed that younger patients (under 65) and older patients (over 75) had higher revision rates than those in-between [1]. The increased risk in younger patients is mainly due to high activity levels whereas in elderly patients the deteriorating health status with comorbidities tends to have a negative effect on outcome.

This was confirmed by Denard et al. [20] who found a 10 year survivorship of only 62.5% for TSA with cemented polyethylene glenoid components in patients younger than 55 years. Higher activity levels and increased infection rates especially with low grade bacteria like Propioni acnes had a negative influence on outcome. Singh et al. [70] showed that men had a 1.72 fold higher risk of revision after TSA. Apparently BMI and comorbidities did not affect the revision rates significantly. Bekerom et al. [83] described the revision rate as being twice as high for men. Recently Johansson et al. [46] reported a significantly increased infection rate involving Propioni species following the insertion of stemless anatomical implants. These had been predominantly implanted in young male patients.

Aetiology

The indication for anatomical shoulder arthroplasty is mainly primary osteoarthritis and rheumatoid arthritis. Instability arthropathy, humeral head necrosis and post-traumatic deformity are less common and when accompanied by rotator cuff insufficiency are better addressed using reverse TSA. The results in osteoarthritis cases with intact rotator cuff and without severe eccentric wear are predictably good or excellent for the majority of patients.

Recently Sowa et al. [73] compared the Constant scores of patients with different aetiologies. They concluded that avascular necrosis (gain of 34 points), rheumatoid arthritis (gain of 37 points) and posttraumatic osteoarthritis (gain of 29 points) showed inferior results in comparison to primary osteoarthritis (gain of 36 points).

Osteoarthritis

The ideal patient for anatomical total shoulder arthroplasty is aged 60–70 in good medical condition with intact rotator cuff, centred mild glenoid wear without significant retroversion or superior inclination, no static subluxation, good bone quality and muscle function without neurological compromise.For the indication of primary osteoarthritis, more than 90% of patients achieve pain free active elevation of at least 150° and good abduction strength can be expected. A Constant score exceeding 70 points (or more than 80% of the age and gender adapted norm value) is documented in large series for at least 5–10 years postoperatively [8].

Rheumatoid Arthritis

In rheumatoid arthritis secondary rotator cuff insufficiency and consecutive superior and medial migration of the head occurs more often than in osteoarthritis [97]. This leads to loss of function and affects the outcome after shoulder replacement significantly [81]. Nevertheless, even in first generation TSA pain reduction was achieved in 92% of patients, though active range of motion remained unfortunately poor [71]. The impaired general medical condition in RA patients with low bone density, rotator cuff dysfunction and increased risk for wound infection is balanced by lower functional demands and reduced activity levels. Therefore in short- to mid-term patient satisfaction is high with complication rates around 8%. For rheumatoid arthritis TSH is delivering better results than hemiarthroplasty. Especially when the rotator cuff is intact [75, 84]. Similar results can be found in resurfacing arthroplasty where Constant scores of 47 points (age and gender adjusted 71%) in HA and 53.4 (adj. 76%) in TSA have been documented [53] (Fig. 15.2).

The Aequalis multicentre study [31] is one of the largest analysing TSA in rheumatoid patients including 172 patients after a minimum follow-up of 2 years (mean 46 months). The complication- (10%) and revision-rate (7.5%) reflected the

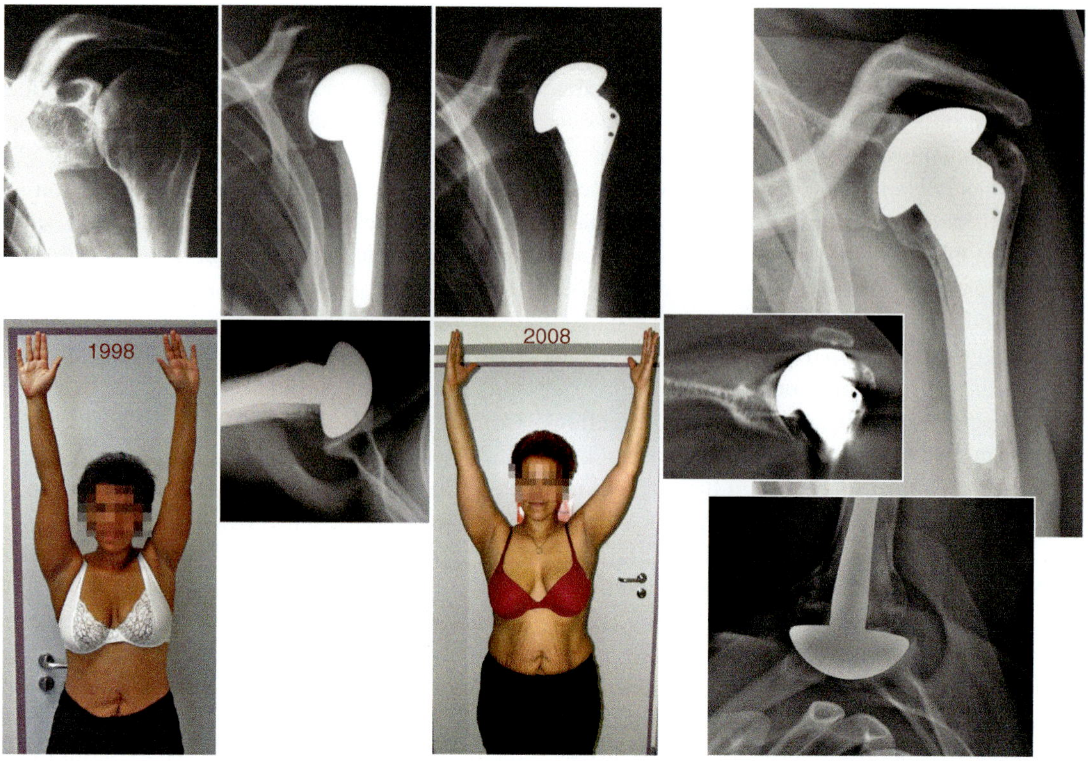

Fig. 15.2 Painful glenoid erosion 19 years after hemiarthroplasty in rheumatoid arthritis

high morbidity with rheumatoid arthritis. With pain relief in 90% of the patients, their adjusted Constant score showed only moderate improvement from 26% to 56%, which is significantly less than in OA cases. Active elevation was improved from 79° to 120° but strength and overhead activity remained poor. 27% of patients could not use their arm above head level, which was correlated to fatty infiltration and atrophy of the rotator cuff in the preoperative CT scans.

Progressive radiolucent lines around the glenoid component, even in the mid-term follow-up, are a common finding in 30–95% of cases [31, 71] and probably related to rotator cuff failure and poor bone quality. Asymptomatic glenoid component loosening, however, was observed only in 5–10% of the cases.

Barlow et al. [2] evaluated the survivorship of 303 consecutive shoulder arthroplasties (108 HA, 195 TSA) with a minimum follow-up of 5 years. The 10-year survival was calculated as 93% for TSA and 88% for hemiarthroplasty. The most common indications for revision were glenoid loosening (5%) and infection (2%) for TSA revision and glenoid wear (7%) for HA revision. 30% of humeral components and 73% of glenoid components showed periprosthetic radiolucency. Although 33% of glenoid components were definitely loose, revision was reported as "uncommon".

Status of the Rotator Cuff (Tear, Atrophy, Fatty Infiltration)

Status of the rotator cuff is along with glenoid deformity the most important preoperative predictor for functional outcome. Before the introduction of reverse shoulder arthroplasty Neer's „limited goals criteria "were used for cuff deficient shoulders. With hemiarthroplasty sufficient pain relief was achieved but active range of motion remained poor, especially when preoperative active elevation was less than 90° [30].

Partial defects and small tears without significant muscular atrophy were shown to deliver good results in TSA with no difference in shoulder outcome scores. Therefore isolated supraspinatus tears were not found to influence the postoperative outcome. Repair did not improve the results [43].

Moderate fatty infiltration or severe degeneration of the infraspinatus both had a negative effect on postoperative outcome scores, as well as subscapularis degeneration, but not as pronounced [22]. Nevertheless rotator cuff deficiency is reported to have a significantly higher risk for revision, 3.7 fold higher than patients with rheumatoid arthritis [70].

In massive rotator cuff tears it was initially recommended to use HA to avoid eccentric loading and early loosening of the glenoid component [96]. Nowadays, however, reverse arthroplasty seems to be the best choice to deliver good functional results.

A rotator cuff tear may occur secondarily after anatomical replacement. 16.8% of secondary rotator cuff insufficiency was shown in mid- to long-term follow-up. Among the factors correlated with secondary rupture was length of follow-up, fatty infiltration of the infraspinatus muscle and superior inclination of the glenoid component [101].

Clinical Pearl
A torn irreparable rotator cuff or the presence of significant muscle atrophy will result in a poor outcome of an anatomic total shoulder replacement.

Glenoid Morphology

Levine et al. [51] demonstrated that hemiarthroplasty in cases with eccentric glenoid wear frequently leads to unsatisfactory results. Preoperative posterior head subluxation was identified as a negative predictor for early glenoid failure in TSA [89] and poor functional outcome [43].

In biconcave posterior glenoid wear high revision rates and glenoid loosening were demonstrated which correlated to depth of erosion, humeral head subluxation, wear ratio and retroversion [89, 90]. This was confirmed by Ho et al. [38] who described an increased risk of osteolysis around the glenoid component's centre peg occurring in the presence of retroversion of more than 15° [38]. After a mid-term follow-up of 49 months Hussey et al. [41] described a more than twofold increase of glenoid component loosening in patients with eccentric wear pattern compared to those with concentric wear. Hill and Norris [37] reported disappointing long-term results with high failure rates when combining TSA with autograft reconstruction of the glenoid. Augmented glenoid components and bone grafting under metal-backed glenoid components have also shown high failure rates in TSA; static posterior displacement was not always corrected [66, 76]. Before the introduction of RSA many surgeons preferred HA instead of TSA where eccentric glenoid reaming was leading to early failure by eccentric loading [39]. TSA was only considered when after corrective reaming more than 80% of seating could be achieved. The limits of excessive reaming (less than 15° of correction in posterior bone loss) without compromising the remaining bone stock were described by Clavert et al. [12] and recently confirmed by Chen et al. [10] in a 3D reconstruction study.

How far superior tilt of the glenoid influences postoperative outcome or loosening has not been shown in clinical studies. Favard et al. [24] recently outlined the limits of anatomical implants and the principles of reconstruction in cases with superior inclination of more than 10°.

Outcome Factors Related to Complications and Surgical Technique

Periprosthetic chronic infections, nerve injuries, instability and stiffness have a clear impact on the clinical outcome of shoulder arthroplasty. Fracture patients were shown to have a higher risk of complications and a mortality rate of 1.3% [23].

Cumulative probability of a complication after 5 years was 12%, in a series from 1990–2000. The main complication was rotator cuff tear followed by instability and intraoperative fracture. This corresponds to complication rates reported as 5–10% in mixed aetiology [3, 16].

Unexplained pain after shoulder replacement is always suspicious for occult nerve lesions and neuropathy or low grade infections [57].

Surgeon-Related Outcome Factors

The rate of technical errors was estimated to be 23% in a failure analysis of revised implants by Hasan et al. [34]. Therefore the selection of the proper component size, soft tissue balancing, glenoid preparation and the technique of subscapularis detachment are certainly influential for postoperative performance and longevity of the implant. Analysis of the French multicentre data identified glenoid preparation with removal of the subchondral cortical sclerosis and underlying cancellous bone as risk factors for early glenoid loosening [78, 89, 90]. Proper pre-operative planning may therefore reduce malpositioning and poor implant selection, especially for low volume surgeons. CT scans are helpful in analysing glenoid morphology, humeral head subluxation and fatty infiltration of the rotator cuff muscles. Computer based 3-D planning, virtual implantation and targeting devices have been recently developed. With these, prediction of implant positioning, size of the implants, glenoid version as well as lateral offset when adding bone graft can be achieved.

In a prospective study a significant benefit of patient-specific targeting devices for placement of glenoid components in retroversion of more than 20° was demonstrated [44]. However, the impact on loosening rates or functional outcome remains unclear.

Hammond et al. [33] examined the effect of high and low operative volumes on the outcome of shoulder arthroplasty. High-volume surgeons had half the risk for complications of low-volume surgeons and were three times more likely to get their patients discharged after less than six days. Jain et al. [45] reported similar results showing that complication rates are lower in high volume-surgeons.

Clark et al. [13] showed that high volume surgeons had shorter operative times than low volume surgeons. The risk for hospital readmission increased with longer operative times.

Design-Related Outcome Factors

Humeral Component: Short Versus Standard Stem, "Stemless" Metaphyseal Fixation, Resurfacing

Over decades the use of cemented versus cementless diaphyseal stem fixation has remained controversial. Higher rates of intraoperative complications in cementless press-fit stems and lower loosening rates in cemented fixation were the reasons for the majority of European surgeons preferring cementation, especially in patients with reduced or poor bone quality. The Mayo Clinic showed increased likelihood of humeral component failure in uncemented shafts with 2.7 times less revision after cementation. However, it was argued that the surgeon would be more reluctant to remove a cemented humeral component [11]. The last Mayo registry review of Werthel et al. [95] found survival at 20 years of 98% for cemented stems and 92.4% for uncemented. The 2012 Australian Joint Registry Report showed significantly higher revision rates in uncemented stems.

In Europe this discussion has been bypassed by the trend to use "stemless" implants since their introduction in 2004. Advantages have been summarized as decreased surgical time, less blood loss, bone preservation, and a lower risk of periprosthetic fractures [18]. Early results are promising with clinical and radiological outcomes comparable to stemmed TSA [35]. Long-term results especially survivorship data are only available for few designs [18, 36].

The longest follow-up for resurfacing arthroplasty was reported by authors who have been involved in the development of the implant [52]. They achieved excellent results with an age/gender-related Constant score of 93.7% in osteoarthritis for TSA and 73.5% for hemiarthroplasty. Only 32.7% of humeral implants showed radiolucency, but 64.4% of the metal backed glenoid components.

Revision was required only in 7.7%. Unfortunately, those excellent results were not confirmed by other authors [50] or national registries [85].

Hemi Versus Total

In the past hemiarthroplasty was preferred when either the glenoid articular surface was intact (e.g. early stage of avascular osteonecrosis of the humeral head) or early glenoid loosening could be expected; in very young and active patients, glenoid dysplasia, rotator cuff insufficiency or rheumatoid arthritis. Today RSA is preferentially used for many indications. Due to this mixed aetiology (with exception of fractures) comparison of clinical results for hemiarthroplasty to those of TSA is often difficult (Fig. 15.3).

In 2012 Levine et al. [51] evaluated the long-term results (mean 17 years) of hemiarthroplasty and noticed that only in 75% of patients was pain relief achieved, function

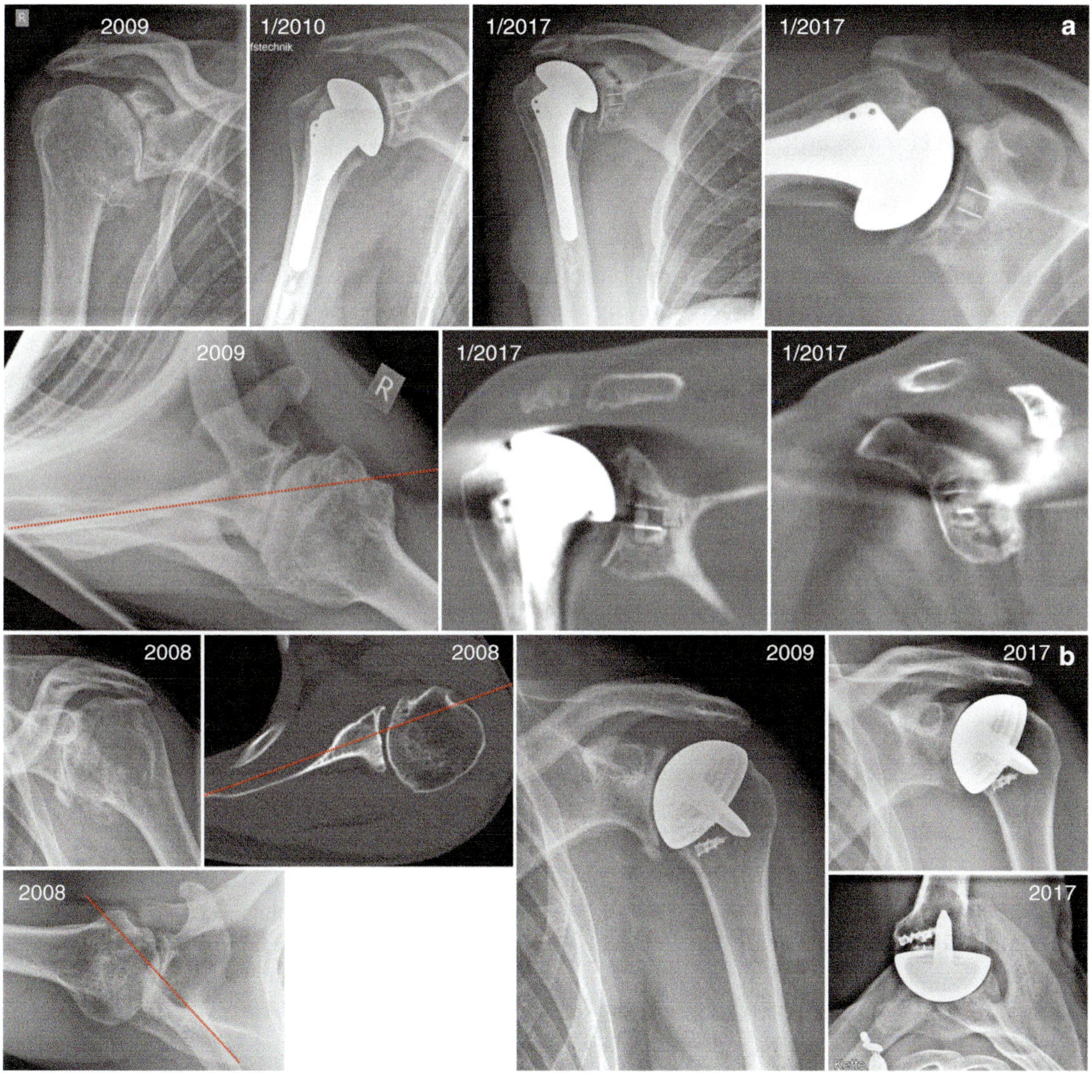

Fig. 15.3 (**a**) Primary TSA at the age of 58 years (manual worker, 190 cm, 91 kg). 7 years after anatomical TSA progressive RLL, increasing moderate pain VAS 3-4, especially after overhead activity and loss of strength from 11.5 kg at 2 years after surgery to 5.6 kg at latest follow-up (**b**) Resurfacing in 40yo- male athletic patient, (122 kg, 188 cm, leisure activity weight lifting), moderate B2 glenoid deformity, 19°Retroversion, 90% posterior subluxation. First 2 years pain VAS 4. 8 years postoperatively no pain, still active with sports, Full ROM. Note the remodelling of the glenoid as result of erosion

deteriorated over time and that the majority were not satisfied with their outcome. Patients with concentric glenoid wear and primary osteoarthritis had better outcomes than those with eccentric glenoid wear and secondary osteoarthritis.

Radnay et al. [63] reviewed 23 studies with a total of 1952 patients and mean follow-up of 43.4 months and concluded that TSA delivers greater pain relief and better active range of motion than HA. The revision rate of TSA (6.5%) was lower than in HA (10.2%). Bekerom et al. [83] reviewed only studies with a follow-up of more than 7 years in a meta-analysis. A higher revision rate of 13% for hemiarthroplasty compared to 7% for TSA was found. However the complication rate was 12% for TSA and 8% in HA. The improvement in range of motion and pain relief were both better in TSA.

The possibility of converting hemiarthroplasty to TSA in case of glenoid erosion unfortunately does not deliver the same results as primary TSA [9].

Whether in young patients the recently introduced pyrocarbon humeral head component provides better results and less symptomatic glenoid erosion, is so far unknown. Recently, the long-term results (mean follow-up 10 years, range 5–16 years) of 176 patients with "ream and run" technique were published. 16% had a subsequent procedure, and 30 patients (17%) had more than 5 years of follow-up. The mean value of the Simple Shoulder Test (SST) was 10 out of 12 points and supported the view that this functional improvement is stable over time [72].

Clinical Pearl
Several studies have now shown that the results of total shoulder arthroplasty are superior to hemi arthroplasty.

Glenoid Design

Cemented Glenoid Component: Keeled Versus Pegged

In a retrospective study Fox et al. [27] evaluated the survival of 1337 different glenoid components. 972 cemented polyethylene (=PE) glenoid components were investigated. The Kaplan-Meier analysis with revision as endpoint showed 95% survival rate after 10 years and 92% after 15 years. The best long-term survival rates for 5, 10 and 15 years were found in 497 components of the Cofield 2 all-poly keeled type with 99%, 94%, and 89% respectively.

In 2013 [28] they re-evaluated 302 all-poly glenoid components of this type with a mean follow-up of 8.6 years and described a concerning high rate (34%) of loosening and a significant increase of radiolucency around the keel after 5 years. The authors stated that "the high frequency of late radiographic changes dictates the need for innovation."

Walch et al. [91] reported on 333 TSA using a pegged cemented all polyethylene glenoid component. Survivorship without revision was 99.7% at 5 years, 98.3% at 10 years. However, radiologic loosening was seen in 0.3% at 5 years and in 48.5% at 10 years. Young et al. [100] presented a retrospective study of 226 TSA using a keeled flat back cemented all-poly glenoid component. Survivorship of the glenoid component was 99.1% at 5 years, 94.5% at 10 years and 79.4% at 15 years. No radiologic loosening was observed in 99.1% at 5 years and 94.5% at 10 years, but only in 33.6% at 15 years. The longest mean follow-up of 15 years in selected patients after TSA was published by [64]. Radiolucency was seen in 74% of all patients. This did not correlate significantly with the clinical results. The survival rate with revision as endpoint was 70% after 20 years. In our experience with the same implant most patients with signs of loosening including altered component position or radiolucency in all zones of the axial X-ray show functional deterioration (especially strength) and at least little to moderate pain. Nuttall et al. [61] using Radio Stereographic Analysis were able to show over a 2 year period migration of a keeled design was significantly greater than that in a pegged design.

As a fact after 10 years the majority of cemented glenoid components are loose, although this does not always have a detrimental effect on the clinical result. Many shoulder surgeons agree that revision as an endpoint in survival analysis has limited importance. There are additional factors including the surgeon's and patient's reluctance to take on the unpleasant task of complex revision surgery with glenoid bone loss and deteriorating general health status which is not reflected in any statistical analysis.

Biomechanical and clinical studies indicate that a curved glenoid component with a radial mismatch of 4-7 mm performs best in regard to longevity. As the glenohumeral joint allows for rotation but also translation, a mismatch where the curvature of the glenoid is slightly larger than the head avoids excessive forces on the edges of the glenoid, thereby decreasing stress between implant and bone. Version has to be correct, the implant fully seated, good cementing technique implemented and the glenoid carefully reamed to have sufficient cortical supporting bone in place [29, 77, 88, 92].

It has been shown that bone impaction into the keel slot and using a smaller amount of cement has the potential to reduce radiolucent lines [29, 78]. In contrast to previous publications, recently published results by Kilian et al. [47] could not show superiority of either keeled or pegged glenoid components.

All-poly ethylene glenoid components with central peg and fins ("anchor peg") have been popularized especially in the USA. Even without evidence for bone ingrowth into the polyethylene surface, excellent short- to mid-term results are reported [56, 98]. The high rate (up to 55%) of osteolysis around the cementless central peg [19, 38, 98] and early migration under radiostereometric analysis [61] is a cause for concern.

Metal-Backed Glenoid Component

Since the first reports of aseptic glenoid loosening it has been proposed that metal-backed glenoid components may help to address the problem by providing better fixation onto bone. Unfortunately, even with improved new designs achieving solid fixation and bone ingrowth, the complication rates remain high. This is attributed to polyethylene wear and consecutive osteolysis [7]. Corresponding biomechanical studies show higher contact stress in more rigidly fixed metal-backed than for all-polyethylene components, which leads to accelerated wear of the polyethylene liner [79].

Taunton et al. [80] described unacceptably high failure rates of the Mayo metal-backed glenoid design. The revision free survival rate dropped between the 5 and 10 years of follow-up from 80% to 52%.

Fox et al. [27] showed a survival rate of only 67% at 15 years for the Neer metal-backed glenoid component compared to 89% for the improved "Cofield-1 design". Loosening was attributed to increased polyethylene wear and subsequent osteolysis. Even the old cemented all-poly Neer glenoid component performed significantly better. Accordingly, data from the New Zealand joint registry revealed a 4.4 times higher revision rate for uncemented glenoid components at short-term follow up of 3.5 years [14].

Boileau et al. [6] reported a revision rate of 46% at 12-year follow-up using the Aequalis metal-backed glenoid component, which has now been withdrawn from the market. This design was associated with significant polyethylene wear and osteolysis which was attributed to inappropriate thickness and insufficient fixation of the polyethylene insert. Overtensioning of the soft tissues by lateralization of the centre of rotation and increased thickness of the glenoid component is felt to cause an increased compression load. Insufficient correction of retroversion or persisting subluxation can lead to eccentric loading followed by excessive polyethylene wear at the glenoid rim.

Papadonikolakis and Matsen [62] analysed the literature and found a significantly higher revision rate for metal-backed glenoid designs in comparison to cemented all-poly components.

Vuillermin et al. [86] reported "catastrophic failure" of the low-profile, cage screw fixed baseplate design with a 29% revision rate after a mean follow-up of 5.5 years. Analysis of the mode of failure of implants identified by robust registries is essential for the development of new prostheses and the pursuit of prosthesis longevity". The authors propose "that any prosthesis withdrawal should be accompanied by appropriate publications to prevent future component design errors".

Clinical Results and Failure Rate after Long-Term Follow-Up

Long-term studies are likely to be the product of interested and expert surgeons in high volume centres. They will not reflect on the performance of the average surgeon undertaking a lower volume of shoulder arthroplasty. Moreover, the first users of an implant are often involved in its development in close cooperation with the manufacturer, which may bias the reported results and complication rate. It was shown that reports by developers of implants exhibited substantially lower revision rates than national joint registry data [48, 49]. Reviews often do not take into consideration that the patients analysed in local series (listed in Table 15.1) are evaluated repeatedly regarding different aspects of their aetiology, morbidity and clinical and radiological outcome.

One of the largest early series with remarkably excellent results was published by Deshmukh et al. [21] who reported on 320 total shoulder arthroplasties using the Neer type standard design with 69% of the patients suffering from rheumatoid arthritis and only 22% from osteoarthritis. Kaplan-Meier survivorship showed 98% at 5 years, 93% at 10 years, 88% at 15 years and 85% at 20 years.

Mayo Experience

The Total Joint Registry of the Mayo Clinic in Rochester was started in 1969 based on the experience of R. Cofield with the Neer design which was modified several times. This local registry has contributed numerous high-quality studies to almost all aspects of anatomical shoulder arthroplasty for more than 40 years. The majority of patients are routinely followed up or at least interviewed using a telephone questionnaire [82]. In 2004 Sperling et al. reported a minimum 15-year follow-up of Neer hemiarthroplasty and TSA in patients younger than 50 years. Radiographs were available for 53 hemiarthroplasties and 25 total shoulder arthroplasties with a minimum 10-year follow-up. Glenoid periprosthetic lucency was present in 19 of 25 total shoulder arthroplasties (76%). The calculated survival rate for total shoulder arthroplasty was 97% at 10 years and 84% at 20 years (Fig. 15.4).

Cil et al. [11] reported on 1584 anatomical shoulder arthroplasties with three different stem designs. Survival of the humeral component without revision or removal was 94.8% after 5 years, 92% after 10 years, 86.7% after 15 years and 82.8% after 20 years. Young age, male gender, replacement due to post-traumatic arthritis, uncemented stems and metal-backed glenoid components increased the likelihood of implant failure.

Singh et al. [70] evaluated a cohort of 1431 humeral head replacements. The implant survival rate was 93.6% after 5 years, 90% after 10 years and 85% after 20 years. Older age and a low BMI were positive predictors for a low risk of revision (Figs. 15.5 and 15.6).

Table 15.1 Long-term results of anatomical shoulder arthroplasty (Hemi and total)

Author (year)	Mean FU (years)	Shoulders/ patients	Type: Hemi/Total	Survival rate	Clinical outcome
Trail and Nuttall [81]	5.1	105, rheumatoid arthritis	65HA/40TSA	8 years: 92%	Constant score Pre 12.3 to Post 33.7
Deshmuk et al. [21]	14	320/367	TSA Neer II(287), various	5y. 98%, 10y. 93%, 15y. 88%, 20y. 85%	Elevation +23°, Ext rot +13°, Pain -4
Sperling et al. (Mayo) [74], Schoch et al. (Mayo) [68]	16.8 21	114 younger 50y 114	78HA/36TSA Neer 78HA/36TSA Neer	HA: 10y. 82%, 20y.75% TSA: 10y.97% 20y. 84% HA 20y. 75,6% TSA 20y. 83.2%	Abduction: HA +36°, TSA +39° Ext rot: HA +19°, TSA +26° Pain HA -2.2 TSA -2.5
Rosenberg et al. [67]	1.:11 2./3.:4	1.90 2.103 3.34	TSA uncemented, metal backed glenoid: 1. Bio Modular 2. Nottingham TSR 3.Nottingham TSR HA	1. 4y. 80.9%, 8y 75.6%, 11y 71.7% 2. 4y. 85.1%, 8y 81.8% 3. 4y. 93.1%	Not reported
Young et al. [100]	10.2	333/295	TSA Aequalis Flat back all-poly glenoid, cemented	5y. 99.1%, 10y. 94.5% 15y. 79.4%	Adjusted Constant score: Pre-OP 36.2% to Post-OP 80%
Walch et al. [91]	7.4	263/247	TSA Aequalis Curved back all-poly glenoid, cemented	5y. 99.7%, 10y 98.3%	Adjusted Constant score: Pre 42.7% Post 97.3%
Denard et al. [20]	9.6	52/49 younger 55y	TSA Aequalis	5y. 98%, 10y. 62.5%	Adjusted Constant score: Pre 37.0% Post 73.4%
Raiss et al. [64]	15	63/58	TSA Aequalis	5y. 98%, 10y. 89%, 15y. 73% 20y. 70%	Adjusted Constant score: Pre 31% post 64%
Barlow et al. [2]	13.8	303	108 HA, 195 TSA Rheumatoid arthritis	HA: 5y.89.2%, 10y. 87.9% TSA. 5y.96%, 10y. 92.9%	Pain: HA -2.4, TSA-2.8 Elevation : HA +32°, TSA +35° Ext rot : HA +16°, TSA +17°
Boileau et al. [6]	8.5	165	TSA Aequalis: Metal-backed glenoid, cementless	8.5 years 63%, 12y. 46%	Adjusted Constant score : Pre-OP 38% Post-OP 94%
Vuillermin et al. [86]	5.5	45	TSA Arthrex, cementless metal-backed glenoid	5.5 years 71%	Not reported
Hawi et al. [36]	9	49	32 HA and 17 TSA Arthrex Eclipse (only stem, glenoid failure excluded)	9y. 100%	Adjusted Constant score: Pre-OP 52% Post-OP 79%

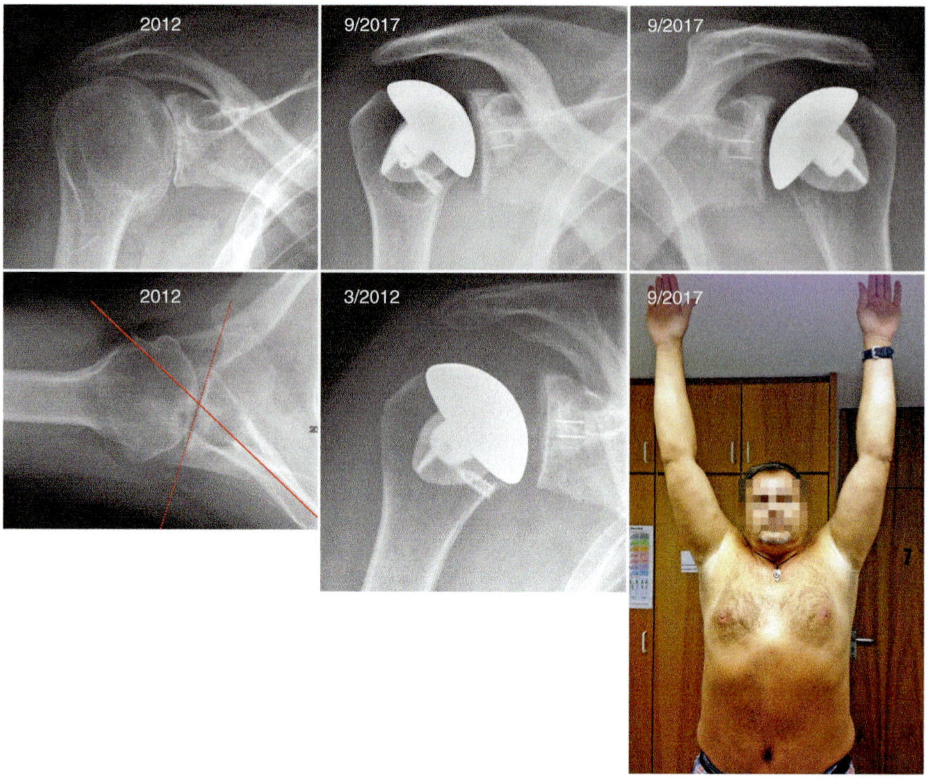

Fig. 15.4 Stemless total shoulder arthroplasty and keeled glenoid component with varying backside radius of curvature

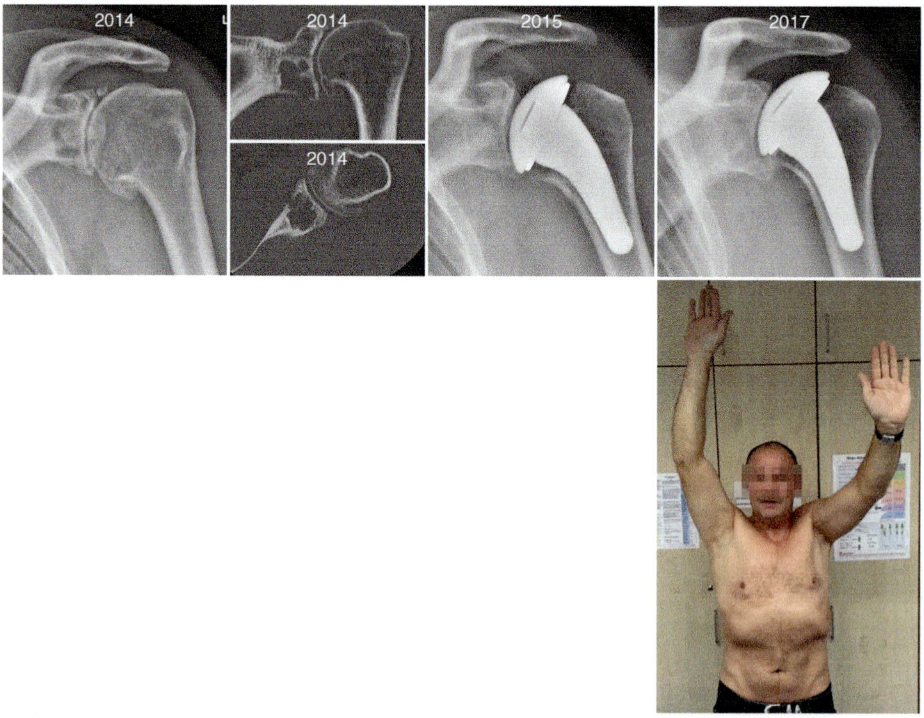

Fig. 15.5 Pyrocarbon hemiarthroplasty in erosive centered osteoarthritis with cystic glenoid bone loss

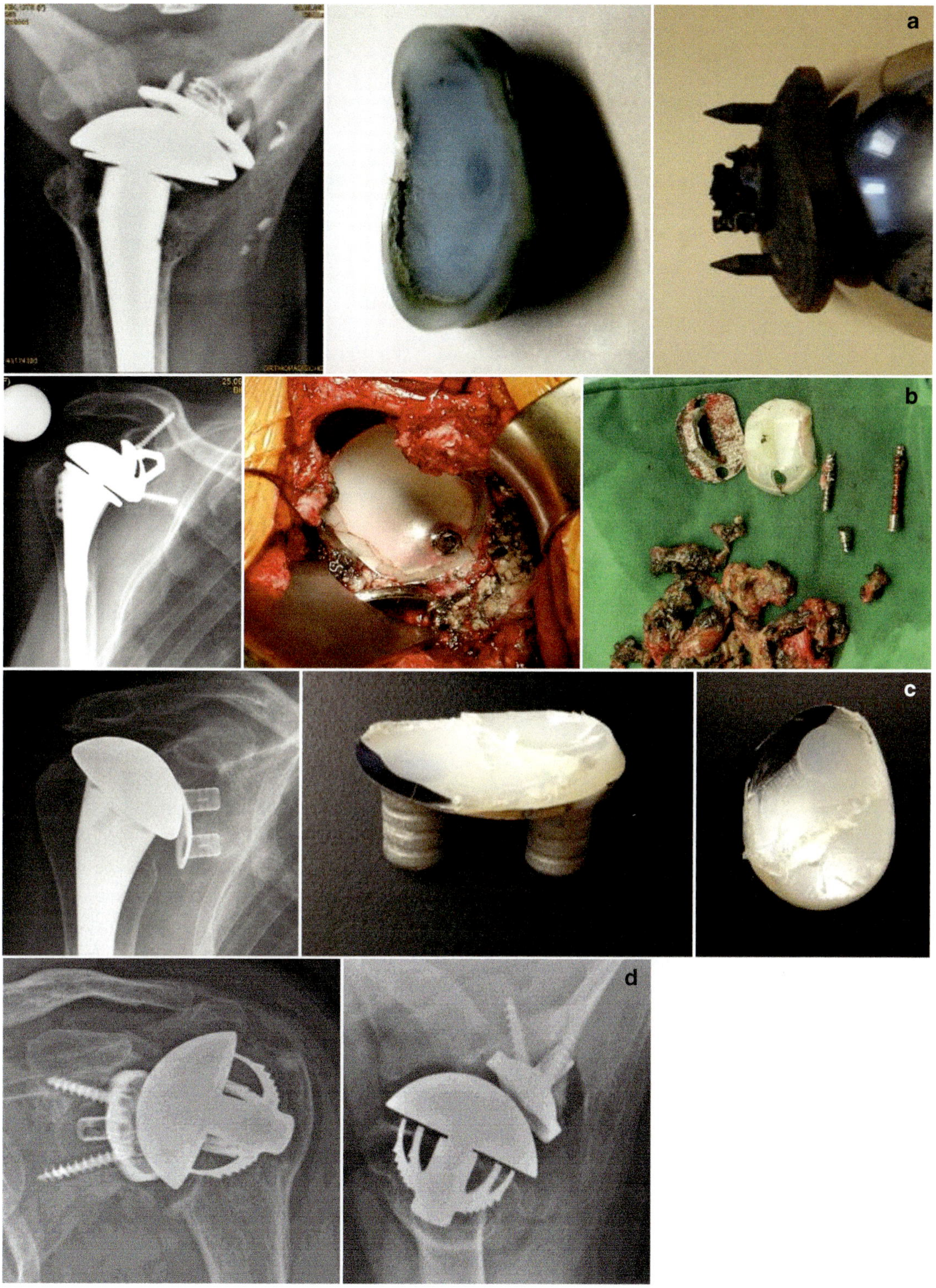

Fig. 15.6 Metal backed glenoid failure after mid-term in different design. (**a**) Premature wear of a PE liner and breakage of cage screw fixation (Arthrex) (**b**) Aequalis expansion screw fixation (**c**) Postero-superior wear and metallosis (Epoca) (**d**) PE liner wear and dissociation (Lima) (**e**) Clinical outcome

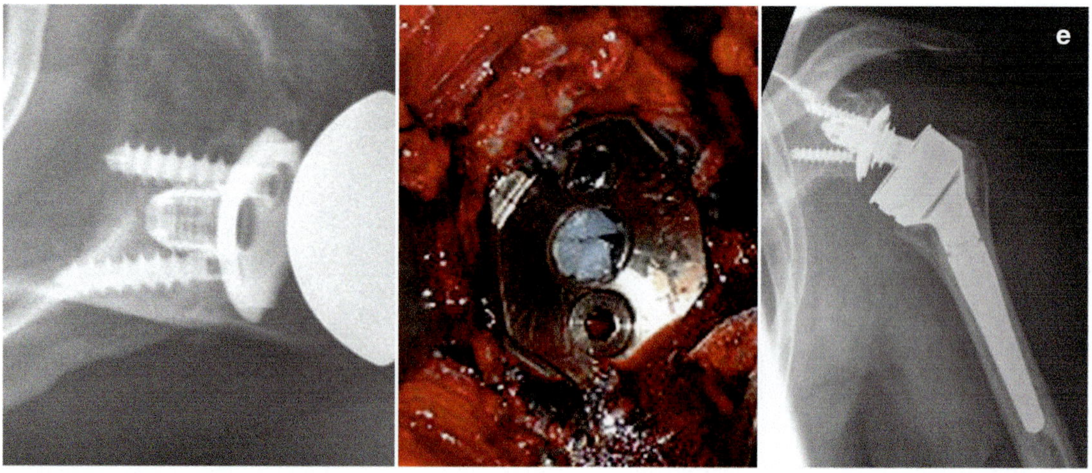

Fig. 15.6 (continued)

Aequalis Multicentre Group

For 20 years French multicentre studies (some including a smaller proportion of data from other European countries including Germany and UK) were supervised by Walch and Boileau. They have mainly focused on clinical and radiological results of the "Aequalis" standard TSA design which represents the third generation of anatomical implants with a short (100 mm), mostly cemented stem and a Neer type polyethylene glenoid component (keeled or pegged). Both components were modified over time and some specific features (e.g. the metal backed glenoid component with extension screws) have been modified or withdrawn.

Summary

- Results of anatomical shoulder arthroplasty depend on numerous factors: patient-related, surgeon-related and, most importantly, aetiology-related. The precondition of the rotator cuff and the amount of glenoid bone loss and deformity are essential for longevity of the implant.
- In cases of centred osteoarthritis and intact rotator cuff without advanced fatty muscle infiltration good or excellent functional results can be expected for the majority of patients with low complication rates for the first 10 years after surgery.
- The trend to preserve bone stock using stemless humeral components has not produced differences in clinical outcome or loosening rates in comparison to stemmed implants yet. However, this needs more long-term survivorship data.
- Glenoid loosening is still the most common failure mode: Caused by aseptic loosening of cemented polyethylene glenoid components after 5–10 years and in metal-backed components due to increased polyethylene wear and dissociation after 4–6 years. A new approach to glenoid resurfacing has to overcome this crucial issue.

References

1. Australian Orthopaedic Association national joint replacement registry annual report 2012.
2. Barlow JD, Yuan BJ, Schleck CD, Harmsen WS, Cofield RH, Sperling JW. Shoulder arthroplasty for rheumatoid arthritis: 303 consecutive with minimum 5-year follow-up. J Shoulder Elb Surg. 2014;23(6):791–9. https://doi.org/10.1016/j.jse.2013.09.016.
3. Bohsali KI, Wirth MA, Rockwood CA Jr. Complications of total shoulder arthroplasty. J Bone Joint Surg Am. 2006;88(10):2279–92.
4. Boileau P, Walch G. Adaptabilité et modularité au cours des prostheses d'épaule [Adaptability and mod-

ulation in shoulder prosthesis]. Acta Orthop Belg. 1995;61(Suppl 1):49–61.

5. Boileau P, Walch G. The three-dimensional geometry of the proximal humerus. Implications for surgical technique and prosthetic design. J Bone Joint Surg Br. 1997;79(5):857–65.
6. Boileau P, Moineau G, Morin-Salvo N, Avidor C, Godenèche A, Lévigne C, Baba M, Walch G. Metal-backed glenoid implant with polyethylene insert is not a viable long-term therapeutic option. J Shoulder Elb Surg. 2015;24(10):1534–43. https://doi.org/10.1016/j.jse.2015.02.012. Epub 2015 Jul 27
7. Boileau P, Baba M, Moineau G, Morin-Salvo N, Avidor C, Godenèche A, Lévigne C, Walch G. Response to Katz et al: the weak link in metal-backed glenoid implants is the polyethylene. J Shoulder Elb Surg. 2016;25(12):e396–8. https://doi.org/10.1016/j.jse.2016.08.010. Epub 2016 Oct 14
8. Carter MJ, Mikuls TR, Nayak S, Fehringer EV, Michaud K. Impact of total shoulder arthroplasty on generic and shoulder-specific health-related quality-of-life measures: a systematic literature review and meta-analysis. J Bone Joint Surg Am. 2012;94(17):e127.
9. Carroll RM, Izquierdo R, Vazquez M, Blaine TA, Levine WN, Bigliani LU. Conversion of painful hemiarthroplasty to total shoulder arthroplasty: long-term results. J Shoulder Elb Surg. 2004;13(6):599–603.
10. Chen X, Reddy AS, Kontaxis A, Choi DS, Wright T, Dines DM, Warren RF, Berhouet J, Gulotta LV. Version correction via eccentric reaming compromises remaining bone quality in B2 Glenoids: a computational study. Clin Orthop Relat Res. 2017;475(12):3090–9. https://doi.org/10.1007/s11999-017-5510-7. Epub 2017 Sep 25
11. Cil A, Veillette CJ, Sanchez-Sotelo J, Sperling JW, Schleck CD, Cofield RH. Survivorship of the humeral component in shoulder arthroplasty. J Shoulder Elb Surg. 2010;19(1):143–50.
12. Clavert P, Millett PJ, Warner JJ. Glenoid resurfacing: what are the limits to asymmetric reaming for posterior erosion? J Shoulder Elb Surg. 2007;16:843–8. https://doi.org/10.1016/j.jse.2007.03.015.
13. Clark JC, Simon P, Clark RE, Christmas KN, Allert JW, Streit JJ, Mighell MA, Hess A, Stone J, Frankle MA. The influence of patient- and surgeon-specific factors on operative duration and early postoperative outcomes in shoulder arthroplasty. J Shoulder Elb Surg. 2017;26(6):1011–6.
14. Clitherow HD, Frampton CM, Astley TM. Effect of glenoid cementation on total shoulder arthroplasty for degenerative arthritis of the shoulder: a review of the New Zealand National Joint Registry. J Shoulder Elb Surg. 2014;23(6):775–81. https://doi.org/10.1016/j.jse.2013.08.022. Epub 2013 Nov 23
15. Cofield RH. Total shoulder arthroplasty with the Neer prosthesis. J Bone Joint Surg Am. 1984;66(6):899–906.
16. Cofield RH, Edgerton BC. Total shoulder arthroplasty: complications and revision surgery. Instr Course Lect. 1990;39:449–62.
17. Constant CR, Gerber C, Emery RJ, Søjbjerg JO, Gohlke F, Boileau PA. Review of the constant score: modifications and guidelines for its use. J Shoulder Elb Surg. 2008;17(2):355–61. https://doi.org/10.1016/j.jse.2007.06.022. Epub 2008 Jan 22
18. Churchill RS, Athwal GS. Stemless shoulder arthroplasty-current results and designs. Curr Rev Musculoskelet Med. 2016;9(1):10–6. https://doi.org/10.1007/s12178-016-9320-4.
19. Churchill RS, Zellmer C, Zimmers HJ, Ruggero R. Clinical and radiographic analysis of a partially cemented glenoid implant: five-year minimum follow-up. J Shoulder Elb Surg. 2010;19:1091–7.
20. Denard PJ, Raiss P, Sowa B, Walch G. Mid- to long-term follow-up of total shoulder arthroplasty using a keeled glenoid in young adults with primary glenohumeral arthritis. J Shoulder Elb Surg. 2013;22(7):894–900. https://doi.org/10.1016/j.jse.2012.09.016. Epub 2013 Jan 9
21. Deshmukh AV, Koris M, Zurakowski D, Thornhill TS. Total shoulder arthroplasty: long-term survivorship, functional outcome, and quality of life. J Shoulder Elb Surg. 2005;14(5):471–9.
22. Edwards TB, Boulahia A, Kempf JF, Boileau P, Nemoz C, Walch G. The influence of rotator cuff disease on the results of shoulder arthroplasty for primary osteoarthritis: results of a multicenter study. J Bone Joint Surg Am. 2002;84-A:2240–8.
23. Farng E, Zingmond D, Krenek L, Soohoo NF. Factors predicting complication rates after primary shoulder arthroplasty. J Shoulder Elb Surg. 2011;20(4):557–63. https://doi.org/10.1016/j.jse.2010.11.005. Epub 2011 Feb 16
24. Favard L, Berhouet J, Walch G, Chaoui J, Lévigne C. Superior glenoid inclination and glenoid bone loss: definition, assessment, biomechanical consequences, and surgical options. Orthopade. 2017;46(12):1015–21. https://doi.org/10.1007/s00132-017-3496-1.
25. Fevang BT, Lie SA, Havelin LI, Skredderstuen A, Furnes O. Risk factors for revision after shoulder arthroplasty: 1,825 shoulder arthroplasties from the Norwegian arthroplasty register. Acta Orthop. 2009;80(1):83–91.
26. Fevang L, Nystad TW, Skredderstuen A, Furnes ON, Havelin LI. Improved survival for anatomical total shoulder prostheses. Acta Orthop. 2015;86(1):63–70.
27. Fox TJ, Cil A, Sperling JW, Sanchez-Sotelo J, Schleck CD, Cofield RH. Survival of the glenoid component in shoulder arthroplasty. J Shoulder Elb Surg. 2009;18:859–63.
28. Fox TJ, Foruria AM, Klika BJ, Sperling JW, Schleck CD, Cofield RH. Radiographic survival in total shoulder arthroplasty. J Shoulder Elb Surg. 2013;22(9):1221–7. https://doi.org/10.1016/j.jse.2012.12.034. Epub 2013 Mar 6
29. Gazielly DF, Scarlet MM, Verborgt O. Long-term survival of the glenoid components in total shoulder replacement for arthritis. Int Orthop. 2015;39(2):285–9.

30. Goldberg SS, Bell JE, Kim HJ, Bak SF, Levine WN, Bigliani LU. Hemiarthroplasty for the rotator cuff-deficient shoulder. J Bone Joint Surg Am. 2008;90(3):554–9. https://doi.org/10.2106/JBJS.F.01029.
31. Gohlke F. Clinical and radiographic results of shoulder arthroplasty in rheumatoid arthritis. In: Walch G, Boileau P, Molé D, editors. Shoulder prosthesis – two to ten year follow-up. Montpellier S: Sauramps Medical; 2001. p. 177–82.
32. Gregory TM, Boukebous B, Gregory J, Pierrart J, Masemjean E. Short, medium and long term complications after total anatomical shoulder arthroplasty. Open Orthopa J. 2017;11(Suppl-6 , M6):1133–41.
33. Hammond JW, Queale WS, Kim TK, McFarland EG. Surgeon experience and clinical and economic outcomes for shoulder arthroplasty. J Bone Joint Surg Am. 2003;85-A(12):2318–24.
34. Hasan, et al. Characteristics of unsatisfactory shoulder arthroplasties. J Shoulder Elb Surg. 2002;11: 431–41.
35. Hawi N, Tauber M, Messina MJ, Habermeyer P, Martetschläger F. Anatomic stemless shoulder arthroplasty and related outcomes: a systematic review. BMC Musculoskelet Disord. 2016;17(1):376. https://doi.org/10.1186/s12891-016-1235-0.
36. Hawi N, Magosch P, Tauber M, Lichtenberg S, Habermeyer P. Nine-year outcome after anatomic stemless shoulder prosthesis: clinical and radiologic results. J Shoulder Elb Surg. 2017;26(9):1609–15. https://doi.org/10.1016/j.jse.2017.02.017. Epub 2017 Apr 11
37. Hill JM, Norris TR. Long-term results of total shoulder arthroplasty following bone grafting of the glenoid. J Bone Joint Surg Am. 2001;83(6):877–83.
38. Ho JC, Sabesan VJ, Iannotti JP. Glenoid component retroversion is associated with osteolysis. J Bone Joint Surg Am. 2013;95:e82. https://doi.org/10.2106/JBJS.L.00336.
39. Hsu JE, Ricchetti ET, Huffman GR, Iannotti JP, Glaser DL. Addressing glenoid bone deficiency and asymmetric posterior erosion in shoulder arthroplasty. J Shoulder Elb Surg. 2013;22(9):1298–308. https://doi.org/10.1016/j.jse.2013.04.014. Epub 2013 Jun 22
40. Hsu JE, Russ SM, Somerson JS, Tang A, Warme WJ, Matsen FA. Is the simple shoulder test a valid outcome instrument for shoulder arthroplasty? J Shoulder Elb Surg. 2017;26(10):1693–700.
41. Hussey MM, Steen BM, Cusick MC, Cox JL, Marberry ST, Simon P, Cottrell BJ, Santoni BG, Frankle MA. The effects of glenoid wear patterns on patients with osteoarthritis in total shoulder arthroplasty: an assessment of outcomes and value. J Shoulder Elb Surg. 2015;24(5):682–90. https://doi.org/10.1016/j.jse.2014.09.043.
42. Hyun YS, Huri G, Garbis NG, McFarland EG. Uncommon indications for reverse total shoulder arthroplasty. Clin Orthop Surg. 2013;5(4):243–55. https://doi.org/10.4055/cios.2013.5.4.243. Epub 2013 Nov 18
43. Iannotti JP, Norris TR. Influence of preoperative factors on outcome of shoulder arthroplasty for glenohumeral osteoarthritis. J Bone Joint Surg Am. 2003;85-A(2):251–8.
44. Iannotti JP, Weiner S, Rodriguez E, Subhas N, Patterson TE, Jun BJ, Ricchetti ET. Three-dimensional imaging and templating improve glenoid implant positioning. J Bone Joint Surg Am. 2015;97(8):651–8.
45. Jain N, Pietrobon R, Hocker S, Guller U, Shankar A, Higgins LD. The relationship between surgeon and hospital volume and outcomes for shoulder arthroplasty. J Bone Joint Surg Am. 2004;86-A(3): 496–505.
46. Johansson L, Hailer NP, Rahme H. High incidence of periprosthetic joint infection with propionibacterium acnes after the use of a stemless shoulder prosthesis with metaphyseal screw fixation - a retrospective cohort study of 241 patients propionibacter infections after eclipse TSA. BMC Musculoskelet Disord. 2017;18(1):203. https://doi.org/10.1186/s12891-017-1555-8.
47. Kilian CM, Press CM, Smith KM, O'Connor DP, Morris BJ, Elkousy HA, Gartsman GM, Edwards TB. Radiographic and clinical comparison of pegged and keeled glenoid components using modern cementing techniques: midterm results of a prospective randomized study. J Shoulder Elb Surg. 2017;26(12):2078–85. https://doi.org/10.1016/j.jse.2017.07.016. Epub 2017 Sep 13
48. Labek G, Thaler M, Janda W, Agreiter M, Stöckl B. Revision rates after total joint replacement: cumulative results from worldwide joint register datasets. J Bone Joint Surg Br. 2011a;93(3):293–7.
49. Labek G, Neumann D, Agreiter M, Schuh R, Böhler N. Impact of implant developers on published outcome and reproducibility of cohort-based clinical studies in arthroplasty. J Bone Joint Surg Am. 2011b;93(Supl 3):55–61.
50. Lebon J, Delclaux S, Bonnevialle N, Rongières M, Bonnevialle P, Mansat P. French Society for Shoulder, Elbow (SOFEC). Orthop Traumatol Surg Res. 2014;100(6Suppl):S327–32.
51. Levine WN, Djurasovic M, Glasson JM, Pollock RG, Flatow EL, Bigliani LU. Hemiarthroplasty for glenohumeral osteoarthritis: results correlated to degree of glenoid wear. J Shoulder Elb Surg. 1997;6(5): 449–54.
52. Levy O, Copeland SA. Cementless surface replacement arthroplasty of the shoulder. 5- to 10-year results with the Copeland mark-2 prosthesis. J Bone Joint Surg Br. 2001;83(2):213–21.
53. Levy O, Funk L, Sforza G, Copeland SA. Copeland surface replacement arthroplasty of the shoulder in rheumatoid arthritis. J Bone Joint Surg Am. 2004;86-A(3):512–8.
54. Mansat P, Coutié AS, Bonnevialle N, Rongières M, Mansat M, Bonnevialle P. Resurfacing humeral prosthesis: do we really reconstruct the anatomy? J Shoulder Elb Surg. 2013;22(5):612–9. https://doi.org/10.1016/j.jse.2012.07.014. Epub 2012 Nov 11
55. Matsen FA 3rd, Tang A, Russ SM, Hsu JE. Relationship between patient-reported assessment of shoulder

function and objective range-of-motion measurements. J Bone Joint Surg Am. 2017;99(5):417–26.
56. Merolla G, Ciaramella G, Fabbri E, Walch G, Paladini P, Porcellini G. Total shoulder replacement using a bone ingrowth central peg polyethylene glenoid component: a prospective clinical and computed tomography study with short- to mid-term follow-up. Int Orthop. 2016;40:2355–63. https://doi.org/10.1007/s00264-016-3255-7.
57. Millett PJ, Yen YM, Price CS, Horan MP, van der Meijden OA, Elser F. Propionibacterium acnes infection as an occult cause of postoperative shoulder pain: a case series. Clin Orthop Relat Res. 2011;469(10):2824–30. https://doi.org/10.1007/s11999-011-1767-4. Epub 2011 Jan 15)
58. Moeckel BH, Dines DM, Warren RF, Altchek DW. Modular hemiarthroplasty for fractures of the proximal part of the humerus. J Bone Joint Surg Am. 1992;74(6):884–9.
59. Neer CS. Articular replacement for the humeral head. J Bone Joint Surg Am. 1955;37:215–28.
60. Neer CS. Replacement arthroplasty for glenohumeral osteoarthritis. J Bone Joint Surg Am. 1974;56(1):1–13.
61. Nuttall D, Haines JF, Trail IA. The early migration of a partially cemented fluted pegged glenoid component using radiostereometric analysis. J Shoulder Elb Surg. 2012;21:1191–6. https://doi.org/10.1016/j.jse.2011.07.028.
62. Papadonikolakis A, Matsen FA 3rd. Metal-backed glenoid components have a higher rate of failure and fail by different modes in comparison with all-polyethylene components: a systematic review. J Bone Joint Surg Am. 2014;96(12):1041–7.
63. Radnay CS, Setter KJ, Chambers L, Levine WN, Bigliani LU, Ahmad CS. Total shoulder replacement compared with humeral head replacement for the treatment of primary glenohumeral osteoarthritis: a systematic review. J Shoulder Elb Surg. 2007;16(4):396–402.
64. Raiss P, Bruckner T, Rickert M, Walch G. Longitudinal observational study of total shoulder replacements with cement: fifteen to twenty-year follow-up. J Bone Joint Surg Am. 2014;96:198–205. https://doi.org/10.2106/JBJS.M.00079.
65. Rees JL, Dawson J, Hand GC, Cooper C, Judge A, Price AJ, Beard DJ, Carr AJ. The use of patient-reported outcome measures and patient satisfaction ratings to assess outcome in hemiarthroplasty of the shoulder. J Bone Joint Surg Br. 2010;92(8):1107–11.
66. Rice RS, Sperling JW, Miletti J, Schleck C, Cofield RH. Augmented glenoid component for bone deficiency in shoulder arthroplasty. Clin Orthop Relat Res. 2008;466(3):579–83. https://doi.org/10.1007/s11999-007-0104-4. Epub 2008 Jan 8
67. Rosenberg N, Neumann L, Modi A, Mersich IJ, Wallace AW. Improvements in survival of the uncemented Nottingham total shoulder prosthesis: a prospective comparative study. BMC Musculoskelet Disord. 2007;8:76.
68. Schoch B, Schleck C, Cofield RH, Sperling JW. Shoulder arthroplasty in patients younger than 50 years: minimum 20-years follow-up. J Shoulder Elb Surg. 2015;24(5):705–10.
69. Sims MT, Detweiler BN, Scott JT, Howard BM, Detten GR, Vassar M. Inconsistent selection of outcomes and measurement devices found in shoulder arthroplasty research: an analysis of studies on ClinicalTrials.gov. PLoS One. 2017;12(11):e0187865. https://doi.org/10.1371/journal.pone.0187865. eCollection 2017.
70. Singh JA, Sperling JW, Cofield RH. Revision surgery following total shoulder arthroplasty: analysis of 2588 shoulders over three decades (1976 to 2008). J Bone Joint Surg Br. 2011;93(11):1513–7.
71. Søjbjerg JO, Frich LH, Johannsen HV, Sneppen O. Late results of total shoulder replacement in patients with rheumatoid arthritis. Clin Orthop Relat Res. 1999;366:39–45.
72. Somerson JS, Matsen FA 3rd. Functional outcomes of the ream-and-run shoulder arthroplasty: a concise follow-up of a previous report. J Bone Joint Surg Am. 2017;99(23):1999–2003. https://doi.org/10.2106/JBJS.17.00201.
73. Sowa B, Bochenek M, Bülhoff M, Zeifang F, Loew M, Bruckner T, Raiss P. The medium- and long-term outcome of total shoulder arthroplasty for primary glenohumeral osteoarthritis in middle-aged patients. Bone Joint J. 2017;99-B(7):939–43. https://doi.org/10.1302/0301-620X.99B7.BJJ-2016-1365.R1.
74. Sperling JW, Cofield RH, Rowland CM. Minimum fifteen-year follow-up of Neer hemiarthroplasty and total shoulder arthroplasty in patients aged fifty years or younger. J Shoulder Elb Surg. 2004;13:604–13. https://doi.org/10.1016/j.jse.2004.03.013.
75. Sperling JW, Cofield RH, Schleck CD, Harmsen WS. Total shoulder arthroplasty versus hemiarthroplasty for rheumatoid arthritis of the shoulder: results of 303 consecutive cases. J Shoulder Elb Surg. 2007;16(6):683–90.
76. Steinmann SP, Cofield RH. Bone grafting for glenoid deficiency in total shoulder replacement. J Shoulder Elb Surg. 2000;9(5):361–7.
77. Strauss EJ, Roche C, Flurin PH, Wright T, Zuckerman JD. The glenoid in shoulder arthroplasty. J Shoulder Elb Surg. 2009;18(5):819–33.
78. Szabo I, Buscayret F, Edwards TB, Nemoz C, O'Connor DP, Boileau P, et al. Radiographic comparison of two glenoid preparation techniques in total shoulder arthroplasty. Clin Orthop Relat Res. 2005;431:104–10.
79. Swieszkowski W, Bednarz P, Prendergast PJ. Contact stresses in the glenoid component in total shoulder arthroplasty. Proc Inst Mech Eng H. 2003;217(1):49–57.
80. Taunton MJ, AL MI, Sperling JW, Cofield RH. Total shoulder arthroplasty with a metal-backed, bone-ingrowth glenoid component. Medium to long-term results. J Bone Joint Surg Am. 2008;90(10):2180–8. https://doi.org/10.2106/JBJS.G.00966.
81. Trail IA, Nuttall D. The results of shoulder arthroplasty in patients with rheumatoid arthritis. J Bone Joint Surg Br. 2002;84(8):1121–5.

82. Torchia ME. Total shoulder arthroplasty with the Neer prosthesis: long-term results. J Shoulder Elb Surg. 1997;6(6):495–505.
83. van den Bekerom MP, Geervliet PC, Somford MP, van den Borne MP, Boer R. Total shoulder arthroplasty versus hemiarthroplasty for glenohumeral arthritis: a systematic review of the literature at long-term follow-up. Int J Shoulder Surg. 2013;7(3):110–5.
84. van de Sande MA, Brand R, Rosig PM. Indications, complications and results of shoulder arthroplasty. Scand J Rheumatol. 2006;35(6):426–34.
85. Voorde PC, Rasmussen JV, Olsen BS, Brorson S. Resurfacing shoulder arthroplasty for the treatment of severe rheumatoid arthritis: outcome in 167 patients from the Danish shoulder registry. Acta Orthop. 2015;86(3):293–7. https://doi.org/10.3109/17453674.2015.1018761. Epub 2015 Feb 12
86. Vuillermin CB, Trump ME, Barwood SA, Hoy GA. Catastrophic failure of a low profile metal-backed glenoid component after total shoulder arthroplasty. Int J Shoulder Surg. 2015;9(4):121–7. https://doi.org/10.4103/0973-6042.167952.
87. Walch G, Boulahia A, Boileau P, Kempf JF. Primary glenohumeral osteoarthritis: clinical and radiographic classification. The Aequalis Group. Acta Orthop Belg. 1998;64(Suppl 2):46–52.
88. Walch G, Edwards TB, Boulahia A, Boileau P, Mole D, Adeleine P. The influence of glenohumeral prosthetic mismatch on glenoid radiolucent lines: results of a multicenter study. J Bone Joint Surg Am. 2002a;84-A(12):2186–91.
89. Walch G, Moraga C, Young A, Castellanos-Rosas J. Results of anatomic nonconstrained prosthesis in primary osteoarthritis with biconcave glenoid. J Shoulder Elb Surg. 2012a;21:1526–33. https://doi.org/10.1016/j.jse.2011.11.030.
90. Walch G, Young AA, Boileau P, Loew M, Gazielly D, Mole D. Patterns of loosening of polyethylene keeled glenoid components after shoulder arthroplasty for primary osteoarthritis: results of a multicenter study with more than five years of follow-up. J Bone Joint Surg Am. 2012b;94:145–50.
91. Walch G, Young AA, Melis B, Gazielly D, Loew M, Boileau P. Results of a convex-back cemented keeled glenoid component in primary osteoarthritis: multicenter study with a follow-up greater than 5 years. J Shoulder Elb Surg. 2011;20(3):385–94. https://doi.org/10.1016/j.jse.2010.07.011. Epub 2010 Nov 5
92. Walch G, Ascani C, Boulahia A, Nove-Josserand L, Edwards TB. Static posterior subluxation of the humeral head: an unrecognized entity responsible for glenohumeral osteoarthritis in the young adult. J Shoulder Elb Surg. 2002b;11:309–14.
93. Werner BS, Gohlke F. Cementless humeral head replacement for dislocation arthropathy of the shoulder joint. Orthopade. 2010;39(11):1036–43. https://doi.org/10.1007/s00132-010-1655-8.
94. Werner BS, Stehle J, Abdelkawi A, Plumhoff P, Hudek R, Gohlke F. Progressive glenoid bone loss caused by erosion in humeral head resurfacing. Orthopade. 2017;46(12):1028–33. https://doi.org/10.1007/s00132-017-3483-6.
95. Werthel JD, Lonjon G, Jo S, Cofield R, Sperling JW, Elhassan BT. Long-term outcomes of cemented versus cementless humeral components in arthroplasty of the shoulder: a propensity score-matched analysis. Bone Joint J. 2017;99-B(5):666–73. https://doi.org/10.1302/0301-620X.99B5.BJJ-2016-0910.R1.
96. Williams GR Jr, Rockwood CA Jr. Hemiarthroplasty in rotator curr-defficient shoulders. J Shoulder Elb Surg. 1996;5(5):362–7.
97. Wirth MA, Rockwood CA. Complications of shoulder arthroplasty. Clin Orth Relat Res. 1994;307:47–69.
98. Wirth MA, Loredo R, Garcia G, Rockwood CA, Southworth C, Iannotti JP. Total shoulder arthroplasty with an all-polyethylene pegged bone-ingrowth glenoid component: a clinical and radiographic outcome study. J Bone Joint Surg Am. 2012;94:260–7.
99. Yian EH, Werner CM, Nyffeler RW, Pfirrmann CW, Ramappa A, Sukthankar A, Gerber C. Radiographic and computed tomography analysis of cemented pegged polyethylene glenoid components in total shoulder replacement. J Bone Joint Surg Am. 2005;87(9):1928–36.
100. Young A, Walch G, Boileau P, Favard L, Gohlke F, Loew M, Molé D. A multicentre study of the long-term results of using a flat-back polyethylene glenoid component in shoulder replacement for primary osteoarthritis. J Bone Joint Surg Br. 2011;93(2):210–6. https://doi.org/10.1302/0301-620X.93B2.25086.
101. Young AA, Walch G, Pape G, Gohlke F, Favard L. Secondary rotator cuff dysfunction following total shoulder arthroplasty for primary glenohumeral osteoarthritis: results of a multicenter study with more than five years of follow-up. J Bone Joint Surg Am. 2012;94(8):685–93. https://doi.org/10.2106/JBJS.J.00727.

Complications in Anatomic Shoulder Replacement

16

Ludwig Seebauer

In the last three decades, there has been exponential growth in the number of anatomic shoulder arthroplasties carried out for primary osteoarthritis, rheumatoid arthritis, avascular necrosis, proximal humeral fracture and even cuff tear arthropathy. There has been an even greater increase in numbers of the reverse shoulder arthroplasties performed for cuff tear arthropathy and complex humeral fractures. In comparison to hip and knee arthroplasty the number of shoulder replacements performed annually continue to rise. However, anatomic shoulder arthroplasty in comparison to total hip or knee replacement probably has lower survival rates together with a relatively high complication rate [1–7].

Complication is an event that results in an adverse outcome for the patient, irrespective of the need for a surgical revision. As with other joint replacements anatomic shoulder arthroplasty can be associated with a multitude of complications. The reported complication rate for anatomic shoulder replacement is highly variable. The most comprehensive analysis of complications in shoulder arthroplasties within the last 3 decades were carried out by Bohsali and Wirth with their three meta-analysis in 1996, 2006 and 2017 [2–4]. The overall complication rate has reduced over the years, although there is an increase in the number of specific complications with long-term follow-up. Bohsali reported in 2006 [3] his meta-analysis of 2810 cases (2810 shoulders; observation period 1996 to 2005) an overall complication rate of 14.7%. Aseptic loosening (39%) was the commonest complication, which increased by 10% at their 1996 review [8] (1858 cases; observation period 1975–1995). In anatomic shoulder arthroplasty, glenoid component loosening represents the most frequent complication; in contrast to total reverse shoulder arthroplasty, where instability is the most frequent complication. In their most recent paper of 2017 (3360 shoulders; observation period 2006–2015) the overall complication rate had decreased to 10.3%, although there has been a paradoxical increase in the number of glenoid component failures within the last decade from 32% to 37.7%. However, it should be noted, that in earlier periods (1975–1995) anatomic shoulder arthroplasties were mostly carried out as a hemiarthroplasty and as a consequence glenoid component failure is mostly a long-term follow-up phenomena [9–11].

Given the increasing numbers of total shoulder carried out accompanied by significant design evolution and instrument and technique improvement in 2006 Chin and co-workers [5] undertook a retrospective study on 431 TSA carried out between 1990 and 2000 to find out, whether complications after TSA are reducing or different. They found an overall complication rate of 12%

L. Seebauer (✉)
Center of Orthopaedics, Traumatology and Sportsmedicine, Klinikum Bogenhausen, München, Germany
e-mail: ludwig.seebauer@klinikum-muenchen.de

I. A. Trail et al. (eds.), *Textbook of Shoulder Surgery*, https://doi.org/10.1007/978-3-319-70099-1_16

with 7.4% major complications, of which 53% requiring revision surgery. The complications in order of frequency were: rotator cuff rupture, postoperative glenohumeral instability and periprosthetic humeral fracture. Developing a complication was unrelated to the initial diagnosis, previous surgery, age, sex, humeral head size, or cementing or not cementing the humeral component. This midterm follow-up study of Chin [5] with a mean follow-up of 4.2 years reported revisions for glenoid or humeral component loosening only for 1 case (0.2%). In comparison to long-term follow-up studies [9, 11, 12] for TSA these results are not surprising, as revision for glenoid component loosening is a long-term problem occurring significantly after 12–15 years. Raiss [10] reported in his 2012-study a 48% rate of radiologic loosening of the glenoid component with 1 case requiring revision for glenoid loosening in a follow-up period of 13 years. At the same time there were no signs of radiologic loosening of any humeral component. In a more recent study in 2014 Raiss [11] reported on implant revision as a consequence of glenoid loosening in 29% of the cases. Survival rate on Kaplan-Meier curve was 89% after 10 years, 73% after 15 years and 70% after 20 years. The same year Raiss [13] reported on the influence of glenoid component erosion on osteolytic changes around the humerus. The author attributes PE-wear debris as the cause of osteolysis. In his study stress-shielding was only observed with cementless stems.

In summary, complications and revisions in anatomic shoulder arthroplasty have to be clearly distinguished as early and late complications and general medical complications (pulmonary infection, renal failure, thromboembolism, longer hospital stay) or shoulder procedure specific complications (component failure, wear, instability, cuff tear, periprosthetic fracture, etc.).

It is crucial to consider the general medical and health status of a patient (age, diabetes, smoking, obesity, osteoporosis, hepatitis C, etc.) to rule out its influence on potential general or shoulder specific complications after anatomic shoulder arthroplasty. Within the last year numerous peer-reviewed papers have been published disclosing significant impact of these conditions on the postoperative outcome and complication rate after anatomic shoulder arthroplasty. In addition it seems that even the insurance status plays a relevant role [14].

Clinical Pearl

Complications following anatomic total shoulder replacement can be classified either into early or late, major or minor and finally medical or surgical.

Influence of General Health Status on Corcmplication Rate

The influence of medical comorbidities and the outcome and complication rate of shoulder arthroplasty is well understood. Leschinger et al. [15] found out that complications after anatomic total shoulder arthroplasty correlate with the patient's overall health status (ASA 3 sign. Worse than ASA 1 + 2; odds ratio 4,28; $p < .01$). Smokers were more prone to a surgical complication (odds ratio, 5.08; $p = .02$). The authors classified complications under 3 categories: Category I: Complications without reoperation / intraoperative complications = Temporary or permanent nerve palsy, intra- or postoperative fractures of the humerus or glenoid, temporary dislocation of the glenohumeral joint, relevant intraoperative bleeding and implant instability. Category II: Complications with soft tissue revision = recurrent dislocation, wound infection, contracture. Category III: Complication with implant revision = painful glenoid erosion, infection, malpositioning of implant, implant loosening.

Age

Wagner [16] et al. ruled out, that there is a strong correlation between elderly patients and decreased rates of revision after shoulder arthroplasty, specially decreased rates of mechanical failures. The risk of revision surgery decreased in a linear fashion between the ages of 40 and 85, with a 3% decreased risk of revision per 1-year increase in age ($p < .01$). Compared with patients aged <50 years, patients aged from 50 to 65 years ($p < .001$) and those >65 years ($p < .001$) have decreased risks of revision surgery. The risk of a revision surgery in a patient aged >50 years was significantly decreased (~13% reduction in risk for each year; $p < .001$). There was a subtle association between older age and decreased rates of infection ($p = .01$). Conversly they found a higher risk for thromboembolic events with a significantly increased risk for venous thromboembolism in patients aged >70 years, with the risk increasing by 15% per year above 70 years. They did not find any correlation with shoulder dislocation or periprosthetic fracture and age.

Diabetes

Diabetes is an established risk factor for higher postoperative morbidity in lower extremity procedures and have already be shown that it is also a significant risk factor for short- term complications after TSA [17]. The impact of insulin dependence in complication rate in anatomic shoulder arthroplasty has only been characterized by a recent study of Fu et al. In this study, after multivariable adjustment for preoperative patient characteristics and comorbidities, patients with non-Insulin dependent diabetes were not at significantly increased risk for postoperative complication relative to nondiabetic patients. In contrast, Insulin-dependent diabetic patients were independently associated with increased odds for 1 or more postoperative complication, having a stroke or CVA, receiving a blood transfusion, and having an extended length of stay. Therefore, in diabetic patients undergoing TSA, insulin dependence should be considered part of preoperative risk assessment.

Obesity: BMI

There are contrasting opinions on the influence of BMI on outcome, complications and revision rates of anatomic shoulder arthroplasties. Anakwenze et al. [18] found in their 2017 retrospective study on 3483 TSA that an increased BMI was only combined with an increased 90-day readmission rate (16% increase per every 5 kg/m^2 increase BMI), but not associated with higher revision-rates, 1-year mortality or 3-year surgical site infections. In contrast to these findings Wagner et al. [19] disclose that an increasing BMI is strongly associated with increased rates of revision surgical procedures and postoperative complications after shoulder arthroplasty. In a multi-variate analysis there is significant association ($p < 0.02$) between BMI and risk for revision for any reason, revision for mechanical failure and risk for reoperation. The most marked association is between BMI and superficial wound infection.

Smoking: Alcohol

Two recent studies [15, 20] demonstrate that smokers have a significant higher risk of complications. Hatta [20] found that current and former smokers have a significantly higher risk of periprosthetic infection (HR 7.27 rsp 4.56) and current smokers additionally have a higher risk for postoperative fractures (HR 6.99). Leschinger [15] reported a significant higher incidence of category I (intraop complications) with nicotine consumption (OR 5.44, $p = .0002$). Interestingly in his study alcohol consumption has no influence on the occurrence of minor or major complications. These findings are in contrast to the results of Ponce et al. [21] in their 2015 publication, were they found, that patients with a preexisting alcohol use disorder (AUD) have a greater likelihood to experience death, pneumonia, deep venous thrombosis, acute renal failure, transfusion, prolonged length of stay, and non-routine discharge irrespective of age, gender, race, and other medical comorbidities. Patients with a preexisting AUD are 2.7 times more likely to experience perioperative complications after shoulder arthroplasty.

Perioperative Transfusion

Grier et al. [22] carried out a retrospective study on 7794 patients who received a perioperative blood transfusion following TSA or RSA. Patients who received a perioperative transfusion had significantly higher rates of myocardial infarction, pneumonia, systemic inflammatory response syndrome or sepsis, venous thromboembolic events, and cerebrovascular accidents at all time points in question. Patients who received a blood transfusion also showed an increased incidence of surgical complications, including periprosthetic infection and mechanical complications, up to 2 years postoperatively. The results highlight the importance of preoperative medical optimization prior to shoulder arthroplasty, particularly in patients with preoperative anemia or multiple medical comorbidities.

Other Medical Conditions

Hepatitis C

A study of Cancienne et al. [23] clearly demonstrated that there is, despite recent advancements in the treatment of hepatitis C, a significant higher complication rate (infection, dislocation, fracture, revision TSA, systemic complications, blood transfusion) in patients with hepatitis C undergoing total shoulder arthroplasty. To explain this by the viral infection alone is unlikely as it is more likely related to higher case complexity and minor postoperative socioeconomic factors.

Shoulder Specific Complications Indications

It is imperative to differentiate the primary underlying pathology for which the anatomic shoulder replacement is carried out. The highest complication and revision rate occurs in the group of anatomic shoulder arthroplasty is for fractures and fracture sequelae [24–28]. The focus of this chapter is on anatomic shoulder replacement for non-traumatic indications (primary osteoarthritis, rheumatoid arthritis and atraumatic avascular necrosis) and complications thereof.

Implants

The traditional stemmed humeral component has recently been overshadowed by the emergence of newer stemless designs. The designs vary from a stemless head replacement prostheses fixed by a huge hollow screw (Arthrex Eclipse™) [29, 30] or by specific metaphyseal cancellous anchoring designs [31–37] (Biomet TESS™, Zimmer Sidus™, Wright Simplicity™, etc.). In the last decade, increasingly the treatment of primary osteoarthritis is by a total shoulder arthroplasty. The use of the humeral head resurfacing (e.g. Biomet Copeland™, Global CAP™, Epoca RH™, etc.) is currently decreasing substantially [38].

For some complications (infection, instability, neurologic, rotator cuff failure) it makes no difference to distinguish between regular stemmed, stemless humeral replacement or humeral head resurfacing and/or whether they are carried out as a total or hemiarthroplasty. Other complications like humeral component loosening, periprosthetic fracture are dependant upon the type of implant used.

Glenoid

In all follow-up studies on anatomic shoulder arthroplasties and all reviews about complications of anatomic arthroplasties the glenoid related complications are the most common one and account for up to 50% of all complications [3, 4, 39–46]. Glenoid component loosening (about 30% of all complications) occur often in combination with rotator cuff failure and/or chronic periprosthetic infections especially if they are present in the early or midterm follow-up period. Glenoid erosion is the most frequent complication of anatomic hemiarthroplasty in more than 20% of all cases [44, 47–53].

Glenoid Component Loosening

Early occurrence of asymptomatic radiolucent lines around the glenoid component after TSA are reported in numerous studies. However the necessity for revision because of loosening is much less [39, 54]. More recent studies have shown that in TSA after 15 years nearly 50% of glenoids are radiologically loose and the glenoid related revision rate increasing [10, 11] (Fig. 16.1).

The reason for early to midterm glenoid loosening is often a combination of several factors. Rotator cuff failure or subscapularis-rupture lead to an eccentric glenoid component loading ("rocking horse phenomena") and secondary glenoid component loosening. Early component loosening from chronic low-grade infection can also present with chronic pain and stiffness [55–57].

Interestingly glenoid component problems are more frequently seen in an osteoarthritic shoulder with significant posterior glenoid erosion [58–62]. The loosening rate even after a midterm follow-up period of average 77 months was reported by Walch [58] at 21% and after a longer term interval of average 112 months by Farvard [12] at 29%. Similar results are reported for other metal-back glenoid components [45, 46, 63, 64], (their implant specific complications will be discussed in details later). Ho et al. [65] clearly demonstrated in a short to mid-term (3.8 ± 1.8 years (range, 2–7 years) follow-up study on 66 shoulders, that postoperative glenoid retroversion greater than 15° is highly correlated with osteolysis around the central peg of a cemented glenoid component (odds ratio = 5.23, 95% CI = 1.31–20.9]). The same group in a short- to mid-term follow-up study on TSA with significant pre exisiting posterior glenoid erosion and retroversion corrected by glenoid bone grafting and a cemented glenoid implant reported good clinical results and a low glenoid associated complication rate. However, this is a low volume series of only 12 shoulders carried out in a high specialized tertiary center and the average patient age (55.8 ± 8.4 years) is significantly lower than in comparison to Walch's 2012 [58] study. Finally, in this study the revision rate for graft associated complications was 17%.

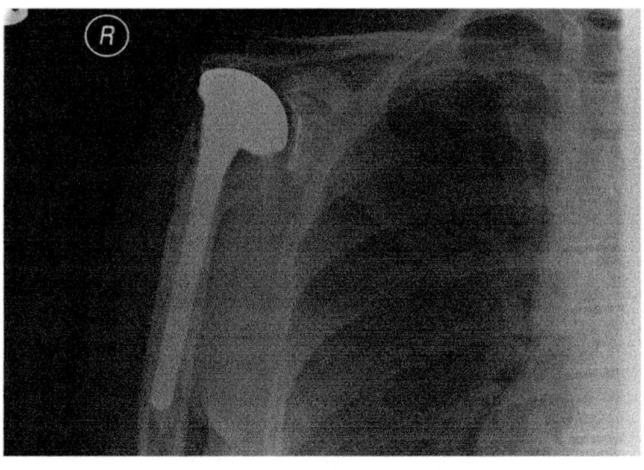

Fig. 16.1 Ten year x-ray of total shoulder arthroplasty showing glenoid component loosening

Long-term studies of anatomic TSA in rheumatoids [66] with a mean follow-up of 20 year in 14 patients report a high rate of radiologic loose glenoid components with superior humeral migration without any influence on ROM and clinical function. A mid- to long term study [54] on 303 rheumatoids with minimum 5 y follow-up by Barlow et al. clearly pointed out the superiority of TSA. However, there were 5% revisions because of glenoid component loosening, 73% peri glenoidal lucencies on x-ray, shift in position of 33% and "at risk" 36%. In comparison, there was a revision rate of 7% in the Hemi group for glenoid erosion; however the need for revision for glenoid erosion occurs earlier, as a rule within the first 5 years postop, than for glenoid component loosening. In contrast, Clement [67] in a long term study of mean 132 months on 36 rheumatoid arthritis shoulders treated with anatomic TSA with a cementless glenoid only reported 1 revision because of a loose glenoid and 4 glenoids with radiolucency; all 5 were associated with significant superior humeral head migration due to rotator cuff insufficiency.

Clinical Pearl
Radiolucent lines around cemented polyethylene glenoid components are frequently seen even in the early postoperative period. Revision for loosening, however, occurs much later.

Uncemented Glenoid Components

The issue of high rates of radiolucency around the glenoid component and later radiological signs of glenoid component loosening led to an attempt to overcome these problems with cementless metal-backed glenoid implants. However, with the exemption of some low volume series [67–69] no mid- to long term studies with higher numbers have proven any benefit of this type of implant. In 2007 Taunton et al. [70] from a series of 124 shoulders with a mean follow-up of 9.4 years using a metal-backed glenoid reported 35% glenoid loosening and polyethylene wear with metal wear of the glenoid component in 21%. More recent publications [46, 71] also pointed out a high rate of component loosening and revision rate at a 2–10-year follow-up interval. Interestingly Papadonikolakis [71] in his meta-analysis on 1571 metal-backed and 3035 all-polyethylene components reported higher rates of radiolucent lines and radiological loosening in cemented all-poly glenoids rather than in cementless metal-backed components. However, the revision rate for metal-backed implants was three times higher within a shorter follow-up period (mean 5.8 years vs. 7.3 years). The reason for revision were not merely component loosening but in 2/3 caused by other factors (screw breakage, component dissociation, polyethylene wear, metal wear, rotator cuff tear) (Fig. 16.2).

In this context it is also interesting, that specifically patients with significant posterior subluxation and glenoid erosion are at higher risk for early failure [43, 58, 63, 72–74].

Boileau et al. [46] reported on a 165 patient with a mean follow-up of 8.5 years a revision rate of 37%. 51% had significant polyethylene wear and 19% glenoid loosening. The 12-year revision free survival only reach 46%. As a consequence this group didn't see uncemented metal-backed glenoid resurfacing as a viable long-term option for glenoid replacement in anatomic TSA. Similarly as in other studies young males with posterior glenoid erosion (biconcave glenoid, posterior subluxation) have the highest risk.

PE-wear associated osteolysis is seen as a major concern in cement less metal-backed glenoid components. Additional problems include achieving minimal PE-thickness (avoiding early wear or brittling) without overstuffing the joint. Therefore, presently the use of a cemented all-poly glenoid is the gold-standard for glenoid resurfacing.

There are currently several designs on the market. A curved back-side is seen beneficial for longtime fixation and stability [75, 76]. Whether peg or keel fixation is superior remains unclear. Work by Nuttall et al. at Wrightington in 2007 using Radio Stereographic Analysis (RSA) were able to show less early motion with pegged components compared to keeled [77]. However, the overall revision rate for component loosening is the same for both designs [78].

There is only one small number (n = 34) series [79] published on a cementless all poly-design with a central bony-ingrowth fluted PE-peg with a short mean follow-up of 28 months. Despite using no cement in an all poly implant, they found in 88% no signs of radiolucency and only 12% of minor or medium radiolucency at the follow-up control by CT. Conversely work by Nuttall et al. (2012) identified using Radio Stereographic Analysis identified significant early motion in the "Anchor peg" (Depuy, Warsaw) and found cystic changes down the central stem in almost 50% of cases [80].

Within recent years specific asymetric glenoid implants have been introduced [6, 60, 81–85], which should reduce the high rate of glenoid loosening especially in significantly posterior eroded glenoids (Type B2, B3 and C according to Walch). Their mid- and long term benefit is currently unproven.

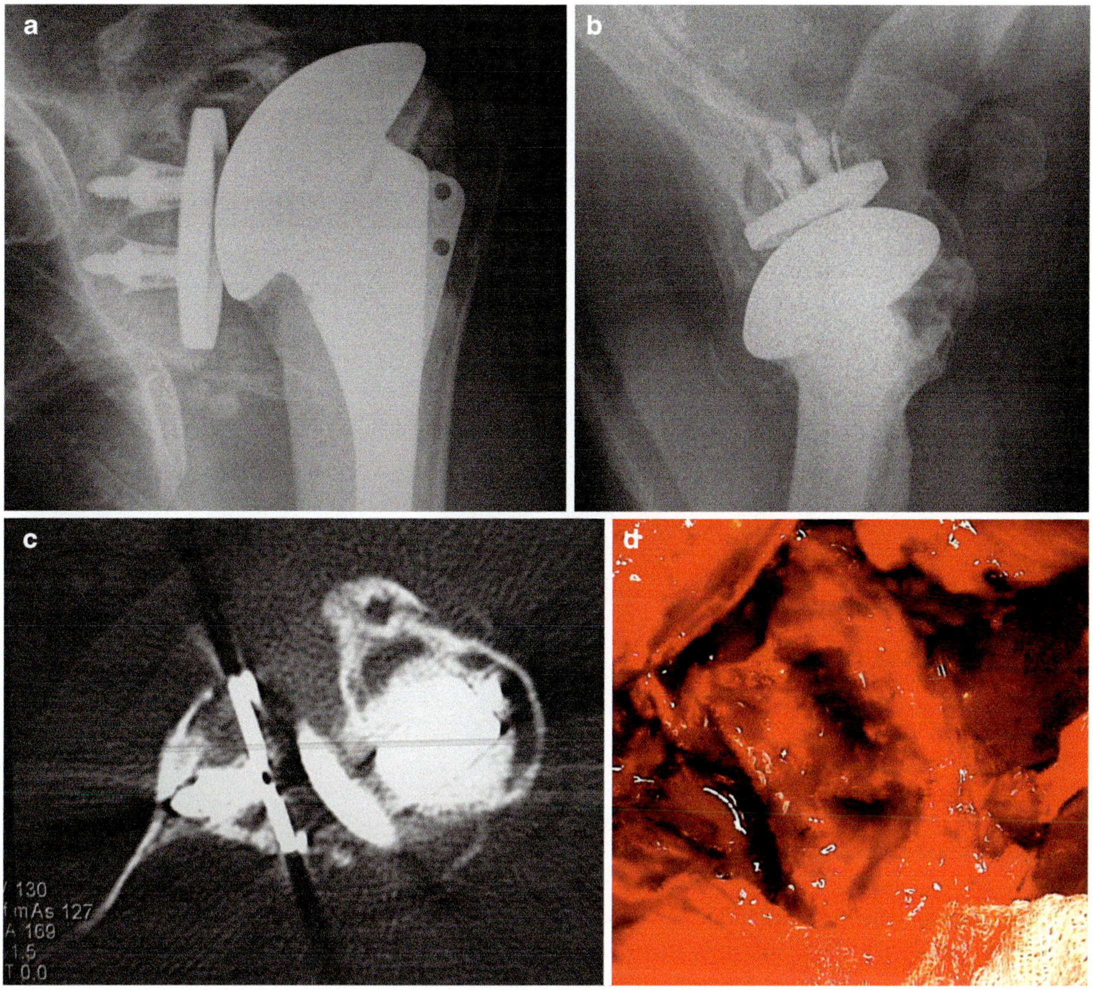

Fig. 16.2 Aseptic early loosening (3 years post) of a metal back glenoid. Revision to hemiarthroplasty with bone grafting of the cavitary glenoid defect. (**a**) ap-view (**b**) axillary view (**c**) CT-scan (**d**) intraop finding: advanced central osteolysis of the glenoid and thining and early destruction of the vault. In the CT-Scan the proximal Polyethylen-wear induced osteolysis at the lesser and greater tuberosity with a thinned cortical wall is also well visible. Intraop finding: advanced central osteolysis of the glenoid and thining and early destruction of the vault. In the CT-Scan the proximal Polyethylen-wear induced osteolysis at the lesser and greater tuberosity with a thinned cortical wall is also well visible (**e**) Revision to hemiarthroplasty by grafting the central defect by cancellous autograft. The cemented stem was well fixed despite beginning Polyethylen-wear induced proximal osteolysis (*) at the humerus

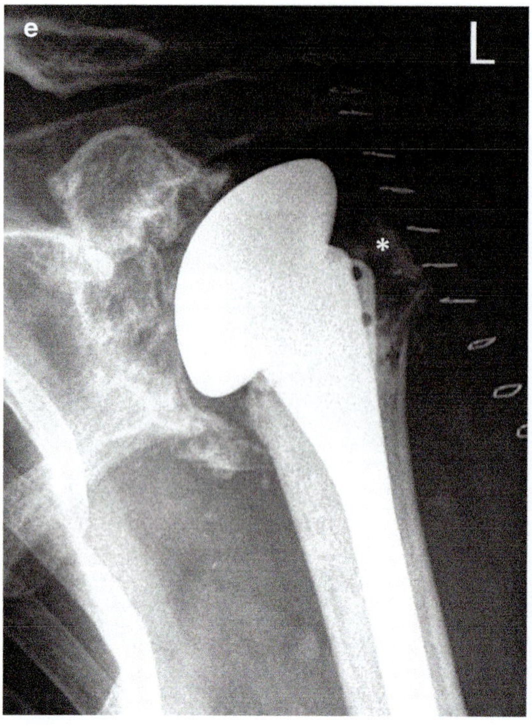

Fig. 16.2 (continued)

Glenoid Erosion

Treating an osteoarthritic shoulder by hemiarthroplasty yields up to 20% unsatisfactory results in the first postoperative years due to progressive eccentric glenoid erosion [47, 86–88]. Bohsali [4] found in his recent most comprehensive analysis on complications in shoulder arthroplasty that 22.6% of complications are related to glenoid wear (Fig. 16.3).

In careful selected cases with a concentric eburnised glenoid surface or a careful concentric reaming of an eccentric glenoid in a 5–10 year follow-up-study Wirth [48] didn't detect an increased rate of glenoid erosion. Similar results are reported by Lynch and Matsen [51, 89], who favoured a hemiarthroplasty for the majority of osteoarthritic patients. It seems therefore that satisfactory clinical and radiologic results can be sustained at least up to mid-term follow-up (Somerson) and that A2 and B2 type glenoids have the most clinical improvement without the influence of medialization [52, 53].

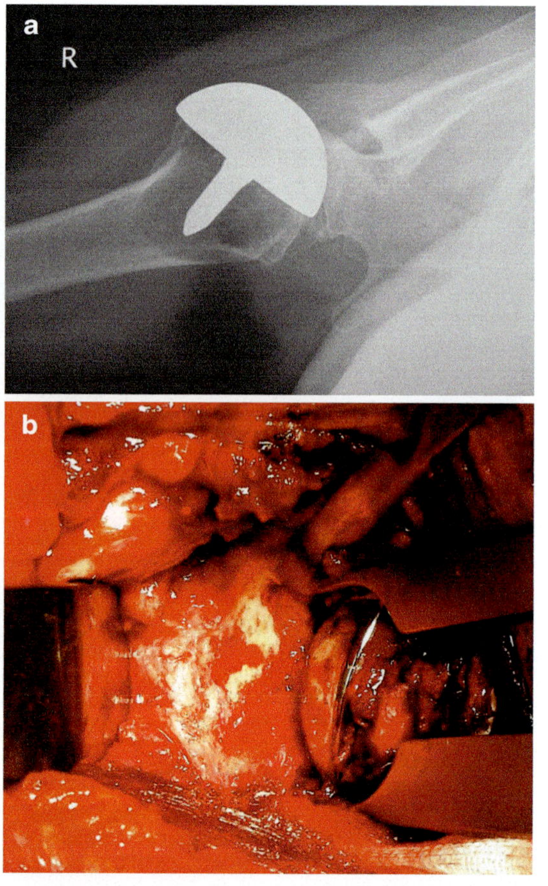

Fig. 16.3 Progressive posterior glenoid erosion and subluxation after Humeral Head Resurfacing hemiarthroplasty (**a**) x-noid erosion (B1 acc. Walch) (**b**) intraoperative finding with significant posterior cartilage and bony erosion

Contrary to the above studies, Herschel et al. reported a 29% moderate and 28% severe glenoid erosion rate at a mean follow-up period of 31 months (5–86 months). 7% of the patients had to be surgically revised (6x TSA, 2x RSA) because of the erosion within this midterm follow-up period. Negative predisposing factors for erosion were glenoid cysts (odds ratio, 5.4; $p < .001$, approximately 3 times more frequent in women), fatty infiltration of the rotator cuff musculature (R, 0.43; $p < .001$), and rheumatoid arthritis (odds ratio, 3.6; $p = .049$). A valgus position of the prosthetic humeral head relative to the glenoid (angle >50°) also appeared to be a negative predictive factor. Interestingly, only 1 patient (of 30) with a fracture-type prosthesis developed progressive glenoid erosion.

It seems, that favourable conditions for resistance to erosion after hemiarthroplasty were lack of glenoid cysts, intact glenoid cartilage, intact rotator cuff musculature, and when hemiarthropasty was performed for a humeral fracture. Interestingly, age, glenoid version, and the size of the prosthetic head seem to have no influence. Hemiarthroplasty should be avoided in conditions of glenoid erosion in female patients with impending osteoarthritis, in rheumatoid arthritis, and if the head is implanted in a valgus position.

Furthermore it seems, that hemiarthroplasty surface replacement develops a higher rate of painful glenoid erosions, with a rate of 20% occurring within the first 2 years postoperatively [90–93]. In midterm follow-up studies recently Verstraelen [94] in a small number (n = 37) reported a 44,6% incidence of radiologically significant glenoid erosion, although didn't identify the clinical impact of the erosion (pain, revision). Werner BS [95] et al. showed in their study with a mean 5 year follow-up period a rate of 37% painful glenoid erosion in patients treated with a surface replacement hemiarthroplasty. Painful glenoid erosion reduces functional outcomes and make revisions necessary in high percentage of cases.

Robinson [96] recently published a long-term study with a minimum 10-years follow-up on 44 patients with osteoarthritis treated with a surface replacement hemiarthroplasty. The rate of moderate to severe glenoid erosion increased from 50% at 5 years postop to 59% at 15 years and finally to 88% at 20 years.

Clinical Pearl
Glenoid associated complications whether it's loosening of the glenoid component, wear or breakage of the polyethylene or glenoid erosion in anatomic arthroplasty is responsible of more than then 50% of all complications in anatomic shoulder arthroplasty.

Instability and Rotator Cuff Failure

These problems stand for nearly 20% of all postoperative complications after anatomic shoulder arthroplasty. The reasons for instability are mainly rotator cuff failure, esp. subscapularis, and malpositioning of the component or significant bony glenoid deficiency (Fig. 16.4).

Early or midterm postoperative subscapularis failure is a major concern producing anterior or anterior-superior instability [97, 98]. The reasons for non-healing or failure of the subscapularis repair are numerous (poor fixation technique, poor tissue quality, excessive humeral head size, traumatic external rotation, inadequate postoperative rehabilitation, etc.). Discussions on subscapularis refixation are still going on without any clear answer2 [99, 100]. However it is obvious that a meticulous repair of the subscapularis over an appropriately anatomically sized humeral head in combination with careful postop regime is beneficial for avoiding this complication.

Posterior instability is rare and mostly caused by insufficient addressing of posterior glenoid bone erosion often in combination with malpositioning of the glenoid and/or humeral component.

The other question is, what impact preexisting rotator cuff lesions have on the postoperative outcome and secondary rotator cuff insufficiency.

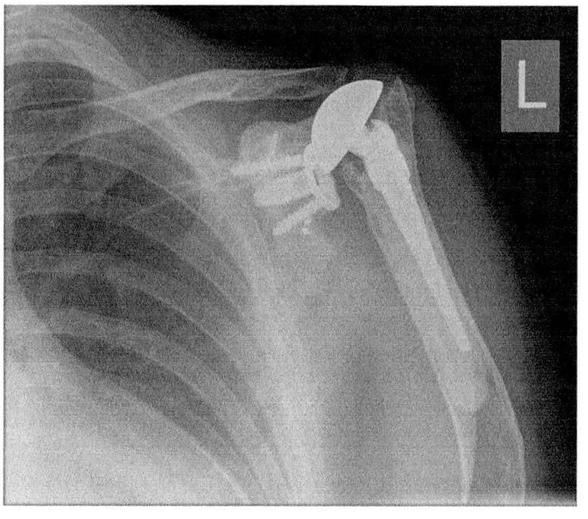

Fig. 16.4 Instability due to secondary cuff failure

In 2002 Godeneche et al. [101] and Edwards et al. [102, 103] 2002 and 2006 pointed out, that a global fatty degeneration index greater or equal to 1 are critical. Especially high degrees of fatty infiltration of the infraspinatus and subscapularis lead to complications and poorer results together with early postoperative rotator cuff failure and superior migration and subluxation with all the subsequent negative effects on the glenoid site (component loosening in TSA or superior glenoid erosion in HA). In a long-term study Young [104] reported similar findings.

In a recent study in 2017 Kany et al. [105] found out that the main reason for instability in unconstrained shoulder arthroplasty is soft tissue deficiency. In their study, they analyzed 27 shoulders with postoperative instability after anatomic shoulder arthroplasty within a decade (2003–2013). These represent an overall incidence of 5%. Most of these complications occurred early within 6 months of surgery (74%). Also, the majority had rotator cuff related reasons for their instability (subscapularis tear 37%, massive rotator cuff tear 22%). There was also hardware associated reasons in 41% of the cases (component malpositioning mostly glenoid 8, component dissociation or loosening 2, humeral shortening 1).

Rotator Cuff Failure

This is the fourth most frequent representing 9% of all complications. In longer follow-up studies this rate is even higher. Young's study [104] revealed a 17% incidence of rotator cuff dysfunction at a mean follow-up of 8.6 years. Preexisting infraspinatus tendon atrophy or fatty infiltration, glenoid malpositioning (superior tilt), inadequate component size (overstuffing) or unaddressed preexisting partial or small complete tears were the most responsible factors. Late-onset rotator cuff dysfunction with moderate or severe superior subluxation is observed after 10 years in 15% and after 15 years in 45% of total shoulder arthroplasties. In the same study, it was not observed at all after 5 years. This occurrence has a significant influence on the clinical and radiographic outcome of total shoulder arthroplasty performed for primary glenohumeral osteoarthritis. Prognostic factors seem to be preexisting fatty infiltration of the infraspinatus muscle and glenoid component positioning with superior tilt [104].

Acute subscapularis tears after anatomic shoulder arthroplasty mostly occur early but do represent a serious complication [106–111]. Without a well-functioning subscapularis, no satisfying clinical result can be expected with anatomic shoulder prosthesis. It has a decisive biomechanical importance in stabilizing the center of rotation of the joint in any phase of glenohumeral joint motion. It is the only anterior partner in the rotator cuff force couple counteracting the superior and anterior dislocation force of the deltoid and pectoralis. Typical symptoms are pain, internal rotational weakness, excessive external rotation with the arm at side, limited active forward flexion and abduction and anterior(superior) instability. Because of its deleterious character timely recognition of this complication is crucial. In the early postoperative period an acute rupture, if detected early can be repaired by a direct repositioning. If missed or in chronic failure situations, direct repair of the subscapularis tendon is rarely possible. Using the pectoralis major transfer as augmentation does not usually result in a satisfactory result [112–114].

Periprosthetic Fracture

Periprosthetic fractures are the fourth most common complication representing 7% of all complications and mainly occur (83%) intraoperatively (Fig. 16.5). The reported prevalence with shoulder arthroplasty is between 1.6% and 2.3% [4, 40, 115]. Main reasons for this complication are patient's inherent status including osteopenia, cortical thinning by osteolysis, but also excessive reaming of the diaphyseal cortex, malpositioning or inadequate size of the humeral component. This problem is more often observed in posttraumatic conditions and in stemmed arthroplasties rather than in stemless prostheses

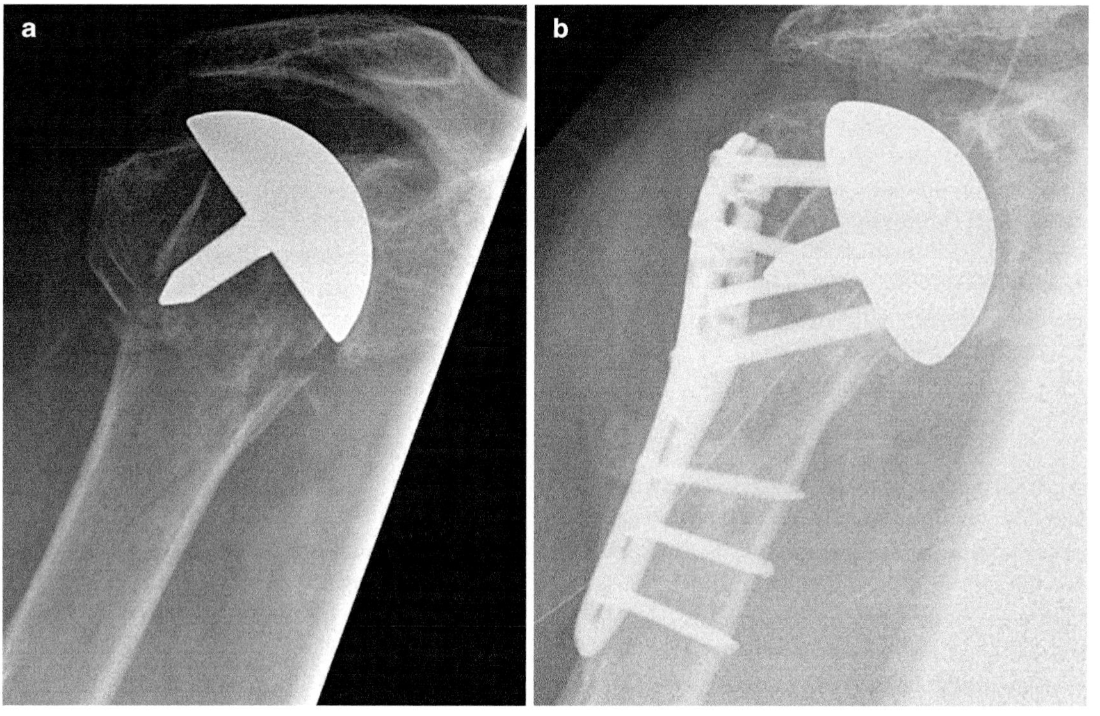

Fig. 16.5 Traumatic periprosthetic fracture (Type B) of a humeral head surface replacement hemiarthroplasty. (**a**) Unstable fracture with well fixed surface replacement component (**b**) treated by ORIF with a locking screw plate (Philos™)

or in surface replacement of the humeral head. It also seems that in the subgroup of postoperative fractures the stemmed anatomic arthroplasty seemed to be at a higher risk. The management of intra- and postoperative periprosthetic fractures are also more difficult and complicated with stemmed arthroplasty. The most frequently used classification was described by Wright and Cofield [116]. Type A fractures occur from the tip of the prosthesis proximally, Type B is at the tip without extension, and type C are extending from the tip distally. There is a modification of this classification by Campbell [117], which is more therapeutically oriented. To our knowledge Athwal G [118] published the largest series of intraoperative fractures with 45 cases. The most common were greater tuberosity fractures, followed by metaphyseal and diaphyseal fractures.

Periprosthetic glenoid fracture is an extremely rare condition in anatomic prosthesis.

Loosening of Humeral Component

Aseptic loosening of the humeral component is also a very rare complication, representing only 1.5% of all complications. It's generally observed in mid- and late follow-up periods. The risk of aseptic loosening is slightly higher with cemented implants. Plainly, however, removal of a well fixed or cemented stem can lead to significant intraoperative complications. Revision to a total shoulder replacement gives better results than to a hemiarthroplasty [119].

Neurologic Complication

Neurological problems following anatomic shoulder arthroplasty represents 6% of all complications; they occur typically intraoperatively or immediately postoperatively. Fortunately, most of these are transient in nature. Alternatively there are studies [120] which point out that neural injury after anatomic shoulder arthroplasty is more common than normally reported. In Nagda's study they carried out intraoperative nerve monitoring in 30 subsequent patients undergoing anatomic shoulder arthroplasty and found in 57% intraoperatively significant nerve alerts. In 23% neither release of retractors nor repositioning of the arm to neutral lead a return to normal nerve signals. In the postoperative follow-up after 1 month 13% still had a pathologic EMG. In an earlier study by Lynch et al. [121] the rate of neurologic complications was reported with an incidence of 4%.

It seems that iatrogenic nerve injury during shoulder arthroplasty is mainly generated by overdue tensioning and traction. Nerves seldom are injured by direct laceration or incorporation in suture repair. Thus in 2/3 of cases neurologic recovery should be expected within a year. Lädermann et al. [122] reported the prevalence of acute postoperative nerve injury was significantly more frequent following reverse shoulder arthroplasty group ($p = 0.002$), with a 10.9 times higher risk. In 23 anatomic shoulder arthroplasties, 1 patient (4.4%) presented with a persistent brachial plexus lesion. Neurologic damage to brachial plexus structure has a worse prognosis than peripheral nerve tractions injuries [123].

There is so far to my knowledge no study carried out, to distinguish between surgeon's related neurologic complications and nerve problems caused by interscalene indwelling catheter or blocks to facilitate anesthesia for intra- and postoperative pain management.

Infection

The infection rate in anatomic shoulder arthroplasty is significantly lower (0.51%) in comparison to RSA (2.9%). The reported incidence of periprosthetic infections appears to have reduced significantly within the last decade [124, 125, 128]. Bohsali [4] reported an incidence of 0.51% in 2017 compared to 0.7% 2006. The Mayo-group reported in their 1900 to 2000-decade series [5] an infection rate of 0.2% in contrast to their 1975 to 1989 series with an infection rate of 1.9% [124]. This infection rate represents obvious postoperative acute deep or superficial infections, mostly caused by pyogenic bacteria like Staph. Aureus, Pseudomonas, etc. The clinical symptoms of the acute infections with putrid effusion, sinus, drainage, erythema, fever, inflammed wounds etc. are obvious.

The incidence and prevalence of chronic low-grade infection is certainly much higher [55, 126]. Matsen [127, 128] reports positive cultures for Propionibacterium in up to two thirds of revisions of TSA. The Propionibacterium infection does not necessarily present with typical infection signs like erythema, swelling, effusion, fever etc. but sometimes with more subtle clinical symptoms like chronic pain, increasing stiffness, early component loosening etc. Unfortunately to date there is still no consensus on harvesting cultures, the number of cultures and the adequate reading and assessment of the results [57, 127, 129, 130]. Blood tests like WBC, sedimentation rate, CRP, Procalcitonin, IL-6, a-Defensin, etc. have significant less sensitivity and normal values do not necessarily exclude infection. Also, synovial fluid IL-6 or a-Defensin does not have high enough specificity. The only absolute test is multiple positive microbiological cultures taken from around the implant. In addition the level of granulocytes in synovial fluid can be helpful. A cell count of more than 2000/μl and/or a granulocyte content of more than 70% are highly predictive [131, 132]. Generally, however, in patients following shoulder arthroplasty who continue to complain of chronic pain, stiffness and reduced function, if all other causes including component malpositioning, soft tissue deficiency, etc. have been excluded, the presence of chronic low-grade infection should be strongly considered [56].

Early and late hematogenous infections are rare, but with an aging population and longer survival rates of last generations of anatomic shoulder arthroplasties there is an increasing risk of occurrence of late metastatic infection. In these cases, it is critical to detect the infection rapidly. If surgical revision is carried out within 3 weeks of onset of the symptom there is a good chance of resolving the problem by surgical debridement, lavage and exchange of not osseous fixed components without removal of the entire prostheses [132].

Hemi Versus Total: Procedure Related Major General Complications

Numerous publication within the last decade have proven, that total shoulder arthroplasties (TSA) yield superior results compared to humeral head replacement (hemiarthroplasty = HA) alone. Conversely, however, there were less intraoperative complications, less operation time and less intraoperative blood loss reported with HA. In a high-volume retrospective study on the survey database of the National Surgical Quality Improvement Program (NSQIP) it was shown, that the rate for all types of perioperative major general complications is the same for TSA as with HA. For example, the transfusion rate is in HA (2.3%) and in TSA 2.9% ($p = .458$). The multivariate analysis in the NSQIP database suggests that patient factors and not the procedure being performed are significant predictors of major complications [133].

Chalmers et al. [134] hypothesized that age, BMI and comorbidity index have a significant influence on the early (minimum 90 day follow-up) postoperative perioperative complication rate after TSA. They found an overall complication of 9.4%, within 3.1% surgical and 6.3% medical complications. Perhaps because their small sample size ($n = 127$) they could not rule out age and BMI as a predictor although significantly the CCI (Charleson Comorbidity Index) impacted on the perioperative complication probability.

In another study [135] also using a high volume nationwide database in the U.S.A. (Nationwide Inpatient Database), comparing perioperative complications between anatomic and reverse total shoulder arthroplasty (RSA) concluded that RSA has a significantly longer length of stay, higher hospital charges that are not completely attributable to increased implant costs alone and increased rates of perioperative complications (blood transfusion, pneumonia, DVT).

Other Complications

Complications like hematoma, deltoid injury or dvt are rarely reported and overall they count of less than 1% of all complications.

Summary

To improve the outcome of anatomic shoulder arthroplasty and avoid complications and revisions due to surgical errors, wrong indications or inappropriate implants it is important to understand the reasons, incidence, probability and time point of occurrence of the most specific shoulder specific complications. Probably glenoid related complications (early, late loosening, glenoid erosion) could be improved by a better understanding, when to do a hemi or a total arthroplasty and when reverse prosthesis would be a better choice rather than an anatomic one. Etiology (atraumatic – traumatic; degenerative – inflammatory), bone quality and defects, rotator cuff herein are decisive factors. Nevertheless, the glenoid will stay the weak link in anatomic shoulder arthroplasty and will be the most common complication. However it is also necessary to understand the importance of the general health of the patient in relation to shoulder specific or general complications. This may be useful for predicting the likelihood of surgical complications and may thus prove important for clinicians to better assess and explain possible risks before surgery. "It is more important to know what patient the disease has than what disease the patient has." (William Osler) [136].

References

1. Gregory T, Hansen U, Emery RJ, Augereau B, Amis AA. Developments in shoulder arthroplasty. Proc Inst Mech Eng H. 2007;221(1):87–96. https://doi.org/10.1243/09544119JEIM167.

2. Wirth MA, Rockwood CA Jr. Complications of shoulder arthroplasty. [Review]. Clin Orthop Relat Res. 1994;307:47–69.
3. Bohsali KI, Wirth MA, Rockwood CA. Complications of total shoulder arthroplasty. J Bone Joint Surg Am. 2006;88:45–9.
4. Bohsali KI, Bois AJ, Wirth MA. Complications of shoulder arthroplasty. [Review]. J Bone Joint Surg Am. 2017;99:256–69.
5. Chin PYK, Sperling JW, Cofield RH, Schleck C. Complications of total shoulder arthroplasty: are they fewer or different? 2006;55902:19–22. https://doi.org/10.1016/j.jse.2005.05.005.
6. Chin PC, Hachadorian ME, Pulido PA, Munro ML, Meric G, Hoenecke HR. Outcomes of anatomic shoulder arthroplasty in primary osteoarthritis in type B glenoids. J Shoulder Elb Surg. 2015;24(12):1888–93. https://doi.org/10.1016/j.jse.2015.05.052.
7. Favard L, Katz D, Colmar M, Benkalfate T, Thomazeau H, Emily S. Total shoulder arthroplasty – arthroplasty for glenohumeral arthropathies: results and complications after a minimum follow-up of 8 years according to the type of arthroplasty and etiology. Orthop Traumatol Surg Res. 2012;98(4 SUPPL):S41–7. https://doi.org/10.1016/j.otsr.2012.04.003.
8. Wirth MA, Rockwood CA Jr. Complications of shoulder arthroplasty. Clin Orthop Relat Res. 1994;307:47–69. https://doi.org/10.2106/JBJS.F.00125.
9. Denard PJ, Raiss P, Sowa B, Walch G. Mid- to long-term follow-up of total shoulder arthroplasty using a keeled glenoid in young adults with primary glenohumeral arthritis. J Shoulder Elb Surg. 2013;22(7):894–900. https://doi.org/10.1016/j.jse.2012.09.016.
10. Raiss P, Schmitt M, Bruckner T, et al. Results of cemented total shoulder replacement with a minimum follow-up of ten years. J Bone Joint Surg Am. 2012;94(23):e1711–0. https://doi.org/10.2106/JBJS.K.00580.
11. Raiss P, Bruckner T, Rickert M, Walch G. Longitudinal observational study of Total shoulder replacement with cement. J Bone Joint Surg Am. 2014;96(3):198–205. https://doi.org/10.2106/JBJS.M.00079.
12. Favard L, Katz D, Colmar M, Benkalfate T, Thomazeau H, Emily S. Total shoulder arthroplasty - arthroplasty for glenohumeral arthropathies: results and complications after a minimum follow-up of 8years according to the type of arthroplasty and etiology. Orthop Traumatol Surg Res. 2012;98(4 SUPPL):S41–7. https://doi.org/10.1016/j.otsr.2012.04.003.
13. Raiss P, Edwards TB, Deutsch A, et al. Radiographic changes around humeral components in shoulder arthroplasty. J Bone Joint Surg Am. 2014;96(e54):1–9.
14. Li X, Veltre DR, Cusano A, et al. Insurance status affects postoperative morbidity and complication rate after shoulder arthroplasty. J Shoulder Elb Surg. 2017;26(8):1423–31. https://doi.org/10.1016/j.jse.2016.12.071.
15. Leschinger T, Raiss P, Loew M, Zeifang F. Total shoulder arthroplasty: risk factors for intra-operative and postoperative complications in patients with primary arthritis. J Shoulder Elb Surg. 2017;26(3):e71–7. https://doi.org/10.1016/j.jse.2016.08.001.
16. Wagner ER, Houdek MT, Schleck CD, et al. The role age plays in the outcomes and complications of shoulder arthroplasty. J Shoulder Elb Surg. 2017;26(9):1573–80. https://doi.org/10.1016/j.jse.2017.01.020.
17. Ponce BA, Menendez ME, Oladeji LO, Soldado F. Diabetes as a risk factor for poorer early post-operative outcomes after shoulder arthroplasty. J Shoulder Elb Surg. 2014;23(5):671–8. https://doi.org/10.1016/j.jse.2014.01.046.
18. Anakwenze O, Fokin A, Chocas M, et al. Complications in total shoulder and reverse total shoulder arthroplasty by body mass index. J Shoulder Elb Surg. 2017;26(7):1230–7. https://doi.org/10.1016/j.jse.2016.11.055.
19. Wagner ER, Houdek MT, Schleck C, et al. Increasing body mass index is associated with worse outcomes after shoulder arthroplasty. J Bone Joint Surg. 2017;99(11):929–37. https://doi.org/10.2106/JBJS.15.00255.
20. Hatta T, Werthel J-D, Wagner ER, et al. Effect of smoking on complications following primary shoulder arthroplasty. J Shoulder Elb Surg. 2017;26(1):1–6. https://doi.org/10.1016/j.jse.2016.09.011.
21. Ponce BA, Oladeji LO, Raley JA, Menendez ME. Analysis of perioperative morbidity and mortality in shoulder arthroplasty patients with preexisting alcohol use disorders. J Shoulder Elb Surg. 2015;24(2):167–73. https://doi.org/10.1016/j.jse.2014.05.019.
22. Grier AJ, Bala A, Penrose CT, Seyler TM, Bolognesi MP, Garrigues GE. Analysis of complication rates following perioperative transfusion in shoulder arthroplasty. J Shoulder Elb Surg. 2017;26(7):1203–9. https://doi.org/10.1016/j.jse.2016.11.039.
23. Cancienne JM, Dempsey IJ, Holzgrefe RE, Brockmeier SF, Werner BC. Is Hepatitis C infection associated with a higher risk of complications after total shoulder arthroplasty? Clin Orthop Relat Res. 2016;474(12):2664–9. https://doi.org/10.1007/s11999-016-4979-9.
24. Gonzalez JF, Alami GB, Baque F, Walch G, Boileau P. Complications of unconstrained shoulder prostheses. J Shoulder Elb Surg. 2011;20(4):666–82. https://doi.org/10.1016/j.jse.2010.11.017.
25. Boileau P, Trojani C, Walch G, Krishnan SG, Romeo A, Sinnerton R. Shoulder arthroplasty for the treatment of the sequelae of fractures of the proximal humerus. J Shoulder Elbow Surg. 2001;10:299–308. https://doi.org/10.1067/mse.2001.115985.

26. Edwards TB, Kadakia NR, Boulahia A, et al. A comparison of hemiarthroplasty and total shoulder arthroplasty in the treatment of primary glenohumeral osteoarthritis: results of a multicenter study. J Shoulder Elb Surg. 2003;12(3):207–13. https://doi.org/10.1016/mse.2003.S1058274602868045\rS1058274602868045. [pii]
27. Boileau P, Baba M, Moineau G, et al. Response to Katz et al: the weak link in metal-backed glenoid implants is the polyethylene. J Shoulder Elb Surg. 2016;25(12):e396–8. https://doi.org/10.1016/j.jse.2016.08.010.
28. Moineau G, McBoileau P. Prognostic factors and limitations of anatomic shoulder arthroplasty for the treatment of posttraumatic cephalic collapse or necrosis. J Bone Joint Surg Am. 2012;94:2186–94.
29. Uschok S, Magosch P, Moe M, Lichtenberg S, Habermeyer P. Is the stemless humeral head replacement clinically and radiographically a secure equivalent to standard stem humeral head replacement in the long-term follow-up ? A prospective randomized trial. J Shoulder Elb Surg. 2017;26(2):225–32. https://doi.org/10.1016/j.jse.2016.09.001.
30. Habermeyer P, Lichtenberg S, Tauber M, Magosch P. Midterm results of stemless shoulder arthroplasty : a prospective study. J Shoulder Elb Surg. 2015;24(9):1463–72. https://doi.org/10.1016/j.jse.2015.02.023.
31. Kadum B, Mukka S, Englund E. Clinical and radiological outcome of the Total Evolutive Shoulder System (TESS ®) reverse shoulder arthroplasty : a prospective comparative non-randomised study. 2014. https://doi.org/10.1007/s00264-013-2277-7.
32. Teissier P, Teissier J, Kouyoumdjian P, Asencio GG. The TESS reverse shoulder arthroplasty without a stem in the treatment of cuff-deficient shoulder conditions: clinical and radiographic results. J Shoulder Elb Surg. 2015;24(1):45–51. https://doi.org/10.1016/j.jse.2014.04.005.
33. Schmidutz F, Agarwal Y, Müller PE, Gueorguiev B, Richards RG, Sprecher CM. Stress-shielding induced bone remodeling in cementless shoulder resurfacing arthroplasty: a finite element analysis and in vivo results. J Biomech. 2014;47(14):3509–16. https://doi.org/10.1016/j.jbiomech.2014.08.029.
34. Bell SN, Coghlan JA. Short stem shoulder replacement. Int J Shoulder Surg. 2014;8(3):72–5. https://doi.org/10.4103/0973-6042.140113.
35. Churchill RS. Stemless shoulder arthroplasty : current status. J Shoulder Elb Surg. 2014;23(9):1409–14. https://doi.org/10.1016/j.jse.2014.05.005.
36. Churchill RS, Athwal GS. Stemless shoulder arthroplasty—current results and designs. Curr Rev Musculoskelet Med. 2016;9(1):10–6. https://doi.org/10.1007/s12178-016-9320-4.
37. Churchill RS. Stemless shoulder arthroplasty : current status. J Shoulder Elb Surg. 2017;23(9):1409–14. https://doi.org/10.1016/j.jse.2014.05.005.
38. Fevang BTS, Nystad TW, Skredderstuen A, Furnes ON, Havelin LI. Improved survival for anatomic total shoulder prostheses. Acta Orthop. 2015;86(1):63–70. https://doi.org/10.3109/17453674.2014.984113.
39. Sperling JW, Hawkins RJ, Walch G, Zuckerman J. Complication in total shoulder arthroplasty. J Bone Joint Surg Am. 2013;62(March 2013):428–35.
40. Herschel R, Wieser K, Morrey ME, Ramos CH, Gerber C, Meyer DC. Risk factors for glenoid erosion in patients with shoulder hemiarthroplasty: an analysis of 118 cases. J Shoulder Elb Surg. 2017;26(2):246–52. https://doi.org/10.1016/j.jse.2016.06.004.
41. Berhouet J, Garaud P, Favard L. Influence of glenoid component design and humeral component retroversion on internal and external rotation in reverse shoulder arthroplasty: a cadaver study. Orthop Traumatol Surg Res. 2013;99(8):887–94. https://doi.org/10.1016/j.otsr.2013.08.008.
42. Clitherow HDS, Frampton CMA, Astley TM. Effect of glenoid cementation on total shoulder arthroplasty for degenerative arthritis of the shoulder: a review of the new Zealand National Joint Registry. J Shoulder Elb Surg. 2014;23(6):775–81. https://doi.org/10.1016/j.jse.2013.08.022.
43. Vuillermin CB, Trump ME, Barwood SA, Hoy GA. Catastrophic failure of a low profile metal-backed glenoid component after total shoulder arthroplasty. Int J Shoulder Surg. 2015;9(4):121–7. https://doi.org/10.4103/0973-6042.167952.
44. Gadea F, Alami G, Pape G, Boileau P, Favard L. Shoulder hemiarthroplasty: outcomes and long-term survival analysis according to etiology. Orthop Traumatol Surg Res. 2012;98(6):659–65. https://doi.org/10.1016/j.otsr.2012.03.020.
45. Boileau P, Avidor C, Krishnan SG, Walch G, Kempf JF, Molé D. Cemented polyethylene versus uncemented metal-backed glenoid components in total shoulder arthroplasty: a prospective, double-blind, randomized study. J Shoulder Elb Surg. 2002;11(4):351–9. https://doi.org/10.1067/mse.2002.125807.
46. Boileau P, Moineau G, Morin-Salvo N, et al. Metal-backed glenoid implant with polyethylene insert is not a viable long-term therapeutic option. J Shoulder Elb Surg. 2015;24(10):1534–43. https://doi.org/10.1016/j.jse.2015.02.012.
47. Herschel R, Wieser K, Morrey ME, Ramos CH, Gerber C, Meyer DC. Risk factors for glenoid erosion in patients with shoulder hemiarthroplasty: an analysis of 118 cases. J Shoulder Elb Surg. 2016;26:1–7. https://doi.org/10.1016/j.jse.2016.06.004.
48. Wirth MA, Tapscott RS, Southworth C, Rockwood CA. Treatment of glenohumeral arthritis with a hemiarthroplasty: a minimum five-year follow-up outcome study. J Bone Joint Surg Am. 2006;88(5):964–73. https://doi.org/10.2106/JBJS.D.03030.
49. Denard BPJ, Wirth MA, Orfaly RM, et al. Management of glenohumeral arthritis in the young adult. J Bone Joint Surg Am. 2011;93(9):885–92. https://doi.org/10.2106/JBJS.J.00960.

50. Matsen FA, Warme WJ, Jackins SE. Can the ream and run procedure improve Glenohumeral relationships and function for shoulders with the arthritic triad? Clin Orthop Relat Res. 2015;473(6):2088–96. https://doi.org/10.1007/s11999-014-4095-7.
51. Matsen FA. The ream and run: not for every patient, every surgeon or every problem. Int Orthop. 2015;39(2):255–61. https://doi.org/10.1007/s00264-014-2641-2.
52. Somerson JS, Neradilek MB, Service BC, Hsu JE, Russ SM, Matsen FA. Clinical and radiographic outcomes of the ream-and-run procedure for primary Glenohumeral arthritis. J Bone Joint Surg Am. 2017;99(15):1291–304. https://doi.org/10.2106/JBJS.16.01201.
53. Somerson JS, MIIIF A. Functional Outcomes of the Ream-and-Run Shoulder Arthroplasty A Concise Follow-up of a Previous Report. J Bone Joint Surg Am. 2017;99:1999–2003. https://doi.org/10.2106/JBJS.17.00201.
54. Barlow JD, Yuan BJ, Schleck CD, Harmsen WS, Cofield RH, Sperling JW. Shoulder arthroplasty for rheumatoid arthritis: 303 consecutive cases with minimum 5-year follow-up. J Shoulder Elb Surg. 2014;23(6):791–9. https://doi.org/10.1016/j.jse.2013.09.016.
55. Franta AK, Lenters TR, Mounce D, Neradilek B, Matsen FA. The complex characteristics of 282 unsatisfactory shoulder arthroplasties. J Shoulder Elbow Surg:555–62. https://doi.org/10.1016/j.jse.2006.11.004.
56. Hsu JE, Somerson JS, Vo KV, Matsen FA. What is a "periprosthetic shoulder infection"? A systematic review of two decades of publications. Int Orthop. 2017;41(4):813–22. https://doi.org/10.1007/s00264-017-3421-6.
57. Lucas RM, Hsu JE, Whitney IJ, Wasserburger J, Matsen FA. Loose glenoid components in revision shoulder arthroplasty: is there an association with positive cultures? J Shoulder Elb Surg. 2016;25(8):1371–5. https://doi.org/10.1016/j.jse.2015.12.026.
58. Walch G, Moraga C, Young A, Castellanos-rosas J. Results of anatomic nonconstrained prosthesis in primary osteoarthritis with biconcave glenoid. J Shoulder Elb Surg. 2012;21(11):1526–33. https://doi.org/10.1016/j.jse.2011.11.030.
59. Hsu JE, Ricchetti ET, Huffman GR, Iannotti JP, Glaser DL. Addressing glenoid bone deficiency and asymmetric posterior erosion in shoulder arthroplasty. J Shoulder Elb Surg. 2013;22(9):1298–308. https://doi.org/10.1016/j.jse.2013.04.014.
60. Sabesan V, Callanan M, Ho J, Iannotti JP. Clinical and radiographic outcomes of total shoulder arthroplasty with bone graft for osteoarthritis with severe glenoid bone loss. J Bone Joint Surg Am. 2013;95:1290–6. https://doi.org/10.2106/JBJS.L.00097.
61. Phipatanakul WP, Norris TR, Linda L, Francisco S. Treatment of glenoid loosening and bone loss due to osteolysis with glenoid bone grafting. J Shoulder Elbow Surg. 2006:84–7. https://doi.org/10.1016/j.jse.2005.06.004.
62. Elkinson I, Giles JW, Boons HW, et al. The shoulder remplissage procedure for hill-Sachs defects : does technique matter ? J Shoulder Elb Surg. 2013;22(6):835–41. https://doi.org/10.1016/j.jse.2012.08.015.
63. Montoya F, Magosch P, Scheiderer B, Lichtenberg S, Melean P, Habermeyer P. Midterm results of a total shoulder prosthesis fixed with a cementless glenoid component. J Shoulder Elb Surg. 2013;22(5):628–35. https://doi.org/10.1016/j.jse.2012.07.005.
64. Fucentese SF, Costouros JG, Ku S, Gerber C. Total shoulder arthroplasty with an uncemented soft-metal-backed glenoid component. J Shoulder Elbow Surg. 2010;19:624–31. https://doi.org/10.1016/j.jse.2009.12.021.
65. Ho JC, Sabesan VJ, Iannotti JP. Glenoid component retroversion is associated with osteolysis. J Bone Joint Surg Am. 2013;82:1–8.
66. Betts HM, Abu-Rajab R, Nunn T, Brooksbank AJ. Total shoulder replacement in rheumatoid disease: a 16- to 23-year follow-up. J Bone Joint Surg Br. 2009;91(9):1197–200. https://doi.org/10.1302/0301-620X.91B9.22035.
67. Clement ND, Mathur K, Colling R, Stirrat AN. The metal-backed glenoid component in rheumatoid disease: eight- to fourteen-year follow-up. J Shoulder Elb Surg. 2010;19(5):749–56. https://doi.org/10.1016/j.jse.2009.11.005.
68. Castagna A, Randelli M, Garofalo R, Maradei L, Giardella A, Borroni M. Mid-term results of a metal-backed glenoid component in total shoulder replacement. J Bone Joint Surg Br. 2010;92-B(10):1410–5. https://doi.org/10.1302/0301-620X.92B10.23578.
69. Clement ND, Duckworth AD, Colling RC, Stirrat AN. An uncemented metal-backed glenoid component in total shoulder arthroplasty for osteoarthritis: factors affecting survival and outcome. J Orthop Sci. 2013;18(1):22–8. https://doi.org/10.1007/s00776-012-0308-7.
70. Taunton MJ, McIntosh AL, Sperling JW, Cofield RH. Total Shoulder Arthroplasty with a Metal-Backed, Bone-Ingrowth Glenoid Component. J Bone Joint Surg Am. 2008;90:2180–8. https://doi.org/10.2106/JBJS.G.00966.
71. Papadonikolakis A, Fa M. Metal-Backed glenoid components have a higher. J Bone Joint Surg Am. 2014;96:1041–7. https://doi.org/10.1016/S0021-9355(14)74242-0.
72. Bonnevialle N, Melis B, Neyton L, et al. Aseptic glenoid loosening or failure in total shoulder arthroplasty: revision with glenoid reimplantation. J Shoulder Elb Surg. 2013;22(6):745–51. https://doi.org/10.1016/j.jse.2012.08.009.
73. Fucentese SF, Costouros JG, Kühnel SP, Gerber C. Total shoulder arthroplasty with an uncemented soft-metal-backed glenoid component. J Shoulder Elb Surg. 2010;19(4):624–31. https://doi.org/10.1016/j.jse.2009.12.021.

74. Gerber C, Costouros JG, Sukthankar A, Fucentese SF. Static posterior humeral head subluxation and total shoulder arthroplasty. J Shoulder Elb Surg. 2009;18(4):505–10. https://doi.org/10.1016/j.jse.2009.03.003.
75. Anglin C, Wyss UP, Pichora DR. Proceedings of the Institution of Mechanical Engineers Part H. J Eng Med. 2000;214:637–44. https://doi.org/10.1243/0954411001535660.
76. Nyffeler RW, Anglin C, Sheikh R, Gerber C. Influence of peg design and cement mantle thickness on pull-out strength of glenoid component pegs. J Bone Joint Surg Br. 2003;85-B:748–52. https://doi.org/10.1302/0301-620X.85B5.12580.
77. Nuttall D, Haines JF, Trail IA. A study of the micromovment of pegged and keeled glenoid components compared using radio Stereometric analysis. J Shoulder Elb Surg. 2007;16(3 Suppl):S65–70. https://doi.org/10.1016/j.jse.2006.01.015.
78. Khazzam M, Argo M, Landrum M, Box H. Comparison of pegged and keeled glenoid components for total shoulder arthroplasty. J Shoulder Elbow Arthroplast. 2017;1:247154921770532. https://doi.org/10.1177/2471549217705323.
79. De Wilde L, Dayerizadeh N, De Neve F, Basamania C, Van Tongel A. Fully uncemented glenoid component in total shoulder arthroplasty. J Shoulder Elb Surg. 2013;22(10):e1–7. https://doi.org/10.1016/j.jse.2013.01.036.
80. Nuttall D, Haines JF, Trail IA. The early migration of a partially cemented fluted pegged glenoid component using radiostereometric analysis. J Shoulder Elb Surg. 2012;21(9):1191–6. https://doi.org/10.1016/j.jse.2011.07.028.
81. Sabesan V, Callanan M, Sharma V, Iannotti JP. Correction of acquired glenoid bone loss in osteoarthritis with a standard versus an augmented glenoid component. J Shoulder Elb Surg. 2014;23(7):964–73. https://doi.org/10.1016/j.jse.2013.09.019.
82. Knowles NK, Ferreira LM, Athwal GS. Augmented glenoid component designs for type B2 erosions: a computational comparison by volume of bone removal and quality of remaining bone. J Shoulder Elb Surg. 2015;24(8):1218–26. https://doi.org/10.1016/j.jse.2014.12.018.
83. Lenart BA, Namdari S, Williams GR. Total shoulder arthroplasty with an augmented component for anterior glenoid bone deficiency. J Shoulder Elb Surg. 2015;25:1–8. https://doi.org/10.1016/j.jse.2015.08.012.
84. Hermida JC, Flores-Hernandez C, Hoenecke HR, D'Lima DD. Augmented wedge-shaped glenoid component for the correction of glenoid retroversion: a finite element analysis. J Shoulder Elb Surg. 2014;23(3):347–54. https://doi.org/10.1016/j.jse.2013.06.008.
85. Jones RB, Wright TW, Roche CP. Bone grafting the glenoid versus use of augmented glenoid baseplates with reverse shoulder arthroplasty. Bull Hosp Jt Dis. 2015;73(1):129–35. Available at: http://www.ncbi.nlm.nih.gov/pubmed/26631209.
86. Puskas GJ, Meyer DC, Lebschi JA, Gerber C. Unacceptable failure of hemiarthroplasty combined with biological glenoid resurfacing in the treatment of glenohumeral arthritis in the young. J Shoulder Elb Surg. 2015;24(12):1900–7. https://doi.org/10.1016/j.jse.2015.05.037.
87. Sandow MJ, David H, Orth MCH, Bentall SJ. Hemiarthroplasty vs total shoulder replacement for rotator cuff intact osteoarthritis : how do they fare after a decade ? J Shoulder Elb Surg. 2013;22(7):877–85. https://doi.org/10.1016/j.jse.2012.10.023.
88. Sperling JW, Cofield RH, Schleck CD, Harmsen WS. Total shoulder arthroplasty versus hemiarthroplasty for rheumatoid arthritis of the shoulder: results of 303 consecutive cases. J Shoulder Elb Surg. 2007;16(6):683–90. https://doi.org/10.1016/j.jse.2007.02.135.
89. Lynch BJR, Franta AK, Jr WHM, Lenters TR, Mounce D, Iii FAM. Shoulder hemiarthroplasty with concentric glenoid reaming. J Bone Joint Surg Am. 2007;89(6):1284–92. https://doi.org/10.2106/JBJS.E.00942.
90. Mansat P, Coutié AS, Bonnevialle N, Rongières M, Mansat M, Bonnevialle P. Resurfacing humeral prosthesis: do we really reconstruct the anatomy? J Shoulder Elb Surg. 2013;22(5):612–9. https://doi.org/10.1016/j.jse.2012.07.014.
91. Thomas SR, Wilson AJ, Chambler A, Harding I, Thomas M. Outcome of Copeland surface replacement shoulder arthroplasty. J Shoulder Elb Surg. 2005;14(5):485–91. https://doi.org/10.1016/j.jse.2005.02.011.
92. Al-Hadithy N, Domos P, Sewell MD, Naleem A, Papanna MC, Pandit R. Cementless surface replacement arthroplasty of the shoulder for osteoarthritis: results of fifty Mark III Copeland prosthesis from an independent center with four-year mean follow-up. J Shoulder Elb Surg. 2012;21(12):1776–81. https://doi.org/10.1016/j.jse.2012.01.024.
93. Raiss P, Pape G, Becker S, Rickert M, Loew M. Der zementfreie oberflächenersatz des humeruskopfes bei patienten unter 55 jahren. Orthopade. 2010;39(2):201–8. https://doi.org/10.1007/s00132-009-1525-4.
94. Verstraelen FU, Horta LA, Schotanus MGM, Kort NP, Samijo SK, Jansen EJP. Clinical and radiological results 7 years after Copeland shoulder resurfacing arthroplasty in patients with primary glenohumeral osteoarthritis: an independent multicentre retrospective study. Eur J Orthop Surg Traumatol. 2017;19(1):1–8. https://doi.org/10.1007/s00590-017-2023-8.
95. Werner BS, Stehle J, Abdelkawi A, Plumhoff P, Hudek R, Gohlke F. Progressive glenoid bone loss caused by erosion in humeral head resurfacing. Orthopade. 2017:1028–33. https://doi.org/10.1007/s00132-017-3483-6.
96. Robinson WA, Wagner ER, Cofield R, Sanchez-Sotelo J, Sperling JW. Long-term outcomes of humeral head replacement for the treatment of osteoarthritis; a report of 44 arthroplasties with minimum

10-year follow-up. J Shoulder Elbow Surg. 2017. https://doi.org/10.1016/j.jse.2017.10.017.
97. Gerber C, Yian EH, CAW P, Zumstein MA. Subscapularis muscle function and structure after total shoulder replacement with lesser tuberosity osteotomy and repair. J Bone Joint Surg Am. 2006;87:1739. https://doi.org/10.2106/JBJS.D.02788.
98. Nyffeler RW, Meyer D, Sheikh R, Koller BJ, Gerber C. The effect of cementing technique on structural fixation of pegged glenoid components in total shoulder arthroplasty. J Shoulder Elbow Surg. 15(1):106–11. https://doi.org/10.1016/j.jse.2005.05.002.
99. Gerber C, Yian E, Pfirrmann C, Zumstein M, Werner C. Subscapularis function and structure after total shoulder replacement with lesser tuberosity osteotomy and repair. J Bone Joint Surg Am. 2005;87:1739–45. https://doi.org/10.2106/JBJS.D.02788.
100. Van Den BGR, Nguyen B, Patil S, et al. A biomechanical evaluation of three surgical techniques for subscapularis repair. J Shoulder Elbow Surg. 17(1):156–61. https://doi.org/10.1016/j.jse.2007.04.016.
101. Godenèche A, Boileau P, Favard L, et al. Prosthetic replacement in the treatment of osteoarthritis of the shoulder: Early results of 268 cases. J Shoulder Elbow Surg. 2002:11–8. https://doi.org/10.1067/mse.2002.120140.
102. Edwards T, Boulahia A, Kempf J, Boilau P, Nemoz C, Walch G. The influence of rotator cuff disease on the results of shoulder arthroplasty for primary osteoarthritis. J Bone Joint Surg Am. 2002;84:2240–8.
103. Edwards TB, Boulahia A, Kempf J, et al. The influence of rotator cuff disease on the results of shoulder arthroplasty for primary osteoarthritis. J Bone Joint Surg Am. 2006;88(10):2279–92.
104. Young A, Walch G, Pape G, Gohlke F, Favard L. Secondary rotator cuff dysfunction following Total shoulder arthroplasty for primary glenohumeral osteoarthritis : results of a multicenter study with more than five years of follow-up. J Bone Joint Surg Am. 2012;94:685–93. https://doi.org/10.2106/JBJS.J.00727.
105. Kany J, Jose J, Katz D, et al. The main cause of instability after unconstrained shoulder prosthesis is soft tissue deficiency. J Shoulder Elb Surg. 2017;26(8):e243–51. https://doi.org/10.1016/j.jse.2017.01.019.
106. Shields E, Ho A, Wiater JM. Management of the subscapularis tendon during total shoulder arthroplasty. J Shoulder Elb Surg. 2017;26(4):723–31. https://doi.org/10.1016/j.jse.2016.11.006.
107. Gobezie R, Denard PJ, Shishani Y, Romeo AA, Lederman E. Healing and functional outcome of a subscapularis peel repair with a stem-based repair after total shoulder arthroplasty. J Shoulder Elb Surg. 2017;26(9):1603–8. https://doi.org/10.1016/j.jse.2017.02.013.
108. Lapner PLC, Sabri E, Rakhra K, Bell K, Athwal GS. Healing rates and subscapularis fatty infiltration after lesser tuberosity osteotomy versus subscapularis peel for exposure during shoulder arthroplasty. J Shoulder Elb Surg. 2013;22(3):396–402. https://doi.org/10.1016/j.jse.2012.05.031.
109. Miller SL, Hazrati Y, Klepps S, Chiang A, Flatow EL. Loss of subscapularis function after total shoulder replacement : A seldom recognized problem. J Shoulder Elbow Surg. 2003;12:29–34. https://doi.org/10.1067/mse.2003.128195.
110. Terrier A, Larrea X, Malfroy Camine V, Pioletti DP, Farron A. Importance of the subscapularis muscle after total shoulder arthroplasty. Clin Biomech. 2013;28(2):146–50. https://doi.org/10.1016/j.clinbiomech.2012.11.010.
111. Buckley T, Miller R, Nicandri G, Lewis R, Voloshin I. Analysis of subscapularis integrity and function after lesser tuberosity osteotomy versus subscapularis tenotomy in total shoulder arthroplasty using ultrasound and validated clinical outcome measures. J Shoulder Elb Surg. 2014;23(9):1309–17. https://doi.org/10.1016/j.jse.2013.12.009.
112. Elhassan B, Ozbaydar M, Massimini D, Diller D, Higgins L, Warner JJP. Transfer of pectoralis major for the treatment of irreparable tears of subscapularis: does it work? J Bone Joint Surg Br. 2008;90(8):1059–65. https://doi.org/10.1302/0301-620X.90B8.20659.
113. Nelson GN, Namdari S, Galatz L, Keener JD. Pectoralis major tendon transfer for irreparable subscapularis tears. J Shoulder Elb Surg. 2014;23(6):909–18. https://doi.org/10.1016/j.jse.2013.12.035.
114. Elhassan BT, Wagner ER. Outcome of transfer of the sternal head of the pectoralis major with its bone insertion to the scapula to manage scapular winging. J Shoulder Elb Surg. 2015;24(5):733–40. https://doi.org/10.1016/j.jse.2014.08.022.
115. Sperling JW, Hawkins RJ, Walch GZJ. Complications in total shoulder arthroplasty. J Bone Joint Surg Am. 2013;62(March 2013):428–35.
116. Wright T, Cofield R. Humeral fractures after humeral arthroplasty. J Bone Joint Surg Am. 1995;77:1340–6.
117. Campbell JT, Moore RS, Iannotti JP, Norris TR, Williams GR. Periprosthetic humeral fractures: mechanisms of fracture and treatment options. J Shoulder Elb Surg. 1998;7(4):406–13. https://doi.org/10.1016/S1058-2746(98)90033-7.
118. Athwal GS, Sperling JW, Rispoli DM, Cofield RH. Periprosthetic humeral fractures during shoulder arthroplasty. J Bone Joint Surg Am. 2009;91(3):594–603. https://doi.org/10.2106/JBJS.H.00439.
119. Cil A, CJH V, Sanchez-Sotelo J, Sperling JW, Schleck C, Cofield RH. Revision of the humeral component for aseptic loosening in arthroplasty of the shoulder. J Bone Joint Surg Br. 2009;91(1):75–81. https://doi.org/10.1302/0301-620X.91B1.21094.
120. Nagda SH, Rogers KJ, Sestokas AK, et al. Neer award 2005: Peripheral nerve function during shoul-

der arthroplasty using intraoperative nerve monitoring. J Shoulder Elbow Surg. 2005:2–8. https://doi.org/10.1016/j.jse.2006.01.016.
121. Lynch NM, Cofield RH, Silbert PL, Hermann RC. Neurologic complications after total shoulder arthroplasty. J Shoulder Elbow Surg. 1996;5:53–61.
122. Lädermann A, Lübbeke A, Melis B, et al. Prevalence of neurologic lesions after. J Bone Joint Surg Am. 2011;93:1288–93. https://doi.org/10.2106/JBJS.J.00369.
123. Carofino BC, Brogan DM, Elhassan BT, Bishop AT, Spinner RJ, Shin AY. Iatrogenic nerve injuries during shoulder surgery: a series of 27 cases. J Bone Joint Surg. 2013;36:6. https://doi.org/10.1016/S0363-5023(11)60006-3.
124. Singh JA, Sperling JW, Schleck C, Harmsen WS, Cofield RH. Periprosthetic infections after total shoulder arthroplasty: a 33-year perspective. J Shoulder Elb Surg. 2012;21(11):1534–41. https://doi.org/10.1016/j.jse.2012.01.006.
125. Tanwar YS, Singh SP, Lal H. Anconeus pedicle olecranon flip osteotomy. Bone Joint J. 1990;96-B:1252–7. https://doi.org/10.1302/0301-620X.96B9.33343.
126. Hasan SS, Leith JM, Campbell B, et al. Characteristics of unsatisfactory shoulder arthroplasties. J Shoulder Elb Surg. 2002;11(5):431–41. https://doi.org/10.1067/mse.2002.125806.
127. Matsen FA, Russ SM, Bertelsen A, Butler-Wu S, Pottinger PS. Propionibacterium can be isolated from deep cultures obtained at primary arthroplasty despite intravenous antimicrobial prophylaxis. J Shoulder Elb Surg. 2015;24(6):844–7. https://doi.org/10.1016/j.jse.2014.10.016.
128. McGoldrick E, McElvany MD, Butler-Wu S, Pottinger PS, Matsen FA. Substantial cultures of Propionibacterium can be found in apparently aseptic shoulders revised three years or more after the index arthroplasty. J Shoulder Elb Surg. 2015;24(1):31–5. https://doi.org/10.1016/j.jse.2014.05.008.
129. Hsu JE, Bumgarner RE, Matsen FA. Propionibacterium in shoulder arthroplasty: what we think we know today. J Bone Joint Surg Am. 2016;98(7):597–606. https://doi.org/10.2106/JBJS.15.00568.
130. Hou C, Gupta A, Chen M, Matsen FA. How do revised shoulders that are culture positive for Propionibacterium differ from those that are not? J Shoulder Elb Surg. 2015;24(9):1427–32. https://doi.org/10.1016/j.jse.2015.01.003.
131. Zappe B, Graf S, Ochsner PE, Zimmerli W, Sendi P. Propionibacterium spp. in prosthetic joint infections: a diagnostic challenge. Arch Orthop Trauma Surg. 2008;128(10):1039–46. https://doi.org/10.1007/s00402-007-0454-0.
132. Zimmerli W, Trampuz A, Ochsner PE. Prosthetic-joint infections. N Engl J Med. 2004;351(16):1645–54. https://doi.org/10.1056/NEJMra040181.
133. Shields E, Iannuzzi JC, Thorsness R, Noyes K, Voloshin I. Perioperative complications after hemiarthroplasty and total shoulder arthroplasty are equivalent. J Shoulder Elb Surg. 2014;23(10):1449–53. https://doi.org/10.1016/j.jse.2014.01.052.
134. Chalmers PN, Gupta AK, Rahman Z, Bruce B, Romeo AAA, Nicholson GP. Predictors of early complications of total shoulder arthroplasty. J Arthroplast. 2014;29(4):856–60. https://doi.org/10.1016/j.arth.2013.07.002.
135. Jiang JJ, Toor AS, Shi LL, Koh JL. Analysis of perioperative complications in patients after total shoulder arthroplasty and reverse total shoulder arthroplasty. J Shoulder Elb Surg. 2014;23(12):1852–9. https://doi.org/10.1016/j.jse.2014.04.008.
136. Bliss M. William Osler: a life in medicine. New York: Oxford University Press; 1999.

Part IV

Arthritis of the Shoulder: II

Design Principles of Reverse Arthroplasty

17

Anders Ekelund and Didier Poncet

Introduction

In the early era of arthroplasty of the shoulder, it was recognized that the results of non-constrained anatomical arthroplasty in cuff-deficient shoulders were inferior to those in shoulders with an intact rotator cuff. In his book, Charles Neer wrote "the combination of painful incongruity of the articular surfaces and massive rotator cuff tear is very difficult to treat" [1]. The pain relief was usually good, but the functional improvement was unpredictable. Attempts were therefore made to develop constrained anatomical arthroplasties or reverse arthroplasties [1, 2]. These early designs had high failure rates and were abandoned. The first successful design of a reverse total shoulder arthroplasty was developed by Paul Grammont in Dijon, France [3–6]. Today, all reverse arthroplasties are based on his principles.

Rotator Cuff-Deficient Shoulder

The centre of rotation in the shoulder is located in the humeral head. In the normal shoulder, the resultant force from the deltoid and rotator cuff muscles is directed into the glenoid fossa, thus keeping the humeral head centred in the glenoid. If the force from the rotator cuff muscles is significantly reduced by a tendon tear or muscle atrophy, the humeral head will move superiorly. This results in shortening of the deltoid muscle. Furthermore, the centre of rotation may be unstable due to less compressive forces. This may result in pain and weakness. Patients may lose the ability to elevate the arm (pseudoparalysis) or to perform external rotation (lack of posterior rotator cuff).

By having a constrained anatomical arthroplasty, it was possible to control the position of the centre of rotation and to prevent superior migration of the humeral head; i.e. the length of the deltoid muscle was restored [2]. The early designs of a reverse arthroplasty used the same concept [1, 2]. The centre of rotation was fixed, with restoration of the length of the deltoid muscle. These early designs failed, usually on the glenoid side [2]. The centre of rotation was away from the glenoid surface, thereby creating a lever arm and shear forces that increased the risk of glenoid component failure. Neer tried three different reverse designs (Mark I, II, and III), but all of them were abandoned [1]. The main concern was the fixation of the glenoid component, since there is limited bone stock in the glenoid vault.

A. Ekelund (✉)
Department of Orthopaedics, Capio St Görans Hospital, Stockholm, Sweden
e-mail: anders.ekelund@capiostgoran.se

D. Poncet
Lyon, France

I. A. Trail et al. (eds.), *Textbook of Shoulder Surgery*, https://doi.org/10.1007/978-3-319-70099-1_17

The Novel Concept from Grammont

While many researchers gave up their attempts to design a reverse arthroplasty, Paul Grammont continued his work. He realized that the key was to change the centre of rotation to improve the strength of the deltoid muscle. After several attempts to place the centre of rotation more medially using anatomical designs, he changed to a reverse concept. In 1981, together with two engineers, Grammont published a report: "Study of a mechanical model for a shoulder total prosthesis: realization of a prototype" [5]. In this article, he wrote that by medializing the centre of rotation, the lever arm for the deltoid muscle would increase and compensate for the lack of activity of the supraspinatus muscle. There were four main principles: (1) that the centre of rotation should be fixed in a medial and inferior position, (2) that the system should be stable, (3) that the lever arm of the deltoid muscle must be effective from the start of the movement, and (4) that the glenosphere and cup should form a semi-constrained articulation. The purpose was to strengthen the abduction moment of the middle deltoid. Grammont had previously tried to achieve this without an arthroplasty, by performing a Translation-Rotation-Elevation osteotomy of the scapular spine [2, 3]. The first reverse arthroplasty with a medialized centre of rotation was the "Trompette" arthroplasty. It was composed of two-thirds of a 44-mm-diameter sphere. The centre of rotation was medialized, but was still not at the glenoid-implant interface (slightly lateralized). The humeral component had a non-anatomical inclination angle of 155 degrees to increase the stability and length of the deltoid muscle. He reported the first eight cases in 1987 [6]. Due to loosening of the cemented large sphere, the design was changed to a metal baseplate with a central peg and screw fixation, upon which a half-sphere was attached (36 or 42 mm in diameter). By having a half-sphere, the centre of rotation was at the bone-implant interface without any lever arm creating shear forces. Grammont called this design the Delta prosthesis, since the concept was based on the deltoid muscle for function and stability [4–7]. The humeral component continued to be a stemmed component with an inclination angle of 155 degrees. The latest version of the Delta reverse ball-and-socket design (Delta Xtend; DePuy Synthes, Warzaw, Indiana, USA) has a curved-back baseplate (Metaglene) with a central peg and four screw holes for locking or non-locking screws (Fig. 17.1). A curved back design allows for reduction in frontal glenosphere size (Fig. 17.2) maintaining the centre of rotation at the bone-implant junction and also allows preservation of more glenoid bone stock by allowing a more anatomical reaming of the glenoid surface. There are two glenosphere sizes: 38 and 42. The centre of rotation is in the glenoid. The humeral component maintains the 155 degrees of inclination. There are three different polyethylene inserts, the difference between them being the depth of the insert. A more shallow insert allows better range of motion before impingement

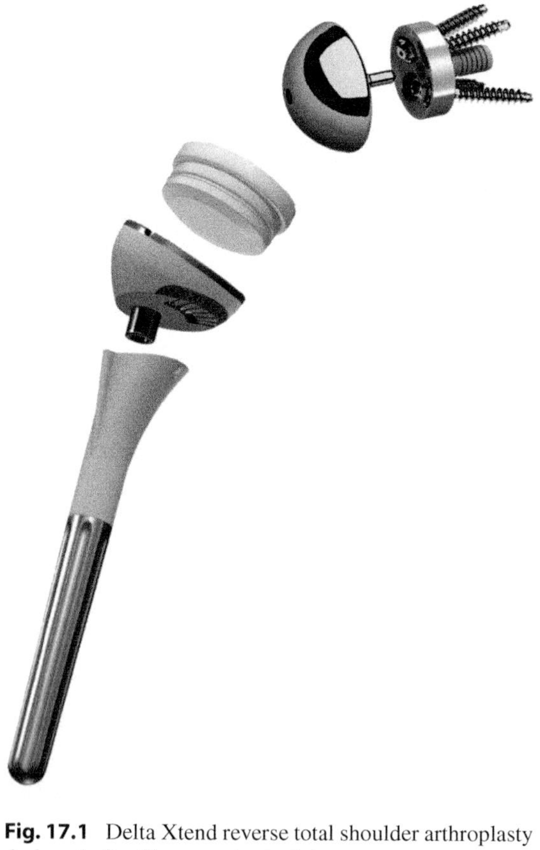

Fig. 17.1 Delta Xtend reverse total shoulder arthroplasty designed after Grammont principles

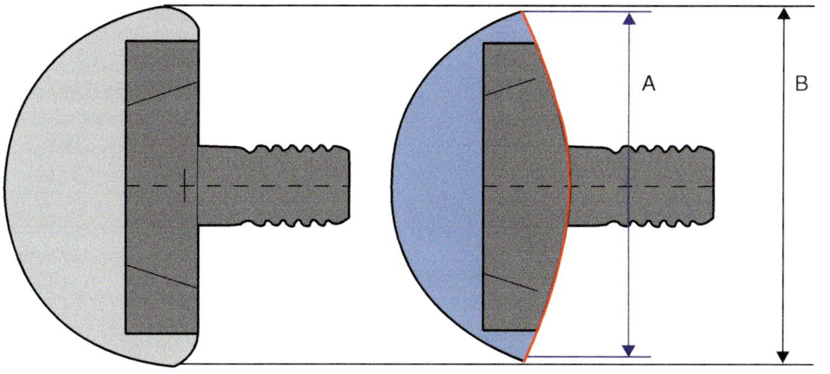

Fig. 17.2 A curved back surface on the metaglene allows for reduction of frontal glenoid size (less than a hemisphere) maintaining the centre of rotation in the glenoid. The diameter of the glenopshere is slightly reduced (Distance A vs B)

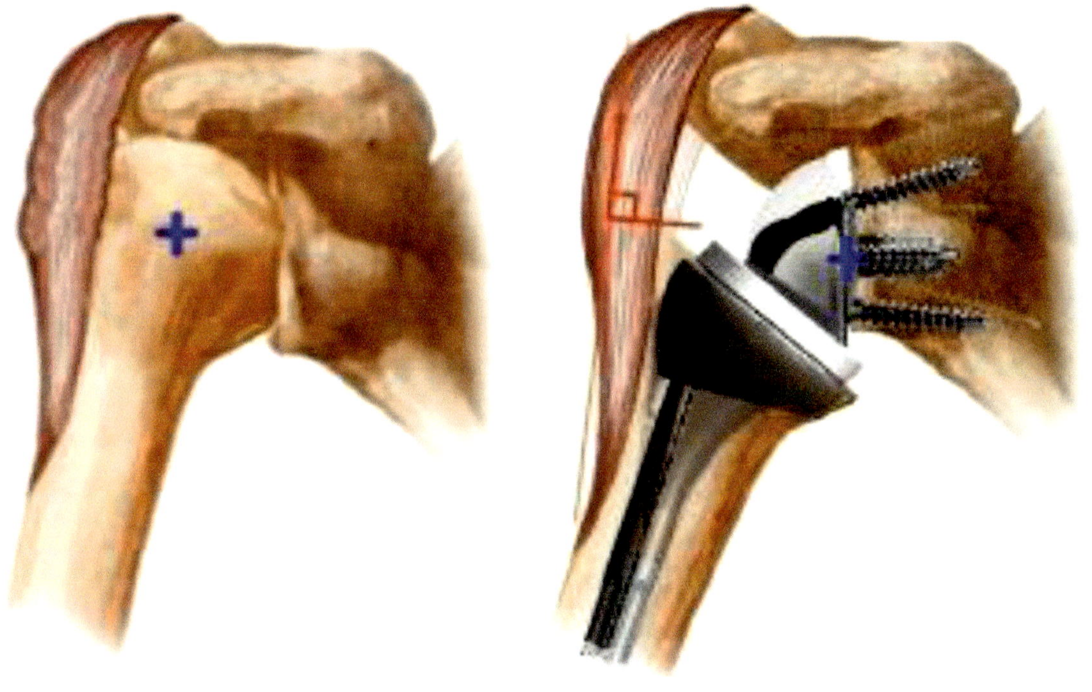

Fig. 17.3 A Grammont type reverse arthroplasty placing the center of rotation (blue cross) medially and inferiorly compared to the normal shoulder. The center of rotation is at the bone implant junction. The length of deltoid muscle is restored

against bone occurs, but the stability is reduced [8]. A deeper, more constrained insert is more stable, but the range of motion is reduced, with an increased risk of polyethylene wear [8, 9]. The Grammont concept has proven to be very successful [10–12].

The Grammont design medializes the centre of rotation and the humerus is medialized and lowered, which changes the contour of the shoulder (making it flatter) (Fig. 17.3) [4, 6, 7, 13–15]. The passive tension in the deltoid muscle is restored; actually, it overtensions the deltoid. The average lengthening of the upper extremity after reverse shoulder arthroplasty has been reported to be 15–27 mm [16]. This may improve the force-generating capacity of the deltoid muscle [17]. Furthermore, more deltoid musclefibres are recruited for abduction (Fig. 17.4) [7]. Ackland et al. [18] showed that the moment arm for abduction increased in the anterior, middle, and

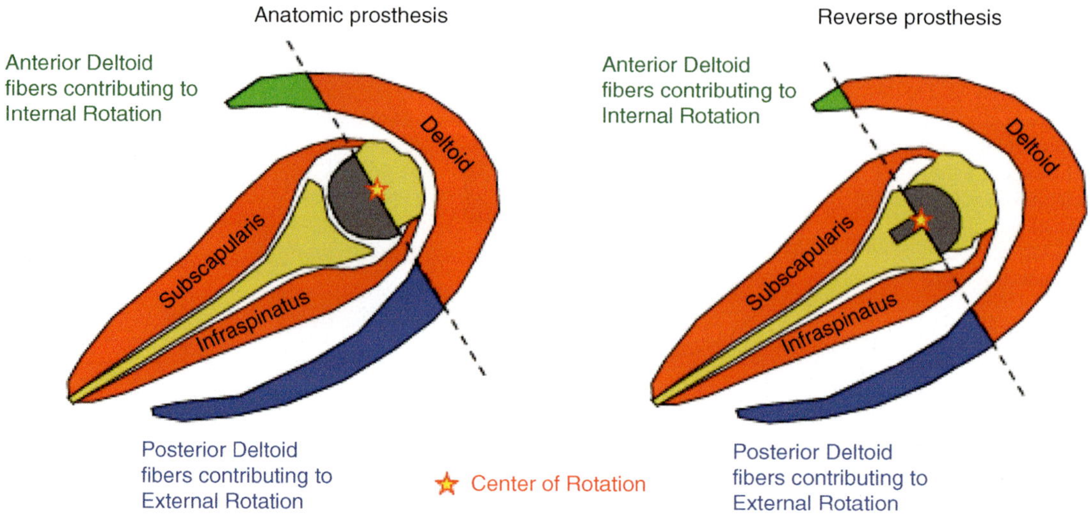

Fig. 17.4 After a reverse arthroplasty more deltoid muscle is recruited for abduction (Red), while the part of the deltoid muscle contributing to external and internal rotation is reduced (Blue and Green)

posterior deltoid after reconstruction with a reverse arthroplasty [18]. Furthermore, the shoulder flexors (the middle and anterior deltoid, the superior part of the pectoralis major) showed greater capacity to initiate flexion. Similar findings were reported by Walker et al. [19], with increased moment arm for anterior and lateral deltoid muscle in abduction [19]. However, more tension in the deltoid muscle may increase the risk of postoperative fracture of the acromion or scapular spine [7, 16]. In platform systems the reverse epiphysis component is sometimes placed on top of the anatomical humeral component. Such a design, with the reverse epiphysis outside the humerus, will put more tension on the deltoid muscle compared to an epiphysis component inside the humerus. The effect of prolonged overtensioning of the deltoid muscle is unknown, but it may result in degenerative changes of the muscle and long-term decline in deltoid function [20]. Furthermore, with this design the humeral component can impinge on the scapula, most commonly seen inferiorly, creating an erosion (notching) (Fig. 17.4) [8, 15, 21–24]. This notching has been a concern—since it may result in loosening, polyethylene wear, and osteolysis [8, 25, 26]. The consequent medialization of the humerus also results in less tension of the remaining rotator cuff, which may lead to reduced strength in external and internal rotation. Ackland et al. [27] reported a decrease in external rotation moment arm of the posterior deltoid muscle and of the infraspinatus and teres minor in abduction after reverse arthroplasty (Fig. 17.4) [27]. Thus, patients undergoing a reverse shoulder arthroplasty can lose external rotational capacity.

To overcome these problems with the Grammont concept, modified implants have been introduced, particularly changes in design to reduce the risk of scapular impingement (notching) (Fig. 17.5). The effect of notching on the long-term clinical outcome remains unclear. Inferior clinical outcome [11, 25] and no clinical effect [10, 12] of notching have been reported. Surgical technique, however, has been shown to be important in reducing the risk of notching [14, 22, 26, 28, 29]. A low placement of the baseplate, creating an inferior overhang, is the most important factor (Fig. 17.6) [22, 26]. Poon et al. [29] reported less notching with an inferior overhang of >3.5 mm [29]. An eccentric glenosphere allows the surgeon to create an inferior overhang, but increases the stress on the glenoid-baseplate junction, which may increase the risk of component loosening [30–32].

Lateralization of the centre of rotation (with the glenosphere being more than a half-sphere), lateralization of the humerus, or a change in the

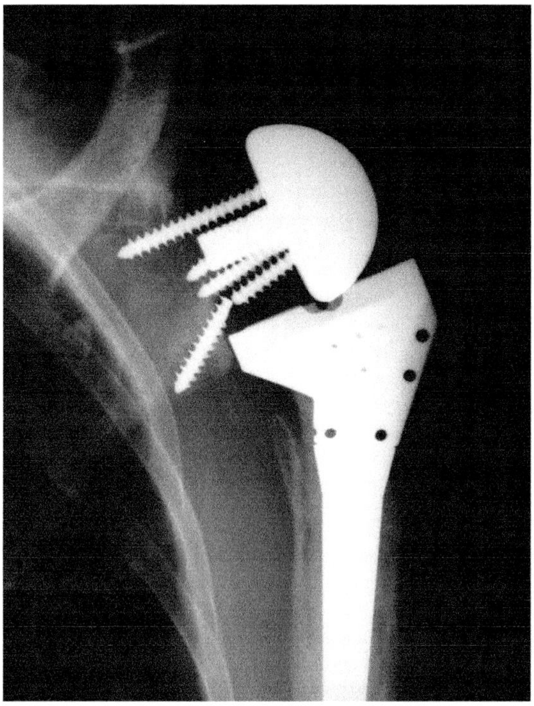

Fig. 17.5 Radiograph showing erosion (notching) with a broken screw inferiorly as a result of impingement between the humeral component and the inferior part of the glenoid

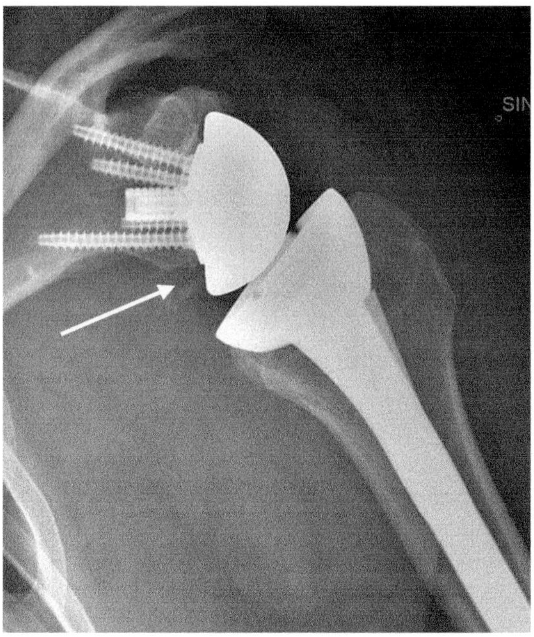

Fig. 17.6 Postoperative radiograph showing a low placement of the metaglene resulting in an inferior overhang of the glenosphere (white arrow) to reduce the risk of notching

humeral inclination angle to a more anatomical design has been suggested [8, 13, 15, 28, 33–42]. This reduces the risk of notching, increases the tension in the remaining cuff, and improves the contour of the shoulder. These different design concepts can be used to classify the different reverse arthroplasties that are available. Routman et al. [38] suggested that a glenoid design with a medialized centre of rotation <5 mm from the bone-implant interface should be called a medialized glenoid (MG) design and a centre of rotation that is more lateral should be called a lateralized glenoid (LG) design [38]. On the humeral side, the horizontal distance from the humeral stem axis to the centre of the liner (offset) is used to classify the humeral design. An offset of greater than 15 mm was called a lateralized humerus (LH) and an offset of less than 15 mm was called a medialized humerus (MH). There has been no scientific support for the numbers selected, but a classification system is valuable and helpful when analyzing different studies of reverse arthroplasties. These changes in design may have potential benefits, but they also increase the risk of complications. Humeral component with shorter stems or metaphyseal fixation are available [43–45]. In 2016 Moroder et al. found no difference in clinical outcome comparing a stemmed with a stemless reverse arthroplasty design [44]. Levy et al. [43] reported excellent clinical outcome in 98 patients with 2–7 years follow-up using a hydroxyapatite coated short stem designed for metaphyseal fixation [43].

Baseplate Design

The present Grammont type of circular HA-(hydroxyapatite-) coated baseplate design (Delta Xtend) of 27 mm with a central peg and the possibility of up to four compression and locking screws has a very low incidence of aseptic loosening. The optimal shape and diameter of the baseplate is not known. Chae et al. [46] found less micromotion with a circular 25-mm baseplate than with a 29-mm baseplate; the smaller baseplate also had a greater impingement-free range of motion [46]. Oval-shaped baseplates have been reported to have less shear displacement than a circular design, while there was no difference between a flat-back or curved-back design [47]. The optimal length of the central peg is yet to be determined. Königshausen et al. [48] found that there was a correlation between the loading capacity of the implant and the length of the peg inside bone [48]. The recommendation was that the central peg should be anchored as deeply as possible into native scapula bone stock. The introduction of long-pegged baseplates has enhanced initial fixation in glenoid deficiencies (Fig. 17.7). The screws are also important for initial fixation, and optimal rotation of the baseplate is necessary in order to place the screws in the coracoid and scapular spine pillar [49, 50]. The central peg has been replaced by a screw in some baseplate designs, which may prevent this ideal baseplate rotation [8]. The number of screws that are necessary to achieve initial stability depends on bone quality and the degree of bone loss. In some cases, two locking screws are sufficient—whereas more fixation points are necessary in glenoids with bone loss or severe osteoporosis [51, 52].

Clinical Pearl
Convex back-side improve contact surface area. No difference in boxplate motion between 2 and 4 screws.

The Glenosphere and Lateralized Centre of Rotation

The glenosphere is connected to the baseplate with a morse taper, which in some designs is augmented with a compression screw (Fig. 17.1). The purpose of the compression screw is to prevent dissociation. However it may facilitate the disconnection of the glenosphere from the metaglene by unscrewing it the glenosphere is pushed away from the metaglene. Cusick et al. [53] reported 13 cases of glenosphere baseplate dissociation in a prosthetic system with a morse taper design [53]. A compression screw decreases the risk of this complication, but concern has been that the hole in the glenosphere can increase polyethylene wear. However, Vaupel et al. [54] reported similar wear rates and total volume loss in glenospheres with and without holes [54]. The design of the glenosphere can also affect the incidence of notching. A larger glenosphere (42 mm) was found to have less notching than a smaller glenosphere (38 mm), and better range of motion [21, 55]. To increase the impingement-free range of motion, various degrees of lateralization of the centre of rotation have been recommended [23, 40–42, 50, 56–58]. The center of rotation is still medialized compared to the native gleno-humeral joint, but less compared to the original Grammont design [59]. Lateralization of the centre of rotation improves shoulder contour and increases the tension of the remaining rotator cuff. However, the lever arm for the deltoid muscle is reduced compared with the design using a hemisphere

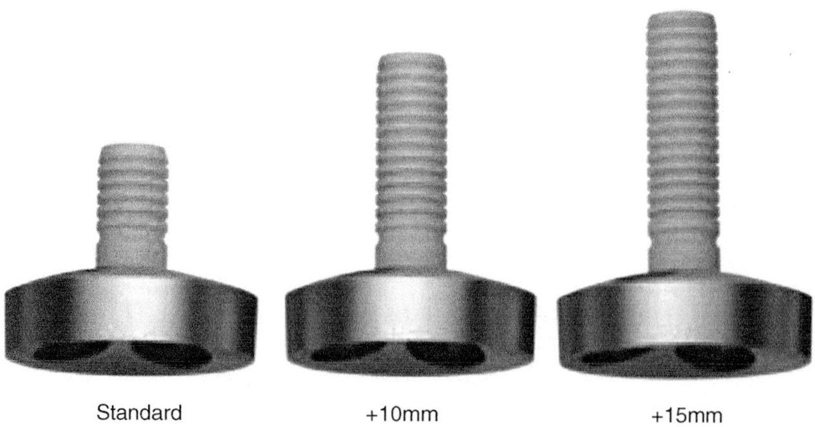

Fig. 17.7 Image of a standard and two long pegged metaglene (+10 and + 15 mm)

[59]. Valenti et al. [41] showed that a less medialized centre of rotation improved external and internal rotation and reduced notching compared to the classic Grammont design [41]. However, when the centre of rotation is away from the glenoid, there will be a lever arm, generating increased shear forces resulting in an increased risk of glenoid component loosening [58–60]. Finite element analysis (FEA) shoulder models have shown increased micromotion with a lateralized design [31, 32]. If a glenosphere with a lateralized centre of rotation is combined with glenosphere eccentricity there will be two lever arms (lateral and inferior) further increasing the risk for glenoid component failure. Current systems available with a lateralized centre of rotation offer different amounts of lateralization. The optimal degree is however unknown. Boileau et al. [61] recommended lateralization with a circular bone graft instead of having a thicker metal glenosphere, to avoid shear forces at the bone-implant interface (BIO-RSA) [61]. A low rate of inferior scapular notching, improved shoulder rotation, and improved shoulder contour were reported. However, in contrast, Athwal et al. [62] found no difference in clinical outcome between bony increased-offset reverse arthroplasty (BIO-RSA) and Grammont-style design, although the incidence of notching was significantly less in the BIO-RSA group (40% vs. 70%) [62]. Lateralization has been shown to increase the load on the acromion and also the risk of postoperative acromial or scapular spine fractures [63]. This is potentially a severe complication, resulting in inferior functional outcome. To reduce polyethylene (PE) wear of the insert, if impingement occurs, a reversal of the bearings has been suggested. Simulated wear models have shown a reduction in wear with a ployethylene glenosphere articulating against a metal insert [64].

> **Clinical Pearl**
> Lateralisation increases joint stability but increases deltoid abduction force.

Inclination Angle

The original Delta design has an inclination angle of 155 degrees. It places the humerus medially and inferiorly, more under the glenosphere. By decreasing the inclination angle, the humerus may be more lateralized (design dependent), which reduces inferior notching and increases impingement-free range of motion [14, 33, 34, 42]. However, superior impingement against the acromion occurs earlier during range of motion [42]. The change in inclination angle can be done in different ways. The PE insert or humeral component can have different angles, and the humeral stem can be placed in a different position in relation to the insert. These different designs will affect the gain in adduction, deltoid force angle, the tension in the deltoid muscle, and the degree of humeral lateralization (Fig 17.8a, b). Lädermann et al. [65] reported that with decreased inclination angle (135 vs 145 degrees) elevation remained unchanged, abduction decreased, while extension, external rotation and adduction improved [65]. By moving the humerus laterally, the contour of the shoulder becomes more rounded and the deltoid wrapping angle is improved. However, Oh et al. [66] showed reduced stability with a reduction in the inclination angle [66]. Erickson et al. [33] performed a systematic review of the influence of inclination angle on clinical outcome and complications [33, 34]. They compared designs with 155-degree and 135-degree inclination angles. They found less notching with 135 degrees of inclination, without any increased incidence of instability. However, the 135-degree design used in the studies also had a lateralization of the centre of rotation. It is therefore difficult to determine the true effect of the different inclination designs. Furthermore, Langohr et al. [67] found that decreasing the inclination angle reduced the contact area of the insert in abduction and increased the maximum contact stress [67]. This may affect long-term wear of the polyethylene insert. Furthermore, since the humerus may be lateralized when the inclination angle is reduced, it may increase the risk of postoperative fracture of the acromion or

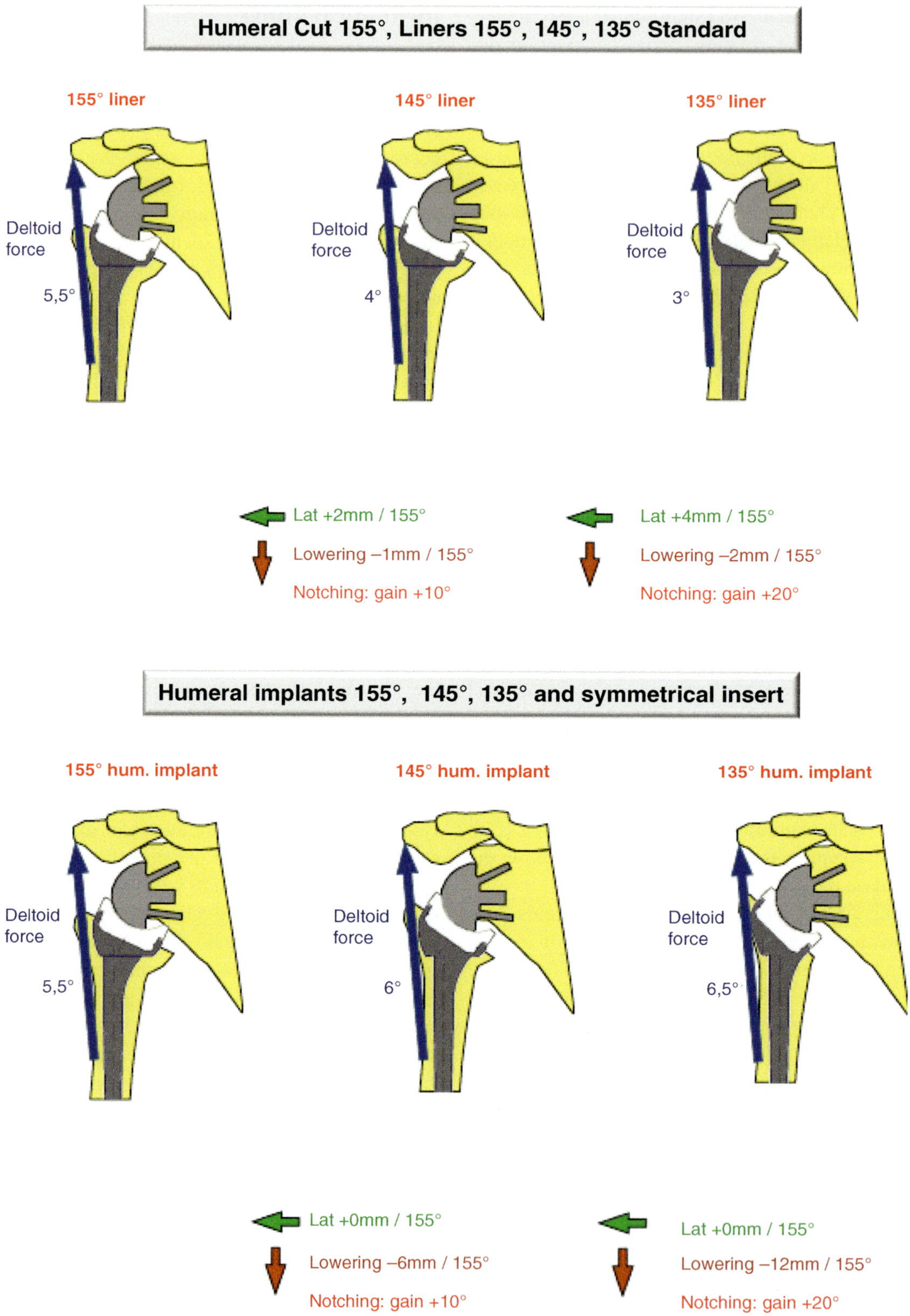

Fig. 17.8 (**a**,**b**) Image showing the effect on Deltoid force angle, degree of inferior and lateral shift of humerus, and gain in adduction angle (notching angle) when the inclination angle is changed in the insert (**a**) or by changing the inclination of the humeral component (humeral cut) (**b**)

scapular spine [63]. Thus, there are advantages and disadvantages with the different inclination angles and the optimal design is still to be determined.

> **Clinical Pearl**
> Increased inferior offset and lateralisation reduces notching. However, both increase stress.
> concentration on glenoid.

The Humeral Component

To improve the deltoid wrapping angle and increase the tension in the remaining rotator cuff, the humeral component is designed to lateralize the humerus [9, 35, 39]. Giles et al. [35] found that lateralization of the humerus improved the joint and muscle loading [35]. Less force from the deltoid muscle was required for abduction than with a lateralized glenosphere. Furthermore, the joint loading angle decreased, creating more compressive forces—thereby reducing the risk of baseplate failure. Humeral lateralization may lead to earlier impingement against the acromion in abduction, which may increase the risk of acromial or scapular spine fractures.

Summary

The Grammont design concept of a reverse arthroplasty to restore the biomechanics of a cuff-deficient shoulder has revolutionized the treatment for many shoulder pathologies. The number of reverse arthroplasties are increasing and the indications are widening. The design with a medialized centre of rotation at the bone-implant interface has a very low risk of aseptic loosening and improves the deltoid function. The non-anatomical inclination angle of 155 degrees restores deltoid length. The negative effects of this design, such as inferior scapular notching, loss of shoulder contour, and reduced force of the remaining rotator cuff have been a concern. Attempts to overcome these problems by reducing the humeral inclination angle, lateralizing the centre of rotation, or lateralizing the humerus are currently being evaluated. Surgical technique is important and a low placement of the baseplate, associated with the use of bigger glenosphere diameter or an eccentric glenosphere creating an inferior overhang of the glenosphere, is the most important factor to reduce the risk of notching. The optimal design in reverse total shoulder arthroplasty remains to be defined, and further studies are required [8, 13, 33, 34]. Changing the position of the centre of rotation, the inclination angle, the size of the glenosphere, the depth of the humeral insert, the humeral position, and the position of the implant in relation to the anatomy affects the biomechanics, the risk of impingement, and the forces generated by the deltoid muscle and remaining rotator cuff. The current literature regarding the design parameters and biomechanics of a reverse arthroplasty are difficult to interpret. However, since the classic Grammont design has shown very good clinical outcome and has a survival rate of over 90% at 10 years, any change in design should be made with caution [10–12].

References

1. Neer CS. Shoulder reconstruction. Philadelphia: WB Saunders Company; 1990.
2. Flatow EL, Harrison AK. A history of reverse total shoulder arthroplasty. Clin Orthop Relat Res. 2011;469:2432–9.
3. Baulot E, Sirveaux F, Boileau P. Grammont's idea. The story of Paul Grammont's functional surgery concept and development of the reverse principle. Clin Orthop Relat Res. 2011;469:2425–31.
4. Grammont PM, Baulot E. Delta shoulder prosthesis for rotator cuff rupture. Orthopaedics. 1993;16:65–8.
5. Grammont PM, Bourgon J, Pelzer P. Study of a mechanical model for a shoulder total prosthesis: realization of a prototype. These de sciences de lÍngénieur. Dijon/Lyon: Université Dijon/ECAM de Lyon; 1981.
6. Grammont PM, Trouilloud P, Laffay JP, Deries X. Study and development of a new shoulder prosthesis (In French). Rhumatologie. 1987;39:407–18.
7. Boileau P, Watkinson DJ, Hatzidakis AM, Balg F. Grammont reverse prosthesis: design, rationale, and biomechanics. J Shoulder Elb Surg. 2005;14:147S–61S.
8. Middernacht B, Van Tongel A, De Wilde L. A critical review of prosthetic features available for reversed total shoulder arthroplasty. Biomed Res Int. 2016.; Article ID 3256931.

9. Carpenter S, Pinkas D, Newton MD, Kurdziel MD, Baker KC, Wiater JM. Wear rates of retentive versus nonretentive reverse total shoulder arthroplasty liners in an in vitro wear simulation. J Shoulder Elb Surg. 2015;24:1372–9.
10. Bacle G, Nové-Josserand L, Garaud P, Walch G. Long-term outcomes of reverse total shoulder arthroplasty. J Bone Joint Surg. 2017;99-A:454–61.
11. Ek ETH, Neukom L, Catanzaro S, Gerber C. Reverse total shoulder arthroplasty for massive irreparable rotator cuff tears in patients younger than 65 years old: results after five to fifteen years. J Shoulder Elb Surg. 2013;22:1199–208.
12. Favard L, Levigne C, Nerot C, Gerber C, De Wilde L, Mole D. Reverse prosthesis in arthropathies with cuff tear. Clin Orthop Relat Res. 2011;469:2469–75.
13. Ackland DC, Patel M, Knox D. Prosthesis design and placement in reverse total shoulder arthroplasty. J Orthop Surg Res. 2015;10:101–9.
14. Berliner JL, Regalado-Magdos A, Ma CB, Feeley BT. Biomechanics of reverse total shoulder arthroplasty. J Shoulder Elb Surg. 2015;24:150–60.
15. Jazayeri R, Kwon YW. Evolution of the reverse total shoulder arthroplasty. Bull Hosp Joint Dis. 2011;69:50–5.
16. Lädermann A, Edwards TB, Walch G. Arm lengthening after reverse shoulder arthroplasty: a review. Int Orthop. 2014;38:991–1000.
17. Jobin CM, Brown GD, Bahu MJ, Gardner TR, Bigliani LU, Levine WN, Ahmad CS. Reverse total shoulder arthroplasty for cuff tear arthropathy: the clinical effect of deltoid lengthening and center of rotation medialization. J Shoulder Elb Surg. 2012;21:1269–77.
18. Ackland DC, Roshan-Zamir S, Richardson M, Pandy MG. Moment arms of the shoulder musculature after reverse total shoulder arthroplasty. J Bone Joint Surg. 2010;92:1221–30.
19. Walker DR, Struk AM, Matsuki K, Wright TW, Banks SA. How do deltoid muscle moment arms change after reverse total shoulder arthroplasty? J Shoulder Elb Surg. 2016;25:581–8.
20. Greiner SH, Back DA, Herrmann S, Perka C, Asbach P. Degenerative changes of the deltoid muscle have impact on clinical outcome after reversed total shoulder arthroplasty. Arch Orthop Trauma Surg. 2010;130:177–83.
21. Berhouet J, Garaud P, Favard L. Evaluation of the role of glenosphere design and humeral component retroversion in avoiding scapular notching during reverse shoulder arthroplasty. J Shoulder Elb Surg. 2014;23:151–8.
22. De Wilde LF, Poncet D, Middernacht B, Ekelund A. Prosthetic overhang is the most effective way to prevent scapular conflict in reverse total shoulder arthroplasty. Acta Orthop Scand. 2010;81:719–26.
23. Huri G, Familiari F, Salari N, Petersen SA, Doral MN, McFarland EG. Prosthetic design of reverse shoulder arthroplasty contributes to scapular notching and instability. World J Orthop. 2016;7:738–45.
24. Krämer M, Bäunker A, Wellmann M, Hurschler C, Smoth T. Implant impingement during internal rotation after reverse shoulder arthroplasty. The effect of implant configuration and scapula anatomy: a biomechanical study. Clin Biomech. 2016;3:111–6.
25. Mollon B, Mahure SA, Roche CP, Zuckerman JD. Impact of scapular notching on clinical outcomes after reverse total shoulder arthroplasty: an analysis of 476 shoulders. J Shoulder Elb Surg. 2017;26:1253–61.
26. Nyffler RW, Werner CM, Gerber C. Biomechanical relevance of glenoid component positioning in reverse delta III total shoulder prosthesis. J Shoulder Elb Surg. 2005;14:524–8.
27. Ackland DC, Richardson M, Pandy MG. Axial rotation moment arms of the shoulder musculature after reverse total shoulder arthroplasty. J Bone Joint Surg. 2012;94:1886–95.
28. Roche CP, Marczuk Y, Wright TW, Flurin P-H, Grey SG, Jones RB, Routman HD, Gilot GJ, Zuckerman JD. Scapular notching in reverse arthroplasty. Bull Hosp Jt Dis. 2013;71(4):278–83.
29. Poon PC, Chou J, Young SW, Astley T. A comparison of concentric and eccentric glenospheres in reverse shoulder arthroplasty. J Bone Joint Surg. 2014;96:e138 (1–7).
30. Di Biase CF, Ziveri G, Delcogliani M, de Caro F, Gumina S, Borroni M, Castagna A, Postacchini R. The use of an eccentric glenosphere compared with a concentric glenosphere in reverse total shoulder arthroplasty: two-year minimum follow-up results. Int Orthop. 2013;37:1949–55.
31. Elwell J, Choi J, Willing R. Quantifying the competing relationship between adduction range of motion and baseplate micromotion with lateralization of reverse total shoulder arthroplasty. J Biomech. 2017;52:24–30.
32. Yang C-C, Lu C-L, Wu CH, Wu J-J, Huang T-L, Chen R, Yeh M-K. Stress analysis of glenoid component in design of reverse shoulder prosthesis using finite element method. J Shoulder Elb Surg. 2013;22:932–9.
33. Erickson BJ, Frank RM, Harris JD, Mall N, Romeo AA. The influence of humeral head inclination in reverse total shoulder arthroplasty: a systematic review. J Shoulder Elb Surg. 2015;24:988–93.
34. Erickson BJ, Harris JD, Romeo AA. The effect of humeral inclination on range of motion in reverse total shoulder arthroplasty: a systematic review. Am J Orthop. 2016;45(4):E174–9.
35. Giles JW, Langohr DG, Johnson JA, Athwal GS. Implant design variations in reverse total shoulder arthroplasty influence the required deltoid force and resultant joint load. Clin Orthop Relat Res. 2015;473:3615–26.
36. Hoenecke HR, Flores-Hernandez C, D'Lima DD. Reverse total shoulder arthroplasty component center of rotation affects muscle function. J Shoulder Elb Surg. 2014;233:1128–35.
37. Jeon B-K, Panchal KA, Ji J-H, Xin Y-Z, Park S-R, Kim J-H, Yang S-J. Combined effect of change in humeral neck-shaft angle and retroversion on shoulder range

of motion in reverse total shoulder arthroplasty- A simulation study. Clin Biomech. 2016;31:12–9.

38. Routman HD, Fluron P-H, Wright TW, Zuckerman JD, Hamilton MA, Roche CP. Reverse shoulder arthroplasty prosthesis design classification system. Bull Hosp Jt Dis. 2015;73(Suppl 1):S5–S14.
39. Sachinis NP, Athanasiadou P. Current designs and trends in reverse shoulder arthroplasty. OA Orthop. 2013;1(3):24.
40. Streit JJ, Shishani Y, Gobezie R. Medialized versus lateralized center of rotation in reverse shoulder arthroplasty. Orthopaedics. 2015;38:e1098–103.
41. Valenti P, Sauzieres P, Katz D, Kalouche I, Kilinc AS. Do less medialized reverse shoulder prosthesis increase motion and reduce notching? Clin Orthop Relat Res. 2011;469:2550–7.
42. Werner BS, Chaoui J, Walch G. The influence of humeral neck shaft angle and glenoid lateralization on range of motion in reverse shoulder arthroplasty. J Shoulder Elb Surg. https://doi.org/10.1016/j.jse.2017.03.032. [Epub ahead of print].
43. Levy O, Narvani A, Hous N, Abraham R, Relwani J, Pradhan R, Bruguera J, Sforza G, Atoun E. Reverse shoulder arthroplasty with cementless short metaphyseal humeral implant without a stem: clinical and radiological outcomes in prospective 2- to 7 years follow-up study. J Shoulder Elb Surg. 2016;25:1362–70.
44. Moroder P, Ernstbrunner L, Zweiger C, Schatz M, Seitlinger G, Skursky R, Becker J, Resch H, Krifter RM. Short to mid-term results of stemless reverse shoulder arthroplasty in a selected patient population compared to a matched control group with stem. Int Orthop. 2016;40:2115–20.
45. Teissier P, Teissier J, Kouyoumdjian P, Asencio G. The TESS reverse shoulder arthroplasty without a stem in the treatment of cuff-deficient shoulder conditions: clinical and radiological results. J Shoulder Elb Surg. 2015;24:45–51.
46. Chae SW, Kim SY, Lee H, Yon JR, Lee J, Han SH. Effect of baseplate size on primary glenoid stability and impingementfree range of motion in reverse shoulder arthroplasty. BMC Musculoskelet Disord. 2014;15:417–22. https://doi.org/10.1186/1471-2474-15-417.
47. Roche CP, Stroud NJ, Flurin PH, Wright TW, Zuckderman JD, DiPaola MJ. Reverse shoulder glenoid base plate fixation: a comparison of flat-back versus curved-back designs and oval versus circular designs with 2 different offset glenospheres. J Shoulder Elb Surg. 2014;23:1388–94.
48. Königshausen M, Jettkant B, Sverdlova N, Ehlert C, Gessman J, Schildhauer TA, Seybold D. Influence of different peg length in glenoid bone loss: a biomechanical analysis regarding primary stability of the glenoid baseplater in reverse shoulder arthroplasty. Technol Health Care. 2015;23:855–69.
49. Stephens BF, Hebert CT, Azar FM, Mihalko WM, Throckmorton TW. Optimal baseplate rotational alignment for locking-screw fixation in reverse total shoulder arthroplasty: a three-dimensional computer-aided design study. J Shoulder Elb Surg. 2015;24:1367–71.
50. Walker M, Brooks J, Willis M, Frankle M. How reverse shoulder arthroplasty works. Clin Orthop Relat Res. 2011;469:2440–51.
51. Formaini NT, Everding NG, Levy JC, Santoni BG, Nayak AN, Wilson C. Glenoid baseplate fixation using hybrid configurations of locked and unlocked peripheral screws. J Orthop Traumatol. 2017; https://doi.org/10.1007/s10195-016-0438-3. [Epub ahead of print].
52. James J, Allison MA, Werner FW, McBride DE, Basu NN, Sutton LG, Nanavati VN. Reverse shoulder arthroplasty glenoid fixation: is there a benefit in using four instead of two screws? J Shoulder Elb Surg. 2013;22:1030–6.
53. Cusick MC, Husey MM, Steen BM, Hartzler RU, Clark RE, Cuff DJ, Cabezas AF, Santoni BG, Frankle MA. Glenosphere dissociation after reverse shoulder arthroplasty. J Shoulder Elb Surg. 2015;24:1061–8.
54. Vaupel ZM, Baker KC, Kurdziel MD, Wiater JM. Wear simulation of reverse total shoulder arthroplasty system: effect of glenosphere design. J Shoulder Elb Surg. 2012;21:1422–9.
55. Torrens C, Guirro P, Miquel J, Santana F. Influence of glenosphere size on the development of scapular notching: a prospective randomized study. J Shoulder Elb Surg. 2016;25:1735–41.
56. Gutiérrez S, Levy JC, Frankle MA, Cuff D, Keller TS, Pupello DR, Lee WE. Evaluation of abduction range of motion and avoidance of inferior scapular impingement in a reverse shoulder model. J Shoulder Elb Surg. 2008;17:608–15.
57. Henninger HB, King FK, Tashjian RZ, Burks RT. Biomechanical comparison of reverse total shoulder arthroplasty systems in soft tissue-constrained shoulders. J Shoulder Elb Surg. 2014;23:e108–17.
58. Lawrence C, Wiliams GR, Namdari S. Influence of glenosphere design on outcomes and complications of reverse arthroplasty: a systematic review. Clin Orthop Surg. 2016;8:288–97.
59. Constantini O, Choi DS, Kontaxis A, Gulotta LV. The effects of progressive lateralization of the joint center of rotation of reverse total shoulder implants. J Shoulder Elb Surg. 2015;24:1120–8.
60. Liou W, Yang Y, Petersen-Fitts GR, Lombardo DJ, Stine S, Sabesan VJ. Effect of lateralized design on muscle and joint reaction forces for reverse shoulder arthroplasty. J Shoulder Elb Surg. 2017;26:564–72.
61. Boileau P, Moineau G, Roussanne Y, O'Shea K. Bony increased-offset reversed shoulder arthroplasty: minimizing scapular impingement while maximizing glenoid fixation. Clin Orthop Relat Res. 2011;469:2558–67.
62. Athwal GS, MacDermid JC, Redy KM, Marsh JP, Faber KJ, Drosdowech D. Does bony increased-offset reverse shoulder arthroplasty decrease scapular notching? J Shoulder Elb Surg. 2015;24:468–73.
63. Wong MT, Langohr DG, Athwal GS, Johnson JA. Implant positioning in reverse shoulder

arthroplasty has an impact on acromial stresses. J Shoulder Elb Surg. 2016;25:1889–95.
64. Kohut G, Dallmann F, Irlenbusch U. Wear induced loss of mass in reversed total shoulder arhroplasty with conventional and inverted bearing materials. J Biomech. 2012;45:469–73.
65. Lädermann A, Denard PJ, Boileau P, Farron A, Deransart P, Terrier A, Ston J, Walch G. Effect of humeral stem design on humeral position and range of motion in reverse arthroplasty. Int Orthop. 2015;39:2205–13.
66. Oh JH, Shin S-J, McGarry MH, Scott JH, Heckmann N, Lee TQ. Biomechanical effects of humeral neck-shaft angle and subscapularis integrity in reverse total shoulder arthroplasty. J Shoulder Elb Surg. 2014;23:1091–8.
67. Langohr GDG, Willing R, Medley JB, Athwal GS, Johnson JA. Contact mechanics of reverse total shoulder arthroplasty during abduction: the effect of neck-shaft angle, humeral cup depth, and glenosphere diameter. J Shoulder Elb Surg. 2016;25:589–97.

Results of the Reverse Total Shoulder Arthroplasty

18

Ian A. Trail

Introduction

The concept of reverse total shoulder arthroplasty has been with us for some time. Most of the earlier designs, however, were unsuccessful. It was not until the work of Paul Grammont in 1981 that the procedure gained widespread acceptance (Fig. 18.1). The initial design was intended for patients with osteoarthritis of the shoulder with a non- functioning or irreparable rotator cuff. So successful, however, was this replacement that the indications have expanded such that reverse total shoulder arthroplasty RTSR now matches anatomical total shoulder arthroplasty in numbers inserted. The purpose of this chapter is to provide an overview of the results for these various indications. In addition, at the end, the results of this implant in uncommon and unique scenarios will also be considered. Currently this implant is commonly used to treat patients with cuff tear arthropathy, older patients with a massive and irreparable rotator cuff but no arthritis, rheumatoid arthritis trauma and in revision surgery. For complications this is the subject of a separate chapter authored by Daniel Mok.

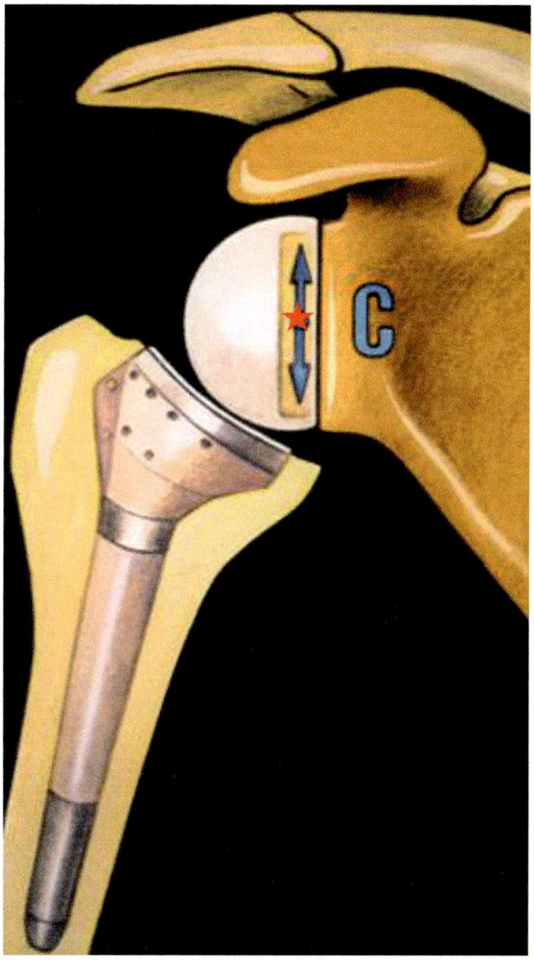

Fig. 18.1 Grammont reverse total shoulder replacement prosthesis

I. A. Trail (✉)
Wrightington Hospital, Wigan, Lancashire, UK
e-mail: upperlimb@wrightington.org.uk

I. A. Trail et al. (eds.), *Textbook of Shoulder Surgery*, https://doi.org/10.1007/978-3-319-70099-1_18

Cuff Tear Arthropathy

The modern concept of cuff tear arthropathy is the combination of arthritis and a massive cuff tear where the shoulder joint may remain concentric (Seebauer type 1) or the humeral head may migrate superiorly (Seebauer type 2) (Fig. 18.2). It has been estimated that between 2% and 5% of all people over 80 years of age suffer from cuff tear arthropathy although many may be asymptomatic. Many of the original studies on reverse shoulder arthroplasty unfortunately have limited numbers and often varied indications. As such, whilst they obviously are of historic interest and indeed show the potential they do not provide much information on long term outcome or survival. Added to that there has been a number of significant changes in design of the implant as well as surgical technique in recent years.

Three studies have been identified that contain a significant number of patients (minimum of 50 patients) and significant follow up (minimum of 2 years).

Naveed et al. [1] looked at 50 replacements in 43 patients treated with a reverse implant with a mean follow up of 39 months. They reported significant improvement in function using both the American Shoulder and Elbow and Oxford scores. The mean maximum elevation improved from 55° pre-operatively to 105° at final follow-up. Abduction was also improved to 85° but

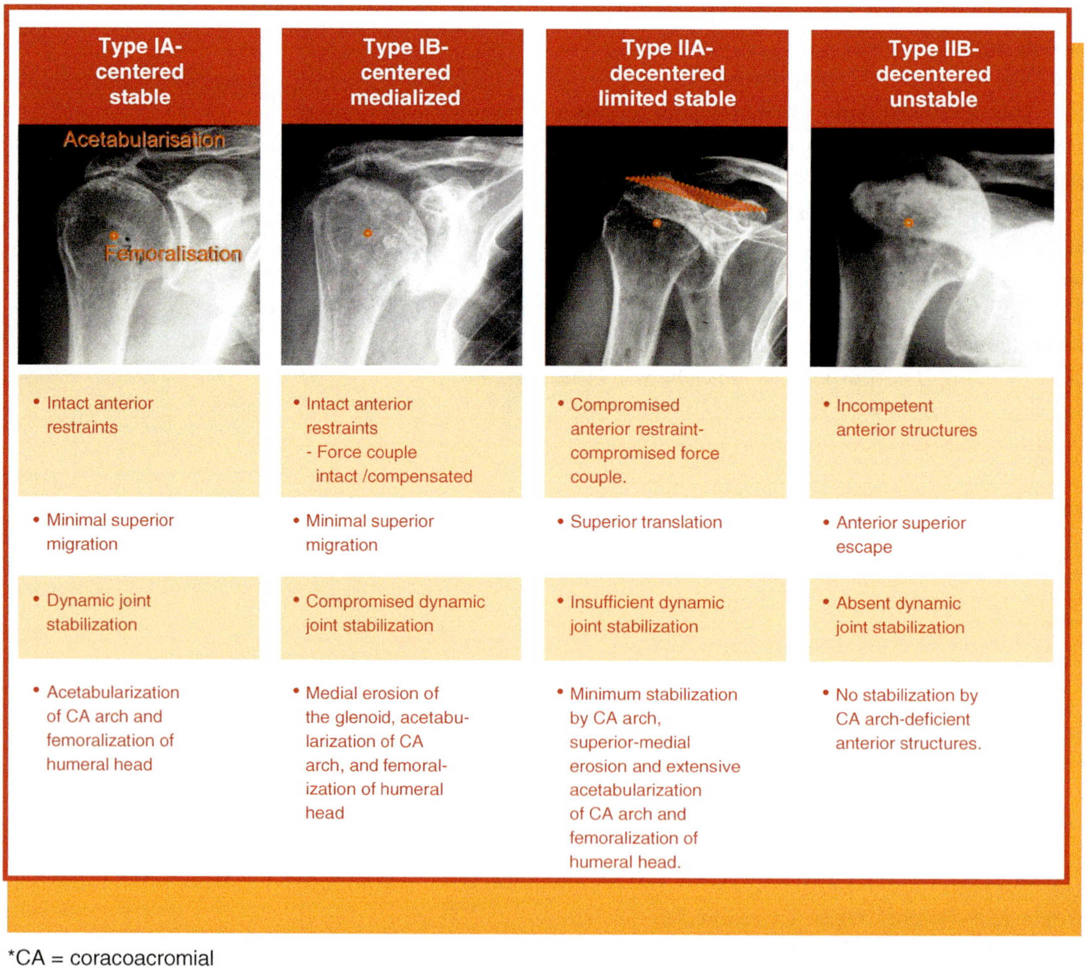

Fig. 18.2 Seebauer classification for cuff tear arthropathy. CA coracoacromial

internal and external rotation remain diminished. Radiologically 70% of patients showed some evidence of scapular notching and eight were described as severe.

Nolan et al. again in 2011 reviewed 67 patients who underwent 71 implants with an average follow-up of 24 months [2]. Again they showed significant improvement in function using both the American Shoulder and Elbow and Constant-Murley scores. Active forward flexion improved from 61° to 121°. There was, however, no improvement in active external rotation. Again 49% of patients showed some evidence of radiographic notching. The overall complication rate was 23%.

The longest review was by Favard et al. again in (2011) and included 464 patients with a minimum follow-up of 2 years [3]. One hundred and forty eight of these patients had a minimum follow-up of 5 years with a range from 5 to 17 years. In this group they reported good ongoing pain relief with active anterior elevation of 129° and active external rotation with the elbow at the side of 11°. A longer term follow-up showed some slight diminution in these ranges. Overall survivalship used a Kaplan-Meier with removal of the implant as the end point was 89% at 10 years. However, when a Constant-Murley score of less than 30 was used as the end point, this was reduced to 72% at 10 years with a marked reduction at 8 years. Radiologically more glenoid notching was seen with longer follow-up although this did not correlate with clinical outcome. There were complications in 89 cases out of 489 (16%). These ranged from infection, glenoid loosening or unscrewing, dislocation as well as haematoma, humeral fractures etc.

In conclusion it does appear that cuff tear arthropathy remains the pre-eminent indication for a reverse total shoulder arthroplasty. The patients can expect significant and continuing pain relief with satisfactory movement, particularly elevation and abduction and as a consequence an improvement in function. Long term studies available show continuing good results for 10 years. There were, however, some concerns with regard to continuing glenoid notching and an ongoing lack of internal and external rotation.

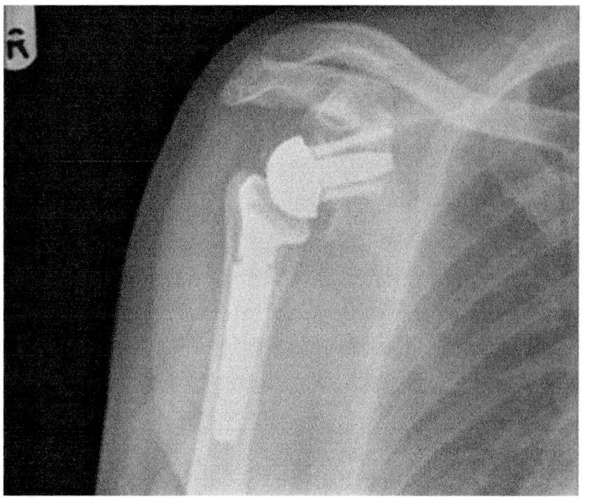

Fig. 18.3 Example of scapular notching

Scapular notching has been noted following a reverse total shoulder arthroplasty really from the very beginning (Fig. 18.3). It often develops early and can be seen in x-rays within 18 months to 2 years from the initial surgery. With regard to aetiology it is now accepted that this is due to impingement of the infero-medial portion with a polyethylene insert on the inferior surface of the bony glenoid (Day et al. [4]). Subsequent research has identified positioning of the glenoid component to be an important factor. Both Simovitch et al. [5] and Roche et al. [6] concluded that the optimum position of the glenoid component should be towards the bottom of the glenoid rather than central. This would have the effect of creating an overhang of the glenosphere. They also concluded that a degree of inferior tilt of the glenosphere would also have a beneficial effect. This has, however, been disputed by Bradley-Edwards et al. [7] in a prospective randomised clinical trial. Of 52 consecutive reverse total shoulder arthroplasties replacing the glenoid component with an inferior tilt did not reduce the incidence of severity of radiographic scapular notching. In addition there was no clinical difference between groups. Torrens et al. [8] concluded that the use of a bigger glenosphere (42 mm) also reduced the development of scapular notching compared with smaller glenospheres (38 mm). More recent work by Werner et al. [9] using computer templating concluded that the lower humeral neck-shaft angle and glenoid lateralization effective for improvement in range of motion after reverse shoulder arthroplasty. The use of the 135° model with 5 mm of glenoid lateralization provided the best results in impingement-free range of motion, with the exception of abduction. Further to that work by Berhouet et al. [10] in a cadaveric study has shown that placing the humeral stem in 20–30° of retroversion avoids inferior impingement. Finally and more recently certain manufacturers have modified their polyethylene inserts in an attempt to again further diminish impingement.

For some time a number of surgeons Boileau et al. [11] have recommended lateralisation of the gleno-sphere using bone graft harvested from the humeral head. Initial basic science research using a shoulder simulator by Henninger et al. [12] revealed that lateralisation does increase joint stability but also increases the deltoid abduction force. Work by Virani et al. [13] using a virtual shoulder model indicated that lateralisation improves motion in all planes. More recent work has shown that the bone graft predictively incorporates into host bone and allows good functional results comparable to those of RSA in the absence of bone graft.

One of the most striking clinical findings after a reverse total shoulder arthroplasty RTSA is a continuing lack of internal and external rotation. That is whilst patients often demonstrate a significant improvement in abduction and flexion they continue to struggle particularly with internal but also external rotation. The reason for this is complex. More careful analysis would indicate that many of these patients have poor internal and external rotation prior to surgery. In addition post-operatively with the rotator cuff removed or dysfunctional the deltoid is not able to compensate. Work by Müller et al. [14] concluded that the increase in glenosphere diameter led to a clinically moderate but significant increase in external rotation.

Finally this deficit in rotation has led some authors to consider combining RTSA with a latissimus dorsi transfer. This transfer of latissimus dorsi allows it to act as an external rotator rather than an internal rotator. Early work by Puskas et al. [15] showed encouraging results. At this time, however, most surgeons would only use this secondarily in patients who continue to complain of a lack of external rotation after primary surgery.

Clinical Pearl

Cuff tear arthropathy remains the pre-eminent indication for a reverse total shoulder arthroplasty. Current evidence indicates good long term clinical results up to at least ten years.

Trauma

The use of reverse total shoulder arthroplasty particularly in elderly patients with unreconstructable or severe fracture dislocation has become more common place. This appears to be as a consequence of the more predictable outcome compared to open reduction and internal fixation or hemi-arthroplasty.

Bufquin et al. [16] published their prospective review of 43 cases in elderly patients who had sustained a three or four part fracture of the upper humerus. The mean follow-up being 22 months. Clinical outcome was satisfactory with a mean active anterior elevation of 97° and a mean active external rotation in abduction of 30°. In addition there was an improvement in modified Constant scores. Post-operative x-rays revealed evidence of peri-prosthetic calcification in 90% of cases, displacement of tuberosity in 53% and notching in 25%. Again they concluded that whilst reverse shoulder arthroplasty can be recommended in this group of patients, longer term follow-up was required.

Gallinet et al. in 2009 compared the outcome in 40 patients treated either by a shoulder hemi-arthroplasty or reverse prosthesis for three or four part displaced fractures of the proximal humerus [17]. They concluded that the reverse prosthesis group showed better results in terms of abduction (mean 91° versus 60°), anterior elevation (mean 97.5° versus 53.5°) and Constant score (mean 53 versus 39). Rotation was, however, better in the hemiarthroplasty group (external rotation, 13.5° versus 9°; internal rotation 54.6° versus 31°. Dash scores were identical in both groups. X-ray analysis showed three abnormal tuberosity fixations in the hemiarthroplasty group and 15 cases of glenoid notching in the reverse implants. They concluded that the reverse implants provided better results providing the patient was no younger than 70 years of age.

Cazeneuve et al. in 2010 reported the clinical and radiological outcome of 36 fractures at a mean of 6.6 years [18]. For this longer term follow-up, there was some diminution in Constant score but 63% of patients had evidence of loosening of a glenoid component.

In conclusion published and ongoing research appears to confirm that reverse total shoulder replacement is the best option in older patients who sustain a severe fracture dislocation of the shoulder. Whilst currently this would apply to patients over 70 years of age, there is no doubt that reverse total shoulder replacement is being used for this indication in younger patients. This should only, however, be undertaken with caution as a long term outcome remains uncertain and does not appear from current data to be as good as for other indications particularly cuff tear arthropathy.

Most manufacturers of reverse total shoulder arthroplasty provide a fracture variant. That is a specifically designed humeral stem (Fig. 18.4). This stem is designed to facilitate cementation but also fixation of the greater and lesser tuberosities. With regard to the latter there is no doubt that theoretically this would have significant advantages, particularly with regard to subsequent internal and external rotation. That said, however, there is no doubt that this can be technically difficult and in many instances tuberosities do not heal and often migrate. As such currently whilst reattachment should be an aim of surgery, there is little hard evidence that this does in fact result in improved outcome.

Clinical Pearl

There seems little doubt that reverse total shoulder replacement gives the best and most consistent results for the treatment of elderly patients with severe fracture dislocation of the shoulder. At this time, however, this should be used with caution in patients under 70 years of age.

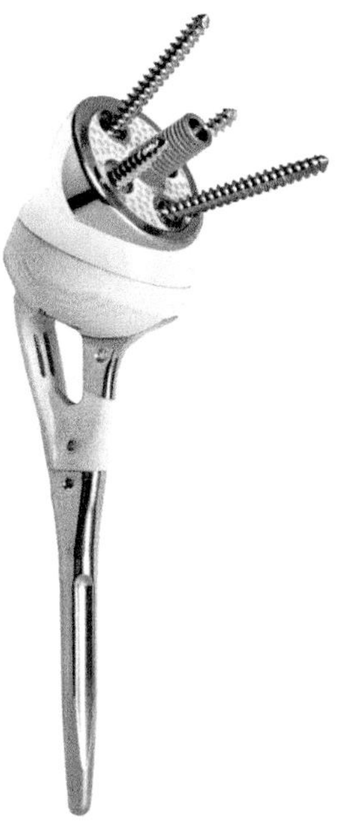

Fig. 18.4 Fracture stem for a reverse total shoulder replacement (Tornier)

Fracture Sequelae

As with acute fractures a reverse shoulder replacement has become increasing used in the sequelae of such injuries, particularly malunion, avascular necrosis, intra-articular disruption, as well as long standing dislocation. As in an acute situation, reverse total shoulder has been shown to give a more predictive outcome when compared to hemi-arthroplasty. Kiliç et al. [19] analysed 55 patients who underwent a delayed prosthesis with ongoing problems. In 36 cases they used an anatomic implant and in 19 a reverse

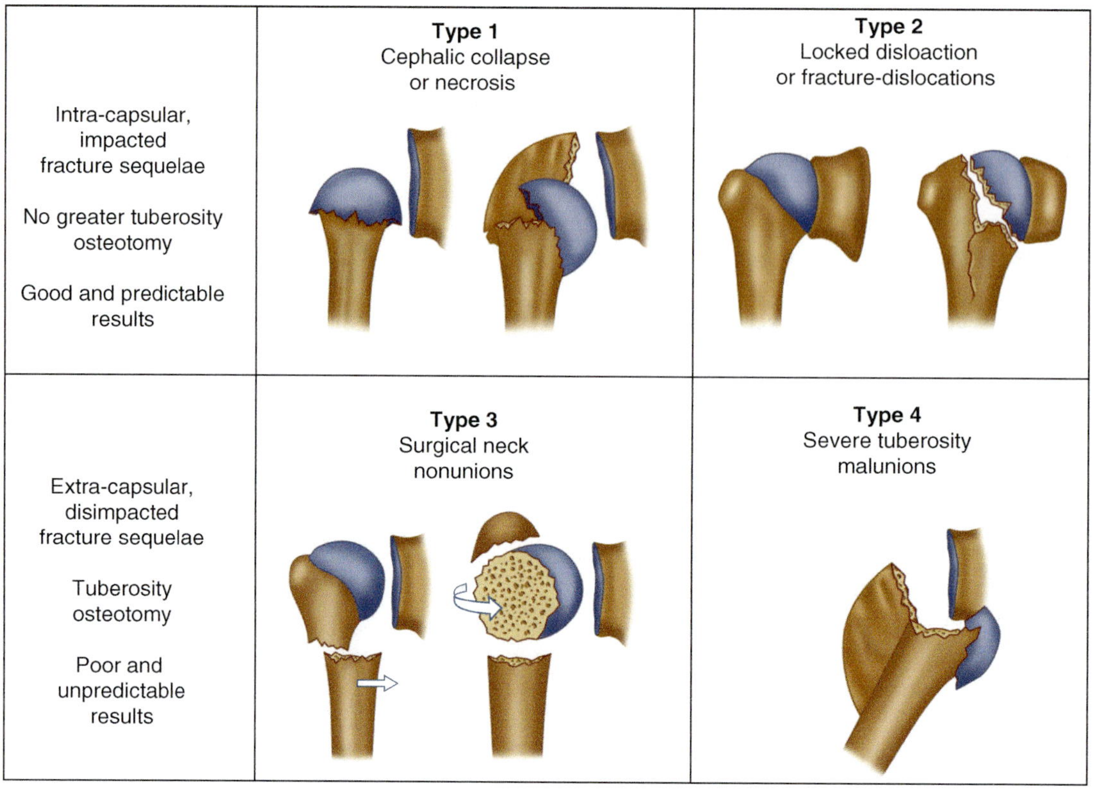

Fig. 18.5 Classification of fractures sequelae of the proximal humerus Boileau and Walch [20]

shoulder replacement. They concluded in the less deformed cases (Boileau and Walch types 1 and 2) (Fig. 18.5) anatomic implants were the better choice. With the more severe types (Boileau and Walch types 3 and 4) the results of reversed implants were superior to anatomic.

Recent studies by Willis et al. [21] looked at 16 patients who were treated with a reverse shoulder arthroplasty for malunion of a proximal humeral fracture. They reported improvement in the ASES score from 28 to 63 and improvement in both pain and function. Forward flexion improved from 53° to 105° and abduction from 48° to 105°. External rotation also improved from 5° to 30° and internal rotation from S1 to L3. They reported no significant complications. Radiologically, however two of the patients had some evidence of notching and one with proximal humeral resorption.

Raiss et al. [22] reported their results in 22 patients followed up for a mean of 3.5 years. These patients had a chronic locked dislocation of the shoulder. Again they reported a significant increase in function with a Constant- Murley score improving from 13.6 to 47.4. Shoulder flexion increasing 37.7°–103°. External rotation from −0.5° to 14.7°. Otherwise six patients (27%) underwent revision surgery. The commonest indication being failure of the glenoid component due to bone defects on the glenoid side.

Finally Shannon et al. [23] compared the outcome of reverse shoulder replacement used in the acute scenario, that is immediately after fracture versus reverse shoulder replacement after failed osteosynthesis. They concluded that clinical outcome and function remained comparable, although there was a higher rate of complications in patients who underwent RTSA after failed ORIF. These included dislocation and aseptic loosening.

By way of conclusion there is no doubt that a reverse shoulder replacement has an important role in the management of sequelae of fractured dislocations of the shoulder. Whilst in the less deformed cases, with an intact functioning rotator cuff, there is a role for an anatomic replacement, in the more severe cases of malunion, cuff deficiency and dislocation a reverse implant provides the most consistent outcome. Results, however, whilst showing some improvement in motion are not as good as in the acute scenario.

Clinical Pearl
A reverse shoulder replacement provides a good and consistent outcome for patients who suffer with significant sequelae following a fracture dislocation of the shoulder (Boileau and Walch types 3 and 4).

Irreparable Massive Cuff Tear Without Osteoarthritis

Whilst repair remains the cornerstone for the treatment for rotator cuff tears. In patients with massive tears this may not be possible. Whilst the use of augments and tendon transfers have been popularised, results to date have been unpredictable. As such, in older patients with a pseudopalsy reverse total shoulder replacement has been popularised. On the downside of course this is a much more invasive procedure with a higher rate of potential complications. As such, this surgery should only be undertaken in patients who are suffering significantly with pain and loss of function. As would be expected publications on this indication are few and far between. However, in 2009 Boileau et al. reported their analysis on 42 implants (40 patients) who underwent a reverse shoulder arthroplasty for a painful or pseudoparalytic shoulder [24]. The mean follow-up was 50 months. Overall they reported an increase in active elevation from 56° to 123° with particular improvement in patients suffering with pseudopalsy. Despite this, approximately one quarter of patients were disappointed or dissatisfied. Added to that there were 5 complications of which 2 patients underwent reoperation.

In 2010 Mulieri et al. reported their experience in 69 patients (72 implants) with a minimum of 2 year follow- up [25]. They reported an improvement in all measures post-operatively both with function and pain relief. Average forward flexion improved from 53° to 134° and abduction from 49° to 125°. Average internal rotation improved from S1 to L2 and average external rotation from 27° to 51°. Overall there were 12 complications (20%). A mean survivorship of 52 months was 90.7%.

Whilst undoubtedly controversial reverse total shoulder replacement does offer a viable option in older patients with a massive irreparable rotator cuff in the absence of osteoarthritis. Early clinical results are optimistic, however there is no doubt that this is a major undertaking with a potential high rate of complications.

Inflammatory Arthritis with Cuff Tears

The use of reverse shoulder replacement in inflammatory arthritis has lagged behind its use in osteoarthritis. The rationale for this being that there was some concern with regard to the quality of the glenoid bone stock and as a consequence glenoid fixation. With time, however, and some satisfactory early results its use has become more common place. This should, however, be contrasted against an overall reduction in the numbers of shoulder replacements being undertaken in patients with inflammatory arthritis as a result of improved medical management (Fig. 18.6).

In 2001 Rittmeister and Kerschbaumer reported their results in 7 patients (8 shoulders) with severe inflammatory arthritis [26]. They reported improvement in the Constant score as well as movement in strength. Complications included sepsis in one shoulder and glenoid loosening in another two. They concluded the results in this type of implant are encouraging however, glenoid loosening remains a problem.

In 2010 Holcomb et al. reported their results of 21 implants in patients who suffered with severe rheumatoid arthritis [27]. They again

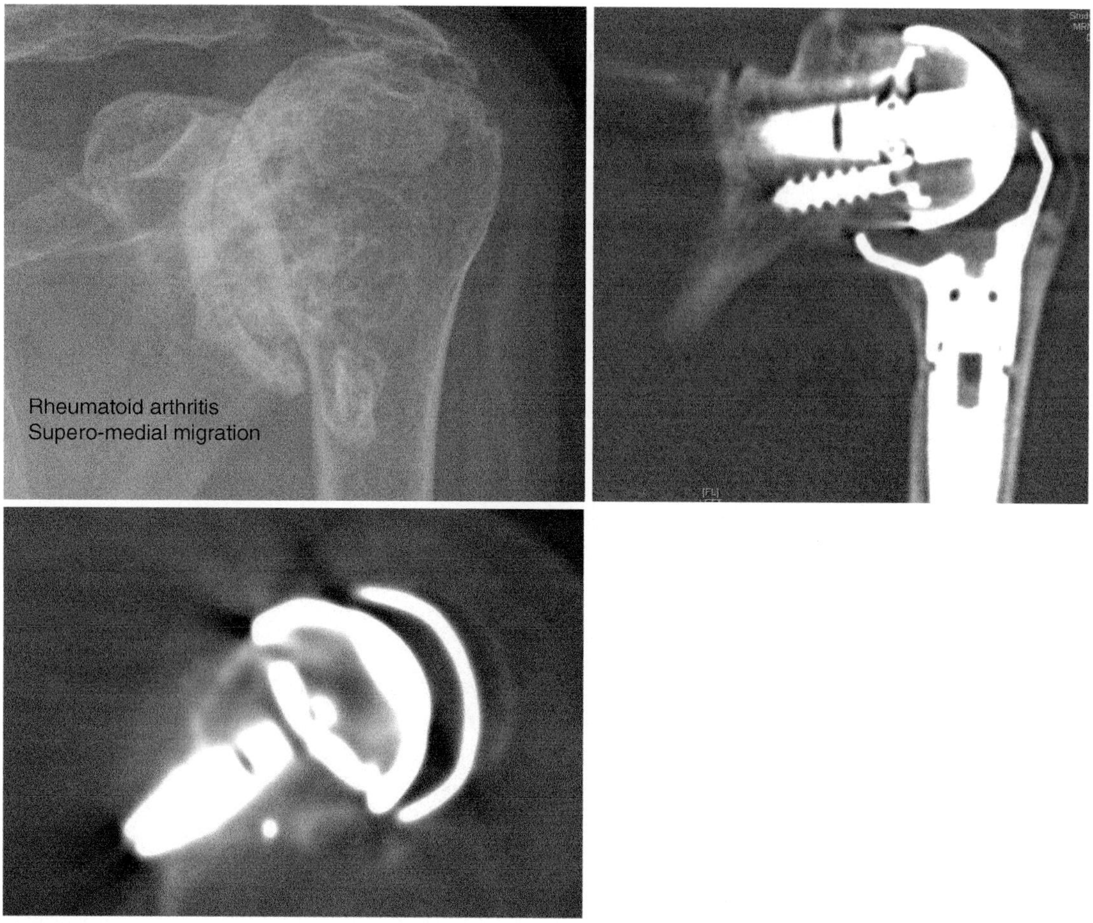

Fig. 18.6 Severe rheumatoid arthritis treated by a reverse total shoulder replacement and bone graft

reported a significant improvement in all outcome measures including American Shoulder and Elbow scores for both pain and function. Added to that, elevation improved from 52° to 126° and abduction from 55° to 116°. External rotation improved from 19° to 33° and internal rotation from S1 to L4. Overall patient satisfaction was high. Three patients (14%) sustained a complication that required reoperation.

Finally in 2011 Young et al. reported their results in 18 reverse shoulder replacements in 16 patients with rheumatoid arthritis [28]. Again they reported an improvement in function as per the Constant score with a high patient satisfaction. Active forward elevation improved from 77.5° to 138.6° and external rotation of the arm in 90°abduction from 16.9° to 46.1°. Scapular notching was observed in 10 of the 18 shoulders. Added to that there was a fracture of the acromion, acromial spine, coracoid, or greater tuberosity in 4 of the 18 shoulders. None of these patients required revision surgery. Again they concluded this type of replacement did have a place in the treatment of patients with inflammatory arthritis of the shoulder although there was an increased risk of intraoperative or postoperative fractures.

By way of a summary it appears that despite initial concerns inflammatory arthritis has now become a recognised indication for a reverse total shoulder arthroplasty. Early results show satisfactory pain relief, movement and function although there is an increased risk of an intra or post-operative fracture. It is likely, however, that the number of such surgeries will be limited given the advent of more successful medical management.

Revision Surgery

Revision surgery can be performed for many and varied reasons. These include aseptic loosening, cuff failure, infection, glenoid erosion etc. In our experience reverse shoulder prosthesis is more commonly used than anatomic in this scenario.

To date, there are a number of publications confirming that reverse shoulder arthroplasty works well in the revision scenario. In 2007 Levy et al. reported their experience using this type of implant for a failed hemiarthroplasty after a proximal humeral fracture [29]. In a series of 29 patients they reported a significant improvement in pain score, function and movement. The forward flexion improved from 38° to 73° and abduction from 34° to 72°. There was, however, a high overall complication rate of 28%. These included a peri-prosthestic fracture together with a dislocation, infection and implant failure.

Similar work by Black et al. [30] who analysed the role of RTSA as a salvage procedure for failed arthroplasty in patients 65 years or younger. In their series of 36 patients there were a number of indications including infection, rotator cuff failure, glenoid component loosening and glenoid erosion. Previous implants included total shoulder arthroplasty, hemiarthroplasty or a cement spacer. Clinical outcome showed a significant improvement in pain and function and forward elevation to 115° and external rotation of 31°. Again, however, there was a high rate of complications at 19% which included instability and base plate failure.

Following infection Cuff et al. [31] reported their results in 21 patients (22 shoulders) who underwent revision surgery for deep infection. At a mean follow-up of 43 months there was no evidence of a recurrent infection. Most patients again noted satisfactory pain relief with a mean abduction improvement from 36° to 76°, forward flexion from 43° to 80° and a mean external rotation of 25°. There were, however, 11 complications in 7 shoulders. These included a periprosthetic scapular fracture, dislocation, base plate loosening, humeral fracture and radial nerve palsy.

For subsequent failure of the rotator cuff Flury et al. [32] reported their experience in 20 consecutive patients who underwent 21 revisions to a reverse implant. These were followed up for a mean of 46 months from surgery. Again clinical results were satisfactory by way of good pain relief and function and flexion improving from 43° to 97° and abduction from 44° to 90°. Unfortunately active external rotation decreased and there was a higher rate of complications. These included fracture of the humerus, radial nerve palsy and infection.

Holcomb et al. [33] reported their results of revision for a failure of the glenoid base plate in 14 patients. Again results were similar in that in the successful patients there was pain relief and improved motion, unfortunately there was again a high rate of complications.

Work from Wrightington Hospital has shown the benefit of the use of autograft either structural or impaction grafting taken either from the humeral head or iliac crest to reconstruct glenoid deficiencies. Malhas et al. [34] in a series of 45 shoulder replacements taken for a range of aetiologies were able to show integration of bone graft in 93% of cases. Integration being to the host bone but also trabecular titanium peg. There were, however, again a number of complications including rotator cuff failure for which revision surgery was required. Further work using allograft and metal augments again to correct for deficiencies have shown encouraging results although the use of allograft in cases of revision for infection is no longer recommended (Figs. 18.7, 18.8, and 18.9).

There is no doubt that a reverse total shoulder replacement has a significant role to play in the revision scenario. The particular advantages are the metal glenoid base plate which facilitates the attachments of augments particularly and allows one composite fixation. Added to that significant soft tissue defect can be addressed as well as any consequent instability.

Clinical Pearl
A reverse total shoulder replacement remains the main stay of revision shoulder arthroplasty in that it allows reconstruction of glenoid defects as well as addressing soft tissue abnormalities around the proximal humerus.

Miscellaneous

The use of reverse shoulder replacement is evolving. As stated previously, indications have expanded to include fracture, massive irreparable cuff tear without arthritis in the elderly patient and revision. Reverse shoulder replacement, however, has been used in other perhaps unique situations. A publication by Otto et al. [35]

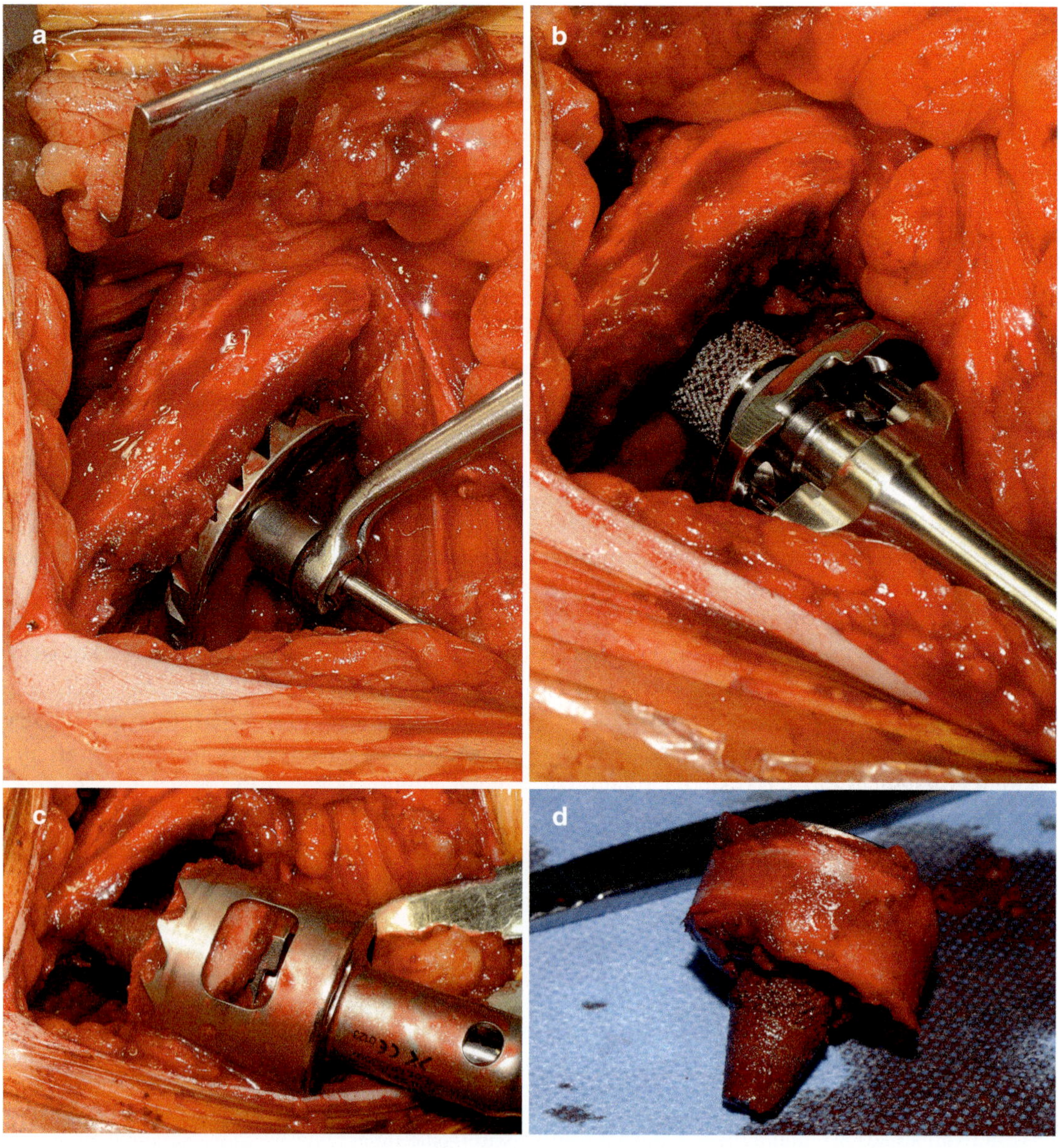

Fig. 18.7 Iliac crest bone used as a structural graft to reconstruct the glenoid

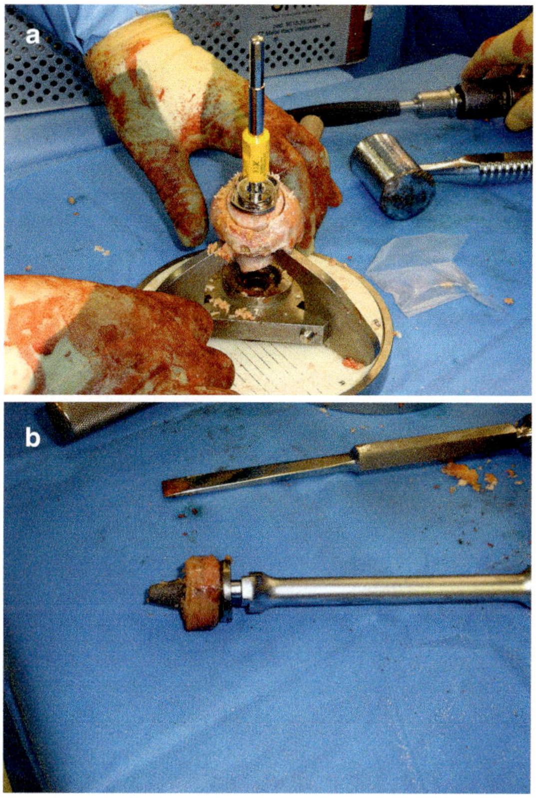

Fig. 18.8 Femoral head allograft used as a structural graft to reconstruct the glenoid

assessed the outcome of RTSA in patients younger than 55 years of age. In their series there were 67 patients with an average age of 48. The average follow-up being 62 months. Within the group, however, there were both primary and revision implants. Both groups showed significant improvements in pain relief, function and movement. In the revision group, however, internal and external rotation did not improve. Overall implant retention was 91% with a total complication rate of 22.4%.

Similar work by Samuelsen et al. again in (2017) reported their experience in 63 patients with a mean age of 60 [36]. In this series there were no revisions. With a mean follow-up of 3 years again there was a significant improvement in pain, active abduction at 132° and external rotation of 39°. Ninety per cent of patients were satisfied with the results and revision free survival was 91% at 5 years. Both these publications, however, emphasize the importance of long term follow-up. Certainly at this stage, use of RTSA should only be used in a young age group with caution.

In 2016 Statz et al. reported their results in patients who were morbidly obese and

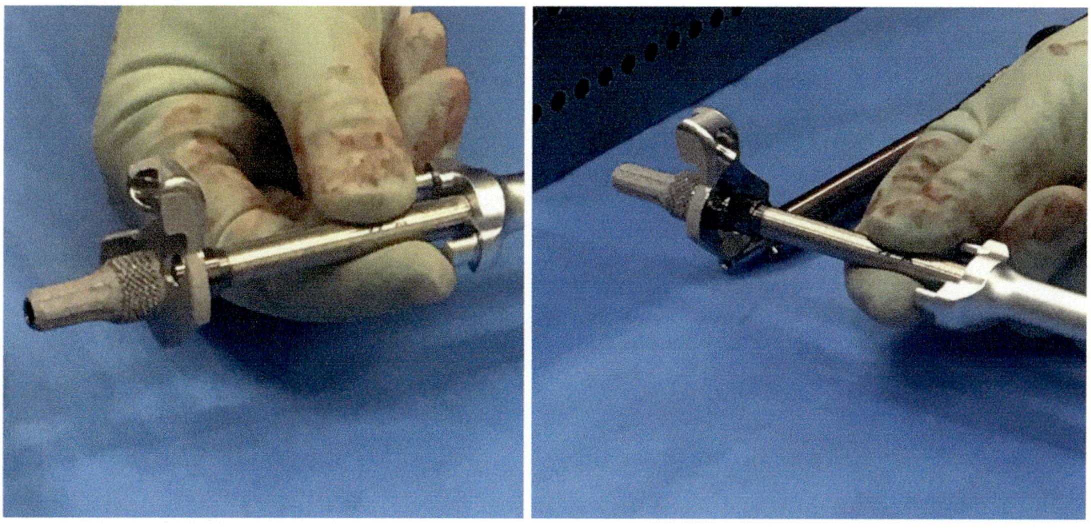

Fig. 18.9 Metal augment to reconstruct the glenoid (Promade, Lima)

underwent primary reverse shoulder arthroplasty [37]. They concluded that this prosthesis can be used in this clinical scenario and that at intermediate follow-up there was good implant survival with a reasonable complication rate.

Finally Aibinder et al. [38] again from the Mayo Clinic reported the outcome of reverse shoulder arthroplasty in patients with an os acromiale. They concluded that the latter did not seem to negatively affect the outcome in that pain around the os acromiale was rare.

Summary

There is no doubt since the initial successful design by Paul Grammont in 1981 the use of reverse total shoulder arthroplasty has become common place. Whilst the initial design demonstrated the clinical value of the procedure, more recent modifications have reduced the potential for complications. Overall reverse total shoulder arthroplasty has equalled and in some instances surpassed the use of anatomic total shoulder arthroplasty. Initial concerns with regard to glenoid notching appear to have been addressed by various techniques including lateralisation, inferior placing of the glenoid plate as well as various implant design changes. As a consequence glenoid plate fixation seems assured. Instability has also been addressed primarily by changes to surgical technique but also changes in implant design. The incidence of dislocation in primary cases seems to have diminished. The only ongoing concerns remain the lack of rotation both internal but particularly external. Whether this can be addressed in the long term remains a topic of great debate. Finally and perhaps more importantly there is little in the literature related to long term survival. That is survivalship of the implant 10 years or more. Hopefully, however, with increasing usage this will be addressed over the next few years. With regard to indications these appear to be solidifying and there is no doubt the use of reverse total shoulder arthroplasty will be with us for many years to come.

References

1. Naveed MA, Kitson J, Bunker TD. The Delta III reverse shoulder replacement for cuff tear arthropathy.: a single-centre study of 50 consecutive procedures. J Bone Joint Surg (Br). 2011;93:57–61.
2. Nolan BM, Ankerson E, Wiater JM. Reverse total shoulder arthroplasty improves function in cuff tear arthropathy. Clin Orthop Relat Res. 2011;469:2476–82.
3. Favard L, Levigne C, Nerot C, Gerber C, De Wilde L, Mok D. Reverse prostheses in arthroplasties with cuff tear: are survivorship and function maintained over time? Clin Orthop Relat Res. 2011;469:2469–75.
4. Day JS, MacDonald DW, Olsen M, Getz C, Williams GR, Kurtz SM. Polyethylene wear in retrieved reverse total shoulder components. J Shoulder Elb Surg. 2012;21:667–74.
5. Simovitch RW, Zumstein MA, Lohri E, Helmy N, Gerber C. Predictors of scapular notching in patients managed with the Delta III reverse total shoulder replacement. J Bone Joint Surg [Am]. 2007;89(3):588–600.
6. Roche CP, Marczuk Y, Wright TW, Flurin PH, Grey S, Jones R, Routman HD, Gilot G, Zuckerman JD. Scapular notching and osteophyte formation after reverse shoulder replacement. Bone Joint J [Am]. 2013;95:530–5.
7. Bradley Edwards T, Trappey GJ, Riley C, O'Connor DP, Elkousy HA, Gartsman GM. Inferior tilt of the glenoid component does not decrease scapular notching in reverse shoulder arthroplasty: results of a prospective randomized study. J Shoulder Elb Surg. 2012;21:641–6.
8. Torrens C, Guirro P, Miquel J, Santana F. Influence of glenosphere size on the development of scapular notching: a prospective randomized study. J Shoulder Elb Surg. 2016;25:1735–41.
9. Werner BS, Chaoui J, Walch G. The influence of humeral neck shaft angle and glenoid lateralization on range of motion in reverse shoulder arthroplasty. J Shoulder Elb Surg. 2017;26:1726–31.
10. Berhouet J, Garaud P, Favard L. Evaluation of the role of glenosphere design and humeral component retroversion in avoiding scapular notching during reverse shoulder arthroplasty. J Shoulder Elb Surg. 2013;23:151–8.
11. Boileau P, Moineau G, Roussanne Y, O'Shea K. Bony increased-offset reversed shoulder arthroplasty: minimizing scapular impingement while maximizing glenoid fixation. Clin Orthop Relat Res. 2011;469:2558–67.
12. Henninger HB, Barg A, Anderson AE, Bachus KN, Burks RT, Tashjian RZ. Effect of lateral offset centre of rotation in reverse total shoulder arthroplasty: a biomechanical study. J Shoulder Elbow Surg. 2012;21(9):1128–35.
13. Virani NA, Cabezas A, Gutiérrez S, Santoni BG, Otto R, Frankle M. Reverse shoulder arthroplasty compo-

nents and surgical techniques that restore glenohumeral motion. J Shoulder Elb Surg. 2013;22:179–87.
14. Müller AM, Born M, Jung C, Flury M, Kolling C, Schwyzer HK, Audigé L. Glenosphere size in reverse shoulder arthroplasty: is larger better for external rotation and abduction strength? J Shoulder Elb Surg. 2018;27:44–52.
15. Puskas GJ, Germann M, Catanzaro S, Gerber C. Secondary latissimus dorsi transfer after failed reverse total shoulder arthroplasty. J Shoulder Elb Surg. 2015;24:e337–44.
16. Bufquin T, Hersan A, Hubert L, Massin P. Reverse shoulder arthroplasty for the treatment of three and four part fracutres in the proximal humerus in the elderly: a prospective review of 43 cases with a short-term follow-up. J Bone Joint Surg [Br]. 2007;89(4):516–20.
17. Gallinet D, Clappaz P, Garbuio P, Tropet Y, Obert L. Three or four parts complex proximal humerus fractures: hemiarthroplasty versus reverse prosthesis: a comparative study of 40 cases. Orthop Traumatol Surg Res. 2009;95:48–55.
18. Cazeneuve JF, Cristofari DJ. The reverse shoulder prosthesis in the treatment of fractures of the proximal humerus in the elderly. J Bone Joint Surg [Br]. 2010;92(4):535–9.
19. Kiliç M, Berth A, Blatter G, Fuhrmann U, Gebhardt K, Rott O, Zenz P, Irlenbusch U. Anatomic and reverse shoulder prostheses in fracture sequelae of the humeral head. Acta Orthop Traumatol Turc. 2010;44(6):417–25.
20. Boileau P, Walch G, Trojani C, Veneau B, Sinnerton R. Sequelae of fractures of the proximal humerus: results of shoulder arthroplasty without greater tuberosity osteotomy. In: Walch G, Boileau P, editors. Shoulder arthroplasty. Berlin/Heidelberg/New York: Springer; 1999. p. 359–69.
21. Willis M, Min W, Brooks JP, Mulieri P, Walker M, Pupello D, Frankle M. Proximal humeral malunion treated with reverse shoulder arthroplasty. J Shoulder Elb Surg. 2012;21:507–13.
22. Raiss P, Bradley Edwards T, Bruckner T, Loew M, Zeifang F, Walch G. Reverse arthroplasty for patients with chronic locked dislocation of the shoulder (type 2 fracture sequela). J Shoulder Elbow Surg. 2017;26:279–87.
23. Shannon SF, Wagner ER, Houdek MT, Cross WW, Sánchez-Sotelo J. Reverse shoulder arthroplasty for proximal humeral fractures: outcomes comparing primary reverse arthroplasty for fracture versus reverse arthroplasty after failed osteosynthesis. J Shoulder Elb Surg. 2016;25:1655–60.
24. Boileau P, Gonzalez JF, Chuinard C, Bicknell R, Walch G. Reverse total shoulder arthroplasty after failed rotator cuff surgery. J Shoulder Elb Surg. 2009;18:600–6.
25. Mulieri P, Dunning P, Klein S, Pupello D, Frankle M. Reverse shoulder arthroplasty for the treatment of irreparable rotator cuff tear without glenohumeral arthritis. J Bone Joint Surg Am. 2010;92:2544–56.
26. Rittmeister M, Kerschbaumer F. Grammont reverse total shoulder arthroplasty in patients with rheumatoid arthritis and nonreconstructible rotator cuff lesions. J Shoulder Elbow Surg. 2001;10(1):17–22.
27. Holcomb JO, Hebert DJ, Mighell MA, Dunning PE, Pupello DR, Pliner MD, Frankle MA. Reverse shoulder arthroplasty in patients with rheumatoid arthritis. J Shoulder Elb Surg. 2010;19:1076–84.
28. Young AA, Smith MM, Bacle G, Moraga C, Walch G. Early results of reverse shoulder arthroplasty in patients with rheumatoid arthritis. J Bone Joint Surg Am. 2011;93:1915–23.
29. Levy J, Frankle M, Mighell M, Pupello D. The use of the reverse shoulder prosthesis for the treatment of failed hemiarthroplasty for proximal humeral fracture. J Bone Joint Surg Am. 2007;89(2):292–300.
30. Black EM, Roberts SM, Siegel E, Yannopoulos P, Higgins LD, Warner JJP. Reverse shoulder arthroplasty as salvage for failed prior arthroplasty in patients 65 years of age or younger. J Shoulder Elb Surg. 2014;23:1036–42.
31. Cuff DJ, Virani J, Levy NA, Frankle MA, Derasari A, Hines B, Pupello DR, Cancio M, Mighell M. The treatment of deep shoulder infection and glenohumeral instability with debridement, reverse shoulder arthroplasty and post-operative antibiotics. J Bone Joint Surg (Br). 2008;90(3):336–42.
32. Flury MP, Frey P, Goldhahn J. Reverse shoulder arthroplasty as a salvage procedure for failed conventional shoulder replacement due to cuff failure – midterm results. Inter Orthop (SICOT). 2011;35:53–60.
33. Holcomb JO, Cuff D, Petersen SA, Pupello DR, Frankle MA. Revision reverse shoulder arthroplasty for glenoid baseplate failure after primary reverse shoulder arthroplasty. J Shoulder Elb Surg. 2009;18:717–23.
34. Malhas A, Brookes-Fazackerley S, Walton M, Bale S, Trail IA. Autologous bone-graft glenoid reconstruction with the SMR TT metal-back prosthesis: the first fifty cases at two years follow-up. The Bone & Joint Journal. 2018.
35. Otto RJ, Clark RE, Frankle MA. Reverse shoulder arthroplasty in patients younger than 55 years: 2 to 12 year follow-up. J Shoulder Elb Surg. 2017;26:792–7.
36. Samuelsen BT, Wagner ER, Houdek MT, Elhassan BT, Sánchez-Sotelo J, Cofield R, Sperling JW. Primary reverse shoulder arthroplasty in patients aged 65 years or younger. J Shoulder Elb Surg. 2017;26:e13–7.
37. Statz JM, Wagner ER, Houdek MT, Cofield RH, Sánchez-Sotelo J, Elhassan BT, Sperling JW. Outcomes of primary reverse shoulder arthroplasty in patients with morbid obesity. J Shoulder Elb Surg. 2016;25:e191–8.
38. Aibinder WR, Schoch BS, Cofield RH, Sperling JW, Sánchez-Sotelo J. Reverse shoulder arthroplasty in patients with os acromiale. J Shoulder Elb Surg. 2017;26:1598–602.

Complications of the Reverse Implant

19

Daniel Mok, Francis Lam, and Ram Chidambaram

Introduction

Reverse shoulder replacements (RSA) is known to have a high complication rate. Werner reported an overall complication rate of 50% for the first series of Delta III prosthesis (DePuy France, Saint Priest CEDEX, France) [1]. In a review of 10,884 shoulder arthroplasties performed in 2011–2013, the overall complication rates of RSA and anatomical total shoulder arthroplasty (TSA) were compared [2]. At 30 days, the overall complication rate for for both types of shoulder arthroplasties was 2.2%. The higher early complication rate of 3% for RSA compared with 1.7% for TSA reached statistical significance. RSA patients had increased risk of infection, dislocation and revision in the early postoperative period. At 2 years, the complication rates for RSA rose to 21.8% compared with TSA at 14.3%. Dislocation and infection remained as significant complication for RSA. The study also found patients younger than 65 years, male sex, patients with anaemia, and those with worker's compensation had a higher risk in developing complications.

There were many reasons for this. The prosthesis was a new design in 1985 and it needed time to evolve and improve after clinical use. In 2005, Boileau reported 31% complications in his initial series of RSA with scapular notching noted in 68% [3]. Frankle changed his design to one with stronger locking screws for his glenosphere baseplate as the earlier design failed [4].

Secondly, the procedure is challenging with a steep learning curve. Most authors experience a learning curve in choosing the right prosthesis and their ideal placement location. Harmsden reported a reduction of complication rate from 17.3% to 8% after the first 75 patients [5].

Thirdly, indications for its use are wide and variable. That is RSA is used to treat a variety of conditions including proximal humeral fractures in the elderly, failed fracture fixation as well as revision arthroplasties. Complications for each indication are different. Werner's high complication rate may be related to the large number of RSA (71%) they used to revise failed arthroplasties [1]. In a literature review of 782 RSA between 1995 and 2008, Zumstein found RSA performed for revision arthroplasties had a complication rate of 33.3% compared with those performed for cuff tear arthropathy at 19.5% [6]. Patients with rheumatoid arthritis did badly with a complication rate of 45% and those after acute fractures had a complication rate of 36%. In order to reduce complications for our RSA, we need to

D. Mok,
FRCSEd, FRCS, FHKCOS, FHKAM (✉)
Hong Kong Shoulder Wrist and Knee Centre,
Hong Kong, China
e-mail: daniel@topshoulder.com.hk

F. Lam, FRCS Ed (Orth)
Adventist Hospital, Hong Kong, China
e-mail: Francis.Lam@hkah.org.hk

R. Chidambaram, Ms Ortho, DNB, FRCS, FRCS Orth
Department of Shoulder and Upper Limb Surgery,
MIOT International Hospitals, Chennai, India

I. A. Trail et al. (eds.), *Textbook of Shoulder Surgery*, https://doi.org/10.1007/978-3-319-70099-1_19

review the causes and adopt the appropriate technique to ensure a good outcome.

Scapular Notching

This is the most common complication after RSA [7]. With medialisation of the centre of rotation, impingement of the humeral component against the scapular neck with the arm by the side of the body is the reason potentially for notching. It has been reported in 44–96% of RSA, usually occurring as early as after 6 months [8]. Sirveaux described four grades of notching based on antero-posterior radiographs (Fig. 19.1a). Grade 1 notching does not involve the inferior screw. Grade 2 notching occurs up to the inferior screw (Fig. 19.1b). Grade 3 notching occurs above the inferior screw and grade 4 extends to the base plate [9].

Anterior and posterior notching can be detected as areas of lucencies under the base plate on axillary radiographs. In 80 first generation reverse shoulder replacements (Delta, DePuy, France) followed up for 44 months, he reported erosions of grade 3 or above were associated with a compromised Constant score. In a larger series of 326 patients followed up for an average of 47 months, Lévigne reported notching increased with time [7]. They attributed two reasons for this progression. The continued impingement of the humeral component and polyethylene debris particles could cause osteolysis of the glenoid rim. Unlike Sirveaux, they did not find notching to be associated with a poor clinical outcome. Although there is a correlation between notching and lucent lines around the glenoid fixation screws, they only had one case of glenoid loosening. The authors also found notching was associated with the superolateral approach. They postulated that the inability to clear soft tissues off the inferior glenoid rim and neck from this approach was to blame for the higher percentage of notching seen when compared with the delto-pectoral approach.

In cuff arthropathy, proximal migration of the humeral head can cause erosion of the superior part of the glenoid. Favard classified this erosion into neutral (E0), concentric (E1), Superior (E2), Global superior (E3) and inferior (E4) (Fig. 19.2). He found that the Superior tilt (E2) glenoid is associated with notching in 83% [10]. His recommendation was to avoid placing the glenosphere with a superior tilt, even though this may have been the "natural orientation" for that patient.

Gerber noted anterior and posterior notching as well as the presence of osteophytes on the inferior scapular neck in his review of 188 Delta

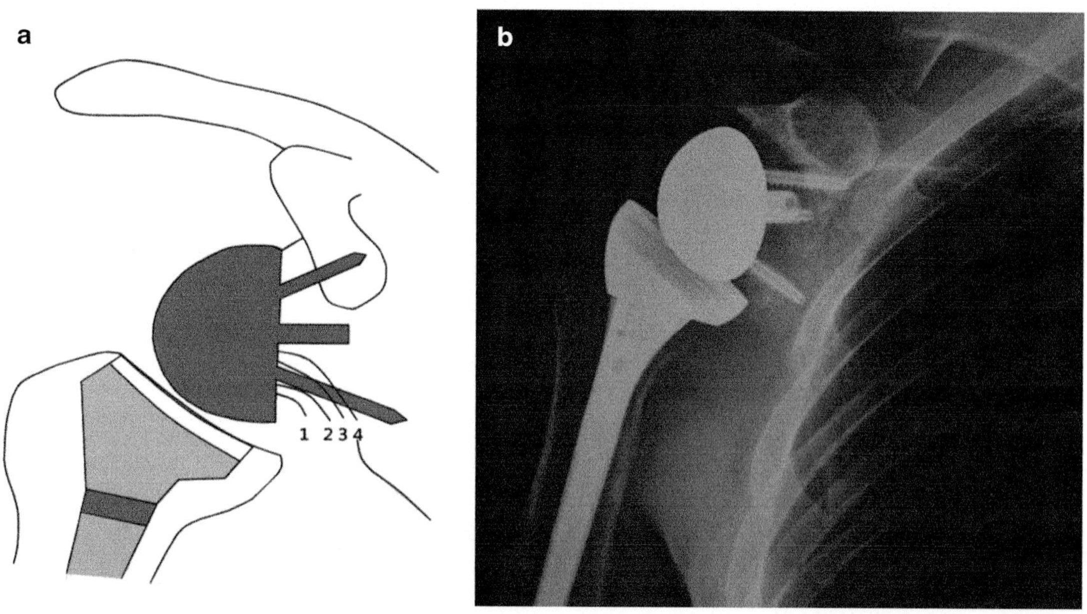

Fig. 19.1 (a) Sirveaux classification of scapular notching. (b) Type 2 notching 2 years post surgery

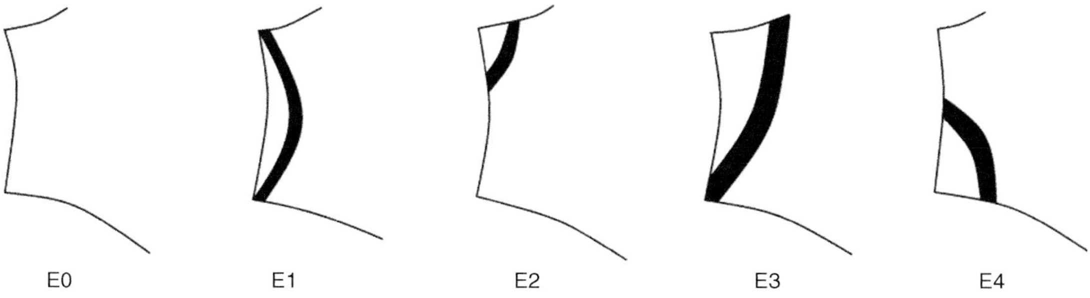

Fig. 19.2 Favard classification of glenoid erosion

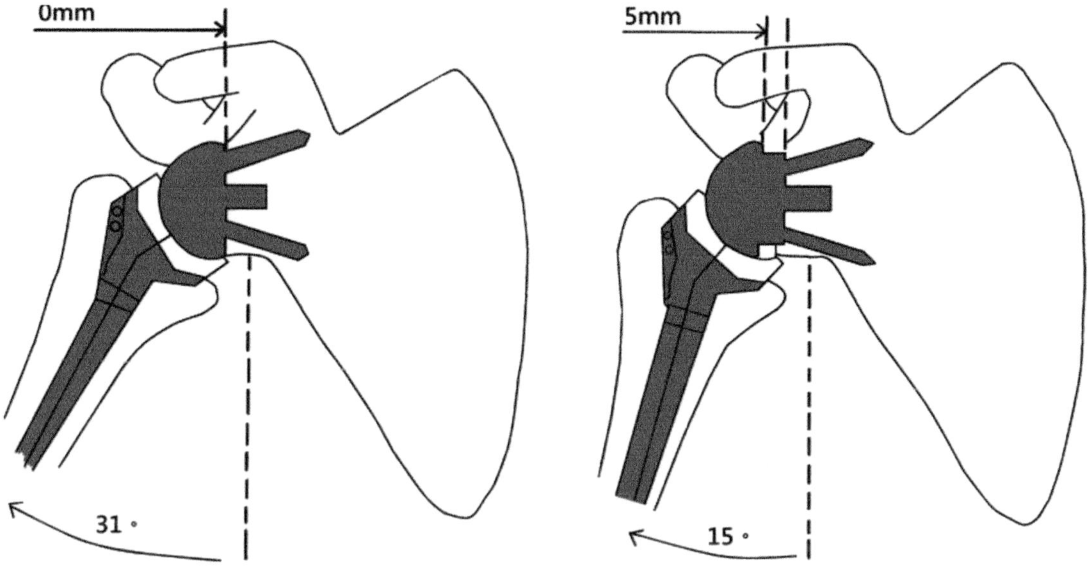

Fig. 19.3 Lateralisation of centre of rotation by 5 mm improves adduction by 16°. (Re-drawn with permission from Dr. L. De Wilder)

III RSA (DePuy Orthopaedics, Warsaw, Indiana) followed up for an average of 44 months [11]. Posterior notching is associated with external rotation. Anterior notching is rare and probably associated with impingement in internal rotation. The osteophytes were probably traction spurs formed after incomplete release of the triceps tendon. None of the observations affected the clinical outcome. He confirmed notching is associated with both a lower Constant score and Subjective Shoulder value.

In order to reduce notching, various technical as well as prosthetic modifications have been introduced.

1. Lateralisation of the centre of rotation by a glenosphere larger than a hemisphere (Fig. 19.3). Theoretically, moving the humeral component away from the scapular neck would allow greater adduction movement at the expense of increased load on the glenoid component, which may induce loosening. Frankle has reported less notching in his first 60 prostheses reviewed at an average of 33 months. It was, however, associated with glenoid loosening in 12% and all required revision [12]. He resolved this by changing the base plate locking screws to 5 mm [13].

2. Lateralisation by extending the scapular neck by insertion of a 10 mm bone block under the base plate (Fig. 19.4). Boileau harvested his graft from the humeral head and fixed it to the glenoid with a 25 mm central peg base plate. (Aequalis Reverse Shoulder Prosthesis, Tornier Inc., Houston, TX) [14]. He only had 19% of 42 shoulders with notching at an average follow up of 28 months. Bone graft incorporation to the neck was observed in 98%. There was no glenoid loosening or instability. Good clinical results were obtained. He attributed the success of this modification because the centre of rotation remained at the base plate bone interface.
3. Increase in the overhang of the glenosphere by moving the humeral component more distal. This can be achieved by the use of an eccentric glenosphere with inferior overhang (Fig. 19.5), tilting the glenosphere inferiorly (Fig. 19.6), or use of a larger glenosphere (Fig. 19.7).

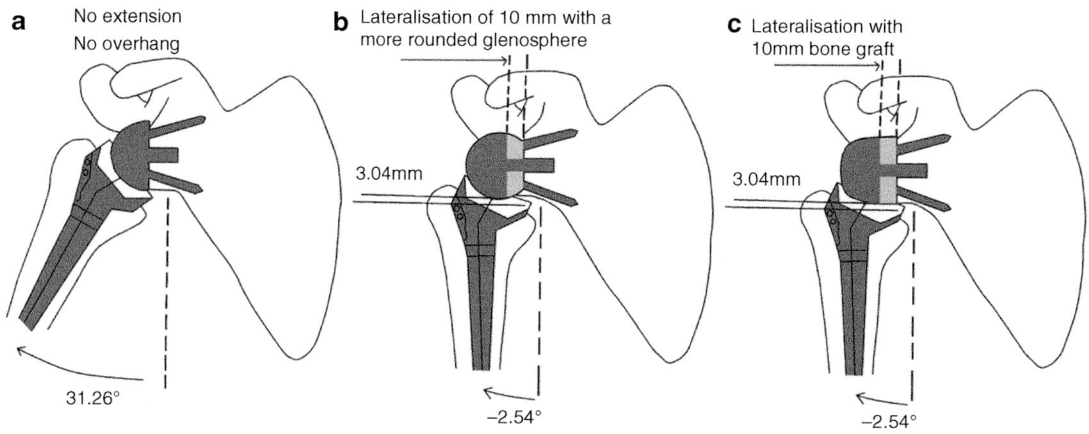

Fig. 19.4 Lateralisation of 10 mm using more rounded glenosphere and bone graft augmentation

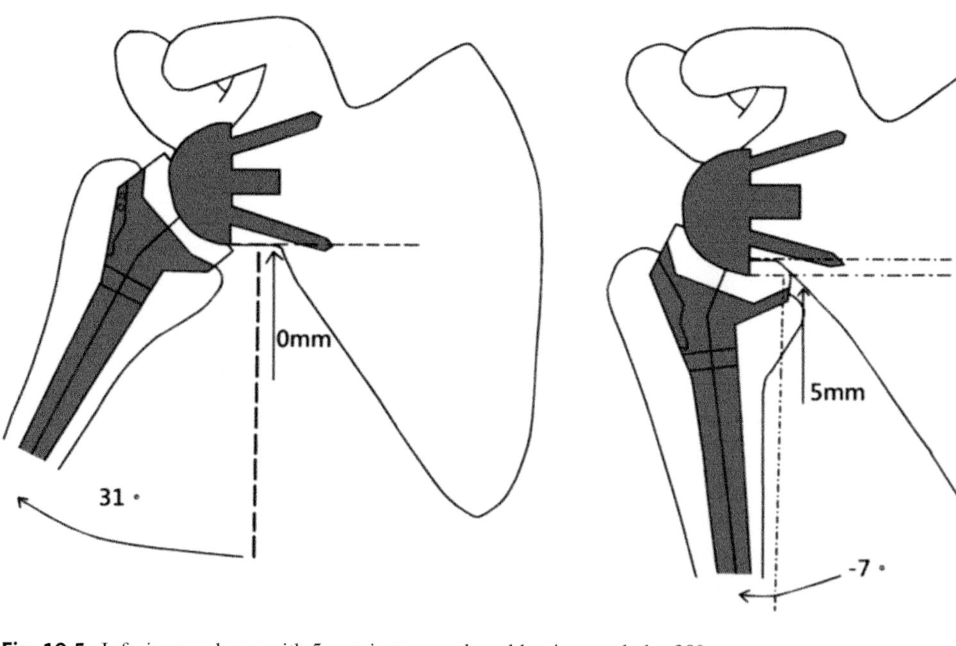

Fig. 19.5 Inferior overhang with 5 mm increases the adduction angle by 38°

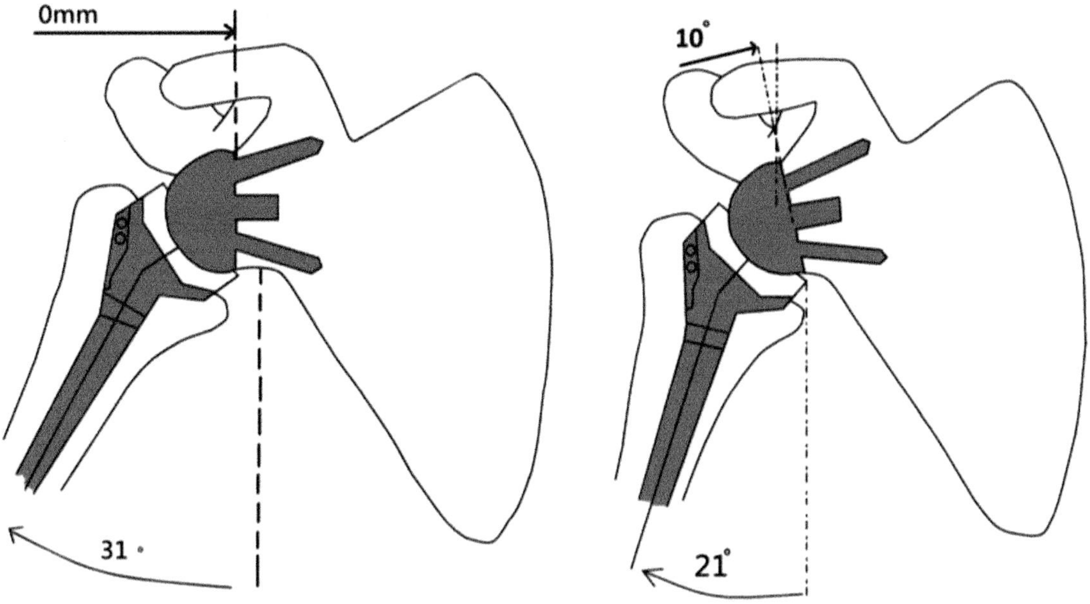

Fig. 19.6 Inferior tilt of 10° improves adduction by 10°

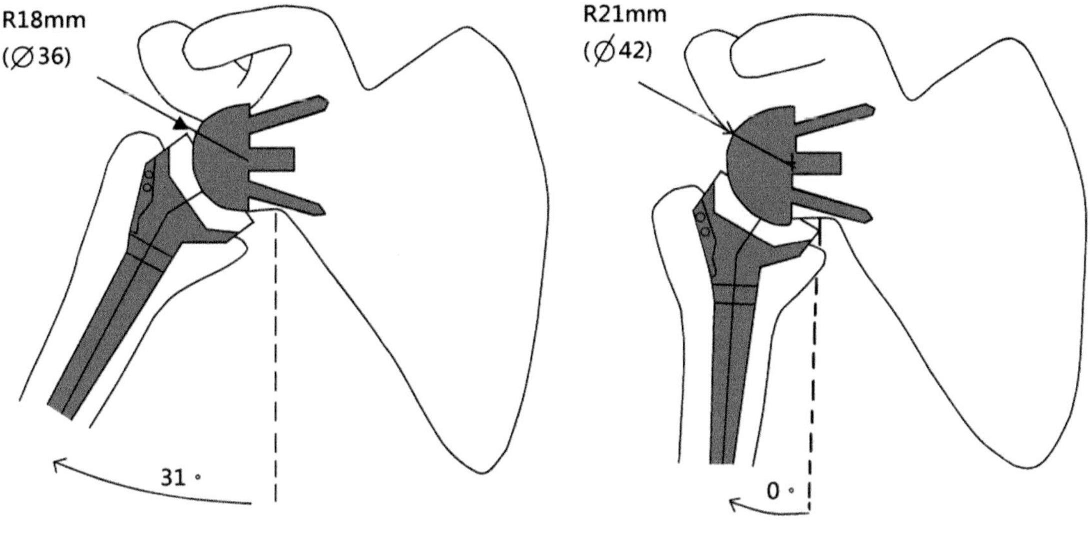

Fig. 19.7 42 mm Glenosphere extra 3 mm overhang reduces scapular notching

Inferior tilt of the glenosphere by 10° only gains 10° of adduction. It medialises the centre of rotation and reduces the inferior locking screw bone purchase as it now has to travel along the inferior part of the glenoid neck rather than down the lateral scapular border. Its beneficial effect is therefore not significant. It is a useful technique to prevent notching in patients with low bmi and those with preoperative evidence of superior glenoid erosion [15]. In a prospective study of 42 RSA, Edwards did not find inferior tilt of the glenosphere reduces notching [16]. Chae found increased micromotion at the bone-glenoid component interface and higher bone stresses in cadaveric specimens with glenospheres fixed with 10° inferior tilt, compared with ones fixed in

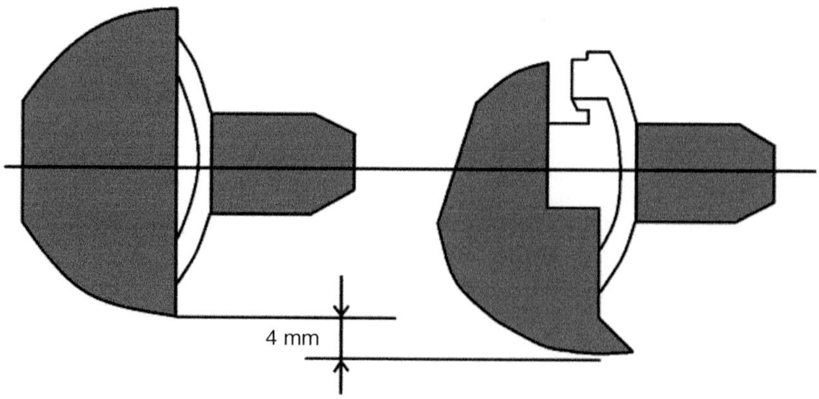

Fig. 19.8 36 mm glenosphere increases inferior offset by 4 mm (right) compared with a standard (left)

neutral tilt [17]. They attributed their findings to exposure of the softer cancellous bone after inferior reaming together with decreased bone-screw purchase resulting in a weakened glenosphere fixation.

Increased overhang of the glenosphere by 3 mm from 18 to 21 mm with a larger glenosphere, increases the adduction angle by 31°. The larger 42 mm glenosphere is therefore the recommended choice as it offers automatic overhang. This computer model study was confirmed by Berhouet in a cadaveric specimen study with 40 Aequalis RSA (Tornier Inc., Edina, Minn, USA) [18]. The authors found a 42 mm glenosphere with 7–10 mm lateralization was the best techniques to reduce notching.

Not all patients with cuff arthropathy have a large body frame to accommodate a 42 mm glenosphere with lateral offset. In a smaller patient, one can consider the use of an eccentric glenosphere with a 2–4 mm inferior offset. DeBiase reported 40 patients who were treated with a 36 mm glenosphere with a 4 mm inferior offset (SMR System, Lima Corporate, San Daniele del-Friuli, Italy) with no scapular notching seen after a minimum of 2 years (Fig. 19.8) [19].

Dislocation

Dislocation of RSA is the most common postoperative complication at 4.7% [6]. There are many causes of instability. Revision arthroplasty surgery has a higher dislocation rate at 9.4% compared with primary arthroplasty at 4.1%. 97.3% of RSA with instability were operated via a deltopectoral approach. The superolateral approach with subscapularis sparing was believed to be the reason behind the apparent lack of dislocation [20]. Damage to the subscapularis muscle after extensive release and its poor repair after has often been quoted as a causative factor [21]. Controversy still exists as to whether it is possible to repair the subscapularis. RSA in shoulders with distorted anatomy secondary to previous fracture also have a high dislocation rate. Martinez reported a dislocation rate of 13.6% in RSA used in the treatment for fracture sequalae [22]. Inadequate deltoid tensioning due to incorrect choice or positioning of the implants is the most common cause of recurrent instability in primary RSA [23].

In an in vivo study, Gerber has shown that if the glenosphere has been retroverted by 20°, significant instability occurs with any humeral version [24]. This can occur in a situation where the posterior glenoid bone is of poor bone quality. In order to obtain good quality bone for fixation, the base plate may have been fixed in a retroverted manner. Of more serious consequence, he found retroversion of the humeral component could lead to instability of the RSA. In his model, if the glenoid is in neutral, and the humeral component is inserted to the anatomical retroversion of 20°, the joint will become unstable when the arm is abducted at 90°. By increasing anteversion of the humeral component to neutral, intrinsic stability returns. His conclusion is that the glenoid component should be fixed without retroversion of more than 10°, and the humeral component should be inserted in neutral or slight anteversion.

In a 2D computer scapula model, de Wilde concluded that overhang of the glenosphere is the most important factor in achieving stability [25]. The extra 3 mm overhang in a 42 mm glenosphere affords more stability when compared with a 38 mm glenosphere. Increasing the thickness of the polyethylene insert increases the contact area of the articular surface, increases the deltoid tension, but decreases the impingement angle. The thicker plastic liner will hit the scapular neck earlier on adduction.

Most dislocations occur early, usually within the first 3 months [26]. Closed reduction should be attempted first. When recurrent, it is likely to be secondary to surgical error and revision of the components may become necessary [7]. Chalmers reviewed 11 of 385 patients (2.9%) who dislocated their RSA within the first 3 months. Ten were Trabecular Metal Reverse Shoulders (Zimmer Inc., Warsaw, IN, USA) and one was Delta III (DePuy Inc., Warsaw, IN, USA). Their patients were mainly male (82%), obese with poor subscapularis muscle. All but one dislocated within the first 5 weeks. They were all dislocated anteriorly. Closed reduction was only successful in 4.7 (56%) required revision surgery. Five required thicker polyethylene liner to increase deltoid tension and 2 were converted to hemiarthroplasty. As their patient shoulders stabilized after insertion of a thicker insert, they believed inadequate tensioning of the deltoid muscles was the primary cause of instability. Also the thicker insert automatically increases the compressive forces across the joint thus making it more stable. This trade off being to decrease the impingement angle of the humeral component against the glenoid neck.

In a recent study, Frankle reported a more successful outcome with closed reduction of his dislocated lateralized prosthesis (DJO Surgical, Austin Tx, USA). In a 10 year period, he had 2.3% dislocations, 30 out of 1293 RSA [27]. 48% of his patients had previous surgery, 80% being revision surgery. He performed his reduction in the outpatient department. With the patient's arm by the side, longitudinal traction was applied while a posteriorly directed force is applied to the upper humerus. Meanwhile, the humerus is gently external rotated. After closed reduction, 62% remained stable. 29% required revision surgery with larger components for both the glenoid and humerus. 9% remained unstable but patients were unfit for further surgery. He concluded that closed reduction, whether early or late in the postoperative period, had an equal good outcome. Secondly, closed reduction results were equally as good as that of revision surgery. After closed reduction, the arm should be rested in a sling for 4–6 weeks, avoiding adduction, internal rotation and extension.

If closed reduction fails, one should prepare for open reduction and revision. Before surgery, it is necessary to assess the positions of the glenosphere by CT scan. New software can reduce metal scatter which blocks assessment of the components position. We suggest looking for the following. Retroversion of the glenosphere should be checked, it should be 10° or less. The humeral component should be in neutral. There should be an overhang of the glenosphere at the scapula neck. During surgery, all soft tissues, including scar tissues, have to be cleared from the inferior margins of the glenoid to ensure the glenosphere has an adequate overhang. This is particularly important if preoperative assessment has shown all the components are in their optimal solution.

The following is an example of a RSA with early recurrent dislocation that illustrates the discussed management.

Fifty year old patient with rheumatoid arthritis developed avascular necrosis of the humeral head (Fig. 19.9a). She also had an eroded glenoid with very poor bone stock (Fig. 19.9b). At initial surgery, the base plate just managed to cover the glenoid. A 36 mm glenosphere was locked into position with apparent stability (Aequalis, Tornier Inc., Bloomington, MN, USA) (Fig. 19.10). She returned 1 week later with an acute anterior dislocation. This was reduced closed under general anaesthesia. Screening of the RSA in theatre showed apparent stability. Patient was discharged home and she was requested to rest her arm in a sling.

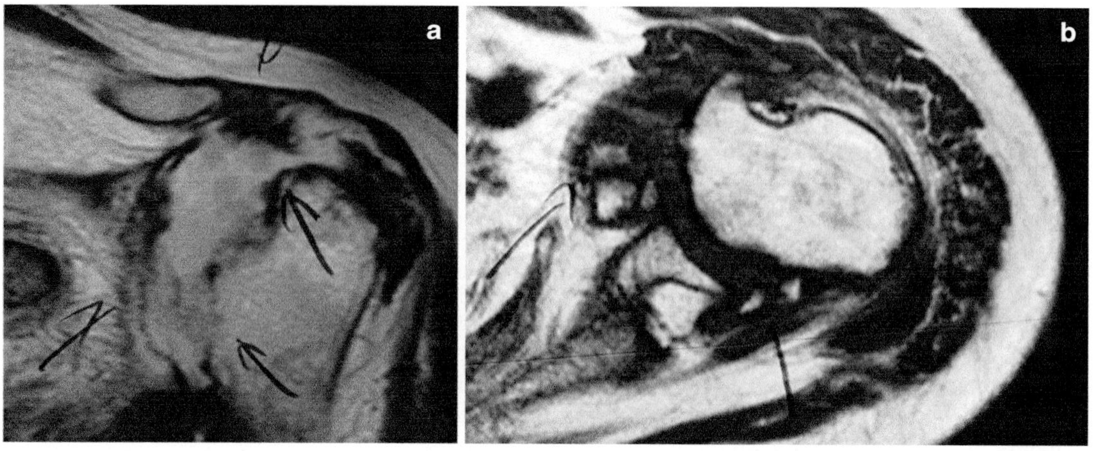

Fig. 19.9 (**a**) MRI shows AVN of left humeral head. (**b**) Axial view shows shallow eroded glenoid

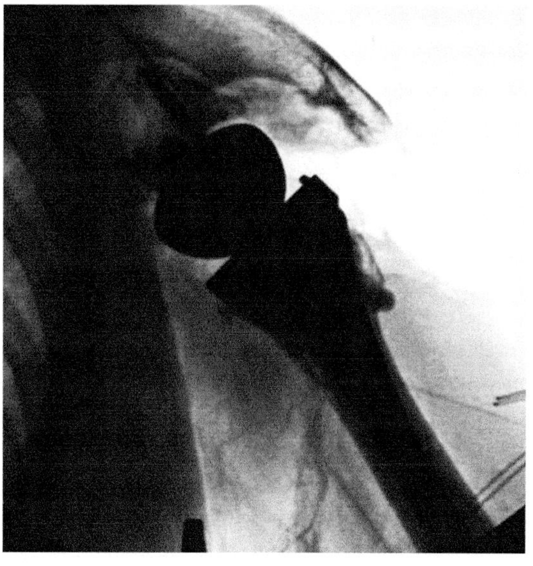

Fig. 19.10 On table radiograph shows apparent stable RSA

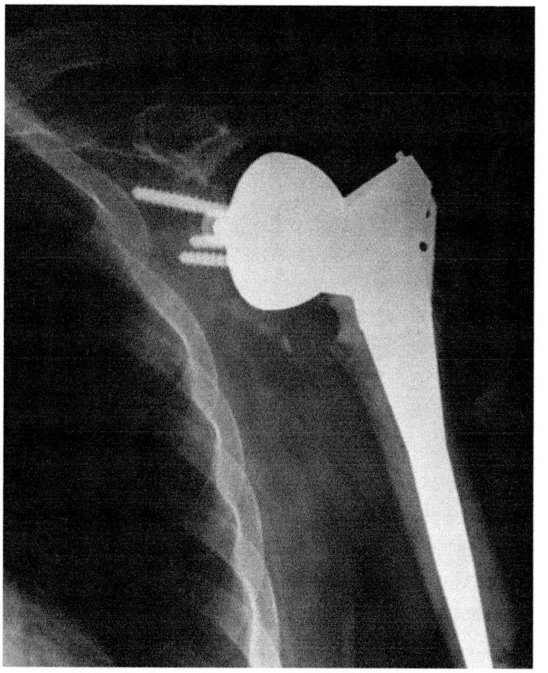

Fig. 19.11 Anterior dislocation of humeral component

Three days later, the shoulder re-dislocated. As it was a second dislocation, her instability was perceived to be secondary to inadequate deltoid tension. The humeral insert was then changed to a thicker variety (Fig. 19.11). After a week, her shoulder dislocated again. On this occasion, she had a CT scan. Careful assessment of the glenoid component showed the lack of overhang in the glenosphere over the scapular neck (Fig. 19.12). The 36 mm glenosphere was exchanged to sized 42 mm. A + 3 mm humeral insert was used. The shoulder felt immediately stable and has remained so since (Fig. 19.13). This case illustrates the importance of Glenoid overhang as the major factor in contribution to RSA stability.

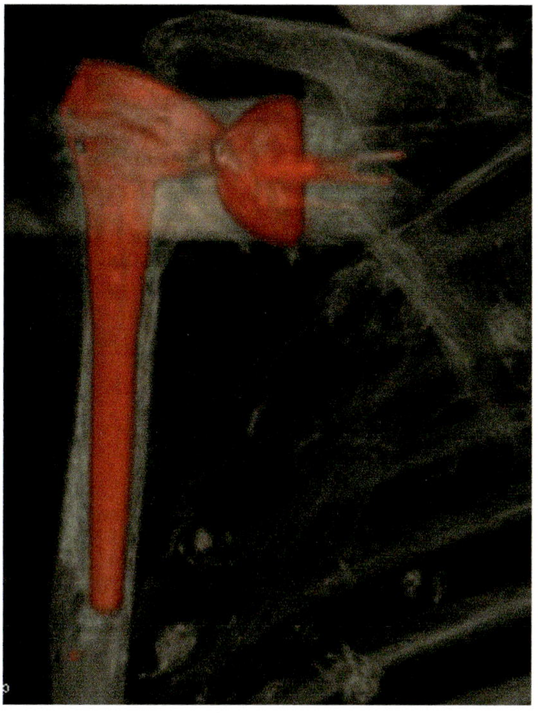

Fig. 19.12 CT scan shows 36 mm glenosphere with no overhang

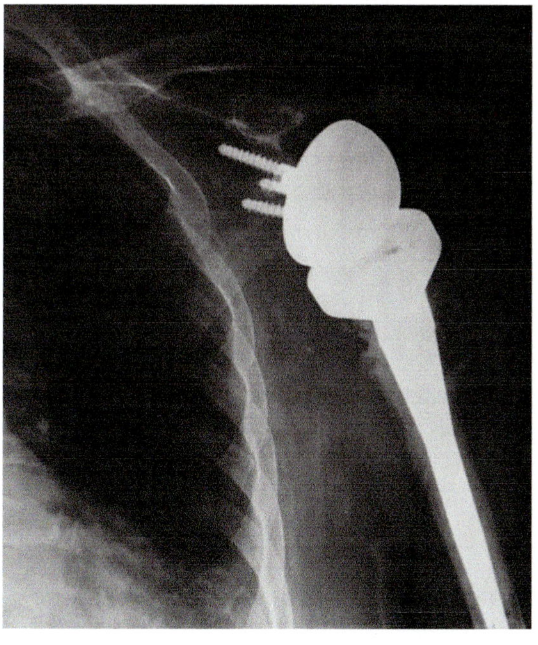

Fig. 19.13 Revision to 42 mm glenosphere with good overhang

Humeral Fractures

The incidence of periprosthetic humeral fracture around shoulder arthroplasties is between 0.6% and 3% [28]. García-Fernández et al. reported an overall incidence of 3.4% in a series of 203 RSA patients with a mean age of 75 years [29].

The fractures can occur during surgery or in the postoperative period, following trauma. Intraoperative fracture increases the operation time, increases blood loss, alters implant choices, increase the need for bone graft or fixation and may have an effect on postoperative outcome. The risk factors associated with increased periprosthetic fractures in shoulder arthroplasty include female sex, osteopenia, Rheumatoid Arthritis, over-reaming of humeral canal, insertion of oversized broach, proximal humeral deformity or malunion and soft tissue contracture requiring excessive external rotation force for dislocation [30].

The incidence of periprosthetic fracture is higher in patients undergoing revision RSA compared to primary RSA [29, 31]. Wagner et al. reported 16% of intraoperative periprosthetic fractures in a series of 224 patients that underwent revision surgery to RSA. Most fractures occurred during humeral component removal. A history of instability and prior hemiarthroplasty were found to be significant risk factors [31]. A few studies also show higher incidence of periprosthetic fractures with the use of press fit uncemented components. King et al. compared 51 uncemented RSA with 32 cemented RSA and reported an incidence of fracture in 6.02% in uncemented group compared to 1.2% in the cemented group [32].

Periprosthetic fractures are classified according to the location of fracture. Wright and Cofield's classification is the most commonly used. This was originally created for postoperative fractures and is limited to those occurring around the tip of humeral stem [33]. Type A fractures include the tip and extend proximally. Type B fractures extends from the tip. Type C fracture occur distal to the end of humeral component.

Campbell proposed a classification system, that included tuberosity and metaphyseal fractures [30] This is more suitable for intra-operative fractures, particularly following the use of press-fit implants. Campbell divided these fractures into four types based on location. Type A include greater and lesser tuberosity fractures. Type B include fracture of the metaphyseal portion or surgical neck of humerus. Type C involves proximal humeral diaphysis. Type D involves the mid and distal diaphysis of humerus.

Worland et al. classified these fractures depending on fracture anatomy and implant stability so as to guide the treatment [34]. Type A fractures involve the tuberosities. Type B fractures occur around the stem and are subclassified into three types, B1 fractures are spiral fractures with a stable implant. B2 fractures are transverse or short oblique fractures about the tip of the stem with a stable implant. B3 fractures are fractures about the stem with an unstable implant. Type C fractures occur distal to the tip of the stem.

As most fractures occur intra-operatively, prevention is the best way to avoid this complication. Special attention should be paid to bone quality especially in elderly patients, osteoporotic and female patients, Rheumatoid Arthritis patients, when using press fit components and in revision surgery [29].

The following preventive measures are useful in reducing the incidence of fracture:

1. Preoperative templating and awareness of proximal humeral geometry like malunion, deformity, canal stenosis and osteopenia to prevent use of oversized reamers, broaches and implants
2. Use of intraoperative fluoroscopy to guide humeral preparation in complex cases
3. Careful exposure and complete soft tissue release to facilitate easy dislocation
4. Systematic approach for removing well fixed humeral components – cortical window, proximal humeral splitting osteotomy and use of implant specific removal device

During surgery, once a fracture has occurred, the surgeon should follow a systematic approach. The surgical approach should be extended if necessary to identify and characterize the fracture. If a distal fracture is suspected, fluoroscopy of the entire arm should be obtained.

Fractures occurring intraoperatively should undergo fixation appropriate to fracture configuration and implant stability. This will allow early mobilization and prevent further displacement of the fracture and therefore a shorter time to union. Outcomes of intraoperative fractures managed with fixation or long stemmed implant are equivalent in terms of range of movement and pain as those primary arthroplasty cases [35].

Fractures involving greater /lesser tuberosity (Campbell Type A) should be assessed for stability. If deemed stable, with the periosteum intact and without displacement, they may be treated with insertion of standard implants without specific fixation. If the fracture is mobile or there is displacement, suture fixation of the fractured tuberosity to the humeral implant and around the proximal part of humerus is recommended. Fractures involving the metaphysis (Campbell Type B) are treated with standard – length implant with cerclage wire fixation (Fig. 19.14). Care should be taken when passing the cerclage wires to avoid iatrogenic nerve damage. The fracture site may be augmented with bone graft from the humeral head to promote union. Fracture involving the proximal part (Campbell Type C) and the middle and distal parts (Campbell Type D) of the humeral shaft are best treated with long stemmed implants with cerclage fixation and in some cases with supplementary plate or allograft cortical strut fixation (Fig. 19.15).

Treatment for postoperative fracture include both conservative and surgical management. This depends on fracture location, displacement, stability of prosthesis and bone quality. If the fracture is undisplaced or minimally displaced, and thes implant is stable, the fracture can be treated by nonoperative methods. For unstable diaphyseal fracture with well-fixed components, it is recommended to fix using multiple cerclage wires or a heavy plate with proximal cerclage wires and distal screws [36] (Fig. 19.16). For diaphyseal fracture with loose stem, revision to

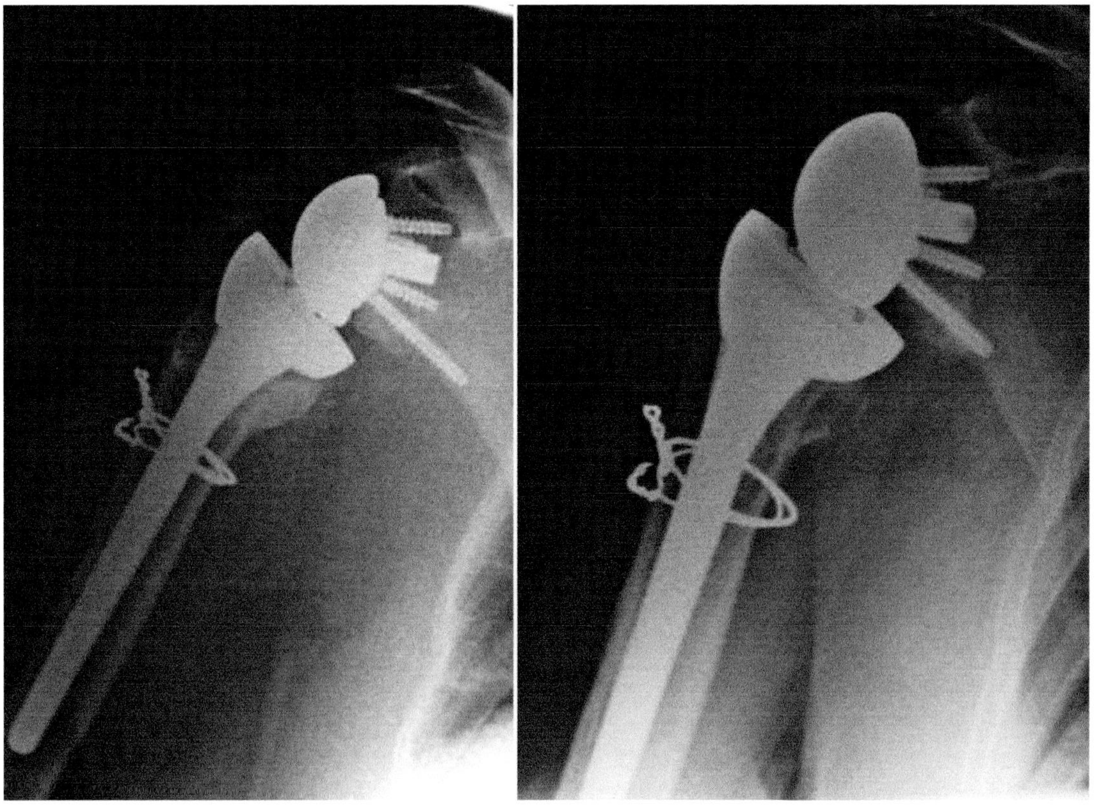

Fig. 19.14 Intra-operative fracture (Campbell Type B) treated by cerclage

long stem prosthesis is recommended [29]. Fractures distal to the prosthesis responds well to conservative treatment, and require fixation in very selected cases only.

Glenoid Complications

These include intraoperative fracture, glenoid baseplate loosening and glenosphere disassembly. In a multicentre study of 1953 cases, glenoid loosening was reported to be 1.7% and glenoid disassembly was observed in 0.5% [37].

Glenoid Fracture

Intraoperative glenoid fractures can occur during reaming or the subsequent fixation. It can be challenging in patients with severe osteoporosis, those with previous glenoid fracture or failed hemiarthroplasty. The reamer should start on full speed before bone contact and only the sclerotic surface is lightly reamed to avoid weakening the subchondral bone. In cases of bone insufficiency, the reaming is best done by hand. A pre-op CT scan is mandatory to assess the position of the triangular cone of bone of the glenoid in relation to its articular surface. This will help the surgeon to determine the best position to drill for the central peg. The humeral head can be used as bone graft to place on the glenoid in cases of bone deficiency. If intraoperative fracture does occur, the use of a longer central peg and redirectioning of the peripheral locking screws may be able to salvage the situation. If fixation is not possible, then a two stage procedure may be performed with bone grafting of the glenoid using either autologous or allograft and once the bone graft has incorporated, the humeral component is inserted as a secondary procedure.

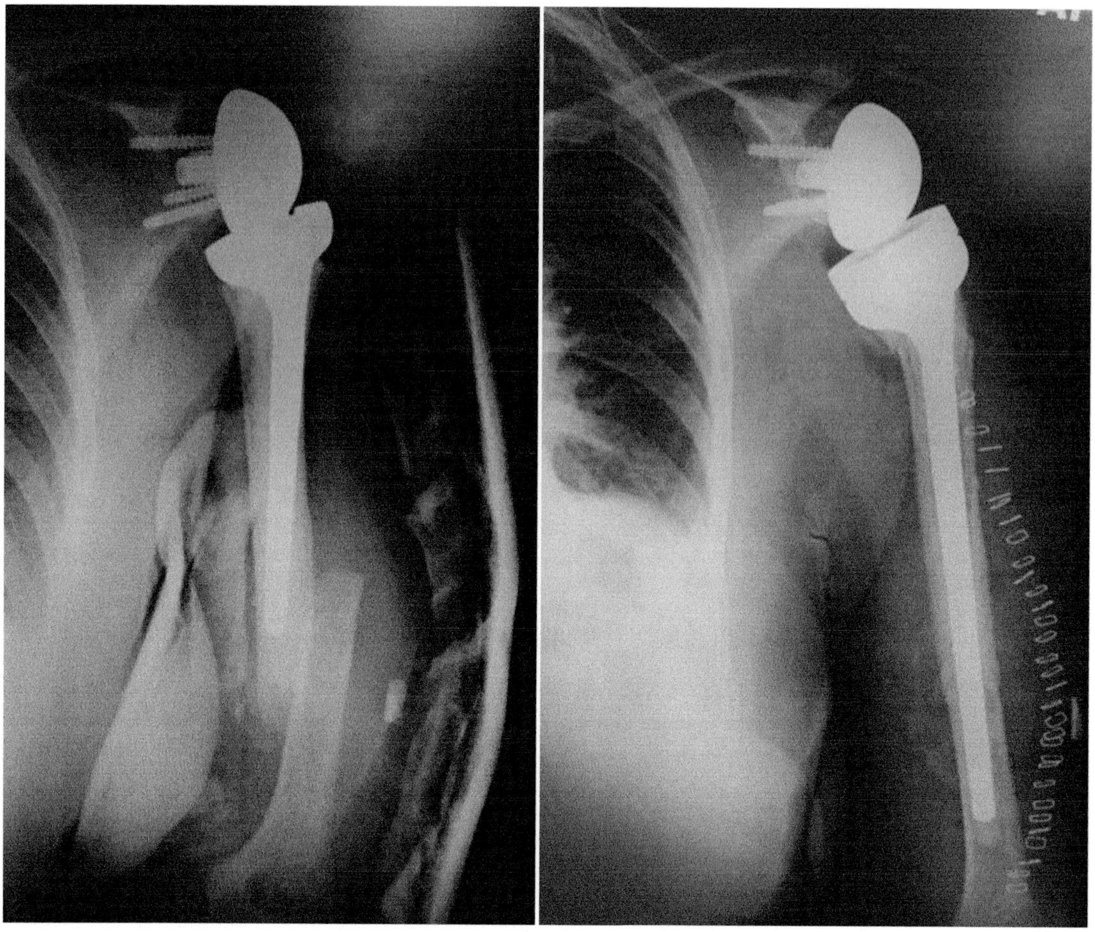

Fig. 19.15 Campbell Type D fracture, treated by long stemmed humerus implant

Glenoid Loosening

The most common causes are infection, failure to achieve adequate fixation at the time of initial surgery, loosening of the screws secondary to osteolysis and technical problems. When the baseplate is loose, it is usually associated with bone loss and screw breakage is often seen. Screw failure is induced by a seesaw movement of the glenosphere onto the baseplate. Middernacht found that the design of the prosthesis, including the use of 5.0-mm locking peripheral screws, and the technique of implantation, incorporating a 15° inferior tilt of the baseplate were the most important factors to prevent mechanical failure of the baseplate fixation [38] (Fig. 19.17).

Three types of bone defects have been described, based on the location and severity on CT namely, Cavity defect (type A), uncontained wall defect (Type B) and Complex defect (Type C).

Small contained defects can be filled with either autograft or allograft, whereas larger defects will require structural support usually with a tricortical iliac crest graft.

Glenoid Disassembly

Disassembly can occur between the baseplate and the glenosphere. In a series of 479 RSA (468 Delta III and 11 Aequalis), the incidence

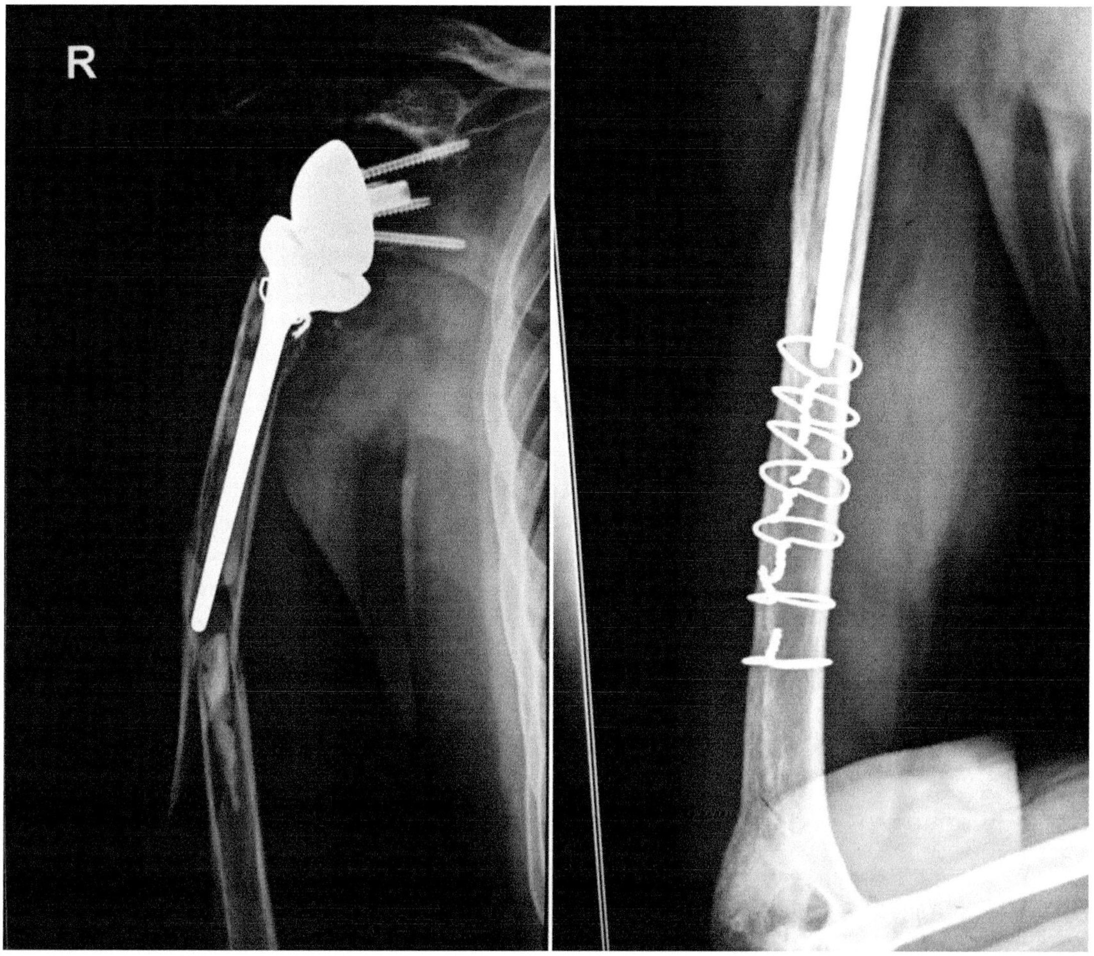

Fig. 19.16 Post-operative fracture 2 years after RSA, treated by multiple cerclage

of glenosphere disengagement was found to be 3.2%. In 13 patients, the disengagement was partial and was not associated with a poor functional outcome [38]. In three patients, the disengagement led to a fracture of the central screw and complete disengagement of the glenosphere from the baseplate. Improper seating of the glenosphere on the baseplate can occur as a result of inadequate reaming of bone around the peripheral edge of the baseplate, interposition of bone or soft tissue between the glenosphere and the baseplate at the time of impaction and failure of the locking mechanism between the central peg and glenosphere. The positioning of the baseplate is also crucial, if the baseplate is being positioned too high or associated with superior tilt, there is excess shear stress which may induce early failure (Fig. 19.18 a, b).

Measures to try and prevent the risk of glenoid loosening include inferior placement of the baseplate in relation to glenoid, placement of locking screws in best quality bone, larger central screw, multiple peripheral screws, and larger diameter screws. Cusick et al. reported a significantly higher likelihood of glenosphere dissociation when larger diameter glenospheres (40 and 44 mm) were implanted; thought to be related to the larger exposed surface area for potential soft tissue or bone impingement [39].

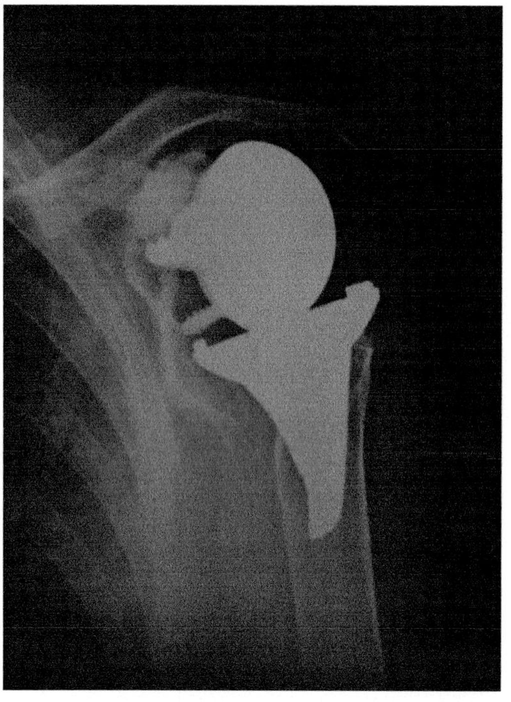

Fig. 19.17 Complete loosening of baseplate and significant glenoid bone loss

Acromial Fracture

The incidence of a fracture of the acromion following RSA varies from 1% to 7% according to the reported series. These fractures can occur at any point after surgery ranging from 1 to 94 months postoperatively.

The exact aetiology of acromion fractures is unclear but it is thought to be due to a combination of bone insufficiency and intra-operative technical factors. Preop risk factors include osteoporosis, os acromiale, acromion erosion, spine non-union. Intra-operative risk factors include excess tension on the deltoid with resultant arm lengthening and the position as well as the length of the glenoid baseplate screws. The superior 12 o'clock and posterior 9 o'clock screws have been implicated as stress risers in the development of scapular spine fractures. Crosby found that three of the four Type III fractures appeared to propagate from the tip of the most superiorly placed metaglene screws and as a

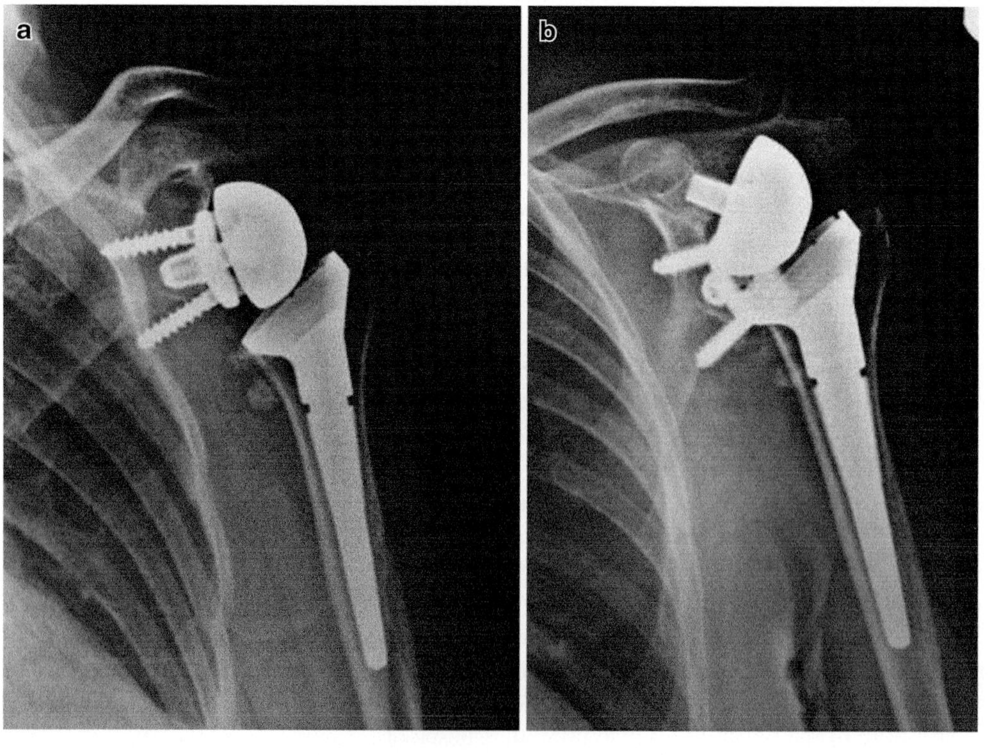

Fig. 19.18 (a) The baseplate is positioned with superior tilt and there is bony impingement superiorly against the glenosphere with partial disengagement from the baseplate. (b) Early failure with glenoid disassembly occurred due to excess shear stress

consequence they no longer use the most superior screw hole for fixation of the metaglene.

It is likely that the reported incidence will increase due to the longer duration of follow up of our patients and better diagnostic techniques. Undisplaced acromial or scapular spine fractures are difficult to diagnose on plain radiographs and the reported accuracy rate is only 78.8% (Otto). The investigation of choice is single photon emission computed tomography (SPECT CT) which has significantly less radiation exposure than conventional CT scans [40] (Fig. 19.19).

There are three classification systems described. Rouleau proposed a classification system which is descriptive and based on the anatomy and functionality of the scapula [41] (Fig. 19.20). Fractures of the tip were those of the most lateral or anterior portion of the acromion. Fractures of the body of the acromion are those medial to the tip of the acromion and lateral to the beginning of the scapular base. The scapular base is the lateral border of the scapular spine, which is smooth and round.

Crosby's classification system was intended to recommend the best choice of treatment [42] (Table 19.1).

Levy proposed a further classification based on the involvement of the deltoid origin. Type I indicated involvement of a portion of the anterior and middle deltoid origin; type II, at least the entire middle deltoid origin with a portion but not all of the posterior deltoid origin; and type III, the entire middle and posterior deltoid origin [43] (Fig. 19.21).

In their series of 16 patients, all were treated non operatively with a shoulder immobiliser for 6 weeks and were instructed to limit activities to pendulum exercises. Teusink et al. reported a series of 25 patients with acromion fractures and all were treated non operatively. The union rate was 57% for acromial fractures and 50% for scapular spine fractures. They found that the location of the fracture (acromion or spine) did not affect the outcome. Overall, patients with acromion fracture still had improved scores but inferior clinical outcome.

Hattrup also managed his series of nine patients with acromial fracture non operatively and concluded that a decision for surgical treatment will need to balance the challenges of internal fixation with the incremental improvement that may occur with improved fracture healing.

Operative treatment is potentially challenging as the bone is soft and the amount of bone that can hold fixation is limited. Furthermore, despite fixation, the rate of non-union and malunion

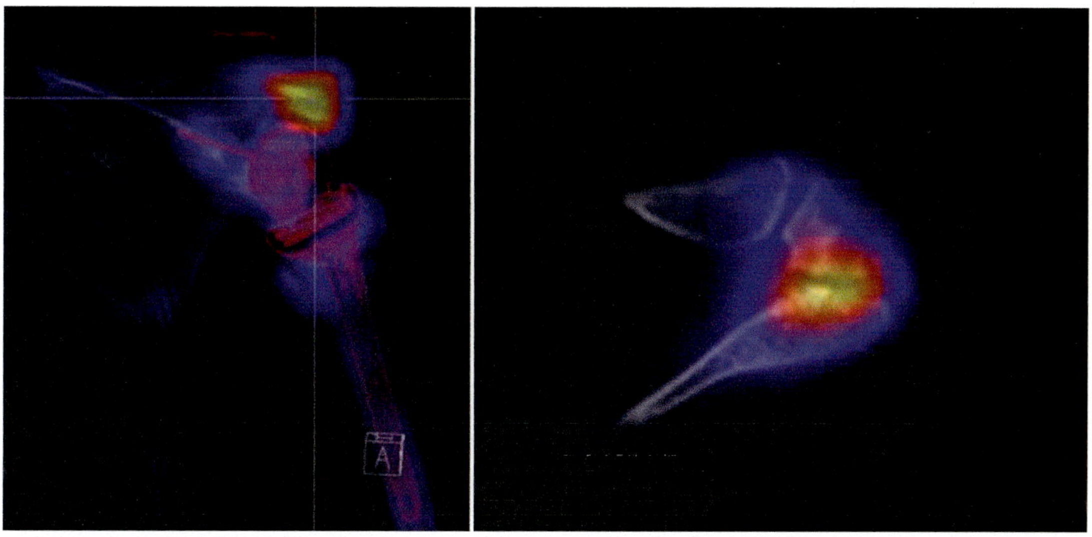

Fig. 19.19 Spect CT showing acromon fracture

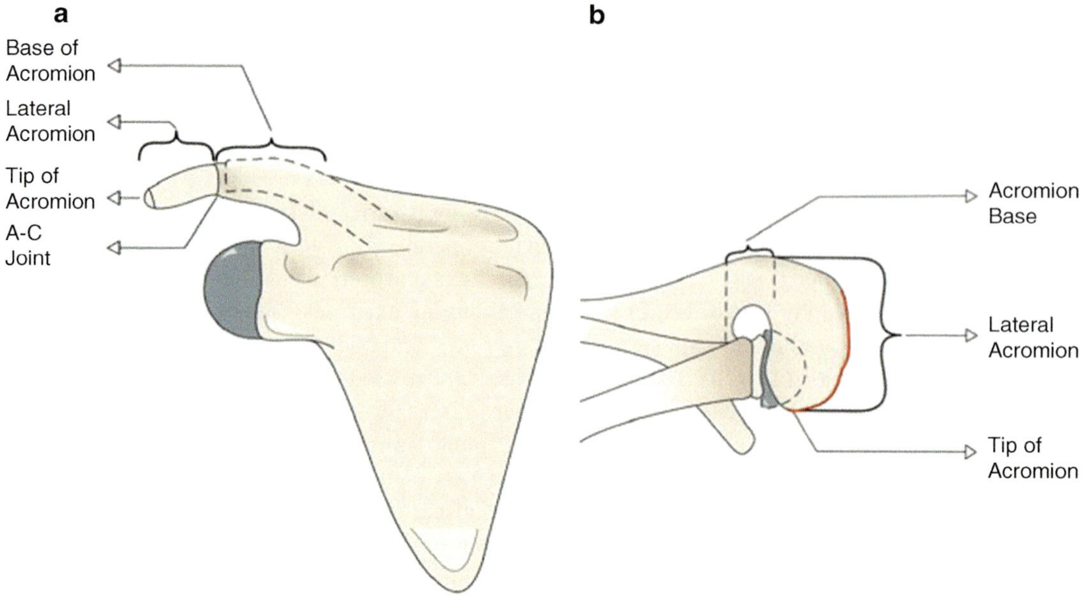

Fig. 19.20 Rouleau's classification of acromion fracture

Table 19.1 Crosby's classification of acromion fractures

Types	Location	Suggested treatment
I	Small fractures of the anterior acromion near to or including the footprint of the coracoacromial ligament	Observation with a likelihood of symptom relief.
II	Fractures of the acromion posterior to the acromioclavicular joint	Acromioclavicular joint resection if stable but open reduction internal fixation if unstable
III	Fractures of the scapular spine	Best treated with open reduction internal fixation.

remains high. There are two surgical techniques described. For distal acromion fractures, the authors recommend the use of tension band wire fixation to control the rotation of the distal fragment and provide compression at the fracture site. However, this technique is not without its problems, notably hardware loosening and failure due to the strong pull of the deltoid. For this reason, De Wilde advocates the use of a second tension band fixation across the acromioclavicular joint (Fig. 19.22 a, b).

Alternatively, the fracture may be fixed with two locking plates with one over the superior superior edge of the scapular spine in a compression mode and the other applied from the posterior acromion to the posterior cortex of the scapular spine, in the infraspinatus fossa (a 90/90 configuration) (Fig. 19.23).

Neurological Injury

The rate of neurological injury following all forms of shoulder arthroplasty is reported to be around 1%. It can occur immediately after surgery as seen in proximal lesions involving axillary, brachial plexus, radial and musculocutaneous nerves. It can also have a delayed presentation, manifesting as nerve entrapment syndromes including carpal tunnel and cubital tunnel syndromes.

Nerve injury can occur intraoperatively due to a variety of reasons including surgical approach,

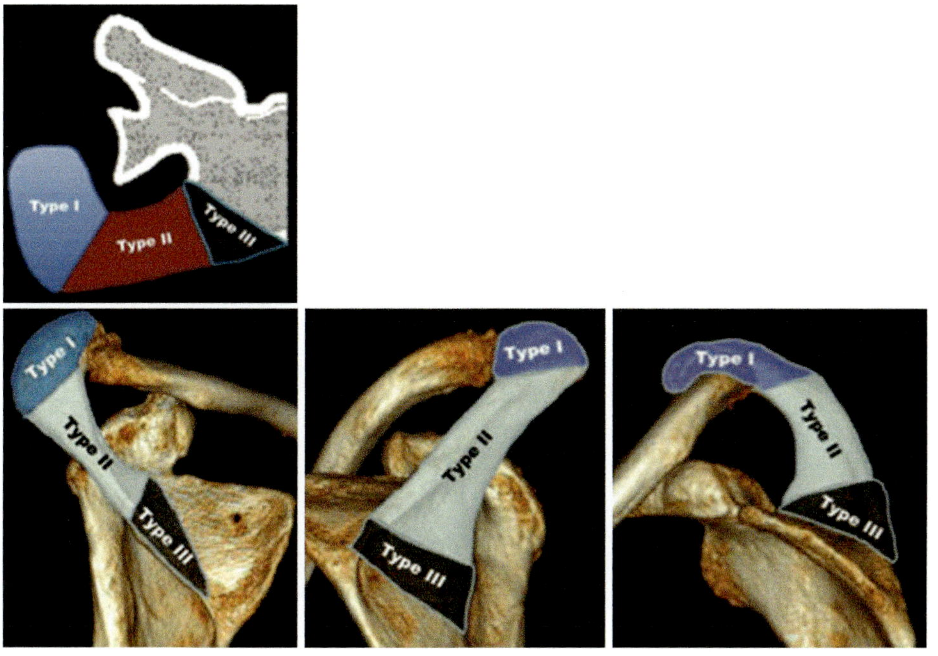

Fig. 19.21 Levy's classification of acromion fracture

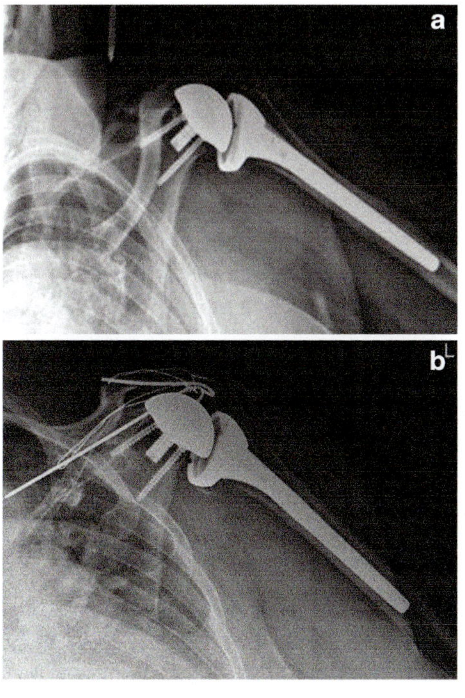

Fig. 19.22 (**a**) Displaced acromion fracture (Figures kindly provided by L De Wilde). (**b**) Double Tension Band fixation (Figures kindly provided by L De Wilde)

placement of retractors, screw malposition, compression from haematoma or cement and injury from interscalene block. The use of a cement removal heat probe can generate high temperature within the humeral canal. This in turn can lead to neurapraxia of the radial nerve. Ladermann found the rate of neurological injury following reverse arthroplasty is 10.9 times higher than anatomical arthroplasty, with the axillary nerve involved in 50%. This is probably related to the design of reverse prosthesis which distalises the centre of rotation. The humerus is lengthened by approximately 2.7 cm (+/− 1.8 cm). This in turn increases the tension on the axillary nerve. An anatomical study has found that when the humerus is lowered, the axillary nerve below the mid glenoid level which corresponds to the highest level of nerve tension, loses its curvature and becomes more vertical and straight. When the humerus is lateralised, there was no evidence of stretching of the nerve. The practical implication of this study is that if the reverse shoulder arthroplasty is found to be unstable intraoperatively, it would be safer to increase the size of the glenosphere, thereby increasing the

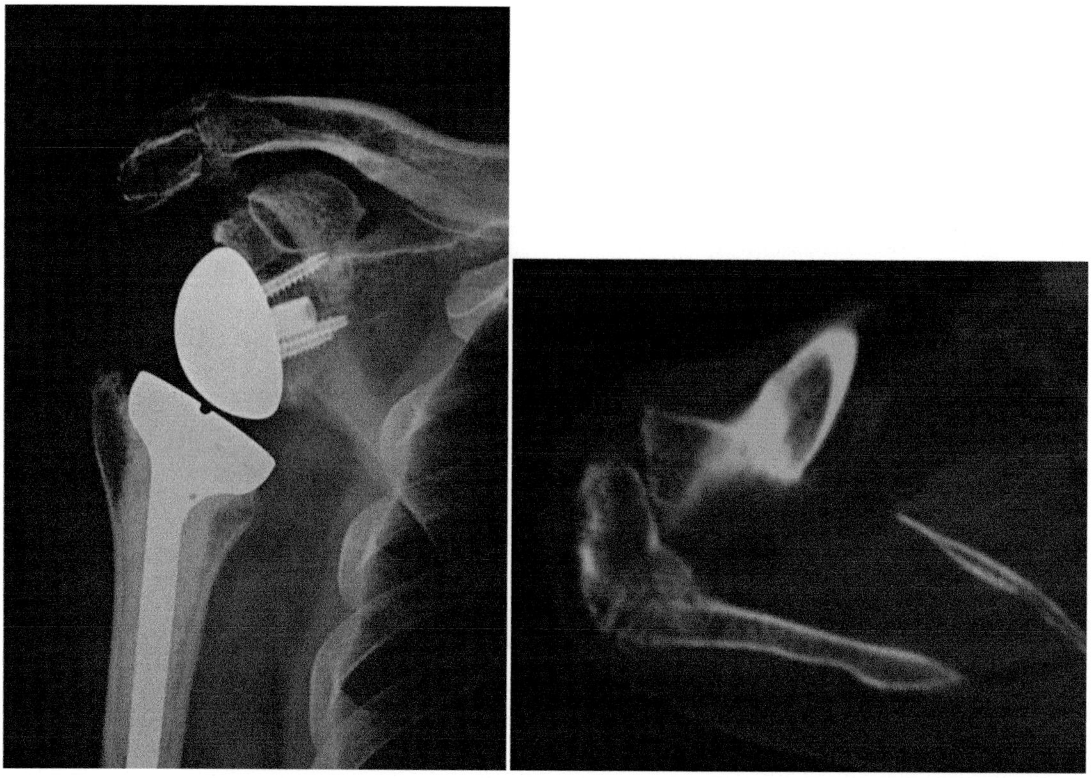

Fig. 19.23 : Patient presented with mild discomfort over acromion, 2 years following RSA. Acromion stress fracture was treated by conservative measures

lateralisation, rather than using a thicker polyethylene insert or metallic spacer which lowers the humerus increasing the risk of brachial plexus stretching [44, 45].

Haematoma

Haematoma formation is relatively common in RSA. In 2005, Gerber reported postoperative haematoma occurred in 20% of his RSA [1] By moving the gleno-humeral articulation medially and distally, a large dead space below the acromion is thus created. Without the tamponade effect of the rotator cuff over this dead space, blood and fluid will accumulate there. Haematoma formation is invariably present after RSA but does not necessarily require intervention. Historically, the concern is that the presence of a haematoma may lead to joint infection [46]. In a literature review in 2011, Zumstein found only 20 cases of haematoma reported in 782 RSA [6]. A much lower reported rate at 2.6%. Nine cases required intervention and five cases were aspirated. None led to infection.

The current practice to reduce haematoma formation is the use of tranexamic acid before surgery to reduce bleeding. During surgery, meticulous attention is paid to control all bleeding points. After surgery, a suction drain is left in the dead space for 24–48 h. Frequently, 400 mls of blood will be drained. Gentle early mobilization is encouraged to allow the deltoid muscle to pump any fluid out of the dead space. If a haematoma is formed, one can monitor its progress before aspiration or rushing in to evacuate it.

Infection

Infection is the third commonest complication following reverse shoulder arthroplasty at 3–6%. This is substantially higher than the 2% rate quoted for anatomical shoulder arthroplasty.

Florschutz found infection rates following primary anatomical and primary reverse shoulder arthroplasty were the same at 2%. When RSA was used in revision arthroplasty, the infection rate was 7%. Morris et al. have found that a history of previous failed arthroplasty and age less than 65 were independent risk factors for infection after RSA. Other factors implicated include an increased subacromial dead space after RSA where haematoma collects; those with poor soft tissue envelope around the prosthesis, as well as in patients with rheumatoid arthritis.

Propionibacterium acnes and staphylococcus epidermidis were the most common organisms identified, accounting for 87.5%. Propionibacterium acnes is a gram positive anaerobic bacillus which is found in the sebaceous glands associated with hair follicles. It is postulated that men have more sebaceous glands and therefore have a higher rate of Propionibacterium acnes infection around the shoulder (Patel et al). Other potential risk factors for Propionibacterium acnes infection include long duration of surgery and age. Lucas et al. recommended that at least 5 explant or tissue specimens should be obtained for microbiologic testing and extended cultures for at least 17 days [47]. Sethi et al. [48] have shown that the positive culture rate for Propionibacterium acnes after 7 days of culture was 8.8% whereas the rate increases to 15.8% after 14 days and 22.8% after 28 days of incubation. Clindamycin is effective against most strains of Propionibacterium and can be considered as suitable prophylactic antibiotics [49]. A dose of 600 mg given iv 30 min before surgery is recommended. Gentamicin impregnated collagen sponge has been found to reduce surgical site infection in orthopaedic surgery [50]. Our practice is to place a small amount inside the glenosphere which may help to reduce possible dead space infection.

For established infection treatment options include early debridement with removal and exchange of liner and glenosphere, one or two stage revision and resection arthroplasty.

If infection occurred at less than 60 days from surgery, we recommend initial debridement, washout and exchange of polyethylene liner and glenosphere. This is on the assumption that the implants are not loose and surrounding soft tissues are healthy. Arthroscopy and lavage may be helpful to obtain a microbiological sample but should not be relied on solely as therapeutic procedure.

If debridement fails to control the infection, the next step would be either a one stage or two stage revision. There is no clear consensus in the published literature as to whether one stage or two stage is better. One stage revision has better functional results with a lower morbidity and complication rate, but with a greater risk of recurrent infection. De Wilde advocated a single stage approach with the advantages of significantly shorter treatment, less patient morbidity, lower costs and avoiding glenoid erosion by the antibiotic spacer [51].

Boileau on the other hand advocates a two stage approach and reported eradication of infection in all cases [52]. It has a higher morbidity but higher success rate for infection eradication. It also allows complex problems such as bone loss to be addressed. The potential benefit of an antibiotic-impregnated cement spacer is controversial. They deliver a high concentration of antibiotics locally at the infected site and maintain soft tissue tension whilst waiting for reimplantation after eradication of infection. Verhelst found no improvement in outcome with the use of antibiotic-impregnated cement spacers after retrieval of the infected prosthesis, compared with resection arthroplasty alone.

Resection arthroplasty remains a salvage option with a high complication rate (33%). A much poorer outcome is to be expected when compared with resection arthroplasty following hemiarthroplasty or anatomical shoulder arthroplasty.

References

1. Werner CM, Steinmann PA, Gilbart M, Gerber C. Treatment of painful pseudoparesis due to irreparable rotator cuff dysfunction with the delta III reverse-ball-and-socket total shoulder prosthesis. J Bone Joint Surg Am. 2005;87(7):1476–86.
2. Villacis D, Sivasundaram L, Pannell W, Heckmann N, Omid R, Hatch GR. Complication rate and implants survival for reverse shoulder arthroplasty versus total

shoulder arthroplasty: results during the initial 2 years. J Shoulder Elb Surg. 2016;25:927–35.
3. Boileau P, Watkinson D, Hatzidakis AM, Hovorka I. Neer award 2005: the Grammont reverse shoulder prosthesis: results in cuff tear arthritis, fracture sequale, and revision arthroplasty. J Shoulder Elb Surg. 2006;15:527–40.
4. Cheung E, Willis M, Walker M, Clark R, Frankle MA. Complications in reverse Total shoulder arthroplasty. J Am Acad Orthop Surg. 2011;19(7):439–49.
5. Harmsen SM, Chang YH, Hattrup SJ. Simple moving average: a method of reporting evolving complication rates. Orthopedics. 2016;23:1–8.
6. Zumstein MA, Pinedo M, Old J, Boileau P. Problems, complications, reoperations, and revisions in reverse total shoulder arthroplasty: a systemic review. J Shoulder Elb Surg. 2011;20:146–57.
7. Farshad F, Gerber C. Reverse total shoulder arthroplasty—from the most to the least common complication. Int Orthop (SICOT). 2010;34:1075–82.
8. Nicholson GP, Srauss EJ, Sherman SL. Scapular nothching: recognition and strategies to minimize clinical impact. Clin Orthop Relat Res. 2011;469(9):2521–30.
9. Sirveaux F, Favard L, Oudet D, Huquet D, Walch G, Molé D. Grammont inverted total shoulder arthroplasty in the treatment of glenohumeral osteoarthritis with massive rupture of the cuff. Results of a multicenter study of 80mshoulders. J Bone Joint Surg Br. 2004;86:388–95.
10. Levigne C, Garret J, Boileau P, Alami G, Favard L, Walch G. Scapular notching in reverse shoulder arthroplasty: is it important to avoid it and how? Clin Orthop Relat Res. 2011;469:2512–20.
11. Simovitch RW, Zumstein MA, Lohri E, Helmy N, Gerber C. Predictors of scapular notching in patients managed with delta III ReverseTotal shoulder replacement. J Bone Joint Surg. 2007;89A(3):588–600.
12. Frankle M, Levy JC, Pupello D, Siegal S, Saleem A, Mighell M, Vasey M. The reverse shoulder prosthesis for glenohumeral arthritis associated with severe rotator cuff deficiency: a minimum two-year follow-up study of sixty patients: surgical technique. J Bone Joint Surg Am. 2006;88(suppl 1):178–90.
13. Cuff D, Pupello D, Virani N, Levy J, Frankle M. Reverse shoulder arthroplasty for the treatment of rotator cuff deficiency. J Bone Joint Surg Am. 2008;90:1244–51.
14. Boileau P, Moineau G, Roussanne Y, O'Shea K. Bony increaed-offset reversed shoulder arthroplasty. Clin Orthop Relat Res. 2011;469:2558–67.
15. Edwards TB, Trappey GJ, Riley C, O'Connor DP, Elkousy HA, Gartsman GM. Inferior tilt of the glenoid component does not decrease scapular notching in reverse shoulder arthroplasty: results of a prospective randomized study. J Shoulder Elb Surg. 2012;21(5):641–6.
16. Falaise V, Levigne C, Favard L, SOFEC. Scapular notching in reverse shoulder arthroplasties: the influence of glenometaphyseal angle. Orthop Traumatol Surg Res. 2011;97(6 supp):S131–7.
17. Chae SW, Lee H, Kim SM, Lee J, Han SH, Kim SY. Primary stability of inferior tilt fixation of the glenoid component in reverse total shoulder arthroplasty: a finite element study. J Orthop Res. 2016;34(6):1061–8.
18. Berhouet J, Garaud P, Favard L. Evaluation of the role of glenosphere design and humeral component retroversion in avoiding scapular notching during reverse shoulder arthroplasty. J Shoulder Elb Surg. 2014;23:151–8.
19. De Biase CF, Delcogliano M, Borroni M, Castagna A. Reverse total shoulder arthroplasty: radiological and clinical result using an eccentric glenosphere. Musculoskelet Surg. 2012;96(Suppl 1):S27–34.
20. Walch G, Wall B, Mottier F. Complications and revision of the reverse prosthesis: a multicenter study of 457 cases. In: Boileau P, editor. Reverse shoulder arthroplasty. Nice: Sauramps; 2006. p. 335–52.
21. Edwards TB, Williams MD, Labriola JE, Elkousy HA, Gartsman GM, O'Connor DP. Subscapularis insufficiency and the risk of shoulder dislocation after reverse shoulder arthroplasty. J Shoulder Elb Surg. 2009;18(6):892–6.
22. Martinez AA, Calvo A, Bejarano C, Carbonel I, Herrera A. The use of the Lima reverse shoulder arthroplasty for the treatment of fracture sequelae of the proximal humerus. J Orthop Sci. 2012;17:141–7.
23. Alentorn-Geli E, Samtier G, Torrens C, Wright TW. Reverse shoulder arthroplasty. Part2: systemic review of reoperations, revisions, problems and complications. Int J Shoulder Surg. 2015;9(2):60–7.
24. Favre P, Sussmann PS, Gerber C. The effect of component positioning on intrinsic stability of the reverse shoulder arthroplasty. J Shoulder Elbow Surg. 2010;19:550–6.
25. De Wilde LF, Poncet D, Middemacht B, Ekelund A. Prosthetic overhang is the most effective way to prevent scaular conflict in a reverse total shoulder shoulder prosthesis. Acta Orthop. 2010;81(6):719–26.
26. Chalmers PN, Rahman Z, Romeo AA, Nicholson GP. Early dislocations after reverse total shoulder arthroplasty. J Shoulder Elb Surg. 2014;23:737–44.
27. Teusink MJ, Pappou IP, Schwarts DG, Cottrell BJ. Frankle MA results of closed management of acute dislocation after reverse shoulder arthroplasty. J Shoulder Elb Surg. 2015;24(4):621–7.
28. Kumar S, Sperling JW, Haidukewych GH, Cofield RH. Periprosthetic humeral fractures after shoulder arthroplasty. J Bone Joint Surg Am. 2004;86-A(4):680–9.
29. García-Fernández C, Lópiz-Morales Y, Rodríguez A, López-Durán L, Martínez FM. Periprosthetic humeral fractures associated with reverse total shoulder arthroplasty: incidence and management. Int Orthop. 2015;39(10):1965–9.
30. Campbell JT, Moore RS, Iannotti JP, Norris TR, Williams GR. Periprosthetic humeral fractures: mechanisms of fracture and treatment options. J Shoulder Elbow Surg Am Shoulder Elbow Surg. 1998;7(4):406–13.

31. Wagner ER, Houdek MT, Elhassan BT, Sanchez-Sotelo J, Cofield RH, Sperling JW. What are risk factors for intraoperative humerus fractures during revision reverse shoulder arthroplasty and do they influence outcomes? Clin Orthop Relat Res. 2015;473(10):3228–34.
32. King JJ, Farmer KW, Struk AM, Wright TW. Uncemented versus cemented humeral stem fixation in reverse shoulder arthroplasty. Int Orthop. 2015;39:291–8.
33. Wright TW, Cofield RH. Humeral fractures after shoulder arthroplasty. J Bone Joint Surg Am. 1995;77(9):1340–6.
34. Worland RL, Kim DY, Arredondo J. Periprosthetic humeral fractures: management and classification. J Shoulder Elbow Surg J Bone Joint Surg. 1999;8(6):590–4.
35. Athwal GS, Sperling JW, Rispoli DM, Cofield RH. Periprosthetic humeral fractures during shoulder arthroplasty. J Bone Joint Surg Am. 2009;91(3):594–603.
36. Cameron B, Iannotti JP. Periprosthetic fractures of the humerus and scapula: management and prevention. Orthop Clin North Am. 1999;30(2):305–18.
37. Molé D, Godeneche A, Laedermann A. Problems & complications related to the Glenoid. Shoulder concepts 2016 – reverse shoulder arthroplasty 20 year anniversary.
38. Middernacht B, De Wilde L, Molé D, Favard L, Debeer P. Glenosphere disengagement: a potentially serious default in reverse shoulder surgery. Clin Orthop Relat Res. 2008;466:892–8.
39. Cusick MC, Hussey MM, Steen BM, Hartzler RU, Clark RE, Cuff DJ, Cabezas AF, Santoni BG, Frankle MA. Glenosphere dissociation after reverse shoulder arthroplasty. J Shoulder Elb Surg. 2015;24(7):1061–8.
40. Teasing MJ, Otto RJ, Cottrell BJ, Frankle MA. What is the effect of postoperative scapular fracture on outcomes of reverse shoulder arthroplasty? J Shoulder Elb Surg. 2014;23(6):782–90.
41. Rouleau DM, Gaudelli C. Successful treatment of fractures of the base of the acromion after reverse shoulder arthroplasty: case report and review of the literature. Int J Shoulder Surg. 2013;7(4):149–52.
42. Crosby LA, Hamilton A, Twiss T. Scapula fractures after reverse total shoulder arthroplasty: classification and treatment. Clin Orthop Relat Res. 2011;469:2544–9.
43. Levy JC, Anderson C, Samson A. Classification of postoperative acromial fractures following reverse shoulder arthroplasty. J Bone Joint Surg Am. 2013;95(15):e104.
44. Lädermann A, Williams M, Mekis B, Hoffmeyer P, Walch G. Objective evaluation of lengthening in reverse shoulder arthroplasty. J Shoulder Elb Surg. 2009;18(4):588–95.
45. Marion B, Leclère FM, Casoli V, Paganini F, Unglaub F, Spies C, Valenti P. Potential axillary nerve stretching during RSA implantation: an anatomical study. Anat Sci Int. 2014;89(4):232–7. Epub 2014 Feb 5.
46. Cheung EV, Sperling JW, Cofield RH. Infection associated with haematoma formation after shoulder arthroplasty. Clin Orthop Relat Res. 2008;466(6):1363–7.
47. Lucas RM, Hsu JE, Whitney IJ, Wasserburger J, Matsen FA III. Loose glenoid components in revision shoulder arthroplasty: is there an association with positive cultures? J Shoulder Elb Surg. 2016;25(8):1371–5.
48. Sethi PM, Sabetta JR, Stuek SJ, Horine SV, Vadasdi KB, Greene RT, Cunningham JG, Miller SR. Presence of Propionibacterium acnes inprimary shoulder arthroscopy: results of aspiration and tissue cultures. J Shoulder Elb Surg. 2015;24(5):796–803.
49. Crane JK, Hohman DW, Nodzo SR, Duquin TR. Antimicrobial susceptibility of propionibacterium acnes isolates from shoulder surgery. Antimicrob Agents Chemother. 2013;57(7):3424–6.
50. Knaepler H. Local application of gentamicin-containing collagen implant in the prophylaxis and treatment of surgical site infection in orthopaedic surgery. Int J Surg. 2012;10(Suppl 1):S15–20.
51. De Wild L, Walch G. Humeral prosthetic failure of reversed total shoulder hemiarthroplasty: a report of three cases. J Shoulder Elbow Surg. 2006;15:261–4.
52. Boileau P, Melis B, Duperron D, Moineau G, Rumian AP, Han Y. Revision surgery of reverse shoulder arthroplasty. J Shoulder Elb Surg. 2013;22(10):1359–70.

Glenoid Bone Augmentation in Shoulder Arthroplasty

20

Steve Bale

Introduction

Expansion of the indications for shoulder arthroplasty has resulted in a huge increase in the numbers being performed [1] and long-term studies document favourable outcomes with respect to pain relief and improved function [2, 3].

Glenoid component failure remains the commonest cause of a poorly performing arthroplasty and may relate to failure to address glenoid bone deficiency or version and associated soft tissue imbalance [4–11]. Certainly, studies have shown poorer results when anatomical prostheses are performed where there is pre-existing posterior glenoid erosion and survivorship analysis shows better results in the absence of posterior glenoid wear [12].

Assessing Glenoid Bone Loss

Preoperative planning is essential. Standard radiographs are essential and help to give an indication to the pattern of wear although axillary views often overestimate the amount of reroversion by 86% [13]. Computed Tomography does provide a more detailed assessment of bone loss, version and vault anatomy [13]. The axial slice at the level of the coracoid tip as described by Friedman is said to give the most reproducible assessment of version with the angle of version measured from a perpendicular line to the scapular line at the level of the joint [14] (Fig. 20.1).

A number of classifications of glenoid wear have been presented [15] but Walch developed the most commonly used classification [16] Fig. 20.2.

Habermeyers classification addresses the superior / inferior bone loss and its use compliments that of Walch [17] (Figs. 20.3 and 20.4).

Rotator cuff arthropathy produces different patterns of wear with the superior migration of the humeral head. This was first described by Sirveaux et al. [18].

E0 49% no erosion
E1 35% concentric erosion
E2 10% superior erosion
E3 6% with inferior erosion

50% of patients will have some degree of glenoid erosion in the antero-posterior plane although this classification does not take into account the coexisting erosion which may be present in the posterior or anterior glenoid.

The assessment of a 3-D deficiency in 2-D has limitations. Atuna et al. [19] described a

S. Bale (✉)
Wrightington Hospital, Wigan, UK

I. A. Trail et al. (eds.), *Textbook of Shoulder Surgery*, https://doi.org/10.1007/978-3-319-70099-1_20

classification based on findings at revision surgery and described the defects as central, peripheral or combined. Page et al. [20] from our institution proposed a similar classification of contained, uncontained incomplete and uncontained complete which has a direct impact on the ability to perform impaction bone grafting.

Further modifications to these 3D classifications have helped us to understand the pathological anatomy of the glenoid defining the site of the defect whether central or eccentric and the extent of the defect [21, 22].

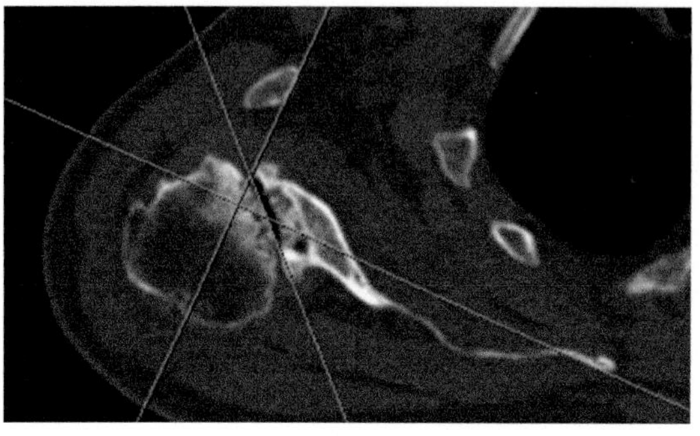

Fig. 20.1 The method of Friedman et al. for assessing glenoid retroversion. The slice is taken at the tip of the coracoid

Full appreciation of the glenoid defect is key to preoperative planning and the introduction of 3D modelling of the defects has helped surgeon's assessment of the defects. Production of patient specific guides have been shown to be useful in defining the best bone available [23].

Some of the most complex glenoid deficiencies come in failed arthroplasties and quality imaging of a loose glenoid component and the associated glenoid defect can be a real challenge particularly in the presence of an artefact -inducing metal humeral component. Metal artefact reduction software has helped with this problem.

> **Clinical Pearl**
> Full appreciation of the glenoid and any deficiencies is the key to adequate preoperative planning. Use of CT scans with metal artefact reduction software is recommended.

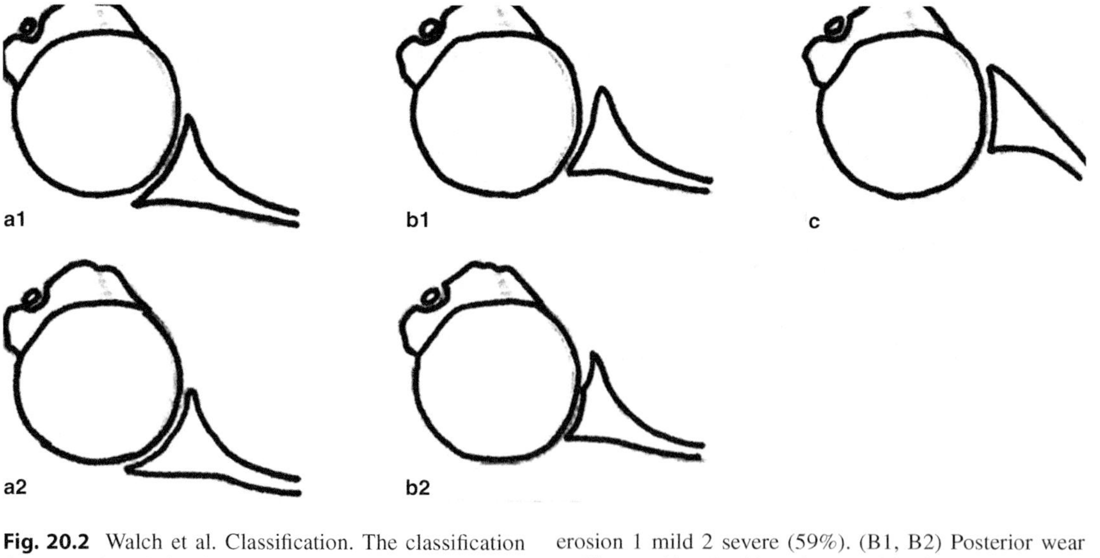

Fig. 20.2 Walch et al. Classification. The classification draws on the relationship between the anterior and posterior glenoid rims and the scapular axis. (A1, A2) Central erosion 1 mild 2 severe (59%). (B1, B2) Posterior wear and humeral head subluxation 1 and 2 with biconcave glenoid (32%). (C1, C2) Greater than 25 deg. retroversion

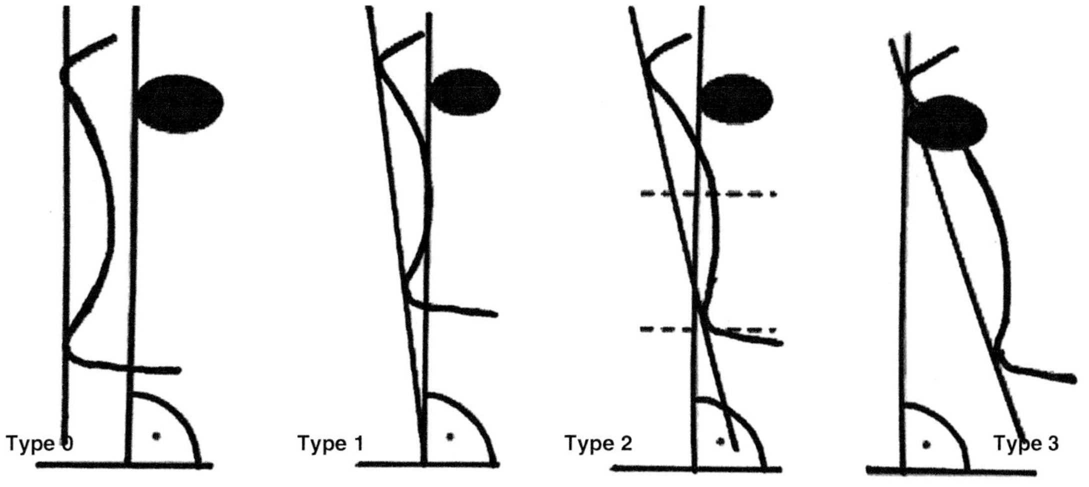

Fig. 20.3 Classification of Habermeyer et al. Type 0, Type 1, Type 2, Type 3. The classification relies on a relationship between a line drawn from superior to inferior glenoid rim and a comparison line drawn vertically at the level of the coracoid

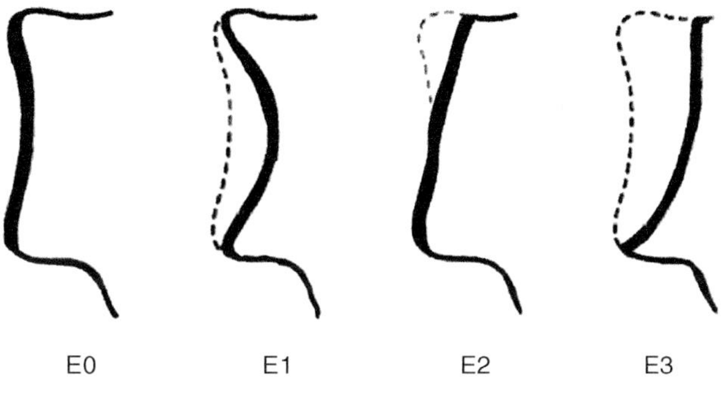

Fig. 20.4 Sirveaux classification of bone loss in cuff arthropathy

What Are the Limits of a Standard Anatomic Glenoid?

Careful preparation of the glenoid is required. The subchondral plate is ideally preserved and reamed carefully to obtain a good backside fit for the glenoid implant. Over-reaming leads to a loss of this plate and the implant then relies on inferior quality bone in the vault. This can be associated with early failure [24].

Glenoid version should be corrected for a long-term favourable outcome [25, 26]. As little as 2.5 degrees of retroversion can result in posterior humeral head subluxation, shifting the joint reaction force posteriorly, leading to eccentric loading with the potential for loosening. Once the retroversion is beyond 10 degrees finite element analysis studies have predicted reduced contact area, increased contact pressures and more than seven fold increase in micro-motion again leading to early loosening. In the clinical setting studies of failed arthroplasties have found 46% incidence of glenoid implants in excessive retroversion [27].

Whilst it appears important to correct glenoid version, how it is achieved is more controversial.

Techniques to realign a retroverted glenoid include high side reaming (HSR). However, excessive reaming for significant defects can lead to medialisation of the joint, loss of vault volume, loss of bone strength, perforation of peg holes, the need to downsize glenoid implants suboptimally and poor soft tissue balancing. HSR can probably correct up to 15 degrees of retroversion without compromising the implant [28, 29].

Walch et al. [10] noted that preoperative posterior humeral head subluxation of 80% is associated with 11% risk of posterior instability. With retroversion greater than 27 degrees there was a 44% rate of implant loosening or posterior head dislocation. Walch reviewed the results of TSA in biconcave glenoids. Loosening had occurred in 20.6% at mean 6 year and revisions were performed in 16.3% in a series of 92 patients. Ho et al. [30] found glenoid osteolysis in patients with15 degrees or more retroversion in a review of 66 patients.

What Are the Limits of a Standard Reverse Glenoid?

Glenoid preparation for reverse geometry prostheses is more invasive and relies on the volume and depth of the vault to accept a central peg and a variable number of locking and non-locking screws depending on the choice of implant [31].

The depth of the vault can be up to 35 mm at the centre point of the inferior glenoid circle [32] and is required to take the peg of all implants. The length of the pegs vary between implants and the optimum peg length is currently not defined. Companies may provide a range of peg lengths which will be considered further when it comes to discussion of complex primary and revisions cases. The vault volume is also important as it will have to accept a varying number and varying angles of screws dependent again on implant.

Hopkins et al. [33] using finite element analysis studies of different screw configurations and sizes found that increasing the length of the screws from 16 mm to 30 mm led to a reduction in micromotion of 30%. Angulation of the screws away from the base plate also had a beneficial effect.

Bone Grafting Techniques

The approach to glenoid defects has traditionally been to address them with a bone graft.

The type of grafting technique chosen will depend on the deficiency present. Central defects can be treated with traditional impaction grafting techniques.

Neer and Morrison [34] reported success where central defects were treated with cancellous fragments and a standard glenoid component. Neyton et al. [35] used iliac crest to fill defects left by failed glenoids but further reimplantation did not take place. Page et al. [20] used impaction grafting to treat contained or containable defects with satisfactory results.

Peripheral defects have proved to be more challenging particularly with attempts to realign B2 glenoids. Steinmann and Cofield [36] used wedge grafts separately fixed behind the glenoid implant in anatomic arthroplasty and while 68% had good or excellent results 14% had complete graft lucency. Similar issues were reported by Hill and Norris [37] where 8 of 17 cases showed either graft failure or resorption or needed revision. In the series from Walch et al. [10] of 92 anatomic arthroplasties 7 needed grafting but only only 2 of this group healed. The reasons for failure may be related to the presence of cement, soft tissue imbalance and the mechanical loading of the glenoid and its effect on bone healing.

Two stage implantation was therefore tried with initial grafting followed by later reimplantation of a glenoid component. However, in a series of 18 cases Iannotti and Frangiamore [38] reported resorption of the structural allograft in 10 of 18 cases and Phipatanakul and Norris [39] reported subsidence of their graft in 50% of cases.

In contrast to the experience in anatomical arthroplasty, the healing of grafts in the mechanical environment generated by the reverse geometry prosthesis has been more promising. Boileau et al. [40] reported the BIO technique to reconstruct offset and reported 98% graft healing. It is likely that the metal back of the prosthesis and the compression of the graft by that component achieved by screw fixation allows a favourable graft healing environment. Neyton et al. [41] reported no graft failures in 9 patients followed to 2 years and we reported the early results in our series of 56 cases with graft implant composites with peg integration of 95% and graft healing of 90% [42]. The success appears to relate to compression of the graft by the convex deep surface of the implant and the osteo-integrative properties of trabecular metal [43, 44]. Two stage implantation has also been carried out with excellent graft incorporation.

Practical Considerations

Source of Bone Graft

Humeral head autograft is the usual source of bone graft in the primary setting and can usually be relied upon to yield good quality material. A preoperative CT is a useful way of assessing the humeral head bone stock for large cysts and marked osteopaenia which may affect the choice of bone source.

There are many techniques for harvesting humeral head bone. We use a technique which involves implantation of the base plate into the humeral head prior to over-reaming to produce the implant/graft composite (Figs. 20.5, 20.6, 20.7 and 20.8).

The graft implant composite is then shaped according to the defect present.

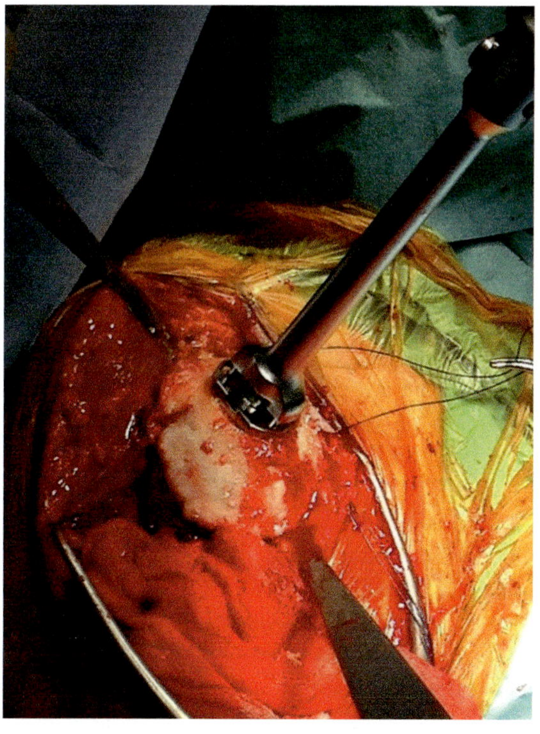

Fig. 20.5 The implant has been impacted into the humeral head

Clinical Pearl
The humeral head usually provides ample quality bone graft for most complex primary situations.

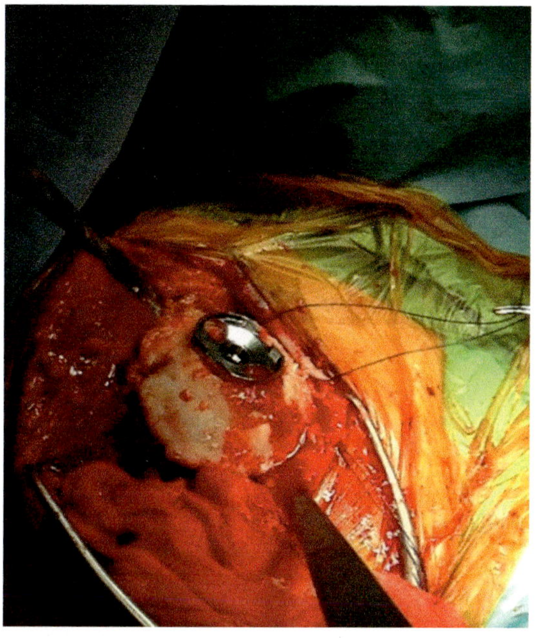

Fig. 20.6 Implant in situ

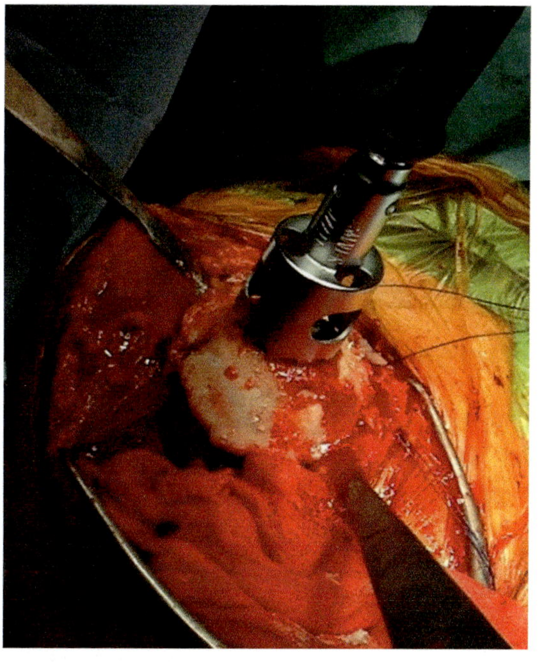

Fig. 20.7 Over-reaming

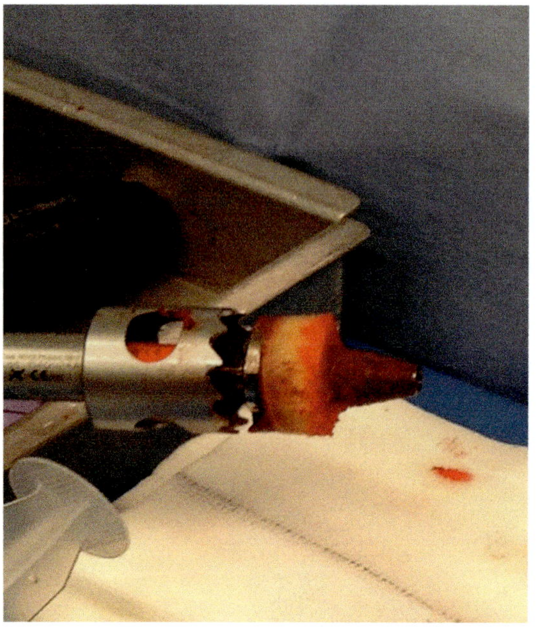

Fig. 20.8 Graft inplant composite

Iliac Crest

Kelly et al. [45] described the use of a composite of the baseplate and structural graft by implanting the baseplate directly into the iliac crest and then fashioning the bone taken according to the defect. They reported a significant improvement in scores in 12 patients. Potential issues with this technique relate to the defect caused to the iliac crest and the potential for this defect to act as a stress riser with the potential for a fracture down into the ilium and the hip joint. Prophylactic plating of the crest deficiency has been advocated to avoid this complication.

Iliac Wing

Given concerns over the implantation technique into the crest, we have used bone from the iliac wing. In partnership with our pelvic surgeons we have been able to identify a column of bone running down from the iliac crest to the acetabulum which yields a good volume of quality bone.

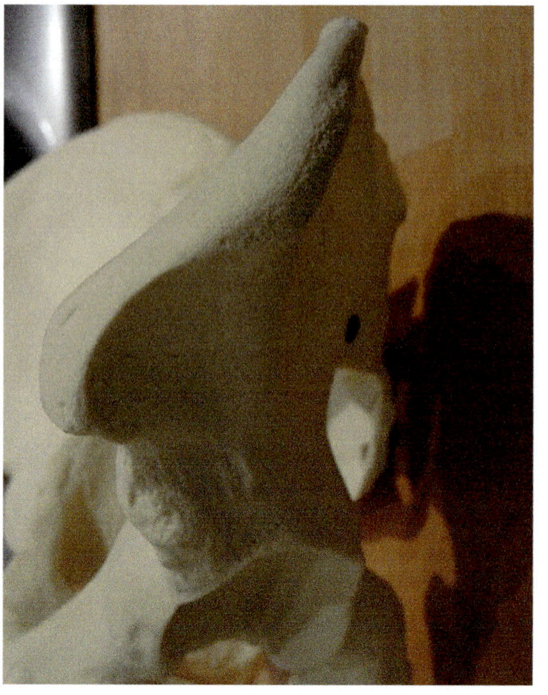

Fig. 20.9 Thick column of quality bone

Careful dissection of the tissue off both tables of the iliac wing allows access to this bone. The procedure can be done supine or if the patient is larger the graft can be harvested as a primary procedure in the lateral position with the table broken to improve access.

Swabs or retractors can be used to protect the internal viscera. Careful wire placement, reaming, implantation of implant and removal of composite can be safely achieved. Bone wax can seal the raw cancellous areas and the wound is closed over a drain.

However, any procedure involving pelvic bone will have an impact on patient mobility and is likely to increase inpatient stay (Figs. 20.9, 20.10, 20.11, 20.12, 20.13, 20.14, 20.15 and 20.16).

One way of avoiding the morbidity associated with utilisation of pelvic bone is to use allograft. There are many sources, the most frequently used being frozen femoral heads. In the shoulder, it is currently unclear as to the long term effectiveness.

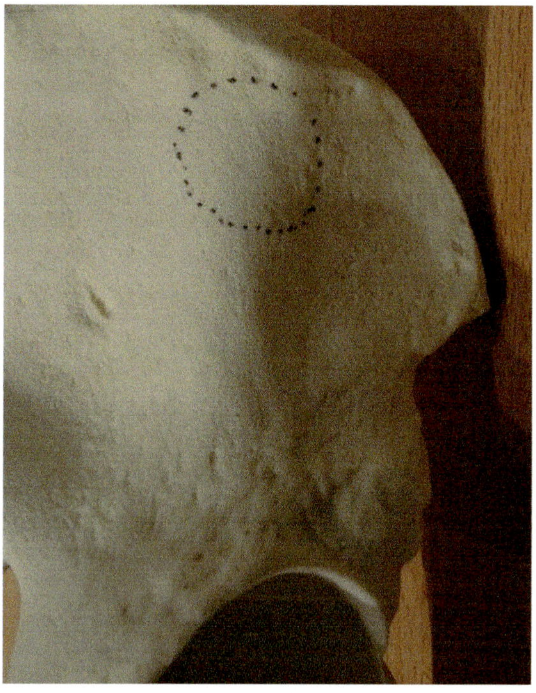

Fig. 20.10 Position of donor bone

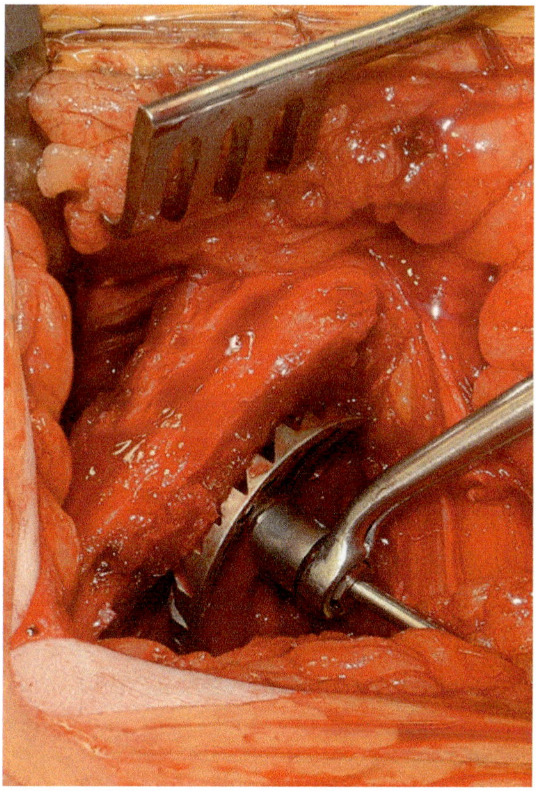

Fig. 20.11 K wire insertion and reaming of outer table

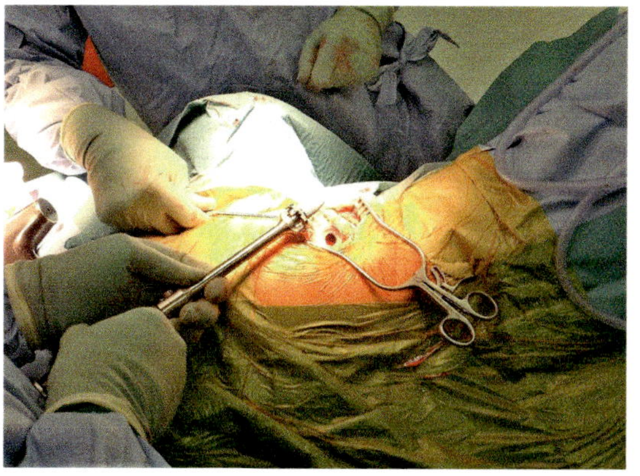

Fig. 20.12 Implantation of baseplate

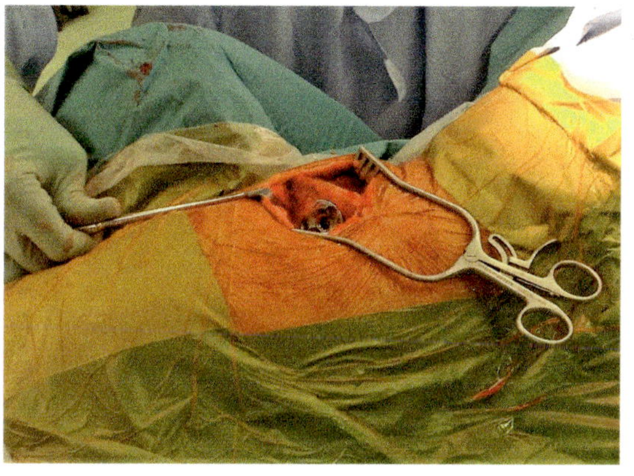

Fig. 20.13 Base plate inserted

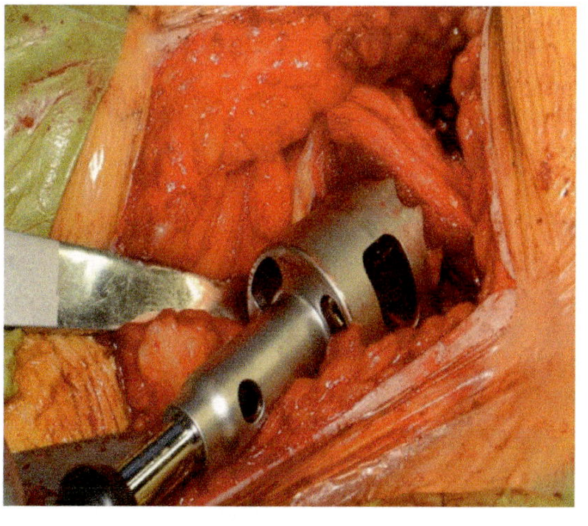

Fig. 20.14 Over-reaming

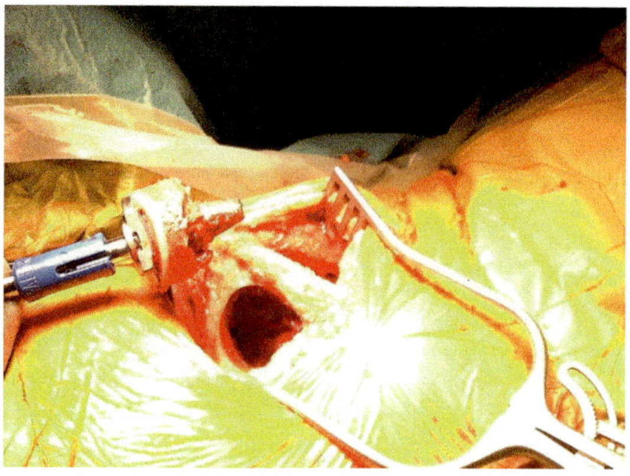

Fig. 20.15 Composite and bony defect

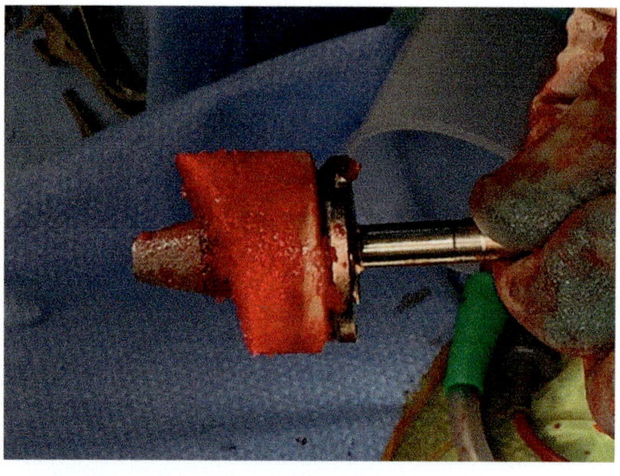

Fig. 20.16 Quality of composite obtaines

In order to avoid large structural grafts Bateman and Donald [46] described a novel technique employing a dual biology approach. The technique centres around the use of appropriately sized femoral neck allograft being used as a method to create a ring of bone rendering a defect containable. The ring of femoral neck and the deep defect are then filled with cancellous graft. Satisfactory results were reported in the first 5 of a 10 patient cohort study followed to 12–36 months with documented incorporation of bone (Fig. 20.16).

The Bateman technique however, does not get away from the need to involve taking the bone from the iliac crest to fill the contained defect and therefore does not confer an advantage in terms of patient mobilisation and therefore post operative stay.

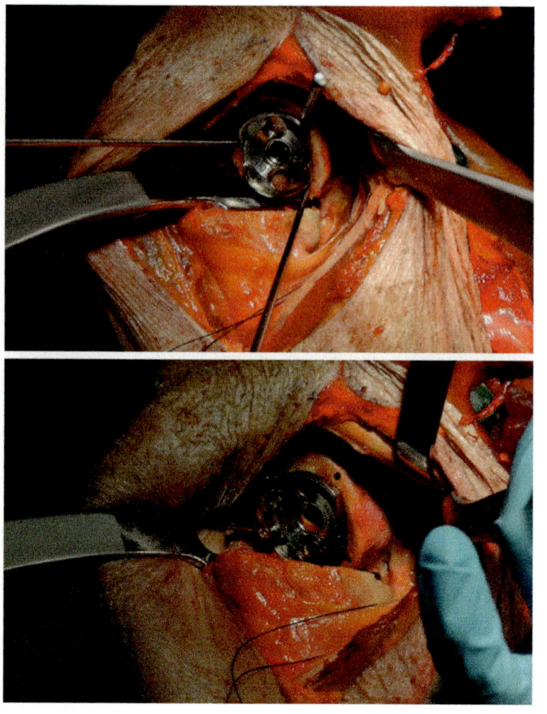

Fig. 20.17 Cadaveric studies using the technique of Bateman and Donald

We have therefore used this technique in a modified way so as to avoid any significant assault on the pelvis. Our dual biology technique involves the use of a reamer/ irrigator/ aspirator (RIA) to obtain graft from a single pass of a reamer down the femur. This technique usually yields copious amounts of quality cancellous graft with no impact on mobilisation post operatively. We have shown bone incorporation on post-operative CT at 4 months (Figs. 20.17, 20.18 and 20.19).

There is other literature to support the use of femoral neck allograft [47].

Whilst we have reported the early results of our first 56 cases using a large structural autograft the only large published series of large structural grafts beyond 2 years has come from Jones et al. [48]. In this multi-centre series of 44 patients there were 29 humeral head autografts,

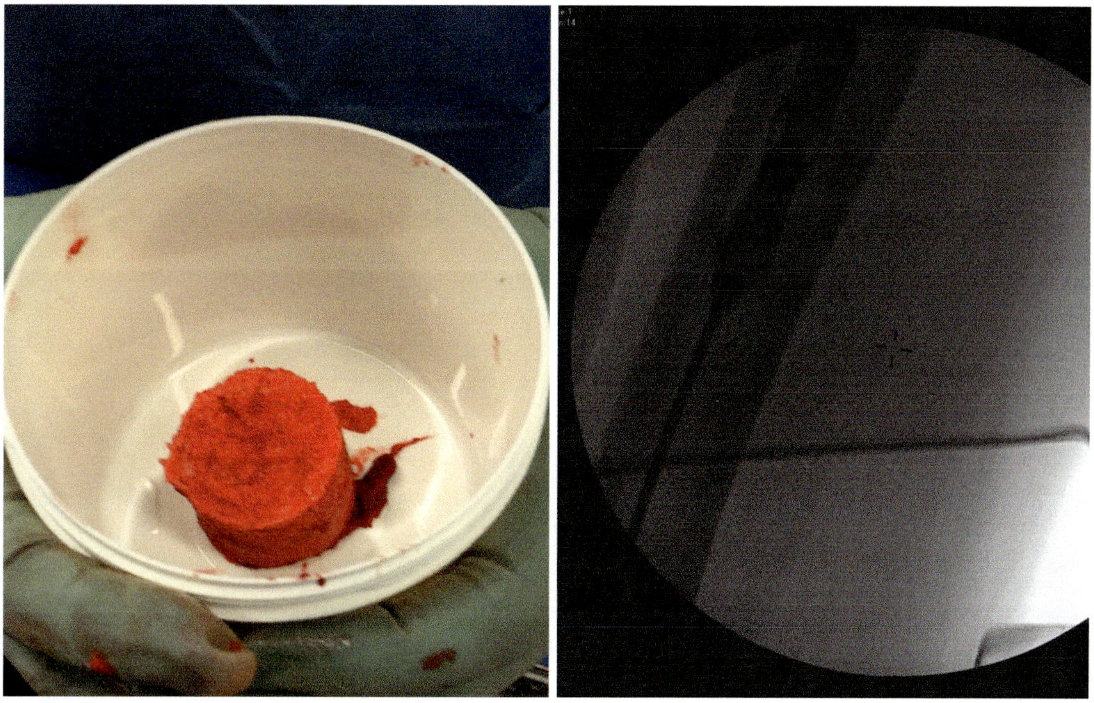

Fig. 20.18 Quantity of cancellous graft and image intensifier of reamer in the femur

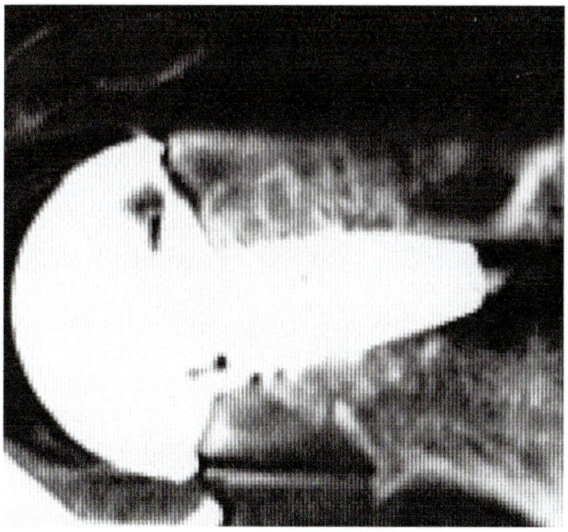

Fig. 20.19 Bone healing at 4 months

1 iliac crest autograft and 14 femoral allografts. Improvements in scores were noted in most cases. Interestingly the cohort needing the graft fared less well generally than the cohort not needing graft. 81% of grafts were thought to be completely or partially incorporated though the assessment of incorporation was based on radiographs and not CT. Overall, there was a complication rate of 36% consistent with the demanding surgery in both the complex primary and revision settings.

> **Clinical Pearl**
> Bone grafts under compression can be left to incorporate and definitive glenosphere implantation can be delayed until healing is confirmed on CT.

Non Bone Grafting Option

In order to avoid bone grafting, particularly in glenoid defects which are only mild to moderate and particularly in relation to B type glenoids, there are now a number of non-standard implants being offered by manufacturers including posterior, anterior and superior augmented metal and all poly glenoids with wedges. Their use is supported by laboratory and finite element analysis studies [49, 50]. Clinical studies have yielded varying results. Rice et al. [51] reported on a posteriorly augmented glenoid. Unfortunately the posterior subluxation was not addressed resulting in unsatisfactory results. Favarito et al. [52] have recently reported on 22 all polyethylene posteriorly augmented glenoids with a mean follow up of 36 months. Outcome scores improved significantly. There were 3 episodes of prosthetic instability. Whilst short term results are encouraging long term date is currently unavailable. Similar results were presented by Lenart et al. [53] in smaller numbers again with an anteriorly augmented glenoid.

Sandow and Schutz [54] reported on the use of separately fixed trabecular metal wedges, to correct the version, used in conjuction with a standard cemented polyethylene glenoid. The 2 year results are encouraging with good metal integration allowing correction of up to 25 deg. retroversion. Longer term studies are required but this work will rekindle debate about the use of uncemented metal backed glenoids with trabecular metal technology in cases of glenoid deficiency in the anatomic shoulder setting avoiding the need for wedge bone grafting.

Bespoke Options

Where destruction of the glenoid is severe, which can be seen in certain primary settings but perhaps more commonly in the revision scenario, the ability to apply a standard glenoid component to the deficiency becomes less likely. This was the situation historically where a hemiarthroplasty for pain relief would have been advocated. The use of a hemiarthroplasty may still have its place but the limits of reconstruction have been reset. These have yet to be redefined but the use of custom implants providing bespoke answers to glenoid deficiencies by providing prostheses specific for each deficiency are now available.

Whilst there is some encouraging evidence in the literature [55] currently again there are no long term studies (Figs. 20.20, 20.21 and 20.22).

Clinical Pearl

As a last resort, if reconstruction of the glenoid appears impossible with standard implants, consider a bespoke augmented implant.

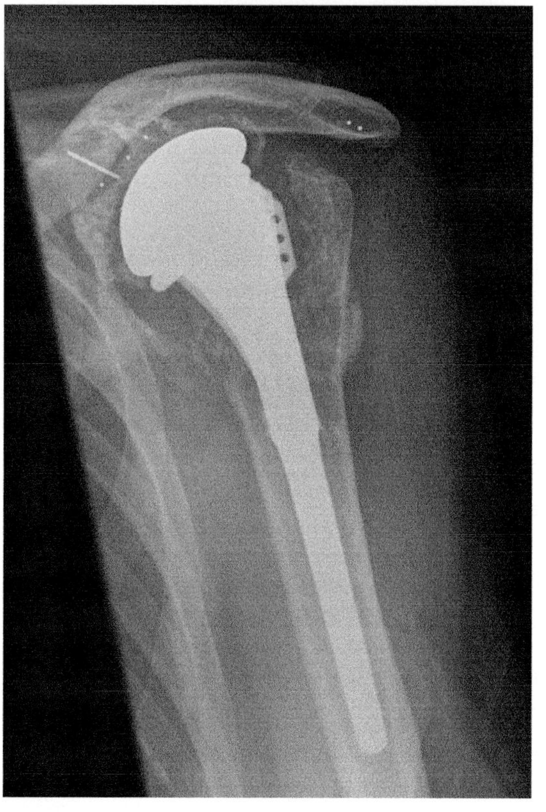

Fig. 20.20 Severe glenoid bone loss associated with failed polyethylene glenoid

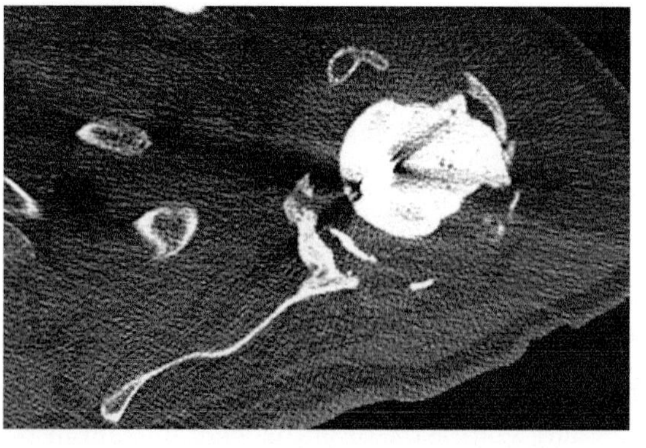

Fig. 20.21 CT demonstrating marked glenoid destruction

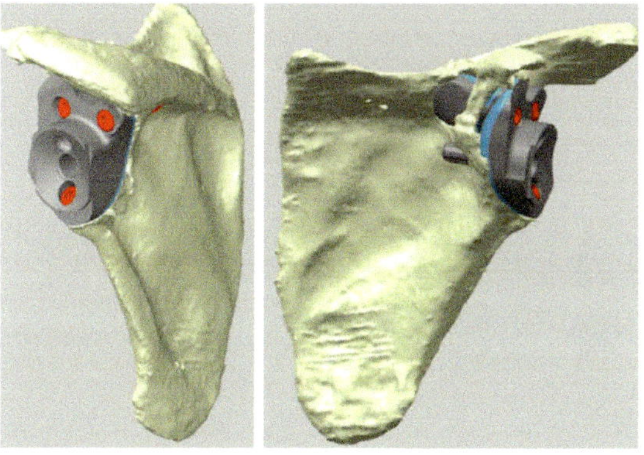

Fig. 20.22 Example of bespoke glenoid implant proposal

Proposed Algorithm

After considering the literature and considering the availability of products and techniques it is possible to propose a reasonable algorithm to aid the decision making process from patient presentation to selection of surgical implant. Given current lack of knowledge however, particularly long term studies' obviously this algorithm may change with time.

For the anatomic replacement with intact cuff the degree of glenoid erosion is the key.

Erosion

- Less than 15 degrees – ream and implant standard implant
- 15 – 20 degrees – consider PSI and implantation of standard implant after reaming
- More than 20 degrees – standard glenoid with metal inserts or augmented poly
  - Metal backed glenoid + graft or wedge augments

Medialisation → Graft baseplate composite or thicker all polyethylene implant

For primary reverse

- No erosion – normal technique
- Medialisation posterior or anterior erosion but more than 10mm native bone – bone graft implant composite
- Less than 10mm or no screw space – custom or hemi

Revision case

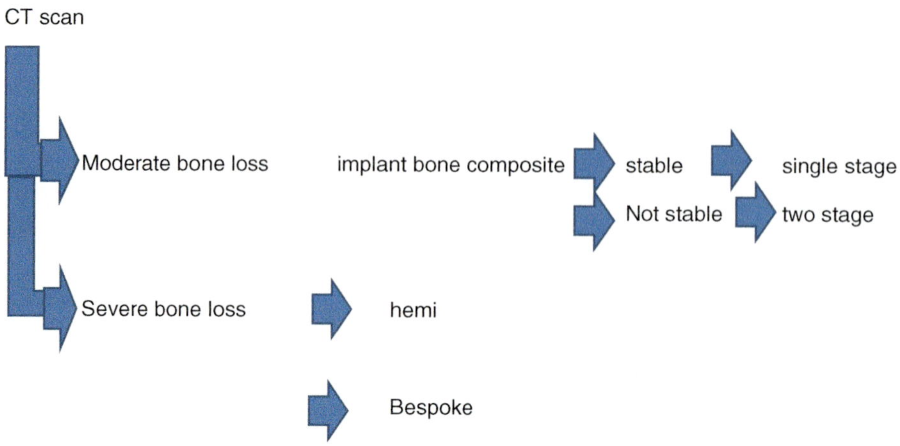

References

1. Day JS, et al. Prevalence and projections of total shoulder and elbow arthroplasty in the United States to 2015. J Shoulder Elb Surg. 2010;19:1115–20.
2. Boileau P, et al. Arthroplasty of the shoulder. J Bone Joint Surg Br. 1996;88:562–75.
3. Cofield RH. Total shoulder arthroplasty with a Neer prosthesis. J Bone Joint Surg Am. 1984;66:899–906.
4. Ianonotti JP, Norris TR. Influence of preoperative factors on outcome of shoulder arthroplasty for glenohumeral arthritis. J Bone Joint Surg Am. 2003;85:251–8.
5. Hasan SS, et al. Characteristics of unsatisfactory shoulder arthroplasties. J Shoulder Elb Surg. 2002;11:431–41.
6. Bohsali KJ, et al. Complications of total shoulder arthroplasty. J Bone Joint Surg Am. 2006;88:2279–92.
7. Franta AK, et al. The complex characteristics of 282 unsatisfactory shoulder arthoplasties. J Shoulder Elb Surg. 2007;16:555–62.
8. Fox TJ. Survival of the glenoid component in shoulder arthroplasty. J Shoulder Elb Surg. 2009;18:859–63.
9. Iannotti JP, et al. Prosthetic positioning in total shoulder arthroplasty. J Shoulder Elb Surg. 2005;14:111–21.
10. Walch G, Moraga C, Young A, Castellanos-Rosas J. Results of anatomic nonconstrained prosthesis in primary osteoarthritis with biconcave glenoid. J Shoulder Elb Surg. 2012;21:1526–33.
11. Matsen FA 3rd, et al. Glenoid component failure in total shoulder arthroplasty. J Bone Joint Surg Am. 2008;90:885–96.
12. Cil A, et al. Survivorship of the humeral component in shoulder arthroplasty. J Shoulder Elb Surg. 2010;19:143–50.
13. Nyffeler RW, et al. Measurement of glenoid version: conventional radiographs versus computed tomography scans. J Shoulder Elb Surg. 2003;12(5):493–6.
14. Friedman RJ, Hawthorne KB, Genez BM. The use of computerized tomography in the measurement of glenoid version. J Bone Joint Surg Am. 1992;74(7):1032–7.
15. Levine WN, et al. Hemiarthroplasty for glenohumeral osteoarthritis: results correlated to degree of glenoid wear. J Shoulder Elb Surg. 1997;6:449–54.
16. Walch G, Badet R, Boulahia A, Khoury A. Morphologic study of the glenoid in primary glenohumeral osteoarthritis. J Arthroplast. 1999;14(6):756–60.
17. Habermeyer P, Magosch P, Luz V, Lichtenberg S. Three-dimensional glenoid deformity in patients with osteoarthritis: a radiographic analysis. J Bone Joint Surg. 2006;88(6):1301–7.
18. Sirveaux F, Favard L, Oudet D, Huquet D, Walch G, Mole D. Grammont inverted total shoulder arthroplasty in the treatment of glenohumeral osteoarthritis with massive rupture of the cuff results of a multicentre study of 80 shoulders. J Bone Joint Surg (Br). 2004;86(3):388–95.
19. Antuna SA, Sperling JW, Cofield RH, Rowland CM. Glenoid revision surgery after total shoulder arthroplasty. J Shoulder Elb Surg. 2001;10(3):217–24.
20. Page RS, Haines JF, Trail I. Impaction bone grafting in revision shoulder arthroplasty: classification, technical description and early results. Should Elb. 2009;1:81–8.
21. Frankle MA, et al. Glenoid morphology in reverse shoulder arthroplasty: classification and surgical implications. J Shoulder Elb Surg. 2009;15:521–6.
22. Visotsky JL, et al. Cuff tear arthropathy: pathogenesis, classification and algorithm for treatment. J Bone Joint Surg Am. 2004;86(Suppl 2):35–40.
23. Hendel MD, Bryan JA, Barsoum WK, Rodriguez EJ, Brems JJ, Evans PJ, Iannotti JP. Comparison of patient-specific instruments with standard surgical instruments in determining glenoid component position. J Bone Joint Surg. 2012;94(23):2167–75.

24. Anglin C, Tolhurst P, Wyss UP, Pichora DR. Glenoid cancellous bone strength and modulus. J Biomech. 1999;32(10):1091–7.
25. Shapiro TA, McGarry MH, Gupta R, Lee YS, Lee TQ. Biomechanical effects of glenoid retroversion in total shoulder arthroplasty. J Shoulder Elb Surg. 2007;16(3 Suppl):S90–5. Epub 2006 Dec 12.
26. Büchler P, Ramaniraka NA, Rakotomanana LR, Iannotti JP, Farron A. A finite element model of the shoulder: application to the comparison of normal and osteoarthritic joints. Clin Biomech. 2002;17(9):630–9.
27. Moskal MJ, Duckworth D, Matsen FA. An analysis of 122 failed shoulder arthroplasties. J Shoulder Elb Surg. 1999;8:554.
28. Gillespie R, Lyons R, Lazarus M. Eccentric reaming in total shoulder arthroplasty: a cadaveric study. Orthopedics. 2009;32(1):21.
29. Clavert P, Millett PJ, Warner JJ. Glenoid resurfacing: what are the limits to asymmetric reaming for posterior erosion? J Shoulder Elb Surg. 2007;16(6):843–8.
30. Ho JC, et al. Glenoid component retroversion is associated with osteolysis. J Bone Joint Surg Am. 2013;95:821–8.
31. Flatow EL, Harrison AK. A history of reverse total shoulder arthroplasty. Clin Orthop Relat Res. 2011;469(9):2432–9.
32. Rispoli DM, Sperling JW, Athwal GS, Wenger DE, Cofield RH. Projection of the glenoid center point within the glenoid vault. Clin Orthop Relat Res. 2008;466(3):573–8.
33. Hopkins AR, Hansen UN, Bull AM, Emery R, Amis AA. Fixation of the reversed shoulder prosthesis. J Shoulder Elb Surg. 2008;17(6):974–80.
34. Neer CS, Morrison DS. Glenoid bone-grafting in total shoulder arthroplasty. J Bone Joint Surg. 1988;70(8):1154–62.
35. Neyton L, Walch G, Nové-Josserand L, Edwards TB. Glenoid corticocancellous bone grafting after glenoid component removal in the treatment of glenoid loosening. J Shoulder Elb Surg. 2006;15(2):173–9.
36. Steinmann SP, Cofield RH. Bone grafting for glenoid deficiency in total shoulder replacement. J Shoulder Elb Surg. 2000;9(5):361–7.
37. Hill JM, Norris TR. Long-term results of total shoulder arthroplasty following bone-grafting of the glenoid. J Bone Joint Surg. 2001;83(6):877–83.
38. Iannotti JP, Frangiamore SJ. Fate of large structural allograft for treatment of severe unconstrained glenoid bone deficiency. J Shoulder Elb Surg. 2012;21:765–71.
39. Phipatanakul WP, Norris TR. Treatment of glenoid loosening and bone loss due to osteolysis with glenoid bone grafting. J Shoulder Elb Surg. 2006;15(1):84–7.
40. Boileau P, Moineau G, Roussanne Y, O'Shea K. Bony increased-offset reversed shoulder arthroplasty: minimizing scapular impingement while maximizing glenoid fixation. Clin Orthop Relat Res. 2011;469(9):2558–67.
41. Neyton L, Boileau P, Nové-Josserand L, Edwards TB, Walch G. Glenoid bone grafting with a reverse design prosthesis. J Shoulder Elb Surg. 2007;16(3):S71–8.
42. Abstracts for the 26th Annual Scientific Meeting, BESS 24–26 June 2015, Sheffield, UK. Should Elb. 2015;7(4):309–32.
43. Christie MJ. Clinical applications of Trabecular metal. Am J Orthop (Belle Mead NJ). 2002;31(4):219–20.
44. Bogle A, Budge M, Richman A, Miller RJ, Wiater JM, Voloshin I. Radiographic results of fully uncemented trabecular metal reverse shoulder system at 1 and 2 years' follow-up. J Shoulder Elb Surg. 2013;22(4):e20–5.
45. Kelly JD, et al. Clinical results of revision shoulder arthroplasty using the reverse prosthesis. J Shoulder Elb Surg. 2012;21(11):1516–25.
46. Bateman E, Donald SM. Reconstruction of massive uncontained glenoid defects using a combined autograft-allograft construct with reverse shoulder arthroplasty: preliminary results. J Shoulder Elb Surg. 2012;21:925–34.
47. De Biase CF, et al. Reverse shoulder arthroplasty using a "L" shaped allograft for glenoid reconstruction in a patient with massive glenoid bone loss: case report. Eur Rev Med Pharmacol Sci. 2014;18:44–9.
48. Jones RB, et al. Reverse total shoulder arthroplasty with structural bone grafting of large glenoid defects. J Shoulder Elb Surg. 2016;25:1425–32.
49. Hermida JC, Flores-Hernandez C, Hoenecke HR, D'Lima DD. Augmented wedge-shaped glenoid component for the correction of glenoid retroversion: a finite element analysis. J Shoulder Elb Surg. 2014;23(3):347–54.
50. Allred JJ, Flores-Hernandez C, Hoenecke HR, D'Lima DD. Posterior augmented glenoid implants require less bone removal and generate lower stresses: a finite element analysis. J Shoulder Elb Surg. 2016;25(5):823–30.
51. Rice RS, Sperling JW, Miletti J, Schleck C, Cofield RH. Augmented glenoid component for bone deficiency in shoulder arthroplasty. Clin Orthop Relat Res. 2008;466(3):579–83.
52. Favarito PJ, et al. Total shoulder arthroplasty for glenohumeral arthritis associated with posterior glenoid bone loss: results of an all-polyethylene, posteriorly augmented glenoid component. J Shoulder Elb Surg. 2016;25:1681–9.
53. Lenart BA, et al. Total shoulder arthroplasty with and augmented component for anterior glenoid bone deficiency. J Shoulder Elb Surg. 2016;25:398–405.
54. Sandow M, Schutz C. Total shoulder arthroplasty using trabecular metal augments to address glenoid retroversion: the preliminary study of 10 patients with minimum 2 – year follow-up. J Shoulder Elb Surg. 2016;25:598–607.
55. Gunther SB, Lynch TL. Total shoulder replacement surgery with custom glenoid implants for severe bone deficiency. J Shoulder Elb Surg. 2012;21(5):675–84.

Polyethylene Augmented Glenoid Components in Anatomic Total Shoulder Arthroplasty

21

Jason C. Ho, Eric T. Ricchetti, and Joseph P. Iannotti

Introduction

Glenohumeral osteoarthritis can cause significant glenoid bone loss. Asymmetric bone loss in advanced osteoarthritis is primarily posterior resulting in increased retroversion. In contrast, patients with instability-related arthritis may develop anterior glenoid wear and increased anteversion. Walch initially described a three group classification of wear patterns in advanced osteoarthritis based on the morphology of the glenoid and humeral head subluxation. In a recent article, Walch described the addition of the B3 and D types to the classification to include posterior and central bone loss without hypoplasia and anteverted glenoids, respectively (Fig. 21.1) [1, 2]. Operative treatment options include anatomic and reverse total shoulder arthroplasty (TSA).

The goals for treatment of advanced glenohumeral arthritis with asymmetric bone loss using anatomic TSA include (1) correction of glenoid bony deformity to restore the patient's native anatomy, particularly native version, (2) restoration of the patient's native joint line, (3) balancing of the soft tissues, and (4) centering of the humeral head. Implant selection and design can significantly influence the achievement of these goals. This chapter will focus on use of the augmented glenoid component and its ability to restore native anatomy in anatomic TSA.

J. C. Ho · E. T. Ricchetti · J. P. Iannotti, MD, PhD (✉)
Department of Orthopaedic Surgery, Orthopaedic and Rheumatologic Institute, Cleveland Clinic, Cleveland, OH, USA
e-mail: iannotj@ccf.org

Challenges of Anatomic TSA with Asymmetric Glenoid Bone Loss

The correction of pathologic version and glenoid bone loss in shoulder arthroplasty has been shown to improve outcomes by balancing forces across the shoulder joint and recreating an anatomic alignment of the humeral head and glenoid [3–12]. In patients with minimal glenoid bone loss, the goals of shoulder arthroplasty can be achieved with a standard symmetric glenoid implant. However, in patients with moderate to severe asymmetric posterior glenoid bone loss, it is difficult to (a) determine the patient's premorbid or native glenoid version, and (b) effectively correct the pathologic deformity [6, 13]. Defining the native or premorbid glenoid version can be done with the use of three-dimensional (3D) computed tomography (CT) modeling and the vault model. The vault model was developed by defining the shape of the glenoid vault in the non-arthritic shoulder and defining the method to virtually place that model into the pathologic glenoid [6, 14–16]. Once positioned in the pathologic glenoid, the vault model defines the area of posterior glenoid bone loss and has been shown

I. A. Trail et al. (eds.), *Textbook of Shoulder Surgery*, https://doi.org/10.1007/978-3-319-70099-1_21

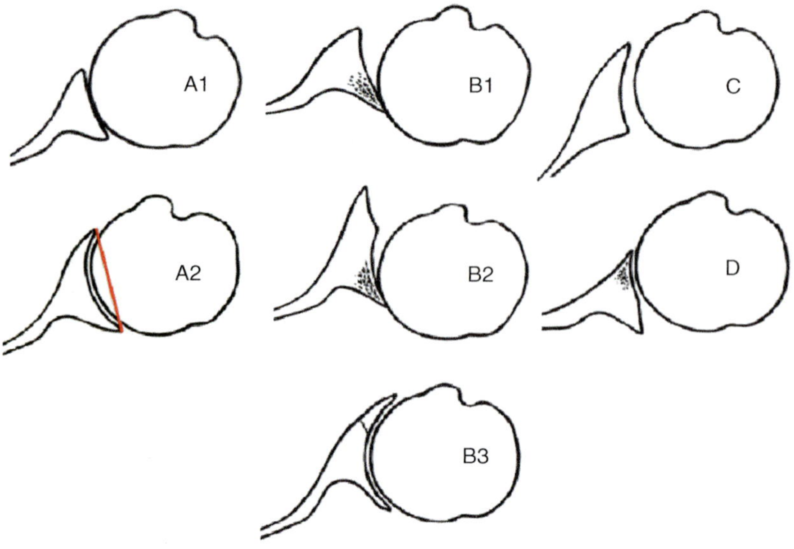

Fig. 21.1 Updated Walch classification of osteoarthritic glenoid bone loss. A1: centered humeral head with minor erosion, a line drawn from the anterior to posterior rim of the native glenoid does not transect the humeral head. A2: centered humeral head, major central glenoid erosion, a line drawn from the anterior to posterior rims of the native glenoid transects the humeral head. B1: posterior subluxated head, no bony erosion. B2: posterior subluxated head, posterior erosion with biconcavity of the glenoid. B3: monoconcave and posteriorly worn, with at least 15° of retroversion or at least 70% posterior humeral head subluxation, or both. C: dysplastic glenoid with at least 25° of retroversion not caused by erosion. D: any level of glenoid anteversion or humeral head subluxation of less than 40% anterior subluxation. (Figure 2 from Bercik et al. [2])

to be predictive of the location of the native glenoid joint line, version, and inclination [6, 14–17]. Therefore, this tool can be used to define patient specific correction of the pathologic glenoid to its pre-morbid condition [18, 19].

Techniques for Addressing Glenoid Bone Loss in Anatomic TSA

Prior to the availability of modern imaging techniques, implants and understanding of glenohumeral relationships, reaming the high side to correct pathologic version had been widely described as the preferred method to manage mild to moderate retroversion [10, 20–23]. Yet reaming the high-side to match native version as retroversion increases can cause significant medialization of the joint-line, narrow the anteroposterior dimensions of the glenoid, and/or lead to possible peg perforation with standard glenoid components in anatomic TSA. Cadaveric and clinical studies have shown that these problems commonly occur with asymmetric reaming when the technique is used to correct 15–20° or more of retroversion [13, 24–26]. However, inadequate correction of glenoid version in anatomic TSA can lead to increased rates of osteolysis of a pegged polyethylene glenoid component [27]. It is likely that early osteolysis in standard pegged components will result in later glenoid component loosening, as demonstrated in keeled glenoid designs where there is a relationship between radiolucencies and pain [28]. Early radiolucent lines around keeled glenoids have also been shown to be predictive of progressive radiolucent lines and worse patient reported outcomes [29]. In addition to clinical studies using standard glenoid components; biomechanical and cadaveric studies have all shown an increase risk of loosening of the glenoid component when placed in >15° of retroversion [21, 24, 30–37].

Another technique described to correct glenoid bone loss and retroversion has been the use of bone graft with a standard symmetric glenoid component. This technique allows both correction of version and maintenance of the joint line. Bone grafts are technically more difficult to obtain stability with a polyethylene component and require bone incorporation to have long term implant stability. Studies have demonstrated good clinical success in several case series, but a high incidence of radiolucency and radiographic concerns, and complications associated with graft preparation, fixation and graft incorporation have been reported [5, 38–41]. Based on the limitations of reaming the high side and the worrisome long-term durability of posterior glenoid bone grafting or placement of a retroverted implant for moderate to severe glenoid bone loss, a more recent alternative to correcting moderate to severe pathologic glenoid deformity during anatomic TSA has been the introduction of the augmented glenoid component.

Polyethylene Augmented Glenoid History and Modern Biomechanics

Historically, a cemented augmented polyethylene wedge glenoid was available from 1995–1999 (Fig. 21.2), but did not demonstrate enough clinical improvement over standard components to warrant continued use in a case series of 14 shoulders with midterm (2–8 year) follow-up [42]. Another study documented "nonstandard glenoids" in 38 patients at 2–19 year follow-up that included an angled keeled, extra thick standard keeled, and wedge augmented metal-back glenoid component. Of the 38 patients, 18 had an angled keel component, 12 had an extra thick standard keeled component, and 8 had augmented metal back components. At 10 years, there was 31% revision-free and removal-free survivorship of the augmented metal back, 73% of the angled keel, and 69% with the extra thick standard keeled component; with 50%, 44%, and 33% unsatisfactory Neer ratings, respectively (Fig. 21.3) [43]. In addition to the high complication rate, there was a failure of correcting the posterior subluxation in this heterogenous cohort. In both of the above studies advanced pre-operative imaging and planning or post-operative assessment of the correction were not performed. More recently, several biomechanical studies have attempted to study the potential advantages of an augmented polyethylene glenoid component to address glenoid retroversion and bone loss [44–48].

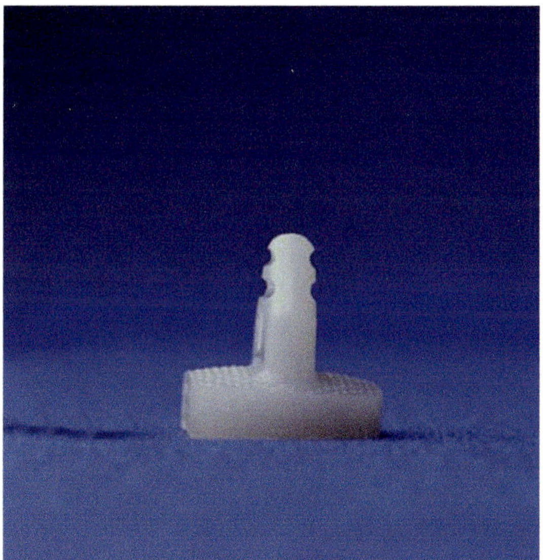

Fig. 21.2 View from bottom to top of a keeled all polyethylene glenoid component. Three component sizes were available that corrected the slope of the glenoid bone by approximately 4°. This implant is no longer available. (Figure 1 from Rice et al. [42])

A variety of augmented polyethylene glenoid designs have been evaluated biomechanically in the recent literature and three are currently commercially available; a stepped design (Steptech, Depuy Synthes, Johnson & Johnson, Warsaw, IN) (Fig. 21.4a), a wedge shaped design (Equinoxe Posterior Augment, Exactech, Gainesville, FL) (Fig. 21.4b), and a posterior wedge shaped design (Cortiloc, Wright Medical Group N.V., Memphis, TN) (Fig. 21.4c). All are currently available commercially in the United States in a variety of augmented sizes, and the stepped design has been in use since 2010. Several biomechanical studies have been conducted to determine which augmented glenoid design is the most biomechanically advantageous in glenoids with severe posterior wear or retroversion.

One study compared the commercially available wedge augmented glenoid to a stepped augmented glenoid, standard glenoid placed in neutral version after reaming the high side, and standard glenoid placed in retroversion using

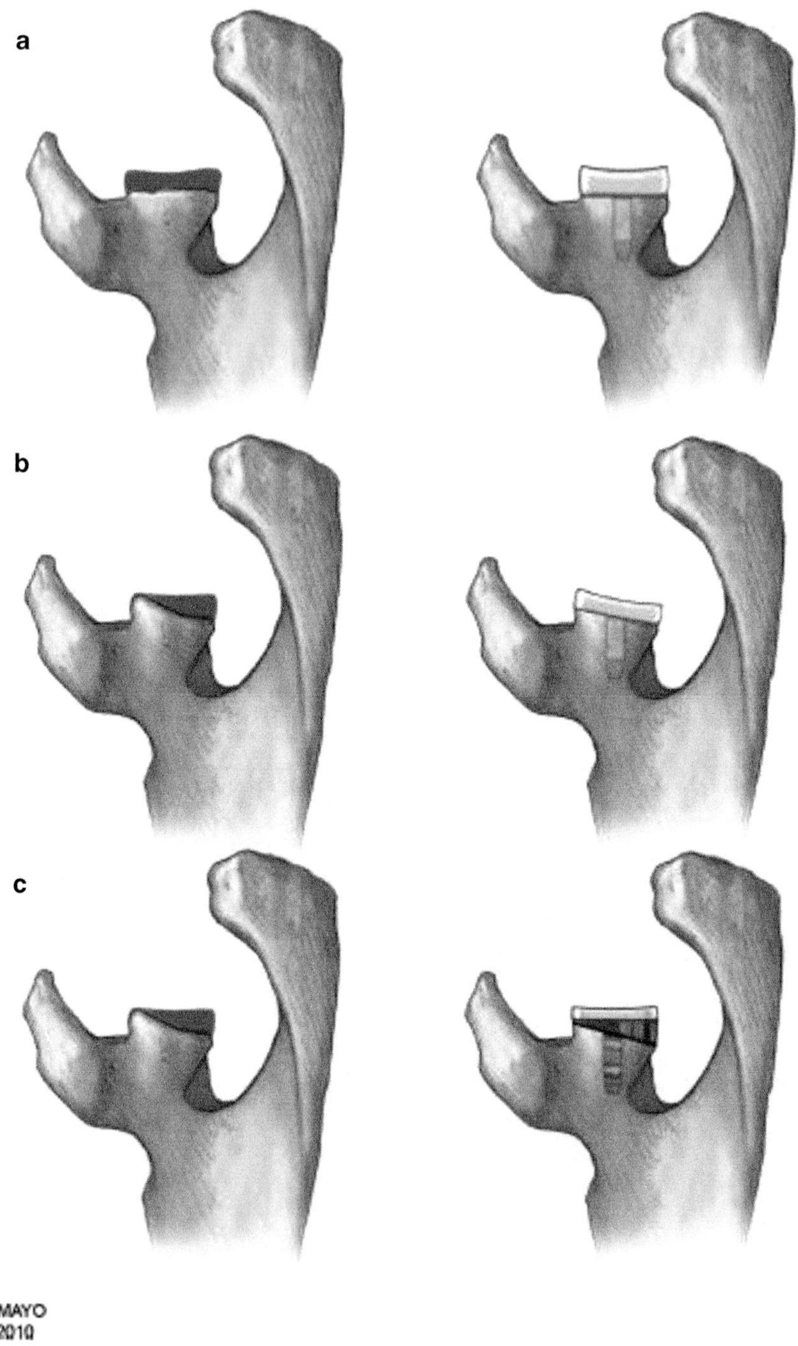

Fig. 21.3 Left column shows glenoid bone deficiencies addressed by custom implants. On the right demonstrates from top to bottom, a thicker polyethylene keeled glenoid, angled keel component, and posteriorly augmented wedge metal-backed glenoid. (Figure 1 from Cil et al. [43])

finite element analysis (FEA). This study found that the wedge design had more backside contact and less volume of bone at risk for strain damage when compared to the standard glenoid after reaming the high side, but did not find differences when compared to the stepped design [48]. Another study compared the wedged augment to a standard component in retroversion and found the wedged augment required a smaller cement mantle and had greater bone fatigue life [47].

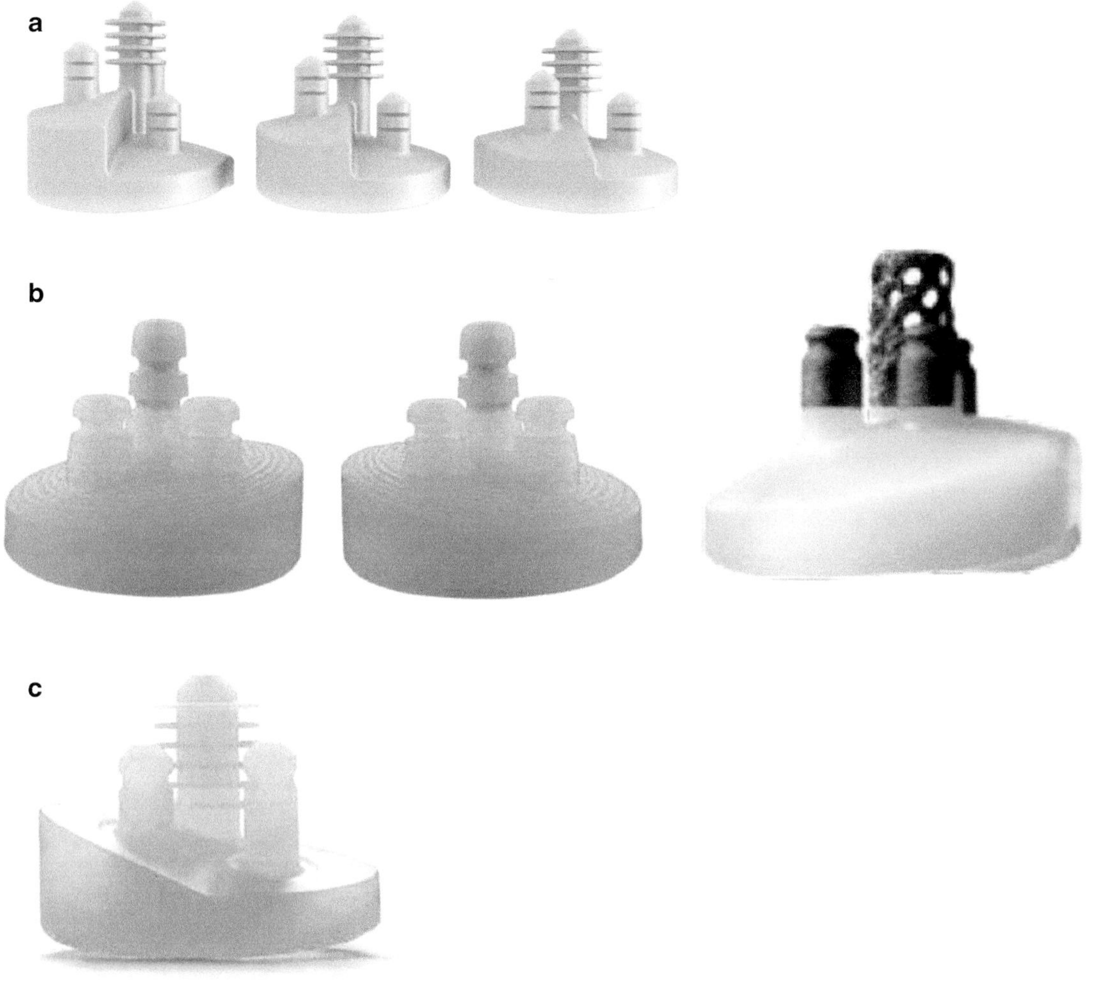

Fig. 21.4 (**a**) From left to right, the +7mm, +5mm, and +3mm posteriorly stepped all polyethylene augments, Step Tech, available from Depuy-Synthes, Johnson & Johnson, Warsaw, IN. (**b**) The wedged all polyethylene augment, Equinoxe Posterior Augment Glenoid, available from Exactech, Gainesville, FL. These come in 8° and 16° side-specific wedges, and also come with hybrid metal pegs with polyethylene (right). (**c**) The Aequalis Perform+ posteriorly wedged augment is available in 15°, 25°, and 35° posterior wedges that are side specific from Wright Medical Group N.V., Memphis, TN

The stepped augment component was compared to four other augment designs – spherical asymmetric, spherical symmetric, flat angled, standard pegged – for resistance to anterior liftoff when posteriorly loaded in a biomechanical study modeling early and late fixation states. This study demonstrated that the stepped augmented had decreased liftoff when compared to all other types, and no different than a standard glenoid (Fig. 21.5) [45]. Another study tested a non-commercial version of a stepped augmented glenoid in cadaveric specimens modeling a B2 glenoid. This study demonstrated strains with a stepped component placed in a B2 glenoid had no significant difference when compared to a standard component in a normal glenoid. These strains were tested in a variety of arm positions in their cadaveric model, with all arm positions showing similar strains. Interestingly, they also tested a titanium based

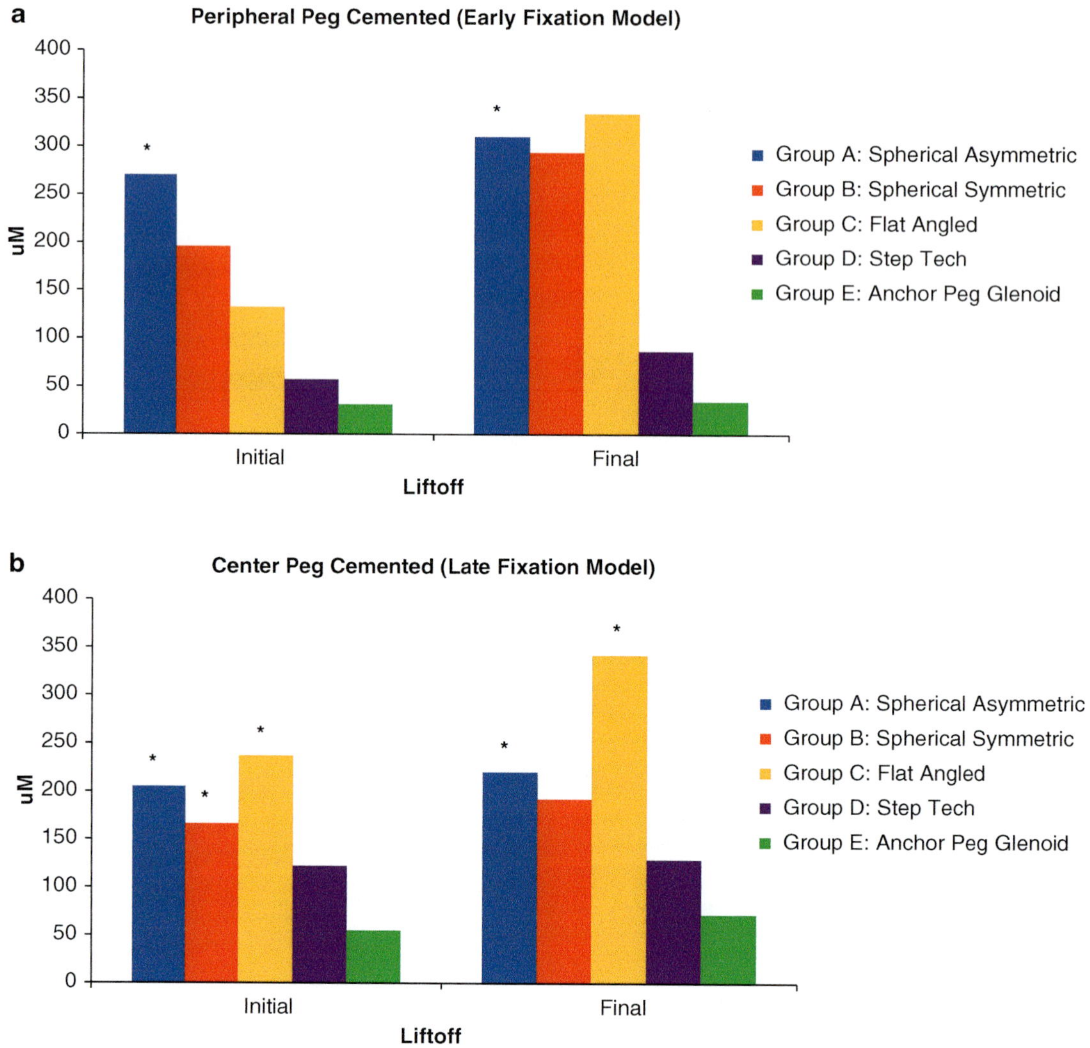

Fig. 21.5 (**a**) Chart showing lift-off of augmented and standard glenoid components with posterior-superior loading with peripheral pegs cemented, modeling early fixation. The bars on the left demonstrate initial lift-off and the right shows after 100,000 cycles. (**b**) Chart showing lift-off of augmented and standard glenoid components with posterior-superior loading with center pegs cemented, modeling late fixation. The bars on the left demonstrate initial lift-off and the right shows after 100,000 cycles. An asterisk (*) notes significant differences in liftoff when compared to the Step Tech glenoid ($P < 0.05$) in both charts. There were no statistically significant differences between the Step Tech and Anchor Peg Glenoid. (Adapted from Iannotti et al. [45])

step on a poly glenoid, but showed increased strain at certain arm position loads in the same study [46]. Another study demonstrated biomechanical superiority of eccentric reaming with a standard component versus an augmented wedge glenoid in a sawbones model, but the biomechanical model presented was done with repetitive superior-inferior loading, rather than the posterior loading seen in patients with severe glenoid bone loss, retroversion, and posterior subluxation of the humeral head [49]. Finally, a computational modeling study compared the commercially available wedge, stepped and posterior wedge components placed in B2 glenoids to assess the amount of bone removal and bone quality remaining.

This study demonstrated the posterior wedge design had less bone removal when compared to the wedge and stepped designs, and that the remaining bone was of a better quality [44, 50].

Polyethylene Augmented Glenoid Clinical Outcomes

Although there have been several biomechanical studies published in the peer-reviewed literature, there have been only a few clinical studies available to date on augmented glenoid components. The posterior wedge augment has no clinical data published to date. The wedge augmented glenoid was studied in patients with posterior glenoid wear and compared to standard glenoids without wear in an age and sex matched cohort study of 48 total patients with an average of 29.4 month follow-up. This study showed significant improvement in pain and functional outcome scores in all patients, and no difference in patient reported outcomes at final follow-up between the wedge augment and standard glenoid groups. There was no quantitative assessment of preoperative bone loss, retroversion, or degree of postoperative pathologic correction reported. Seventeen of twenty augmented glenoids had a centered humeral head postoperatively, three were anteriorly translated, and none were posteriorly translated [51].

The stepped augment has been compared to standard glenoids virtually using 3D CT preoperative planning software in patients with posterior glenoid bone loss. In this study, the stepped glenoid was able to correct larger amounts of pathologic retroversion with less medialization of the joint line when compared to standard components. This study demonstrated +3 mm, +5 mm, and + 7 mm augments being able to correct an average of 9.5°, 17.5°, and 27.9° of retroversion, respectively, to 0° and 6° of retroversion with significantly less medialization when compared to standard glenoids [52]. In a short term clinical series, the stepped augment has been studied at 6–15 month follow-up with 24 cases, all showing significant improvement in range of motion and patient reported outcomes. Eight of these patients had postoperative CT scans that showed stepped glenoids improved retroversion (16.7° vs. 11.3° of correction) and joint line correction (within 0.45 mm vs. 3.56 mm) better than standard glenoids in patients with similar retroversion [53]. Favorito et al. reported on 22 shoulders (20 B2 and 2 C type glenoids) that underwent TSA with a stepped augment at an average of 36 months follow-up. This study demonstrated significant improvements in VAS, WOOS, SF-36, and range of motion postoperatively. The authors also showed low rates of glenoid radiolucency with Lazarus scores of 0–2, 18/22 having a score of 0 or 1, and only one glenoid demonstrated central peg osteolysis.

Our group recently evaluated 88 patients with advanced glenohumeral osteoarthritis who underwent TSA with a standard ($n = 57$) or step augmented ($n = 31$) glenoid component with preoperative CT and a postoperative CT performed within 3 months of surgery [54]. All patients underwent preoperative planning with 3D CT imaging software prior to surgery. Overall, glenoid version correction (pre- to postoperative improvement in retroversion) was significantly greater with stepped compared to standard implants (12.1 ± 6.1° vs. 0.8 ± 3.8°, $P < 0.001$). When specifically comparing Walch B2 glenoids; version correction was significantly greater with stepped compared to standard implants (11.9 ± 6.6° vs. 3.6 ± 3.8°, $P < 0.001$), and stepped implants showed a trend for more closely correcting to premorbid version than standard implants (within −2.2 ± 6.3° vs. −5.2 ± 5.1° of premorbid version, $P = 0.096$). Correction of pathologic joint line was significantly greater with stepped than standard implants (1.1 ± 2.0 mm lateralization vs. 0.7 ± 1.8 mm medialization from the preoperative joint line, $P = 0.005$), and postoperative humeral-glenoid alignment showed a trend for better humeral head centering with stepped than standard implants (0.4 ± 3.2% vs. −1.3 ± 2.7%, $P = 0.083$), with stepped augments showing significantly greater correction of posterior humeral head subluxation relative to premorbid anatomy

(20.4 ± 7.4% versus 13.6 ± 4.9%, P = 0.001) in B2 glenoids. B2 glenoids with stepped implants were also compared to A1 glenoids with standard implants; with correction to premorbid version (within −2.2 ± 6.3° vs. −1.8 ± 4.1° of premorbid version, P = 0.839), joint line correction (1.1 ± 2.0 mm lateralization versus 1.2 ± 1.4 mm lateralization, P = 0.822), and postoperative humeral-glenoid alignment (0.4 ± 3.2% versus −1.1 ± 4.0%, P = 0.154) not significantly different between the groups. Stepped implants did not correct to the premorbid joint line in B2 glenoids as much as standard implants in A1 glenoids (within 1.2 ± 2.2 mm medial vs. 0.9 ± 1.0 mm lateral of premorbid joint line, P < 0.001).

In addition to the step augmented glenoid being used for posterior wear, a case series of 5 patients with anterior glenoid deficiencies have been treated with this implant. At an average of 33.2 months (range 21.9–43.2 months) follow-up, no patient had undergone revision surgery, and had an average postoperative Penn shoulder score of 84.4 (range 58–100) [55].

Augmented Glenoid Conclusions and Future Directions

The biomechanical and computational data available is supportive of the use of augmented polyethylene glenoids when addressing significant glenoid wear and deformity. There is support for both stepped and wedge designs that are commercially available, but clinical outcomes are still sparse in the literature. Prior literature has shown a high (16%) revision rate in biconcave B2 glenoids treated with standard glenoid components [56]. We believe an augmented glenoid component is a reliable option for joint line restoration, version correction, and centering of the humeral head for B2 glenoids, and there is early literature supporting this claim [53, 54]. However, longer term clinical follow-up will be needed to assess the longevity of the augmented glenoids, including maintenance of the pathologic glenoid correction and centering of the humeral head, patient-reported outcomes, component failure rates and variables associated with these failures.

Currently, we use 3D CT imaging for preoperative planning in cases of moderate or severe posterior glenoid bone loss, as this allows more precise determination of the optimal implant choice based on the degree of pathologic correction and joint line restoration that is possible with augmented or standard glenoid components. Prior studies have shown that using 3D CT preoperative planning can help predict the amount of correction achievable using standard and augmented glenoids and improves glenoid implant positioning postoperatively [18, 52, 57]. The B2 glenoid is the most common pattern of moderate to severe bone loss in which we utilize an augmented glenoid component (Fig. 21.6). However, even with the advances in preoperative planning and implant designs, there may be limitations to the use of augmented glenoids when bone loss is very severe (B3 or C type glenoids, for example). In these cases of advanced bone loss or pathology, reverse TSA with or without bone grafting may be a more reliable option for implant stability and longevity.

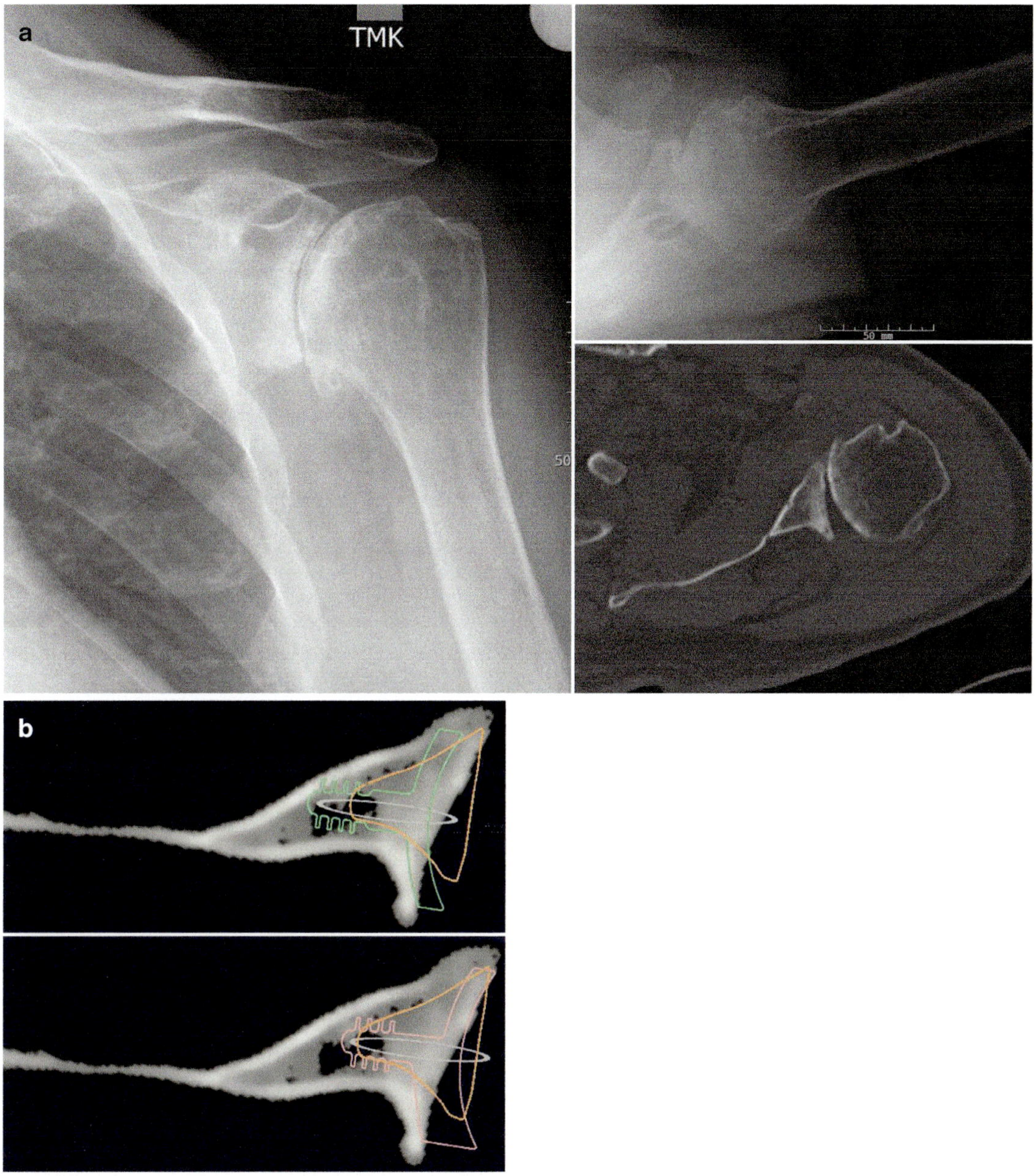

Fig. 21.6 Use of pre-operative planning with an augmented glenoid component. (**a**) Pre-operative True AP and axillary x-rays and axial computed tomography (CT) image of a B2 glenoid. Glenoid biconcavity and posterior subluxation of the humeral head are seen on the axillary radiograph and axial CT. (**b**) Axial cuts of glenoid with three-dimensional (3D) CT pre-operative planning showing pathologic correction with a standard (left) vs. a posterior stepped glenoid component (right). The glenoid vault model (orange template) demonstrates the pre morbid glenoid version and joint line. In this example, version is corrected from −24.9° to −7° with both the standard and the augmented (+5 mm step) component, however, the posterior stepped component is able to restore the pre-morbid joint line while the standard component requires excessive bone removal and joint line medialization for the same version correction. (**c**) Post-operative x-rays showing pathologic correction, with centering of the humeral head on the True AP and axillary view

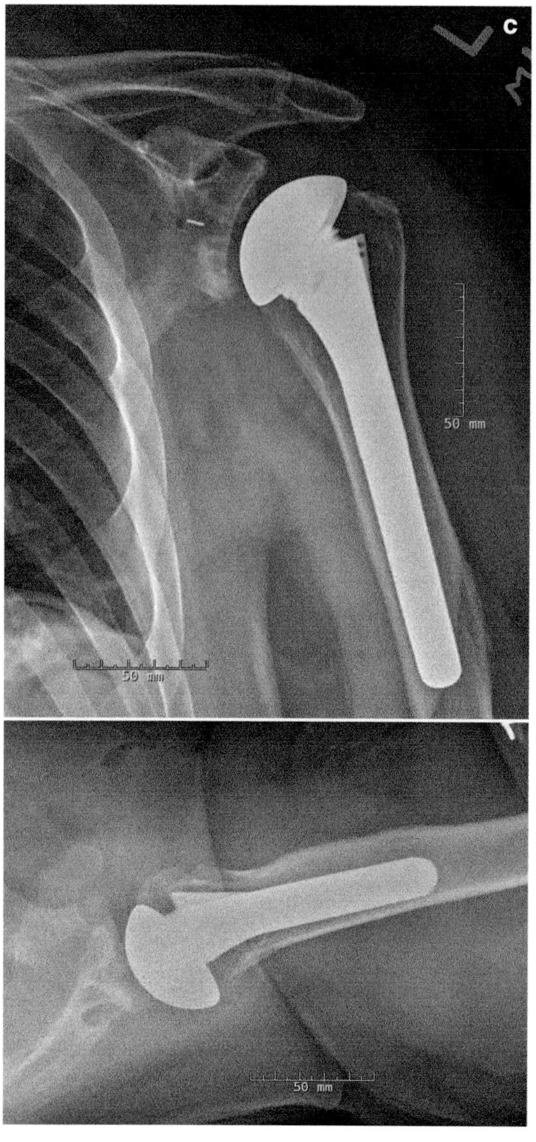

Fig. 21.6 (continued)

References

1. Walch G, Badet R, Boulahia A, Khoury A. Morphologic study of the glenoid in primary glenohumeral osteoarthritis. J Arthroplast. 1999;14(6):756–60.
2. Bercik MJ, Kruse K, Yalizis M, Gauci M-O, Chaoui J, Walch G. A modification to the Walch classification of the glenoid in primary glenohumeral osteoarthritis using three-dimensional imaging. J Shoulder Elb Surg. 2016;25(10):1601–6.
3. Iannotti JP, Norris TR. Influence of preoperative factors on outcome of shoulder arthroplasty for glenohumeral osteoarthritis. J Bone Joint Surg Am. 2003;85–A(2):251–8.
4. Levine WN, Djurasovic M, Glasson JM, Pollock RG, Flatow EL, Bigliani LU. Hemiarthroplasty for glenohumeral osteoarthritis: results correlated to degree of glenoid wear. J Shoulder Elb Surg. 1997;6(5):449–54.
5. Norris TR, Iannotti JP. Functional outcome after shoulder arthroplasty for primary osteoarthritis: a multicenter study. J Shoulder Elb Surg. 2002;11(2):130–5.
6. Scalise JJ, Codsi MJ, Bryan J, Iannotti JP. The three-dimensional glenoid vault model can estimate normal glenoid version in osteoarthritis. J Shoulder Elb Surg. 2008;17(3):487–91.
7. Sperling JW, Cofield RH, Rowland CM. Neer hemiarthroplasty and Neer total shoulder arthroplasty in patients fifty years old or less. Long-term results. J Bone Joint Surg Am. 1998;80(4):464–73.
8. Wirth MA, Tapscott RS, Southworth C, Rockwood CA. Treatment of glenohumeral arthritis with a hemiarthroplasty: a minimum five-year follow-up outcome study. J Bone Joint Surg Am. 2006;88(5):964–73.
9. Sperling JW, Cofield RH, Rowland CM. Minimum fifteen-year follow-up of Neer hemiarthroplasty and total shoulder arthroplasty in patients aged fifty years or younger. J Shoulder Elb Surg. 2004;13(6):604–13.
10. Habermeyer P, Magosch P, Lichtenberg S. Recentering the humeral head for glenoid deficiency in total shoulder arthroplasty. Clin Orthop. 2007;457:124–32.
11. Gutiérrez S. CORR Insights(®): posterior glenoid wear in total shoulder arthroplasty: eccentric anterior reaming is superior to posterior augment. Clin Orthop. 2015;473(12):3937–9.
12. Yian EH, Werner CML, Nyffeler RW, Pfirrmann CW, Ramappa A, Sukthankar A, Gerber C. Radiographic and computed tomography analysis of cemented pegged polyethylene glenoid components in total shoulder replacement. J Bone Joint Surg Am. 2005;87(9):1928–36.
13. Iannotti JP, Greeson C, Downing D, Sabesan V, Bryan JA. Effect of glenoid deformity on glenoid component placement in primary shoulder arthroplasty. J Shoulder Elb Surg. 2012;21(1):48–55.
14. Ganapathi A, McCarron JA, Chen X, Iannotti JP. Predicting normal glenoid version from the pathologic scapula: a comparison of 4 methods in 2- and 3-dimensional models. J Shoulder Elb Surg. 2011;20(2):234–44.
15. Codsi MJ, Bennetts C, Gordiev K, Boeck DM, Kwon Y, Brems J, Powell K, Iannotti JP. Normal glenoid vault anatomy and validation of a novel glenoid implant shape. J Shoulder Elb Surg. 2008;17(3):471–8.
16. Scalise JJ, Bryan J, Polster J, Brems JJ, Iannotti JP. Quantitative analysis of glenoid bone loss in osteoarthritis using three-dimensional computed tomography scans. J Shoulder Elb Surg. 2008;17(2):328–35.
17. Ricchetti ET, Hendel MD, Collins DN, Iannotti JP. Is premorbid glenoid anatomy altered in patients with glenohumeral osteoarthritis? Clin Orthop. 2013;471(9):2932–9.

18. Hendel MD, Bryan JA, Barsoum WK, Rodriguez EJ, Brems JJ, Evans PJ, Iannotti JP. Comparison of patient-specific instruments with standard surgical instruments in determining glenoid component position: a randomized prospective clinical trial. J Bone Joint Surg Am. 2012;94(23):2167–75.
19. Iannotti JP, Ricchetti ET, Rodriguez EJ, Bryan JA. Development and validation of a new method of 3-dimensional assessment of glenoid and humeral component position after total shoulder arthroplasty. J Shoulder Elb Surg. 2013;22(10):1413–22.
20. Bell RH, Noble JS. The management of significant glenoid deficiency in total shoulder arthroplasty. J Shoulder Elb Surg. 2000;9(3):248–56.
21. Farron A, Terrier A, Büchler P. Risks of loosening of a prosthetic glenoid implanted in retroversion. J Shoulder Elb Surg. 2006;15(4):521–6.
22. Kelly JD, Norris TR. Decision making in glenohumeral arthroplasty. J Arthroplast. 2003;18(1):75–82.
23. Clinton J, Franta AK, Lenters TR, Mounce D, Matsen FA. Nonprosthetic glenoid arthroplasty with humeral hemiarthroplasty and total shoulder arthroplasty yield similar self-assessed outcomes in the management of comparable patients with glenohumeral arthritis. J Shoulder Elb Surg. 2007;16(5):534–8.
24. Clavert P, Millett PJ, Warner JJP. Glenoid resurfacing: what are the limits to asymmetric reaming for posterior erosion? J Shoulder Elb Surg. 2007;16(6):843–8.
25. Gillespie R, Lyons R, Lazarus M. Eccentric reaming in total shoulder arthroplasty: a cadaveric study. Orthopedics. 2009;32(1):21.
26. Nowak DD, Bahu MJ, Gardner TR, Dyrszka MD, Levine WN, Bigliani LU, Ahmad CS. Simulation of surgical glenoid resurfacing using three-dimensional computed tomography of the arthritic glenohumeral joint: the amount of glenoid retroversion that can be corrected. J Shoulder Elb Surg. 2009;18(5):680–8.
27. Ho JC, Sabesan VJ, Iannotti JP. Glenoid component retroversion is associated with osteolysis. J Bone Joint Surg Am. 2013;95(12):e82.
28. Torchia ME, Cofield RH, Settergren CR. Total shoulder arthroplasty with the Neer prosthesis: long-term results. J Shoulder Elb Surg. 1997;6(6):495–505.
29. Collin P, Tay AKL, Melis B, Boileau P, Walch G. A ten-year radiologic comparison of two-all polyethylene glenoid component designs: a prospective trial. J Shoulder Elb Surg. 2011;20(8):1217–23.
30. Mansat P, Briot J, Mansat M, Swider P. Evaluation of the glenoid implant survival using a biomechanical finite element analysis: influence of the implant design, bone properties, and loading location. J Shoulder Elb Surg. 2007;16(3 Suppl):S79–83.
31. Nuttall D, Haines JF, Trail II. A study of the micromovement of pegged and keeled glenoid components compared using radiostereometric analysis. J Shoulder Elb Surg. 2007;16(3 Suppl):S65–70.
32. Lacroix D, Murphy LA, Prendergast PJ. Three-dimensional finite element analysis of glenoid replacement prostheses: a comparison of keeled and pegged anchorage systems. J Biomech Eng. 2000;122(4):430–6.
33. Schamblin M, Gupta R, Yang BY, McGarry MH, McMaster WC, Lee TQ. In vitro quantitative assessment of total and bipolar shoulder arthroplasties: a biomechanical study using human cadaver shoulders. Clin Biomech (Bristol, Avon). 2009;24(8):626–31.
34. Shapiro TA, McGarry MH, Gupta R, Lee YS, Lee TQ. Biomechanical effects of glenoid retroversion in total shoulder arthroplasty. J Shoulder Elb Surg. 2007;16(3 Suppl):S90–5.
35. Hopkins AR, Hansen UN, Amis AA, Emery R. The effects of glenoid component alignment variations on cement mantle stresses in total shoulder arthroplasty. J Shoulder Elb Surg. 2004;13(6):668–75.
36. Nyffeler RW, Sheikh R, Atkinson TS, Jacob HAC, Favre P, Gerber C. Effects of glenoid component version on humeral head displacement and joint reaction forces: an experimental study. J Shoulder Elb Surg. 2006;15(5):625–9.
37. Terrier A, Büchler P, Farron A. Influence of glenohumeral conformity on glenoid stresses after total shoulder arthroplasty. J Shoulder Elb Surg. 2006;15(4):515–20.
38. Sabesan V, Callanan M, Ho J, Iannotti JP. Clinical and radiographic outcomes of total shoulder arthroplasty with bone graft for osteoarthritis with severe glenoid bone loss. J Bone Joint Surg Am. 2013;95(14):1290–6.
39. Steinmann SP, Cofield RH. Bone grafting for glenoid deficiency in total shoulder replacement. J Shoulder Elb Surg. 2000;9(5):361–7.
40. Neer CS, Morrison DS. Glenoid bone-grafting in total shoulder arthroplasty. J Bone Joint Surg. 1988;70(8):1154–62.
41. Klika BJ, Wooten CW, Sperling JW, Steinmann SP, Schleck CD, Harmsen WS, Cofield RH. Structural bone grafting for glenoid deficiency in primary total shoulder arthroplasty. J Shoulder Elb Surg. 2014;23(7):1066–72.
42. Rice RS, Sperling JW, Miletti J, Schleck C, Cofield RH. Augmented glenoid component for bone deficiency in shoulder arthroplasty. Clin Orthop. 2008;466(3):579–83.
43. Cil A, Sperling JW, Cofield RH. Nonstandard glenoid components for bone deficiencies in shoulder arthroplasty. J Shoulder Elb Surg. 2014;23(7):e149–57.
44. Knowles NK, Ferreira LM, Athwal GS. Augmented glenoid component designs for type B2 erosions: a computational comparison by volume of bone removal and quality of remaining bone. J Shoulder Elb Surg. 2015;24(8):1218–26.
45. Iannotti JP, Lappin KE, Klotz CL, Reber EW, Swope SW. Liftoff resistance of augmented glenoid components during cyclic fatigue loading in the posterior-superior direction. J Shoulder Elb Surg. 2013;22(11):1530–6.
46. Kirane YM, Lewis GS, Sharkey NA, Armstrong AD. Mechanical characteristics of a novel posterior-step prosthesis for biconcave glenoid defects. J Shoulder Elb Surg. 2012;21(1):105–15.

47. Hermida JC, Flores-Hernandez C, Hoenecke HR, D'Lima DD. Augmented wedge-shaped glenoid component for the correction of glenoid retroversion: a finite element analysis. J Shoulder Elb Surg. 2014;23(3):347–54.
48. Allred JJ, Flores-Hernandez C, Hoenecke HR, D'Lima DD. Posterior augmented glenoid implants require less bone removal and generate lower stresses: a finite element analysis. J Shoulder Elb Surg. 2016;25(5):823–30.
49. Wang T, Abrams GD, Behn AW, Lindsey D, Giori N, Cheung EV. Posterior glenoid wear in total shoulder arthroplasty: eccentric anterior reaming is superior to posterior augment. Clin Orthop. 2015;473(12):3928–36.
50. Knowles NK, Ferreira LM, Athwal GS. The arthritic glenoid: anatomy and arthroplasty designs. Curr Rev Musculoskelet Med. 2016;9(1):23–9.
51. Wright TW, Grey SG, Roche CP, Wright L, Flurin P-H, Zuckerman JD. Preliminary results of a posterior augmented glenoid compared to an all polyethylene standard glenoid in anatomic total shoulder arthroplasty. Bull Hosp Joint Dis 2013. 2015;73(Suppl 1):S79–85.
52. Sabesan V, Callanan M, Sharma V, Iannotti JP. Correction of acquired glenoid bone loss in osteoarthritis with a standard versus an augmented glenoid component. J Shoulder Elb Surg. 2014;23(7):964–73.
53. Youderian AR, Napolitano LAJM, Davidson IUM, Iannotti JP. Management of glenoid bone loss with the use of a new augmented all-polyethylene glenoid component. Tech Should Elb Surg. 2012;13(4):163–9.
54. Ricchetti ET, Jun BJ, Patterson TE, Iannotti JP. CT analysis of pathologic correction in total shoulder arthroplasty using a standard or augmented glenoid component. Presentation presented at: American Academy of Orthopaedic Surgeons 83rd Annual Meeting; 2016 Mar 3; Orlando, FL.
55. Lenart BA, Namdari S, Williams GR. Total shoulder arthroplasty with an augmented component for anterior glenoid bone deficiency. J Shoulder Elb Surg. 2016;25(3):398–405.
56. Walch G, Moraga C, Young A, Castellanos-Rosas J. Results of anatomic nonconstrained prosthesis in primary osteoarthritis with biconcave glenoid. J Shoulder Elb Surg. 2012;21(11):1526–33.
57. Iannotti JP, Weiner S, Rodriguez E, Subhas N, Patterson TE, Jun BJ, Ricchetti ET. Three-dimensional imaging and templating improve glenoid implant positioning. J Bone Joint Surg Am. 2015;97(8):651–8.

22 Metal Augments in Shoulder Arthroplasty

Ian P. Mayne and Peter C. Poon

Introduction

Severe glenoid bone loss in shoulder arthroplasty is a challenge for the shoulder reconstructive surgeon due to the difficulty of restoring the normal glenoid anatomy [9, 14, 16, 25, 37], stable fixation of the glenoid prosthesis [19, 37] and increased complications and poor clinical outcomes [13, 15, 43]. Current strategies for the correction of glenoid bone loss and deformity such as eccentric reaming and/or bone grafting have their limitations in severe cases [19, 25].

Porous metal augments (PMA's) have been used in other Orthopaedic sub-specialties to provide a structural substitute to bone graft with favourable results [17, 23, 35, 40]. Continued improvements in manufacturing and biomaterial technology have lead to a push to integrate PMA's into shoulder arthroplasty with the aim of solving the paucity of solutions for severe bone loss in primary and revision shoulder arthroplasty. In this chapter, we will describe the potential uses of PMA's in shoulder arthroplasty for severe glenoid bone loss/deformity and will review the current literature.

I. P. Mayne (✉) · P. C. Poon
Department of Orthopaedic Surgery, North Shore Hospital, Auckland, New Zealand

Assessment of Bone Loss in Shoulder Arthroplasty

The workup of bone loss/deformity starts with a thorough history and physical examination. In the primary arthroplasty setting this includes the diagnosis of the shoulder pathology (i.e. Osteoarthritis, cuff tear arthropathy, inflammatory or post-traumatic arthritis) which will provide the surgeon with an idea of the location and type of bone loss (e.g. Horizontal versus vertical bone deficiency).

In the revision setting, the surgeon must inquire about the previous surgical history (i.e. surgical approach, prosthesis, complications) and current clinical issues relating the shoulder (e.g. infection, pain, instability, impingement).

The physical examination starts with inspection of the shoulder for the presence of previous surgical scars and/or muscle atrophy. Active and passive range of motion (ROM) are then assessed. Deficits in motion are assessed for the underlying etiology (e.g. contracture, bony or implant impingement, instability). Muscle power in the upper extremity specifically focusing on the rotator cuff and deltoid is examined. In addition, a detailed neurologic examination is performed and any deficits can be further assessed with electrodiagnostic studies.

Standard shoulder radiographs (Anteroposterior (AP), axillary views) provide initial information regarding the underlying pathology, pattern of bone loss in the native shoulder or abnormal position/loosening of the previous shoulder arthroplasty.

I. A. Trail et al. (eds.), *Textbook of Shoulder Surgery*, https://doi.org/10.1007/978-3-319-70099-1_22

We order a pre-operative Computed Tomography (CT) scan with 3D reconstruction views in all primary anatomic total shoulder arthroplasty, revision shoulder arthroplasty or whenever there is evidence of severe bone loss/deformity (Table 22.1). It is important that the CT scan images are parallel and perpendicular to the scapular plane in order to accurately assess the glenoid anatomy. Preoperatively, the CT scan is scrutinized for the following measurements/variables: Glenoid version (Freidman Method [11]), Glenoid Inclination (Reverse Shoulder Angle [37]), Location of bone loss (i.e. Glenoid rim, sub-chondral bone, or vault [42]), Type of Glenoid/Humeral Bone Loss (i.e. Peripheral, Contained/Uncontained, Combined [42]). In the setting where a patient specific implant (PSI) is being considered, a detailed CT scan protocol is required by the manufacturer (Promade, Lima Corporate Medical Systems, Villanova San Daniele del Friuli, Italy) as shown in Fig. 22.1.

Table 22.1 Severe glenoid bone loss/deformity encountered in primary and revision shoulder arthroplasty

Glenoid bone loss/deformity
Glenoid retroversion >15°
Joint line medialization to or medial to the foot of the coracoid
Glenoid superior bone loss/inclination: Favard E2 and E3 (Lévigne et al. [27])
Revision shoulder arthroplasty Uncontained glenoid bone loss (sub-chondral bone, rim, vault)

Porous Metal Augments

Porous metal augments have been frequently used in hip and knee arthroplasty for the management of bone defects and/or deformities since the 1980s [29]. The integration of porous metals to the prosthesis and augments was hypothesized to improve the bond between the implant and bone thereby improving the longevity and decreasing mechanical failure [29]. Matassi et al. described characteristics of an ideal porous metal: biocompatible (i.e. osteoinductive/osteoconductive), mechanical properties similar to host bone, ease of reproducibility, porosity (60–80%), and pore size (100–600 μm) (Fig. 22.2) [30]. Titanium and Tantulum alloys are commonly used due to their high specific strength, low weight, and biocompatibility [30] in addition to ideal characteristics mentioned above. Porous Tantalum and Titanium both have a low modulus of elasticity similar to cancellous bone that is thought to decrease stress shielding [2, 33]. In addition, a high coefficient of friction allows for an improved initial stabilization of implants in host bone [2, 30].

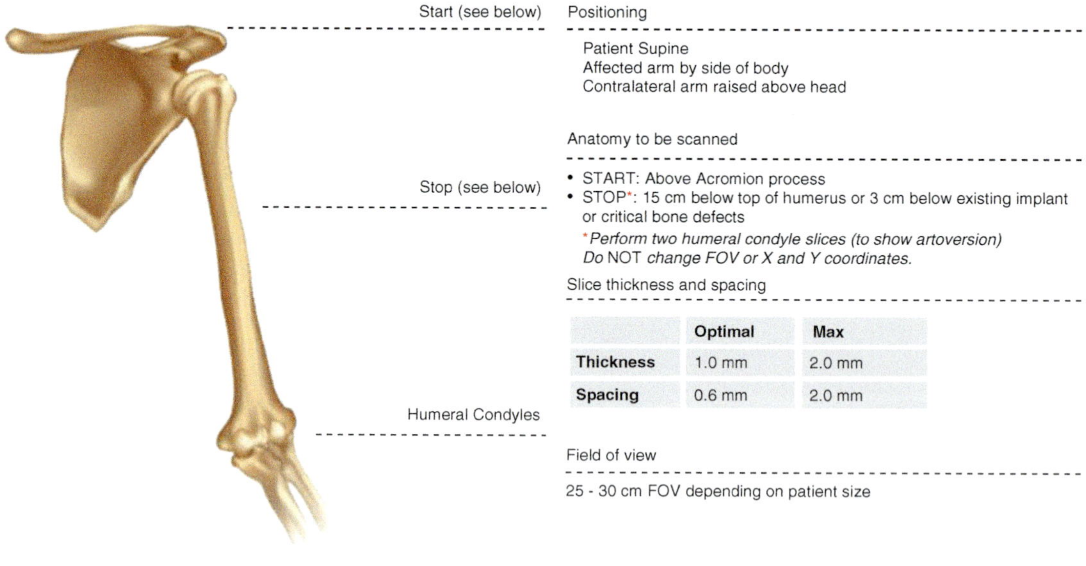

Fig. 22.1 CT Scan protocol for patient specific implant (Promade, Lima Corporate Medical Systems, Villanova San Daniele del Friuli, Italy)

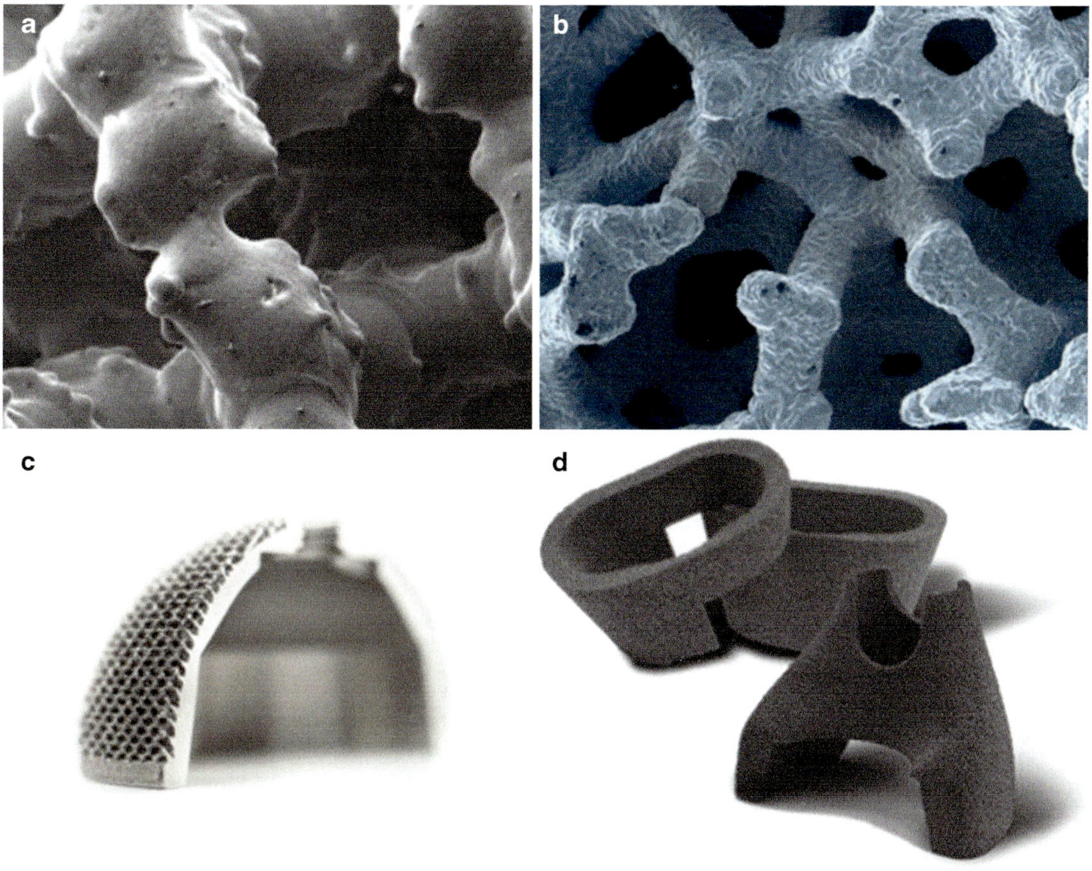

Fig. 22.2 3D microscopic structure of (**a**) Trabecular Titanium™ (Lima Corporate Medical Systems, Villanova San Daniele del Friuli, Italy) and (**b**) Trabecular Metal™ (Zimmer® Biomet, Warsaw, Indiana, USA). (**c**) Lima Delta Trabecular Titanium™ Cup (*Courtesy:* Lima Corporate Medical Systems, Villanova San Daniele del Friuli, Italy) (**d**) Zimmer® Trabecular Metal™ tibial and femoral cone augments (*Courtesy:* Zimmer Biomet (Warsaw, Indiana, USA))

These newer generation "open-celled" porous metals have individual cells that are interconnected similar to the trabecular pattern of cancellous bone. In vivo and In vitro studies have shown excellent osteointegration and osetogenic properties of Trabecular Titanium™ [1, 8].

The utilization of PMA's in orthopaedic surgery initially started in hip and knee arthroplasty with recent use in spine and foot and ankle surgery. Intermediate term results (5–10 years) of PMA's for reconstruction of bone defects in both hip [40] and knee [7, 23] arthroplasty has shown high survival, consistent bone ingrowth, and low revision rates. Porous tantalum augments have been used as an alternative to structural bone graft in ankle arthrodesis with reliable fusion rates [35]. Furthermore, porous tantalum augments have been used in anterior cervical and lumbar spine fusion procedures with favourable short-term results [17]. Due to the success of PMA's in other orthopaedic sub-specialties there is optimism that these results can be adapted to shoulder arthroplasty.

Metal Augments in Primary Anatomic Shoulder Arthroplasty

Primary shoulder osteoarthritis is the most common indication for primary anatomic shoulder arthroplasty [21]. Glenoid component loosening has been shown to be the most common long-term complication, occurring in up to 24% of patients [13]. Ho et al. [19] showed that the rate of osteolysis surrounding the central peg of a cemented glenoid component increased by five-fold with retroversion >15° when compared to neutral version. Furthermore, inadequate restoration of glenoid version is associated with decreased shoulder function and range of motion [15, 43].

Walch et al. [38] classified the morphology of the glenoid in osteoarthritis. Horizontal glenoid deficiency with posterior erosion and biconcavity (Type B2) and hypoplasia with retroversion >25° (Type C) have received the most attention in the literature due to the difficulty in restoring neutral version and a stable glenoid component. The current strategies to correct glenoid version and/or reconstruct glenoid bone loss include eccentric reaming [20], bone grafting [18], augmented all-polyethylene (stepped versus wedge) components [26], or conversion to reverse shoulder arthroplasty [31]. Each reconstruction method has been described in literature with mixed success and/or limited long-term results [14]. In severe glenoid bone loss, the current gold standard is bone grafting, but is technically difficult, fixation is challenging in deficient glenoid bone with high rates of graft failure and/or non-union [25]. Further discussion of this surgical technique can be found within Chap. 20 – *Bone Augmentation in Shoulder Arthroplasty*.

Rheumatoid arthritis is the second most common indication for primary shoulder arthroplasty and is associated with central erosion of the glenoid (Walch Type A2 [39]). We consider the central erosion to be severe if the glenoid is medial to the foot of the coracoid which Lévigne and Francheschi have previously described [28]. However, there is no consensus in the literature that dictates the amount of the central erosion before deleterious effects on the post-operative clinical outcome. Expert consensus has suggested that joint medialization >1 cm affects the length-tension relationship of the rotator cuff/soft-tissues and may also lead to increased post-operative shoulder arthroplasty instability [6].

Indications for Metal Augments in Anatomic Shoulder Arthroplasty

We consider the use of PMA's in primary anatomic shoulder arthroplasty for severe glenoid bone loss/deformity secondary to osteoarthritis (Walch B2/C with retroversion >15°) or rheumatoid arthritis (Walch A2 with glenoid at or medial to foot of coracoid) or post-traumatic OA with non-contained defects that are unable to be adequately reconstructed with bone graft. Our goal is to restore ≤10° of retroversion while preserving glenoid bone stock and maximizing contact between the bone and glenoid component. Humeral bone loss is generally not an issue and will not be discussed in this section.

Metal-Backed Glenoid Component

In the cases where the patient has one of the aforementioned severe glenoid deformities, we utilize a metal-backed augmented glenoid (Lima SMR™ liner and augmented baseplate). We believe that this component provides a stable base for deformity reconstruction with immediate fixation achieved with a central peg and two screws, porous metal backing for bone ingrowth, and the modularity to allow an anatomic or reverse shoulder arthroplasty. In cases of severe glenoid deformity, optimal soft tissue balance can be difficult to achieve. Walch et al. reported late posterior subluxation despite adequate correction of glenoid deformity [39]. A modular augmented metal baseplate provides the surgeon the "bail out" option of a reverse shoulder arthroplasty if the anatomic shoulder arthroplasty in the index surgery is unstable or in revision of a failed anatomic shoulder arthroplasty. However, we recognize the potential negatives associated with metal-back glenoid components including polyethylene wear and early failure [3]. Our experience with the Lima SMR™ prosthesis has been similar to Castagna et al. [4] with no prosthesis related complications (i.e. Polyethylene-glenoid disassembly, loosening, or severe polyethylene wear). We reserve the use of this component for lower demand patients with severe glenoid deformity requiring a metal augment.

Key Steps in the Surgical Technique

Patient Position

The patient is positioned on the T-Max Shoulder Positioner (Smith & Nephew, London, UK) in a supine position. Operative arm draped free and placed on a padded Mayo stand.

Deltopectoral Approach/Releases

A "4-Direction" release is then performed: CA ligament complete release, superior 1 cm of Pectoralis Major tendon, lateral aspect of conjoint tendon, sub-deltoid bursa. Long head of biceps tenotomy. Subscapularis tenotomy or lesser tuberosity osteotomy performed if we are using a stemless or stemmed humeral component respectively. Humeral head osteophytes removed and neck cut performed according to implant design and protector applied.

Glenoid Exposure and Preparation

Adequate glenoid exposure is essential for the visualization of the severe glenoid deformity, preparation of glenoid and insertion of the augmented baseplate and polyethylene liner. Further release of the anterior, superior and posterior aspects of the subscapularis is performed to increase exposure and mobility for later repair. Glenoid retractors inserted: Sonnabend retractor inserted over proximal humerus and under the posteroinferior glenoid, double-pronged glenoid retractor inserted on anterior and inferior glenoid rim. A 270° capsulolabral release is performed off the glenoid rim, sparing the posterior aspect. If further exposure is required, the remaining posterior capsule is released and/or a clavicular osteotomy is performed.

For the insertion of the central guide wire, corrective guides in increments of 5° are available for 10–35° of correction. The preoperative CT scan is used to determine the severity of the glenoid deformity and the extent of correction required. The chosen corrective guide is used to insert the central guide wire, which is over drilled to produce the central peg hole (Fig. 22.3). This

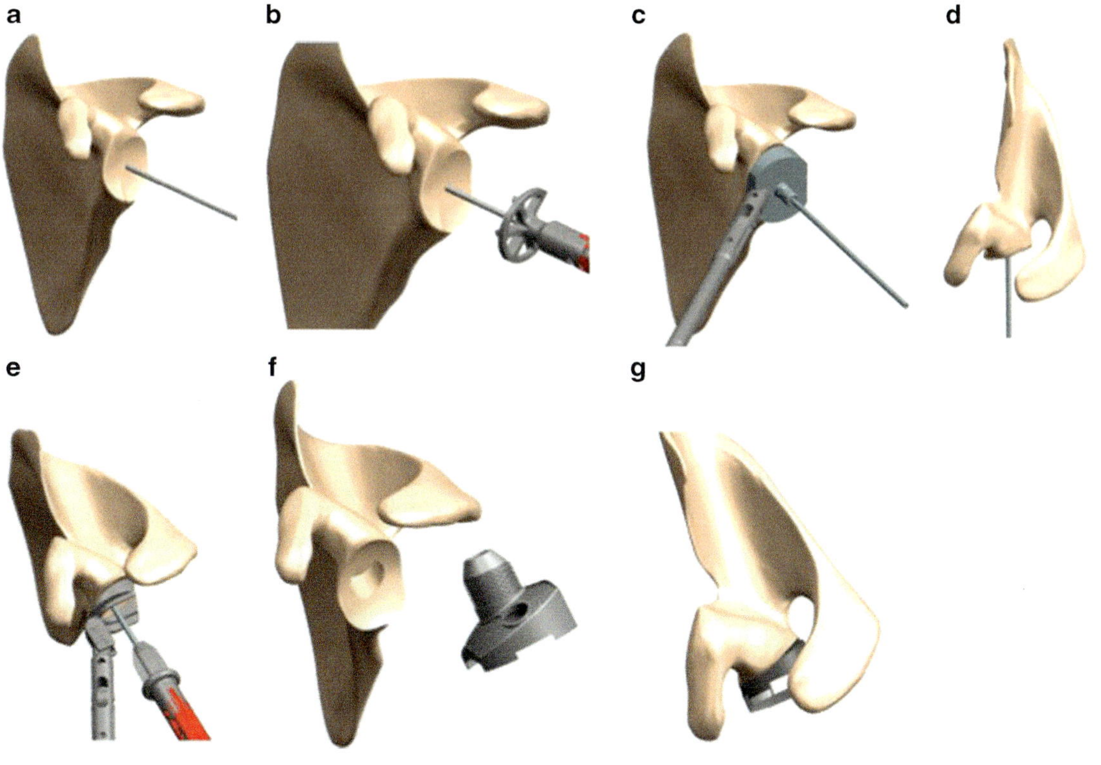

Fig. 22.3 Surgical technique for correction of a biconcave glenoid deformity with a posterior wedged porous metal augment. (**a**) Guidewire placed in anticipated corrected version. (**b**) Eccentric reaming performed to convert the B2 to a C Glenoid. (**c/d**) Guidewire re-inserted using posterior wedge guide. (**e**) Central peg drill hole completed. (**f**) Posterior augmented baseplate inserted. (**g**) Final posterior augmented baseplate with correction of version

Table 22.2 Deformities encountered in primary anatomic shoulder arthroplasty with correction strategies and metal augments

Deformity	Reconstruction strategy	Metal augment
Biconcave glenoid with posterior Erosion (Walch B2) Dysplastic retroverted glenoid (Walch C)	1. Surface of glenoid prepared free hand with high speed burr 2. Posterior wedged metal-back component 3. 2 × 6.5 mm screw fixation	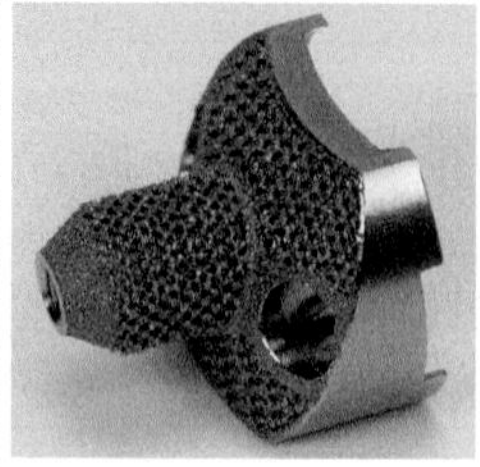 *Courtesy: Lima*
Rheumatoid Arthritis with severe central erosion (Walch A2)	1. Humeral head autograft 2. Metal backed glenoid with long porous Trabecular Titanium™ central peg 3. 2 × 6.5 mm screw fixation	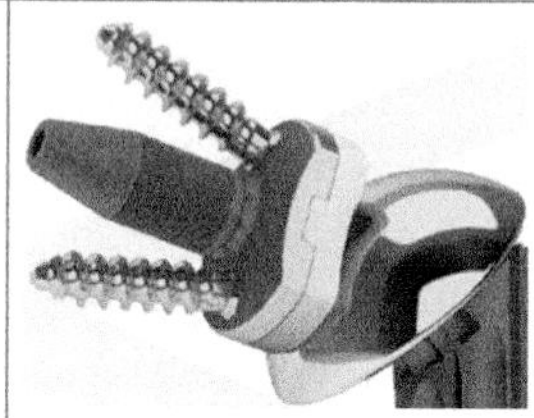 *Courtesy: Lima*

will determine the alignment of the glenoid prosthesis. The surface of the glenoid is then prepared free hand with a high speed burr to produce a bleeding surface. As the porous metal backing can embed into the glenoid, the preparation of the glenoid surface does not have to exactly match the backside geometry of the baseplate. The wedged baseplate with porous metal backing is implanted to full seating. Further fixation of the glenoid component is achieved with two 6.5 mm screws into the base of the coracoid and lateral scapular pillar. Table 22.2 describes the techniques and metal augments used for the common deformities encountered in primary anatomic shoulder arthroplasty.

Metal Augments in Anatomic Shoulder Arthroplasty

The results of PMA's in anatomic shoulder arthroplasty is extremely limited. Sandow et al. reported on 10 patients with glenohumeral osteoarthritis and glenoid retroversion >15° and posterior head subluxation >60% [36]. The Bigliani-Flatow anatomic shoulder arthroplasty system (Zimmer, Warsaw, IN, USA) was used. A posterior Trabecular Metal™ Wedge (15° or 30°) was inserted according to the severity of retroversion to achieve a neutral glenoid. The wedge was fixed to the glenoid with two screws and the polyethylene liner was cemented onto the wedge (Fig. 22.4). At a minimum of 24-month follow-up there were no complications/revisions or lucency surrounding the pegs. Glenoid retroversion of ≤10° was achieved in all patients with no residual posterior subluxation. This design of metal augment is only for use in anatomic shoulder arthroplasty and not for reverse arthroplasty. Cil et al. [5] retrospectively examined eight patients with posteriorly augmented metal-backed glenoid (Cofield glenoid components (Smith & Nephew, Memphis, TN, USA). Four patients required reoperation for infection ($n = 2$), posterior instability, and polyethylene wear and synovitis.

Our unpublished experience of PMA's in anatomic shoulder arthroplasty is limited to seven cases with an example in Fig. 22.5. All patients had primary osteoarthritis with a Walch Type B2 glenoid and retroversion ≥25°. Mean patient age was 77.5 years old (67–85) with at least 1-year follow-up. Our results have been positive with only one complication involving a subscapularis tenotomy repair failure. This patient subsequently underwent a conversion to a reverse shoulder

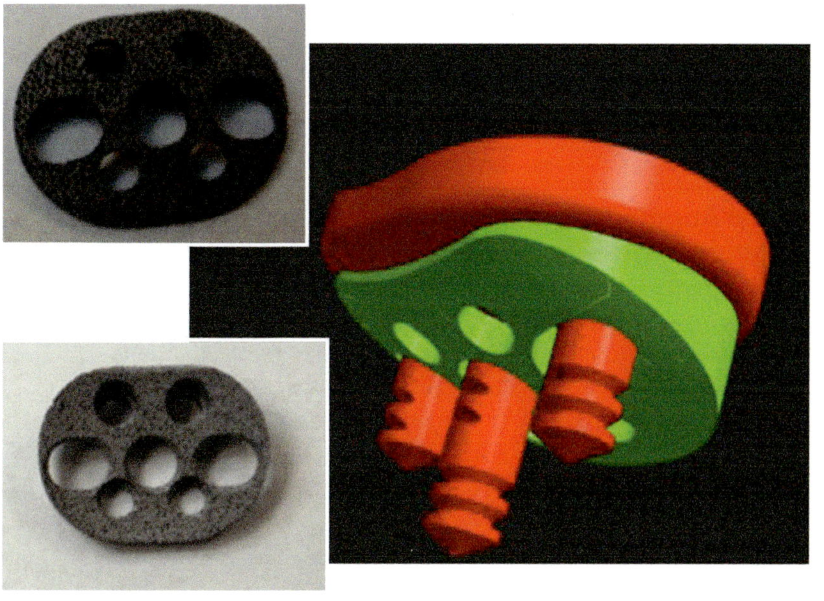

Fig. 22.4 (*Left*) Trabecular Metal wedge augments. (*Right*) 3D model showing the insertion of the 3-pegged polyethylene liner into the trabecular metal wedge. (*Courtesy* of Sandow et al. 2016) [36]

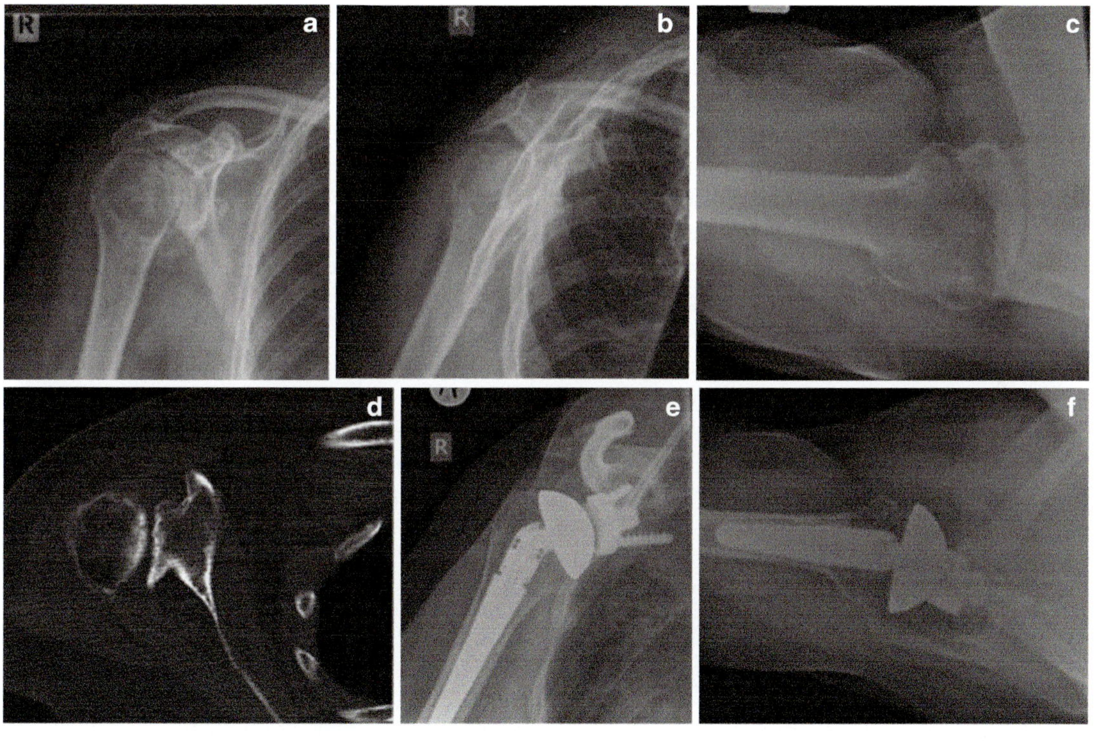

Fig. 22.5 Case example of a 74 year-old female with right shoulder osteoarthritis. Underwent an uncemented Right Anatomic Shoulder arthroplasty (Lima SMR™) with a 15° posterior wedge. (**a**–**c**) Pre-operative X-rays showing severe osteoarthritis and a Walch Type B2 glenoid. (**d**) Pre-operative Axial CT Scan showing 35° of retroversion. (**e**, **f**) Post-operative (14 months) x-rays showing restoration of glenoid version, no evidence of posterior humeral subluxation or surrounding the glenoid baseplate/screws

arthroplasty at 13 months after the index procedure. The augmented modular baseplate allowed easy conversion of an anatomic glenoid to a reverse glenosphere.

Metal Augments in Primary Reverse Shoulder Arthroplasty

Reverse shoulder arthroplasty (RSA) utilization has continued to increase with a progressive expansion of surgical indications [21]. However, cuff tear arthropathy (CTA) remains the most common indication [21, 37]. The bone loss pattern in CTA is a vertical deficiency of the superior glenoid. Posterior (Walch B2/C) and centralized (Walch A2) glenoid bone loss are also encountered in RSA [37]. Frankle et al. found that 37.5% of RSA's in a series had an abnormal glenoid due to bone loss [10]. Furthermore, in a series of 216 RSA's, Klein et al. found that 56 (25.9%) had glenoid bone loss with 22 patients requiring a bone graft [24] during the index RSA. Favard et al. described a classification of bone loss in CTA with the E2 and E3 types representing erosion of the superior glenoid rim and superior and inferior glenoid respectively [27]. Superior glenoid bone loss increases the likelihood of inserting the glenoid baseplate with a superior tilt which has been shown to increase the rate of aseptic loosening by increasing the shear forces and decreasing the compressive forces [9, 16]. Therefore, the proposed optimal position of the glenoid is a slight inferior tilt of approximately 10° [24, 32].

Current strategies to address superior glenoid bone loss in RSA include eccentric reaming with/without a lateralized glenoid component, bone grafting (Humeral head [37], Iliac Crest autograft or allograft), or PMA's [12]. Eccentric reaming has been proposed as a cost-effective and technically simple option. However, there is a concern for the loss of subchondral bone, medialization of the joint line, and perforation of the central glenoid peg [37]. In anatomic shoulder arthroplasty, this technique is limited to glenoid retroversion <15°. However, the upper limit of superior glenoid bone loss that can be addressed with this technique has not been established in the literature. The technique of humeral head autograft (Angled Bony Increase Offset – RSA) has been described for asymmetric glenoid bone loss up 25 mm and version ≤50° [37]. Boileau et al. have used this technique in 54 patients with a minimum 2 years follow-up and observed 98% complete graft healing in vertical (Favard E2/E3/E4) and/or horizontal (Walch B2/C) plane bone defects [3].

Indications for Metal Augments in Reverse Shoulder Arthroplasty

The authors have not currently used PMA's for reverse shoulder arthroplasty. However, as we continue to integrate PMA's into our surgical strategy for addressing glenoid bone loss in RSA we believe there are several potential scenarios listed in Table 22.3.

Table 22.3 Deformities encountered in reverse shoulder arthroplasty and potential applications of metal augments

Deformity	Reconstruction strategy	Metal augment
CTA with severe vertical bone deficiency (Favard E3)	1. Minimal eccentric inferior reaming 2. Insertion of superior augmented (10°) glenoid baseplate +/− humeral head autograft 3. Screw fixation	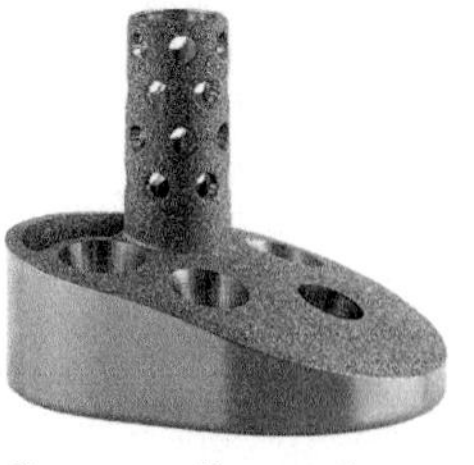 *Courtesy: Exactech*

Table 22.3 (continued)

Deformity	Reconstruction strategy	Metal augment
Rheumatoid Arthritis with severe central erosion (Walch A2)	1. Minimal concentric reaming of glenoid 2. Humeral head autograft, Long pegged glenoid baseplate +/– lateralized glenosphere 3. Screw fixation	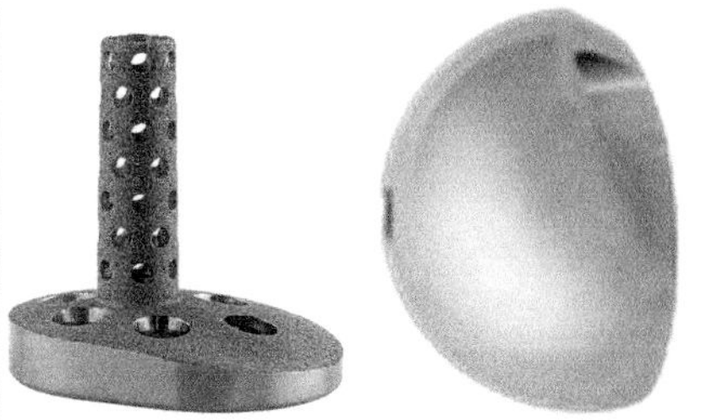 *Courtesy: Exactech* 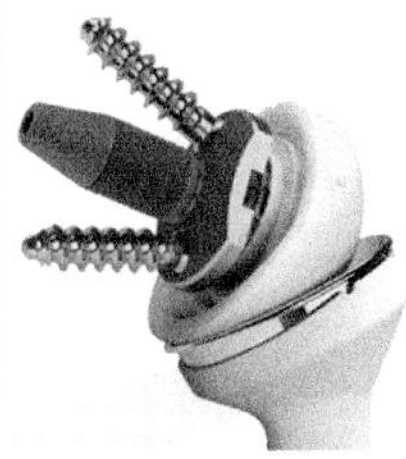 *Courtesy: Lima*
Biconcave glenoid with posterior Erosion (Walch B2) Dysplastic retroverted glenoid (Walch C)	1. Minimal eccentric anterior reaming 2. Insert posterior augmented glenoid baseplate 3. Screw fixation	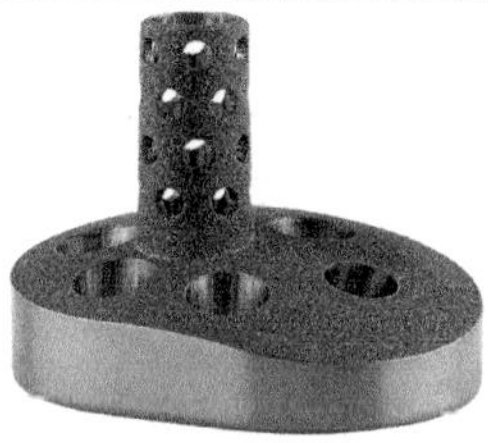 *Courtesy: Exactech* 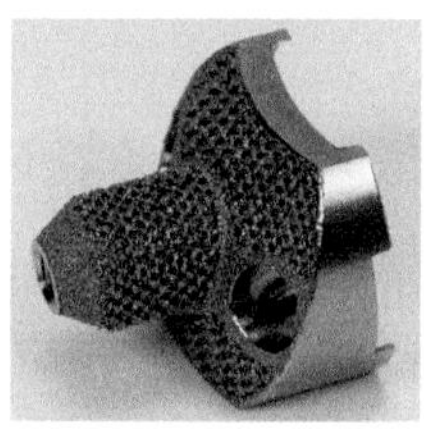 *Courtesy: Lima*

Metal Augments in Reverse Shoulder Arthroplasty

There is limited literature on PMA's in RSA as well as Orthopaedic Implant manufacturers that offer metal augments in the primary setting. Roche et al. [34] examined two techniques of addressing superior glenoid tilt (Favard E2): eccentric reaming and standard glenoid baseplate versus off-axis reaming with a 10° superior augmented glenoid baseplate (Exactech Inc. Gainesville, Florida, USA) in a composite scapula model. They assessed the fixation of the glenoid baseplate after 10,000 cycles and found that there was no significant difference between the reaming techniques/implants. The same group of authors performed a multicentre retrospective study on patients undergoing RSA with glenoid bone loss requiring an augmented baseplate (n = 39, (24 patients with a 8° posterior augment baseplate and 15 patients with a 10° superior augment baseplate)) or bone graft ($n = 41$, (5 allograft and 36 autograft)) [22]. The pre-operative severity of the glenoid retroversion or inclination was not recorded for either group. There were no post-operative differences with respect to clinical outcomes at 2-year follow-up. There was a 14.6% complication rate in the bone graft (two glenoid loosening, two graft failures) and 0% in the metal augment group. It must be noted that the authors in both of these papers are either employees or consultants for Exactech.

Metal Augments in Revision Anatomic and Reverse Shoulder Arthroplasty

Revision shoulder arthroplasty presents a unique set of challenges related to soft-tissue contractures, muscle deficit, and bone loss. In meta-analyses, the revision rate of anatomic [13] and reverse shoulder arthroplasty [44] was 11.2% and 13.4% respectively in studies with at least a 2-year follow-up. The detailed workup, challenges and techniques of revision shoulder arthroplasty will be examined in Chap. 24 – *Revision Techniques in Anatomic Shoulder Arthroplasty.* In revision arthroplasty, the characteristic bone loss patterns observed in the primary setting are absent and therefore depend upon the previous implant used, reason for failure, and technique used to remove the prosthesis. There is currently no literature on the use of PMA's in revision shoulder arthroplasty and therefore this section will focus on potential scenarios where the author's believe metal augments will be useful.

Pre-operative Planning

The preparation for the revision shoulder arthroplasty is essential in order to successfully expose the shoulder, remove the previous implants and insert a new prosthesis in order to the provide the patient with an optimal outcome. A detailed assessment of the patient is essential to determine the underlying etiology of failure keeping in mind that it may be multifactorial. The shoulder radiographs and CT scan are carefully scrutinized for location, size and type of bone loss [42]. Humeral bone loss is generally managed with conventional revision stems and therefore will not be discussed in this section.

We favour revision to RSA as it provides improved stability where soft-tissue loss is common and stable fixation of the glenoid baseplate in native bone when PMA's and/or patient specific implants are utilized. Glenoid bone loss and revision implant fixation are the major concern once the component is removed. On the humeral side, the improved modularity of shoulder prostheses has decreased the requirement of humeral stem removal, which is associated with increased blood loss, surgical time and intra-operative complications [41]. However, if the humeral stem is loose and/or precludes the successful revision we will remove the implant (Table 22.4).

Patient Specific Implants

We have had successful experience with the web-based platform Promade (Promade, Lima Corporate Medical Systems, Villanova San Daniele del Friuli, Italy) to plan and design the patient specific implant. The process is outlined in Fig. 22.6 and a case example in Fig. 22.7.

Table 22.4 Glenoid Bone Loss encountered in revision shoulder arthroplasty and reconstruction strategies

Glenoid Bone Loss Williams and Iannotti [43]	Reconstruction strategy	Metal augment
Central		
Contained (S+/−, R+, V+)	1. Minimal concentric reaming 2. ICBG in contained defect 3. Long central-pegged (26.6 mm) glenoid baseplate 4. Screw fixation	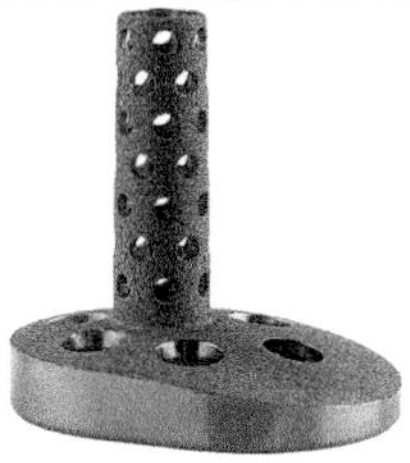 *Courtesy: Exactech* 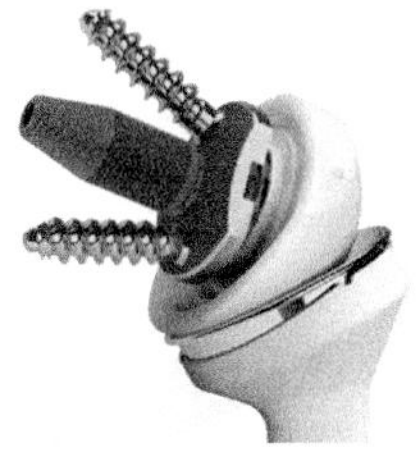 *Courtesy: Lima*
Uncontained (S+/−, R+, V−)	1. Patient specific implant with porous metal backing 2. Screw fixation	
Peripheral		
Symmetric (S+, R−, V+/−)	1. Minimal concentric reaming 2. Long central-pegged glenoid baseplate +/− lateralized glenosphere 3. Screw fixation	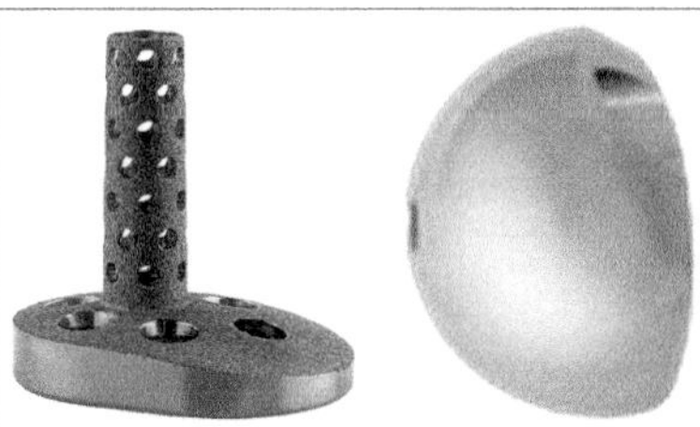 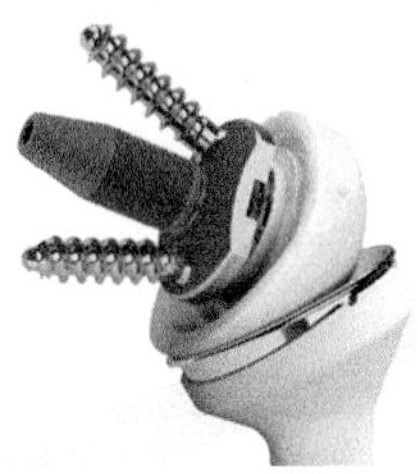 *Courtesy: Lima*
Asymmetric (S+, R−, V+/−)	1. Minimal eccentric reaming 2. Augmented glenoid baseplate (anterior or posterior) or patient specific implant 3. Screw fixation	

(continued)

Table 22.4 (continued)

Glenoid Bone Loss Williams and Iannotti [43]	Reconstruction strategy	Metal augment
Combined		
Asymmetric/symmetric (S− R−, V−)	1. Patient specific implant with porous metal backing	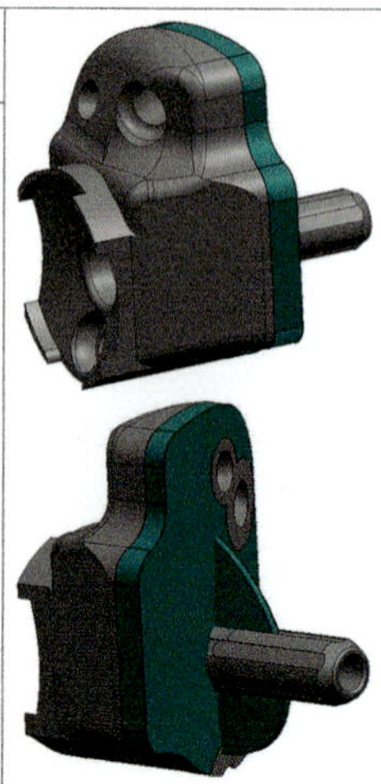
	2. Screw fixation	*Courtesy: Lima*

S sub-chondral bone, *R* glenoid rim, *V* glenoid vault
+ Intact, – deficient

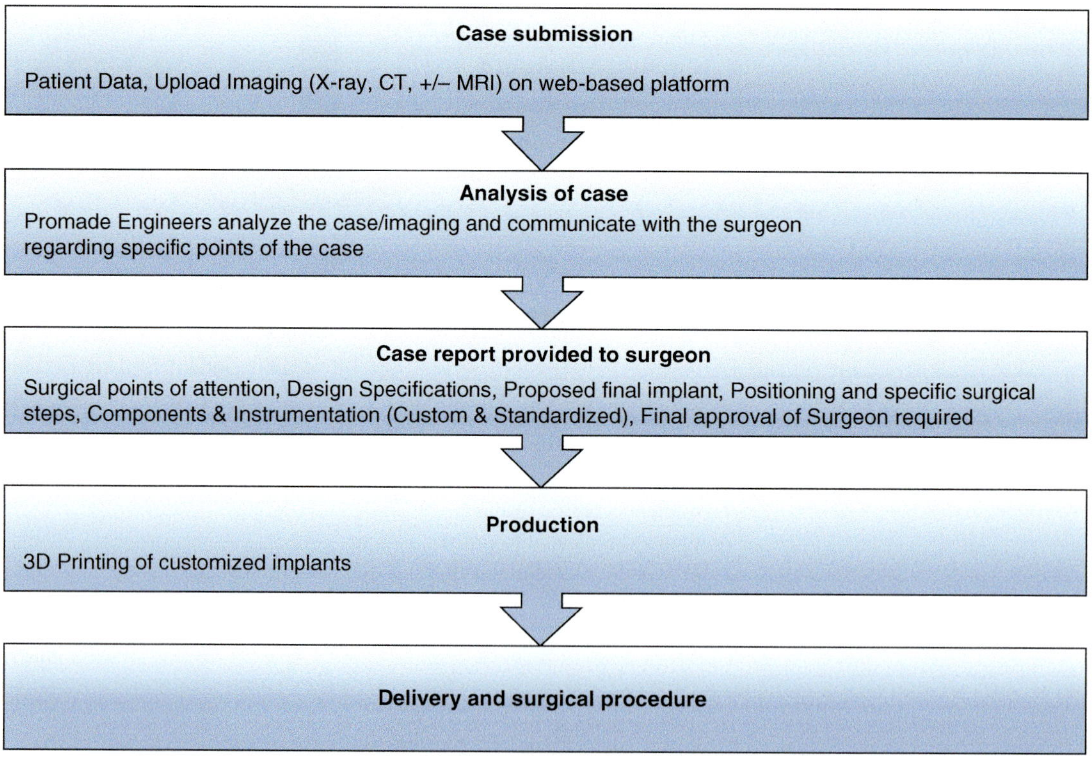

Fig. 22.6 Patient specific implant design process

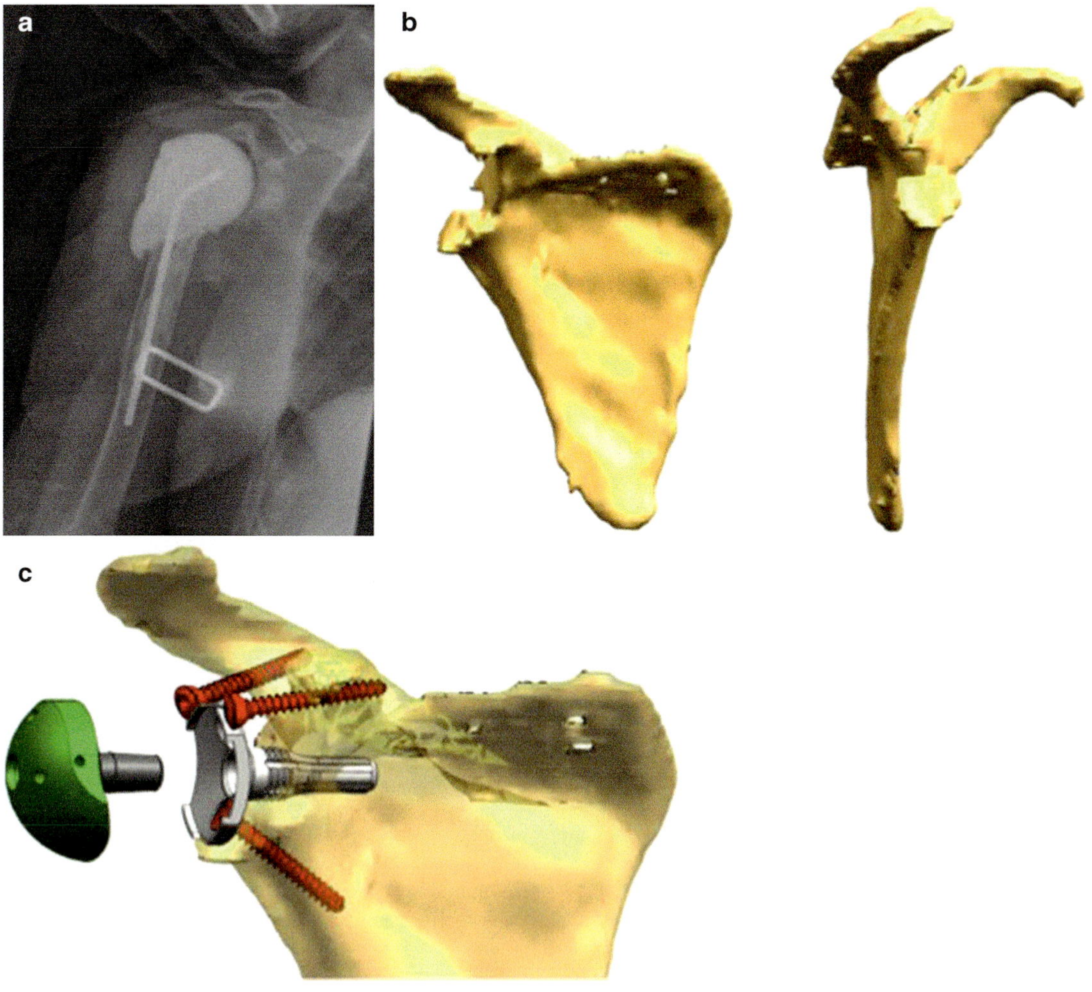

Fig. 22.7 71 year-old female. Underwent right total shoulder arthroplasty in 2009. Infected in 2014 with Streptococcus pyogenes. (**a**) Subsequently underwent First Stage Revision Arthroplasty and insertion of cement spacer. Infection treated with IV antibiotics and inflammatory markers returned to normal. (**b**) Pre-operative 3D reconstruction of scapula showing severe uncontained glenoid bone loss (**c**) Pre-operative ProMade custom glenoid component

Limitations/Complications

Currently, there is a paucity of shoulder literature on this topic to fully support the use of PMA's and we believe it is too early to draw conclusions. However, we are optimistic that the positive clinical outcomes in other Orthopaedic sub-specialties will be observed in shoulder arthroplasty. Several limitations and potential complications must be considered. The PMA provides immediate correction of the bone deformity but does not restore the native bone stock. Therefore, we still advocate the use of conventional reconstruction strategies when there is moderate glenoid bone loss. The rate of polyethylene wear and dissociation has not been examined, but we believe it is low with more recent and improved implant designs. Osteointegration of the native glenoid bone to the PMA in shoulder arthroplasty requires further assessment as well.

Conclusion

Porous metal augments in shoulder arthroplasty is an emerging area that is currently in its infancy. We believe that there is a defined spectrum of clinical pathologies that PMA's provide a useful adjunct to addressing severe bone loss. However, with very limited literature on the success of the current PMA's we have a guarded outlook in the complete integration into routine shoulder arthroplasty. We are optimistic that with increased research, improved biomaterials and prostheses, PMA's will provide Shoulder Surgeons with a valuable tool to solve severe glenoid bone loss and deformity in shoulder arthroplasty.

References

1. Benazzo F, Botta L, Scaffino MF, Caliogna L, Marullo M, Fusi S, et al. Trabecular titanium can induce in vitro osteogenic differentiation of human adipose derived stem cells without osteogenic factors. J Biomed Mater Res A. 2014;102A:2061–71. https://doi.org/10.1002/jbm.a.34875.
2. Bobyn JD, Stackpool GJ, Hacking SA, Tanzer M, Krygier JJ. Characteristics of bone ingrowth and interface mechanics of a new porous tantalum biomaterial. J Bone Joint Surg Br. 1999;81B:907–14.
3. Boileau P, Moineau G, Morin-Salvo N, Avidor C, Godenèche A, Lévigne C, et al. Metal-backed glenoid implant with polyethylene insert is not a viable long-term therapeutic option. J Shoulder Elb Surg. 2015;24:1534–43. https://doi.org/10.1016/j.jse.2015.02.012.
4. Castagna A, Randelli M, Garofalo R, Maradei L, Giardella A, Borroni M. Mid-term results of a metal-backed glenoid component in total shoulder replacement. J Bone Joint Surg Br. 2010;92:1410–5. https://doi.org/10.1302/0301-620X.92B10.23578.
5. Cil A, Sperling JW, Cofield RH. Nonstandard glenoid components for bone deficiencies in shoulder arthroplasty. J Shoulder Elb Surg. 2014;23:e149–57. https://doi.org/10.1016/j.jse.2013.09.023.
6. Clavert P, Millett PJ, Warner JJ. Glenoid resurfacing: what are the limits to asymmetric reaming for posterior erosion? J Shoulder Elb Surg. 2007;16:843–8.
7. Derome P, Sternheim A, Backstein D, Malo M. Treatment of large bone defects with trabecular metal cones in revision total knee arthroplasty: short term clinical and radiographic outcomes. J Arthroplast. 2014;29:122–6. https://doi.org/10.1016/j.arth.2013.04.033.
8. Devine D, Arens D, Burelli S, Bloch HR, Boure L. In vivo evaluation of the osteointegration of new highly porous Trabecular Titanium™. J Bone Joint Surg Br. 2012;94-B(Supp 37):201.
9. Frankle MA, Siegal S, Pupello DR, Gutierrez S, Griewe M, Mighell M. Coronal plane tilt angle affects risk of catastrophic failure in patients treated with a reverse shoulder prosthesis. J Shoulder Elb Surg. 2007;16:e46. https://doi.org/10.1016/j.jse.2007.02.096.
10. Frankle M, Teramoto A, Luo ZP, Levy JC, Pupello D. Glenoid morphology in reverse shoulder arthroplasty: classification and surgical implications. J Shoulder Elb Surg. 2009;18:874–85. https://doi.org/10.1016/j.jse.2009.02.013.
11. Friedman RJ, Hawthorne KB, Genez BM. The use of computerized tomography in the measurement of glenoid version. J Bone Joint Surg Am. 1992;74:1032–7.
12. Gilot GJ. Addressing glenoid erosion in reverse total shoulder arthroplasty. Bull Hosp Jt Dis. 2013;71(Suppl 2):51–3.
13. Gonzalez JF, Alami GB, Baque F, Walch G, Boileau P. Complications of unconstrained shoulder prostheses. J Shoulder Elb Surg. 2011;20:666–82. https://doi.org/10.1016/j.jse.2010.11.017.
14. Gowda A, Pinkas D, Wiater JM. Treatment of glenoid bone deficiency in Total shoulder arthroplasty a critical analysis review. JBJS Rev. 2015;3:3–11. https://doi.org/10.2106/jbjs.rvw.n.00097.
15. Gregory TM, Sankey A, Augereau B, Vandenbussche E, Amis A, Emery R, et al. Accuracy of glenoid component placement in total shoulder arthroplasty and its effect on clinical and radiological outcome in a retrospective, longitudinal, monocentric open study. PLoS One. 2013;8:e75791. https://doi.org/10.1371/journal.pone.0075791.
16. Gutierrez S, Greiwe RM, Frankle MA, Siegal S, Lee WE III. Biomechanical comparison of component position and hardware failure in the reverse shoulder prosthesis. J Shoulder Elb Surg. 2007;16(Suppl 3):9–12.
17. Hanc M, Fokter SK, Vogrin M, Molicnik A, Recnik G, Hill JM, et al. Porous tantalum in spinal surgery: an overview. Eur J Orthop Surg Traumatol. 2016;26:1–7. https://doi.org/10.1007/s00590-015-1654-x.
18. Hill JM, Norris TR. Long-term results of total shoulder arthroplasty following bone-grafting of the glenoid. J Bone Joint Surg Am. 2001;83:877–83.
19. Ho JC, Sabesan VJ, Iannotti JP. Glenoid component retroversion is associated with osteolysis. J Bone Joint Surg Am. 2013;95:e82. https://doi.org/10.2106/JBJS.L.00336.
20. Iannotti JP, Greeson C, Downing D. Effect of glenoid deformity on glenoid component placement in primary shoulder arthroplasty. J Shoulder Elb Surg. 2012;21:48–55. https://doi.org/10.1016/j.jse.2011.02.011.
21. Jain NB, Yamaguchi K. The contribution of reverse shoulder arthroplasty to utilization of primary shoulder arthroplasty. J Shoulder Elb Surg. 2014;23:1905–12. https://doi.org/10.1016/j.jse.2014.06.055.
22. Jones RB, Wright TW, Roche CP. Bone grafting the glenoid versus use of augmented glenoid baseplates

with reverse shoulder arthroplasty. Bull Hosp Jt Dis. 2015;73(Suppl 1):129–35.
23. Kamath AF, Lewallen DG, Hanssen AD. Porous tantalum metaphyseal cones for severe Tibial bone loss in revision knee arthroplasty: a five to nine-year follow-up. J Bone Joint Surg Am. 2015;97:216–23. https://doi.org/10.2106/JBJS.N.00540.
24. Klein SM, Dunning P, Mulieri P, Pupello D, Downes K, Frankle MA. Effects of acquired glenoid bone defects on surgical technique and clinical outcomes in reverse shoulder arthroplasty. J Bone Joint Surg Am. 2010;92:1144–54. https://doi.org/10.2106/JBJS.I.00778.
25. Klika BJ, Wooten CW, Sperling JW, Steinmann SP, Schleck CD, Harmsen WS, et al. Structural bone grafting for glenoid deficiency in primary total shoulder arthroplasty. J Shoulder Elb Surg. 2014;23:1066–72. https://doi.org/10.1016/j.jse.2013.09.017.
26. Knowles NK, Ferreira LM, Athwal GS. Augmented glenoid component designs for type B2 erosions: a computational comparison by volume of bone removal and quality of remaining bone. J Shoulder Elb Surg. 2015;24:1218–26. https://doi.org/10.1016/j.jse.2014.12.018.
27. Lévigne C, Boileau P, Favard L, Garaud P, Mole D, Sirveaux F, et al. Scapular notching in reverse shoulder arthroplasty. J Shoulder Elb Surg. 2008;17:925–35. https://doi.org/10.1016/j.jse.2008.02.010.
28. Lévigne C, Franceschi J. Rheumatoid arthritis of the shoulder: radiological presentation and results of arthroplasty. In: Walch G, Boileau P, editors. Shoulder arthroplasty. Berlin: Springer-Verlag; 1999. p. 221–30.
29. Levine B, Della Valle CJ, Jacobs JJ. Applications of porous tantalum in total hip arthroplasty. J Am Acad Orthop Surg. 2006;14:646–55.
30. Matassi F, Botti A, Sirleo L, Carulli C, Innocenti M. Porous metal for orthopedic implants. Clin Cases Miner Bone Metab. 2013;10:111–5.
31. Mizuno N, Denard PJ, Raiss P, Walch G. Reverse total shoulder arthroplasty for primary glenohumeral osteoarthritis in patients with a biconcave glenoid. J Bone Joint Surg Am. 2013;95(14):1297–304. https://doi.org/10.2106/JBJS.L.00820.
32. Nam D, Kepler CK, Neviaser AS, Jones KJ, Wright TM, Craig EV, et al. Reverse total shoulder arthroplasty: current concepts, results, and component wear analysis. J Bone Joint Surg Am. 2010;92(Suppl 2):23–35. https://doi.org/10.2106/JBJS.J.00769.
33. Regis M, Marin E, Fedrizzi L, Pressacco M. Additive manufacturing of Trabecular Titanium orthopedic implants. MRS Bull. 2015;40:137–44. https://doi.org/10.1557/mrs.2015.1.
34. Roche CP, Stroud NJ, Martin BL, Steiler CA, Flurin PH, Wright TW, et al. Achieving fixation in glenoids with superior wear using reverse shoulder arthroplasty. J Shoulder Elb Surg. 2013;22:1695–701. https://doi.org/10.1016/j.jse.2013.03.008.
35. Sagherian BH, Claridge RJ. Porous tantalum as a structural graft in foot and ankle surgery. Foot Ankle Int. 2012;33(3):179–89.
36. Sandow M, Schutz C. Total shoulder arthroplasty using trabecular metal augments to address glenoid retroversion: the preliminary result of 10 patients with minimum 2-year follow-up. J Should Elbow Surg. 2016;25:598–607. https://doi.org/10.1016/j.jse.2016.01.001.
37. Seidl AJ, Williams GR, Boileau P. Challenges in reverse shoulder arthroplasty: addressing glenoid bone loss. Orthopedics. 2016;39:14–23. https://doi.org/10.3928/01477447-20160111-01.
38. Walch G, Badet R, Boulahia A, Khoury A. Morphologic study of the glenoid in primary glenohumeral osteoarthritis. J Arthroplast. 1999;14:756–60.
39. Walch G, Moraga C, Young A, Castellanos-Rosas J. Results of anatomic nonconstrained prosthesis in primary osteoarthritis with biconcave glenoid. J Shoulder Elb Surg. 2012;21:1526–33. https://doi.org/10.1016/j.jse.2011.11.030.
40. Whitehouse MR, Masri BA, Duncan CP, Garbuz DS. Continued good results with modular trabecular metal augments for acetabular defects in hip arthroplasty at 7 to 11 years. Clin Orthop Relat Res. 2015;473:521 7. https://doi.org/10.1007/s11999-014-3861-x.
41. Wieser K, Borbas P, Ek ET, Meyer DC, Gerber C. Conversion of stemmed hemi- or total to reverse total shoulder arthroplasty: advantages of a modular stem design. Clin Orthop Relat Res. 2015;473:651–60. https://doi.org/10.1007/s11999-014-3985-z.
42. Williams GR Jr, Iannotti JP. Options for glenoid bone loss: composites of prosthetics and biologics. J Shoulder Elb Surg. 2007;16(Suppl 5):267–72.
43. Yian EH, Werner CML, Nyffeler RW, Pfirrmann CW, Ramappa A, Sukthankar A, et al. Radiographic and computed tomography analysis of cemented pegged polyethylene glenoid components in total shoulder replacement. J Bone Joint Surg Am. 2005;87:1928–36.
44. Zumstein MA, Pinedo M, Old J, Boileau P. Problems, complications, reoperations, and revisions in reverse total shoulder arthroplasty: a systematic review. J Shoulder Elb Surg. 2011;20:146–57. https://doi.org/10.1016/j.jse.2010.08.001.

Part V

Arthritis of the Shoulder: III

23 Complications of Shoulder Arthroplasty

Michael Walton, Daoud Makki,
and Steven Brookes-Fazakerley

Introduction

The volume of shoulder arthroplasty (SA) has increased significantly over the last decade. Techniques and indications are evolving which poses a challenge to surgeons. As we have learned from our lower limb colleagues, increasing volume and complexity of arthroplasty necessitates a subsequent increase in revision surgery. A detailed understanding of the principles of primary arthroplasty in order to minimise complication rates, but also an understanding of the management of those complications when they occur, is essential for a practising shoulder arthroplasty surgeon.

Accurate positioning of the implants in order to restore the near normal biomechanics of the shoulder joint in principle, should improve survival of prostheses. In order to achieve this, adequate joint exposure is paramount during shoulder arthroplasty. Difficult joint exposure, distorted anatomy from previous trauma and bone loss from severe wear or previous surgery can all increase the likelihood of complications in shoulder arthroplasty procedures.

Complications can be divided into those that occur intraoperatively with immediate or delayed declaration and those that develop in the postoperative period and are more related to implant survival.

Intraoperative Complications

Nerve Injuries

It is crucial that patients are thoroughly examined preoperatively for any pre-existing discrete neurological deficit. These may occur in the form of a radiculopathy or individual peripheral nerve involvement for example, carpal tunnel syndrome. Shoulder pain can be distracting from a neurological deficit which might become more prominent following the pain relief after arthroplasty.

The most common intraoperative nerve injury during shoulder arthroplasty is to the nerves of the brachial plexus particularly the axillary nerve [1]. The plexus is at risk from traction injuries with over zealous retraction but also from direct iatrogenic injury during glenoid exposure. When releasing soft tissue inferiorly care must be taken to avoid the axillary nerve. The axillary nerve originates from the posterior cord of the brachial plexus. It passes over the antero-inferior surface of the subscapularis and then travels posteriorly, closely related to the inferior capsule of the glenohumeral joint and then though the quadrangular space. The nerve should either be formally

M. Walton (✉) · D. Makki · S. Brookes-Fazakerley
Upper Limb Unit, Wrightington Hospital, Wigan, UK

I. A. Trail et al. (eds.), *Textbook of Shoulder Surgery*, https://doi.org/10.1007/978-3-319-70099-1_23

identified or consciously avoided in all procedures. The nerve can usually be palpated with the tip of the finger as it emerges from under the subscapularis muscle. In cases where there has been a previous fracture or in the case of severe deformity, distortion of the anatomical landmarks predisposes to nerve injuries.

Direct injury to the radial nerve is rare given that it is not in a close vicinity to the operative field. However, humeral shaft fractures during revision procedures can lead to radial nerve injury by nerve entrapment or from cement spillage through diaphyseal perforation in cemented stems. Overzealous retraction on the conjoined tendon can predispose the musculocutaneous nerve to traction injuries [2].

Some nerve injuries relate to the design of arthroplasty itself. In reverse geometry prostheses, the lever arm for rotation is moved laterally and inferiorly which may place strain on the brachial plexus. In the literature, there have been few reports on musculocutaneous; median; radial; and ulnar nerve injuries following reverse shoulder arthroplasty (RSA) [3–5].

Overall, nerve injuries in shoulder arthroplasty often resolve spontaneously but might well halt recovery and impede rehabilitation. If an injury has been identified and failed to resolve over 6 weeks, electrophysiological studies can help determine the extent and site of injury and can also be repeated to identify any potential sign of reinnervation. If, however, there is no recovery, then the opinion of experts specialising in nerve injury should be sought.

Rotator Cuff Injury

The principal role of rotator cuff is to maintain the glenohumeral joint centre of rotation through range of motion and to balance the strong forces of the muscles around the shoulder girdle. The success of anatomical shoulder replacements, total or hemiarthroplasty, therefore rely on the functional integrity of the rotator cuff tendons. Care must be taken to both, identify and protect the posterior cuff tendons and repair the subscapularis (if detached) during surgery. Injury to supraspinatus can occur during exposure of the joint or at the cuff insertion during the humeral cut. The rotator interval should be identified using the biceps tendon, if present, as a landmark to guide the exposure between the supraspinautus and subscapularis. The cuff insertion should be identified, prior to making the humeral osteotomy. This acts as a guide to anatomical version and to ensure that the saw blade does not directly damage the tendon. Insufficiency of the rotator cuff following total anatomical shoulder replacement can occur as a result of tendon attrition and eventually leads to superior instability and limits the success of the arthroplasty procedure [6].

Implant Malpositioning

Correct positioning of the components in shoulder replacement surgery is essential to ensure a well balanced shoulder with good function and maximal longevity. Whilst the humerus is relatively straightforward to expose, achieving adequate glenoid exposure can be technically demanding and is of critical importance to obtain satisfactory positioning of glenoid implant.

Incorrect height and version of the humeral component may predispose to impingement and instability respectively. The height of the cut in total anatomical replacement should spare the cuff insertion but should likewise be low enough to avoid impingement and attrition against the supraspinatus tendon. The natural humerus is retroverted with the articular surface offset posteriorly in relation to the medullary axis. The latest designs have been adjusted accordingly to allow for this [7, 8]. The mean humeral retroversion is approximately 30 degrees. However there is significant variation and the axis of the rotator cuff insertion is an excellent landmark for patient specific anatomy. Incorrect humeral version can predispose to attrition of the subscapularis if there is anterior overhang. The effect of humeral version is dependant on the overall relationship between the humeral and the glenoid components. In contrast to the humerus, accurate positioning of the glenoid is demanding as the local anatomy is more difficult to visualise. The glenoid anatomy is frequently abnormal due to excessive asymmetrical wear and previous trauma which can result in an incorrect version of the glenoid implant or baseplate. Preoperative investigations using CT or MRI scanning can help surgeons identify the available bone stock, plan the glenoid preparation technique and identify the need for any reconstructive techniques. In certain cases, imaging may guide the surgeon as to suitable prosthesis and increasingly, in the form of patient specific implants(PSI). Malposition of the humeral and/or glenoid implants leads to abnormal eccentric loading resulting in increased wear, early loosening or joint instability [9].

Clinical Pearl

Time spent pre-operatively planning the shoulder arthroplasty, in particular the glenoid anatomy is as important as the surgery itself.

Fractures

Perioperative fractures in primary surgery are rare and should be minimised by careful surgical technique. However the risks are increased in osteopaenic individuals especially when using uncemented press-fit humeral prostheses. It is therefore essential to obtain appropriate imaging that outlines the patient's bony anatomy preoperatively and to weigh this risk when making implant choices. The principles of management of periprosthetic fractures have been well described in the femur depending on the relationship of the fracture to the prosthesis (Vancouver Classification). Fixation with a combination of plates, cerclage wires and unicortical screws is required with allograft strut augmentation when necessary. The fracture is then bypassed with the use of a long-stemmed humeral component by a minimum of 2 cortical diameters.

Glenoid fractures occur less commonly in comparison to humeral fractures but can occur during glenoid reaming in osteopaenic patients. The goal of management is to obtain a stable vault for glenoid prosthesis implantation. This is often not possible with cemented polyethylene components. The advent of metal backed stemmed revision glenoid components has provided more options. Fractures can be bypassed by redirecting the insertion of the central peg or screws and if appropriate the use of longer stems. In severe cases, structural bone graft harvested from the humeral head in primary procedures or from the iliac crest or allografts in revision procedures can be used to reconstruct the glenoid. In cases where the glenoid defect is too large or the bone quality too poor to obtain sufficient initial stability, surgeons should consider a two-stage procedure whereby bone grafting is carried out first and allowed to integrate first before considering glenoid implantation at a secondary stage.

Postoperative Complications

Infection

Deep infection of total shoulder arthroplasty (TSA) is estimated around 2.2% [11] and that of RSA 3.8% [12]. The risk of infection increases following revision procedures and may be higher than reported due to undiagnosed low grade infections (Figs. 23.1 and 23.2).

Inoculation of microorganisms usually occurs at the time of surgery and deep infection, declares itself later and depend on the hosts risk factors that can be local (previous surgery and the

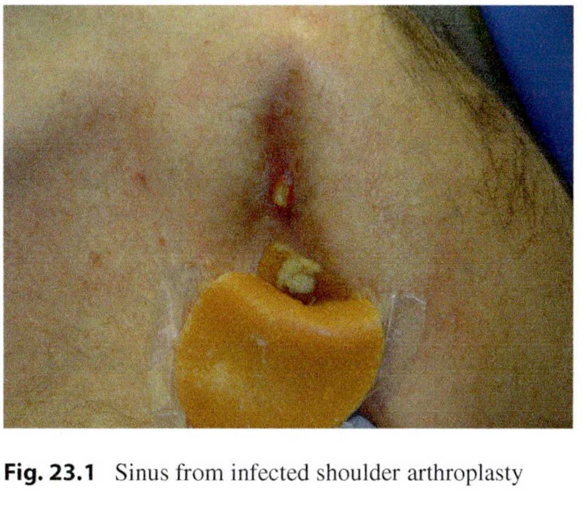

Fig. 23.1 Sinus from infected shoulder arthroplasty

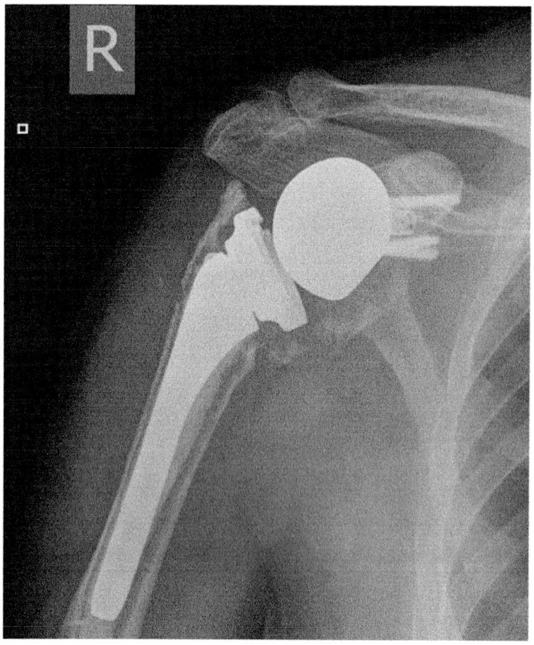

Fig. 23.2 Humeral stem loosening from infected reverse arthroplasty

presence of implants) or systemic such as diabetes or the immunocompromised patient. Microorganisms are usually skin commensals most commonly coagulase negative Staphylococcus Aureus, Staphylococcus Epidermidis and Propionibacterium Acnes. The diagnosis is made from clinical presentation, inflammatory markers and with joint aspiration or biopsy, under sterile conditions. In low grade infections, in particular with P. Acnes, the clinical picture can be vague and blood tests may be normal. In this situation, multiple tissue samples taken from different sites (around glenoid components, from the implants and from the humeral shaft) with prolonged culturing period are required to confirm the diagnosis.

Treatment involves a multidisciplinary team approach. Liaison with a specialist musculoskeletal microbiologist with regards to the best antibiotic regimen and duration of treatment is essential.

Unless there are specific contraindications, an infected arthroplasty requires prosthesis and cement removal and extensive debridement. This can be technically challenging surgery and the surgeon will require experience of humeral osteotomies in the case of well-fixed components. Additional care needs to be taken to avoid iatrogenic neurovascular injury, as there is often abnormal and scarred anatomy. When infection is suspected during a revision procedure, the authors usual approach is to adopt a two-stage revision procedure involving the extraction of the pre-existing prosthesis along with the cement mantle, a thorough debridement and the insertion of antibiotic impregnated cement spacer. The second stage is then carried out when inflammatory markers have normalised combined with a satisfactory clinical progression along with a negative culture on joint aspirate under sterile condition. It is also recommended to have an antibiotic window of 2 weeks before aspirating the joint and performing serial blood tests. There is however, conflicting evidence in the literature regarding single stage versus two-stage revision procedures as most reports are limited by the level of evidence (case series), sample size and the variation in outcome measures.

While some authors [14, 15] have adopted the two-stage revision strategy and claimed that it reduced reinfection rate, others have [16, 17] supported single-stage revision procedures that consisted of removal of the infected implant, thorough debridement and the use of antibiotic-impregnated cement which is effective against the implicated bacteria. They argued that such an approach can reduce cost and is also associated with a low rate of recurrence of infection. Cuff et al. [13] found that single and two stage revision procedures had comparable results with regards to reinfection rate and the shoulder function.

While two-stage revision procedures are regarded by most surgeons as the safer option in dealing with infected shoulder arthroplasty. Strickland et al. [18] have warned that such an approach can have detrimental effects on shoulder function, patient satisfaction and is associated with more surgical complications.

Clinical Pearl

If in doubt use multi-stage surgery. Whilst there is no doubt this increases the risks of surgery, the most important factor in longevity of revisions is eradicating the infection.

Dislocation

Anatomical total shoulder replacements, like the normal glenohumeral joint, are inherently unstable. Stability is maintained by the correct version relationship between the prosthetic glenoid and humerus and a well functioning rotator cuff. Extensive release of the posterior capsule, which is required for adequate glenoid exposure, can predispose to posterior instability. Anterior instability can be as a result of component malposition or subscapularis deficiency. A careful assessment of stability and soft tissue balance is mandatory when trialling anatomical components.

Reverse geometry shoulder replacements in contrast are semi-constrained by their nature and as such are considered inherently more stable. However, there are various factors which could lead to instability and dislocation. The incidence of dislocation has been estimated to be 5% following primary procedures increasing to around 8% in the revision setting [10, 14]. Stability is maintained by soft tissue tension between the humeral cup and glenosphere. Medialisation of the glenoid component and or an exuberant humeral cut reduces the tension in the deltoid fibres and joint compression forces. Stability can be improved by increasing the thickness of the humeral insert, lateralisation of the glenosphere, by bone or metal, or by increasing the diameter of the glenosphere. Instability can also be as a result of impingement of the humerus on the scapula neck. Care must be taken to place the glenosphere low on the glenoid to minimise the risk of inferior scapula notching but care must also be taken to avoid anterior and posterior impingement which is addressed by increasing glenosphere diameter (Fig. 23.3).

The preservation and repair of subscapularis tendon is believed to add to the stability of the implant by exerting adduction forces mainly at the inferior part of the tendon [19]. However, the clinical significance of this concept and the role of subscapularis tendon in reducing the risk of dislocation remain debatable [20]. An unbalanced soft tissue envelop secondary to previous trauma or surgeries might also account for increased risk instability and dislocation [21].

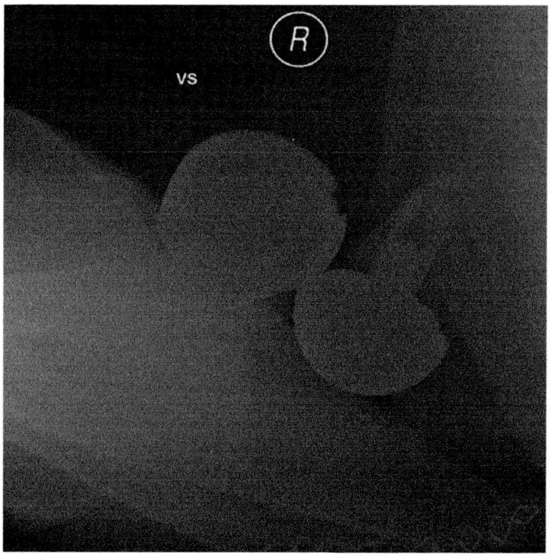

Fig. 23.3 Posterior dislocation of reverse arthroplasty

An attempt to manage dislocations initially with closed reduction is appropriate and satisfactory outcomes have been reported. However, in recurrent instability, surgical management becomes inevitable and options include constrained trays, thicker polyethylene inserts and larger eccentric, or more lateralised glenospheres.

> **Clinical Pearl**
> Many reverse arthroplasty dislocations occur anteriorly when axial load is placed in an internally rotated position (getting out of a chair). Carefully check stability in this position intra-operatively. The other important factor is posterior impingement on external rotation which leads to anterior gapping of the joint. This can be reduced by inserting a larger glenosphere which allows overhang in the AP dimension not just inferiorly.

Implant Specific Complications

Rotator Cuff Deficiency

Rotator cuff tearing following anatomical TSA has a reported prevalence ranging from 1.3% to

7.8% [22]. Rotator cuff tears are associated with prosthesis oversizing, pre-operative tendinopathy, fatty infiltration (seen on MRI scan), multiple previous surgeries and aggressive rehabilitation protocols [23]. Subscapularis tears occur most commonly in around 50% of these cases [24]. This can be traumatic or atraumatic in origin. Its occurrence is often underestimated due to its presence being asymptomatic and not diagnosed until clinical examination reveals weakness in internal rotation, excessive external rotation or axillary radiographs show anterior subluxation of the humeral head. Avoiding subscapularis tears can be facilitated by careful mobilisation of the tendon with release of subcoracoid adhesions together with the middle and inferior glenohumeral ligaments. Particular attention to a sturdy repair is critical as is keeping post-operative external rotation in the early stages (weeks 1–6) to a safe zone which will be determined during surgery. If tears do occur, then primary repair of subscapularis is indicated, if the patient is symptomatic and if the tendon is of good quality. In the presence of muscle belly fatty infiltration and tendon retraction, augmentation with pectoralis major can be considered with some benefit reported [25]. In patients with minimal symptoms and chronic tears, non-operative treatment is preferable as repairs with or without a pectoralis major transfer have poor outcome [24].

Posterosuperior rotator cuff tears can involve the supraspinatus, infraspinatus and/or the teres minor tendons. Posterosuperior cuff dysfunction results in a loss of the dynamic stabilisation function of the glenohumeral joint. Consequently, during abduction there is unopposed upward pull by deltoid resulting in superior subluxation of the humeral head. Increased humeral head translation diminishes glenohumeral contact area leading to point loading and subsequent polyethylene deformation and wear. Eccentric glenoid component loading by the humeral head can also lead to accelerated glenoid loosening by means of the "rocking horse phenomenon" [26].

Pre-operative risk factors for posterosuperior rotator cuff tears include rheumatoid arthritis, fatty infiltration of the muscle on MRI scan, superior tilt of the glenoid component and longer post-operative follow-up [27]. Symptoms include weakness in forward elevation and external rotation. On antero-posterior (AP) radiograph there is anterosuperior escape of the humeral head with reduction of the acromiohumeral distance.

An intact, functioning rotator cuff is essential for a well functioning TSA with clinical outcomes (Constant score, subjective score and range of motion) and radiological outcomes (radiolucent lines, loosening and glenoid component migration) being significantly worse in the presence of secondary rotator cuff dysfunction (defined as >25% superior migration of the humeral component on a true AP radiograph of the glenohumeral joint) [23] (Fig. 23.4). Attempted primary repair of the posterosuperior rotator cuff has demonstrated poor outcome with one study showing a success in only 4 of 18 patients [6]. Consequently, in minimally symptomatic patients a non-operative approach should be adopted, whilst in symptomatic patients either latissimus dorsi/teres major transfer or revision to RSA should be considered [22]. More recently the arthroscopic superior capsular reconstruction technique [28] using biological scaffolds (fascia lata patch) to recreate the posterosuperior cuff may be an option, however there is no evidence supporting this as yet.

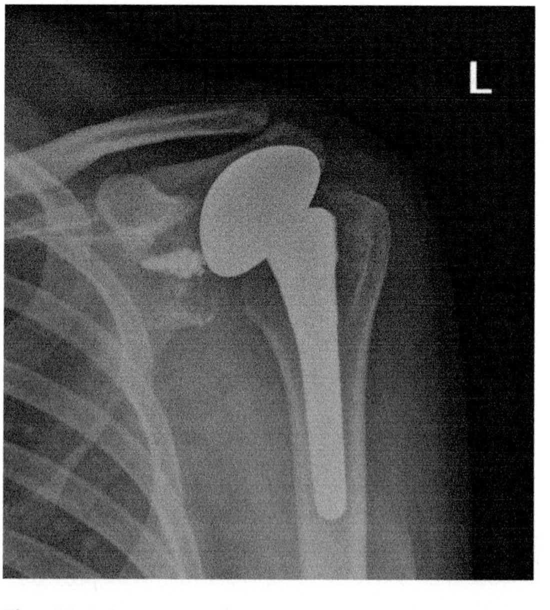

Fig. 23.4 Rotator cuff failure with superior migration following anatomic shoulder arthroplasty

Notching

Notching describes a phenomenon unique to RSA whereby there is impingement of the humeral prosthetic cup against the scapular neck upon adduction of the arm. Notching is a very common complication with a reported incidence ranging from 50% to 96% patients [29]. Its mechanism relates to relative medialisation of the centre of rotation of the Grammont design prosthesis. This AP radiographic observation can result in an osseous defect of the lateral-inferior scapular pillar and can result in glenoid component loosening. The original classification for scapular notching was described by Sirveaux with four progressive grades [30]. Grade 1 shows a notch limited to the scapular pillar, Grade 2 shows a notch reaching the inferior screw of the base plate, Grade 3 shows a notch extending beyond the inferior screw, and Grade 4 shows a notch reaching the base-plate's central peg.

Notching can be reduced by several techniques. Firstly, and most importantly, inferior placement of the glenosphere base plate so that its inferior edge is tangential with the inferior native glenoid rim [31]. Secondly, biomechanical studies have suggested that pre-operative superior glenoid erosion is associated with notching due to it pre-disposing to a superiorly tilted, valgus, glenoid base plate [32]. Consequently, a neutral (0 degrees) or slight inferior tilt (10 degrees) of the base plate is optimal to help avoid notching. More recently, humeral prosthesis design has been modified to create the concept of an "onlay" humeral prosthesis with the aim of limiting scapular notching by lateralising the centre of rotation. The traditional Grammont prosthesis humeral stem has an intraosseous metal inlay that medialises the humerus. RSAs with a lateralising, extraosseous "onlay" usually have a reduced inclination angle (145 degrees rather than 155 degrees) which consequently not only increases length but also lateralises the humerus [33]. Finally, lateralisation of the glenosphere will also have an indirect effect of reducing notching. A few millimetres can be achieved by increasing the glenosphere diameter e.g. using 42 mm rather than 36 mm. However, lateralising the glenosphere itself can be performed using an increased offset glenosphere prosthesis (metallic lateralising) or by adding bone graft to the base plate (bony lateralisation). Both have shown significant reductions in scapula notching rates, but bony lateralisation has the added advantage of maintaining the prosthetic centre of rotation at the prosthesis-bone interface thus reducing torque on the glenoid component and potential loosening [34].

The clinical significance of scapular notching remains to be fully determined. Studies have implicated it with glenoid component loosening and poorer outcome scores [10]. However, the largest and most comprehensive study found no clinical effect and only 1 case of notching leading to glenoid loosening [29].

Stiffness

Stiffness following shoulder arthroplasty can be an extremely problematic complication leading to significant patient impairment and dissatisfaction. Along with recalcitrant pain, stiffness is the most common symptom in patients with failed shoulder arthroplasty [35]. Stiffness can be a multifactorial process and careful elucidation of its primary aetiology is essential to ensure appropriate treatment. Common causes include implant malpositioning and/or inappropriate size, incomplete soft tissue release, heterotopic ossification, infection, previous proximal humerus fracture and inadequate post-operative rehabilitation.

"Overstuffing" the glenohumeral joint (GHJ) with an oversized humeral prosthesis predisposes to stiffness by over-tensioning the soft-tissue envelope. Cadaveric studies have shown that for every 1 mm of oversizing there is a loss of 3–4 degrees of GHJ [36]. Component malposition including incorrect version and height can induce stiffness through indirect capsular shortening and painful acromiohumeral impingement respectively.

Infection with chronic pain will lead to gradual loss of range of motion. The incidence of infection is around 1% with the majority of these being caused by *P. acnes* [37]. *P. acnes* is a low virulence organism causing chronic low grade infection with atypical signs and symptoms of a periprosthetic infection [38]. Instead symptoms of isolated instability and stiffness may occur. For that reason, the surgeon must always be aware of infection as a cause of chronic stiffness and investigate appropriately.

Treating a stiff shoulder arthroplasty should first exclude infection and component malposition. From there the evidence base guiding the treatment is limited. Romeo advised that if a patient has completed a comprehensive physiotherapy regimen and forward elevation is greater than 90 degrees with external rotation more than 20 degrees then conservative, non-operative treatment is appropriate [40]. With significant active and passive loss of motion, operative treatment should be considered. Arthroscopic management of failed shoulder arthroplasty for a variety of causes including pain and stiffness has been advocated by two case series involving 13 and 29 patients reporting significant improvement of post-operative clinical outcome scores and range of motion [39, 41]. Manipulation under anaesthetic should only be considered once a thorough surgical (arthroscopic or open) release has been performed to reduce the risk of periprosthetic fracture [40].

If active motion is lost but passive motion retained, deltoid and/or rotator cuff dysfunction should be considered. Deltoid dysfunction in RSA is a devastating complication with catastrophic loss of shoulder function being the natural outcome. Transfer of the deltoid to trapezius muscle initially described by Saha [42] has shown improvement in abduction and forward elevation [43]. Loss of external rotation in RSA due to deficient infraspinatus and teres minor causes decidedly poorer functional results. Transfer of the latissimus dorsi with or without teres major to the posterolateral side of the humerus (L'Episcopo procedure) has been shown to significantly improve patients' ability to hold the hand in space in external rotation and abduction such as when holding a toothbrush or comb [44].

Heterotopic Ossification

Heterotopic ossification (HO) is a relatively common phenomenon in both RSA and TSA. Retrospective studies have quoted incidence rates between 15% and 29.5%. Identical rates were seen in both male and female groups of patients, although Its occurrence was more frequently seen in patients undergoing RSA for cuff tear arthropathy (29.5% and 36.4%). Patients undergoing hemiarthroplasty and anatomical TSA showed no increased incidence of HO compared to RSA and nonsteroidal anti-inflammatory drugs (NSAIDs) had no effect on its occurrence. Patients with osteoarthritis and rheumatoid arthritis had an insignificant decrease in the incidence of HO being seen in only 14.5% patients [45, 46]. The clinical significance of HO and its relationship to both post-operative pain and stiffness is yet to be fully determined. However, significantly lower Constant scores were reported in patients with grade 2 HO or greater [46].

Thromboembolism

Venous thromboembolism (VTE) after shoulder arthroplasty is generally considered to be a rare event. Multiple incidence rates have been quoted varying from 0.2% to 16% of patients [47]. Sperling and Cofield described the prevalence of symptomatic pulmonary embolism (PE) following shoulder arthroplasty to be 0.17% [48] and Lyman et al. report a deep venous thrombosis (DVT) incidence of 0.5% [49]. The incidence of VTE in an urban population is quoted at 0.05%, hence the incidence following shoulder arthroplasty is increased at least five-fold [50]. The incidence of asymptomatic VTE has been reported as high as 13%, however the clinical significance of this remains debatable [51].

Common risk factors for VTE for a patient undergoing shoulder arthroplasty are the same as for any other patient undergoing major surgery [52]. In the United Kingdom (UK), the National Institute for Health and Care Excellence (NICE) recommend that all patients undergoing shoulder arthroplasty be risk assessed and stratified independently. Those who are at increased risk of VTE should be offered mechanical prophylaxis on admission and pharmacological prophylaxis started within 6–12 h post-operatively [52]. Likewise, the British Elbow and Shoulder Society (BESS) have published VTE guidelines for patients undergoing shoulder and elbow surgery [53]. They advise that any patient who is at high or very high risk be commenced on pharmacological prophylaxis and continued for a month, and those at low or medium risk have mechanical prophylaxis. The risk of bleeding must also be assessed when prescribing VTE prophylaxis to determine the co-existence of any contraindications [52].

Glenoid Loosening

Glenoid component loosening is one of the most frequently seen complications and has been termed the weak link of TSA. Multiple studies have reported varying rates of loosening including a rate of 44% at 12 years of follow-up [54]. Radiolucent lines around the glenoid are frequently seen with Torchia and Cofield reporting them in 75 of 89 TSA glenoids [54]. Evaluation of glenoid loosening requires radiological assessment with plain film and CT scanning. Progression of a radiolucent line around the perimeter of a component or widening of the line on serial radiographs exceeding 1.5–2 mm, associated with frank signs of migration, shift or tilting will provide more concern for true symptomatic loosening [55].

Multiple factors are associated with aseptic glenoid loosening including poor surgical technique, deficient glenoid bone stock, glenoid morphology, rotator cuff deficiency, prosthesis design (round versus flat-back, pegged versus keeled), all polyethyelene or metal backed glenoid components in RSA, length of the baseplate central peg and its surface covering. Key surgical factors to reduce loosening and the presence of immediate postoperative radiographic periprosthetic lines are the use of sharp reamers and saline lavage to avoid thermal osteonecrosis, pulsatile lavage to remove bone and clot debris, careful drying of the glenoid, and the use of vacuum prepared, diminished porosity cement with pressurisation on insertion and insertion of only a very thin layer [22].

Careful planning of the primary surgery is essential in the prevention of glenoid loosening. Pre-operative assessment of glenoid morphology with a CT scan will help determine neck length, bone loss, version and inclination guiding the direction of reaming and subsequent prosthesis position avoiding eccentric loading. Magnetic resonance scanning will determine rotator cuff and subscapularis integrity both essential to avoid eccentric loading too. Failure to anticipate wear direction can result in a reamed glenoid with suboptimal support of the implant in either the AP or inferosuperior directions or both. Consequent eccentric loading of the implanted glenoid component by the humeral head results in development of the "rocking horse" phenomenon. This causes loading of one edge of the component and lift off of the opposite edge from the bone leading to premature glenoid loosening [56]. Importance of preservation of the subchondral plate and concentric loading was demonstrated by Walch et al. where anterior reaming or bone grafting of a retroverted glenoid in TSA for osteoarthritis although providing satisfactory therapeutic outcomes was associated with revision rates of between 16% and 21% of patients suffering glenoid loosening at 6 years [9]. However, multiple studies have now shown that a constrained RSA prosthesis in this situation provides excellent outcome without the need for eccentric reaming or bone grafting [57]. Hence decision on type of prosthesis should be carefully rationalised pre-operatively.

Aseptic loosening of the glenoid can also be as a result of osteolysis. Wear of the glenoid component creates polyethylene wear particles. Sub-micron particles are phagocytised by macrophages and osteoblasts initiating a pro-inflammatory cell signalling pathway culminating in activation of osteoclasts resulting in osteolysis. Osteolysis is less commonly seen in the shoulder compared to the hip and is postulated to be due to wear particles being less round in shape and larger in size stimulating a less vivid pro-inflammatory response [58].

Multiple studies have demonstrated that glenoid component design is essential in reducing loosening rates. Round-backed, all polyethylene components with peg fixation do better than flat-backed, metal-backed or keeled components. Pegged glenoids undergo less loosening and radiolucent line development when compared to keeled constructs [59, 60]. Metal-backed glenoid implants were introduced with the aim of reducing all polyethylene glenoid component aseptic loosening. Initial results reported lower rates of radiolucent lines and loosening [61]. Further studies have however, consistently shown higher rates of failure with increased rates of revision. The added metal-polyethylene bearing surface creates another interface for wear, loosening and disarticulation. Fixation of the base plate with screws introduces another relative joint space for osteolysis to happen around and metal fatigue can result in screw fracture. Not surprisingly therefore reports of failure include massive osteolysis, dissociation of the metal and polyethylene components, catastrophic wear, screw fracture and high rates of radiolucent line progression and aseptic loosening. In two series by Boileau and Martin et al., they found rates of 25% and 37.8% respectively for the occurrence of radiolucent lines around the uncemented glenoid component in patients at three and 7 years follow-up with revision rates of 20% and 11% respectively [62, 63]. More recently Fox et al. reported on the 20 year Mayo clinic experience of 1542 primary TSAs [64]. The revision rate for all polyethylene cemented glenoids was 15% compared to 62% for a metal-back component.

Clincial Pearl

Less is more with glenoid cement. Pressurised cement in the peg or keel holes is sufficient. Avoid putting cement on the back side of the prosthesis.

The introduction of newer technology to prosthesis design has now demonstrated more promising results with metal-back glenoids. The addition of a central, hydroxyappatite coated peg for bone ingrowth, knowledge of preferential articular surface radial mismatch values and curved-back glenoids have reduced loosening rates and produced prostheses with better outcomes. Castagna et al. showed that in a series of 35 consecutive TSAs they had radiolucent lines in only 8 patients with no disassembly or fracture at a mean follow-up of 75.4 months [65].

Revision of a loose glenoid can be technically demanding and requires meticulous attention to maintaining bone stock. If enough bone is present then reimplantation of a new glenoid is possible, however, if not conversion to hemiarthroplasty is all that is possible. Cheung et al., described a series of 68 TSAs with 33 having a new glenoid component and the remaining 35 being bone grafted and converted to hemiarthroplasty. At 5 years post-operative, 91% of the glenoid re-implants and 78% of the hemiarthroplasty group had a satisfactory result [66]. In contrast to this however, Bonnevialle et al. had a recurrent re-loosening rate of 67% of 42 revised glenoids with a re-revision rate of 17% and complication rate of 45% [67]. The same group also demonstrated the importance of RSA in the management of aseptic glenoid loosening with the results of 37 patients having 86% satisfied or very satisfied outcomes when revised from TSA to RSA [68].

Glenoid component loosening in RSA is much rarer than that for conventional TSA. It has a prevalence of 2.5% in the Grammont style prosthesis [69] but increases up to 11.7% in the new lateralised centre of rotation prosthesis [70]. Like TSA, radiolucent lines around the base-plate are much more common than true baseplate loosening. Glenosphere component premature loosening is nearly always due to technical error with malposition (too high or in superior inclination) being the most common occurrence resulting in significant superior shear stresses. Aggressive reaming or implant insertion can also lead to unrecognised glenoid fracture and early loosening due to non-union. If bone graft has been used, failure to insert a long enough central peg (require at least 8 mm of peg in native bone) into the native scapula is associated with non-union of the graft to the native bone and will result in early loosening and failure [33]. Scapular notching although postulated to be a factor in glenoid baseplate loosening has yet to be confirmed. This could be due to the fact that the glenoid central peg is key in initial fixation of the baseplate [71].

Glenoid Erosion

Hemiarthoplasty of the humerus attempts to avoid the known risk of glenoid component loosening by not inserting a glenoid component. Results, especially with resurfacing hemiarthoplasty, were shown to be comparable to total shoulder replacement in some series with good long term symptomatic and functional results [72]. However persistent pain secondary to glenoid erosion has proved problematic and the leading cause of revision. Favourable conditions for resistance to erosion are lack of glenoid cysts, intact glenoid cartilage, intact rotator cuff musculature and use in the fracture situation. The use in females, rheumatoid arthritic and valgus head position is particularly associated with glenoid destruction [73].

Managing the painful hemiarthroplasty usually involves conversion to a total shoulder replacement. If the glenoid bone loss in minimal and the rotator cuff intact then revision to an anatomic shoulder replacement is a good option especially *in* the younger patient. If however the glenoid bone stock has been compromised then revision to a reverse geometry prosthesis is more predictable. In severe cases of glenoid erosion the glenoid requires reconstruction in order to achieve sufficient lateralisation of the glenosphere to maintain stability. Lateralisation can be achieved with bone or metal augmentation (Figs. 23.5 and 23.6).

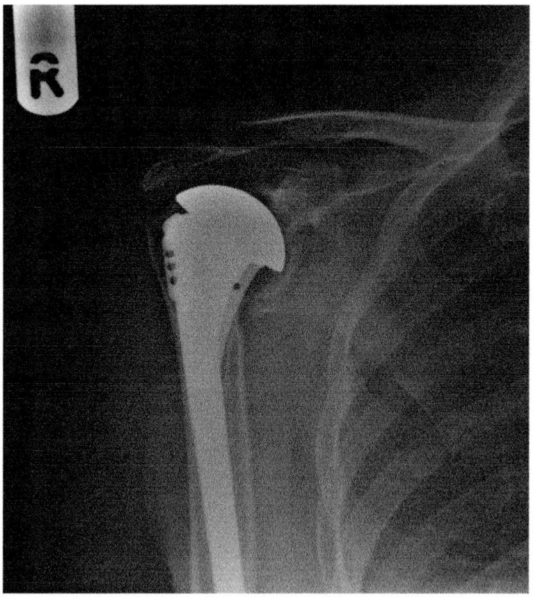

Fig. 23.5 Severe superomedial glenoid erosion in a female rheumatoid patient

Other Rare Complications

Humeral Stem Loosening

Clinically significant humeral stem loosening in TSA is a much less common occurrence than that of the glenoid prosthesis with an overall prevalence of 1.1% [74]. However, radiographic lucent lines around the stem are common although their correlation with clinical symptoms and signs of loosening is poor [75]. Revision due to loosening is rarely reported [74], even after a minimum of 15 years follow-up in young patients [76]. Radiological rates of aseptic loosening occur more often in uncemented press-fit stems (49–55.6% patients at 4.2–12 years) [54, 77] than in uncemented porous coated stems (10% at to 3–5 years) [78, 79] and cemented prostheses (2% at 6 years) [78]. Stress shielding secondary to large areas of uncemented stems having a porous coat is thought to play a significant role in the presence of these clinically insignificant radiolucent lines being seen in 63% of uncemented stems [81].

Determining the clinical significance of radiographic lucency has been clarified by Sperling et al., in both cemented and uncemented stems. They defined the "at risk" humeral prosthesis to be one with subsidence, tilt and at least 2 mm of radiolucency in 3 or more of the 8 zones around the prosthesis when seen by a minimum of 2 out of 3 observers [77, 80].

Studies have also shown the significance of polyethylene wear particles on humeral stem loosening. A significantly higher incidence (65%

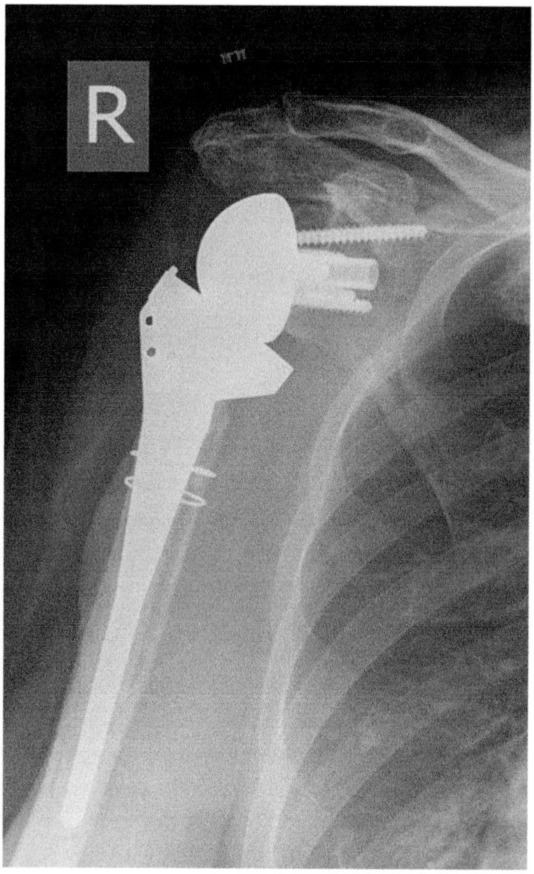

Fig. 23.6 Revision of patient from to a reverse shoulder with glenoid bone reconstruction using long pegged glenoid baseplate

of TSA versus 13% hemiarthroplasty patients) of osteolysis was seen around the proximal part of the humerus after TSA, compared to hemiarthroplasty, this being attributed to the associated glenoid component polyethylene wear [82].

Humeral stem loosening in RSA was surprisingly found to be more common (21% cause of revision) than glenosphere loosening in a recent study by Boileau and colleagues [83]. Proximal humeral bone loss was the main risk factor for humeral loosening being seen more commonly after RSA for fracture or fracture sequelae, due to lysis or posterior migration of the greater tuberosity. Without the greater tuberosity, the humeral component is fixed distally only and as such is put under significant rotational stress. Such mechanical factors are compounded by polyethylene wear debris from metaphyseal component notching against the scapula. In relation to humeral stem fixation and loosening, similar findings in RSA have been seen to that of TSA. A recent systematic review showed that uncemented prostheses on the whole had a significantly higher incidence of early humeral stem migration and non-progressive radiolucent lines when compared to cemented ($p < 0.001$, RR 18.1). However, there was no difference in the risk of stem loosening or revision between the two groups [84].

Conclusions

Shoulder arthroplasty is becoming increasing common. A greater understanding of shoulder biomechanics has allowed the development of more anatomic designs which hopefully, will facilitate better function and greater longevity. The advent of the reverse geometry designs has revolutionised our ability to manage the cuff deficient shoulder. However, with increasing numbers inevitably comes an increasing revision burden. It is beholden on us to take meticulous care in both, our pre-operative preparation for shoulder arthroplasty and our subsequent surgical technique to minimise these potentially devastating complications. When they do occur a multidisciplinary team approach, in a specialist centre, is essential to maximise the resultant function.

References

1. Scarlat MM. Complications with reverse total shoulder arthroplasty and recent evolutions. Int Orthop. 2013;37(5):843–5.
2. Cheung E, Willis M, Walker M, Clark R, Frankle MA. Complications in reverse total shoulder arthroplasty. J Am Acad Orthop Surg. 2011;19(7):439–4.
3. Van Hoof T, Gomes GT, Audenaert E, Verstraete K, Kerckaert I, D'Herde K. 3D computerized model for measuring strain and displacement of the brachial plexus following placement of reverse shoulder prosthesis. Anat Rec (Hoboken). 2008;291(9):1173–85.
4. Boileau P, Watkinson DJ, Hatzidakis AM, Balg F. Grammont reverse prosthesis: design, rationale, and biomechanics. J Shoulder Elbow Surg. 2005;14(1 Suppl S):147S–61S.

5. Wingert NC, Beck JD, Harter GD. Avulsive axillary artery injury in reverse total shoulder arthroplasty. Orthopedics. 2014;37(1):e92–7.
6. Hattrup SJ, Cofield RH, Cha SS. Rotator cuff repair after shoulder replacement. J Shoulder Elb Surg. 2006;15(1):78–83.
7. Roberts SN, Foley AP, Swallow HM, Wallace WA, Coughlan DP. The geometry of the humeral head and the design of prostheses. J Bone Joint Surg (Br). 1992;73-B:647–50.
8. Wallace AL, Phillips RL, MacDougal GA, Walsh WR. Sonnabend DH. Resurfacing of the glenoid in total shoulder arthroplasty: a comparison, at a mean of five years, of prostheses inserted with and without cement. J Bone Joint Surg Am. 1999;81-A:510–8.
9. Walch G, Moraga C, Young A, Castellanos-Rosas J. Results of anatomic non-constrained prosthesis in primary osteoarthritis with biconcave glenoid. J Shoulder Elb Surg. 2012;21(11):1526–33.
10. Zumstein MA, Pinedo M, Old J, Boileau P. Problems, complications, reoperations, and revisions in reverse total shoulder arthroplasty: a systematic review. J Shoulder Elb Surg. 2011;20(1):146–57.
11. Jahoda D, Pokomy D, et al. Infectious complications of total shoulder arthroplasty. Acta Chir Orthp Traumatol Cech. 2008;75(6):422–8.
12. Zimmerli W, et al. Prosthetic joint infections. N Engl J Med. 2004;351(16):1645–54.
13. Cuff DJ, Virani NA, Levy J, Frankle MA, Derasari A, Hines B, Pupello DR, Cancio M, Mighell M. The treatment of deep shoulder infection and glenohumeral instability with debridement, reverse shoulder arthroplasty and postoperative antibiotics. J Bone Joint Surg Br. 2008;90:336–42.
14. Sabesan VJ, Ho JC, Kovacevic D, Iannotti JP. Two-stage reimplantation for treating prosthetic shoulder infections. Clin Orthop Relat Res. 2011;469(9): 2538–43.
15. Sperling JW, Kozak TK, Hanssen AD, Cofield RH. Infection after shoulder arthroplasty. Clin Orthop Relat Res. 2001;382:206–16.
16. Coste JS, Reig S, Trojani C, Berg M, Walch G, Boileau P. The management of infection in arthroplasty of the shoulder. J Bone Joint Surg Br. 2004;86:65–9.
17. Ince A, Seemann K, Frommelt L, Katzer A, Loehr JF. One-stage exchange shoulder arthroplasty for peri-prosthetic infection. J Bone Joint Surg Br. 2005;87:814–8.
18. Strickland JP, Sperling JW, Cofield RH. The results of two-stage re-implantation for infected shoulder replacement. J Bone Joint Surg Br. 2008;90: 460–5.
19. Ackland DC, et al. Moment arms of the shoulder musculature after reverse total shoulder arthroplasty. J Bone Joint Surg Am. 2010;92(5):1221–30.
20. Edwards TB, Williams MD, Labriola JE, Elkousy HA, Gartsman GM, O'Connor DP. Subscapularis insufficiency and the risk of shoulder dislocation after reverse shoulder arthroplasty. J Shoulder Elb Surg. 2009;18:892–6.
21. Trappey GJ IV, O'Connor DP, Edwards TB. What are the instability and infection rates after reverse shoulder arthroplasty? Clin Orthop Relat Res. 2011;469:2505–11.
22. Sperling JW, Hawkins RJ, Walch G, Zuckerman JD. Complications in total shoulder arthroplasty. J Bone Joint Surg Am. 2013;95-A(6):563–9.
23. Young AA, Walch G, Pape G, Gohlke F, Favard L. Secondary rotator cuff dysfunction following total shoulder arthroplasty for primary glenohumeral osteoarthritis: results of a multicenter study with more than five years of follow-up. J Bone Joint Surg Am. 2012;94(8):685–93.
24. Elhassan B, Ozbaydar M, Massimini D, Diller D, Higgins L, Warner JJ. Transfer of pectoralis major for the treatment of irreparable tears of subscapularis: does it work? J Bone Joint Surg (Br). 2008;90(8):1059–65.
25. Miller BS, Joseph TA, Noonan TJ, Horan MP, Hawkins RJ. Rupture of the subscapularis tendon after shoulder arthroplasty: diagnosis, treatment, and outcome. J Shoulder Elb Surg. 2005;14(5):492–6.
26. Franklin JL, Barrett WP, Jackins SE, Matsen FA 3rd. Glenoid loosening in total shoulder arthroplasty. Association with rotator cuff deficiency. J Arthroplast. 1988;3:39–46.
27. Edwards TB, Boulahia A, Kempf JF, Boileau P, Nemoz C, Walch G. The influence of rotator cuff disease on the results of shoulder arthroplasty for primary osteoarthritis: results of a multicenter study. J Bone Joint Surg Am. 2002;84-A(12):2240–8.
28. Mihata T, Lee TQ, Watanabe C, Fukunishi K, Ohue M, Tsujimura T, Kinoshita M. Clinical results of arthroscopic superior capsule reconstruction for irreparable rotator cuff tears. Arthroscopy. 2013;29(3):459–70.
29. Levigne C, Boileau P, Favard L, Garaud P, Mole D, Sirveaux F, et al. Scapular notching in reverse shoulder arthroplasty. J Shoulder Elb Surg. 2008;17(6):925–35.
30. Sirveaux F, Favard L, Oudet D, Huquet D, Walch G, Mole D. Grammont inverted total shoulder arthroplasty in the treatment of glenohumeral osteoarthritis with massive rupture of the cuff. Results of a multicentre study of 80 shoulders. J Bone Joint Surg Br. 2004;86:388–95.
31. Nyffeler RW, Werner CM, Gerber C. Biomechanical relevance of glenoid component positioning in the reverse Delta III total shoulder prosthesis. J Shoulder Elb Surg. 2005;14:524–8.
32. Lévigne C, Garret J, Boileau P, Alami G, Favard L, Walch G. Scapular notching in reverse shoulder arthroplasty: is it important to avoid it and how? Clin Orthop Relat Res. 2011;469(9):2512–20.
33. Boileau P. Complications and revision of reverse total shoulder arthroplasty. Orthop Traumatol Surg Res. 2016;102:S33–43.
34. Boileau P, Moineau G, Roussanne Y, O'Shea K. Bony increased-offset reversed shoulder arthroplasty: minimizing scapular impingement while maximizing glenoid fixation. Clin Orthop Relat Res. 2011;469(9):2558–67.

35. Franta AK, Lenters TR, Mounce D, Neradilek B, Matsen FA. The complex characteristics of 282 unsatisfactory shoulder arthroplasties. J Shoulder Elb Surg. 2007;16:555–62.
36. Harryman DT, Sidles JA, Harris SL, Lippitt SB, Matsen FA 3rd. The effect of articular conformity and the size of the humeral head component on laxity and motion after glenohumeral arthroplasty. A study in cadavera. J Bone Joint Surg Am. 1995;77: 555–63.
37. Singh JA, Sperling JW, Schleck C, Harmsen WS, Cofield RH. Periprosthetic infections after total shoulder arthroplasty: a 33-year perspective. J Shoulder Elb Surg. 2012;21:1534–41.
38. Topolski MS, Chin PY, Sperling JW, Cofield RH. Revision shoulder arthroplasty with positive intraoperative cultures: the value of preoperative studies and intraoperative histology. J Shoulder Elb Surg. 2006;15(4):402–6.
39. Hersch JC, Dines DM. Arthroscopy for failed shoulder arthroplasty. Arthroscopy. 2000;16:606–12.
40. Thorsness RJ, Romeo AA. Stiffness in shoulder arthroplasty: to manipulate or not? Sem Shoulder Arthropl. 2016;27:104–7.
41. Tytherleigh-Strong GM, Levy O, Sforza G, Copeland SA. The role of arthroscopy for the problem shoulder arthroplasty. J Shoulder Elb Surg. 2002;11: 230–4.
42. Saha AK. Surgery of the paralysed and flail shoulder. Acta Orthop Scand. 1967;97(Suppl):5–90.
43. Rühmann O, Schmolke S, Bohnsack M, Carls J, Wirth CJ. Trapezius transfer in brachial plexus palsy. Correlation of the outcome with muscle power and operative technique. J Bone Joint Surg Br. 2005;87(2):184–90.
44. Boileau P, Chuinard C, Roussanne Y, Neyton L, Trojani C. Modified latissimus dorsi and teres major transfer through a single delto-pectoral approach for external rotation deficit of the shoulder: as an isolated procedure or with a reverse arthroplasty. J Shoulder Elb Surg. 2007;16(6):671–82.
45. Boehm TD, Wallace WA, Neumann LJ. Heterotopic ossification after primary shoulder arthroplasty. J Shoulder Elb Surg. 2005;14(1):6–10.
46. Verhofste B, Decock T, Van Tongel A, De Wilde L. Heterotopic ossification after reverse total shoulder arthroplasty. Bone Joint J. 2016;98-B(9):1215–21.
47. Saleh HE, Pennings AL, ElMaraghy AW. Venous thromboembolism after shoulder arthroplasty: a systematic review. J Shoulder Elb Surg. 2013;22(10):1440–8.
48. Sperling JW, Cofield RH. Pulmonary embolism following shoulder arthroplasty. J Bone Joint Surg Am. 2002;84-A(11):1939–41.
49. Lyman S, Sherman S, Carter T, Bach P, Mandl L, Marx R. Prevalence and risk factors for symptomatic thromboembolic events after shoulder arthroplasty. Clin Orthop Relat Res. 2006;448:152–6.
50. Nordstrom M, Lindblad B, Bergqvist D, Kjellstrom T. A prospective study of the incidence of deep-vein thrombosis within a defined urban population. J Intern Med. 1992;232:155–60.
51. Willis AA, Warren RF, Craig EV, et al. Deep vein thrombosis after reconstructive shoulder arthroplasty: a prospective observational study. J Shoulder Elb Surg. 2009;18:100–6.
52. NICE clinical guideline 92 (NICE 2010) Venous thromboembolism: Reducing the risk of venous thromboembolism (deep vein thrombosis and pulmonary embolism) in patients admitted to hospital. http://www.nice.org.uk/nicemedia/live/12695/47197/47197.pdf. Assessed 26 Sept 2013.
53. British Elbow and Shoulder Society. http://bess.org.uk/media/VTEdraft.pdf. Assessed 26 Sept 2013.
54. Torchia ME, Cofield RH. Total shoulder arthroplasty with the Neer prosthesis: long- term results. Orthop Trans. 1994–1995;18:977.
55. Brems J. The glenoid component in total shoulder arthroplasty. J Shoulder Elb Surg. 1993;2(1):47–54.
56. Collins D, Tencer A, Sidles J, Matsen F. Edge displacement and deformation of glenoid components in response to eccentric loading. The effect of preparation of the glenoid bone. J Bone Joint Surg Am. 1992;74:501–7.
57. Gallusser N, Farron A. Complications of shoulder arthroplasty for osteoarthritis with posterior glenoid wear. Orthop Traumatol Surg Res. 2014;100(5):503–8.
58. Wirth MA, Agrawal CM, Mabrey JD, Dean DD, Blanchard CR, Miller MA, Rockwood CA Jr. Isolation and characterization of polyethylene wear debris associated with osteolysis following total shoulder arthroplasty. J Bone Joint Surg Am. 1999;81:29–37.
59. Gartsman GM, Elkousy HA, Warnock KM, Edwards TB, O'Connor DP. Radiographic comparison of pegged and keeled glenoid components. J Shoulder Elbow. 2005;14:252–7.
60. Lazarus MD, Jensen KL, Southworth C, Matsen FA 3rd. The radiographic evaluation of keeled and pegged glenoid component insertion. J Bone Joint Surg Am. 2002;84:1174–82.
61. Wirth MA, Rockwood CA Jr. Complications of total shoulder-replacement arthroplasty. J Bone Joint Surg Am. 1996;78:603–16.
62. Boileau P, Avidor C, Krishnan SG, Walch G, Kempf JF, Molé D. Cemented polyethylene versus uncemented metal-backed glenoid components in total shoulder arthroplasty: a prospective, double-blind, randomized study. J Shoulder Elb Surg. 2002;11:351–9.
63. Martin SD, Zurakowski D, Thornhill TS. Uncemented glenoid component in total shoulder arthroplasty. Survivorship and outcomes. J Bone Joint Surg Am. 2005;87:1284–92.
64. Fox TJ, Cil A, Sperling JW, Sanchez-Sotelo J, Schleck CD, Cofield RH. Survival of the glenoid component in shoulder arthroplasty. J Shoulder Elb Surg. 2009;18:859–63.
65. Castagna A, Randelli M, Garofalo R, Maradei L, Giardella A, Borroni M. Mid-term results of a metal-backed glenoid component in total shoulder replacement. J Bone Joint Surg Br. 2010;92(10):1410–5.

66. Cheung EV, Sperling JW, Cofield RH. Revision shoulder arthroplasty for glenoid component loosening. J Should Elbow Surg. 2008;17(3):371–5.
67. Bonnevialle N, Melis B, Neyton L, Favard L, Molé D, Walch G, Boileau P. Aseptic glenoid loosening or failure in total shoulder arthroplasty: revision with glenoid re-implantation. J Should Elbow Surg. 2013;22(6):745–51.
68. Melis B, Bonnevialle N, Neyton L, Favard L, Molé D, Walch G, Boileau P. Glenoid loosening and failure in anatomical total shoulder arthroplasty: is revision with a reverse shoulder arthroplasty a reliable option? J Should Elbow Surg. 2012;21(3):342–9.
69. Boulahia A, Edwards TB, Walch G, Baratta RV. Early results of a reverse design prosthesis in the treatment of arthritis of the shoulder in elderly patients with a large rotator cuff tear. Orthopedics. 2002;25:129–33.
70. Frankle M, Siegal S, Pupello D, Saleem A, Mighell M, Vasey M. The reverse shoulder prosthesis for glenohumeral arthritis associated with severe rotator cuff deficiency. A minimum two-year follow-up study of sixty patients. J Bone Joint Surg Am. 2005;87:1697–705.
71. Nyffeler RW, Werner CM, Simmen BR, Gerber C. Analysis of a retrieved delta III total shoulder prosthesis. J Bone Joint Surg Br. 2004;86:1187–91.
72. Levy O, Tsvieli O, Merchant J, Young L, Trimarchi A, Dattani R, Abraham R, Copeland SA, Narvani A, Atoun E. Surface replacement arthroplasty for glenohumeral arthropathy in patients aged younger than fifty years: results after a minimum ten-year follow-up. J Shoulder Elb Surg. 2015;24(7):1049–60. https://doi.org/10.1016/j.jse.2014.11.035. Epub 2015 Jan 16
73. Herschel R, Wieser K, Morrey ME, Ramos CH, Gerber C, Meyer DC. Risk factors for glenoid erosion in patients with shoulder hemiarthroplasty: an analysis of 118 cases. J Shoulder Elb Surg. 2017;26(2):246–52. https://doi.org/10.1016/j.jse.2016.06.004. Epub 2016 Aug 18
74. Bohsali KI, Wirth MA, Rockwood CA Jr. Complications of total shoulder arthroplasty. J Bone Joint Surg Am. 2006;88:2279–92.
75. Matsen FA 3rd, Iannotti JP, Rockwood CA Jr. Humeral fixation by press-fitting of a tapered metaphyseal stem: a prospective radiographic study. J Bone Joint Surg Am. 2003;85:304–8.
76. Cil A, Veillette CJ, Sanchez-Sotelo J, Sperling JW, Schleck C, Cofield RH. Revision of the humeral component for aseptic loosening in arthroplasty of the shoulder. J Bone Joint Surg Br. 2009;91(1):75–81.
77. Sanchez-Sotelo J, Wright TW, O'Driscoll SW, Cofield RH, Rowland CM. Radiographic assessment of uncemented humeral components in total shoulder arthroplasty. J Arthroplast. 2001;16(2):180–7.
78. McElwain JP, English E. The early results of porous-coated total shoulder arthroplasty. Clin Orthop Relat Res. 1987;218:217–24.
79. Weiss AP, Adams MA, Moore JR, Weiland AJ. Unconstrained shoulder arthroplasty: a five-year average follow-up study. Clin Orthop Relat Res. 1990;257:86–90.
80. Sanchez-Sotelo J, O'Driscoll SW, Torchia ME, Cofield RH, Rowland CM. Radiographic assessment of cemented humeral components in shoulder arthroplasty. J Shoulder Elb Surg. 2001;10:526–31.
81. Sperling JW, Cofield RH, O'Driscoll SW, Torchia ME, Rowland CM. Radiographic assessment of ingrowth total shoulder arthroplasty. J Should Elbow Surg. 2002;9:507–13.
82. Raiss P, Edwards TB, Deutsch A, Shah A, Bruckner T, Loew M, Boileau P, Walch G. Radiographic changes around humeral components in shoulder arthroplasty. J Bone Joint Surg Am. 2014;96(7):e54.
83. Boileau P, Melis B, Duperron D, Moineau G, Rumian AP, Han Y. Revision surgery of reverse shoulder arthroplasty. J Shoulder Elb Surg. 2013;22(10):1359–70.
84. Phadnis J, Huang T, Watts A, Krishnan J, Bain GI. Cemented or cementless humeral fixation in reverse total shoulder arthroplasty? a systematic review. Bone Joint J. 2016;98 B(1):65–74.

Revision Shoulder Arthroplasty 24

Adam Seidl, Derek Axibal, Mikaël Chelli, and Pascal Boileau

Introduction

Described in 1983, Dr. Jules-Emile Pean performed the first glenohumeral joint arthroplasty to replace a shoulder damaged by tuberculosis [1, 2]. Since then, the indications for shoulder arthroplasty have expanded, including primary osteoarthritis, rotator cuff arthropathy, acute trauma, post-traumatic arthritis, inflammatory disease, osteonecrosis and tumors. In their epidemiological study of shoulder arthroplasty in the United States (US), Jain et al. found that primary shoulder arthroplasties increased from ~52,000 in 2009 to ~67,000 in 2011. In 2011, anatomic shoulder arthroplasties accounted for ~29,000 (44%), reverse shoulder arthroplasties comprised ~22,000 (32%), and hemiarthroplasties comprised ~16,000 (23%) [3]. Westermann et al. found similar numbers in the US in 2011 [4]. As the number of shoulder replacements continues to grow, so do the complications and need for subsequent revision surgeries. Unfortunately, complications after shoulder arthroplasty are not uncommon and oftentimes require revision surgery. Bohsali et al. found 404 complications in their analysis of 2540 shoulder arthroplasties (15.9%) [2]. Others have reported similar complication rates [5, 6]. Jain found that the number of revision cases increased from 5070 in 2009 to 6028 in 2011 in the US, accounting for ~8% of all cases. Labek found revision rates of 8% in Norway and 6% in New Zealand [7]. Slightly higher numbers were seen in Farvard's study in France, with a 11.2% revision rate in anatomic arthroplasties and 13.4% in reverse implants [8]. With an increase in the numbers of shoulder arthroplasties performed each year, it is important that shoulder surgeons recognize the common modes of failure and have strategies to address this failure with revision shoulder arthroplasty. This chapter outlines the different modes of failure for shoulder arthroplasty, including patient presentation and necessary investigations. Furthermore, this chapter discusses strategies and surgical techniques for revision shoulder arthroplasty and associated results.

A. Seidl (✉)
Division of Sports Medicine and Shoulder Surgery, University of Colorado, Aurora, CO, USA
e-mail: adam.seidl@ucdenver.edu

D. Axibal
Resident Physician, Department of Orthopaedic Surgery, University of Colorado, Aurora, CO, USA

M. Chelli
Department of Orthopaedics and Traumatology, University Hospital of Nice, Nice, France

P. Boileau
Department of Orthopaedics, University Institute of Locomotion and Sports, Pasteur 2 Hospital, Nice, France

I. A. Trail et al. (eds.), *Textbook of Shoulder Surgery*, https://doi.org/10.1007/978-3-319-70099-1_24

Background/Etiology

There are many possible causes of failure of shoulder arthroplasty that will lead to a need for revision surgery. These causes of failure can broadly be categorized in the following groups: infection, instability, aseptic loosening, rotator cuff insufficiency, arthrosis of the native glenoid in hemiarthroplasty, and periprosthetic fracture.

Infection

Although uncommon, infection after shoulder arthroplasty is a dreadful complication. The majority of infections after primary shoulder arthroplasty develop in the situation of previous shoulder surgery [9, 10], immunosuppression, such as diabetes, obesity, smoking [11], and alcoholism [12]. Other risk factors of infection include male gender, chemotherapy, systemic corticosteroid therapy, repeated intra-articular steroid injections, radiotherapy, rheumatoid arthritis, systemic lupus erythematosus, breach in sterile technique and hematoma [2, 13]. The prevalence of infection after total shoulder arthroplasty is about 1%, while the prevalence is between 3–5% for reverse total shoulder arthroplasty [2, 14]. There may be an even higher rate (0–19%) of infection following revision arthroplasty [15–18]. The most frequent organisms include *Propionibacterium acnes*, *Staphylococcus aureus*, and coagulase-negative Staphylococcus. While most species are identified in three to 4 days, *Propionibacterium acnes* species may require 10–14 days to ensure proper identification [13].

Instability

Stability of shoulder arthroplasty is conferred by appropriate soft tissue tensioning and correct implant sizing and positioning. Looking at anatomic shoulder arthroplasty, Bohsali found a prevalence of instability of 4% (124 of 3081 shoulders), comprising 30% of all complications [2].

Anterior instability after anatomic arthroplasty can be due to anterior glenoid deficiency, anterior deltoid muscle dysfunction, incorrect humeral component version, but most often is a result of subscapularis insufficiency [2, 6]. Subscapularis tears account for approximately half of all muscular/ tendon tears in anatomic shoulder arthroplasty [2]. In a report of 119 shoulder arthroplasties, Miller et al. found ruptures in seven patients (5.8%), all of which required surgical management [6]. Factors associated with subscapularis rupture include numerous previous surgeries, aggressive post-operative activity or rehabilitation (specifically external rotation), and overstuffing the joint. Excessive humeral anteversion can also lead to anterior instability [19]. This can lead to eccentric loading, wear, glenoid loosening, and subscapularis failure.

Posterior instability after anatomic arthroplasty can be the result of several factors. It can be caused by excessive glenoid retroversion [20], excessive humeral retroversion, posterior glenoid loss and soft-tissue imbalances [2].

Although uncommon, inferior instability in anatomic arthroplasty can result from failure to reestablish humeral length [2, 21]. Shortening the proximal humerus results in weakening of the deltoid lever arm, and leads to pain and loss of motion [19].

The rate of instability following reverse shoulder arthroplasty has been reported from 2.4% to 31% [13]. In describing instability after reverse shoulder arthroplasty, Affonso divided causes into three categories: patient factors, surgical factors, and design factors [22]. Patient factors that lead to instability include previous surgery, deltoid dysfunction, and those unable to comply with post-operative instructions. Surgical factors include approach and inadequate tensioning of the implants [22]. Though reports are variable, the rate of instability may be influenced by the surgical approach; Boileau et al. showed the deltopectoral approach results in a 6% rate of instability while a superolateral approach results in a 0% rate of instability [23]. Design factors such as glenosphere offset and size, humeral neck-shaft angle, and thickness of the humeral insert can also effect stability [13].

Rotator Cuff Insufficiency

The spectrum of rotator cuff pathology ranges from single tendon tear to massive tear, and is a major cause of failure in anatomic total shoulder arthroplasty and hemiarthroplasty.

Rotator cuff insufficiency may be present preoperatively, or may be iatrogenic occurring intra-operatively during the more technical aspects of surgery. Specifically, the rotator cuff is at risk during excision of the humeral head; especially if an exceedingly large fragment is excised, or excision of the head occurs in too much retroversion [14].

Rotator cuff insufficiency leading to failure of anatomic arthroplasty is characterized by large or massive rotator cuff tear, loss of the cuff force vector compressing the humeral head, superior migration of the humeral head and resultant loosening of the glenoid component [14, 24]. The imbalance between (1) the loss of compressive force of the rotator cuff and (2) a continued deltoid contraction force leads to superior migration of the humeral head, eccentric loading on the glenoid and subsequent glenoid loosening [2]. Franklin et al. described the "rocking horse" phenomena: superior displacement of the humeral head causing tipping and subsequent loosening of the glenoid component [25]. In their study, they found an association between rotator cuff deficiency and glenoid loosening.

Implant Loosening

Glenoid Component

Glenoid component failure may range from distortion of the polyethylene surface to minimal loosening to significant migration with subsequent bone loss [26]. It is the most common complication of total shoulder arthroplasty and is the cause of the majority unsatisfactory results [27]. In an analysis of 2540 shoulder arthroplasties, glenoid loosening comprised 5.3% of all shoulders and 32% of all complications [2]. There are many causes for the failure of the glenoid component. In his review article of glenoid component failure, Matsen et al. categorized this as failure of the component itself, failure of seating and fixation, failure the glenoid bone, or failure to manage eccentric loading [27].

Failure of the component includes distortion of the surface. Distortion can occur when the prosthetic and humeral articular surfaces are nonconforming (humeral component diameter is smaller compared to glenoid component), causing a concavity of the glenoid component. If the surfaces are conforming (have the same diameter of curvature), loading and flattening of the glenoid component occurs. Distortion caused by pitting (secondary to particles of bone, polyethylene or cement) can also occur. With the use of a metal-backed glenoid prosthesis, there is increased wear compared to all polyethylene components, possibly due to higher contact stresses. Furthermore, there is a risk of separation of the polyethylene surface from the metal backing. Fracture of any parts of the glenoid component (poly, pegs, keel, metal backing, or fixation screws) also cause failure of the component [27].

Failure of the component seating can occur with inadequate bone surface preparation resulting in wobble (movement) and warp (bending) of the component. Concentric reaming minimizes the effects of eccentric loading, and can therefore minimize wobble and warp. Malpositioning and cement failure both may cause seating failure. Studies have suggested that component seating can also be more problematic with keeled components compared to pegged components [27]. In Anglin et al.'s study comparing glenoid prosthesis designs after cycling a humeral head 100,000 times, pegged designs showed less displacement and outperformed keeled glenoids [28]. In Lazarus et al.'s radiographic evaluation of 328 shoulder arthroplasties, radiolucencies and incompetent seating were more frequently associated with keel designs compared to pegged designs [29].

Failure of component fixation occurs with suboptimal cement techniques (such as unsuccessfully penetrating into cancellous bone, or retained fluid or clot between the cement and bone). Poor bone quality also limits fixation. This is seen with disuse, age, inflammatory disease, excessive reaming, and previous arthroplasty [27].

Glenoid bone loss can occur with resorption from micromotion, infection, or heat produced by drilling or cement [27]. It has also been hypothesized that an immunological response to the polyethylene can cause increased bone resorption. Furthermore, polyethylene wear particles can lead to osteolysis [27].

Glenoid component failure can also occur with an inability to manage eccentric loading. As previously mentioned, conforming surfaces refer to when the glenoid and humeral articular surfaces have the same diameter of curvature. When these conforming surfaces are in contact, translational and eccentric forces are transmitted to the glenoid-bone interface. Furthermore, eccentric loading at the humeral head- glenoid interface can lead to the previously discussed rocking-horse phenomenon: inferior placement of the glenoid component, superior placement of the humeral component or superior subluxation seen with rotator cuff deficiency leads to eccentric loading, and thus tipping and loosening of the glenoid component. Any alteration in component version (retroversion, anteversion, superior or inferior tilt) or glenohumeral instability (rotator cuff/ subscapularis deficiency or other reasons) cause eccentric loading, as well [27].

Humeral Component

In an analysis of 2540 shoulder arthroplasties, humeral loosening comprised only 1% of all shoulders but 7% of all complications [27]. In their study of 127 shoulders, Matsen found radiolucent lines in seventy-seven (61%) patients, with seventy-five of those appearing at the distal tip of the humeral step. At 3 years postoperatively, no shoulders demonstrated subsidence or a shift [30]. Sperling studied sixty-two total shoulder prostheses, and classified humeral components as “at risk” if they demonstrated radiographic tilt, subsidence or 2.0 millimeter radiolucent lines. With 4.6 years follow-up, six (9.6%) were considered to be “at risk.” Only one of these sixty-two (0.016%) required revision due of symptomatic humeral component loosening [31].

Periprosthetic radiolucent lines are more frequently seen with press-fit humeral stems [30, 32]. In a study of forty humeral replacements, radiolucent lines were seen in twenty. Surgical approach, humeral component position, implant design or glenoid resurfacing were not correlated with the presence of radiolucent lines or with a component loosening. Cementless fixation was the only factor statistically correlated with the presence of radiolucent lines: all eleven of the cementless, press-fit humeral stems displayed radiolucent lines. However, no revisions were necessary [32].

In reverse arthroplasties, the main risk factor for humeral loosening is proximal bone loss, frequently seen after arthroplasty for acute fracture, fracture sequelae, or tumor resection. Indeed, the greater tuberosity may be migrated posteriorly or absent, due to lysis or resection. The humeral stem is then fixed only distally into the shaft and undergoes considerable rotational stress, leading to loosening and/or modular implant unscrewing [18].

Arthrosis of Native Glenoid After Hemiarthroplasty

Glenoid erosion is one of the main concerns specific to shoulder hemiarthroplasty [33]. It occurs secondary to the hard metallic prosthetic component eroding into the softer bone of the glenoid [26]. In their series of 118 hemiarthroplasties, Hershel et al. found unfavorable factors for glenoid erosion to be the presence of glenoid cysts, fatty infiltration of the rotator cuff and damaged glenoid cartilage. Glenoid erosion was also associated with female patients (three times more frequent in women), rheumatoid arthritis, and a valgus prosthetic head relative to the glenoid (>50°). They also found that fracture situation was favorable: only one of thirty patients with a fracture-type prosthesis developed progressive glenoid erosion. Age, glenoid version, and the size of the head showed no importance [33].

Erosion of the glenoid can be peripheral or central. If the rotator cuff is not intact, the erosion is most commonly superior, or less commonly if the subscapularis is deficient, then erosion is anterior [26].

Periprosthetic Fracture

Periprosthetic fractures can be classified as intraoperative and postoperative fractures. Bohsali et al. reported a combined rate of 1.8% periprosthetic fractures from 1996–2005. This comprises about 11% (forty-six) of the total 414 complications. Of these forty-six perioperative fractures, intraoperative fractures accounted for 59% (27) postoperative fractures accounted for 41% (19) [2]. Cofield et al. found similar results regarding intraoperative rates (62%) and postoperative rates (38%). They also reported that the vast majority of fractures involved the humerus (86%) while a smaller number of fractures involve the glenoid (12%) [14].

Intraoperative humeral fractures may occur with excessive manipulation or during instrumentation. Humeral spiral fractures occur secondary to significant torsional influences produced during humeral external rotation. After the humeral head is resected, cortical perforation may occur with incorrect placement of the reamer or prosthetic if the arm is not fully extended off the side of the operating table. If the initial reamer or trial stem is not eccentrically positioned in the superolateral aspect of the proximal humerus, then medial cortex perforation can result [2, 24]. Overzealous reaming and aggressive impaction can also cause intraoperative humeral fracture [14].

In a study of 2588 shoulder arthroplasties, seventy-seven glenoid fractures were initially identified from the joint registry. However, after further chart review, sixty of those were found to be glenoid fenestration. Twelve glenoid fractures occurred intraoperatively while five glenoid fractures occurred postoperatively [34]. The majority of intraoperative glenoid fractures are caused by failure to start the reamer before making contact with the glenoid bone, and reaming osteoporotic glenoid beyond the subchondral bone [13].

Postoperative periprosthetic humeral fractures have been classified by Worland et al. as type A: about the tuberosity; type B, about the stem; and type C, distal to the stem tip. Subclassification includes B1 fractures, spiral fractures with a stable implant; B2 fractures, transverse or short oblique fractures about the tip of the stem with a stable implant; and B3 fractures, fractures about the stem with an unstable implant [19].

> **Clinical Pearl**
> Primary shoulder arthroplasty surgery is not without risk, as complications are relatively common (6–16%) and oftentimes require revision surgery.

Presentation, Investigations and Treatment Options

Infection

The initial clinical symptom of shoulder periprosthetic infection is usually pain, but could also include fevers, chills, nightsweats, erythema, drainage, induration, fluctuance, or effusion. It is recommended to obtain laboratory work including white blood cell count, C-reactive protein level, and erythrocyte sedimentation rate. If clinical suspicion warrants, guided joint aspiration must be performed or a biopsy specimen collected.

Unfortunately, negative pre-operative laboratory data and aspiration results do not exclude infection. In fact, multiple studies have shown the rate of positive intra-operative cultures at the time of revision for a failed arthroplasty presumed not to be infected is quite high [35]. Topolski et al. looked at tissue samples from 439 revision cases with no clinical suspicion of infection and normal pre-operative lab values and discovered 17% of cases had at least one positive culture (out of six performed) [36].

Infections of shoulder arthroplasty may be classified as acute (occurring less than 3 months after surgery), subacute (occurring 3 months to 1 year), or late (occurring more than 1 year after surgery) [2].

Following suit of the total knee and hip arthroplasty guidelines, acute infection is can be managed with irrigation, débridement, and polyethylene or prosthetic exchange. Chronic infection is usually treated with a two-stage revision. The first stage consists of hardware removal, irrigation and débridement, and placement of an antibiotic spacer. The patient is given a minimum of 6 weeks of IV antibiotics. After an "antibiotic holiday," or a short period of time when the IV antibiotics are not administered, the patient is then reevaluated with blood markers and/or aspiration. If the patient is determined to be eradicated of the infection, the patient undergoes stage two: prosthesis reimplantation [13].

Instability

In most cases of instability, patients present with pain and weakness with or without gross instability. In the setting of a subscapularis rupture, physical exam reveals excessive external rotation, weakness or pain with internal rotation, and a positive lift-off or belly-press test. In the case of posterior instability, examination may reveal excessive internal rotation. With inferior instability, patients are unable to raise their arm above the horizontal plane secondary to the inadequate humeral length [2]. Establishing a diagnosis requires elevated clinical suspicion. MRI is not reliable secondary to metal artifact. Computed Tomography with arthrogram is our preferred study and can help determine soft tissue compromise, implant loosening or malpositioning in the horizontal plane (humeral/ glenoid version) or vertical plane (too high humeral/ glenoid component) [23].

In the setting of subscapularis rupture, timing of diagnosis relative to the arthroplasty helps dictate treatment. If detected early and quality tissue and a mobile subscapularis are present, then a direct repair can be performed. Without a sufficient lateral tendinous stump to allow direct soft-tissue repair, then a repair into a bony trough can be performed. If diagnosed late, poor tissue and anterior instability is often present. In this situation a pectoralis major tendon transfer can be used to augment the repair, but results of this strategy, in general, have been poor [37]. In Miller's study of seven patients with subscapularis ruptures after shoulder arthroplasty, four patients needed a pec major transfer secondary to tissue quality and anterior instability [6]. In Elhassan et al.'s study of subscapularis failures after shoulder arthroplasty, all eight failures revealed irreparable tissue which he also treated with pec major transfers [38]. A bone-Achilles allograft has been described as a second revision option [37]. In the setting of posterior instability, correction of the instability can include revision of malpositioned implants with restoration of the normal humeral retroversion, and/or posterior capsuloprraphy [39]. In the setting of inferior instability, it is necessary to restore humeral length.

Instability of reverse shoulder arthroplasty is more common than anatomic arthroplasty. If dislocation occurs early (with the first 6 weeks) without concern for malpositioned components, closed reduction should be attempted. If malpositioning or loosening of the humeral or glenoid component is suspected, it must be revised. In the setting of late or recurrent instability with well-placed components, inadequate tension is often the issue. Options to increase tension and stability include: use of thicker or more constrained polyethylene, and/or use of a larger or more lateralized glenosphere [23].

Rotator Cuff Insufficiency

Patients with rotator cuff insufficiency present with pain, decreased strength, decreased motion, and anterior-superior escape. MRI once again is less reliable secondary to artifact, so physical exam and a high degree of suspicion are required. In their systematic review of rotator cuff tears after total shoulder arthroplasty, Levy et al. found that after 6.6 years, about 30% of patients showed superior humeral head migration and about 18% migrated a distance more than 25% of the humeral head. They found that a radiographic superiorly migrated humeral head was the most commonly reported indicator of rotator cuff integrity [40]. CT scan and x-ray may show glenoid loosening, while CT scan also reveals atrophy of the rotator cuff muscle bellies.

If the rotator cuff is injured during surgery, an attempt to repair the injured tendon is necessary. Tearing of the rotator cuff following shoulder arthroplasty in the post-operative period is said reflect the natural history of rotator cuff disease in the general population. In their study of 268 shoulder arthroplasties with post-operative rotator tears, Godeneche et al. found that these tears or fatty degeneration was inversely related to strength, motion and satisfaction [41]. Therefore, an attempt to treat these tears is made, whether operative or nonoperative [14].

In the case of superior instability or glenoid loosening in a patient with a hemiarthroplasty or total shoulder, revision to a constrained, reverse total shoulder arthroplasty may be indicated.

Implant Loosening

Patients with glenoid or humeral loosening present with pain and loss of function and possibly an audible or sense of clunking [42, 43]. With high quality radiographs and acknowledging patient symptoms and presentation, it is often feasible to diagnose glenoid or humeral component failure without the need to obtain more invasive studies. CT, however, is undoubtedly helpful in the analysis: it can assess bone loss around the implants [8]. Arthrography may be helpful. Arthrography can not only delineate the rotator cuff and display synovitis, but the dye can trace between any loose inter-faces. Shoulder arthroscopy has also been proposed a way to directly visualize and diagnose component loosening [44].

Glenoid Component

In the setting of glenoid loosening, standard x-rays of the shoulder do not always show the bone/implant interfaces well, especially if there is metal backing. However, the forty-degree posterior oblique view can help evaluate the bone/implant interface. As with most pathology, change in component position can be seen best with a sequence of radiographs, rather than a single x-ray taken at one point in time [44]. Although progressive glenoid radiolucent lines are alleged to be indicators of component loosening, these radiolucent lines are not definitive indicators of ultimate loosening or poor outcomes [45]. Imaging that reveals migration, tilt, shift of the component or compete radiolucent lines greater than 1.5 millimeters in thickness have been used as markers of glenoid failure [46].

Options for glenoid loosening include isolated glenoid removal without reimplantation, isolated glenoid bone grafting, glenoid component reimplantation in one or two stages, and reverse total shoulder arthroplasty. When the glenoid component has failed, revision surgery options are highly contingent upon the glenoid bone stock and surrounding soft tissue integrity [45]. Therefore, the surgeon must first decide whether or not to reconstruct the osseous glenoid. In a debilitated patient whose main goal is pain relief without significant concern for function, isolated removal of the glenoid component without osseous reconstruction is a reasonable option. In other patients, glenoid reconstruction (i.e.- with iliac crest bone graft) is indicated. In the setting of revision surgery with an unconstrained prosthesis, Gartsman et al. reconstructed the glenoid with bone graft in the first stage. Six months later in the second stage, after complete incorporation of the bone graft, a new glenoid component was placed. In the setting of revision surgery with a reverse total shoulder prosthesis, glenoid reconstruction and revision may be performed in one stage, on condition that the revision glenoid component central post is confidently seated in native glenoid bone [26].

The above techniques have been accomplished via open procedures. In 2005, O'Driscroll et al. described five patients who underwent arthroscopic conversion of TSA to hemiarthroplasty via removal of symptomatic loose glenoid components and the underlying cement mantle. Each patient had relative contraindications to reimplantation or performance of a major surgery (massive obesity, severe medical comorbidities, difficult exposure at primary surgery, and large rotator cuff tear/ superior instability) [47]. In 2011, Namdari et al. described arthroscopic conversion of TSA to hemiarthroplasty with removal of the glenoid component along with bone grafting of the glenoid defect [48].

Humeral Component

Standard shoulder x-rays may not reveal loosening. Cil et al. described a 40-degree posterior oblique radiograph with the humerus in external rotation, 40-degree posterior oblique radiograph with the humerus in internal rotation, and an axillary view for analysis [49]. Furthermore, humeral loosening may be best seen with sequential radiographs. Imaging may reveal migration, subsidence, tilting or a combination of the three [49]. Sperling et al. classified humeral components as "at risk" for loosening if they demonstrated radiographic tilt, subsidence or 2.0 millimeter radiolucent lines [31].

Similar to glenoid loosening, when the humeral component has failed, revision surgery options are highly contingent upon bone stock. Contained defects in bone stock of the proximal humerus can be effectively treated with bone grafts. Filling bone defects with cement may also help add security to the fixation of the humeral component. However, extensive humeral deficiency and uncontained proximal humeral bone loss may require a proximal humeral replacement [49].

Arthrosis of Native Glenoid After Hemiarthroplasty

Initially, the only and main complaint in glenoid erosion may be pain. However, as the erosion advances medially, the rotator cuff length-tension relationship changes and ends in significant weakness. Radiographs will demonstrate osseous glenoid erosion, but CT will help with preoperative planning [26].

Similar to the situation of glenoid component loosening, glenoid erosion options depend on the glenoid bone stock. If there is sufficient native glenoid bone, then resurfacing of the glenoid with a glenoid component is reasonable; the humeral head component may be exchanged for a smaller head size. If the rotator cuff function is compromised and there is insufficient glenoid bone stock, then revision to a reverse prosthesis is indicated. As stated earlier, reverse shoulder arthroplasty provides the ability to providing stability and the option to reconstruct glenoid bone stock in one stage.

Periprosthetic Fractures

In general, most intraoperative fractures during shoulder arthroplasty can be prevented. With preoperative planning, osteopenia and potential stress-risers should be acknowledged. Forces across the osseous structures can be reduced by appropriate release of scar and capsular contractures [31].

For intraoperative humeral fractures, cerclage wiring has been recommended for fractures proximal to the stem tip. Fractures that occur distal to the implant tip require a long-stemmed prosthesis. The prosthesis should extend at least two humeral cortical diameters beyond the most distal aspect of the fracture [2].

For postoperative periprosthetic humeral fractures, fractures proximal to the stem tip, fractures with acceptable alignment at the tip of a well-fixed humeral stem, and fractures distal to the stem with appropriate alignment, should have a trial of nonoperative management. It has been recommended that fractures at the stem tip that do not heal within 3 months be treated with open reduction internal fixation. If the humeral component is loose/ unstable, revision with a long stem is advised [2, 50].

Revision Shoulder Arthroplasty Surgical Technique

Pre-operative Planning

Specific pre-operative imaging studies have been described in the previous section. Particular attention should be paid to bone deficiencies that are present or may be present after implant removal. If severe bone loss is expected, allograft bone must be readily available. In situations with glenoid bone loss, patient must be educated and prepared for iliac crest autogenous grafting. With regard to revision equipment, it is important to have knowledge of the implant being removed and have available implant-specific instrumentation for extraction. Humeral stem removal can be very difficult and necessary equipment may include: flexible osteotomes, oscillating saw, a high speed burr, cerclage wires, and cement extraction tools. In the setting of removing a well-fixed cemented, it is important to have long humeral stems available in case a periprosthetic fracture occurs or when segmental bone loss is present.

Surgical Exposure

Revision shoulder arthroplasty is performed with the patient in the beach-chair position with the cervical spine in neutral position. General and regional anesthesia are used in all cases. In cases where infection is suspected, antibiotics are held until adequate fluid and tissue samples are collected, otherwise antibiotics are administered within 30 min of incision. Choice of incision location can be difficult in the revision setting, as one or more previous incisions may be present. There is typically a scar from previous deltopectoral approach that can be incorporated. If it is felt that the previous incision is far from the desired location, it is generally safe to make another incision as wound healing complications are rare given the excellent vascularity of the shoulder girdle.

In our practice, the deltopectoral approach is used for all revision arthroplasty exposures. Others have described and advocated an anterosuperior approach with release of anterior deltoid off the clavicle and acromion for more complex cases, but in our experience this is rarely necessary [51].

In the revision setting, the deltopectoral interval is not always apparent due to scar tissue and the possibility of a diminutive cephalic vein. In this situation, we advocate using the coracoid process proximally to establish the interval. Additionally, there is typically an area devoid of muscle on the anterior clavicle at the proximal extent of the incision that can be identified. Dissection is then carried distally with care taken to identify and retract laterally the cephalic vein, if patent. Often times there is significant scarring and the vein cannot be identified if it was injured during previous surgical exposures. A portion of pectoralis major tendon can be released to help exposure.

Once deltopectoral interval has been established, subdeltoid and subacromial space is developed. This is often much more difficult in the revision setting and requires meticulous dissection through scar tissue. The deltoid is often adhered to underlying bone or bursal tissue. It is often easiest to define the subdeltoid space distally in the incision along the lateral humerus and carry dissection proximally. Great care must be taken to avoid dissection into the deltoid as the axillary nerve and posterior humeral circumflex artery sit on the undersurface to the muscle. Establishing the subacromial space proximally can also be difficult given dense adhesions often present. It is important to correctly develop the planes to avoid injury to any intact underlying rotator cuff. Complete release of the subdeltoid and subacromial space is crucial for successful revision arthroplasty.

Deep exposure starts with releasing the clavipectoral fascia. Careful blunt dissection is then performed to develop the plane between the conjoined tendon superficially and the deep subscapularis and/or capsular tissue. Establishing this interval allows for localization of the axillary nerve. Patience and cautious dissection should be utilized to clearly identify the axillary nerve and allow for palpation throughout the case.

Once the axillary nerve has been identified, the bicipital groove is identified and defined to identify its borders, the greater and lesser tuberosities. Using these landmarks, dissection is carried through the rotator interval until the glenoid is reached. The subscapularis is then released to expose the prosthesis and glenohumeral joint. Subscapularis release can be performed with a peel, tenotomy, or osteotomy of the lesser tuberosity. In our experience, a subscapularis peel allows the most flexibility for repair in the revision setting, especially when converting from an anatomic implant to a reverse shoulder arthroplasty.

Humeral-sided capsular release is performed as the arm is externally rotated, adducted, and flexed to visualize the entire humeral calcar. This release can be extended distally, staying directly on bone, to the level of latissimus tendon. Once proper release has been performed, the humeral

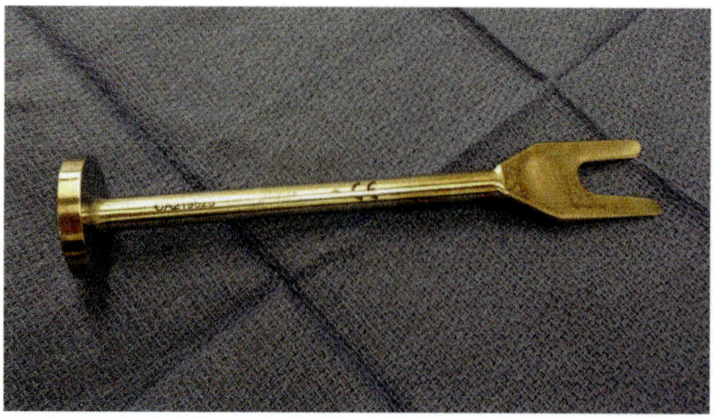

Fig. 24.1 Tuning-fork instrument to remove the modular humeral head

prosthesis can be dislocated for humeral head removal. The majority of modern humeral implants are modular, allowing for removal of the humeral head and permitting the surgeon to retain the humeral stem, either temporarily or definitively. A tuning-fork instrument (Fig. 24.1) and/or osteotomes are used for removal of the modular humeral head.

Removal of Humeral Component

Several contemporary implants were designed to be convertible (from anatomic to RSA or RSA to hemiarthroplasty), so removal of the humeral stem is not always necessary. Given the relatively recent introduction of convertible implants, most revisions today involve non-convertible implants and humeral stem removal is required.

It is crucial to have available proper instruments for successful humeral stem removal and to minimize bone loss and chance of fracture. These instruments include: flexible osteotomes, oscillating saw, a high-speed burr, cerclage wires, and cement extraction tools. Aseptic loosening of the humeral stem is rare; most stems encountered are relatively well-fixed and can be extremely difficult to remove.

Initial steps for humeral stem removal are aimed at disrupting the bonds at the cement-stem or bone-stem interface. This can be accomplished using thin flexible osteotomes. Care should be taken to stay directly adjacent to the implant with the osteotome in order to avoid cortical perforation or iatrogenic fracture. Circumferential freeing of the stem is necessary before implant extraction is attempted. Implant extraction is performed using the implant-specific extraction tool when possible. Alternatively, use of a mallet and tamp placed at the medial aspect of a collared implant can help in extracting the stem. If using this technique, it is critical to avoid a rotational force through the tamp and mallet, as this can lead to fracture of the humerus.

In situations where the aforementioned techniques are unsuccessful for stem extraction, an osteotomy is necessary. Several different techniques have been described for creating an osteotomy for humeral stem removal. Our preference is to create a single osteotomy placed 2–3 mm posterior to the bicipital groove using a micro-saggital saw. The osteotomy should extend superiorly to exit the greater tuberosity and inferiorly to the top of the deltoid insertion. This osteotomy is then expanded using an osteotome until it makes contact with the metal of the prosthesis. The osteotome is taken to this depth throughout the entire length of the osteotomy and the prosthesis is extracted as previously described with a tamp and mallet.

Rarely, a single osteotomy as described is unsuccessful in removing the humeral stem. In these situations, a cortical window is required. To make a cortical window, a transverse cut is made in the humerus starting at the previously placed osteotomy is extending posteriorly. A large osteotome is then used with a twisting motion along its long axis to dilate the osteotomy (Fig. 24.2). Finally, a Cobb elevator is placed into the osteotome at multiple levels and twisted, allowing the humerus to crack longitudinally and hinge open to allow adequate access to loosen the prosthesis.

In the case of an aseptic cemented humeral stem that was removed without requiring an osteotomy, cementing a smaller stem into the previous cement mantle is preferred. In cases where an osteotomy or window was used, or cases of infection, cement will need to be removed. Cement removal can be performed using standard instruments and/or an ultrasonic cement

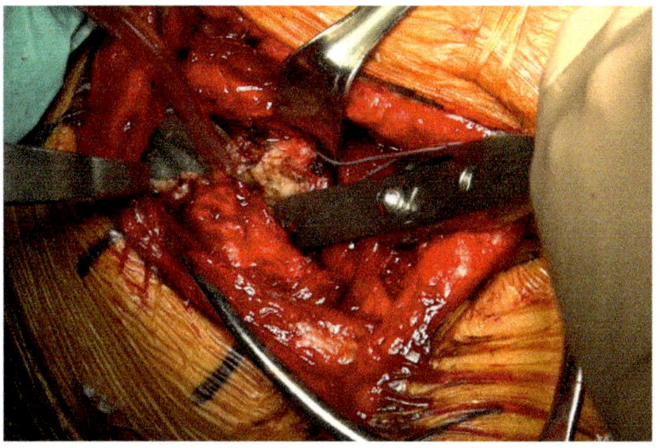

Fig. 24.2 Humeral osteotomy

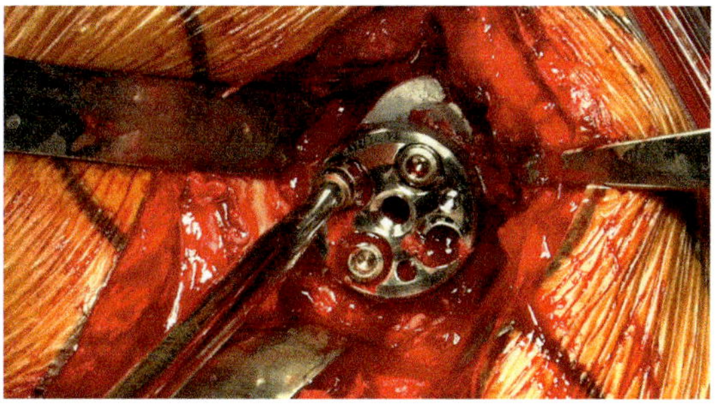

Fig. 24.3 RSA screwed in TSA glenoid and native glenoid bone

removal device. Care should be taken when using this device below the level of the deltoid insertion as thermal injuries to the radial nerve have been reported [52]. Intraoperative radiographs are useful when removing cement to confirm intramedullary placement of instrument and complete removal of cement.

In the setting of either a single osteotomy or a cortical window, we find it useful to pass multiple heavy double-limbed sutures around the humerus prior creating the osteotomy. This allows for easy repair of the osteotomy or cortical window once the implant is extracted. Alternatively, one can use cerclage wires for repair.

Depending on the indication for revision surgery, extensive glenoid exposure may or may not be necessary. In the setting of an aseptic well-fixed glenoid component, humeral revision alone may be performed. However, this situation represents the minority of revision cases and glenoid exposure is often required.

Removal of Glenoid Component

Though arthroscopic glenoid removal in conversion from anatomic total shoulder to hemiarthroplasty has been described in the literature [47, 48], this section will focus on open revision. Once the humeral head or entire humeral prosthesis has been removed, glenoid exposure can commence. Prior dissection and localization of the axillary nerve allows safe retractor placement for protection of the nerve during capsular release. The anterior and inferior joint capsule and corresponding glenohumeral ligaments (superior, middle, inferior) are released. If prolonged glenoid work is anticipated, it is important to periodically change the arm position to neutral and remove retractors to release tension on the brachial plexus. It may be beneficial to have available multiple options for glenoid retractors as subtle differences can help optimize exposure and visualization.

The most common scenario will be revision for failed anatomic arthroplasty with an all-polyethylene glenoid component. When removing a glenoid component, care should be taken to preserve as much glenoid bone stock as possible. In most situations, a small, thin osteotome can be used to shear the glenoid face from its underlying keel or pegs. Remaining polyethylene and cement can then be removed using a combination of osteotomes and currettes. In the setting of aseptic revision to reverse shoulder arthroplasty, it is not always necessary to remove polyethylene or cement that is outside planned baseplate peg or screw trajectory (Fig. 24.3). If any concern for infection exists, all material must be removed.

Revision to Anatomic Shoulder Arthroplasty

Critical assessment of glenoid bone loss and remaining bone stock must be performed. Additionally, evaluation of the rotator cuff should take place as a lack of a functional rotator cuff precludes re-implantation of an anatomic implant.

In patients with glenoid erosion after hemiarthroplasty and a functional rotator cuff, implantation of a glenoid component can be performed using similar methods to primary unconstrained arthroplasty. It is recommended that cemented polyethylene components have 100% bony support to prevent early loosening [53]. In situations of moderate to severe glenoid bone loss, the surgeon may deem in impossible to re-implant a polyethylene glenoid. In these scenarios, options include: bone grafting of the glenoid and conversion to hemiarthroplasty, reverse shoulder arthroplasty, or resection arthroplasty.

Management of glenoid bone loss and re-implantation of a polyethylene component can be performed in a single-stage or two-stage fashion. In patients with very small, manageable bone defects, single stage re-implantation may be possible. In all other cases, our preference is to perform two-stage re-implantation allowing time for bone graft incorporation and confirmation with computed tomography. Depending on the location of the defect, iliac crest autograft, allograft chips, or bulk allograft can be used. Our preference is to use structural autogenous iliac crest graft in most situations, as use of allograft results in a high rate of graft subsidence and medialization of the humeral head [54, 55]. Methods for glenoid reconstruction depend largely on the area of bone deficiency, and whether the defect is contained or uncontained.

In cases with central, contained bone loss, it is often possible to fashion the bone graft for interference fit and, thus, eliminate the need for internal fixation. For contained defects with planned interference-fit bone grafting, the remaining glenoid surface is defined and lightly abraded with a burr to provide a surface that will promote graft incorporation. Tricortical iliac crest bone graft is fashioned with a rongeur to obtain a shape to match the defect. The cancellous bone is placed medially in the defect with the cortical surface facing laterally. The bone graft is then impacted until it sits flush with the intact glenoid surface.

In cases with peripheral, uncontained bone loss, it is necessary to secure the bone graft with internal fixation to prevent migration and failure. In these situations, the tricortical iliac crest is again contoured to fit the defect and positioned with the cortical surface facing laterally. Given the absence of bony support for the graft, screw fixation is necessary. Cannulated screws can be useful as they allow provision fixation and assessment of graft placement with their guide wires. Care is taken to place the screws outside the central portion of the glenoid vault, which could prohibit later placement of a glenoid component. Addressing bone loss involving the posterior rim of the glenoid may necessitate percutaneous placement of screws through the bone graft into native glenoid, whereas bone loss involving the anterior glenoid rim typically involves placement of screws through the deltopectoral incision.

We routinely avoid simultaneous implantation of an anatomic glenoid component when performing bone graft reconstruction of the glenoid. Staged implantation of the glenoid component only occurs after graft incorporation and restoration of sufficient bone stock is confirmed by computed tomography, which is typically ordered at 6 months.

An additional alternative option for revision to anatomic arthroplasty involves the use of an uncemented in-growth component with screw fixation. Yet, this implant design is rarely used in primary arthroplasty due to accelerated polyethylene wear and high loosening rates [56], it may serve a role in the revision setting when other options are not practical.

Revision to Reverse Shoulder Arthroplasty

Reverse shoulder arthroplasty (RSA) affords an excellent option to surgeons dealing with failed shoulder arthroplasty. Previously, there was not a reliable option for patients with failed arthroplasty in the setting of rotator cuff dysfunction and/or significant bone loss. The increased constraint of the reverse prosthesis allows for function even in the face of significant soft tissue compromise. In most situations, the robust fixation and in-growth potential of the baseplate allows for single-stage reconstruction with bone grafting. Additionally, baseplate fixation and stability does not require 100% bony support that is necessary for an anatomic glenoid component. One contraindication for revision to reverse shoulder arthroplasty is deltoid dysfunction, either in the setting of deltoid dehiscence or axillary nerve injury. In patients with dysfunctional anterior deltoid but competent middle and posterior deltoid, reverse shoulder arthroplasty may still be an option, but expectations of optimal functional results should be tempered [57].

The surgical technique for revision of failed arthroplasty to reverse shoulder involves the same principles for exposure described earlier. With RSA, release of the supraspinatus tendon, when present, can significantly improve exposure. With regard to glenoid exposure, the capsule must be released at the inferior glenoid to the level of the triceps origin. Thorough release allows for visualization of the true inferior glenoid rim for appropriate baseplate placement.

Glenoid Bone Loss

Glenoid bone loss is frequently encountered when performing RSA for revision arthroplasty. Unlike primary arthroplasty cases with bone loss, in the revision setting, autograft humeral head is not available. In cases with mild bone central bone loss, non-structural autograft or allograft bone can be used. In cases of moderate or severe bone loss, often involving one or more of the glenoid walls, structural bone graft is necessary. In these cases, options include iliac crest autograft and various types of allograft [58–60]. When performing single-stage RSA with glenoid bone grafting, it is crucial to have the baseplate central post or screw penetrate and capture native glenoid bone. Surgeons must have available a long stem or screwed baseplate option to ensure this is possible (Fig. 24.4).

Once the glenoid is exposed, a threaded guidewire is inserted into the glenoid vault, a step aided with preoperative image templating (possibly patient specific instrumentation). The guidewire is inserted at a level where baseplate will sit flush with the inferior border of the glenoid or slightly lower, and our preference is to angle inferiorly by 10°. A small reamer is then used to abrade the glenoid until the subchondral plate is reached (typically about 5 mm), taking care not to ream excessively. In cases of severe glenoid bone loss, the circular reamer will often not be flush with the glenoid; in these scenarios, unreamed areas are abraded with a burr. The central peg hole is then drilled and small peripheral drill holes are made using the threaded guidewire to attain a complete bleeding bone surface. The goal of the glenoid preparation is to reach cancellous bleeding bone to provide an environment for bone graft incorporation and healing. Once glenoid preparation is completed, bone graft is fashioned and implanted with the baseplate.

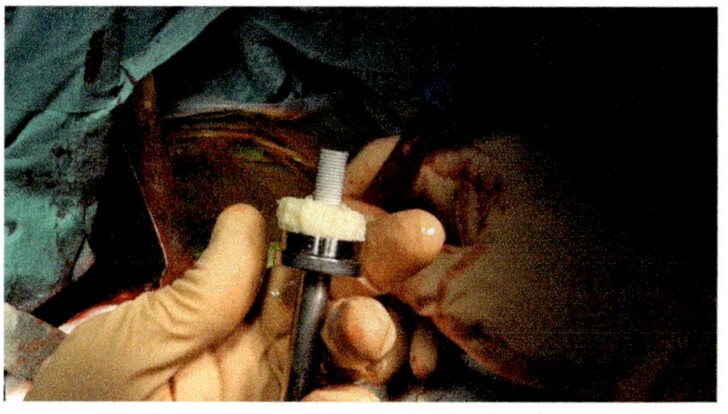

Fig. 24.4 Long peg glenoid baseplate

Our preferred technique for harvesting and contouring iliac crest has been described by Norris et al. [60]. This technique involves implanting the long peg baseplate (25 or 30 mm) directly on the crest prior to harvesting the bone graft. The benefit of this strategy is immediate, solid fixation of the baseplate to the TICBG. After the bone is harvested using an osteotome or oscillating saw, it is contoured to fill the glenoid defect and the baseplate bone graft construct is fixed to the native scapula. A cortical aspect of the graft should be placed superiorly to ensure a solid superior wall and avoid superior tilt of the baseplate.

Allograft can be used in place of or in combination with autograft for large glenoid defects encountered during revision RSA. The patient and/or the surgeon may choose to avoid the morbidity associated with harvesting iliac crest bone and elect to use allograft. Although rare, previous surgeries or body habitus may also preclude use of iliac crest autograft. When selecting allograft, our current preference is to use femoral neck as it has dimensions that mimic the native glenoid [59]. Our institution has available pre-prepared circular femoral neck allograft, which eliminates much of the process and time associated with shaping and contouring a graft from allograft proximal humerus or femur (Fig. 24.5). If pre-prepared graft is unavailable, our preferred method for obtaining and preparing allograft

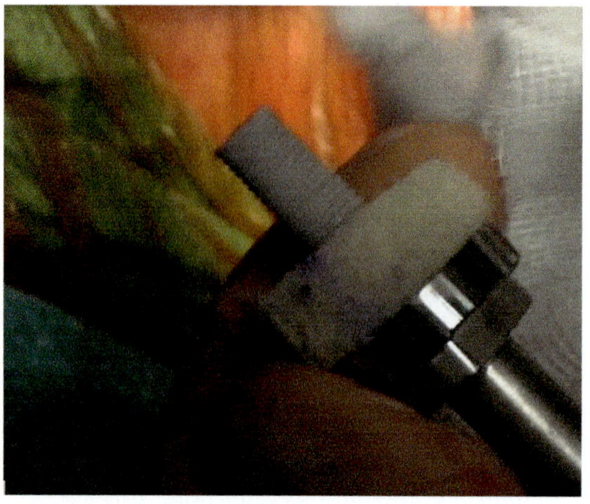

Fig. 24.5 Osteopure on peg

bone graft is similar to that described for collecting humeral autograft for a bony increased-offset reverse shoulder arthroplasty (BIO-RSA) [61]. Using either allograft femoral or humeral head, a small amount of bone is removed at the summit of the head to provide a flat surface. A threaded guidewire is then placed perpendicular to this cut and driven to the lateral cortex. Next, a cannulated drill is used to bore a central hole and a bell saw with the diameter corresponding to the planned baseplate dimensions (generally 25 mm for females and 29 mm for males) is passed to the desired depth. A small osteotome can be passed distally to free the bone graft at the desired depth. The bone graft is removed and inserted over the baseplate peg and a freehand sawcut is performed to modify the angle or thickness of the graft to fit the defect.

Regardless of amount and type of bone graft used, the baseplate should be aligned to allow peripheral screws to be directed toward areas with the best bone quality, such as the coracoid base, and the scapular spine.

Humeral Bone Loss

Significant humeral bone loss can be encountered in cases of failed arthroplasty being revised to RSA. This is most often seen in the setting of previous infection, fracture sequelae, or multiple failed surgeries. Reconstruction in this scenario should only occur after thorough discussion and review of potential complications and limited functional expectations. If not addressed, proximal humeral bone loss has been shown to lead to high rates of instability and humeral stem loosening.

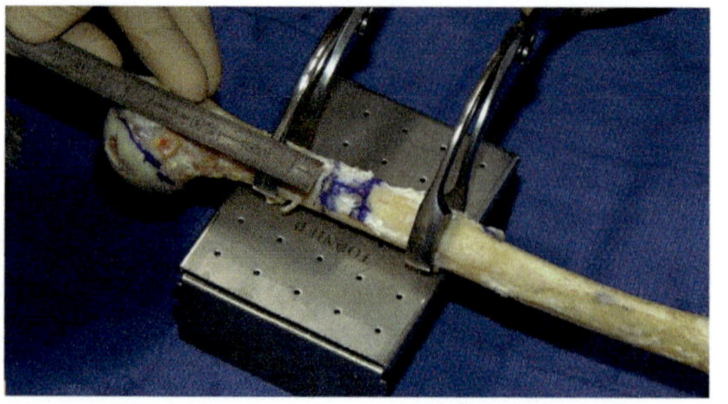

Fig. 24.6 Proximal humerus allograft preparation

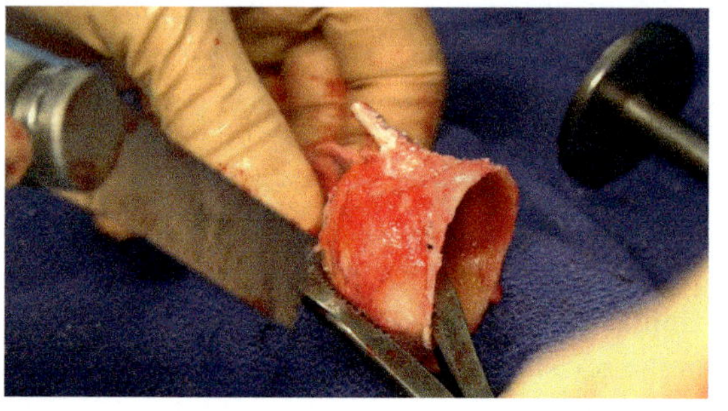

Fig. 24.7 Proximal humerus allograft step-cut

Prosthesis-allograft composite with RSA can be used in the setting of profound humeral bone loss. This technique involves the use of a proximal humeral allograft selected to match the approximate size of the patient. Length of defect is determined based on pre-operative imaging, including full length humerus films of the contralateral arm. On the back table, the articular surface is cut from the allograft, which is then prepared with epiphyseal reamers in standard fashion for long-stem RSA implant. Prior to cementing the prosthesis, the allograft is cut using a step-cut at the appropriate height and the native humerus is prepared with a corresponding step-cut and the canal carefully reamed. Once the prosthesis is secured in the allograft the construct is inserted in 20 to 30° of retroversion. In most situations, we choose to cement the prosthesis both proximally (in the allograft) and distally (in the native humerus) (Figs. 24.6, 24.7, 24.8, and 24.9).

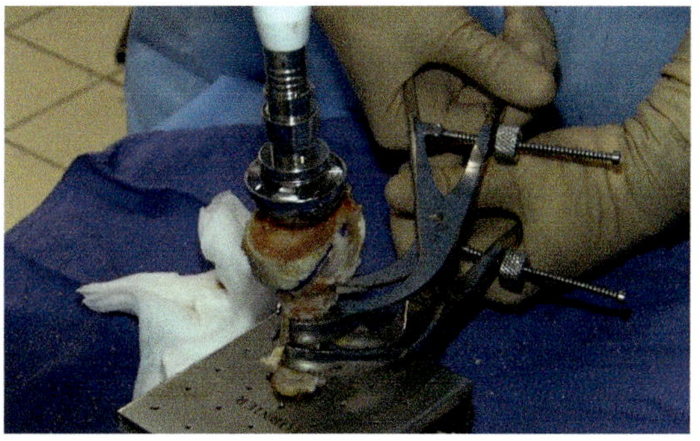

Fig. 24.8 Proximal humeral allograft reaming

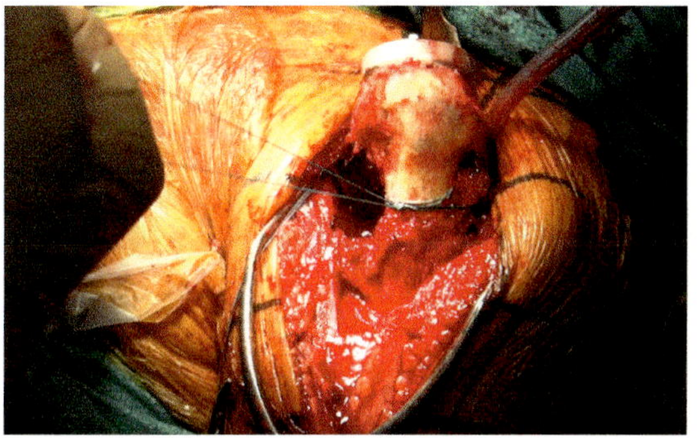

Fig. 24.9 Proximal humerus allograft secured with Nice Loops

Results

The results of revision arthroplasty are largely dependent on the indication for revision. Below you will find the published results of revision arthroplasty for specific indications.

Infection

Many case series have been reported on shoulder periprosthetic infection treatments, with very little direct comparison of outcomes. Nelson et al.'s systematic review compared the outcomes of thirty articles. With resection arthroplasty, one-stage, and two-stage revision all resulting in greater than 90% success rates, they found no statistical difference in success rates between the three options. Although one-stage revisions generated the highest mean Constant score at 48.1, all scores were less than 50, suggesting limited outcomes. Of note, this review did not compare success rates or functional outcomes of the different treatment regimens when stratified by acuity. Ultimately, most authors of the thirty studies preferred the traditional complete component explant, antibiotic spacer placement, and second stage revision arthroplasty [12].

In George et al.'s systematic review of thirty-five articles relating to delayed or chronic infections (6 weeks or later), a comparison of one-stage, two-stage, resection arthroplasty and permanent spacer implant revisions found no statistical difference in infection eradication. Although one-stage revision resulted in statistically significant better postoperative Constant scores, when comparing pre- and post-operative Constant scores, there was no statistical significance [62].

In Cuff et al.'s study of twenty-two shoulders with deep infections (seventeen hemiarthroplasties and five open rotator cuff repairs), he compared the results of extensive debridement with conversion to a reverse shoulder prosthesis in one or two-stage procedures. There was no significant difference in outcome measures when comparing between one or two-stage procedures, and no patients had evidence of recurrent infection [63].

Stine et al. compared the results of two-stage revision to permanent antibiotic spacer placement in the treatment of a chronic infected shoulder. There was no significant difference in the DASH score, Simple Shoulder Test score, forward flexion abduction, or external rotation. The authors suggested that prolonged implantation of an articulating antibiotic spacer is a reasonable option in select low-demand patients with comoborbidities [64].

Codd et al. compared the results of resection arthroplasty vs antibiotic spacer placement for deep shoulder arthroplasty infections. There was no significant difference between the two groups in the infection control, or Visual Analog, Constant, Simple Shoulder Test, or DASH scores. The authors concluded that resection arthroplasty may be offered to patients with chronic shoulder infections, as spacers provided no benefit in this study [65].

Dodson et al. reported on shoulder prosthesis infection caused by P. acnes. There were eleven cases, all with at least two intraoperative cultures positive for P. acnes. Group I patients (five) had an initial diagnosis of infection and underwent two-stage revision. These patients received antibiotics for an average of 6.3 weeks, with three patients additionally receiving oral antibiotics for an average 3.3 weeks. Two of these five patients had recurrent infections and required additional procedures. Group II patients (six) had no preoperative suspicion of infection, underwent revision arthroplasty which revealed at least two intraoperative cultures positive for P. acnes, and therefore received an extended course of postoperative IV antibiotics. Although recurrence nor the length of intravenous antibiotic treatment was reported, five patients received additional oral antibiotics for an average 9.0 weeks, while one patient remained on lifelong suppressive oral antibiotics [66].

Instability

In Miller's study of seven patients that underwent repair of subscapularis failures after anatomic shoulder arthroplasties with or without augmentation using the pectoralis major tendon, patient satisfaction scores and outcome scores were quite low. The mean American Shoulder and Elbow Surgeons shoulder score was 63.2 points at 2.3 years follow-up [6]. Augmentation of repair with pectoralis major tendon transfer did not improve these results as two of four patients continued to have anterior instability and failed, requiring an additional surgery [6]. In Elhassan et al.'s study of pectoralis major transfers for irreparable subscapularis failures after shoulder arthroplasty, only one of eight patients reported significant improvement in the shoulder subjective score and pain [38].

Sanchez-Sotelo et al. studied thirty-three total shoulder arthroplasties with instability, nineteen shoulders with anterior instability and fourteen with posterior instability. Revision surgery was performed in all cases, and only restored stability in nine of the shoulders. Eleven shoulders had recurrent instability and had additional surgery [67].

In Farshad's study of 67 reverse shoulder arthroplasties who underwent revision, twelve patients did so because of instability. Five patients underwent closed reduction in the early period (mean of 101 days), while seven patients underwent operative treatment in the late period (mean of 781 days). Of the five patients who underwent initial closed reduction, two patients required later operative intervention. Of the seven patients who underwent initial operative intervention, three required even further surgical intervention. Additionally, two of the twelve patients developed brachial plexus injuries [68].

Rotator Cuff Insufficiency

Looking at outcomes for intraoperative cuff tears during total shoulder arthroplasty, one study found that if the full thickness tears of the supraspinatus are amenable to repair, the outcome is not affected [2].

In situations of rotator cuff tear after shoulder arthroplasty, Hattrup et al. evaluated 18 patients who underwent repair with an average of 9 years follow-up. Fourteen shoulders had unsuccessful results while four shoulders had successful results. Three patients had moderate pain, five patients had occasionally moderate pain, six had slight pain, and four shoulders had no pain. The average final forward elevation was 78° [69]. Complications include re-tearing or continued superior instability.

The use of a revision constrained shoulder arthroplasty in the setting of a failed anatomic shoulder arthroplasty for rotator cuff deficiency may help to improve function and pain, but not without risk of complications. In Kelly et al.'s study of thirty failed hemi- or anatomic shoulder arthroplasties treated with reverse shoulder arthroplasty, all had significant rotator cuff deficiency without glenoid bone loss. The Constant score improved from 24% to 65% and the ASES score improved from 55 to 72. Forward flexion increased from 42° to 106°, and the pain score improved from 6.6. to 1.6. 80% of the shoulders were satisfied or very satisfied. However, the complication rate was 50% [70]. Flury et al. studied 21 shoulders who underwent revision to a reverse shoulder prosthesis secondary to a painful loss of function with rotator cuff insufficiency in the anatomic shoulder arthroplasty. Pain decreased from 8.7 to 3.0, active flexion increased from 23° to 97°, and abduction increased from 44° to 90°. The Constant score improved from 16.7 to 55.9, and 84% rated their shoulder as much better or better than before. However, external rotation decreased from 26° to 12°, and there was a 43% intraoperative and 38% postoperative complication rate [71]. These studies reveal that in the setting of a failed anatomic shoulder arthroplasty secondary to rotator cuff deficiency, a reverse shoulder arthroplasty may help to improve function and pain, but not without risk of complications.

Implant Loosening

Glenoid Component

In Bonnevialle et al.'s study of 42 total shoulder arthroplasties with failed glenoid components revised with reimplantation of an all-polyethylene, cemented glenoid component, they reported poor results after component reimplantation, with a 67% rate of recurrent loosening. They concluded that revision of a total shoulder with reimplantation of an all-poly cemented glenoid component does not solve the problem of glenoid loosening, and that soft-tissue failure and instability are underestimated and may partly explain the elevated rate of recurrent glenoid loosening [72].

In a study of thirty-seven anatomic total shoulders revised with reverse total shoulders for glenoid loosening with or without rotator cuff failure, 86% of patients were satisfied, despite a 20% subsequent reoperation rate. Complications included recurrent glenoid loosening (3), and new complications of anterior instability (3) and humeral subsidence (2) [73].

In O'Driscoll's case series of five patients who underwent arthroscopic conversion of TSA to hemiarthroplasty by removal of loose glenoid component, the operations were technically and clinically successful. Glenoid loosening was confirmed by probing/ lifting the component away from the underlying bone, and successfully removed. At an average of 49 months, complete pain relief was seen in three patients, with 40–50% pain relief in two patients. No complications were encountered, and no additional surgeries were needed. Furthermore, each patient stated the procedure was worthwhile and s/he would undergo the procedure if needed to in the future [47].

Humeral Component

Humeral loosening is very rare. As stated earlier, Sperling classified humeral components as "at risk" if they demonstrated radiographic tilt, subsidence or 2.0 millimeter radiolucent lines. In sixty-two shoulder prostheses, only six (9.6%) were considered to be "at risk." However, only one of these sixty-two (0.016%) required revision due of symptomatic humeral component loosening [31]. Revision surgery of aseptic humeral loosening may provide pain relief and improvements in motion, but not without complications. In one study of thirty-eight revision arthroplasties performed for aseptic loosening of the humeral component, there was a significant decrease in pain and significant improvement in active abduction. Excellent or satisfactory results were achieved in twenty-five of the patients (71%). However, intraoperative complications included cement extrusion in eight patients, humeral shaft fracture in two patients, and tuberosity fracture in four patients. Four-reoperations were needed [49].

Arthrosis of Native Glenoid After Hemiarthroplasty

When glenoid arthrosis occurs after shoulder hemiarthroplasty, revision to a total shoulder arthroplasty may be necessary. This can result in pain relief and improved motion; however unsatisfactory results are not uncommon. Sperling et al. studied twenty-two revision total shoulder arthroplasties for the treatment of painful glenoid arthrosis in the setting of a hemiarthroplasty. The pain score improved from 4.3 to 2.2, active abduction improved from 94° to 124°, and external rotation improved from 32° to 58°. However, seven patients (38%) had unsatisfactory results secondary to a limited range of motion or need for subsequent operation [74]. Hattrup et al. reviewed the results of seventeen hemiarthroplasty patients with a painful humeral head replacement and glenoid arthrosis and a painful humeral head replacement who were revised with a total shoulder arthroplasty. At an average of 56 months, flexion improved from 73° to 124°, abduction improved from 63° to 115°, and external rotation improved from 12° to 46° [75].

Periprosthetic Fracture

In Athwal et al.'s study of intraoperative periprosthetic humeral fractures, twenty-eight fractures occurred during primary total shoulder arthroplasty, three occurred during primary hemi arthroplasty, and fourteen occurred during revision arthroplasty. The mean fracture healing time was 17 weeks. The greater tuberosity fractures that required reduction and fixation healed at a mean of 13.5 weeks, nondisplaced greater tuberosity fractures healed at a mean of 6.5 weeks, combined tuberosity and shaft fractures healed at a mean of 9.7 weeks, and humeral shaft fractures healed at a mean of 22.5 weeks. Thirty-one patients were rated as having an excellent or satisfactory result, while fourteen patients were rated as having unsatisfactory results. There were no significant differences between displaced greater tuberosity fractures requiring fixation compared to nondisplaced/stable fractures in regards to forward elevation, external rotation, Simple Shoulder Test, and ASES score. Eighteen complications were seen including: six nerve injuries, two malunion greater tuberosity fractures treated nonoperatively, one hematoma, one with extensive fracture blisters, loss of shaft fracture reduction treated nonoperatively, and refracture of a shaft fracture after a fall, which required open reduction internal fixation [76].

In a study of sixteen postoperative periprosthetic humeral fractures, six healed with nonoperative management at an average of 180 days post-injury. Ten required operative intervention: five had immediate surgery while the other five had surgery at an average of 123 days post-injury. All ten operative cases healed [2, 50]. Complications include nonunion of fractures initially trialed with nonoperative management and subsequent surgical delay of those nonunions.

Clinical Pearls

1. Revision shoulder arthroplasty presents a challenging scenario due to loss of bone stock and risk of fracture.
2. Knowledge of techniques for implant removal focused on minimizing bone loss and risk of fracture are crucial for successful revision surgery.
3. Surgeons undertaking revision arthroplasty should be familiar with strategies for managing bone loss that is encountered at the time of revision.

Complications

In general, there is a significant risk of complications in revision shoulder arthroplasty. Many of these complications have been summarized above in the results section.

Farshad presented data on thirty-seven patients who underwent a primary RSA and later required revision surgery. Of these thirty-seven revisions, twenty-one needed a second intervention (56%), nine needed a third intervention (24%), and four required a fourth intervention (10%). The most common reason for an additional intervention was instability [68]. In the setting of revision shoulder arthroplasty using the reverse prosthesis, Kelly found a 50% complication rate while Flury found a 43% intraoperative and 38% postoperative complication rate [70, 71].

Boileau et al. reported on forty-five patients with reverse shoulder arthroplasty, comparing the results and complications based on indication for surgery: cuff tear arthritis, fracture sequelae and failed arthroplasty. Although all three groups had significant increases in active elevation and Constant scores, complications were higher in the revision group (47%) compared to the cuff tear arthritis group (5%) [18].

In Levy et al.'s study of twenty-nine patients who underwent reverse shoulder prosthesis for the treatment of failed hemiarthroplasty the complication rate was 28%. In another study of thirty reverse shoulder arthroplasties for revision of twenty-five failed hemiarthroplasties and five total shoulder arthroplasties, the complication rate was 26.6%, including four cases of scapular notching [77, 78].

Clinical Pearl

The outcomes of revision arthroplasty are highly dependent on the indication for revision, with complications reported in up to 50% of cases.

Conclusion

Revision shoulder arthroplasty is a challenging problem for both the patient and surgeon. Detailed evaluation of the patient's presenting symptoms and appropriate imaging studies is paramount for successful management. Mode of failure must be elicited to correctly determine and plan treatment. Meticulous surgical exposure and careful implant removal are necessary for any attempted revision surgery. The surgeon must have knowledge of techniques for addressing both glenoid and humeral bone loss, but also understand the limitations of each technique. The role of reverse shoulder arthroplasty in the revision setting has allowed for development and implementation of new techniques to address cases of failed shoulder arthroplasty.

Clinical Pearls

1. Primary shoulder arthroplasty surgery is not without risk, as complications are relatively common (6%–16%) and oftentimes require revision surgery.
2. Revision shoulder arthroplasty presents a challenging scenario due to loss of bone stock and risk of fracture.
3. Knowledge of techniques for implant removal focused on minimizing bone loss and risk of fracture are crucial for successful revision surgery.
4. Surgeons undertaking revision arthroplasty should be familiar with strategies for managing bone loss that is encountered at the time of revision.
5. The outcomes of revision arthroplasty are highly dependent on the indication for revision, with complications reported up to 50%.

References

1. Lugli T. Artificial shoulder joint by Péan (1893): the facts of an exceptional intervention and the prosthetic method. Clin Orthop Relat Res. 1978;1978(133):215–8.
2. Bohsali KI, Wirth MA, Rockwood CA Jr. Complications of total shoulder arthroplasty. J Bone Joint Surg Am. 2006;88(10):2279–92.
3. Jain NB, Yamaguchi K. The contribution of reverse shoulder arthroplasty to utilization of primary shoulder arthroplasty. J Shoulder Elb Surg. 2014;23(12):1905–12.
4. Westermann RW, Pugely AJ, Martin CT, Gao Y, Wolf BR, Hettrich CM. Reverse Shoulder Arthroplasty in the United States: A Comparison of National Volume, Patient Demographics, Complications, and Surgical Indications. Iowa Orthop J. 2015;35:1–7.
5. Chin PY, Sperling JW, Cofield RH, Schleck C. Complications of total shoulder arthroplasty: are they fewer or different? J Shoulder Elbow Surg/Am J Shoulder Elbow Surg [et al.]. 2006;15(1):19–22.
6. Miller BS, Joseph TA, Noonan TJ, Horan MP, Hawkins RJ. Rupture of the subscapularis tendon after shoulder arthroplasty: diagnosis, treatment,

and outcome. J Shoulder Elbow Surg/Am J Shoulder Elbow Surg [et al.]. 2005;14(5):492–6.
7. Labek G, Thaler M, Janda W, Agreiter M, Stöckl B. Revision rates after total joint replacement: cumulative results from worldwide joint register datasets. J Bone Joint Surg Br. 2011;93(3):293–7.
8. Favard L. Revision of total shoulder arthroplasty. Orthop Traumatol Surg Res. 2013;99(1 Suppl):S12–21.
9. Morris BJ, O'Connor DP, Torres D, Elkousy HA, Gartsman GM, Edwards TB. Risk factors for periprosthetic infection after reverse shoulder arthroplasty. J Shoulder Elb Surg. 2015;24(2):161–6.
10. Coste JS, Reig S, Trojani C, Berg M, Walch G, Boileau P. The management of infection in arthroplasty of the shoulder. J Bone Joint Surg Br. 2004;86(1):65–9.
11. Hatta T, Werthel JD, Wagner ER, et al. Effect of smoking on complications following primary shoulder arthroplasty. J Shoulder Elb Surg. 2017;26(1):1–6.
12. Nelson GN, Davis DE, Namdari S. Outcomes in the treatment of periprosthetic joint infection after shoulder arthroplasty: a systematic review. J Shoulder Elb Surg. 2016;25(8):1337–45.
13. Cheung E, Willis M, Walker M, Clark R, Frankle MA. Complications in reverse total shoulder arthroplasty. J Am Acad Orthop Surg. 2011;19(7):439–49.
14. Cofield RH, Sperling JW. Revision and complex shoulder arthroplasty. Philadelphia: Wolters Kluwer Health/Lippincott William & Wilkins; 2010.
15. Cisneros LG, Atoun E, Abraham R, Tsvieli O, Bruguera J, Levy O. Revision shoulder arthroplasty: does the stem really matter? J Shoulder Elb Surg. 2016;25(5):747–55.
16. Antoni M, Barthoulot M, Kempf JF, Clavert P. Revisions of total shoulder arthroplasty: Clinical results and complications of various modalities. Orthop Traumatol Surg Res. 2016;102(3):297–303.
17. Zumstein MA, Pinedo M, Old J, Boileau P. Problems, complications, reoperations, and revisions in reverse total shoulder arthroplasty: a systematic review. J Shoulder Elb Surg. 2011;20(1):146–57.
18. Boileau P, Watkinson D, Hatzidakis AM, Hovorka I. Neer Award 2005: The Grammont reverse shoulder prosthesis: results in cuff tear arthritis, fracture sequelae, and revision arthroplasty. J Shoulder Elb Surg. 2006;15(5):527–40.
19. Williams GR. Shoulder and elbow arthroplasty. Philadelphia: Lippincott Williams & Wilkins; 2005.
20. Walch G, Moraga C, Young A, Castellanos-Rosas J. Results of anatomic nonconstrained prosthesis in primary osteoarthritis with biconcave glenoid. J Shoulder Elb Surg. 2012;21(11):1526–33.
21. Lädermann A, Edwards TB, Walch G. Arm lengthening after reverse shoulder arthroplasty: a review. Int Orthop. 2014;38(5):991–1000.
22. Affonso J, Nicholson GP, Frankle MA, et al. Complications of the reverse prosthesis: prevention and treatment. Instr Course Lect. 2012;61:157–68.
23. Boileau P. Complications and revision of reverse total shoulder arthroplasty. Orthop Traumatol Surg Res. 2016;102(1 Suppl):S33–43.
24. Rockwood CA. The shoulder. 3rd ed. Philadelphia: Saunders; 2004.
25. Franklin JL, Barrett WP, Jackins SE, Matsen FA. Glenoid loosening in total shoulder arthroplasty. Association with rotator cuff deficiency. J Arthroplast. 1988;3(1):39–46.
26. Gartsman GM, Edwards TB. Shoulder arthroplasty. Edinburgh: Saunders; 2008. http://www.clinicalkey.com/dura/browse/bookChapter/3-s2.0-B9781416038573X50017
27. Matsen FA, Clinton J, Lynch J, Bertelsen A, Richardson ML. Glenoid component failure in total shoulder arthroplasty. J Bone Joint Surg Am. 2008;90(4):885–96.
28. Anglin C, Wyss UP, Nyffeler RW, Gerber C. Loosening performance of cemented glenoid prosthesis design pairs. Clin Biomech (Bristol, Avon). 2001;16(2):144–50.
29. Lazarus MD, Jensen KL, Southworth C, Matsen FA. The radiographic evaluation of keeled and pegged glenoid component insertion. J Bone Joint Surg Am. 2002;84-A(7):1174–82.
30. Matsen FA, Iannotti JP, Rockwood CA. Humeral fixation by press-fitting of a tapered metaphyseal stem: a prospective radiographic study. J Bone Joint Surg Am. 2003;85-A(2):304–8.
31. Sperling JW, Cofield RH, O'Driscoll SW, Torchia ME, Rowland CM. Radiographic assessment of ingrowth total shoulder arthroplasty. J Shoulder Elb Surg. 2000;9(6):507–13.
32. Maynou C, Petroff E, Mestdagh H, Dubois HH, Lerue O. Clinical and radiologic outcome of humeral implants in shoulder arthroplasty. Acta Orthop Belg. 1999;65(1):57–64.
33. Herschel R, Wieser K, Morrey ME, Ramos CH, Gerber C, Meyer DC. Risk factors for glenoid erosion in patients with shoulder hemiarthroplasty: an analysis of 118 cases. J Shoulder Elb Surg. 2016; 26(2):246–52.
34. Singh JA, Sperling J, Schleck C, Harmsen W, Cofield R. Periprosthetic fractures associated with primary total shoulder arthroplasty and primary humeral head replacement: a thirty-three-year study. J Bone Joint Surg Am. 2012;94(19):1777–85.
35. Kelly JD, Hobgood ER. Positive culture rate in revision shoulder arthroplasty. Clin Orthop Relat Res. 2009;467(9):2343–8.
36. Topolski MS, Chin PY, Sperling JW, Cofield RH. Revision shoulder arthroplasty with positive intraoperative cultures: the value of preoperative studies and intraoperative histology. J Shoulder Elb Surg. 2006;15(4):402–6.
37. Moeckel BH, Altchek DW, Warren RF, Wickiewicz TL, Dines DM. Instability of the shoulder after arthroplasty. J Bone Joint Surg Am. 1993;75(4):492–7.
38. Elhassan B, Ozbaydar M, Massimini D, Diller D, Higgins L, Warner JJ. Transfer of pectoralis

major for the treatment of irreparable tears of subscapularis: does it work? J Bone Joint Surg Br. 2008;90(8):1059–65.
39. Wirth MA, Rockwood CA Jr. Complications of shoulder arthroplasty. Clin Orthop Relat Res. 1994;307:47–69.
40. Levy DM, Abrams GD, Harris JD, Bach BR, Nicholson GP, Romeo AA. Rotator cuff tears after total shoulder arthroplasty in primary osteoarthritis: A systematic review. Int J Shoulder Surg. 2016;10(2):78–84.
41. Godeneche A, Boileau P, Favard L, et al. Prosthetic replacement in the treatment of osteoarthritis of the shoulder: early results of 268 cases. J Shoulder Elbow Surg/Am J Shoulder Elbow Surg [et al.]. 2002;11(1):11–8.
42. Buckingham BP, Parsons IM, Campbell B, Titelman RM, Smith KL, Matsen FA. Patient functional self-assessment in late glenoid component failure at three to eleven years after total shoulder arthroplasty. J Shoulder Elb Surg. 2005;14(4):368–74.
43. Hawkins RJ, Greis PE, Bonutti PM. Treatment of symptomatic glenoid loosening following unconstrained shoulder arthroplasty. Orthopedics. 1999;22(2):229–34.
44. Iannotti JP, Williams GR. Ovid Technologies Inc. Disorders of the shoulder diagnosis and management. 2nd ed. Philadelphia: Lippincott Williams & Wilkins; 2007. http://ovidsp.ovid.com/ovidweb.cgi?T=JS&MODE=ovid&NEWS=n&PAGE=booktext&D=books&AN=01257005
45. Pinkas D, Wiater B, Wiater JM. The glenoid component in anatomic shoulder arthroplasty. J Am Acad Orthop Surg. 2015;23(5):317–26.
46. Martin SD, Zurakowski D, Thornhill TS. Uncemented glenoid component in total shoulder arthroplasty. Survivorship and outcomes. J Bone Joint Surg Am. 2005;87(6):1284–92.
47. O'Driscoll SW, Petrie RS, Torchia ME. Arthroscopic removal of the glenoid component for failed total shoulder arthroplasty. A report of five cases. J Bone Joint Surg Am. 2005;87(4):858–63.
48. Namdari S, Glaser D. Arthroscopically assisted conversion of total shoulder arthroplasty to hemiarthroplasty with glenoid bone grafting. Orthopedics. 2011;34(11):862–5.
49. Cil A, Veillette CJ, Sanchez-Sotelo J, Sperling JW, Schleck C, Cofield RH. Revision of the humeral component for aseptic loosening in arthroplasty of the shoulder. J Bone Joint Surg Br. 2009;91(1):75–81.
50. Kumar S, Sperling JW, Haidukewych GH, Cofield RH. Periprosthetic humeral fractures after shoulder arthroplasty. J Bone Joint Surg Am. 2004;86-A(4):680–9.
51. Foruria AM, Oh LS, Sperling JW, Cofield RH. Anteromedial approach for shoulder arthroplasty: current indications, complications, and results. J Shoulder Elbow Surg/Am J Shoulder Elbow Surg [et al.]. 2010;19(5):734–8.
52. Goldberg SH, Cohen MS, Young M, Bradnock B. Thermal tissue damage caused by ultrasonic cement removal from the humerus. J Bone Joint Surg Am. 2005;87(3):583–91.
53. Neer CS 2nd, Morrison DS. Glenoid bone-grafting in total shoulder arthroplasty. J Bone Joint Surg Am. 1988;70(8):1154–62.
54. Phipatanakul WP, Norris TR. Treatment of glenoid loosening and bone loss due to osteolysis with glenoid bone grafting. J Shoulder Elbow Surg/Am J Shoulder Elbow Surg [et al.]. 2006;15(1):84–7.
55. Scalise JJ, Iannotti JP. Bone grafting severe glenoid defects in revision shoulder arthroplasty. Clin Orthop Relat Res. 2008;466(1):139–45.
56. Gonzalez JF, Alami GB, Baque F, Walch G, Boileau P. Complications of unconstrained shoulder prostheses. J Shoulder Elbow Surg/Am J Shoulder Elbow Surg [et al.]. 2011;20(4):666–82.
57. Whatley AN, Fowler RL, Warner JJ, Higgins LD. Postoperative rupture of the anterolateral deltoid muscle following reverse total shoulder arthroplasty in patients who have undergone open rotator cuff repair. J Shoulder Elbow Surg/Am J Shoulder Elbow Surg [et al.]. 2011;20(1):114–22.
58. Wagner E, Houdek MT, Griffith T, et al. Glenoid Bone-Grafting in Revision to a Reverse Total Shoulder Arthroplasty. J Bone Joint Surg Am. 2015;97(20):1653–60.
59. Bateman E, Donald SM. Reconstruction of massive uncontained glenoid defects using a combined autograft-allograft construct with reverse shoulder arthroplasty: preliminary results. J Shoulder Elbow Surg/Am J Shoulder Elbow Surg [et al]. 2012;21(7):925–34.
60. Norris TR, Kelly JD, Humphrey SC. Management of glenoid bone defects in revision shoulder arthroplasty: a new application of the reverse total shoulder prosthesis. Tech Should Elbow Surg. 2007;8(1):37–46.
61. Boileau P, Moineau G, Roussanne Y, O'Shea K. Bony increased-offset reversed shoulder arthroplasty: minimizing scapular impingement while maximizing glenoid fixation. Clin Orthop Relat Res. 2011;469(9):2558–67.
62. George DA, Volpin A, Scarponi S, Haddad FS, Romanò CL. Does exchange arthroplasty of an infected shoulder prosthesis provide better eradication rate and better functional outcome, compared to a permanent spacer or resection arthroplasty? a systematic review. BMC Musculoskelet Disord. 2016;17:52.
63. Cuff DJ, Virani NA, Levy J, et al. The treatment of deep shoulder infection and glenohumeral instability with debridement, reverse shoulder arthroplasty and postoperative antibiotics. J Bone Joint Surg Br. 2008;90(3):336–42.
64. Stine IA, Lee B, Zalavras CG, Hatch G, Itamura JM. Management of chronic shoulder infections utilizing a fixed articulating antibiotic-loaded spacer. J Shoulder Elb Surg. 2010;19(5):739–48.
65. Verhelst L, Stuyck J, Bellemans J, Debeer P. Resection arthroplasty of the shoulder as a salvage procedure for deep shoulder infection: does the use of a cement

spacer improve outcome? J Shoulder Elb Surg. 2011;20(8):1224–33.
66. Dodson CC, Craig EV, Cordasco FA, et al. Propionibacterium acnes infection after shoulder arthroplasty: a diagnostic challenge. J Shoulder Elb Surg. 2010;19(2):303–7.
67. Sanchez-Sotelo J, Sperling JW, Rowland CM, Cofield RH. Instability after shoulder arthroplasty: results of surgical treatment. J Bone Joint Surg Am. 2003;85-A(4):622–31.
68. Farshad M, Grögli M, Catanzaro S, Gerber C. Revision of reversed total shoulder arthroplasty. Indications and outcome BMC Musculoskelet Disord. 2012;13:160.
69. Hattrup SJ, Cofield RH, Cha SS. Rotator cuff repair after shoulder replacement. J Shoulder Elb Surg. 2006;15(1):78–83.
70. Kelly JD, Zhao JX, Hobgood ER, Norris TR. Clinical results of revision shoulder arthroplasty using the reverse prosthesis. J Shoulder Elb Surg. 2012;21(11):1516–25.
71. Flury MP, Frey P, Goldhahn J, Schwyzer HK, Simmen BR. Reverse shoulder arthroplasty as a salvage procedure for failed conventional shoulder replacement due to cuff failure–midterm results. Int Orthop. 2011;35(1):53–60.
72. Bonnevialle N, Melis B, Neyton L, et al. Aseptic glenoid loosening or failure in total shoulder arthroplasty: revision with glenoid reimplantation. J Shoulder Elbow Surg/Am J Shoulder Elbow Surg [et al.]. 2013;22(6):745–51.
73. Melis B, Bonnevialle N, Neyton L, et al. Glenoid loosening and failure in anatomical total shoulder arthroplasty: is revision with a reverse shoulder arthroplasty a reliable option? J Shoulder Elbow Surg/Am J Shoulder Elbow Surg [et al.]. 2012;21(3):342–9.
74. Sperling JW, Cofield RH. Revision total shoulder arthroplasty for the treatment of glenoid arthrosis. J Bone Joint Surg Am. 1998;80(6):860–7.
75. Hattrup SJ. Revision total shoulder arthroplasty for painful humeral head replacement with glenoid arthrosis. J Shoulder Elb Surg. 2009;18(2):220–4.
76. Athwal GS, Sperling JW, Rispoli DM, Cofield RH. Periprosthetic humeral fractures during shoulder arthroplasty. J Bone Joint Surg Am. 2009;91(3):594–603.
77. Valenti P, Kilinc AS, Sauzières P, Katz D. Results of 30 reverse shoulder prostheses for revision of failed hemi- or total shoulder arthroplasty. Eur J Orthop Surg Traumatol. 2014;24(8):1375–82.
78. Levy J, Frankle M, Mighell M, Pupello D. The use of the reverse shoulder prosthesis for the treatment of failed hemiarthroplasty for proximal humeral fracture. J Bone Joint Surg Am. 2007;89(2):292–300.

Part VI

Arthritis of the Shoulder: IV

The Anatomic Stemless Humeral Prosthesis

25

Nael Hawi and Peter Habermeyer

Introduction

Since 1951, early applications of shoulder arthroplasty underwent a complete transition in the development of humeral and glenoidal components, towards a more anatomical, modular, revisable, or convertible design (Figs. 25.1 and 25.2). The very first stemless humeral head prosthesis was implanted in 2004. Currently, most manufacturers offer stemless prostheses. The anchorage is cementless and metaphyseal. Thus, one can differentiate between a purely metaphyseal press fit anchorage and a metaphyseal press fit combined with epiphyseal bracing with a compression screw and a collar-bearing baseplate (trunion), to maintain additional primary stability. The advantages of this technique are that it saves intraoperative time, employs a stemless implant, produces less blood loss, incurs less trauma to the humeral shaft, and carries a lower risk of periprosthetic fracture. Additionally the access to the glenoid is compared to resurfacing arthroplasty much easier.

The stemless prosthesis design is applicable even to post-traumatic cases with existing deformities. Moreover, when revision surgery is necessary, this type of prosthesis is much easier to explant than a stemmed prosthesis. After

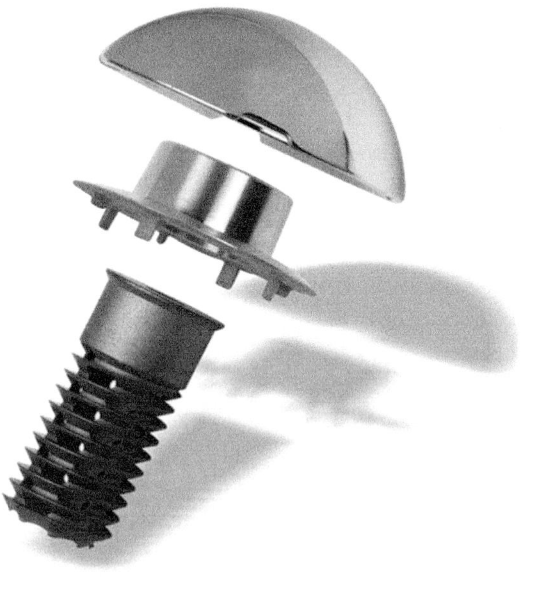

Fig. 25.1 Anatomic stemless prosthesis (Eclipse, Arthrex Inc.)

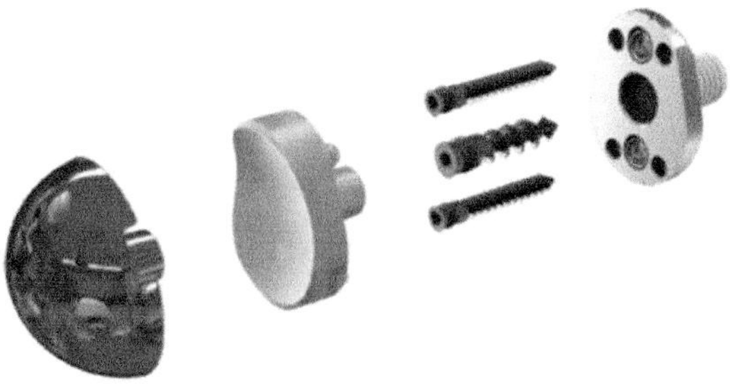

Fig. 25.2 Metalback convertible socket (Universal, Arthrex Inc.)

N. Hawi (✉) · P. Habermeyer
Department of Shoulder and Elbow Surgery, ATOS Clinic Munich, Munich, Germany

I. A. Trail et al. (eds.), *Textbook of Shoulder Surgery*, https://doi.org/10.1007/978-3-319-70099-1_25

explantation, it is possible to use a standard-sized, stemmed prosthesis.

Indications and Contraindications

The indication is basically the same for a stemless prosthesis and for the usual stemmed prosthesis. Contraindications are the presence of space-occupying cysts at the metaphysis, osteopenia, osteoporosis, or other metabolic bone disorders. It should be noted that, to date, we lack an objective tool for measuring bone quality, either pre- or intra-operatively. Other contraindications are fresh fractures and a history of epilepsy.

Preoperative Planning

Biomechanical Principles

Understanding normal three-dimensional anatomy provides the basis for successful joint replacement. In addition, changes in soft tissues, with respect to limb shortening, must be included in the planning. Upon implantation of the metaphyseal anchored prosthesis described here, attention must be focused on placing the baseplate (trunion) utmost anatomical by fitting it to the circular cortical rim for stable fixation. Proper positioning can minimize the load at the cap-trunion-bone-interface and forestall migration of the prosthesis. In addition, contact between the fixing hollow screw and the lateral cortex should be avoided to reduce bending stress on the hollow screw and to achieve uniform loading at the cap-bone interface.

Pathomechanics

Osteoarthritis of the Humeral Head

This condition causes loss of sphericity, with:

- disturbance of the rolling-sliding mechanism
- medialization of the center of rotation
- shortening of the lateral humeral offset
- development of caudal osteophytes, with growth rates according to the stage (classification according to Samilson and Prieto)
- Tensioning of the inferior capsule by bulging osteophytes
- reduction of the articular surface angle, which limits the range of motion
- shortening of the M. subscapularis and increased capsular tension with increasing dorsal decentering of the humeral head

Osteoarthritis of the Glenoid

This condition causes the following:

- medialization of the glenoid surface
- retroversion of the glenoid by posterior/inferior glenoid wear
- inferior tilt of the glenoidal inclination angle; the type of inclination depends on the stage (classification according to Habermeyer)
- enlargement of the glenoidal surface by osteophytes

Course of Primary Humeral Osteoarthritis

The typical course of primary humeral omarthrosis can be divided into three stages, as follows:

Stage 1

The initial shape of the humeral head in the coronal plane remains round and spherical. No substantial decentralization of the apex of the humeral head can be detected in the transverse plane. The cartilage wear primarily takes place in the inferior portion of the humerus. There is no posterior decentering of the humeral head. At this stage, osteophytes are generally shorter, though all stages according to Samilson and Prieto can occur. Regarding the glenoid morphology at this stage in the coronal plane, an inclination of 0–1 according to Habermeyer is mainly observed.

Stage 2

At this stage, there is a flattening of the humeral head in the coronal plane. Furthermore, an increasing deformation can be observed in the transverse plane, with displacement of the apex, primarily posteriorly. An extension of cartilage wear occurs superiorly. In addition, an incipient posterior subluxation can be observed. Moreover, there is growth of caudal osteophytes and an increase in the glenoidal type of inclination.

Stage 3

At this stage, an aspherical humeral head is observed in the coronal plane, and a decentered apex is observed in the transverse plane. Extensive cartilage damage extending superiorly is apparent. The humeral head is subluxated dorsally. In addition, caudal osteophytes and glenoidal inclinations are primarily higher grade.

Medical History

The patient history should cover the overall situation of the patient, including all medical, psychological, and social aspects (social environment). The medical aspects should include information on major complaints, typical pain symptoms, restrictions in the range of movement, and loss of strength.

Clinical Findings

The clinical examination should include evaluations of the following parameters:

- efflorescence of the skin
- signs of an infection
- swelling
- atrophic changes
- active and passive movements
- functionality of the rotator cuff
- neurological function (optionally extended neurological examination)
- increases in function scores (Constant-Murley Score)
- in case of a metallosis, perform a skin test

Instrument-Based Diagnostics

Diagnostic assessments tools:

(i) ***Sonography (use standard sonographical section planes)***
  - Assess the rotator cuff, including effusion

(ii) ***Radiography/X-Ray (true antero-posterior (AP), axial)***
  - Assess narrowing of the joint gap
  - X-Ray AP: Assess the humeral head curvature, the caudal humeral osteophyte (according to Samilson and Prieto), centering, lateral humeral offset, medial glenoidal protrusion, and the type of glenoidal inclination (according to Habermeyer). Estimation of bone density and cyst formation.
  - X-Ray AXIAL: Assess flattening of the humeral head, concentric or eccentric glenoidal wear, humeral centering, and the constellation of osteophytes

(iii) ***Computed tomography:***
  - Assess the posterior subluxation-position (according to Walch) and glenoidal inclination and wear
  - Assess any atrophic changes and determine the presence of any fatty infiltrations in the rotator cuff
  - Preferably use 3 D reconstruction and software planning in order to measure retroversion- and inclination angles and determine if glenoid bone stock is sufficient to guarantee 80% of glenoid component bone contact and a retroversion angle $<15°$.

(iv) ***Magnetic resonance tomography:***
  - Assess the rotator cuff, fatty infiltrations, or muscular atrophies
  - Assess glenoidal and humeral morphology

Surgical Technique

Patient Positioning

The patient is placed in a flat beach chair position (30°). The head and neck are secured with a ring headrest, which is helpful for maintaining the head and neck in the correct position throughout the procedure. The upper body is brought to the lateral edge of the operating table to allow full extension of the arm, which is essential for exposure of the proximal humerus. The arm is positioned on an additional hand table, which is adjustable in height. The shoulder and arm are prepared in sterile conditions, and the body is draped appropriately, to allow full exposure and free movement of the entire limb (Fig. 25.3).

Approach

The deltopectoral approach requires an incision, which starts above the coracoid process and terminates above the insertion of the pectoralis major on the humeral shaft. The skin incision often lies directly over the course of the cephalic vein, between the deltoid and pectoralis major muscles. After ensuring preservation of the cephalic vein, the clavipectoral fascia is split. This allows visualization of the pectoralis major muscle (Fig. 25.4).

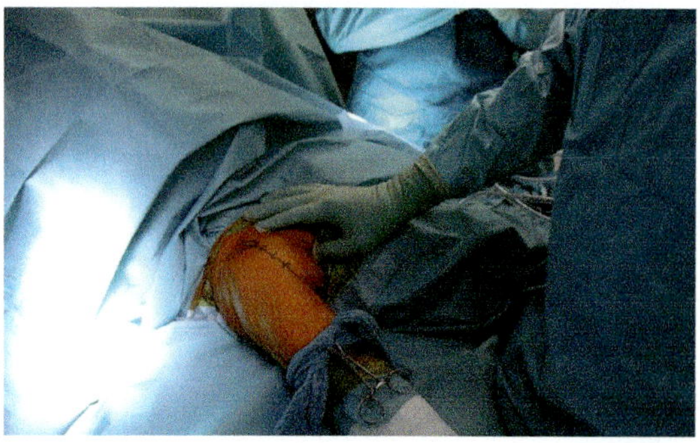

Fig. 25.3 Flat beach-chair position. The patient is draped in that way to allow free intra-operative mobility of the upper extremity

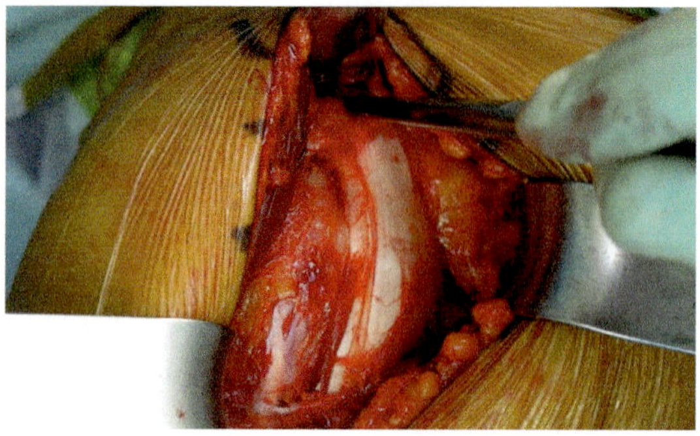

Fig. 25.4 The deltopectoral approach. The incision to expose the humeral shaft starts at the coracoid process and ends at the insertion of the pectoralis major. The forceps point to the surface of the coracoid process; directly below, the conjoint tendon extends vertically; at the lower edge of the image, the tendon of the M. pectoralis major crosses transversely

Next, the subfascial preparation of the proximal humerus beneath the fornix humeri is performed. When severe subacromial and subdeltoid bursitis is present, it is necessary to perform a resection of the bursae. The rotator cuff is preserved. Existing adhesions are removed. Then, tenolysis is performed to release the supraspinatus and infraspinatus tendons. To restore adequate gliding, the entire rotator cuff is mobilized. Furthermore, tenolysis of the subscapularis tendon is performed to release it from adhesion beneath the conjoined tendon. Here, due to the proximity of the posterior axillary gap, it is important to pay particular attention to the safety limits of the axillary nerve. In cases of nerve adhesions, a neurolysis should be performed.

Tenodesis of the Long Head of the Biceps Tendon

During tenodesis of the subpectoral biceps tendon, tension is maintained on the long head of the biceps tendon; also, two inverse U-stitches must be placed at the tendon edge of the pectoralis major, at the crista humeri. After capsular release, the intra-articular portion of the long head of the biceps tendon is completely excised, back to the level of the sulcus intertubercularis (Fig. 25.5).

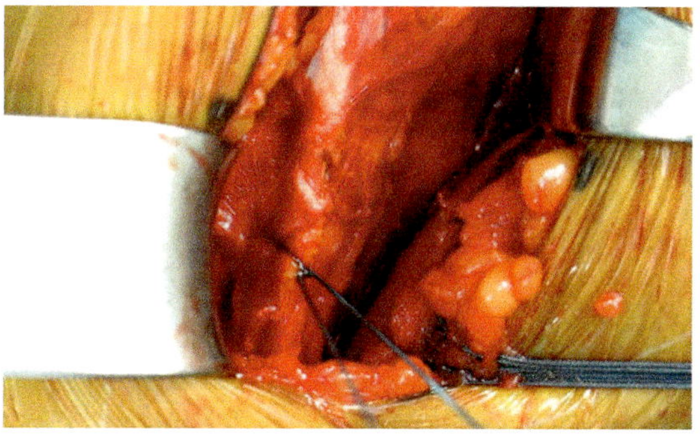

Fig. 25.5 Performing tenodesis of the long head of the biceps with inverse U sutures (upper suture). The insertion of the M. pectoralis major was incised, in this case, at its proximal end, and it has been reinforced with sutures to refix (lower right corner)

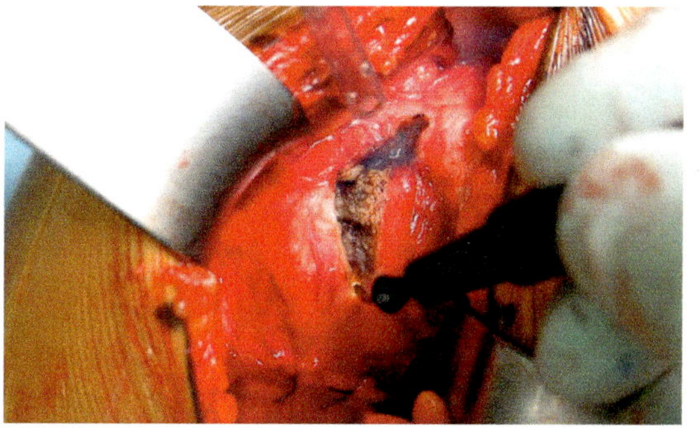

Fig. 25.6 The detachment of the tendon of the subscapularis takes place at the tuberculum minus (lesser tuberosity of the humerus), leaving a tendon stump to repair

Preparation of the Subscapularis Muscle

The rotator cuff interval is opened to perform the tenolysis. Thus, the coraco-humeral ligament is cut, at its base, at the coracoid process. Synovial fluid may be observed. Detachment of the subscapularis muscle tendon is performed at the tuberculum minus (lesser tuberosity of the humerus; Fig. 25.6). Upon detachment, a tendon edge remains attached to facilitate reattachment. Next, the humeral circumflex artery and vein are ligated. Then, a sharp dissection is performed to separate the muscular portion of the subscapularis muscle from the humeral calcar. Special attention should be paid to the safety limits of the axillary nerve. Next, the subscapularis muscle is completely dissected to the height of the latissimus dorsi muscle, and subsequently, it is reinforced with holding threads, in a modified Mason-Allen suture technique (Fig. 25.7).

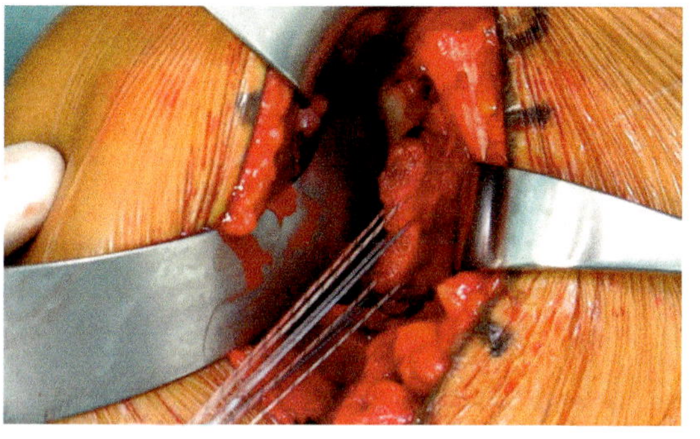

Fig. 25.7 Preparing reinforcement of the subscapularis tendon. Holding threads are placed in a modified Mason-Allen suture technique

Preparation of the Glenohumeral Joint Capsule

First, an inferior humeral capsulotomy is performed. The humeral capsule attachment must be completely cut at the anatomical neck, in a semicircular manner, from antero-superior to postero-inferior. Here also, attention must be paid to the safety limits of the axillary nerve.

Next, a retractor is inserted into the joint space, and the space must be opened until the ventral joint capsule and the subscapularis muscle can be visualized. In cases of subscapularis shortening, a tendon lengthening procedure must be performed, with a 270° release, according to Matsen. Next, a juxta-glenoidal capsulotomy is performed, with release of the subscapularis muscle. Further preparation of the subscapularis muscle up to the coracoid process, keeping the safety limits of the nerval structures in mind.

Preparation of the Humeral Head

A gentle dislocation of the humeral head is necessary. During this procedure, the arm is adducted and externally rotated (Fig. 25.8). A retractor is inserted to visualize the humeral

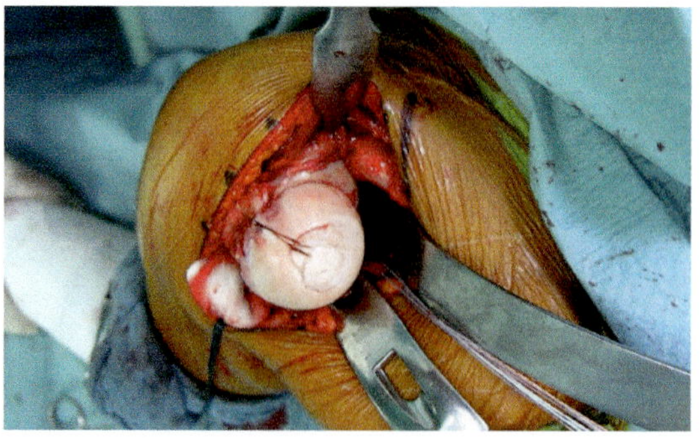

Fig. 25.8 Cautious dislocation of the humeral head, The upper arm is adducted and externally rotated, with the aid of a side table

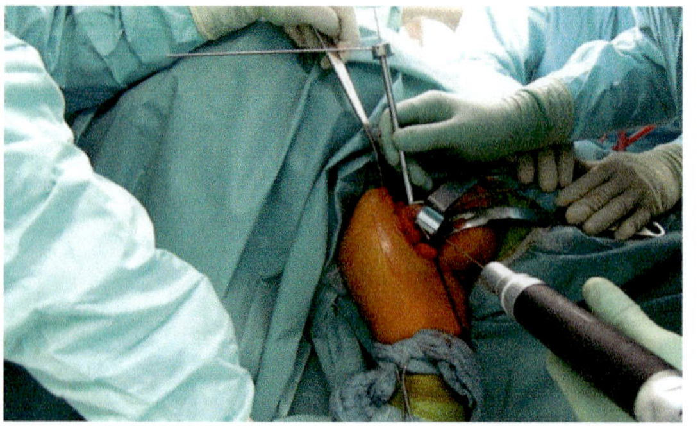

Fig. 25.10 The targeting instrument is fixed, and two K-wires are inserted into the anatomic neck

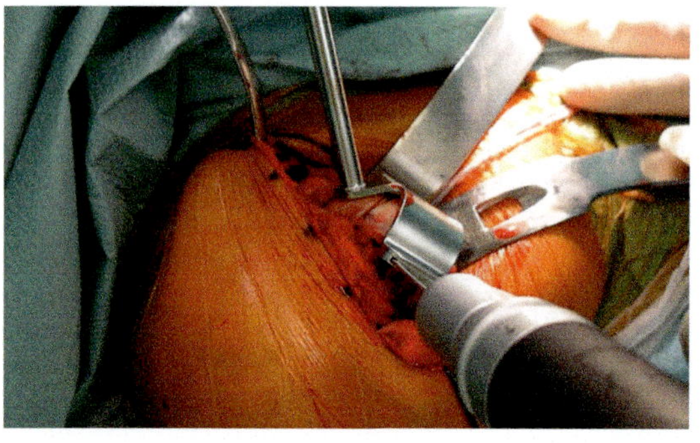

Fig. 25.9 The target instrument is placed to guide resection of the humeral head. The original anatomical neck of the humerus serves for orientation

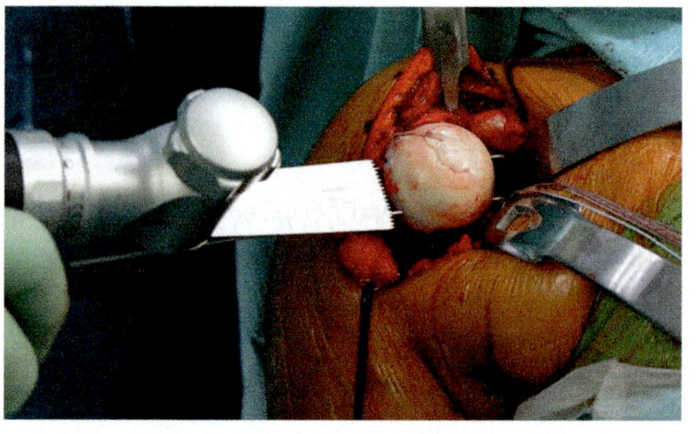

Fig. 25.11 The osteotomy is performed across the anatomical neck with an oscillating saw. The K-wires serve to guide the saw angle

joint surface, with osteophytes. Using a chisel, the antero-inferior and postero-inferior osteophytes along the anatomical neck are carefully removed. This allows visualization of the anatomical neck.

Humeral Head Resection

The target instrument is placed to guide resection of the humeral head (Fig. 25.9). The metaphyseal axis is marked. The retrotorsion is oriented along the anatomical neck. Under pre-drilling of two K-wires, the target instrument is attached in the area of the anatomical neck (Fig. 25.10). Then, the drilling jig is removed, and an osteotomy at the anatomic neck is performed with an oscillating saw. The saw orientation is guided by the K-wires (Fig. 25.11).

The resected humerus head cap is measured to determine the AP diameter and resection height (Fig. 25.12). The size of the baseplate (trunion) is determined with a template, placed directly on the resected anatomical neck. This should sit on the circular face of the resected humerus, flush with the cortical bone (Fig. 25.13).

A crown cutter is placed inside the drilling jig to prepare the thread for receiving the hollow screw (Fig. 25.14). To determine the length of the hollow screw, an insertion device is placed in the drilling jig, and a laser-marked drill wire is used as a depth gauge for drilling to the lateral cortex (Fig. 25.15). Caution: The opposite cortex should not be pierced. If the measured length lies between two laser markings, the shorter screw length should be selected. Finally, the drilling jig and insertion device are removed. A resection

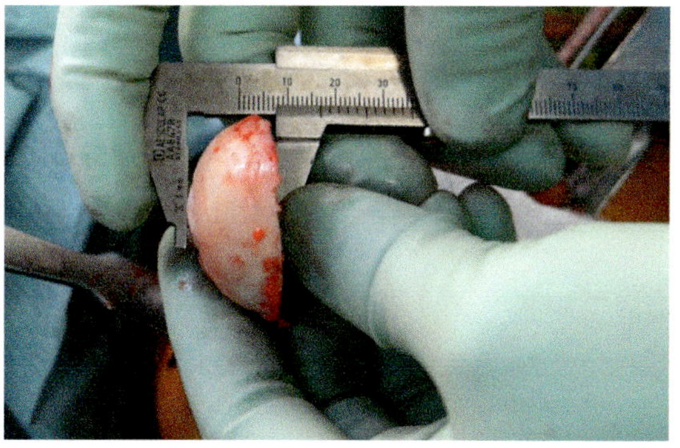

Fig. 25.12 The resected humerus head cap is measured to determine its AP diameter and the height of resection

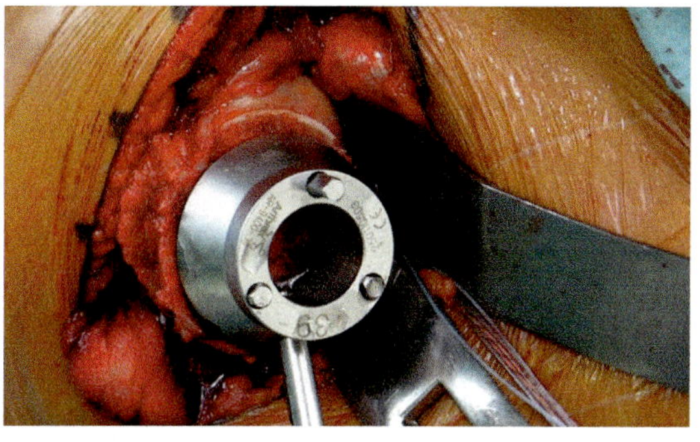

Fig. 25.13 The size of the trunnion (baseplate) is determined directly at the resected anatomical neck with a template

protection is placed during preparation of the glenoid.

Implantation of the Humeral Component (Eclipse, Arthrex)

The humerus is re-exposed, and the resection protection is removed. When necessary, the resection can be filled with cancellous bone and compacting it. The cancellous bone may be acquired from the resected humeral head. With the centering device in place, the baseplate is placed according to the predetermined location (Fig. 25.16). The impactor is placed over the centering device, and the baseplate is fixed by stiking the impactor to achieve a press fit (Fig. 25.17). Next, the centering device is removed, and the hollow screw, of the predetermined length, is inserted through the conus of the impactor (Fig. 25.18). The baseplate is pressed firmly against the resected bone to achieve adequate compression during screw fixation and to ensure primary stability. Next, a trial

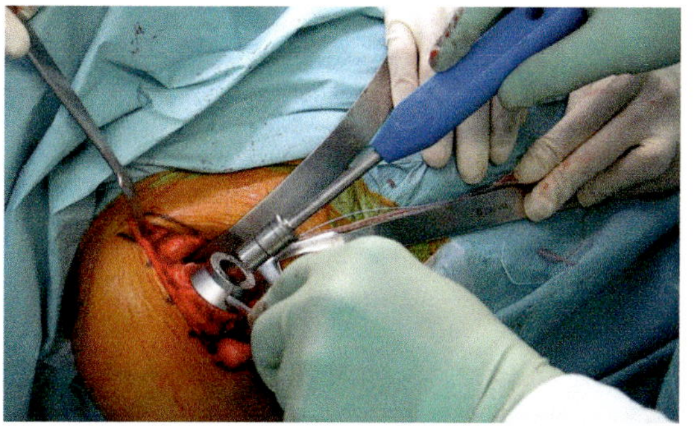

Fig. 25.14 Using the crown cutter, the thread is prepared to receive the hollow screw

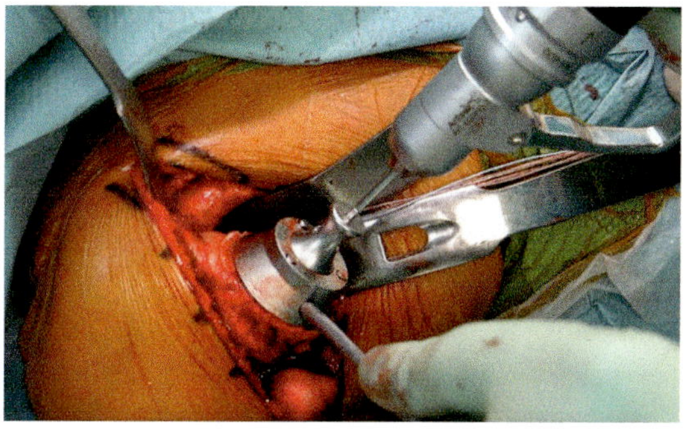

Fig. 25.15 Using the centering device and a graduated cage screw sizer, the length of the screw hole is determined by drilling the cage screw sizer until it reaches the lateral cortex

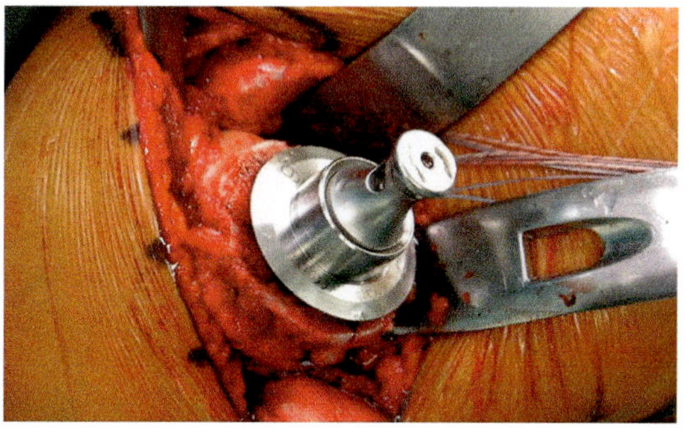

Fig. 25.16 The trunion (baseplate) is inserted over the centering device, in the predetermined location

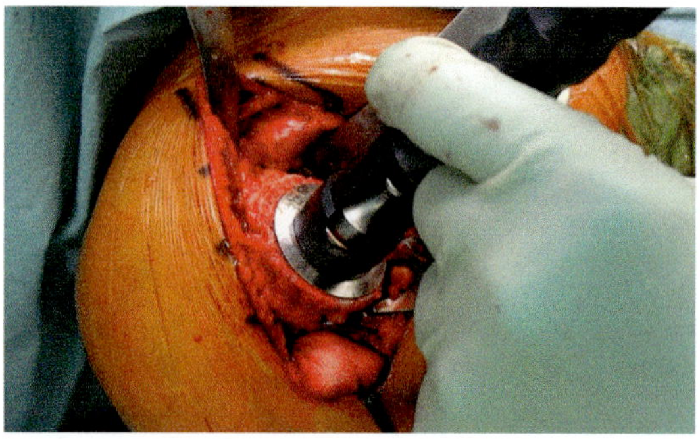

Fig. 25.17 The impactor is placed over the trunion (baseplate), and the impactor is struck to achieve a press fit

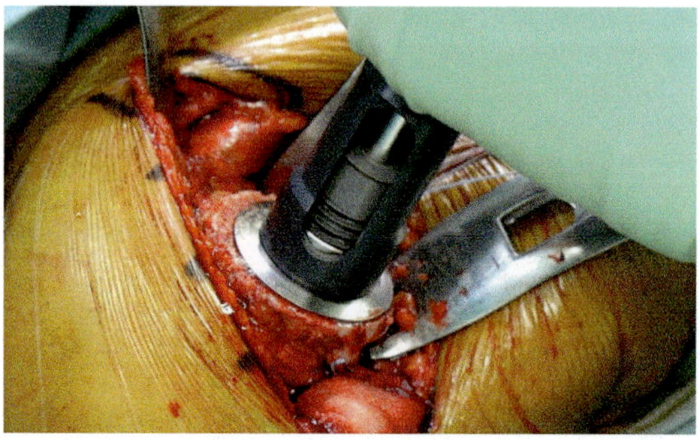

Fig. 25.18 The centering device is removed, and the hollow screw is inserted into to impactor, and screwed into the bone. In this case, the trunion (baseplate) is pressed firmly against the resected face of the proximal humerus

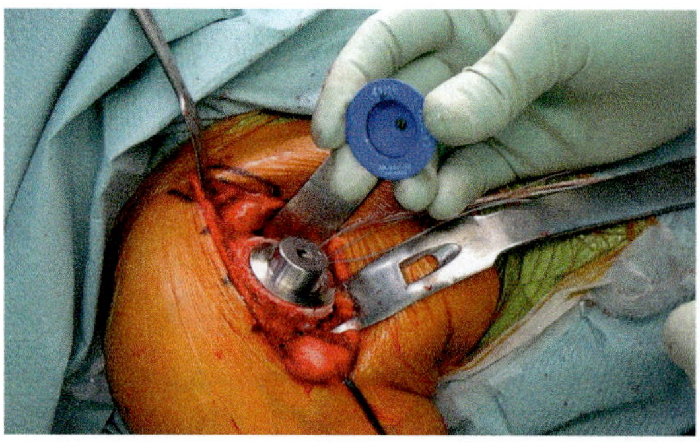

Fig. 25.19 Fitting a trial head for trial positioning

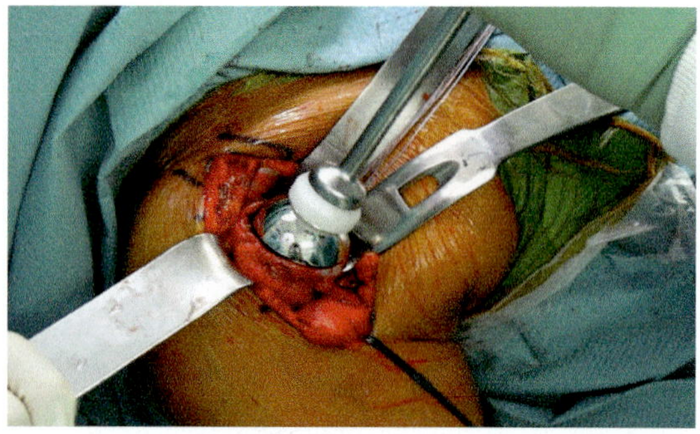

Fig. 25.20 The definitive humeral head prosthesis is struck with an impactor to achieve a press fit

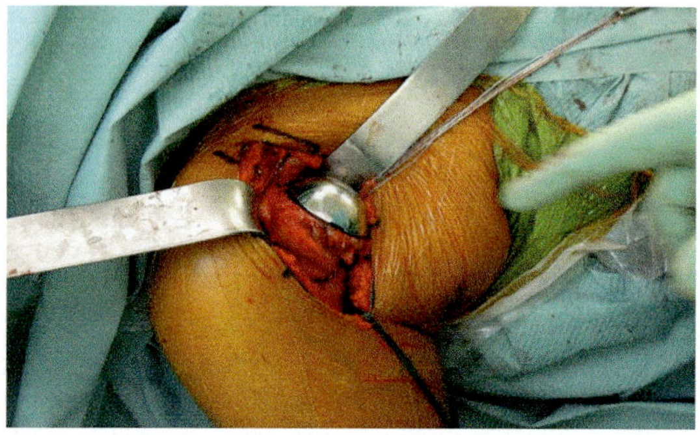

Fig. 25.21 After final implantation, the prosthesis is repositioned to observe "joint play"

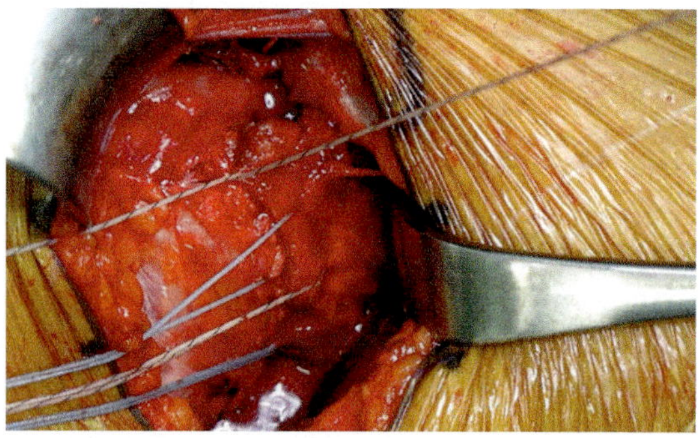

Fig. 25.22 Reattachment of the previously reinforced subscapularis tendon. A tension-free suture is recommended for the rotator cuff interval

positioning is performed with a trial head cap to confirm the correct size of the humeral head cap (Fig. 25.19). Finally, the prosthetic head cap is implanted. Therefore the head cap is chipped (Figs. 25.20 and 25.21).

Next, the subscapularis tendon is reattached according to the Mason-Allen suture technique, with the stitches prepared prior to implantation (Fig. 25.22). A tension-free suture is advised for the rotator cuff interval. An appropriate wound closure is performed, and a drain is inserted.

Figures 25.23, 25.24 and 25.25 show the 2-year follow-up after implantation of a stemless humeral head prosthesis in combination with a metal-back socket. The prosthesis was implanted to repair an avascular humeral head necrosis with deformity of the tubercles. These disorders occurred after a fixed-angle plate osteosynthesis was applied to repair a humeral

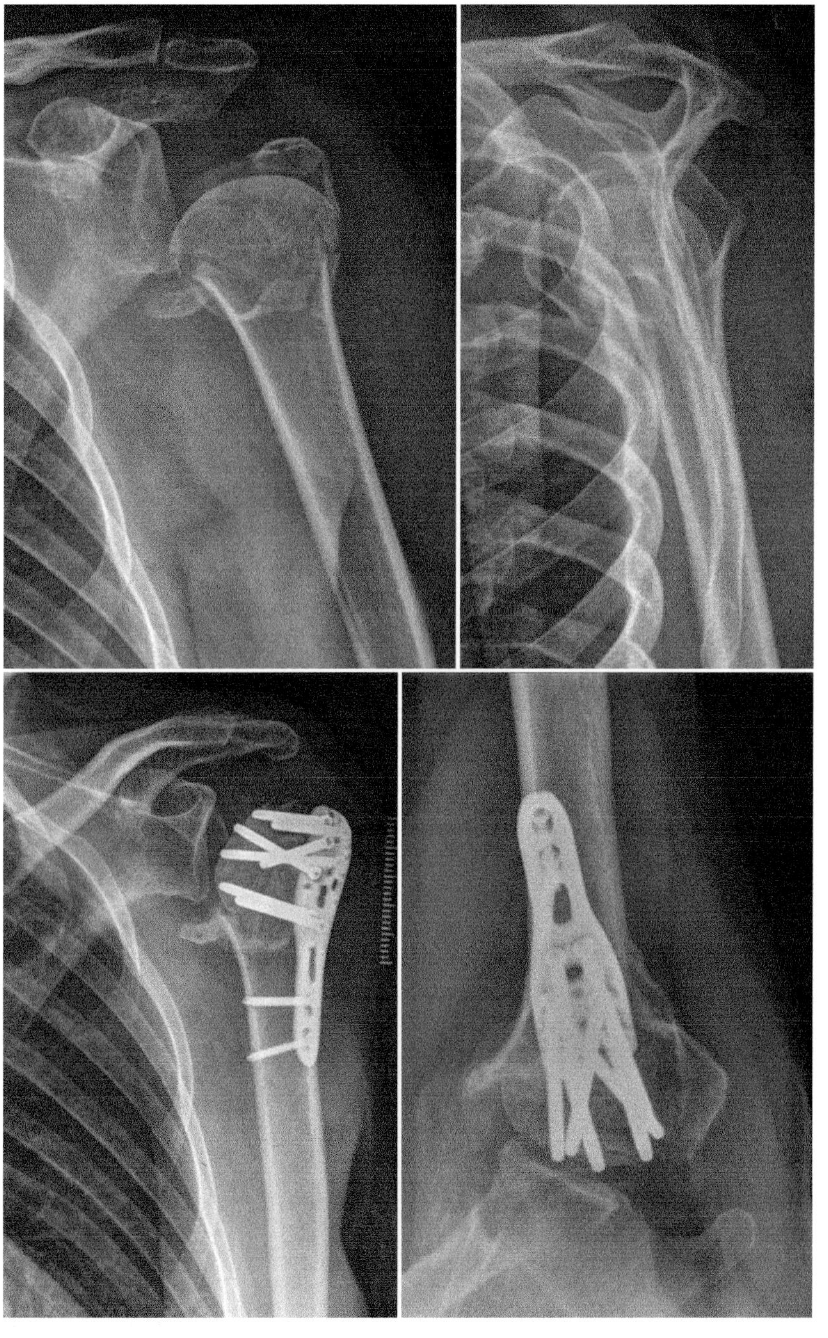

Figs. 25.23, 25.24, 25.25 Two-year follow-up after a stemless humeral head prosthesis was implanted, in combination with a metal-back socket. The prosthesis was implanted to repair an avascular humeral head necrosis with deformity of the tubercles. These disorders occurred after a fixed-angle plate osteosynthesis had been performed, in an attempt to repair a humeral head 4-segment-fracture

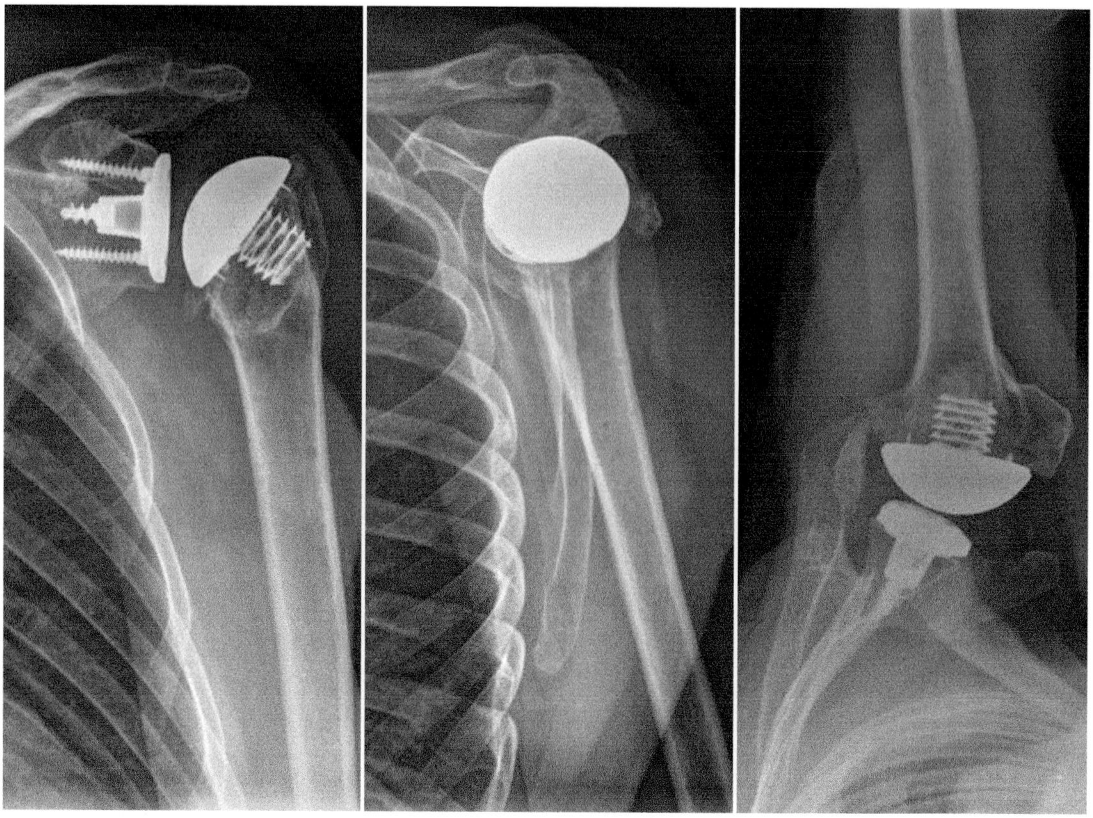

Figs. 25.23, 25.24, 25.25 (continued)

head 4-segment-fracture (Figs. 25.23, 25.24 and 25.25).

Postoperative Management

The major goal of therapy is to achieve a centralized humeral head. For the best possible integration into everyday life, the prosthesis should allow pain-free mobility, coordination, and the ability to exert sufficient and adequate force levels.

Phase 1 (1–3 Postoperative Weeks)

The arm is initially placed in a shoulder brace. The brace is maintained day and night, until the end of the third postoperative week. During the day a short-term positioning on a pillow is possible. The patient is given instructions on isometric exercises for the hand and elbow.

The shoulder is passively mobilized at the scapula level, in a pain-free manner. Mobilization is stopped gently, with a maximal flexion of 90°, abduction of 60°, internal rotation of 45°, and external rotation of 10°.

The adjacent joints are mobilized with instructions to perform gentle isometric centering exercises (joint-near only), under consideration of the scapula level. The scapula is mobilized gently, with assistance. Gentle detoning measures are performed in the areas of the shoulder and neck, with bilateral, assisted flexion, applied in the supine position. The patient is instructed in performing controlled passive pendulum exercises, with posture correction under scapula control. The patient is trained to complete activities of daily life, including getting up, dressing, washing, self-reliance, and gently applying the shoulder brace.

Phase 2 (4–6 Postoperative Weeks)

After three weeks, the patient is advised to undergo follow-up inpatient rehabilitation for a period of 3 weeks.

Focus: mobilization and coordination training

Patients undergo passive mobilization in all planes of motion, painlessly. Mobilization should stop gently, at a maximum flexion of 90°, abduction of 70°, internal rotation of 70°, and external rotation of 20°. The patient should slowly transition to assisted mobilization. Exercises should be performed to strengthen the scapula-fixators (serratus anterior m. and trapezius m.). Light, painless, isometric measures should be applied to the rotator cuff with a small lever. Soft tissue techniques should be applied. A home plan or instructions for independent mobilization should be worked out.

After week 4, the patient should perform active-assisted mobilization.

Goal: 6 weeks post-operatively: painless crest grip and apron grip until the trochanter major.

Phase 3 (7–12 Postoperative Weeks)

Focus: Active mobilization, coordination training, and strengthening

Patients should perform terminal, passive, and active range of motion exercises. With respect to the pain threshold range of motion should be increased. To achieve glenohumeral centering and stabilization, patients should perform isometric and dynamic activity at the rotator cuff. The glenohumeral rhythm should improve at all joint positions. Active counterforce should be applied between the scapula and humerus for flexion, abduction, external rotation, and internal rotation.

Coordination and stabilization exercises for the scapula should be performed (in particular, they should receive training in recruiting the M. serratus anterior and M. lower trapezius). Patients should focus on posture correction.

The home plan should be expanded, and the arms should be integrated into daily life.

After the 9th week, patients should increase dynamic training of the rotator cuff, with both concentric and eccentric exercises at the scapula level. For example, they could employ a Thera band (yellow-red) and light weights (maximum 1 kg).

Patients should focus on improving coordination quality. They should perform complex activation of the shoulder muscles in closed chain movements. Later, they can perform the overhead position (wiping exercise), light lifting exercises, and resume professional activities that require low shoulder strain; typically, it is possible to drive.

Goal at 12 weeks post-op: Apron and crest grip.

Phase 4 (After the 12th Week)

Focus: strengthening and integration into everyday life

Patients should intensify muscular strengthening with closed-system devices. They should perform stabilized closed chain movements with higher intensity. Dynamic stabilization exercises should be performed with increasing loads, based on core stability. They should perform specific, progressive resistance exercises for the rotator cuff (particularly eccentric) and the other shoulder muscles. They should perform reactive exercises, with low intensity, below the shoulder level (supporting exercises, cable, Theraband, catching and throwing exercises). They should receive training in functional activities with increased loads. They can resume professional activities with increased loads.

Phase 5 (After the 21st Week)

Focus: resumption of sports and other active shoulder burdens

Patients should increase the intensity of the previous exercises, and perform power training, when appropriate. They should perform reactive exercises with higher intensity, and gradually increase movements to above shoulder height. They should resume professional activities with intense loads on the shoulders. They can perform independent athletic training, at a slowly increasing intensity, with occasional supervision from a therapist. Even in the late stages of rehabilitation, exercise can lead to overload responses; therefore, an accurate, symptom-based load control remains necessary in everyday life, work, and sports.

Results

The stemless arthroplasty of the shoulder joint is a relatively new concept. The currently available literature has reported 929 cases that employed stemless prostheses from different manufacturers. All authors described a significant improvement, and no cases reported loosening that required revision of the shaft. However, it must be noted that, currently, only two studies have reported results with follow-ups of more than 3 years. Our workgroup applied the described type of humeral prosthesis, and we included follow-ups of 6 and 9 years. We observed functional and radiological outcomes comparable to those achieved with third and fourth generation stem prostheses. Furthermore, in the available literature, comparative studies did not distinguish between stem and stemless prostheses in terms of the outcome.

Complications

Complications associated with the use of stemless prostheses were reported by Huguet et al. In 5 of 63 cases, they noted lateral cortical disruption in the immediate postoperative imaging, with the TESS prosthesis (Biomet). All those cases received conservative treatment. Consolidation was noted within 2 months. However, those cases were considered part of the learning curve.

Brunner et al. reported that one of 233 cases showed an extensive resorption-margin below the baseplate and around the screw in 24-month postoperative x-ray images. That case was evaluated as aseptic loosening, and it was treated conservatively (Eclipse, Arthrex).

The 6- and 9-year results from our workgroup did not show any loosening with the described prosthesis.

Literature

1. Habermeyer P, Lichtenberg S, Tauber M, Magosch P. Midterm results of stemless shoulder arthroplasty: a prospective study. J Shoulder Elb Surg. 2015;24(9):1463–72.
2. Churchill RS, Chuinard C, Wiater JM, Friedman R, Freehill M, Jacobson S, et al. Clinical and radiographic outcomes of the simpliciti canal-sparing shoulder arthroplasty system: a prospective two-year multicenter study. J Bone Joint Surg Am. 2016;98(7):552–60.
3. Brunner UH, Fruth M, Rückl K, Magosch P, Tauber M, Resch H, et al. Die schaftfreie Eclipse-Prothese – Indikation und mittelfristige Ergebnisse. Obere Extrem. 2012;7(1):22–8. German
4. Athwal GS. Spare the canal: stemless shoulder arthroplasty is finally here: commentary on an article by R. Sean Churchill, MD, et al.: "clinical and radiographic outcomes of the simpliciti canal-sparing shoulder arthroplasty system. A prospective two-year multicenter study". J Bone Joint Surg Am. 2016;98(7):e28.
5. Maier MW, Lauer S, Klotz MC, Bulhoff M, Spranz D, Zeifang F. Are there differences between stemless and conventional stemmed shoulder prostheses in the treatment of glenohumeral osteoarthritis? BMC Musculoskelet Disord. 2015;16:275. Pubmed Central PMCID: PMC4591701
6. Kadum B, Hassany H, Wadsten M, Sayed-Noor A, Sjödén G. Geometrical analysis of stemless shoulder arthroplasty: a radiological study of seventy TESS total shoulder prostheses. Int Orthop. 2016;40(4):751–8.
7. Samilson RL, Prieto V. Dislocation arthropathy of the shoulder. J Bone Joint Surg Am. 1983;65(4):456–60.
8. Habermeyer P, Magosch P, Luz V, Lichtenberg S. Three-dimensional glenoid deformity in patients with osteoarthritis: a radiographic analysis. J Bone Joint Surg Am. 2006;88(6):1301–7.
9. Walch G, Badet R, Boulahia A, Khoury A. Morphologic study of the glenoid in primary glenohumeral osteoarthritis. J Arthroplast. 1999;14(6):756–60.

10. Churchill RS. Stemless shoulder arthroplasty: current status. J Shoulder Elb Surg. 2014;23(9):1409–14.
11. Magosch P, Habermeyer P, Bachmaier S, Metcalfe N. Biomechanics of metaphyseal fixed humeral head replacement. Obere Extrem. 2012;7(1):11–6.
12. Hawi N, Tauber M, Messina MJ, Habermeyer P, Martetschlager F. Anatomic stemless shoulder arthroplasty and related outcomes: a systematic review. BMC Musculoskelet Disord. 2016;17(1):376. Pubmed Central PMCID: PMC5006279
13. Hawi N, Magosch P, Tauber M, Lichtenberg S, Martetschlager F, Habermeyer P. Glenoid deformity in the coronal plane correlates with humeral head changes in osteoarthritis: a radiographic analysis. J Shoulder Elb Surg. 2016; https://doi.org/10.1016/j.jse.2016.07.007.

Patient Specific Instrumentation

26

Kyong S. Min, Henry M. Fox, and Jon J. P. Warner

Introduction

Shoulder arthroplasty has become a reliable and effective method to treat arthritis, fracture, nonunion, malunion, tumor and rotator cuff arthropathy. According to the Agency of Healthcare Research and Quality, in 2011there were 53,000 shoulder replacement procedures performed in the United States. The prevalence of these procedures continues to increase [1, 2]. Between 1993 and 2007 the annual growth rate for total shoulder arthroplasty was 10.6%, with an annual growth rate in revision of 14.0% [1]. These increasing rates of shoulder arthroplasty are in contrast with rates of lower extremity arthroplasty. Between 1990 and 2002, primary and revision total knee arthroplasty volumes were shown to grow annually at rates of 6–7%. Primary and revision total hip arthroplasties increased yearly at rates of 4.5% and 2.5%, respectively [3].

As the popularity of total shoulder arthroplasty (TSA) and reverse shoulder arthroplasty (RSA) increase, more surgeons are providing this service. But as opposed to knee and hip arthroplasty, most orthopaedic surgery residency programs provide limited experience in shoulder arthroplasty. This deficiency in training results in most orthopaedic surgeons having limited skill in shoulder arthroplasty. Furthermore, there is a steep learning curve to achieve reliable outcomes with shoulder arthroplasty [4, 5]. As expected, there is a direct correlation between surgical volume and patient outcomes [6, 7]. Surgeons with higher volumes (more experience) have lower complication rates. This is evidenced in the lower complication rates with hip and knee replacement surgery compared to total shoulder arthroplasty.

Despite the steep learning curve and increasing demand for shoulder replacement surgery, approximately 85% of all shoulder replacement procedures are performed by surgeons who perform fewer than five shoulder replacements per year [8]. Considering that the majority of shoulder arthroplasties are performed by low volume surgeons, a guidance tool to assist with this complex procedure would be highly desirable. Such a tool might provide enormous value by bending the learning (experience) curve to help surgeons avoid common surgical errors.

Computerized planning software and patient-specific instrumentation have been utilized in various areas of orthopedics. There have been conflicting reports of the efficacy of planning and patient-specific implantation in both orthopaedic trauma surgery and total knee arthroplasty. While

K. S. Min
Department of Orthopaedics,
Tripler Army Medical Center, Honolulu, HI, USA

Department of Orthopaedics,
Massachusetts General Hospital, Boston, MA, USA

H. M. Fox · J. J. P. Warner (✉)
Department of Orthopaedics,
Massachusetts General Hospital, Boston, MA, USA
e-mail: jwarner@partners.org

I. A. Trail et al. (eds.), *Textbook of Shoulder Surgery*, https://doi.org/10.1007/978-3-319-70099-1_26

some studies have shown more anatomic implant positions with both computerized planning and patient-specific instrumentation, no significant improvements in patient reported outcomes or implant survival have been demonstrated [9, 10]. Since consistent improvements have not been demonstrated in patient-reported outcomes using patient-specific instruments, as compared to outcomes with traditional instruments, these technologies have not yet been heavily adopted. However, the current endpoint of measurement may not be wholly accurate, as durability may be affected and most available studies have only evaluated initial short-term outcomes.

Shoulder arthroplasty differs significantly from knee and hip arthroplasty. Arguably, the surgical approaches to the arthritic shoulder are more technically difficult and visualization can be a significant issue, especially with significant glenoid deformities. Moreover, many of the landmarks and reference points used to guide glenoid implantation are obscured by soft tissues. In addition, the scapula moves on the chest wall, making it difficult to place the component in the anatomic position. In comparison to patient-specific planning and instrumentation in hip and knee arthroplasty, these innovations in shoulder arthroplasty likely present a higher relative benefit due to these factors.

Reasons for Failure

Total Shoulder Arthroplasty

In anatomic total shoulder arthroplasty, glenoid component malpositioning is the most common reason for failure (Table 26.1). Boileau et al. performed a review of all complications associated in total shoulder arthroplasty; glenoid component accounts for 24% of all complications in total shoulder arthroplasty [15]. In an analysis of glenoid-specific failure, Matsen et al. conducted a review of twenty-seven articles reporting on 3853 total shoulder arthroplasties. Asymptomatic radiolucent lines were encountered at a rate of 7.3% per year, while symptomatic loosening occurred at 1.2% per year. These findings contributed to a revision rate of 0.8% per year [16].

Table 26.1 Five golden rules for the glenoid component

1. The glenoid retroversion should be kept below 10° [11]
2. The superior glenoid inclination should be less than 10° [12]
3. Posterior humeral head subluxation greater than 80% cannot be corrected with asymmetric reaming [13]
4. The seating of the glenoid component must be greater than 80% contact; seating less than 80% will lead to early loosening [14]
5. Excessive reaming leads to early loosening due to loss of bony support [14]

Malpositioning of the glenoid component generates abnormal forces across the glenoid. This causes what Matsen and colleagues have called the "rocking horse phenomenon," leading to glenoid loosening [11, 17–19]. Farron et al. performed a finite element modeling study and determined that micromotion at the bone-cement interface was significantly influenced by retroversion. The authors determined that there was an exponential increase in micromotion for internal and external rotation when the component was placed in greater than 10° of retroversion [11]. Shapiro performed a cadaveric biomechanical study and determined that the placement of a glenoid component in 15° of retroversion decreased the glenohumeral contact area and increased the contact pressure, as compared to 0° retroversion [20]. Thus, glenoid component retroversion will lead to eccentric loading, component loosening, increased glenoid component wear and osteolysis [13, 20, 21].

Clinical Pearl 1
Preoperative planning cannot account for soft tissue restrictions. Whether performing total shoulder arthroplasty or reverse shoulder arthroplasty, obtain the best possible visualization of the glenoid by making the necessary soft tissue releases.

In addition to these undesirable outcomes, Young et al. showed that with malpositioning of the glenoid, there is a progressive failure of the rotator cuff [18]. The authors showed that at 15 years of follow-up after anatomic TSA, only

45% of the study patients had evidence of an intact rotator cuff. Placement of the glenoid component in retroversion and superior inclination has been associated with rotator cuff tear [12, 22]. Without a functional rotator cuff, eccentric forces will be placed on the glenoid and the arthroplasty will fail. Boileau found that the majority of failures in total shoulder arthroplasty are avoidable; these failures are largely due to a diagnostic error, a technical error, or a combination thereof [15]. If the surgical plan and the technical execution are inadequate, an operation may fail before the patient goes to the operating room, or before they leave the operating room.

In 2012, Walch et al. showed that when a total shoulder arthroplasty is used in a B2 or C glenoid, there is a higher failure rate [23] (Fig. 26.1). In patients that underwent a TSA with a B2 or C glenoid, at 77 months of follow-up, only 66% of patients were happy with their outcome and there was a 16.3% revision rate due to glenoid loosening and instability. Walch showed that patients with biconcave glenoids can do well for a short time, but after 6 years they have a 21% rate of glenoid loosening [23] (Fig. 26.2).

Clinical Pearl 2
In total shoulder arthroplasty, severely retroverted glenoids may not be correctable with reaming. Such retroversion may require a posterior augemented glenoid or a posterior bone graft to build up the glenoid. If placing a bone graft, the graft should be no smaller than 8 mm.

In the context of glenoid component failure, an understanding of glenoid morphology and accurate measurement of glenoid retroversion are essential to crafting the appropriate surgical plan. Commonly, the Friedman method is used to calculate glenoid retroversion [25, 26]. Using a 2-dimentional CT, the transverse axis of the scapula is determined by a line drawn from the midpoint of the glenoid fossa

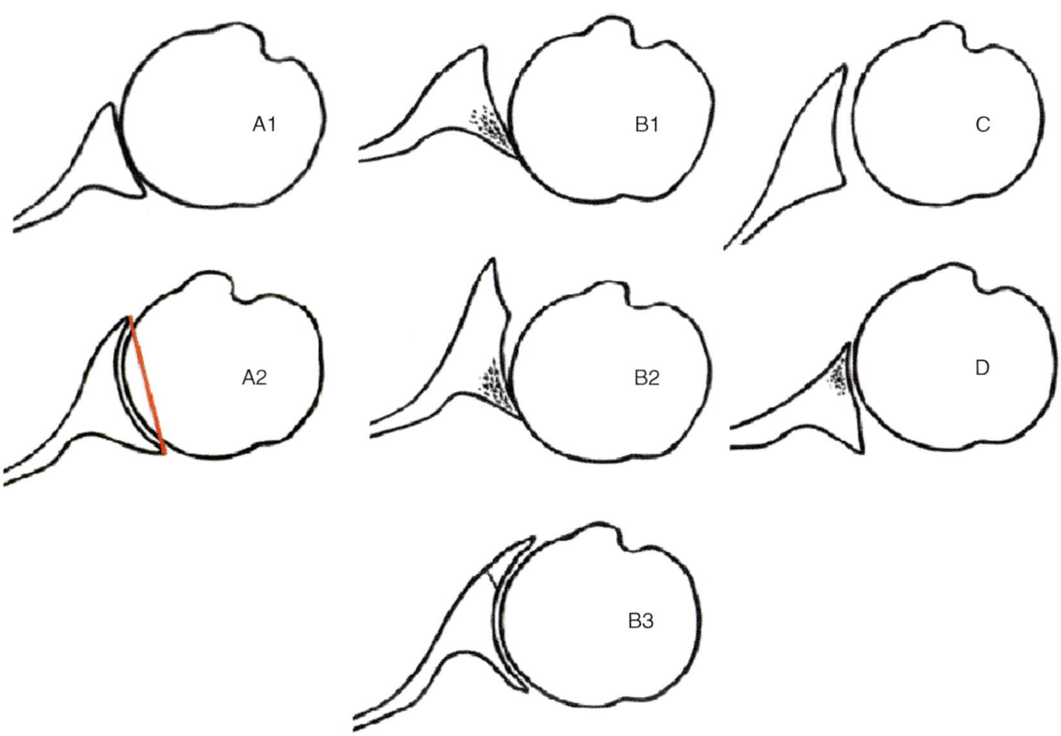

Fig. 26.1 Modified Walch classification. (Source: Bercik et al. [24] (Used with Permission from Elsevier))

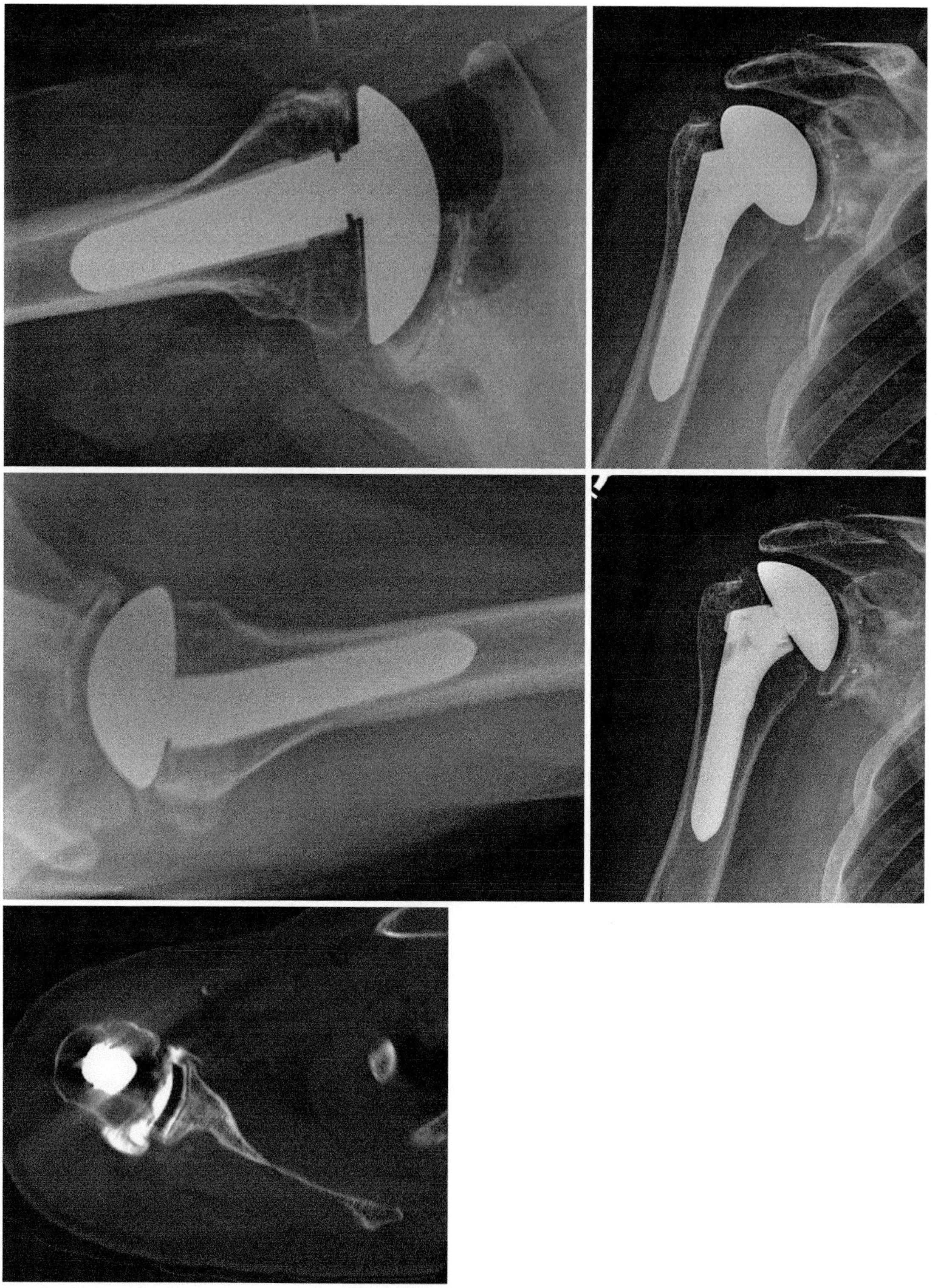

Fig. 26.2 Anatomic total shoulder with progressive loosening of glenoid component. (**a**) 1 year post-op. (**b**) 23 months post-op. When a glenoid is placed in a suboptimal position (retroversion greater than 10°) Walch has shown that with time there can be progressive loosening

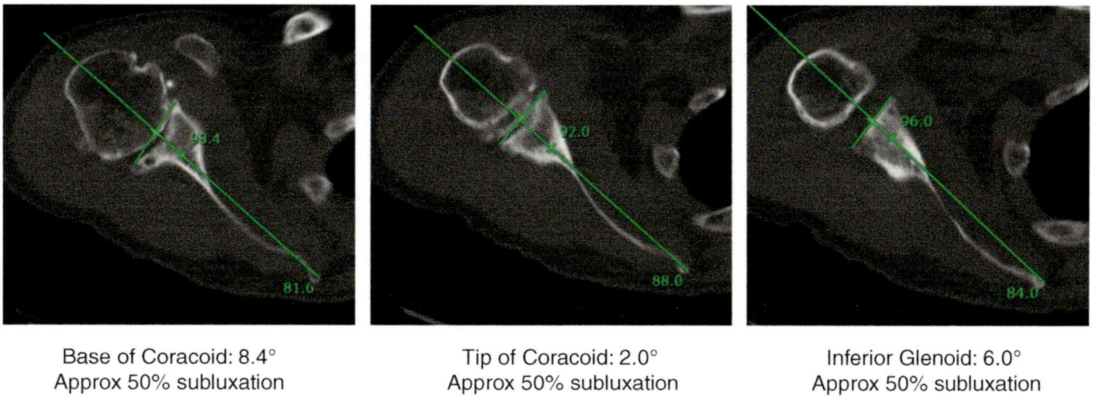

Fig. 26.3 CT retroversion. When using the Friedman method to calculate retroversion, the degree or retroversion measured is dependent upon the level at which it is measured

to the medial edge of the scapula. The line drawn perpendicular to the transverse axis is defined as the line of neutral version. To calculate glenoid version, a line is drawn between the anterior and posterior margins of the glenoid. The angle between the line of neutral version and the line connecting the anterior and posterior margins of the glenoid determines the amount of glenoid version (Fig. 26.3). Rouleau et al. demonstrated that the Friedman method is the most reproducible method of measuring glenoid version on a 2-dimensional CT [25, 26]. While the study demonstrated that there is excellent interobserver and intraobserver reliability with this method, subsequent studies have demonstrated that glenoid retroversion cannot be adequately measured on a 2-dimensional CT [24, 27, 28].

Randelli demonstrated that glenoid retroversion depends greatly on at what level the glenoid is measured [27]. This is because the position of the scapula cannot be controlled when taking a CT; therefore, there is no consistent reference for measure. Recent studies have shown that a 3-dimensional reconstruction is a more accurate tool to measure glenoid retroversion [24, 28]. Scalise et al. showed that 3-dimensional reconstructions of the shoulder improved surgical decisions regarding glenoid preparation and component fit [29]. Furthermore, Budge et al. demonstrated that axial 2-dimensional measurements of retroversion range from 5° to 15° different than those of 3-dimensional measurements [30]. Two-dimensional measurements of glenoid version are less reliable than 3-dimensional reconstructions which analyze the scapula as a free body [30–32]. The 3-dimensional reconstructions provide corrected axial 2-dimensional images that are strictly on the plane of the scapula, allowing for more accurate assessments of version and subluxation.

Reducing glenoid retroversion to less than 10° is the goal in total shoulder arthroplasty [11]. Both clinical and biomechanical data support increased risk of glenoid component loosening if the glenoid is placed in retroversion greater than 10°. Denard and Walch demonstrated that patients with greater than 80% posterior humeral head subluxation and a retroversion greater than 27° will have a higher rate of failure [13]. In order to make the appropriate operative plan, the surgeon must understand glenoid morphology.

As previously stated, most surgeons have limited experience with shoulder arthroplasty as compared to hip and knee arthroplasty, and visualization is quite often a problem. A critical step in shoulder arthroplasty is accurate placement of the glenoid guidewire. Most arthroplasty systems utilize a guidewire, which is placed as a reference point for correction of the glenoid deformity; however, there are no reliable anatomic landmarks that inform the surgeon about the glenoid version during surgery. Therefore, placement of this guidewire, and thus the glenoid component, is highly variable.

Commonly, the glenoid component positioning in a total arthroplasty is determined by either (a) the surgeon's eye, without attention to correction of version or (b) by placing a guidewire, by hand, perpendicular to the plane of the scapula in the axial and sagittal plane and parallel to the plane of the scapula and the coronal plane. Visualization through a deltopectoral or superolateral approach may be difficult due to soft-tissue contractures, bony deformity of the glenoid, or failure to appreciate the plane of the scapula. Therefore, proper orientation of the glenoid component may be difficult to achieve.

Studies have demonstrated that when using this conventional technique, surgeons may deviate 8–10° from their intended position [33, 34]. Thus difficult exposure and lack of anatomic landmarks commonly lead to malpositioning the glenoid component [15]. From insufficient preoperative evaluation of glenoid morphology to improper execution of the surgery itself, many potential pitfalls exist in anatomic total shoulder arthroplasty.

Reverse Shoulder Arthroplasty

Total shoulder arthroplasty allows the rotator cuff and deltoid to function normally in an unconstrained fashion; however, in the setting of a dysfunctional rotator cuff, the reverse shoulder arthroplasty provides reliable pain relief and functional improvement. When there is severe glenoid deformity, a total shoulder arthroplasty may not be the ideal surgical solution. If the glenoid cannot be corrected to a retroversion of 10° or less, there is greater than 80% posterior humeral head subluxation, or there is retroversion greater than 27°, a reverse shoulder replacement should be considered.

Since its FDA approval in 2004, there has been a steady increase in the utilization of reverse shoulder arthroplasty. Reverse shoulder arthroplasty designs have changed over the years, from early lateral center of rotation designs to a more medialized center of rotation [35]. More recently, many systems have shifted back to a more lateralized center of rotation as this geometry has been shown to reduce scapular notching and improve range of motion. Improved baseplate fixation in these updated lateral centers of rotation systems have dramatically reduced the failures observed with the earlier designs of lateralized systems. With these design improvements, the indications for reverse shoulder arthroplasty have expanded to include severe glenoid deformity, revision shoulder arthroplasty, proximal humerus fractures and rotator cuff tear arthropathy [36].

Optimizing baseplate and glenosphere position is paramount to achieving a successful result with reverse shoulder arthroplasty. Currently, consensus is still lacking on the ideal size and position of glenosphere placement. There are arguments for inlay versus onlay humeral designs; medialization versus lateralization of the glenosphere; and neutral tilt versus inferior tilt of the glenosphere. The goal of these variables is to achieve optimum component positioning, to achieve appropriate deltoid tension and ensure satisfactory range of motion. Optimal positioning will also reduce the incidence of scapular notching. In a yet-to-be published study, Walch demonstrated excellent greater than 10-year follow-up in more than 250 reverse shoulder replacements; however, his study demonstrated that there was a direct correlation with scapular notching and failure of the reverse replacement. The size and position of the glenosphere was found to directly influence stability, range of motion and scapular notching.

The reverse shoulder arthroplasty is used when the patient does not have a functional rotator cuff and/or has severe deformity. In situations like inflammatory arthropathy, fracture malunion or revision surgery, significant glenoid erosion and/or humeral deformity may be encountered. In some circumstances, the glenoid vault is compromised to the degree that bony reconstruction is required in addition to reverse shoulder arthroplasty. For the ultimate success and durability of the operation, the orthopedic surgeon must anticipate this problem prior to the surgery. Failure to recognize such deformities may lead to malpositioning of the base plate and glenosphere orientation will be poor. This can result in limited motion, structural failure or significant scapular notching—all factors which negatively affect the longevity of the implant.

The technical steps of reverse shoulder arthroplasty are somewhat different than conventional nonconstrained total shoulder replacement; achieving proper soft-tissue tensioning and component orientation may be quite complex in some patients. Similar to the total shoulder arthroplasty, a reverse shoulder arthroplasty is performed using the deltopectoral or superolateral approach. It is critical that a 360-degree view of the entire glenoid is achieved. In addition, it is important to be conscious of the location of the axillary nerve, particularly in revision cases with asymmetric erosion of the glenoid. Moreover, with such deformity there may be even fewer landmarks for guidewire placement, which is required to orient the baseplate accurately.

Once the components are positioned and implanted, the surgeon can clinically test for stability of the prosthesis and adjust deltoid tension to increase stability. However, it is very difficult to appreciate the degree of perimeter impingement, which may result in scapular notching.

Clinical Pearl 3
In reverse shoulder arthroplasty, the ideal component position and size may not be possible due to soft tissue restrictions. When planning a difficult reverse shoulder arthroplasty, create multiple surgical plans with varying implant sizes, positions, lateralizations and eccentricities.

Patient Specific Planning

Patient specific planning and patient specific instrumentation can significantly help orthopaedic surgeons avoid diagnostic and technical errors in shoulder arthroplasty, which may otherwise occur due to failing to appreciate the pathoanatomy. By using virtual surgery methodology on the computer, the surgeon can potentially perform trial without error. This is akin to the aeronautics industry in training pilots with a flight simulator—pilots learn how to fly without the fear of an actual crash. Virtual surgery provides an accurate map of the shoulder anatomy, thereby allowing the surgeon to anticipate problems and be prepared to navigate these obstacles with the necessary tools. In a yet-to-be published study, the Codman Shoulder Society® conducted a survey that assessed the influence of patient specific planning in surgical decision making. The study clearly demonstrated that patient specific planning provides statistically significant information and guides the surgeon's treatment plan. This information and surgical planning was particularly impactful for lesser experienced surgeons, in allowing them to more accurately identify the anatomy and select the best treatment option. Thus, patient-specific planning may ultimately bend the experience curve and improve surgeon decision-making and technical execution.

Total Shoulder Arthroplasty

Computerized planning software and patient specific instrumentation can assist the surgeon in managing these difficult cases. By utilizing computerized planning software, the surgeon can understand the glenoid orientation and deformity. Conventional 2-dimensional CTs are dependent upon patient positioning and scapulothoracic orientation. Patient specific planning software provides 3-dimensional reconstruction of the glenoid and corrected axial 2-dimensional images that are on the plane of the scapula. These corrected images allow for more accurate assessments of glenoid version and humeral subluxation (Figs. 26.4 and 26.5).

These tools will allow the surgeon to better understand the shoulder and anticipate potential pitfalls in reconstruction for each patient. Possessing accurate information about the glenoid version and posterior subluxation will help the surgeon decide if a total shoulder arthroplasty is a viable option, or whether the plan should change to a reverse shoulder arthroplasty. By implementing the "Five Golden Rules of Glenoid Component Positioning" (Table 26.1) and the

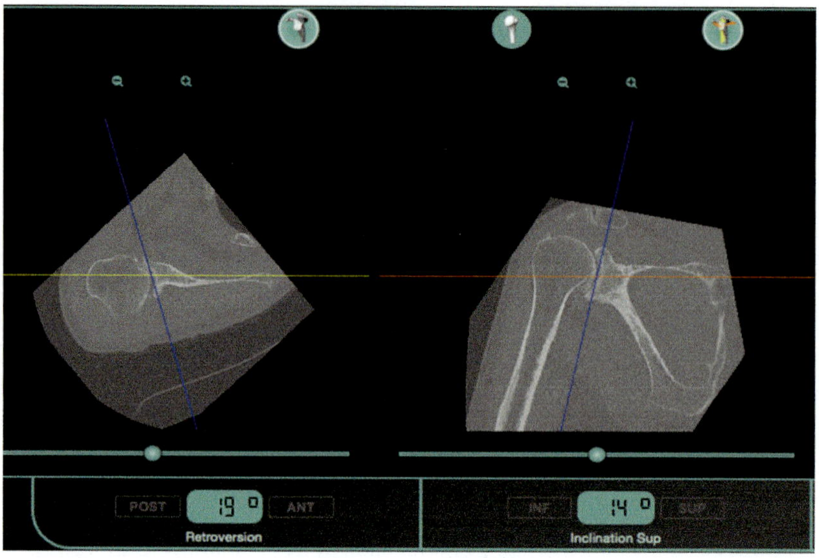

Fig. 26.4 PSP retroversion. Patient specific planning creates a 3-dimensional reconstruction of the scapula and provides a corrected axial 2-dimensional images that are strictly on the plane of the scapula. This allows for a more accurate measurement of retroversion and inclination

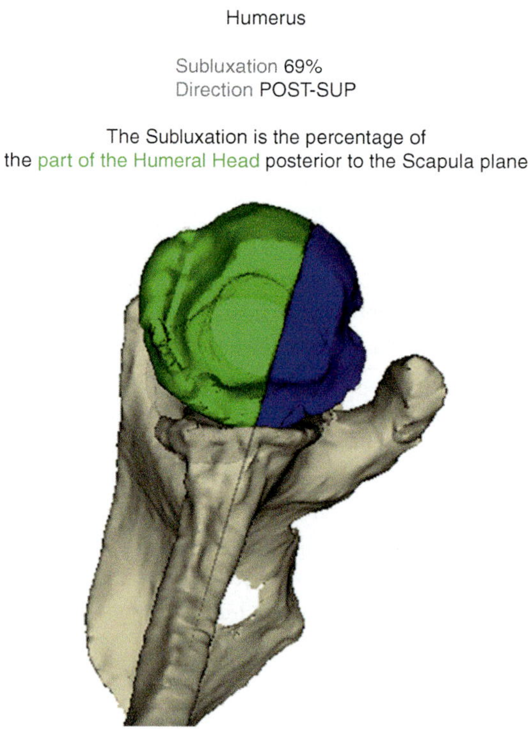

Fig. 26.5 Subluxation. Patient specific planning visualizes the glenohumeral joint in 3-dimension; therefore, it provides a more accurate calculate of subluxation

information provided by the patient specific planning, the surgeon can avoid diagnostic error.

Furthermore, in situations where the glenoid is severely deformed, the computer planning software can be used to create patient specific instrumentation. Specifically, a patient specific guide can be created to accurately place the glenoid guidewire in the optimum position, which properly orients the implant (Fig. 26.6). Walch et al. performed a cadaver study and showed excellent correlations between the guide pin position on preoperative planning and those placed at the time of implantation using patient specific instrumentation [37]. Throckmorton et al. performed a cadaver study by randomizing scapulae to either conventional or patient specific instrumentation for implantation of an anatomic total shoulder arthroplasty [34]. They encountered significantly more malpositioned components in the conventional instrument group compared to the patient specific group. Hendel et al. reported on clinical data of anatomic shoulder arthroplasty performed using patient specific instrumentation [33]. They performed a randomized controlled trial using conventional instrumentation versus patient specific instrumentation for glenoid placement during anatomic shoulder arthroplasty. Their study found that patient specific instrumentation significantly reduced the average deviation of implant position in both inclination and mediolateral offset, compared to conventional instrumentation. The authors reported the largest benefit was seen in patients with presurgical retroversion in excess of 16°. In those patients with retroversion greater than 16° preoperatively, the average devia-

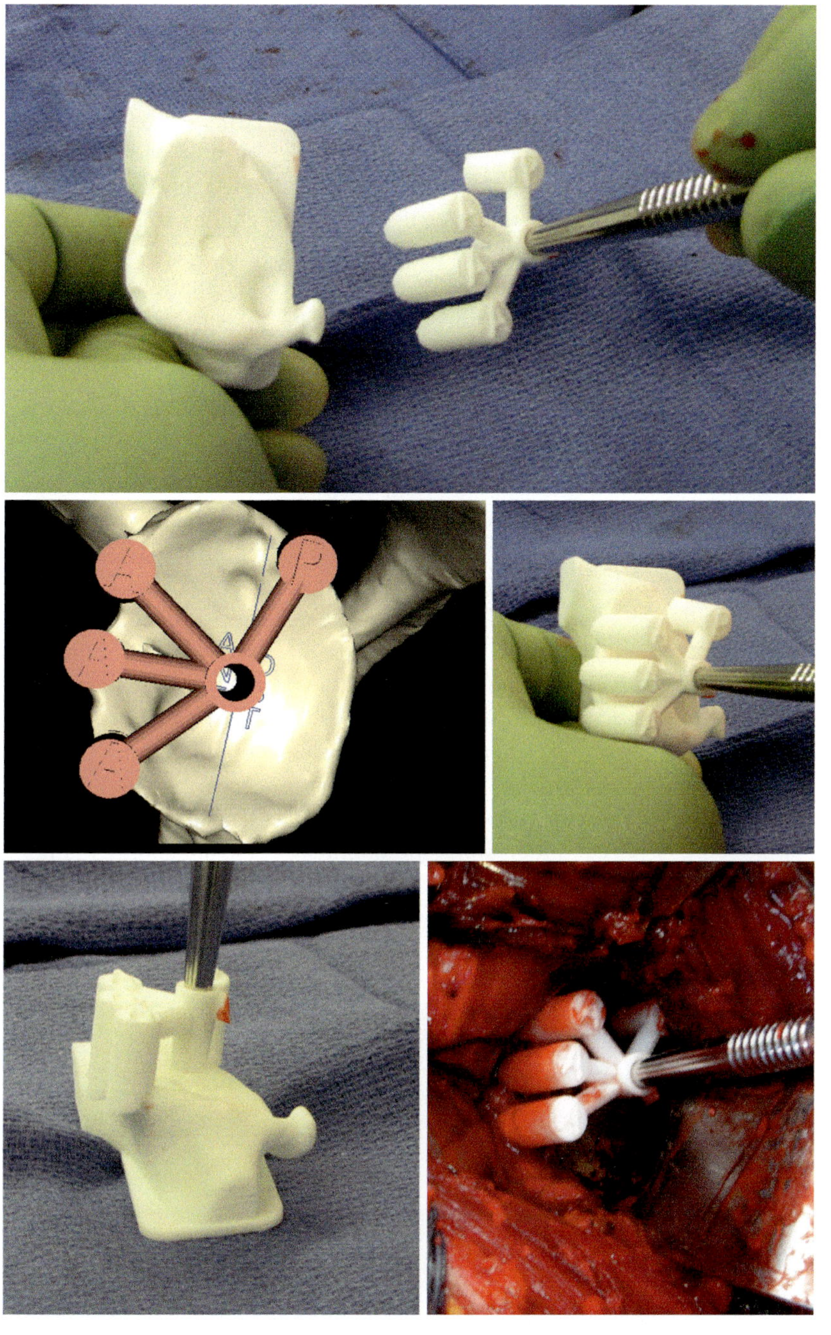

Fig. 26.6 Patient specific instrumentation—from planning to the OR. By obtaining a 3-dimensional print of the scapula and utilizing a patient-specific pin guide, the surgeon can trial and place the guidewire in the ideal position

tion in the conventional method group was 10°, while the average deviation was 1.2° in the patient specific instrumentation group [33]. Patient specific instrumentation resulted in a lower incidence of malpositioned glenoid components, and significantly improved selection of the optimal implant type for the specific glenoid anatomy.

Reverse Shoulder Arthroplasty

Many recent studies have investigated the benefits of glenosphere lateralization in reverse shoulder replacement. Boileau and colleagues have shown that with lateralization and inferior tilt of the glenosphere, there is improved range of motion and decreased notching [38]. Several studies have also recently shown that a high rate of bone graft incorporation is achieved when a graft is utilized to achieve lateralization of the base plate and glenosphere [38, 39]. Furthermore, Frankle has demonstrated that lateralization of the glenoid improves the function of the posterior rotator cuff, which will improve internal rotation [40]. While some component designs achieve lateralization through augmentation of the component, others use a bone graft to correct deformity thus reducing the degree of reaming and preserving glenoid bone stock. Patient specific planning allows the surgeon to calculate the exact size and shape of bone graft necessary to create the desired lateralization (Fig. 26.7).

With greater deformity, conventional placement of the guide-pin for the glenosphere becomes more inaccurate, but this can be improved with patient specific guides. Levy et al. performed a cadaver study where patient specific guides were used during glenoid baseplate placement. The authors demonstrated that these patient-specific guides are very accurate at reproducing a three dimensional preoperative plan [41]. Heylen et al. evaluated the influence of patient specific instrumentation on baseplate inclination after reverse shoulder arthroplasty [42]. They performed 24 reverse total shoulder arthroplasties in which half of the cases utilized preoperative planning and patient specific guides, and half used conventional instrumentation. The investigators reported that extreme inclination angles—deviating from optimum position—were more likely to occur with conventional instrumentation. The use of planning and patient specific instrumentation convincingly reduced variability of baseplate placement.

Some patient specific planning tools exist, which can reduce notching and increase range of motion. By simulating motion of the components, the tool can calculate the point at which the components will develop perimeter impingement. This impingement may result in notching and thus give an assessment of range of motion. This tool will allow the surgeon to trial and select optimum base plate positioning. Various components, sizes, bone grafts and positions can be trialed to determine the optimum combination for the arthroplasty (Fig. 26.8).

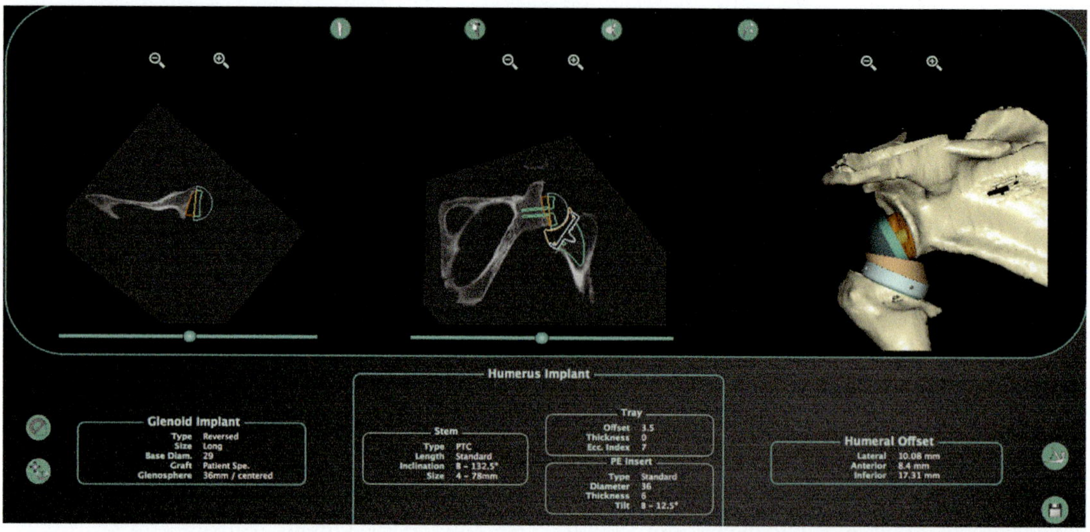

Fig. 26.7 Demonstration of 3D planning for BIORSA. The tool allows utilization of bone graft to augment the glenoid baseplate

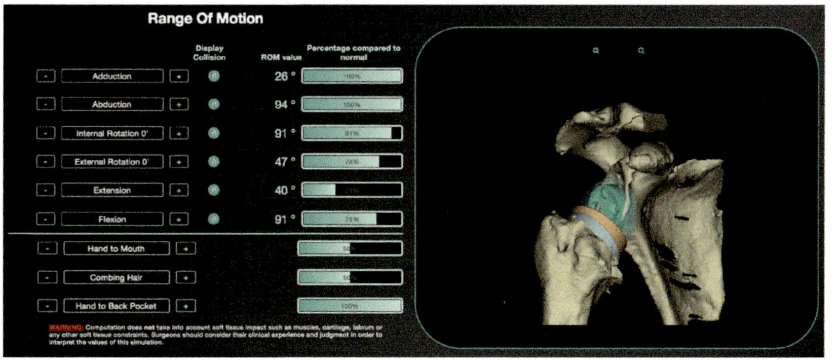

Fig. 26.8 ROM assessment. Using the bony anatomy, this tool can determine the potential points of impingement and calculate the projected range of motion

Value

We live in a world where healthcare costs are increasing at an extraordinary pace. Within the United States, the per capita health expenditure is $9403 and the total national health expenditure is over $3 trillion [43]. Some of this cost is attributed to unneeded or ineffective treatment. Thus, there has been a recent emphasis on achieving value in both surgical and medical care by (a) controlling costs and (b) reducing variation in treatment which may result in poor outcomes. As defined by Professor Michael Porter and Professor Robert Kaplan, value is outcome divided by cost [44–46]. In terms of healthcare economics, the cost effectiveness of a procedure is defined by the Incremental Cost Effectiveness Ratio (ICER); this metric compares the value provided by two different treatment modalities. The ICER is equaled to the difference in cost between two treatment options divided by the difference in outcomes of these options. By improving the placement of the components, patient specific planning and patient specific instruments can increase the cost effectiveness of shoulder arthroplasty and deliver greater value.

Patient specific planning will help the surgeon to provide a more reliable solution and potentially avoid problems. This reduction in unnecessary treatment variation will lower costs by several mechanisms. First, by anticipating potential obstacles and necessary equipment, the surgeon can effectively convey the surgical plan to the entire operative team. This will minimize trial and error, decrease surgical time, improve the flow of the operating room and reduce technical errors. Second, by pre-planning the appropriate components required for surgery, improved inventory management will further drive down costs. This will benefit not only the implant vendor but also the hospital, the surgeon, and the patient.

In summary, patient-specific planning effectively aligns all stakeholders in providing value. Patients receive a more reliable operation, with diminished variability and reduced risk for error and complication. Inventory management improves for the vendor, which drives down prices for the hospital. Finally, the surgeon improves efficiency and time management, and avoids errors during surgery.

Case Example

History and Physical Exam

The patient is a 75-year-old, right hand dominant, male, who presents with a 2-year history of right shoulder pain. He has no history of trauma and no history of previous shoulder surgeries. He rates his pain as 2/10 at rest but 8/10 with overhead activities. His subjective shoulder value is 40%.

On exam, he has painful active forward elevation from 0° to 160°. He can actively abduct 90° and actively externally rotate 30°. Internal rotation is to L5. Active and passive range of motion is symmetric. On strength assessment, using a hand-held force gauge, he has 12 kg of force with abduction, 8 kg of force with resisted external rotation at neutral abduction, and 10 kg of force with resisted internal rotation at neutral abduction. He has good strength but pain with resisted empty can, resisted bear-hugger & belly press. Hornblowers exam is normal.

He is otherwise healthy and has no significant past medical or surgical history. He denies tobacco use.

Plain radiographs demonstrate severe osteoarthritis and the humeral head is well centered on the glenoid. A CT was obtained, which demonstrates an A1 glenoid with 2° of retroversion.

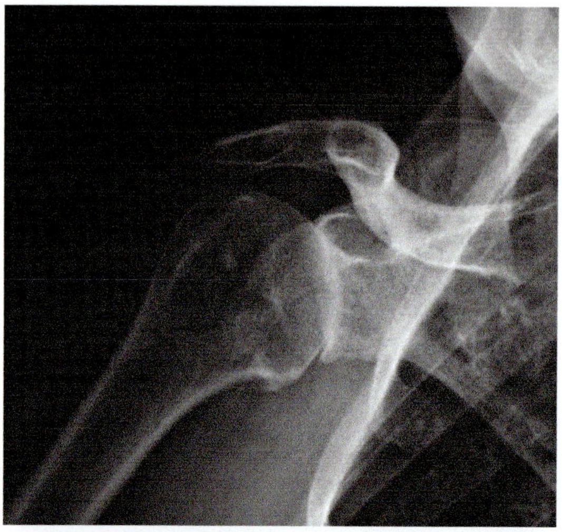

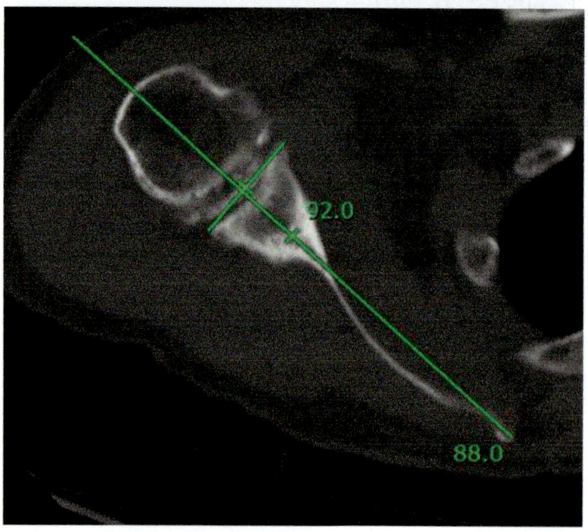

Assessment & Plan

The patient has severe osteoarthritis and an intact rotator cuff. The plan is to perform a total shoulder arthroplasty.

Patient Specific Planning

Using patient specific planning, virtual surgery was planned for this patient. The patient specific planning demonstrated a B2 glenoid, retroversion of 19° and 14° of superior inclination. In addition, he has 69% posterior subluxation.

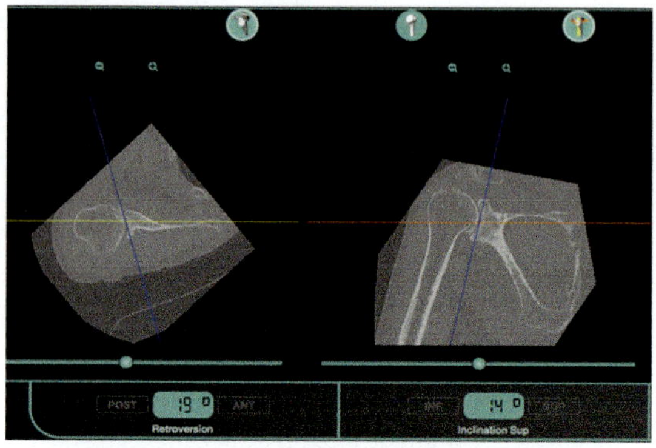

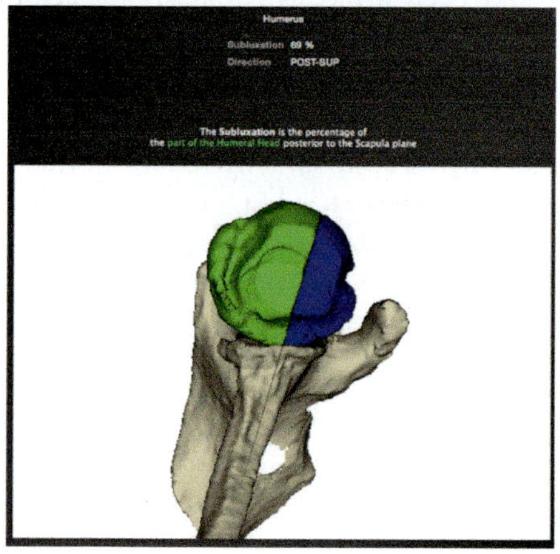

The conventional 2-dimensional CT scan under-recognized the level of deformity. He has osteoarthritis and an intact rotator cuff. However, considering his level of deformity, patient specific planning was performed for both a conventional total shoulder arthroplasty and a reverse shoulder arthroplasty.

The patient specific planing tool allows us to calculate the patient's premorbid anatomy (known as Michaelangelos David's Scapula). For this patient, his premorbid retroversion is 6° with 0° of superior inclination.

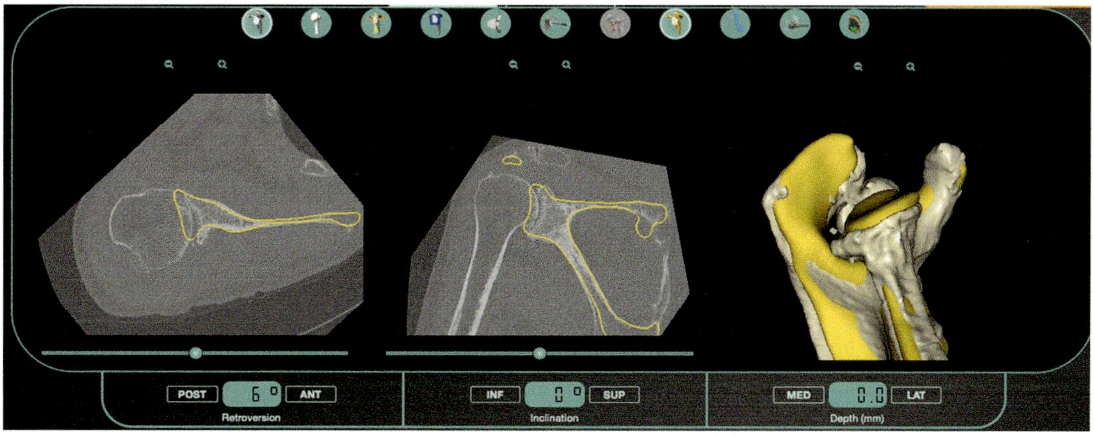

Given the information provided by David's Scapula and using the tools provided with patient specific planning, the optimal implant, size, position and reaming for the glenoid is determined.

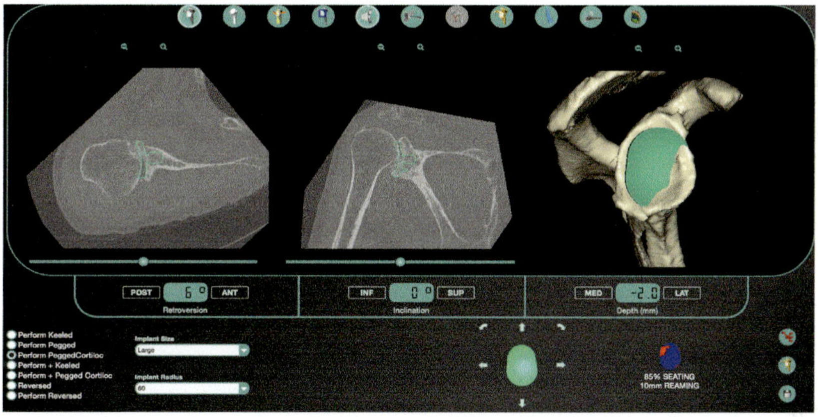

Patient specific planning is also available for the humerus.

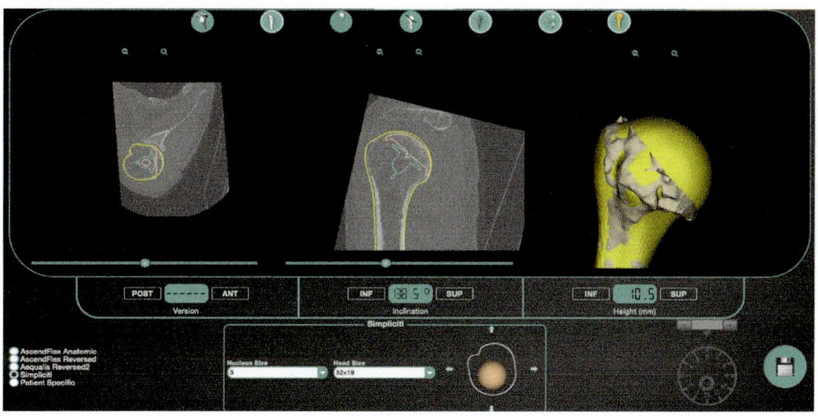

In order to optimize the glenoid placement and accurately place the guide-pin, a patient specific guide has been generated.

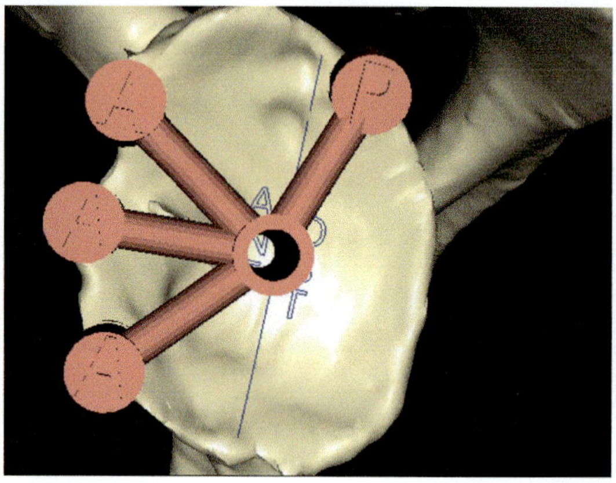

For this patient, the plan is to perform a stemless humeral component with a size 3 nucleus and 52 × 19 mm head; he will get a locking-pegged, large glenoid with a 60 mm radius of curvature. The glenoid will be placed at 6° of retroversion and neutral superior inclination. In order to obtain our corrected version, the guide pin will be placed using the patient specific guide and reamed 2 mm anteriorly. The planning tool shows that 2 mm of reaming may result in some softer bone exposure.

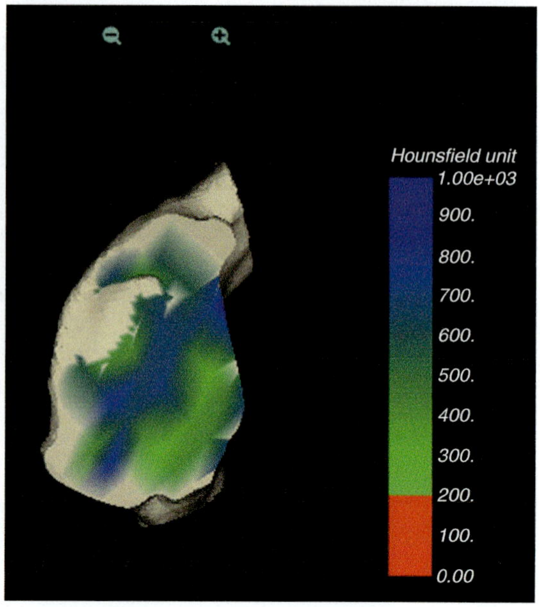

Therefore, a reverse shoulder arthroplasty patient specific plan was also performed as a back-up.

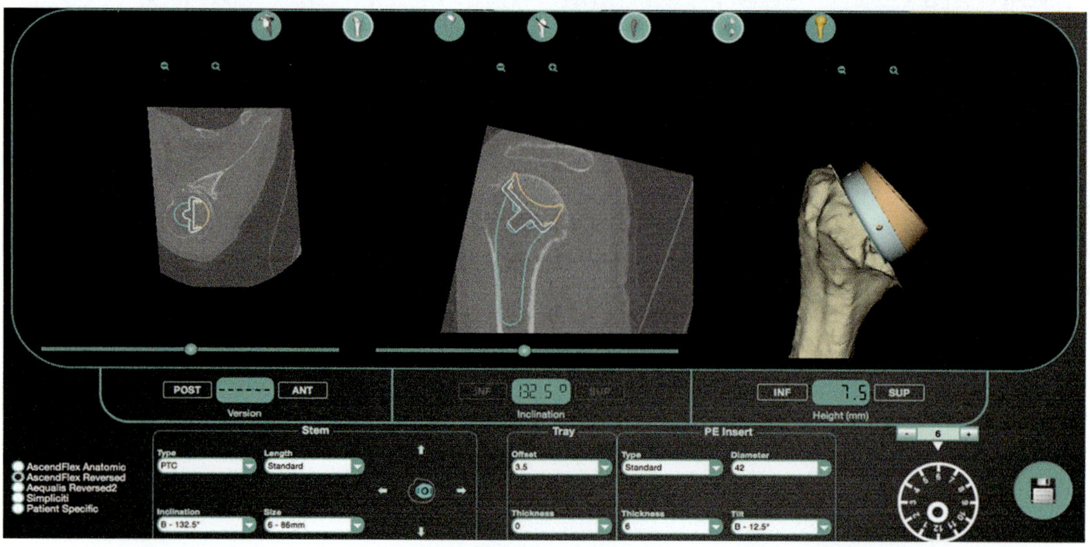

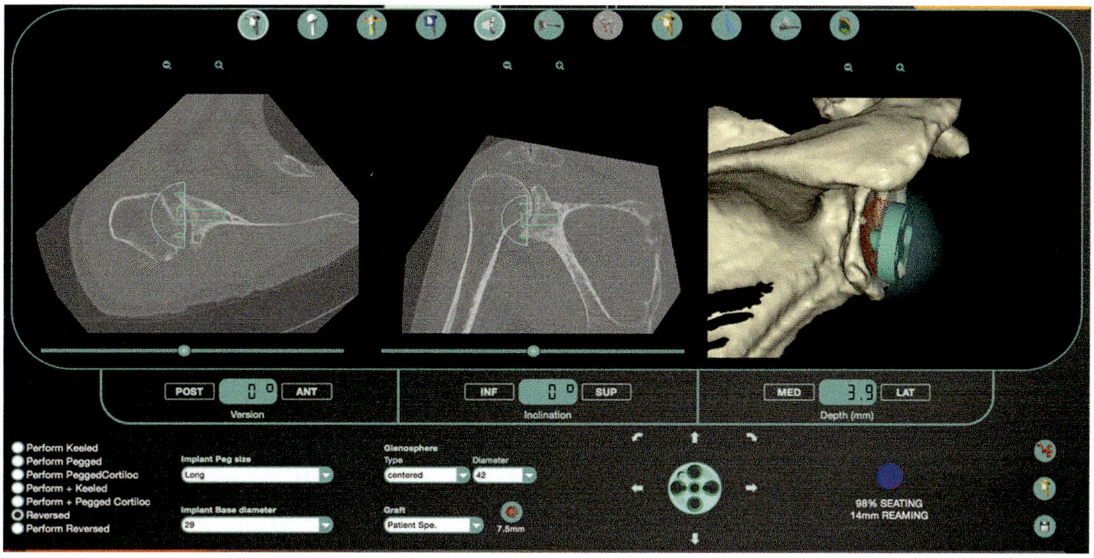

The appropriate size and position of glenosphere was determined. In order to lateralize the glenosphere and place in neutral position, a 7.5 mm bone graft is required.

Once the plan is completed, a range of motion analysis can be performed.

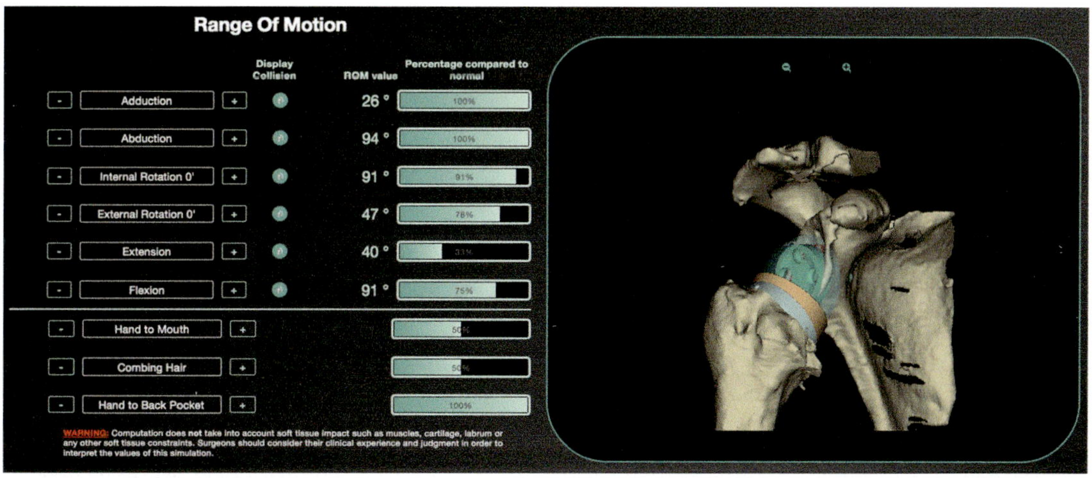

If a reverse shoulder replacement is performed, the patient would have a standard size 6–132.5° stem with a 6 mm polyethylene insert. The 42 mm glenosphere would be placed in neutral version and tilt with a 7.5 mm bone graft and 29 mm baseplate with long post.

Preoperative Counseling

During his preoperative evaluation, the surgical options were discussed. The patient understood that the primary plan would be to perform a total shoulder replacement.

In our practice, we collect all of our outcomes and have created expected recovery curves for our patients. Using this information, the patient was educated on what we expect for his pain levels and function at various stages of his recovery.

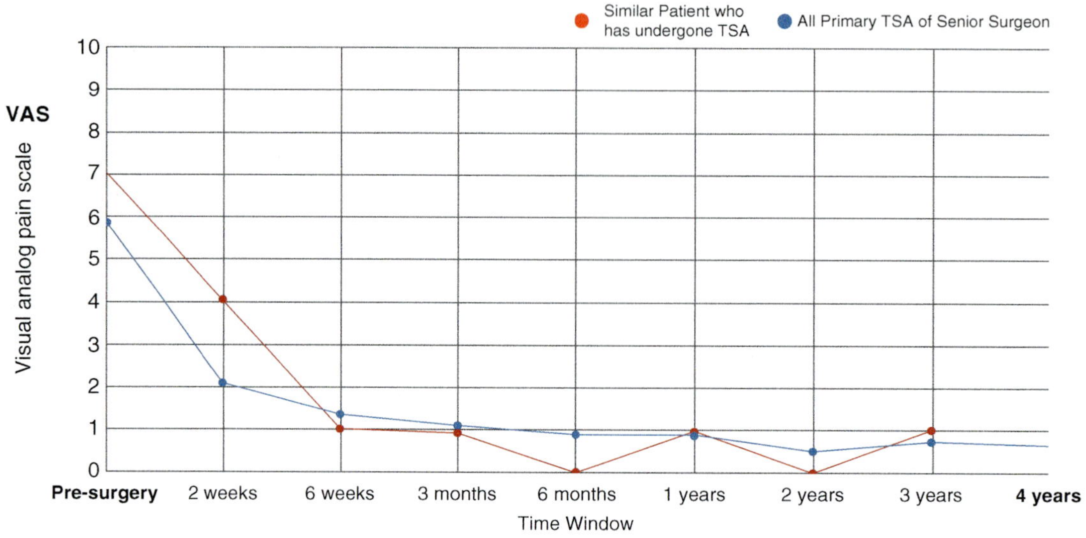

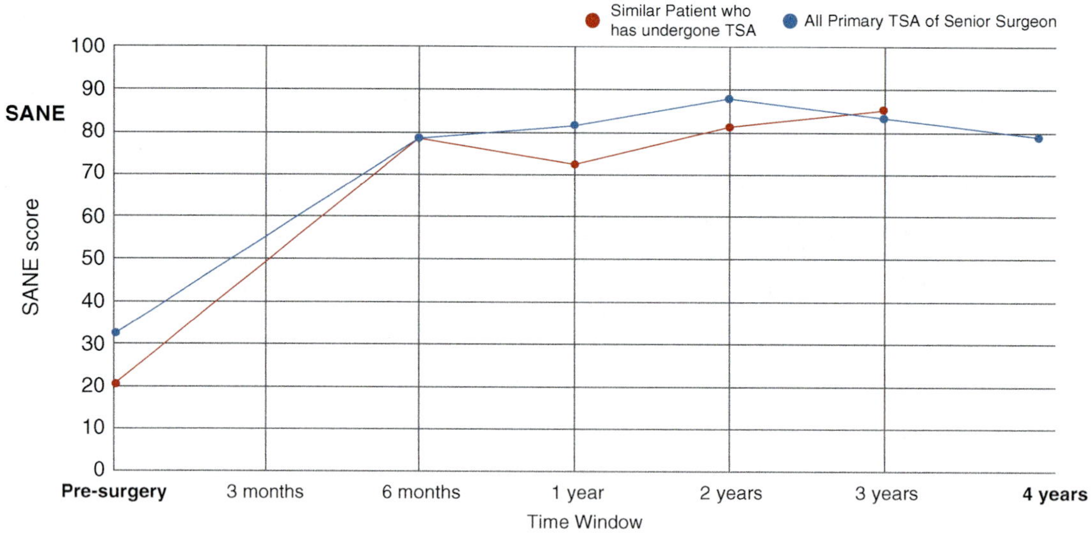

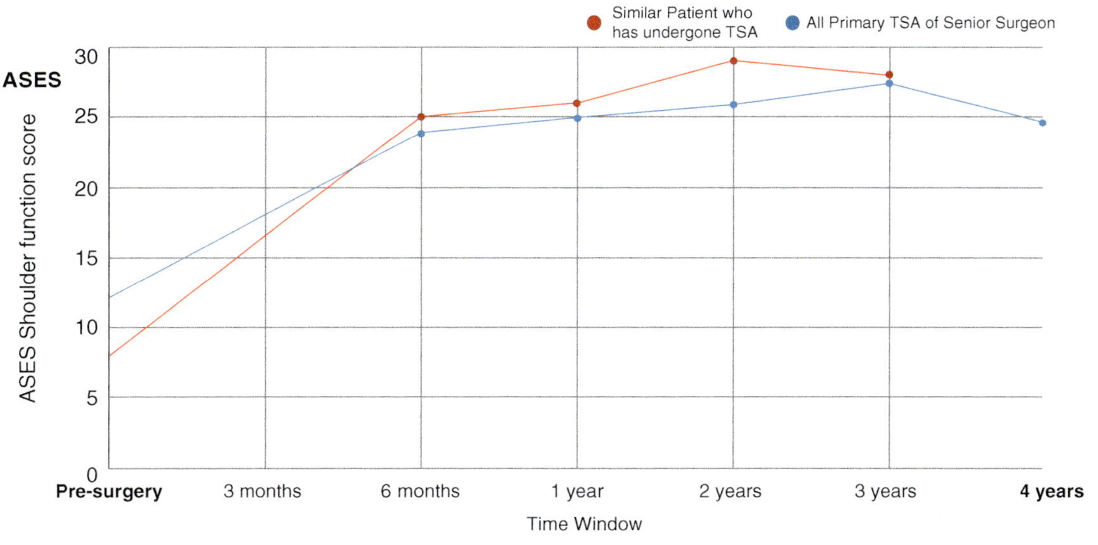

Post-operative Evaluation

The patient's procedure went according to plan. A primary total shoulder arthroplasty was performed. He had excellent bone quality. A stemless humeral component with a size 3 nucleus and 52 × 19 mm head was anatomically placed and the locking-pegged, large glenoid with a 60 mm radius of curvature was placed in 6° of retroversion.

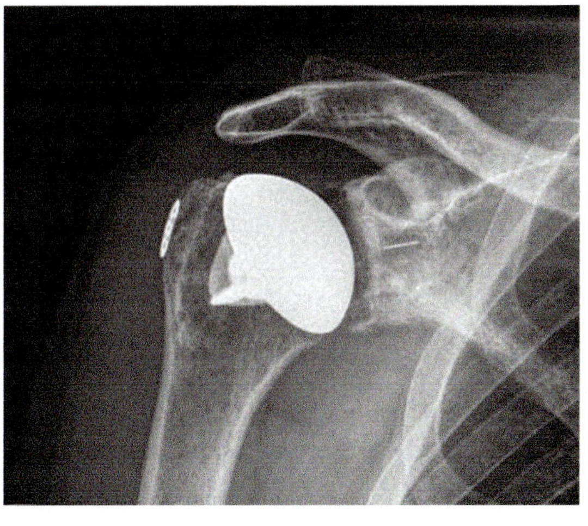

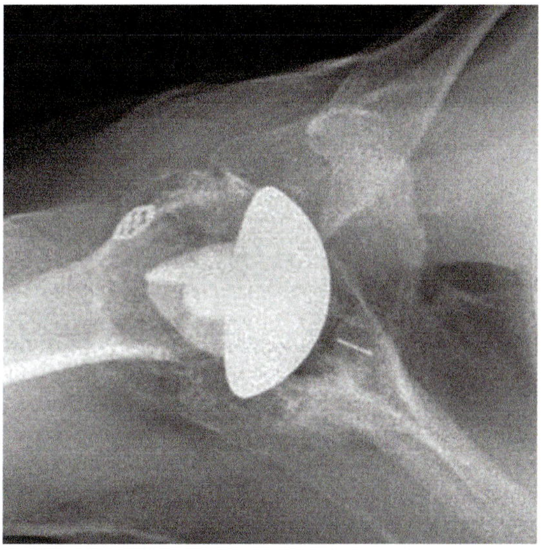

Restoration of glenoid retroversion to 10° can be accomplished by asymmetric glenoid reaming. But cadaveric and computer simulation studies suggest that about 15° of correction can be obtained prior to a glenoid vault violation [47–49]. Also, excessive reaming may increase the risk for glenoid loosening if the subchondral bone of the glenoid has been violated [14].

References

1. Day JS, Lau E, Ong KL, Williams GR, Ramsey ML, Kurtz SM. Prevalence and projections of total shoulder and elbow arthroplasty in the United States to 2015. J Shoulder Elb Surg. 2010;19(8):1115–20.
2. Kim SH, Wise BL, Zhang Y, Szabo RM. Increasing incidence of shoulder arthroplasty in the United States. J Bone Joint Surg Am. 2011;93(24):2249–54.
3. Kurtz S, Mowat F, Ong K, Chan N, Lau EHM. Prevalence of primary and revision total hip and knee arthroplasty in the United States from 1990 through 2002. J Bone Joint Surg Am. 2005;87(7):1487.
4. Kempton LB, Ankerson E, Wiater JM. A complication-based learning curve from 200 reverse shoulder arthroplasties. Clin Orthop Relat Res. 2011;469(9):2496–504.
5. Riedel BB, Mildren ME, Jobe CM, Wongworawat MD, Phipatanakul WP. Evaluation of the learning curve for reverse shoulder arthroplasty. Orthopedics. 2010;16:237–41.
6. Jain N, Pietrobon R, Hocker S, Guller U, Shankar AHL. The relationship between surgeon and hospital volume and outcomes for shoulder arthroplasty. J Bone Joint Surg Am. 2004;86(3):496–505.
7. Singh A, Yian EH, Dillon MT, Takayanagi M, Burke MF, Navarro RA. The effect of surgeon and hospital volume on shoulder arthroplasty perioperative quality metrics. J Shoulder Elb Surg. 2014;23(8):1187–94.
8. Hasan SS, Leith JM, Smith KLMF. The distribution of shoulder replacement among surgeons and hospitals is significantly different than that of hip or knee replacement. J Shoulder Elb Surg. 2003;12(2):164–9.
9. Sassoon A, Nam D, Nunley R, Barrack R. ystematic Review of Patient-specific Instrumentation in Total Knee Arthroplasty: New but Not Improved. Clin Orthop Relat Res. 2015;473(1):151–8.
10. Venkatesan M, Mahadevan D, Ashford R. Computer-assisted navigation in knee arthroplasty: a critical appraisal. J Knee Surg. 2013;26(5):357–62.
11. Farron A, Terrier A, Büchler P. Risks of loosening of a prosthetic glenoid implanted in retroversion. J Shoulder Elb Surg. 2006;15(4):521–6.
12. Moor BK, Bouaicha S, Rothenfluh DA, Sukthankar A, Gerber C. Is there an association between the individual anatomy of the scapula and the development of rotator cuff tears or osteoarthritis of the glenohumeral joint?: A radiological study of the critical shoulder angle. Bone Joint J. 2013;95–B(7):935–41.
13. Denard PJ, Walch G. Current concepts in the surgical management of primary glenohumeral arthritis with a biconcave glenoid. J Shoulder Elb Surg. 2013;22(11):1589–98.
14. Walch G, Young AA, Boileau P, Loew M, Gazielly D, Molé D. Patterns of loosening of polyethylene keeled glenoid components after shoulder arthroplasty for primary osteoarthritis. J Bone Joint Surg Am. 2012;94(2):145–50.
15. Gonzalez J-F, Alami GB, Baque F, Walch G, Boileau P. Complications of unconstrained shoulder prostheses. J Shoulder Elb Surg. 2011;20(4):666–82.
16. Papadonikolakis A, Neradilek MB, Matsen FA. Failure of the glenoid component in anatomic total shoulder arthroplasty. J Bone Joint Surg Am. 2013;95(24):2205–12.
17. Karelse A, Van Tongel A, Verstraeten T, Poncet D, De Wilde LF. Rocking-horse phenomenon of the glenoid component: the importance of inclination. J Shoulder Elb Surg. 2015;24(7):1142–8.
18. Young AA, Walch G, Pape G, Gohlke F, Favard L. Secondary rotator cuff dysfunction following total shoulder arthroplasty for primary glenohumeral osteoarthritis: results of a multicenter study with more than five years of follow-up. J Bone Joint Surg Am. 2012;94(8):685–93.
19. Nyffeler RW, Sheikh R, Atkinson TS, Jacob HAC, Favre P, Gerber C. Effects of glenoid component version on humeral head displacement and joint reaction forces: an experimental study. J Shoulder Elb Surg. 2006;15(5):625–9.
20. Shapiro TA, McGarry MH, Gupta R, Lee YS, Lee TQ. Biomechanical effects of glenoid retroversion in total shoulder arthroplasty. J Shoulder Elb Surg. 2007;16(3):S90–5.
21. Ho JC, Sabesan VJ, Iannotti JP. Glenoid component retroversion is associated with Osteolysis. J Bone Joint Surg Am. 2013;95(12):e82. 1–8.
22. Tetreault P, Krueger A, Zurakowski D, Gerber C. Glenoid version and rotator cuff tears. J Orthop Res. 2004;22(1):202–7.
23. Walch G, Moraga C, Young A, Castellanos-Rosas J. Results of anatomic nonconstrained prosthesis in primary osteoarthritis with biconcave glenoid. J Shoulder Elb Surg. 2012;21(11):1526–33.
24. Bercik MJ, Kruse K, Yalizis M, Gauci M-O, Chaoui J, Walch G. A modification to the Walch classification of the glenoid in primary glenohumeral osteoarthritis using three-dimensional imaging. J Shoulder Elb Surg. 2016;25(10):1601–6.
25. Friedman RJ, Hawthorne KBGB. The use of computerized tomography in the measurement of glenoid version. J Bone Joint Surg Am. 1992;74(7):1032–7.
26. Rouleau DM, Kidder JF, Pons-Villanueva J, Dynamidis S, Defranco M, Walch G. Glenoid version: how to measure it? Validity of different methods in two-dimensional computed tomography scans. J Shoulder Elb Surg. 2010;19(8):1230–7.
27. Randelli MGP. Glenohumeral osteometry by computed tomography in normal and unstable shoulders. Clin Orthop Relat Res. 1986;208:151–6.
28. Iannotti JP, Weiner S, Rodriguez E, Subhas N, Patterson TE, Jun BJ, et al. Three-dimensional imaging and templating improve glenoid implant positioning. J Bone Joint Surg Am. 2015;97(8):651–8.
29. Scalise JJ, Codsi MJ, Bryan J, Brems JJ, Iannotti JP. The influence of three-dimensional computed tomography images of the shoulder in preoperative

planning for total shoulder arthroplasty. J Bone Joint Surg Am. 2008;90(11):2438–45.
30. Budge MD, Lewis GS, Schaefer E, Coquia S, Flemming DJ, Armstrong AD. Comparison of standard two-dimensional and three-dimensional corrected glenoid version measurements. J Shoulder Elb Surg. 2011;20(4):577–83.
31. Jacxsens M, Van Tongel A, Willemot LB, Mueller AM, Valderrabano V, De Wilde L. Accuracy of the glenohumeral subluxation index in nonpathologic shoulders. J Shoulder Elb Surg. 2015;24(4):541–6.
32. Terrier A, Ston J, Farron A. Importance of a three-dimensional measure of humeral head subluxation in osteoarthritic shoulders. J Shoulder Elb Surg. 2015;24(2):295–301.
33. Hendel MD, Bryan JA, Barsoum WK, Rodriguez EJ, Brems JJ, Evans PJ, et al. Comparison of patient-specific instruments with standard surgical instruments in determining glenoid component position. J Bone Joint Surg Am. 2012;94(23):2167–75.
34. Throckmorton TW, Gulotta LV, Bonnarens FO, Wright SA, Hartzell JL, Rozzi WB, et al. Patient-specific targeting guides compared with traditional instrumentation for glenoid component placement in shoulder arthroplasty: a multi-surgeon study in 70 arthritic cadaver specimens. J Shoulder Elb Surg. 2015;24(6):965–71.
35. Boileau P, Watkinson DJ, Hatzidakis AM, Balg F. Grammont reverse prosthesis: design, rationale, and biomechanics. J Shoulder Elb Surg. 2005;14(1):S147–61.
36. Boileau P, Watkinson D, Hatzidakis AM, Hovorka I. Neer award 2005: the Grammont reverse shoulder prosthesis: results in cuff tear arthritis, fracture sequelae, and revision arthroplasty. J Shoulder Elb Surg. 2006;15(5):527–40.
37. Walch G, Vezeridis PS, Boileau P, Deransart P, Chaoui J. Three-dimensional planning and use of patient-specific guides improve glenoid component position: an in vitro study. J Shoulder Elb Surg. 2015;24(2):302–9.
38. Boileau P, Moineau G, Roussanne Y, O'Shea K. Bony increased-offset reversed shoulder arthroplasty: minimizing scapular impingement while maximizing glenoid fixation. Clin Orthop Relat Res. 2011;469(9):2558–67.
39. Lopiz Y, García-Fernández C, Arriaza A, Rizo B, Marcelo H, Marco F. Midterm outcomes of bone grafting in glenoid defects treated with reverse shoulder arthroplasty. J Shoulder Elbow Surg. 2017;26:1581–8.
40. Virani NA, Cabezas A, Gutiérrez S, Santoni BG, Otto R, Frankle M. Reverse shoulder arthroplasty components and surgical techniques that restore glenohumeral motion. J Shoulder Elb Surg. 2013;22(2):179–87.
41. Levy JC, Everding NG, Frankle MA, Keppler LJ. Accuracy of patient-specific guided glenoid baseplate positioning for reverse shoulder arthroplasty. J Shoulder Elb Surg. 2014;23(10):1563–7.
42. Heylen S, Van Haver A, Vuylsteke K, Declercq G, Verborgt O. Patient-specific instrument guidance of glenoid component implantation reduces inclination variability in total and reverse shoulder arthroplasty. J Shoulder Elb Surg. 2016;25(2):186–92.
43. Yu S, Zuckerman JD. Orthopedics in US Health Care. Am J Orthop (Belle Mead NJ). 2015;44(12):538–41.
44. Porter ME, Lee TH. The strategy that will fix health-care. Harv Bus Rev. 2013;91(10):50–70.
45. Porter ME, Lee TH. From volume to value in health care. JAMA. 2016;316(10):1047–8.
46. Porter ME, Kaplan RS. How to pay for health care. Harv Bus Rev. 2016;94:1–13.
47. Gillespie R, Lyons R, Lazarus M. Eccentric reaming in total shoulder arthroplasty: a cadaveric study. Orthopedics. 2009;32(1):21–6.
48. Clavert P, Millett PJ, Warner JJP. Glenoid resurfacing: what are the limits to asymmetric reaming for posterior erosion? J Shoulder Elb Surg. 2007;16(6):843–8.
49. Nowak DD, Bahu MJ, Gardner TR, Dyrszka MD, Levine WN, Bigliani LU, et al. Simulation of surgical glenoid resurfacing using three-dimensional computed tomography of the arthritic glenohumeral joint: the amount of glenoid retroversion that can be corrected. J Shoulder Elb Surg. 2009;18(5):680–8.

Rehabilitation Following Shoulder Arthroplasty

27

Julia Walton, Sonya Spencer, and Michael Walton

Introduction

The success of a shoulder arthroplasty is dependant, not only on the surgical procedure itself, but in conjunction with a well performed and logical rehabilitation program.

It is 3 party process, involving the patient, the surgeon and the physiotherapist. The patient is an active participant not a passive recipient [1]. It is imperative that a post-operative rehabilitation plan is in place and that the surgeon communicates effectively with the therapy team. Knowledge of the stability of the implants, soft tissue quality of any repairs, associated procedures and any important additional perioperative findings allows the therapist to make informed rehabilitation decisions during the rehabilitation process [2]. See Fig. 27.1.

Shoulder arthroplasty surgery includes a variety of options including humeral hemiarthroplasty, anatomical total shoulder arthroplasty, reverse total shoulder arthroplasty and revision procedures. The principal indication is gleno-humeral joint arthrosis secondary to osteoarthritis or cuff tear arthropathy but the success of surgery has led to expansion of the indications to include trauma and functional loss due to massive cuff tears. All these scenarios share the same basic principles for rehabilitation but with differing considerations relating to the individual surgical procedure.

This chapter is not intended as a practical guide to rehabilitation but as a review of the principals and considerations which should be taken into account when designing a patient specific plan.

J. Walton (✉) · S. Spencer · M. Walton
Wrightington Hospital, Wigan, UK
e-mail: julia.walton@wwl.nhs.uk

Background

Rehabilitation following a shoulder arthroplasty always balances protection and enhancement of tissue healing whilst allowing implant integration and progression of movement. Rehabilitation should be a logical process which initially prevents the deterioration of the musculoskeletal system. It should then progress to addressing post-operative pain then increasing work on functional range of movement, control, strength and endurance. The programme must continually focus on the patient specific, functional and realistic goals. The process requires patient compliance with a home exercise programme guided and supported by their physiotherapist [3]. For anatomical total shoulder arthroplasty, this process involves the restoration of normal functional biomechanics. However, in the case of reverse geometry shoulder arthroplasty, where there is an alteration of normal functional anatomy, new strategies of functional muscle recruitment must be addressed [4].

I. A. Trail et al. (eds.), *Textbook of Shoulder Surgery*, https://doi.org/10.1007/978-3-319-70099-1_27

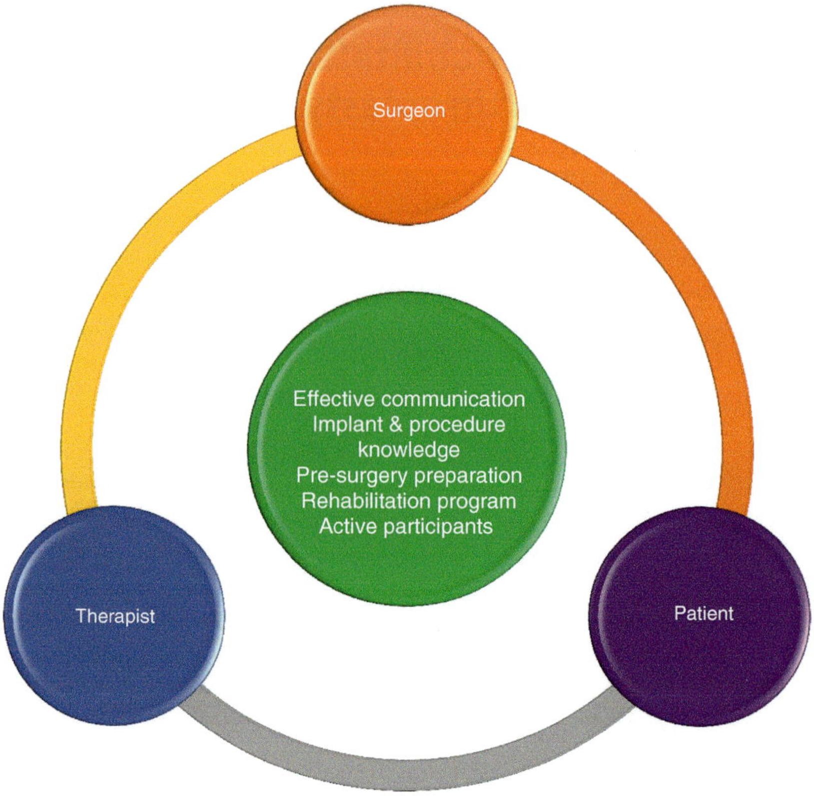

Fig. 27.1 Effective multi-disciplinary communication

Factors Affecting Shoulder Arthroplasty Rehabilitation

There are many rehabilitation challenges that may be encountered following shoulder arthroplasty surgery. The indications for shoulder arthroplasty varies from trauma to joint degenerative disease, congenital deformity or ortho-oncology surgery. A patent may have isolated single joint arthrosis or the shoulder may be part of a widespread musculoskeletal disease. A patient may present with few or many of these rehabilitation challenges (Table 27.1). These challenges need consideration and may greatly influence the patient's management, engagement, and ultimately, their outcome.

General health concerns are particularly relevant, as the majority of arthroplasties are performed in the older patient demographic [5]. This may affect a patient's ability to perform particular rehabilitation activities. The rehabilitation programme should always be tailored to cater for the individual needs and restrictions of the patient, to enable the best outcome following their surgery.

Table 27.1 Rehabilitation challenges for consideration

Rehabilitation challenges
Soft tissue adaptation
Maladaptive movement strategies
Fear
Post-operative pain
Proprioceptive deficits
Fitness
Comorbidities
Cognitive deficits
Joint restriction and/or pain
Compliance

Principles of Rehabilitation Following Shoulder Arthroplasty

Pre-operative Assessment

Active engagement with all patients pre-operatively may improve a patient's shoulder symptoms and performance. There is a possibility that this can affect, delay or even avoid the requirement for shoulder arthroplasty surgery. This preoperative intervention is multi-factorial

Table 27.2 Factors to be addressed preoperatively

Intrinsic factors	Extrinsic factors
Optimisation of ipsilateral upper limb Rotator cuff function Anterior deltoid function	Home environment
Upper limb involvement during ambulation with possible walking aid use	Social and domestic support
Function of the contralateral upper limb	Caring responsibilities to others
Fear avoidance and anxiety	Occupation
Unrealistic expectations	Recreational activities
Lower limb strength and conditioning during ADL function e.g. Sit to stand	

and includes intrinsic and extrinsic factors. Addressing these issues pre-operatively can reduce in-patient hospital stay by facilitating earlier discharge (Table 27.2).

Intrinsic Factors

All patients embarking on shoulder arthroplasty surgery for joint arthrosis should have had undergone a course of physiotherapy to maximise their functional strength, range of movement and strategies to address their pain. This process in invaluable to ensure they have maximised their potential for conservative management but also maintained and reached their shoulder rehabilitation potential on which the post-operative rehabilitation can build on. Understanding a patient's pre-operative status is invaluable in facilitating realistic functional goals and enhances the rehabilitation process.

Developing a relationship with the physiotherapist builds trust and confidence with the clinician and the post-operative process, and also introduces familiarity with exercises and concepts which will continue and be built on post operatively. Importantly it allows time to set realistic expectations of both the surgery and rehabilitation. From a clinician's perspective, it allows more realistic expectations to be set of the patient, as time has been spent understanding the individual's capabilities and abilities, motivations and functional demands.

When patients require upper limb assistance and support to assist in activities of daily living and activities such as sit to stand, addressing the actual technique and lower limb strength can reduce the functional demand on the shoulder arthroplasty. This is particularly vital during the protection phase immediately post-operatively.

Kinesiophobia is a fear of movement, usually due to anticipation of pain or symptoms. A patient presenting with kinesiophobia pre-operatively may be associated with a poorer outcome post arthroplasty. Strategies to improve this fear avoidance behaviour will be invaluable to the patient's surgical outcome [6]. Treatments such as hydrotherapy have been shown to be effective in these cases [7].

Addressing rotator cuff function in an arthritic shoulder is a challenging process. It balances the demands of paced exercise around a painful stiff joint and challenges tendonopathic structures. The key is to address this process in a comfortable range of movement so to avoid muscle pain inhibition and thus provocation of symptoms [8].

In a rotator cuff deficient shoulder, focus on optimising the anterior deltoid to compensate can be enough to provide a patient with enough functional strength and range of movement to delay or even avoid shoulder arthroplasty surgery [9]. However, if this is not the case, a well-conditioned deltoid is fundamental to the success of reverse geometry arthroplasty [10]. See Fig. 27.2.

Global pre-operative fitness and conditioning will enhance the patient's confidence and coping ability post arthroplasty.

Extrinsic Factors

Patients preparing for arthroplasty surgery benefit from guidance regarding their home environment. This should be undertaken by a therapist who is familiar with the expected limitations of the surgical intervention during the rehabilitation phases. Assessing and modifying the height of surfaces to stand from (chair, bed, toilet facilities) reduces the demand to utilise the operated arm to complete these transfers. Environmental adaptations may include short-term equipment provision or long-term home modifications, which could impact on surgical schedules.

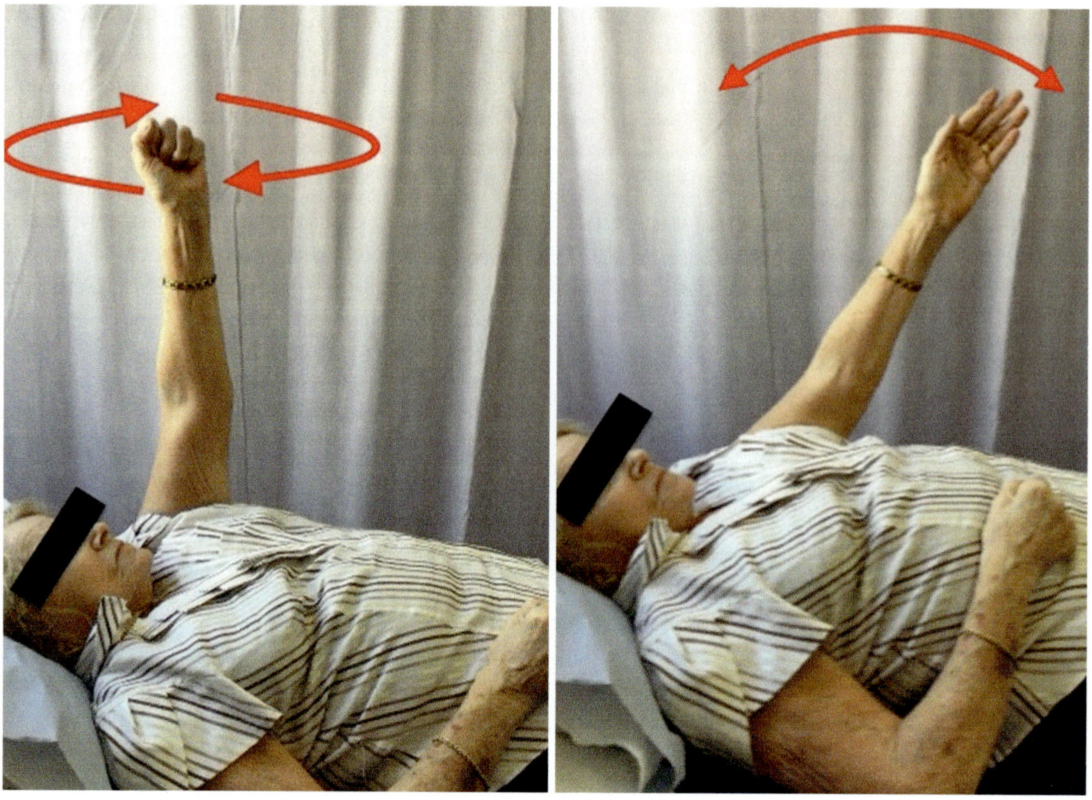

Fig. 27.2 Examples of anterior deltoid training

Consideration and discussion of hand dominance for domestic duties such as meal preparation, cleaning and functional tasks of dressing and hygiene care should be common practice. It can affect the level of additional care support needed for the patient during the post-operative period. Patients who provide care for others will need to schedule alternative care for their dependants. A surgeon/therapist team can more accurately advise on duration on an individual basis.

Recreational activities and care giving can substitute the patient's occupation in the absence of a formal role and will therefore trigger rehabilitation goals specifically related to these tasks.

> **Clinical Pearl**
> The decision to progress to surgery should include more than anatomical and clinical factors. Patient suitability should be approached holistically, considering all intrinsic and extrinsic factors, with the patient as an active participant.

Phases of Rehabilitation Following Shoulder Arthroplasty

It is important to structure a rehabilitation programme. There will inevitably be time considerations in place. These are usually surgically directed to allow bony and soft tissue healing and adaptation to surgery. Determining the rate of progression can be a multifactorial process and should a facilitated by an experienced physiotherapist working in close relation with the surgical team.

Specific guidelines or protocols offer evidence informed recommendations for clinicians and can provide robust support to the multidisciplinary teams rehabilitating these patients. These guidelines should ideally be based on critical evaluation of the highest level of evidence available at that time, reviewed regularly and applied in combination with clinical experience.

Commonly, the phases of rehabilitation are described as 'early, intermediate and late'.

Early phases focus on pain control, protected mobilisation within physiological safe zones, controlled muscle activation and return to basic self-care tasks. Progression into intermediate phases indicates suitability to increase joint ranges of motion beyond the initial safe zones, muscle control through available ranges, and re-introduction of appropriate movements in multiple and combined planes of motion.

The late phase rehabilitation can indicate progressing to loaded activity, an increase in resistive forces and functional independence. Sporting and recreational specific training also ensures a robust rehabilitative process.

The main guiding principle to rehabilitation progression should be largely patient specific, milestone and progress led.

Education

At all times, the clinician and patient must consider the tissue healing time frames and respect these. Patient compliance can only be expected with adequate patient education and guidance by clinicians [11]. The decision to progress to arthroplasty includes patient education as a core value to the consent process [12]. Education is the combined responsibility of the clinical team.

Formal pre-surgery education sessions are common practice in the hip and knee arthroplasty fields. The documented positive benefits should be transferrable to shoulder arthroplasty, specifically the reduction in patient anxiety levels pre-surgery [13]. A variety of learning styles should be considered to maximise patient retention of information, written, audio-visual and practical. The relative benefits of one-to-one or group settings should be considered, acknowledging the potential for peer support within a group format [14]. Content of upper limb pre-surgery education can range from; statistical evidence regarding surgical complication rates, understanding of the concept of safe zones in different movement planes, practical pre-surgery coaching of early rehabilitative exercises, home environment preparation, shoulder immobiliser use, axillary hygiene techniques and detailed discussion of individualised expectations.

Surgeon/Surgical Considerations for Rehabilitation

The surgeon plays an integral role in the rehabilitation process but it is one that is often overlooked. There are many aspects of the surgical procedure which will have direct impact upon the process of rehabilitation and one of the key roles of the treating surgeon is to accurately and clearly convey this information to the rest of the multidisciplinary team. Direct communication is ideal but is best substituted for by clear post-operative notes and instructions.

The goal of all arthroplasty surgery is to create an immediate secure construct which can begin early mobilisation. However, this is not always the case and information regarding any areas of concern need to be accurately communicated. Of particular importance is knowledge of surgical approach utilised as this will have implications on soft-tissue protection post-surgery. The most commonly utilised surgical approach is via the deltopectoral interval and via the subscapularis. The subsequent subscapularis repair will often need protecting in the early phases of the rehabilitation in order to heal. Many surgeons will therefore place a restriction in external rotation to facilitate this but information regarding the quality/strength of the repair will help guide an experienced therapist. Early mobilisation has been shown to lead to a more rapid return of motion but concerns still exist with regard to subscapularis healing [15]. It is our practice to establish "safe zones" for movement. Intraoperatively, the range of movement, particularly external rotation, is established that can occur before any tension is placed upon the tendon repair. This zone is then established to allow the physiotherapists to begin earlier movement in a safe, controlled manner.

As our population ages, the use of arthroplasty in the presence of bone loss i.e. revision surgery or trauma, is becoming more frequent. In these specific situations, a period of reduced mobilisation to allow bony healing may be required. In trauma arthroplasty, this is to facilitate tuberosity and cuff healing. In revision surgery, there may be humeral bone loss which compromises initial implant stability or increasingly bone graft reconstruction of the glenoid. In these situations, implant stability increases over time with osseo-integration. This must be respected and movement rehabilitation restricted to allow the process to occur.

Pain Management

It is imperative to ensure adequate pain management throughout the whole rehabilitation process. Initially post op, this may be managed with a regional interscalene blockade. This is an effective form of post op analgesia but presents an early challenge post op. It is vital that motor activity returns to the deltoid before the commencement of any early rehabilitation exercise due to its stabilising role. This is especially the case with a reverse geometry shoulder arthroplasty [16]. Post-operative pain can then can be managed with medication, activity modification and pacing, and importantly by reassurance and ongoing education from the clinicians involved in this process. Patients that have been well informed, through preoperative education, addressing post-operative expectations and patient anxiety, may have better post-operative pain experiences [17]. Ensuring a comfortable rehabilitation process limits the presence of pain inhibition [8], muscle guarding and kinesophobia, thus allowing quality movement and optimal muscle recruitment.

Adjuvant therapies, such as post-operative cryotherapy, are often beneficial in the early post-operative stage. Studies have found a reduction in post-operative pain swelling and discomfort during movement following the application of ice to the operated shoulder [18].

Clinical Pearl
The clinical team is strengthened by good channels of communication between surgeon and therapist. It facilitates appropriate pace of rehabilitation and a coordinated approach to milestone based progression.

Movement and Strength

Following shoulder arthroplasty, the neuromuscular system will take time to adjust. It initially has to recover from the operative procedure, but also has to respond to the alteration in new shoulder joint mechanics. Proprioception of the shoulder has to be re-established following surgery. This will continue to improve with appropriate facilitation by the physiotherapist using functional movement patterns, through the theory of motor relearning [19].

Soft tissue contractures that have developed during the progression of shoulder joint degenerative disease will affect the range of movement. Intra-operatively, surgical releases are performed in order to balance the joint biomechanically. One of the key components to success following shoulder arthroplasty is ensuring the restoration in soft tissue tension, allowing humeral head centralisation which restores the normal forces across the gleno-humeral joint. Despite this soft tissue balancing, post-operative movement may still be limited by soreness, but also by possible maladaptive movement strategies which may have evolved over years as a result of arthritic pain and arthrogenic restriction [2].

The shoulder does not function in isolation but as part of a sequential activation of body segments. This starts with establishing a stable base of support for which the lower limbs and trunk can generate force, channelling to the shoulder complex producing functional upper limb power. This activation sequence is termed the kinetic chain (see Fig. 27.3) [20].

Other joint problems may result in compensatory measures elsewhere along the kinetic chain. These often present as a stiff thoracic spine kyphosis or arthritic lower limb joints and will affect the generation of functional power and stability, thus increasing the load and demand on the shoulder girdle complex and upper limb. Optimal restoration of the shoulder following arthroplasty must involve optimal activation of all the kinetic chain segments. Personalised assessment of these movement strategies allows a specific rehabilitation programme to address or to accommodate these as part of the patient's rehabilitation process [20].

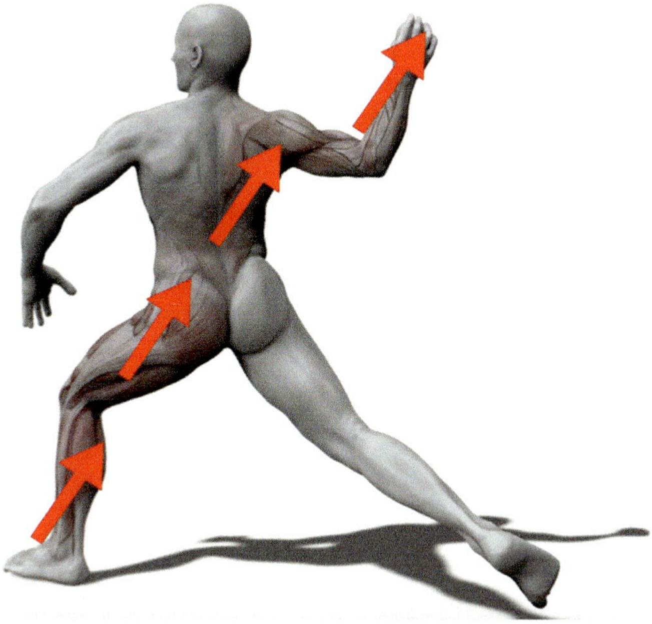

Fig. 27.3 The kinetic chain

> **Clinical Pearl**
> High quality rehabilitation recognises the shoulder complex is not an isolated quadrant of the body. Therapists should address the shoulder as a part of a wider kinetic chain of movement, integrating treatment for the whole chain in addition to the operated shoulder.

Return to Function, Recreational Activities and Sport

The combination of high loaded activity and repetitive overuse leading to osteoarthritic changes in the athletic shoulder present the patient and the clinical team with challenges. Early arthritis detection and management, coupled with advances in arthroplasty surgery and components, have led to achieving higher levels of function [21].

However, expectations should be clearly discussed and set prior to surgery fully informing the patient of the risks of the potential of non-attainment of these goals and of increased wear rates of the prosthesis with higher levels of activity. Young, active candidates for total shoulder arthroplasty not only demand longevity and improved function, but they also desire a return to physical activities [22].

Initial post-surgery treatment focuses on functional return, leading into athletic activity return as rehabilitation progresses. It is vital that realistic strategies for achieving these functional goals are explored, patients' may require task adaptation and therefore occupational therapy input to assist this process. Appropriate patient specific outcome measures are an important tool to gauge success following shoulder arthroplasty [4].

Generally, low demand activities are permitted by most surgeons postoperatively and generally have higher return rates than contact sports or high-demand activities. Patients undergoing shoulder arthroplasty should be counselled that there is a high probability that they will be able to return to their preoperative activity level within 6 months postoperatively [23], but that higher levels of demand may take longer and is less predictable.

As the indications for shoulder arthroplasty procedures expand and life expectancy increases, the goals of shoulder replacement are changing, and many patients are now prioritizing the ability to resume sports postoperatively [23]. While activity levels after hip and knee replacements have been extensively reported in the literature, the number of studies on this topic in the field of shoulder arthroplasty are relatively limited.

Following shoulder arthroplasty, patients have been able to return to one or more sports (including swimming, golf, tennis and fitness sports), with anatomic total shoulder arthroplasty having the highest rate of return [24]. Longevity of return and level of ability remains unclear.

Early and continued discussions about returning to recreational and sporting activities should be encouraged. Some activities can be precluded by the presence of an arthroplasty and some delayed by sub-optimal rehabilitative progression. Patients' expectations are often set in response to return to activity not range of motion or strength testing results [25]. Experienced clinicians should assist the patient to correlate both these findings to measure success.

Conclusion

The volume of shoulder arthroplasty is increasing exponentially. Increasing knowledge of the biomechanics of the shoulder and implants has led to better surgical technique. Outcomes however, are not only a result of optimal surgery, but also as a result of the combined efforts of surgeon, patient and therapist. The shoulder is unique in its requirement of muscle balance to facilitate movement. It is therefore imperative that we, as a shoulder community, place as much importance on soft tissue improvement through effective rehabilitation, as we do on surgery. It is only by increasing the scientific knowledge base of physiotherapy that we will truly achieve the best outcome of shoulder arthroplasty.

Clinical Pearl

Patient satisfaction is frequently reported in relation to functional, recreational and sporting return. Range of motion and muscle power are additional clinician indicators for a successful arthroplasty.

References

1. Brems JJ. Rehabilitation after total shoulder arthroplasty: current concepts. Semin Arthroplast. 2007;18(1):55–65. WB Saunders.
2. Gibson J, Jaggi A, Walton J. Rehabilitation strategies–shoulder disorders. In: Hutson M, Ward A, editors. Oxford textbook of musculoskeletal medicine. Oxford: Oxford University Press; 2015. p. 344–53.
3. Cahill JB, Cavanaugh JT, Craig EV. Total shoulder arthroplasty rehabilitation. Tech Should Elbow Surg. 2014;15(1):13–7.
4. Payne C, Jaggi A, Le Leu A, Garofalo R, Conti M. A rehabilitation for shoulder arthroplasty. Orthop Trauma. 2015;29(5):313–23.
5. NJR. http://www.njrcentre.org.uk/njrcentre/Portals/0/Documents/England/Reports/13th%20Annual%20Report/07950%20NJR%20Annual%20Report%202016%20ONLINE%20REPORT.pdf.
6. Hegedus E, Lewis J. Shoulder assessment. In: Jull G, Moore A, Falla D, Lewis J, McCarthy C, Sterling M, editors. Grieve's modern musculoskeletal physiotherapy. 4th ed. Edinburgh: Elsevier; 2015. p. 557–63.
7. Speer KP, Cavanaugh JT, Warren RF, Day L, Wickiewicz TL. A role for hydrotherapy in shoulder rehabilitation. Am J Sports Med. 1993;21(6):850–3.
8. Ben-Yishay A, Zuckerman JD, Gallagher M, Cuomo F. Pain inhibition of shoulder strength in patients with impingement syndrome. Orthopedics. 1994;17(8):685–8.
9. Ainsworth R. Physiotherapy rehabilitation in patients with massive, irreparable rotator cuff tears. Musculoskelet Care. 2006;4(3):140–51.
10. Boudreau S, Boudreau ED, Higgins LD, Wilcox RB III. Rehabilitation following reverse total shoulder arthroplasty. J Orthop Sports Phys Ther. 2007;37(12):734–43.
11. Jin J, Sklar GE, Oh VM, Li SC. Factors affecting therapeutic compliance: a review from the patient's perspective. Ther Clin Risk Manag. 2008;4(1):269–86.
12. Waljee J, McGlinn EP, Sears ED, Chung KC. Patient expectations and patient-reported outcomes in surgery: a systematic review. Surgery. 2014;155(5):799–808.
13. Giraudet-Le Quintrec JS, Coste J, Vastel L, Pacault V, Jeanne L, Lamas JP, Kerboull L, Fougeray M, Conseiller C, Kahan A, Courpied JP. Positive effect of patient education for hip surgery: a randomized trial. Clin Orthop Relat Res. 2003;414:112–20.
14. Coulter A, Ellins J. Effectiveness of strategies for informing, educating, and involving patients. BMJ. 2007;335(7609):24–7.
15. Denard PJ, Lädermann A. Immediate versus delayed passive range of motion following total shoulder arthroplasty. J Shoulder Elb Surg. 2016;25(12):1918–24.
16. Blacknall J, Neumann L. Rehabilitation following reverse total shoulder replacement. Should Elb. 2011;3(4):232–40.

17. Louw A, Diener I, Butler DS, Puentedura EJ. Preoperative education addressing postoperative pain in total joint arthroplasty: review of content and educational delivery methods. Physiother Theory Pract. 2013;29(3):175–94.
18. Speer KP, Warren RF, Horowitz L. The efficacy of cryotherapy in the postoperative shoulder. J Shoulder Elb Surg. 1996;5(1):62–8.
19. Boudreau SA, Farina D, Falla D. The role of motor learning and neuroplasticity in designing rehabilitation approaches for musculoskeletal pain disorders. Man Ther. 2010;15(5):410–4.
20. Kibler WB, McMullen J, Uhl T. Shoulder rehabilitation strategies, guidelines, and practice. Oper Tech Sports Med. 2000;8(4):258–67.
21. Ellenbecker TS, Bailie DS. Shoulder arthroplasty in the athletic shoulder, in: the athletic shoulder. Philadelphia: Churchill Livingstone; 2009. p. 315–24.
22. Garcia GH, Liu JN, Sinatro A, Wu HH, Dines JS, Warren RF, Dines DM, Gulotta LV. High satisfaction and return to sports after Total shoulder arthroplasty in patients aged 55 years and younger. Am J Sports Med. 2017;1:0363546517695220.
23. Johnson CC, Johnson DJ, Liu JN, Dines JS, Dines DM, Gulotta LV, Garcia GH. Return to sports after shoulder arthroplasty. World J Orthop. 2016;7(9):519–26.
24. Liu JN, Steinhaus ME, Garcia GH, Chang B, Fields K, Dines DM, Warren RF, Gulotta LV. Return to sport after shoulder arthroplasty: a systematic review and meta-analysis. Knee Surg Sports Traumatol Arthrosc. 2017;13:1–3.
25. McCarty EC, Marx RG, Maerz D, Altchek D, Warren RF. Sports participation after shoulder replacement surgery. Am J Sports Med. 2008;36(8):1577–81.

Part VII

The Paediatric Shoulder

Paediatric Trauma Around the Shoulder

28

Abdulaziz F Ahmed and Talal Ibrahim

Clavicle Fractures

The clavicle is one of the most commonly fractured bones in children, constituting up to 15% of all bone fractures in children [1]. The incidence of clavicle fracture is 29–64 per 100,000 person among the paediatric population [2]. The majority of clavicle fractures in children occur in the midshaft (i.e. middle third), which comprise 80% of clavicle fractures and the remaining 20% occurs in the lateral or medial thirds of the clavicle (Fig. 28.1) [1]. Among newborns, the clavicle is the most commonly fractured bone and is associated with difficult deliveries such as shoulder dystocia [3]. In children, the clavicle possesses a remarkable potential for remodeling even in the presence of considerable displacement [4]. Therefore, non-surgical treatment is considered as the treatment of choice in clavicle fractures provided that such injuries are not associated with open wounds, skin compromise, neurologic and/or vascular compromise. However, recent trends are growing in favour of surgical treatment in older children approaching skeletal maturity [5].

A. F. Ahmed
Section of Orthopaedic Surgery,
Hamad General Hospital, Doha, Qatar

T. Ibrahim (✉)
Department of Surgery, Division of Orthopaedic Surgery,
Sidra Medical and Research Center, Doha, Qatar

Anatomy

The clavicle is a S-shaped cylindrical bone that is convex medially and concave laterally. It forms a link between the axial skeleton at the sternoclavicular joint and upper extremity at the acromioclavicular joint. Another important role of the clavicle is the protection of the neurovascular bundle that courses its posterior surface. The clavicle is the first bone to ossify at 7 weeks during the foetal period, and is the only long bone to ossify through intramembranous ossification [6]. The medial clavicular epiphysis fuses in adulthood around the age of 25, thereby the last bone to fuse [6]. As a result, injuries involving the medial and lateral thirds of the clavicle are usually physeal separations rather than a fracture.

The midshaft of the clavicle is the narrowest portion and lacks muscular insertions, thus, making the midshaft the most commonly injured segment of the clavicle [7]. Different forces act upon the clavicle through numerous muscles that can explain the displacement configuration of the fractured clavicle (Fig. 28.2). The sternocleidomastoid muscle inserts on the superomedial aspect of the clavicle leading to superior and posterior displacement of the medial fragment of the fractured clavicle. The trapezius inserts superiorly on the lateral aspect of the clavicle which acts as a superior displacement force, however, the lateral fragment is displaced inferiorly due to the weight of the arm, inferolaterally due to the

I. A. Trail et al. (eds.), *Textbook of Shoulder Surgery*, https://doi.org/10.1007/978-3-319-70099-1_28

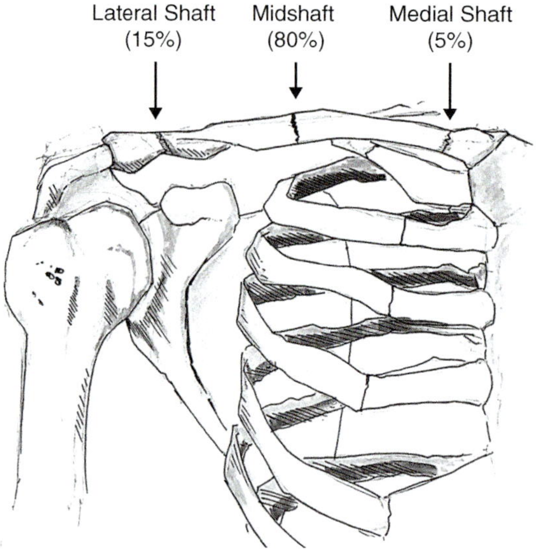

Fig. 28.1 The different patterns of paediatric clavicle fractures

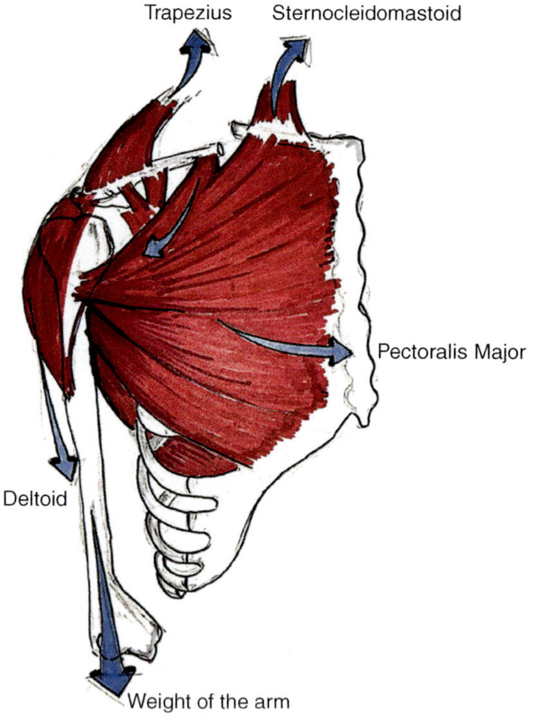

Fig. 28.2 Displacement forces on the fractured clavicle

action of the deltoid muscle and inferomedially due to the pectoralis major muscle. Posteriorly displaced clavicle fracture poses a risk of injury to the subclavian vessels and brachial plexus.

Mechanism of Injury

The vulnerability of the clavicle is accountable to its superficial position. Clavicle fractures result most commonly from direct fall onto the shoulder [8]. Common mechanisms in young individuals include motor vehicle accidents and sport activities [9]. To a lesser extent, clavicle fractures can result as a direct blow to the clavicle by an object or from indirect trauma such as falling onto an outstretched hand [8].

Clinical Evaluation (Pearl 1.1)

Patients with clavicle fractures present with localized pain over the clavicle that is exacerbated by movement of the arm, swelling and/or deformity. It is important to inquire about the inciting event, as such fractures result from moderate to high-energy trauma such as sport activities and motor vehicle accidents. Sport activities implicated in clavicle fractures are contact sports such as soccer and hockey, and those with activities associated with high risk for falls such as horse riding, bicycling and skating [10]. The presence of clavicle fractures warrants examining the patient for further bony or organ injuries that may have been produced by the inciting traumatic event. Low-energy trauma can lead to clavicle fractures where a pathological underlying condition is present such as tumors or metabolic bone disease [11]. The presence of respiratory symptoms such as dyspnoea and chest pain are indicative of lung injury. Upper limb weakness and paraesthesia may indicate damage to the brachial plexus. Esophageal and tracheal injury can result from clavicle fractures involving the medial segment and may be reflected by dysphagia and hoarseness of the voice especially if posteriorly displaced.

On physical examination, it is important to assess the skin condition over the clavicle for an open wound, abrasion or ecchymosis. Open wounds indicate the possibility of an open fracture which may alter the strategy of treatment. Additionally, skin tenting over the clavicle may hint to an impending open fracture and significant angulation of the fracture. Localized tenderness over the clavicle is typically noted on palpation and may be associated with crepitus. Palpation of the nearby bony structures and the chest wall may indicate a concomitant injury. The proximity of the clavicle to the brachial plexus, subclavian vessels and lung parenchyma mandates a thorough neurovascular and chest examination. Neurological status is assessed through sensation, muscle strength and deep tendon reflexes testing. Vascular status is assessed through inspection of skin colour changes, capillary refill and palpation for pulses. It is important to compare the findings of the injured limb with that of the uninjured limb for an objective assessment.

Pearl 1.1 The Key Points in Clinical Assessment of Paediatric Clavicle Fractures

Taking History:

- Mechanism of injury and sport activities.
- Analysis of pain.
- Chest pain and/or dyspnoea (indicative of lung injury).
- Stridor and/or hoarseness of voice (indicative of tracheal injury).
- Dysphagia and/or odynophagia (indicative of oesophageal injury).
- Upper limb numbness and/or weakness (indicative of neurological injury).

Physical Examination:

- Inspect the skin condition for ecchymosis, swelling, wounds and skin tenting (displaced fractures).
- Inspect shoulder for deformity by comparing the injured shoulder to its uninjured counterpart.
- Palpate to illicit crepitation, tenderness and palpate other nearby structures for coexisting injury.
- Range of motion is restricted due to pain and/or deformity.
- Special test: neurological and vascular examination of upper limbs.

Imaging (Pearl 1.2)

Similar to any suspected musculoskeletal injury, radiography is the initial imaging modality in achieving the diagnosis of clavicle fractures (Fig. 28.3). Anteroposterior and serendipity views (35–45° cephalic tilt view) allow for visualization of the clavicle fracture and the degree of displacement [12]. Additionally, chest radiographs should be obtained to exclude concurrent lung injury such as pneumothorax or hemothorax if suspected. Computed tomography (CT) scan may be required to differentiate medial clavicle fractures from true sternoclavicular joint disruptions especially in conditions where fractures are not evident on radiographs but pain and swelling are marked clinically [13]. This distinction is imperative because the method of treatment is vastly different between these two injuries [14]. Another use of CT scans is to assess for co-existing injury of mediastinal structures.

Pearl 1.2 Imaging in Paediatric Clavicle Fractures

- Plain radiography for the clavicle:
  - Anteroposterior view
  - Serendipity view (35–45° cephalic tilt)
- Plain chest radiography to assess for chest injury.
- Computed Tomography (CT) scan to assess for coexisting injury and to differentiate from sternoclavicular joint disruption.

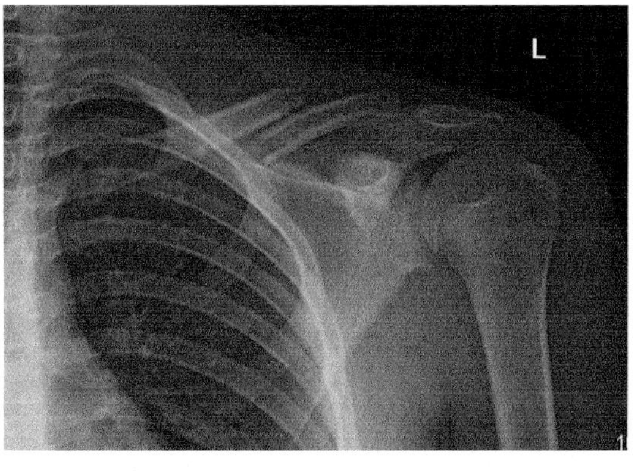

Fig. 28.3 A radiograph of a displaced midshaft clavicle fracture

Management

Non-Surgical Treatment

Non-surgical treatment is considered as the treatment of choice in clavicle fractures due to the substantial growth potential and remodeling of the clavicle. Studies have suggested that non-unions in clavicle fractures are uncommon and do not affect clavicle long-term ability for remodeling [15, 16].

Surgical Treatment

Surgical treatment of clavicle fractures is rarely indicated in children. Absolute indications (Pearl 1.3) of surgical treatment include skin tenting, open fractures, floating shoulder injuries, severe shortening of the shoulder girdle, complete displacement of the fractured clavicle, neurovascular injury and mediastinal structure injury [17–19]. Surgical treatment of clavicle fractures includes the use of Kirschner wire, open reduction and internal fixation (ORIF) with plates and screws and elastic stable intramedullary nailing (Fig. 28.4).

Medial Clavicle Fractures

In medial clavicle fractures, substantial remodeling is anticipated and these fractures are generally managed non-surgically with a figure-of-8 sling for a period of 4 weeks [14]. In the presence of posteriorly displaced fractures or the presence of sternoclavicular dislocations that impose a risk of injury to mediastinal structures, closed reduction could be attempted using a towel clip. Open reduction using suture fixation may be required in failed attempts of closed reduction and this mandates the availability of a cardiothoracic surgeon in the event of major blood vessel injury.

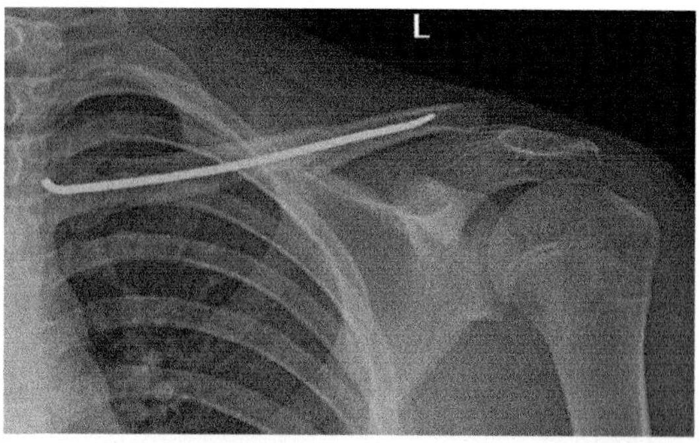

Fig. 28.4 Post-operative radiograph of elastic stable intramedullary nailing treatment of a displaced midshaft clavicle fracture

Lateral Clavicle Fractures

In lateral clavicle fractures, the presence of an intact periosteal sleeve is important in preventing displacement and promoting marked remodeling. Thus, these fractures are universally treated with a sling for 3 weeks, and surgical management is still debated even in the presence of considerable displacement.

Middle Clavicle Fractures

In midshaft clavicle fractures, healing occurs in almost all cases with a rare incidence of complications, which if occurs does not affect shoulder function significantly. Therefore, fractures of the midshaft of the clavicle can be treated non-surgically with a broad arm sling or a figure-of-8-sling for a period of 4–6 weeks. Studies have reported that non-surgical treatment in adolescents with midshaft clavicle fractures had satisfactory union with significant remodeling [15, 20]. Additionally, no significant difference was found in pain, shoulder function when comparing the injured shoulder to the un-injured counterpart. Despite the general agreement of non-surgical treatment in the paediatric age group, recent trends are in support of surgical treatment of adolescents with displaced midshaft clavicle fractures [5]. Surgical treatment using ORIF or elastic stable intramedullary nailing is reserved for severely displaced or shortened midshaft fractures in adolescents. This recommendation has been influenced from the literature on the management of adult displaced midshaft clavicle fractures [21, 22].

Three studies exist in the literature that compare surgical and non-surgical treatment of adolescents with displaced midshaft clavicle fractures; however, all three are retrospective studies. The first study was conducted by Vander Have et al. [16] on 42 patients with a mean age of 15.4 years. They found that the mean time to radiographic fracture union was shorter for those who underwent plate fixation treatment compared to non-surgical treatment. Surgical treatment was successful with no major complications and patients regained full range of motion and mean fracture union time was 88 days [23]. Furthermore, return to activity time was 12 weeks in the surgical patients compared to 16 weeks in the non-surgical patients. Thereafter, Hagstrom et al. [18] reviewed 78 patients and reported no significant difference between both groups in terms of return to activity, fracture healing and disabilities of arm, shoulder and hand (DASH) scores, although approximately 40% and 60% of patients who underwent non-surgical and surgical treatment were lost to follow-up, respectively. These findings were supported 2 years later with a study on 16 patients by Parry et al. [23], who conducted single time follow-up visits retrospectively. They found no significant difference between the surgical and non-surgical treatment with regards to range of motion, strength and fatigue testing, Constant-Murley and QuickDASH scores. However, they had a small sample size of 16 patients and a follow-up period ranging from 10 to 41 months. Therefore, the literature on the treatment of adolescent displaced midshaft clavicle fractures remains controversial with conflicting results being derived from level III evidence studies.

Pearl 1.3 The Absolute Indications of Surgical Treatment of Paediatric Clavicle Fractures

- Skin tenting
- Open fractures
- Floating shoulder
- Severe shortening of the shoulder girdle
- Complete displacement of the fractured clavicle
- Neurovascular injury
- Mediastinal structures injury

Complications

Complications of non-surgical treatment such as malunion and nonunion are rare for clavicle fractures in children and if occurr do not affect shoulder function significantly [15]. However, posteriorly displaced medial third clavicle fractures can pose a considerable risk of damage to mediastinal structures and should be taken into consideration. Surgical treatment is associated with infection, incisional numbness, skin irritation due to implants, necessity for further surgical procedures such as implant removal and increased risk of malunion especially in midshaft fractures [24].

Acromioclavicular Joint Injuries

Acromioclavicular (AC) joint injuries are common in sport injuries that can range from a sprain of the AC ligament to a widely-displaced injury with tears in the AC and coracoclavicular (CC) ligaments. Complete AC joint separation usually occurs in children older than 13 years of age, in contrast, children younger than 13 years sustain distal shaft clavicle fractures instead of AC joint separations [25].

Anatomy

The AC joint is a diarthrodial joint with a markedly limited range of motion of 8 degrees of rotation. The AC joint connects the lateral end of the clavicle with the acromion of the scapula with its articular surfaces lined by fibrocartilage. Within the joint there is an intra-articular fibrocartilage disc that varies in size and shape among individuals [26]. The AC joint capsule is synovium-lined and fibrous in structure and covers the articulating surfaces of the clavicle and acromion.

The stability of the AC joint is provided through the AC and CC ligaments. The AC ligament provides anteroposterior stability. The CC ligament provides stability in the superoposterior aspect and has two components; the conoid part which connects the coracoid process to the conoid tubercle of the clavicle; and the trapezoid part which connects the coracoid process to the trapezoid line of the clavicle.

Mechanism of Injury

In children, true AC joint dislocation due to ligamentous injury is rare. Children rather develop AC joint pseudo-dislocations which are due to lateral clavicle physis injuries while the AC joint ligaments remain intact due to their marked strength. Therefore, the superiorly displaced clavicle end resembles a true AC dislocation, hence the term pseudo-dislocation [27]. In adolescents and young adults, separation of the AC joint is produced by a direct force to the point of the shoulder when falling to the ground while the shoulder is adducted, or as a result of indirect forces such as falling onto an outstretched hand which is transmitted to the AC joint. Upon falling onto the point of the shoulder, the acromion of the scapula is driven inferiorly while the clavicle remains fixed in its position by the sternoclavicular ligaments [28]. The AC and CC ligaments are attached to the periosteal sleeve of the lateral end of the clavicle. During AC injuries and distal clavicle fractures, the ligaments remain attached to the sleeve while the clavicle is driven superiorly.

Clinical Evaluation

Children with AC joint injuries usually present with a history of shoulder pain, swelling and limitation in the range of motion of the shoulder after sustaining shoulder trauma. One should inquire about the physical activity of the patient as wrestling, football, hockey and rugby are the most common precipitating contact-sport activities associated with AC joint separations.

Physical examination should begin with inspection of both shoulders to determine any swelling, deformity or skin tenting which may indicate a fracture with impending skin perforation. Palpation may reveal point tenderness over the lateral end of the clavicle and/or the AC joint, bony defects and crepitus. Passive and active range of motion of the shoulder may illicit pain over the separated AC joint. O'Brien's active compression test may aid in establishing the diagnosis of an AC injury [29]. Another more recent special test is the Bell-van Riet test (BvR) [30], where the shoulder is passively elevated to 90 degrees and then full adducted, thereafter, the elbow is extended with internal rotation of the shoulder. Inability to maintain the arm in an adducted and elevated position reflects a positive BVR test, indicating AC injury.

The stability of the AC joint should be examined by assessing the AC ligament for horizontal stability and the CC ligaments for vertical stability. Finally, in displaced AC joint separations it is important to determine if the joint is reducible as an irreducible joint indicates a more severe injury which dictates the type of treatment to restore the integrity of the AC joint.

Imaging and Classification

Radiography is essential in establishing the diagnosis and classification of AC injuries. Bilateral true AP radiograph for comparison of both acromioclavicular joints is required. An axillary lateral radiograph is required to establish Rockwood type IV AC injury. Zanca views are obtained when the x-ray beam is directed at the AC joint while the patient is in 10-degree cephalic tilt and helpful to visualize the AC joint. Stress views of the AC joints are reported to help in differentiating Rockwood type I and II AC injuries. However, such views are cumbersome on the injured patient and are no longer utilized.

The classification of AC injuries in adults is based on the integrity of the AC joint ligaments, joint reducibility and degree of displacement. The first classification systems were described by Tossy [31] in 1962 and Allman [32] in 1967, the classification systems stratified the AC injuries into three grades. In 1984, Rockwood [33] expanded the classification of AC injuries into six types which remains to be up to this moment as the most widely used classification for AC injuries. Similarly, Rockwood classified AC injuries in paediatrics (Table 28.1) that was based on the position of the clavicle in relation to the acromion and the state of the clavicular periosteal sleeve (Fig. 28.5) [34].

Rockwood type I is a mild sprain of the AC ligament with intact clavicular periosteal sleeve,

Table 28.1 Rockwood classification system for paediatric acromioclavicular injuries

Type	Radiographic features	AC ligaments	Periosteal sleeve
Type I	None	Sprain	Intact
Type II	Slightly widened AC joint	Sprain	Partial disruption
Type III	CC interspace increased by 25–100%	Rupture	Moderate disruption
Type IV	Posteriorly displaced clavicle	Rupture	Full disruption
Type V	Superiorly displaced clavicle and subcutaneous in position CC interspace >100%	Rupture	Full disruption
Type VI	Inferiorly displaced clavicle in subcoracoid or subacromial position	Rupture	Full disruption

AC Acromioclavicular, *CC* Coracoclavicular

the sprain is characterized by tenderness and swelling over the AC joint.

Rockwood type II indicates slight widening of the AC joint with partial disruption of the clavicular periosteal sleeve.

Rockwood type III is complete rupture of both the AC and CC ligaments, and significant disruption of the periosteal sleeve. Anteroposterior and superoinferior instability renders the distal segment of the clavicle unstable. Physical examination reveals a prominent lateral end of the clavicle that is tender to palpation, and a reducible AC joint when applying upward pressure on the elbow joint. Radiographically, the AC joint is dislocated with 25% to 100% increase in the CC interspace compared to the uninjured side. Rockwood type III includes pseudo-dislocations of the AC joint that involve metaphyseal or physeal fractures of the lateral clavicle.

Rockwood type IV is similar to type III with displacement of the clavicle posteriorly seen on axillary radiographs. Physical examination shows a prominent clavicle over the scapula spine, and an irreducible AC joint.

Rockwood type V (Fig. 28.6) is similar to type III as well, however, there is gross displacement of the AC joint with complete periosteal sleeve disruption and 100% increase in the CC interspace compared to the uninjured side. Clinically, the lateral end of the clavicle is found subcutaneously and the AC joint is irreducible.

Rockwood type VI is a rare injury as a result of high-energy trauma. This injury is characterized by the clavicle being displaced in a subacromial or sub-coracoid position. Irreducible AC joint is found on physical examination.

Management (Pearl 2.1)

Non-surgical Treatment

Most paediatric AC injuries represent lateral physeal or metaphyseal clavicle fractures rather than AC separation, thus termed with pseudo-dislocation of the AC joint [27]. According to certain reports in the literature, non-surgical treatment is advocated in young children due to the significant remodeling potential even in the presence of more severe injuries such as Rockwood types IV to VI.

In adolescents, Rockwood type I and II injuries are generally treated non-surgically with immobilisation using a sling or shoulder immobiliser and analgesia usually for a period of 1–2 weeks [35]. Physical therapy should ensure early range of motion and strengthening exercises with avoidance of contact-sport activities. Return to activity is expected within 3 months.

Surgical Treatment

The treatment of Rockwood type III injuries remains controversial. Recently, Korsten et al. [36] conducted a systematic review on surgical and non-surgical treatment of Rockwood type III. Patients who were treated surgically had comparable shoulder functional outcomes to those who were treated non-surgically, however, young athletes had better functional outcomes when treated surgically. Cosmetic results were significantly better in the surgical group (18%) compared to the non-surgical group (84%) who had worse deformities. Surgical treatment had a higher rate of complications such as infection, scars,

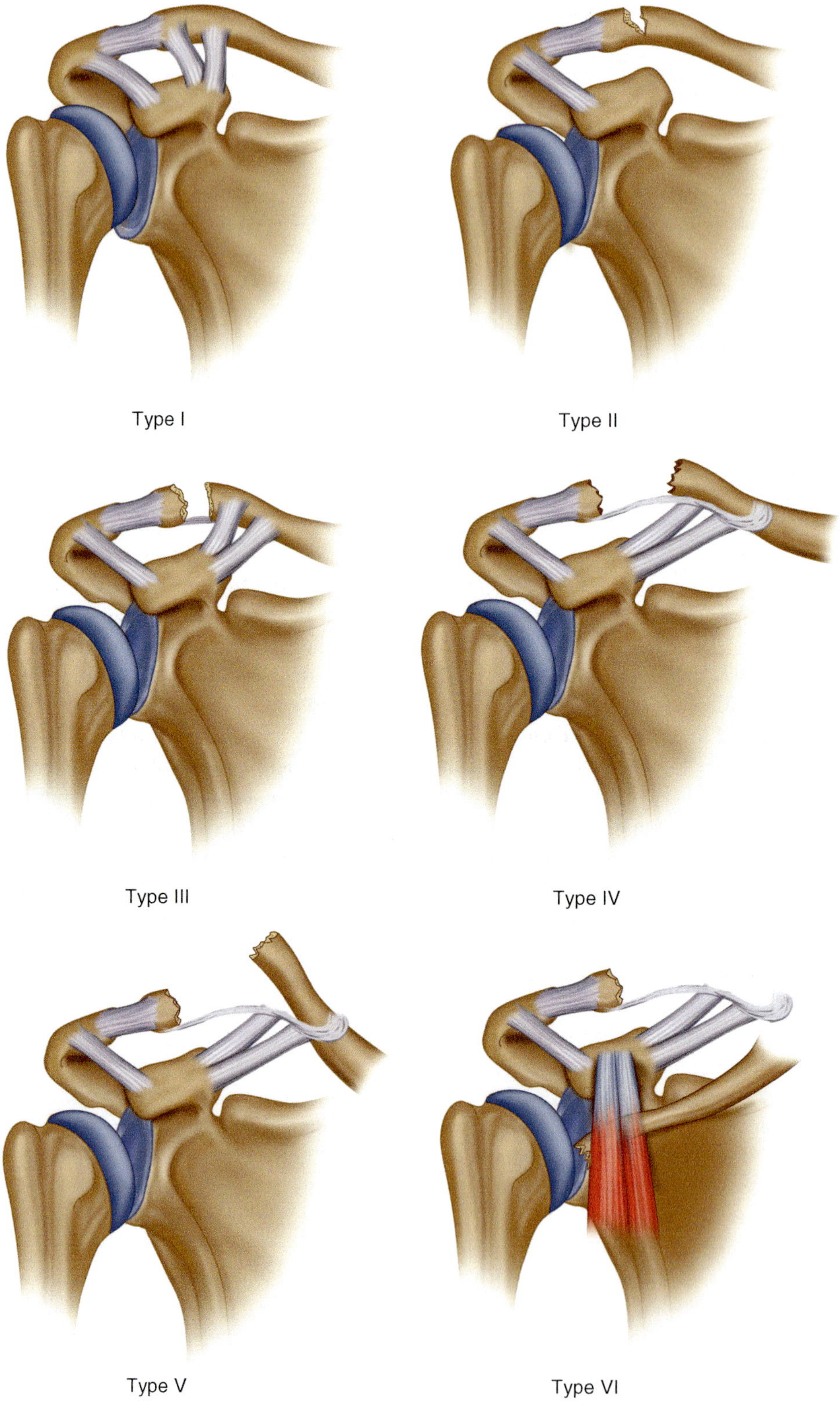

Fig. 28.5 Morphological illustration of the Rockwood classification system for paediatric acromioclavicular injuries

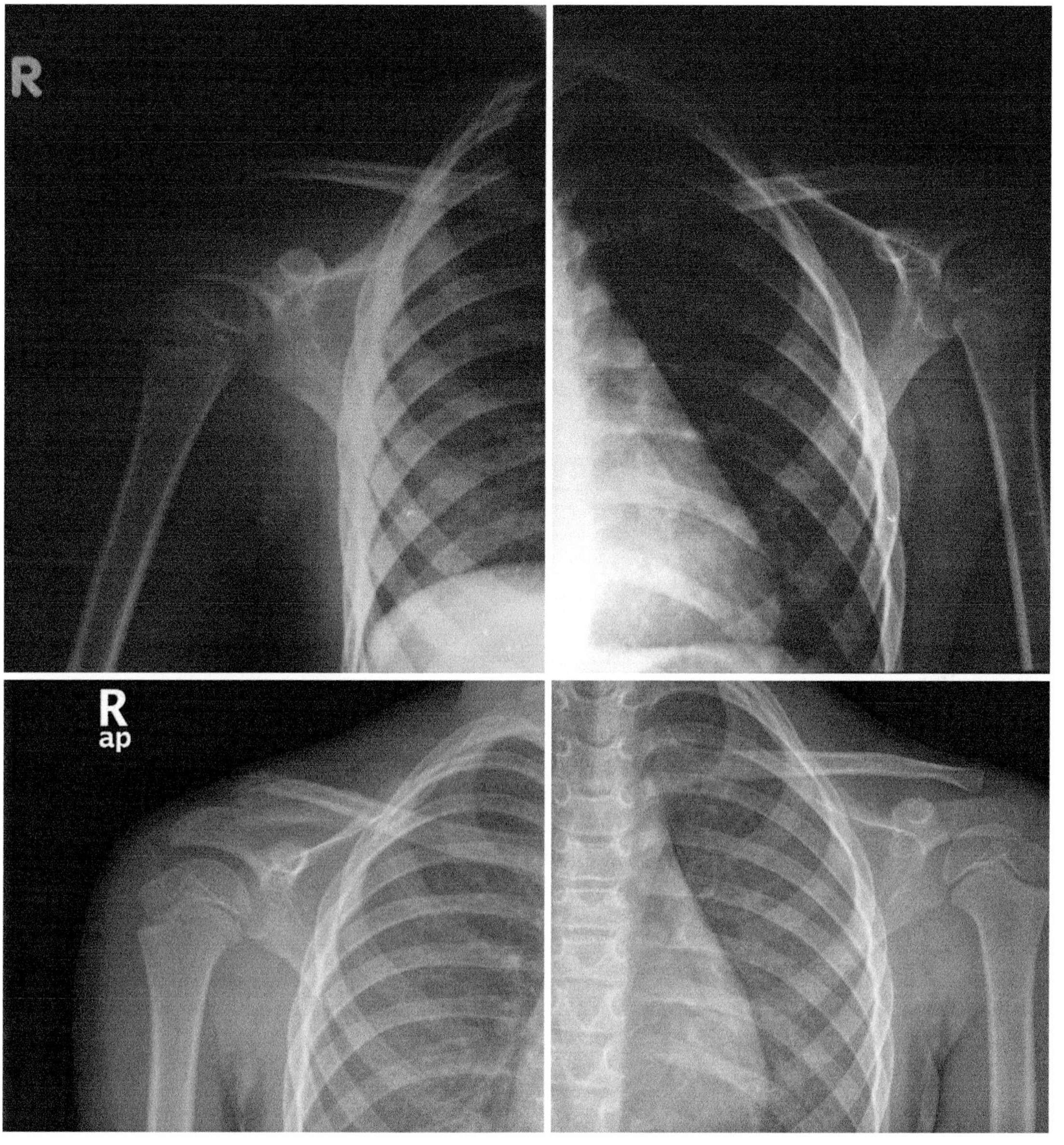

Fig. 28.6 The top radiographs show a 6-year-old female with a right Rockwood type V acromioclavicular injury compared to the left acromioclavicular joint at the time of injury. The bottom radiographs show healing of the right acromioclavicular joint injury after two months of non-operative treatment

keloids and pin migration. Therefore, surgical treatment in Rockwood type III injury may be recommended in athletes and those with cosmetic concerns.

For Rockwood type IV-VI injuries, surgical treatment is indicated in all age groups [37]. Surgical treatment includes AC and/or CC screw fixation or ligament reconstruction.

Pearl 2.1 The Principles of Treatment of Paediatric Acromioclavicular Joint Injuries

- **Non-surgical treatment**
  - Children and adolescents with Rockwood type I and II injuries
- **Controversial**
  - Rockwood type III injuries, treatment generally remains controversial.
- **Surgical treatment**
  - Rockwood type III injury may be recommended in athletes and those with cosmetic concerns.
  - Rockwood type IV-VI injuries in all age groups.

Scapula Fractures

Scapula fractures are uncommon in children and account for 1% of all bone fractures and up to 5% in shoulder injuries [38]. Fractures involving the scapula are produced by high injury mechanisms such as motor vehicle accidents and occasionally are associated with other injuries [39]. In a recent review of 1986 paediatric patients by Shannon et al. [40], 39 children were found to have scapula fractures. Moreover, these patients had a higher rate of concomitant spine, skull, rib and upper extremity fractures compared to patients without scapula fractures. Thus, the presence of a scapula fracture should warrant careful survey for other serious injuries. Additionally, scapula fractures in children should raise the suspicion of non-accidental trauma [41].

Anatomy

The scapula is a flat triangular shaped bone that connects the upper extremity to the axial skeleton and serves as an attachment to 18 muscles. The anterior surface of the scapula contains the subscapular fossa where the subscapularis muscle originates. Posteriorly the scapula is divided by the scapula spine into two fossae; the supraspinous and infraspinous fossae where the supraspinatus and infraspinatus muscles of the rotator cuff originate, respectively. The scapula has two projections; the coracoid process anteriorly and the acromion laterally. The coracoid process is a hook-like structure that serves as an insertion of the pectoralis minor and the origin of the coracobrachialis and biceps brachii. The acromion is a projection that articulates with the clavicle, thus forming the AC joint, which is one of two articulations of the scapula. The lateral aspect of the scapula contains the glenoid cavity which forms the glenohumeral joint articulating with the humerus and provides two-thirds of the shoulder range of motion. The scapula body ossification center begins in foetal life at 8 weeks, whereas, the coracoid, glenoid and acromion start to ossify at 12–18 months of age. The suprascapular notch is a gap found medial to the base of the coracoid process on the superior aspect of the scapula and is covered by the superior transverse ligament; its clinically important as the suprascapular nerve passes beneath the ligament while the suprascapular artery passes from above.

Mechanism of Injury

High-energy trauma is responsible for fractures of the scapula where direct blunt trauma in motor vehicle accidents account for the majority (approximately 80%) of the inciting events, while falls onto an outstretched extremity account for 11% of all scapula fractures [42].

Considering the increased forces in such fractures, other injuries throughout the body may exist. According to Shannon et al. [40], thoracic trauma is the most common associated injury which constitutes 79% of all associated injuries with scapula fractures. Upper extremity injury accounts for the majority of associated bony injury (58%), and is followed by vertebral, skull, rib and clavicle fractures.

Clinical Evaluation

One should be aware of the high-energy that is involved in producing scapula fractures.

Therefore, evaluation of patients should be systematic according to trauma protocols such as the Advanced Trauma Life Support (ATLS) algorithm to manage life-threatening conditions and subsequently limb-threatening conditions.

Detailed history should be acquired by inquiring about the mechanism of injury and other associated symptoms such as shoulder and/or back pain, limited range of motion, weakness, paraesthesia, and respiratory symptoms. Inconsistent history provided by the care-giver or radiographic findings should illicit the suspicion of non-accidental trauma.

On physical examination, localized tenderness over a specific part of the scapula may indicate a fracture. Tenderness over the scapula body may represent a scapula body fracture, tenderness over the acromion may indicate an acromion fracture and coracoid fractures may be represented by tenderness over the coracoid. Other findings may include limited range of motion of the shoulder due to pain or deformity, open wounds and abrasions, ecchymosis over the shoulder area, subcutaneous emphysema and signs of respiratory distress. Patients with scapula fractures should be examined carefully for neurovascular injury through assessment of distal limb pulses, and signs of suprascapular and axillary nerve injuries such as weakness and altered sensation. Injury to the suprascapular nerve at the suprascapular notch leads to weakness of the supraspinatus and infraspinatus muscles. The suprascapular nerve can lead to isolated infraspinatus muscle weakness if injured at the sphenoglenoid notch.

Imaging and Classification

Scapula fractures are investigated through standard radiography by true anteroposterior (Grashey), axillary lateral and scapula Y views. The glenopolar angle and fragment displacement (i.e. lateral border offset) is measured on the Grashey view, acromion and coracoid fractures are determined through the lateral view, and angulation is assessed on the scapula Y view. These radiographic parameters are important in determining the method of treatment. For example, markedly increased angulation, lateral border offset and glenopolar angle mandate surgical treatment. Plain chest radiographs are equally important in the evaluation of scapula fractures and detect any co-existing lung injury and rib fractures.

Computed tomography (CT) scans provide better visualization of the fracture pattern in significantly displaced fractures and/or the presence of intra-articular fragments. Moreover, CT scans allow for proper assessment of other injuries and three-dimensional reconstruction of the scapula which is beneficial for surgical planning.

Classification of scapula fracture is based on imaging findings, and several classification systems exist based on the fracture location. The Ogawa [43] classification describes coracoid process fractures; the Kuhn [44] classification concentrates on acromion fractures; the Ada and Miller [45] classification describes different scapula body fractures; and the Ideberg [46] classification is based on glenoid fractures which has been modified by Mayo et al. [47] by adding fractures that involve the body, acromion and coracoid.

Management (Pearl 3.1)

Non-Surgical Treatment

The treatment of scapula fractures in children is similar to that in adults, as the majority of fractures are minimally displaced, thus, favouring non-surgical treatment through immobilisation for a period of 1–2 weeks followed by range of motion exercises. In adult displaced scapula body fractures, Dimitroulias et al. [48] treated 49 patients non-surgically with early mobilization. Patients were followed for a mean period of 15 months, all patient fractures healed with no complications and satisfactory clinical outcomes using the DASH score.

Surgical Treatment

There is a paucity of evidence in the literature on the surgical treatment of paediatric scapula fractures, and one can only derive treatment strategy from adult studies.

Scapula body fractures are treated surgically when there is double disruption of the superior shoulder suspensory complex [49], floating shoulder fractures [50], greater than 2 cm lateral border offset, 20° or less of the glenohumeral angle and 45 ° or more of angulation on scapula Y views [51].

Scapula neck fractures should be surgically managed if there is more than 1 cm displacement and/or if more than 40-degrees of angulation exists [45].

Scapula coracoid and acromion processes fractures are generally managed non-surgically with the exception of displacement of at least 1 cm or the presence of a concomitant clavicle fracture [38]. Acromion fractures that are depressed may impinge on the rotator cuff, thus requires surgical fixation [51].

Glenoid rim and fossa fractures are managed surgically if the fracture translation is more than 10 mm and 5 mm, respectively [38]. Additionally, scapula fractures with intra-articular glenoid fractures, glenohumeral instability or dislocation are indicated for surgical fixation [51].

Pearl 3.1 The Principles of Treatment of Paediatric Scapula Fractures

- **Non-surgical treatment**
  - In the vast majority of scapula fractures as they are minimally displaced.
- **Surgical treatment**
  - Superior shoulder suspensory complex disruption
  - Floating scapula fractures
  - Lateral border offset >2 cm
  - Glenohumeral angle ≤20°
  - Scapula angulation ≥45 °
  - Scapula neck with displacement >1 cm
  - Coracoid and acromion processes with displacement ≥1 cm or clavicle fracture
  - Depressed acromion fractures impinging on rotator cuff muscles
  - Glenoid rim and fossa fractures translation >10 mm and 5 mm, respectively
  - Intra-articular glenoid fractures
  - Co-existing glenohumeral instability or dislocations

Proximal Humerus Fractures

Fractures of the proximal humerus are comprised of metaphyseal and physeal fractures in 70% and 30% of cases of paediatric proximal humerus fractures respectively [52]. These fractures are not common as they constitute up to 2% of all fractures and up to 7% of all physeal injuries in children [53, 54]. Metaphyseal fractures usually occur at the humeral surgical neck or metaphyseal-diaphyseal junction [3]. Fractures of the physis can have different patterns depending on skeletal maturity. Salter-Harris type I fractures occur in children less than 5 years old, while physeal fractures extending to the metaphysis (i.e. Salter Harris type II) are common among adolescents. Salter-Harris type III and IV fractures are rare injuries. Neonates who endure birth-related proximal humerus injuries mainly sustain Salter-Harris type I fractures [55]. Eighty percent of the humeral growth is attributed to the proximal humerus [56]. Therefore, an ample potential for remodeling in proximal humerus fractures allows for excellent prognosis with non-surgical treatment.

Anatomy

The proximal humerus is composed of the humeral head, an anatomic and surgical neck, greater and lesser tuberosities, and proximal shaft. The humeral head articulates with the glenoid of scapula forming the glenohumeral joint.

The development of the proximal humerus is characterized by three ossification centers; the head appears at 3 months of age; the greater tuberosity at 3 years of age; and the lesser tuberosity at 5 years of age. The proximal humerus epiphysis fuses by the age of 21 and contributes to 80% of the humeral growth, leading to exceptional remodeling potential.

The humerus has a thick periosteum which limits displacement of the proximal humerus fracture and ensures adequate blood flow, thus, allowing for satisfactory remodeling.

Fracture patterns of the proximal humerus are explained by the forces exerted by the rotator cuff, deltoid and pectoralis major muscles. The supraspinatus, infraspinatus and teres minor displace the proximal fragment posteromedially, while the deltoid pulls the fragment upwards. The pectoralis major leads to medial displacement of the distal fragment.

The axillary nerve is a direct continuation of the posterior cord of the brachial plexus. It courses inferiorly and posteriorly to the shoulder joint capsule along with the posterior circumflex artery.

The axillary nerve provides sensory innervation to the lateral proximal arm and motor innervation to the deltoid and teres minor muscles. Injuries to the axillary nerve after proximal humerus fractures are uncommon. The axillary artery is another important structure that runs nearby the humeral head and is rarely injured in proximal humeral fractures.

Mechanism of Injury

In neonates, humerus fractures are considered to be the second most common fractures. Proximal humeral fractures result from upper limb hyperextension during difficult vaginal births such as shoulder dystocia.

Among the paediatric age group, falling onto an outstretched hand is the most common cause of proximal humeral fractures, and less commonly due to a direct fall onto the shoulder. Most of these fractures are due to motor vehicle accidents and contact sport injuries such as soccer and hockey.

Stress fractures of the proximal humerus, "little league shoulder" typically occurs in young baseball and tennis players due to repetitive overuse of the shoulder.

Trivial injuries leading to proximal humerus fractures should raise the suspicion of pathological fractures or child abuse. Bone cysts such as unicameral bone cysts commonly occur in the proximal humerus and weaken the bone resulting in pathological fractures [57].

Clinical Evaluation (Pearl 4.1)

Neonates with proximal humerus fractures may present with pseudo-paralysis. Children with proximal humerus fractures present with shoulder pain of sudden onset that is aggravated by attempting shoulder movement. Additionally, patients may complain of accompanying deformity, swelling or ecchymosis over the fracture site. Upper limb weakness and paraesthesia indicate axillary nerve damage that is usually due to stretching of the nerve and results in a neuropraxia.

On physical examination, patients typically have point tenderness with or without ecchymosis over the proximal humerus fracture site. Non-displaced fractures may be accompanied with swelling, while displacement may be associated with severe swelling and deformity. Patients usually have limited range of motion due to pain or co-existing deformity. Neurovascular examination should be conducted carefully to assess for axillary nerve or vascular injury. Axillary nerve damage presents with paraesthesia over the lateral aspect of the arm and weakness in the deltoid muscle which is manifested by decreased shoulder abduction.

Pearl 4.1 The Key Points in Clinical Assessment of Paediatric Proximal Humerus Fractures

History Taking:
- Mechanism of injury and sport activities.
- Analysis of pain.

- Upper limb numbness and/or weakness (indicative of neurological injury).
- Pseudo-paralysis maybe reported in neonates by their caregivers.

Physical Examination:

- Inspect for skin condition such as ecchymosis, mild to severe swelling and wounds
- Inspect shoulder for deformity by comparing the injured shoulder to its uninjured counterpart.
- Palpate to illicit tenderness and palpate other nearby structures for coexisting injury.
- Range of motion is restricted due to pain and/or deformity.
- Special test: neurological and vascular examination of upper limbs.

Imaging and Classification (Pearl 4.2)

The diagnosis of proximal humerus fractures is established through radiography of the shoulder which includes AP and lateral views, scapula Y and axillary views. Radiographs are important to assess the configuration of the fracture and degree of displacement (translation and angulation), assess if a lesion co-exists at the fracture site indicating a pathological fracture and evaluate the physis especially for the presence of subtle injuries such as Salter-Harris type I fractures in neonates and adolescents with little league shoulder. Ultrasonography is helpful in neonates with birth trauma to the proximal humerus; the visualization of epiphysis separations are hindered on radiographs as the ossification centers are yet to develop [55]. The Neer and Horwitz classification (Table 28.2) is the most commonly used classification system for proximal humerus fractures in the paediatric age group (Fig. 28.7) [54]. This system is based on the degree of displacement. Grade I indicates less than 5 mm displacement, grade II indicates displacement less than one-third of the humeral shaft width, grade III refers to displacement equal to two-thirds of the shaft width and grade IV is displacement more than two-thirds of the shaft width (Fig. 28.8). Fractures involving the physis are commonly described by the Salter-Harris classification system [58]. Salter-Harris type I fractures commonly occurs in neonates due to birth injuries and children less than 5 years old. Athletic adolescents who suffer from little league shoulder manifest as Salter Harris type I fractures of the proximal humerus. Salter Harris type II fractures are common among adolescents, while Salter-Harris type III and IV fractures are rare injuries [59].

Table 28.2 Neer-Horwitz Classification for proximal humerus fractures [54]

Grade	Radiographic features
I	Displacement less than 5 mm
II	Displacement less than 1/3 of the humeral shaft width
III	Displacement less than to 2/3 of humeral shaft width
IV	Displacement more than 2/3 of humeral shaft width

Pearl 4.2 Imaging for Paediatric Proximal Humerus Fractures

- Plain Radiography of the shoulder joint:
  - Anteroposterior view
  - Lateral view
  - Scapula Y view
  - Axillary view
- Ultrasonography in neonates with birth trauma to the proximal humerus

Management (Pearl 4.3)

The majority of proximal humerus fracture are managed non-surgically due to the remarkable remodeling potential of proximal humerus fractures even in the presence of considerable displacement [60].

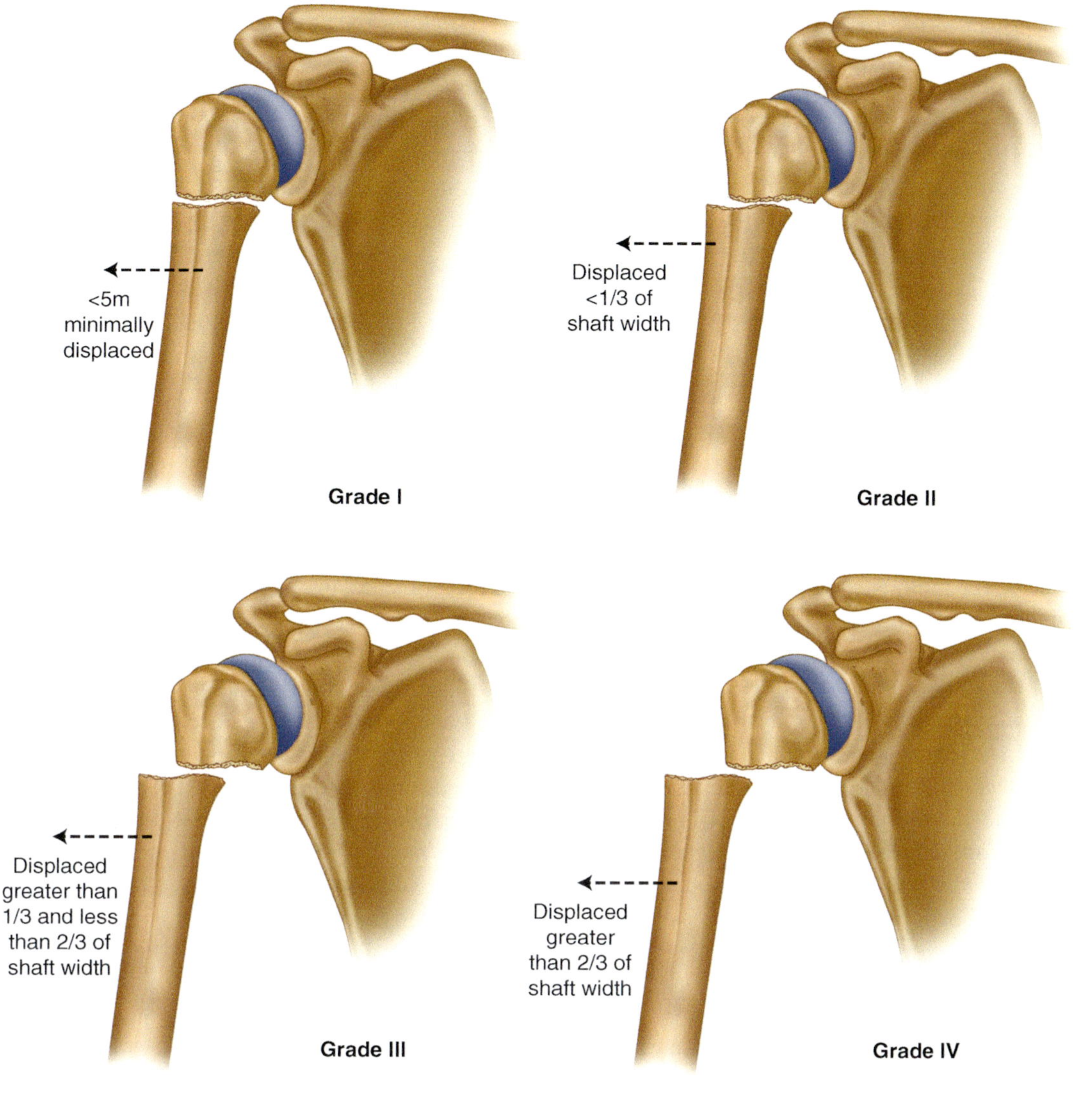

Fig. 28.7 Morphological illustration of the Neer-Horwitz Classification for proximal humerus fractures

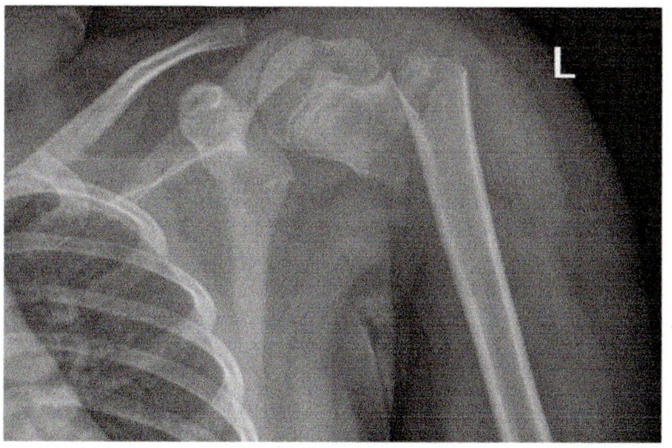

Fig. 28.8 An anteroposterior radiograph of a 13-year-old male with a Neer-Horowitz type IV left proximal humerus fracture

Non-Surgical Treatment

Immobilisation of proximal humerus fractures with a sling and swathe, collar and cuff, hanging arm cast or coaptation splint are accepted methods of treatment if acceptable displacement exists. Birth injuries fairly heal rapidly and usually require no more than 2 weeks of immobilisation.

Children and adolescents with Neer-Horowitz grade I and II fractures can be treated with immobilisation due to the aforementioned excellent remodeling [61]. In addition, patients younger than the age of 10 years with Neer-Horowitz grade III and IV fractures can be managed non-surgically

[62]. This has been supported by a recent study by Chaus et al. [63] where they studied surgical and non-surgical treatment of proximal humerus fracture among children with Neer-Horowitz grade III and IV fractures. They reported no difference in terms of complication rates, functional outcomes, return to activity time and cosmetic results between both groups. Nonetheless, patients who were older than 12 years of age had worse outcomes among the non-surgical group.

For angulated fractures, children younger than the age of 10 years with angulated fractures up to 60 ° can be managed with immobilisation [64], while those who are 12 years and older can be managed through immobilisation if the fracture angulation is up to 45° [65]. However, closed reduction is seldom successful in maintaining the reduced fracture. Non-surgical treatment of the proximal humerus is supplemented with range of motion exercises after 1 week from the time of injury.

Treatment for adolescent athletes with little league shoulder should include rest and refrainment of shoulder use for a period of 12 weeks combined with physical therapy for rotator cuff strengthening and glenohumeral capsular stretching and gradual return to activity.

Surgical Treatment

Rarely is adequate reduction achieved through non-surgical treatment in older children with severe displacement which is attributed to the limited potential for remodeling. Surgical treatment is indicated in children older than 13 years of age with Neer-Horowitz grade III and IV fractures. Whereas, the management of children between the age of 10–13 years should be individualised. This age-dependent surgical treatment indications were clarified by Pahlavan et al. in a systematic review on paediatric proximal humerus fractures [62]. Failure of closed reduction warrants surgical treatment as the reduction may be blocked by interposed soft tissue at the fracture site such as the deltoid muscle, long head of biceps or the shoulder joint capsule. Other indications for surgical treatment regardless of the patient's age include open fractures, associated neurovascular compromise and polytrauma.

One way to treat proximal humerus fractures is to utilise open or closed reduction and pinning. However, recent studies have indicated increased rate of complications such as pin site infection and pin migration. To prevent nail migration, the operating surgeon should allow for pins to be longer and bent outside the skin. Open reduction and pinning is specifically indicated in the presence of interposed soft tissue at the fracture site. Other methods of surgical treatment include cannulated screw fixation, elastic stable intramedullary nailing and plate fixation.

The use of elastic stable intramedullary nailing has recently been favoured as a surgical treatment for proximal humerus fractures. As opposed to percutaneous pinning, elastic stable intramedullary nailing avoids the complications of pins site infection and pin migration. However, it may expose the patient to potential anaesthesia related complications as nail removal requires a subsequent surgical procedure under anaesthesia. Hutchinson et al. [66] conducted a study on 50 patients who were treated either by elastic stable intramedullary nailing or percutaneous pinning. They concluded that both treatments were equally effective and whether one treatment should be preferred over the other is dependent on the surgeon's preference. Additionally, patients who were treated with elastic stable intramedullary nailing had lower angulation and lower complications despite being subjected to longer operative time that was associated with increased estimated blood loss. Similarly, Kraus et al. [67] reported favourable outcomes in 40 adolescent with Neer-Horowtiz grades III and IV fractures who underwent surgical treatment using either elastic stable intramedullary nailing or pinning by Kirschner wires (Fig. 28.9).

Pearl 4.3 The Principles of Treatment of Paediatric Proximal Humerus Fractures

- **Non-surgical treatment**
  - Children and adolescents with Neer-Horowitz grade I and II fractures.
  - Age < 10 years with Neer-Horowitz grade III and IV fractures.

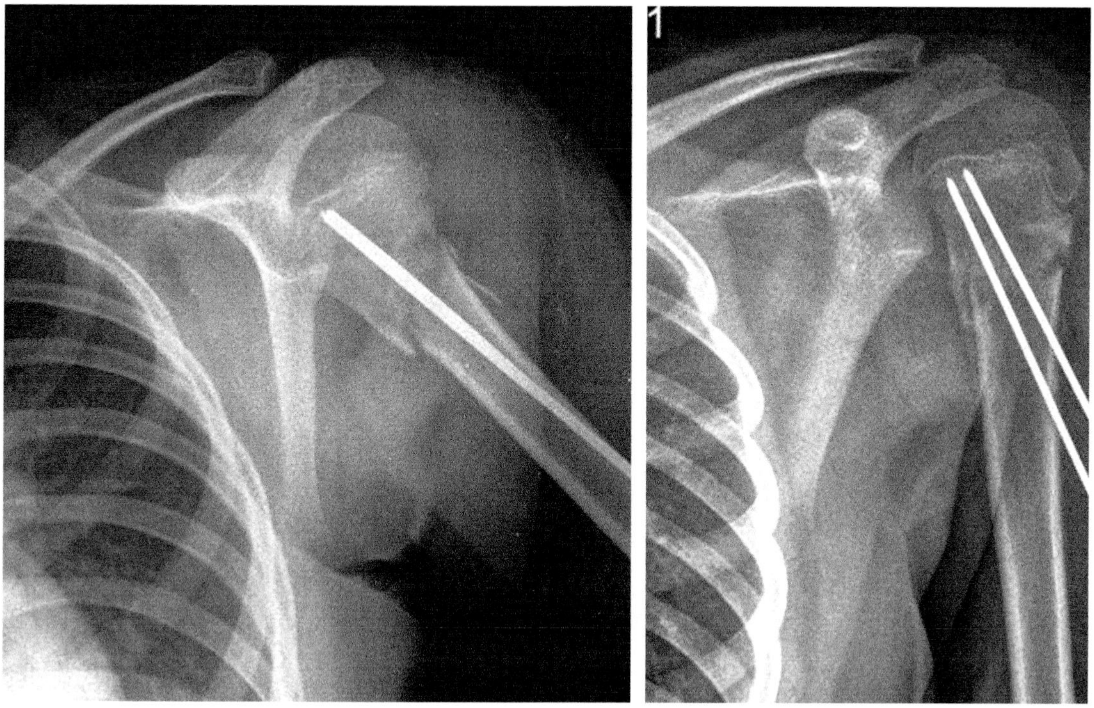

Fig. 28.9 Radiographs demonstrating surgical fixation of a Neer-Horowitz type IV fracture using Kirschner wires at the time of surgery (left), and bone healing with callus formation three weeks post-surgery (right)

  - Age < 10 years with angulated fractures up to 60 °.
  - Age ≥ 12 years with angulated fractures up to 45°.
- **Controversial**
  - Age between 10 and 13 years, the treatment should be individualised.
- **Surgical treatment**
  - Age ≥ 13 years with Neer-Horowitz grade III and IV fractures.
  - Open fractures
  - Neurological and vascular injury
  - Polytrauma

Complications

Despite the reported excellent outcomes of proximal humerus fractures, it is not without complications. Displaced fractures of the proximal humerus are unstable and closed reduction can be lost but can be prevented with percutaneous pinning of the fracture.

Another complication of proximal humerus fracture is malunion which is rarely of functional significance. Malunion in such fractures has been reported to result in humeral varus malalignment and glenohumeral impingement [68].

Brachial plexus injuries are uncommon complications affecting 0.7% of all children who sustain proximal humerus fractures [69]. This injury is usually a neuropraxia that lasts for at least 6 months and most patients recover fully within a period of 5–9 months with no functional disability.

Acknowledgment We thank Ali Farouk Ahmed B.Arch, for his generous contribution to this chapter by providing us with original high quality illustrations.

References

1. Postacchini F, Gumina S, De Santis P, Albo F. Epidemiology of clavicle fractures. J Shoulder Elb Surg. 2002;11(5):452–6.
2. Nordqvist A, Petersson C. The incidence of fractures of the clavicle. Clin Orthop Relat Res. 1994;300:127–32.
3. Lam M, Wong G, Lao T. Reappraisal of neonatal clavicular fracture: relationship between infant size and neonatal morbidity. Obstet Gynecol. 2002:100–15.
4. McGraw MA, Mehlman CT, Lindsell CJ, Kirby CL. Postnatal growth of the clavicle: birth to 18 years of age. J Pediatr Orthop. 2009;29(8):937–43.
5. Carry PM, Koonce R, Pan Z, Polousky JD. A survey of physician opinion: adolescent midshaft clavicle fracture treatment preferences among POSNA members. J Pediatr Orthop. 2011;31(1):44–9.
6. Toogood P, Horst P, Samagh S, Feeley BT. Clavicle fractures: a review of the literature and update on treatment. Phys Sportsmed. 2011;39(3):142–50.
7. Rowe CR. An atlas of anatomy and treatment of midclavicular fractures. Clin Orthop Relat Res. 1968;58:29–42.
8. Stanley D, Trowbridge EA, Norris SH. The mechanism of clavicular fracture. A clinical and biomechanical analysis. J Bone Joint Surg Br. 1988;70(3):461–4.
9. Robinson CM. Fractures of the clavicle in the adult. Epidemiology and classification. J Bone Joint Surg Br. 1998;80(3):476–84.
10. Nowak J, Mallmin H, Larsson S. The aetiology and epidemiology of clavicular fractures. A prospective study during a two-year period in Uppsala, Sweden. Injury. 2000;31(5):353–8.
11. McKee M. Clavicle fractures. In: Bucholz R, Heckman J, Court-Brown C, Tornetta P, editors. Rockwood and green's fractures in adults. Philadelphia: Lippincott Williams & Wilkins; 2010. p. 1106–43.
12. Pandya NK, Namdari S, Hosalkar HS. Displaced clavicle fractures in adolescents: facts, controversies, and current trends. J Am Acad Orthop Surg. 2012;20(8):498–505.
13. El Mekkaoui MJ, Sekkach N, Bazeli A, Faustin JM. Proximal clavicle physeal fracture-separation mimicking an anterior sterno-clavicular dislocation. Orthop Traumatol Surg Res. 2011;97(3):349–52.
14. van der Meijden OA, Gaskill TR, Millett PJ. Treatment of clavicle fractures: current concepts review. J Shoulder Elb Surg. 2012;21(3):423–9.
15. Bae DS, Shah AS, Kalish LA, Kwon JY, Waters PM. Shoulder motion, strength, and functional outcomes in children with established malunion of the clavicle. J Pediatr Orthop. 2013;33(5):544–50.
16. Vander Have KL, Perdue AM, Caird MS, Farley FA. Operative versus nonoperative treatment of midshaft clavicle fractures in adolescents. J Pediatr Orthop. 2010;30(4):307–12.
17. Kubiak R, Slongo T. Operative treatment of clavicle fractures in children: a review of 21 years. J Pediatr Orthop. 2002;22(6):736–9.
18. Hagstrom LS, Ferrick M, Galpin R. Outcomes of operative versus nonoperative treatment of displaced pediatric clavicle fractures. Orthopedics. 2015;38(2):e135–8.
19. Rapp M, Prinz K, Kaiser MM. Elastic stable intramedullary nailing for displaced pediatric clavicle midshaft fractures: a prospective study of the results and patient satisfaction in 24 children and adolescents aged 10 to 15 years. J Pediatr Orthop. 2013;33(6):608–13.
20. Schulz J, Moor M, Roocroft J, Bastrom TP, Pennock AT. Functional and radiographic outcomes of nonoperative treatment of displaced adolescent clavicle fractures. J Bone Joint Surg Am. 2013;95(13):1159–65.
21. Canadian Orthopaedic Trauma S. Nonoperative treatment compared with plate fixation of displaced midshaft clavicular fractures. A multicenter, randomized clinical trial. J Bone Joint Surg Am. 2007;89(1):1–10.
22. Robinson CM, Goudie EB, Murray IR, Jenkins PJ, Ahktar MA, Read EO, et al. Open reduction and plate fixation versus nonoperative treatment for displaced midshaft clavicular fractures: a multicenter, randomized, controlled trial. J Bone Joint Surg Am. 2013;95(17):1576–84.
23. Parry J, Van Straaten M, Luo T. Is there a deficit after nonoperative versus operative treatment of shortened Midshaft clavicular fractures in adolescents? J Pediatr Orthop. 2017;37(4):227–3.
24. Wijdicks FJ, Van der Meijden OA, Millett PJ, Verleisdonk EJ, Houwert RM. Systematic review of the complications of plate fixation of clavicle fractures. Arch Orthop Trauma Surg. 2012;132(5):617–25.
25. Eidman DK, Siff SJ, Tullos HS. Acromioclavicular lesions in children. Am J Sports Med. 1981;9(3):150–4.
26. Renfree KJ, Wright TW. Anatomy and biomechanics of the acromioclavicular and sternoclavicular joints. Clin Sports Med. 2003;22(2):219–37.
27. Black GB, McPherson JA, Reed MH. Traumatic pseudodislocation of the acromioclavicular joint in children. A fifteen year review. Am J Sports Med. 1991;19(6):644–6.
28. Rios CG, Arciero RA, Mazzocca AD. Anatomy of the clavicle and coracoid process for reconstruction of the coracoclavicular ligaments. Am J Sports Med. 2007;35(5):811–7.
29. O'Brien SJ, Pagnani MJ, Fealy S, McGlynn SR, Wilson JB. The active compression test: a new and effective test for diagnosing labral tears and acromioclavicular joint abnormality. Am J Sports Med. 1998;26(5):610–3.
30. van Riet RP, Bell SN. Clinical evaluation of acromioclavicular joint pathology: sensitivity of a new test. J Shoulder Elb Surg. 2011;20(1):73–6.

31. Tossy JD, Mead NC, Sigmond HM. Acromioclavicular separations: useful and practical classification for treatment. Clin Orthop Relat Res. 1963;28:111–9.
32. Allman FL Jr. Fractures and ligamentous injuries of the clavicle and its articulation. J Bone Joint Surg Am. 1967;49(4):774–84.
33. Rockwood CJ. Fractures and dislocations of the shoulder. In: Rockwood CJ, editor. Fractures in adults. Philadelphia: Lippincott; 1984. p. 860–910.
34. Rockwood C. Fractures of outer clavicle in children and adults. J Bone Joint Surg Br. 1982;64:642–9.
35. Sarwark J, King E, Luhmann S. Proximal humerus, scapula, and clavicle. In: Beaty J, Kasser J, editors. Rockwood and Wilkin's fractures in children. 6th ed. Philadelphia: Lippincott-Raven; 2006. p. 704–11.
36. Korsten K, Gunning AC, Leenen LP. Operative or conservative treatment in patients with Rockwood type III acromioclavicular dislocation: a systematic review and update of current literature. Int Orthop. 2014;38(4):831–8.
37. Kocher M, Waters P, Micheli L. Upper extremity injuries in the pediatric athlete. Sports Med. 2000;30:117–35.
38. Goss TP. Scapular fractures and dislocations: diagnosis and treatment. J Am Acad Orthop Surg. 1995;3(1):22–33.
39. Baldwin KD, Ohman-Strickland P, Mehta S, Hume E. Scapula fractures: a marker for concomitant injury? A retrospective review of data in the National Trauma Database. J Trauma. 2008;65(2):430–5.
40. Shannon SF, Hernandez NM, Sems SA, Larson AN, Milbrandt TA. High-energy pediatric scapula fractures and their associated injuries. J Pediatr Orthop. 2017; https://doi.org/10.1097/BPO.0000000000000969. [Epub ahead of print].
41. Carty HM. Fractures caused by child abuse. J Bone Joint Surg Br. 1993;75(6):849–57.
42. McGahan JP, Rab GT, Dublin A. Fractures of the scapula. J Trauma. 1980;20(10):880–3.
43. Ogawa K, Naniwa T. Fractures of the acromion and the lateral scapular spine. J Shoulder Elb Surg. 1997;6(6):544–8.
44. Kuhn JE, Blasier RB, Carpenter JE. Fractures of the acromion process: a proposed classification system. J Orthop Trauma. 1994;8(1):6–13.
45. Ada JR, Miller ME. Scapular fractures. Analysis of 113 cases. Clin Orthop Relat Res. 1991;269:174–80.
46. Ideberg R, Grevsten S, Larsson S. Epidemiology of scapular fractures. Incidence and classification of 338 fractures. Acta Orthop Scand. 1995;66(5):395–7.
47. Mayo KA, Benirschke SK, Mast JW. Displaced fractures of the glenoid fossa. Results of open reduction and internal fixation. Clin Orthop Relat Res. 1998;347:122–30.
48. Dimitroulias A, Molinero KG, Krenk DE, Muffly MT, Altman DT, Altman GT. Outcomes of nonoperatively treated displaced scapular body fractures. Clin Orthop Relat Res. 2011;469(5):1459–65.
49. Goss TP. Double disruptions of the superior shoulder suspensory complex. J Orthop Trauma. 1993;7(2):99–106.
50. Herscovici D Jr, Fiennes AG, Allgower M, Ruedi TP. The floating shoulder: ipsilateral clavicle and scapular neck fractures. J Bone Joint Surg Br. 1992;74(3):362–4.
51. Cole PA, Freeman G, Dubin JR. Scapula fractures. Curr Rev Musculoskelet Med. 2013;6(1):79–87.
52. Lefevre Y, Journeau P, Angelliaume A, Bouty A, Dobremez E. Proximal humerus fractures in children and adolescents. Orthop Traumatol Surg Res. 2014;100(1 Suppl):S149–56.
53. Landin LA. Epidemiology of children's fractures. J Pediatr Orthop B. 1997;6(2):79–83.
54. Neer CS 2nd, Horwitz BS. Fractures of the proximal humeral epiphysial plate. Clin Orthop Relat Res. 1965;41:24–31.
55. Broker FH, Burbach T. Ultrasonic diagnosis of separation of the proximal humeral epiphysis in the newborn. J Bone Joint Surg Am. 1990;72(2):187–91.
56. Baxter MP, Wiley JJ. Fractures of the proximal humeral epiphysis. Their influence on humeral growth. J Bone Joint Surg Br. 1986;68(4):570–3.
57. Pretell-Mazzini J, Murphy RF, Kushare I, Dormans JP. Unicameral bone cysts: general characteristics and management controversies. J Am Acad Orthop Surg. 2014;22(5):295–303.
58. Salter RB, Harris WR. Injuries involving the epiphyseal plate. J Bone Joint Surg Am. 1963;45(3): 587–622.
59. Lee SH, Lee DH, Baek JR. Proximal humerus salter type III physeal injury with posterior dislocation. Arch Orthop Trauma Surg. 2007;127(2):143–6.
60. Larsen CF, Kiaer T, Lindequist S. Fractures of the proximal humerus in children. Nine-year follow-up of 64 unoperated on cases. Acta Orthop Scand. 1990;61(3):255–7.
61. Popkin CA, Levine WN, Ahmad CS. Evaluation and management of pediatric proximal humerus fractures. J Am Acad Orthop Surg. 2015;23(2):77–86.
62. Pahlavan S, Baldwin KD, Pandya NK, Namdari S, Hosalkar H. Proximal humerus fractures in the pediatric population: a systematic review. J Child Orthop. 2011;5(3):187–94.
63. Chaus GW, Carry PM, Pishkenari AK, Hadley-Miller N. Operative versus nonoperative treatment of displaced proximal humeral physeal fractures: a matched cohort. J Pediatr Orthop. 2015;35(3):234–9.
64. Bahrs C, Zipplies S, Ochs BG, Rether J, Oehm J, Eingartner C, et al. Proximal humeral fractures in children and adolescents. J Pediatr Orthop. 2009;29(3):238–42.
65. Dobbs MB, Luhmann SL, Gordon JE, Strecker WB, Schoenecker PL. Severely displaced proximal

humeral epiphyseal fractures. J Pediatr Orthop. 2003;23(2):208–15.
66. Hutchinson PH, Bae DS, Waters PM. Intramedullary nailing versus percutaneous pin fixation of pediatric proximal humerus fractures: a comparison of complications and early radiographic results. J Pediatr Orthop. 2011;31(6):617–22.
67. Kraus T, Hoermann S, Ploder G, Zoetsch S, Eberl R, Singer G. Elastic stable intramedullary nailing versus Kirschner wire pinning: outcome of severely displaced proximal humeral fractures in juvenile patients. J Shoulder Elb Surg. 2014;23(10):1462–7.
68. Ellefsen BK, Frierson MA, Raney EM, Ogden JA. Humerus varus: a complication of neonatal, infantile, and childhood injury and infection. J Pediatr Orthop. 1994;14(4):479–86.
69. Hwang RW, Bae DS, Waters PM. Brachial plexus palsy following proximal humerus fracture in patients who are skeletally immature. J Orthop Trauma. 2008;22(4):286–90.

Neuromuscular Shoulder Reconstruction in Children

29

Peter M. Waters and Carley Vuillermin

Introduction

Shoulder reconstruction in children with neuromuscular conditions is most common in brachial plexus birth palsy; however, there are also a group of less common conditions that surgical care of the shoulder can improve pain and function. This chapter shall address the shoulder in brachial plexus birth palsy, facioscapulohumeral dystrophy, cerebral palsy and amyloplasia. In addition to these paediatric specific conditions, children are also affected by posttraumatic brachial plexus injuries and mononeuropathies. In young children treatment of these conditions follow many of the principles of management of the birth-associated injuries and in older children the adult management and shall therefore be addressed elsewhere in this book.

P. M. Waters · C. Vuillermin (✉)
Department of Orthopaedic Surgery,
Boston Childrens Hospital, Harvard Medical School,
Boston, MA, USA
e-mail: carley.vuillermin@childrens.harvard.edu

Brachial Plexus Birth Palsy

Introduction

Brachial plexus birth palsy is relatively common and occurs during the process of birth with an incidence between 0.5 and 2 per 1000 births [1, 2]. It is associated with foetal macrosomia (large for gestational age, maternal diabetes), shoulder dystocia and assisted deliveries.

The severity and pattern of the nerve injury determines the clinical prognosis for the infant. Many birth palsies are mild neuropraxias; however, there is a complete spectrum of more severe injuries up to and including avulsions of the nerve roots from the spinal cord. Determining the anatomic injury pattern early is difficult and requires serial assessment.

Development of shoulder dysfunction and displacement relates to the initial injury pattern as well as the natural recovery and treatment of the primary plexus injury. For those infants who have persistent motor deficits beyond three to 6 months of age, 60–80% will develop glenohumeral deformity [3–5].

The earliest presentation is that of infantile dislocation, with older patients showing progressive glenohumeral dysplasia and eventual dislocation [6–8].

I. A. Trail et al. (eds.), *Textbook of Shoulder Surgery*, https://doi.org/10.1007/978-3-319-70099-1_29

Aetiology and Pathoanatomy

Shoulder displacement in brachial plexus birth palsy is a secondary developmental event. Fairbanks drew attention to this in his lecture in 1913 [6] noting a common observation of posterior subluxation or dislocation of the shoulder and attributed it to be as a result of muscle paralysis and imbalance. However, it has become clear that it is not simply weakness but a combination of contracture, muscle imbalance and abnormal growth that leads to shoulder deformity.

Basic science research has contributed greatly to this area in recent years. This research has come from St Louis [9], Cincinnati [10] and Wake Forrest [11, 12]. Creating a brachial plexus injury in the rat model leads to typical shoulder deformities. In the rat model there is reduced muscle mass, shorter muscle fibres and impaired growth of the affected muscles. The expression of myogenic and adipogenic genes is upregulated.

This basic science research is supported by clinical studies [13–15]. MRI has shown that the cross-sectional area of the affected muscles is reduced and subscapularis muscle biopsy has shown reduced fibre length and diameter.

The morphologic changes in the glenohumeral joint tend to be more severe with age [3]. In infantile dislocation the morphology of the glenoid is less disrupted and this represents a different group of patients to the older patients with persistent deficits. Patients with infantile dislocation still have the potential for neurologic recovery.

In patients with persistent deficits morphologic changes progress from glenoid retroversion to posterior humeral head subluxation to formation of a pseudoglenoid and then onto humeral head deformity [3].

Clinical Presentation

Presentation of brachial plexus birth palsy is with reduced upper extremity motion in the neonatal period and must be distinguished from neonatal sepsis, birth associated fractures (humerus and clavicle) and central neurologic causes.

The injury is characterised by the number of nerve roots affected and classified simply by the Narakas Classification [16], traditionally at 3 weeks of age. The most common pattern is that of an upper trunk injury involving C5-6 (Narakas 1), classically known as an Erb's palsy. This results in a lack of elbow flexion and shoulder abduction/external rotation. This pattern carries with it the best prognosis; however, in those infants that do not recover fully it also accounts for the greatest number of infants with shoulder displacement and dysfunction. C5-7 (Narakas 2) palsies are the next most common with deficits in elbow and wrist extension and pan plexus injuries C5-T1 (Narakas 3), affecting hand function, the least common; and when associated with a Horner's syndrome (ptosis, miosis and anhydrosis) portends the worst prognosis as it indicates a proximal avulsion of the lower nerve roots (Narakas 4). Although patients with persistent panplexus injuries will have shoulder dysfunction, the shoulder displaces less commonly than in more proximal lesions due to less imbalance and overall they represent a smaller absolute number of patients.

Clinical Assessment

Clinical assessment is by serial examination with a multidisciplinary team approach. Physical examination is the key to assessing both the neurologic injury and the shoulder function.

The status of the neurologic injury can be evaluated using the Active Movement Scale (AMS) [17], this is a systematic assessment of 15 active movements with positioning of the infant in order to assess range of motion with and without gravity and achieved through observation and play (Fig. 29.1). The Toronto Test Score (TTS) [18] is an abbreviated version of the AMS scoring system and only grades 5 movements against gravity. Each movement is graded out of 2 and a combined score of less than 3.5 at 3 months predicts a poor natural recovery at 12 months and indicates microsurgery should be considered. This assessment occurs monthly until the need for microsurgery is determined.

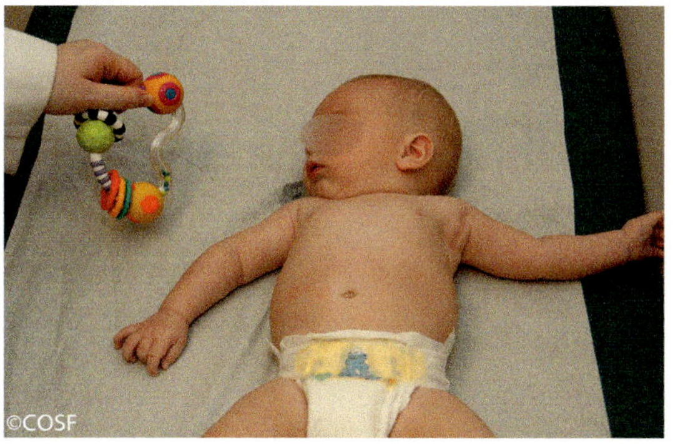

Fig. 29.1 Examination of an infant through play with gravity eliminated. ©Children's Orthopaedic Surgery Foundation

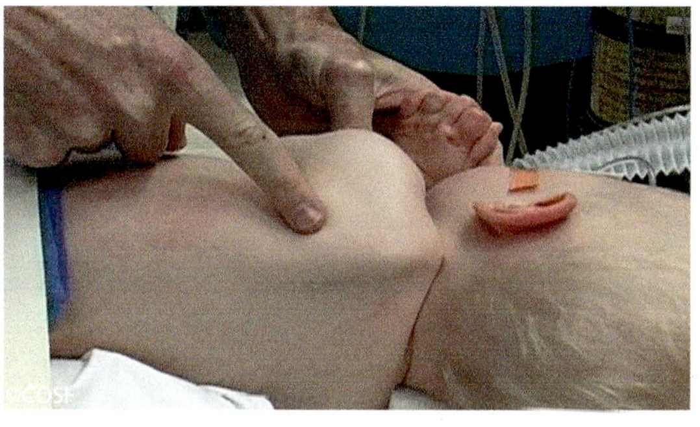

Fig. 29.2 Posterior prominence of the humeral head with the scapular moving as one due to fixed glenohumeral dislocation. ©Children's Orthopaedic Surgery Foundation

The shoulder needs to be independently assessed at each clinic visit. The humeral head may be palpated posteriorly when dislocated and at times discrete instability is detectable by exam. A posteriorly dislocated humeral head may reduce with external rotation and abduction of the arm and dislocate with internal rotation in adduction (Fig. 29.2). Internal rotation contracture (by passive external rotation) is assessed both with the shoulder in the adducted position and abducted to 90 degrees – this can help to assess for contracture of the subscapularis and pectoralis major respectively. Loss of passive external rotation has been shown to be the most sensitive examination finding for shoulder displacement.

Being able to bring the hand to the mouth without a significant trumpet sign (abduction) is a sensitive test of global external rotation. Assess for abduction contracture with a Putti sign by bringing the arm to the side and observing for prominence of the superomedial angle of the scapula. Always be mindful that children may develop significant scapulothoracic compensation, truncal sway or throw and catch manoeuvres to mask shoulder dysfunction. In the older child assessing strength and arc of external and internal rotation assists with clinical decision making when considering tendon transfer and humeral osteotomy procedures.

The Mallet Score [19] is an assessment of global shoulder function and should be performed once the child is old enough to follow directions.

Imaging

More subtle findings of dislocation and dysplasia may not always be appreciated on clinical examination.

The use of ultrasound for assessment of the shoulder in BPBP has become widespread and is now a well-established technique [20–22]. It is a low cost, effective assessment tool that does not require sedation and can provide accurate diagnosis of shoulder displacement and some information regarding glenoid morphology.

Ultrasound can be performed in a sitting or lying position. The arm is imaged both statically and dynamically. Initial static images are performed with the arm adducted by the side and internally rotated. Alpha (α) angles and posterior humeral head displacement (PHHD) are measured (Fig. 29.3). The alpha angle is measured as the angle formed by a line along the posterior scapular margin and a line tangent to the humeral head. PHHD as the percentage of the humeral head posterior to the line along the posterior scapular margin at the greatest diameter of the humeral head.

Next dynamic screening is performed if the shoulder is dislocated or subluxated. This is to determine if the humeral head is reducible. Static measurements in external rotation are then also recorded.

Ultrasound is most useful in the first year of life; however, the correlation between MRI and US for glenoid morphology is not high [23]. When assessing glenoid morphology in

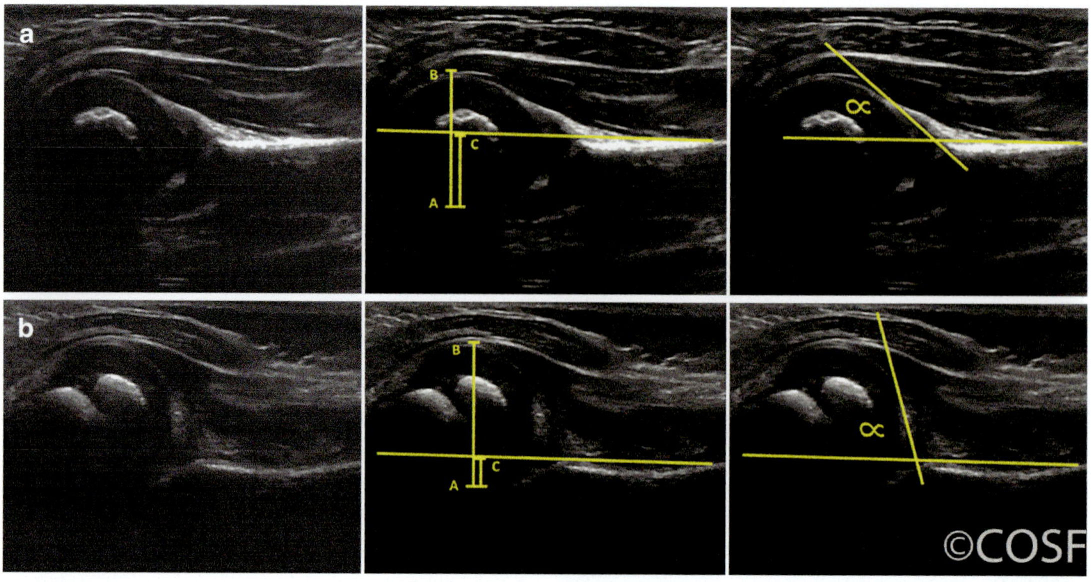

Fig. 29.3 Ultrasound of the glenohumeral joint demonstrating (**a**) A normal shoulder. PHHA is measured using the distance AC/AB and α as demonstrated and (**b**) A dislocated shoulder with demonstration of the changes that occur with migration of the humeral head. ©Children's Orthopaedic Surgery Foundation

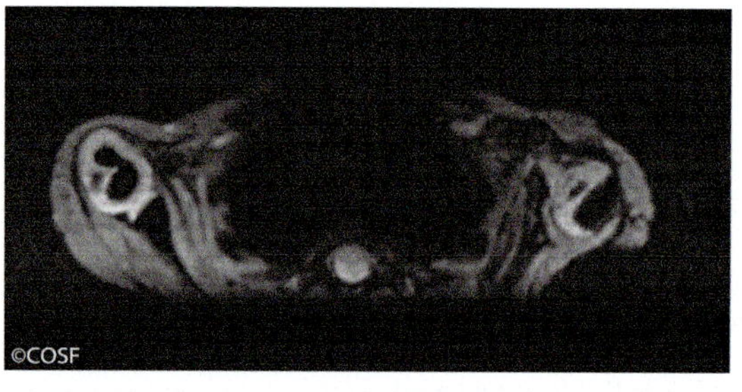

Fig. 29.4 MRI of both shoulders demonstrating a normal right shoulder and dislocated left shoulder with pseudo-glenoid formation. ©Children's Orthopaedic Surgery Foundation

Clinical Pearls: BPBP Assessment

- Repeated independent assessments
- Active Movement Scale and Toronto Test score in neonates
- Mallet score in older children
- Assess for dislocated humeral head and internal rotation contracture
- Trumpet sign assesses for loss of global external rotation
- Ultrasound or MRI can assess for posterior humeral head dislocation

preoperative planning MRI is superior, in particular cartilage sensitive sequences (Fig. 29.4). It is important the MRI aligned in the plane of the scapular.

The Waters' Classification [3] is used to grade the deformity on MRI (Table 29.1). This assesses the glenoid version, percentage of the humeral head anterior to the middle of the glenoid (PHHA) and the morphology of the glenoid and humeral head on MRI.

Management of the Shoulder

Decisions around the most appropriate management of the shoulder depends on several factors including the likelihood of natural recovery of neurologic function, re-innervation, muscular balance about the joint, morphology of the joint and age of the patient. These decisions should be made concurrently with microsurgical care of the upper limb.

Table 29.1 Waters' classification of glenohumeral deformity

	Deformity severity	Description
Type I	Normal glenoid	<5° difference in retroversion compared to the normal side
Type II	Minimal deformity	>5° difference in retroversion, no posterior subluxation
Type III	Moderate deformity	<35% humeral head anterior to the bisecting line of the scapular blade
Type IV	Severe deformity	Presence of a false glenoid
Type V	Humeral head deformity	Flattening of the humeral head and glenoid with progressive or complete dislocation of the humeral head
Type VI	Infantile dislocation	Dislocation of the glenohumeral joint in infancy
Type VII	Growth arrest	Growth arrest of the proximal humerus

Non-Operative Intervention

Ideally passive range of motion will commences at 2–3 weeks of age in order to prevent contracture development whilst observing for neurologic recovery.

All joints with a reduced range of motion should be passively taken through a full range of motion several times per day. Range of motion for the shoulder should include abduction with the scapular stabilised (Fig. 29.5) and external rotation with the elbow flexed and supinated to protect the radial head.

The parents perform therapy with regular review by physical or occupational therapy providers. Therapy providers in addition to performing range of motion and checking family technique, also monitor for contracture formation and joint subluxation.

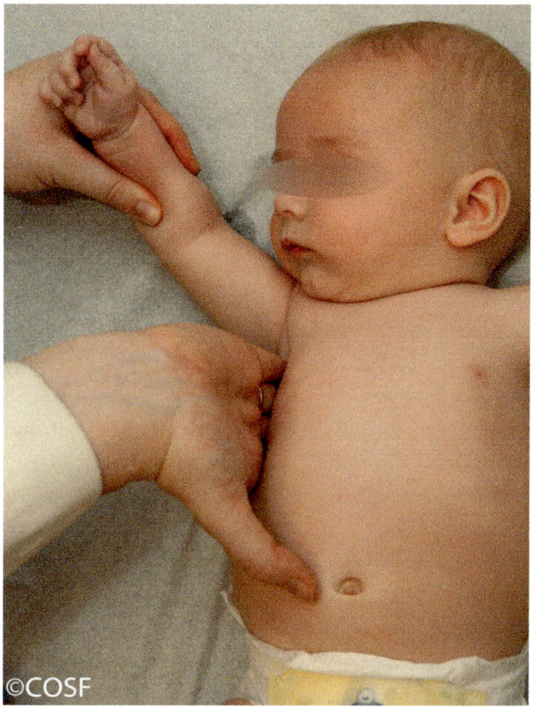

Fig. 29.5 Therapist performing an abduction stretch with the scapular stabilized. ©Children's Orthopaedic Surgery Foundation

Splinting

The role for splinting is less well established. Several devices have been designed and are used in some centres. Splinting aims to hold the forearm in supination and the shoulder in external rotation, initially regaining range of motion and then being worn for nights and naps so as to allow daytime development of appropriate hand function [24]. The goal of splinting is to keep the humeral head reduced and allow the development of normal glenoid morphology.

Reinnervation

Although patient selection and a comprehensive review of the clinical decision making is outside the scope of this text re-innervation either by neurologic recovery or through intervention with neuroma resection and grafting or nerve transfers is an important consideration for the outcome of the shoulder and it's function.

Neurologic recovery may occur with re-innervation along intact pathways in minor injuries. With more marked injuries, internal disruption occurs and then reinnervation may result in cross innervation.

Neuroma excision and nerve grafting is generally considered under 12mo of age, ideally around 5 months of age and beyond the scope of this chapter. Nerve grafting requires intact nerve roots to graft from. Nerve transfers are becoming more common and offer several advantages especially where there is loss of proximal donors to graft from, as occurs in spinal cord avulsions. It is also becoming the standard of care in a group of older patients with either plateaued recovery or late presentation, as the distance to the motor end plate is shorter. Nerve transfers in neonatal brachial plexus palsy have been shown to be safe and effective [25].

The most commonly utilized nerve transfer for reanimation of the shoulder is the partial spinal accessory (CNXI) to suprascapular nerve transfer. This is commonly combined with a partial median and/or ulnar nerve transfer to the biceps and/or brachialis (Oberlin transfer). Partial spinal accessory to suprascapular nerve transfer has been shown to be equivalent to C5 nerve grafting. This transfer can also be used to allow plexal roots to graft other recipients or when C5 is avulsed and therefore not available as a donor [26]. Re-innervation of the suprascapular nerve will restore abduction and external rotation function.

Less commonly a partial radial nerve transfer to the axillary nerve may be performed however this relies on there being sufficient radial nerve functional recovery. This transfer will aid abduction more than external rotation.

Botulinum Toxin

The use of botulinum toxin in management of the shoulder in patients with neonatal brachial plexus birth palsy is primarily to provide reversible weakening of the internal rotators of the glenohumeral joint to allow ongoing therapy or closed reduction whilst neurologic recovery is expected to occur. It is generally considered in infantile shoulder dislocation with the potential for ongoing neurologic recovery. In this group of patients upto 60% of patients will maintain a reduction with a single dose of botox and period of spica casting [27].

Consideration can be given for repeat injection; however, there is some concern that repeat injections may lead to irreversible weakening of the muscles and this must be kept in mind especially if a muscle is potentially a donor for transfer or needed for maintenance of midline function.

TECHNIQUE: Botulinum Injections with Closed Reduction of the Shoulder and Spica Casting

Following induction of general anaesthesia an examination under anaesthetic is performed to determine if the shoulder may be reduced following muscle relaxation. If not, a slow steady manipulation is performed, the elbow is held at 90degrees of flexion and in the supinated position to protect the collateral ligaments and radial head, the shoulder is adducted and then slowly externally rotated. The humeral head can be palpated to slide anteriorly, aiming in the reduced position for >60 degrees of external rotation. If this can be achieved then botulinum toxin is utilised and a spica cast. If not, then the patient is indicated for open shoulder releases to achieve shoulder reduction.

The use of Botox (Botulinum toxin A, Allergan, Irvine, California) in this group of patients is considered off label use and families should be informed of this and the potential for prolonged weakness including respiratory complications. Dosing should be limited to 10 IU per kg. Dosing is specific to the brand preparation. Dilution should be to 50 IU per ml for most small children, as the total dose is 70–80 IU. A tuberculin syringe is ideal and each injection site should receive less than 0.5 ml of injectate and where possible multiple sites per muscle used. Commonly treated muscles are the pectoralis major (anterior axillary fold), teres major (posterior axillary fold from the inferior angle of the scapular) and subscapularis (shoulder abducted, to deliver scapular with subscapularis on the anterior surface). The muscle is palpated and nerve stimulation performed to confirm intramuscular location. Dose per muscle should be equally divided from the total dose. This is commonly 2–3 IU/kg/muscle [27].

A spica cast is applied in two sections. A well-padded long arm cast in full supination with the elbow at 90 degrees and a bellyband. The bellyband should ensure that there is sufficient room for the abdomen to expand and a bolster placed during application to allow this expansion. Felt is placed over the sacrum and iliac crests for the abdominal band to rest on and then generous webril padding prior to casting material. Immobilization is in the adducted and externally rotated position. Two options exist for connecting the arm and abdominal portions, a strut connection (either dowels or a casting material twisted splint) or a solid wrap. The solid connection allows of moulding into the posterior shoulder to support the reduced humeral head however the strut connection allows confirmatory ultrasound to be performed at the conclusion of the procedure.

Glenohumeral Joint Reduction and Rebalancing

Once neurologic recovery is no longer anticipated then glenohumeral joint reconstruction with shoulder reduction and rebalancing is indicated for persistent shoulder dysfunction.

When there is joint deformity or fixed contractures then releases are required to achieve adequate reduction and remodelling. This can be achieved either with an open approach or arthroscopically. It has been shown that once glenohumeral deformity exists then joint remodelling can't be expected with tendon transfers alone [28]. Arthroscopic release can address the contracture of the capsule and the superior tendinous portion of the subscapularis. This technique requires arthroscopic skill however has become more wide spread in recent years [29]. Open joint release can be achieved through an anterior or axillary approach and readily combined with other open procedures particularly tendon transfers. The axillary nerve is protected and commonly the capsule, pectoralis major and subscapularis are fractionally lengthened.

When performing the release it is important to perform it in an al a carte fashion taking care not to over release the subscapularis. Over release can lead to internal rotation weakness and loss of midline function.

Tendon transfer of the latissimus dorsi and teres major is indicated when external rotation weakness exists. It is most commonly combined with joint and musculotendinous releases. As an isolated procedure this is reserved for those patients without joint deformity, this tends to be an older group of patients with isolated external rotation weakness. Patients who also have relative internal rotation weakness may benefit from an isolated transfer of either teres or latisimus to avoid the complication of external rotation contracture.

The key to achieving joint remodelling and improving function is joint reduction and rebalancing (Fig. 29.6).

TECHNIQUE: Open Reduction and Tendon Transfers

The procedure is performed with the patient in a lateral decubitus position and the affected extremity up. A beanbag or gel rolls are used for positioning and great care taken to pad all bony prominences and avoid pressure or traction on neurovascular structures (Fig. 29.7).

After induction an examination under anaesthesia is performed. Joint reduicability, scapulohumeral angle and external rotation in the adducted and abducted position are assessed.

A axillary crease incision is utilized (Fig. 29.8). Skin and subcutaneous flaps are elevated; there are often a number of fascial bands that need to be released. Dissection is initially carried down anteriorly to the pectoralis major tendon, a musculotendinous lengthening can be performed as the posterior tendinous fibres are released and the anterior muscle preserved. This aims to improve external rotation in abduction. (This anterior interval can also be utilised to access the Subscapularis musculotendinous junction and anterior capsule).

Posterior dissection can then be carried out down to the latissimus dorsi and teres major insertions into the humerus. Axillary nerve must be protected and lies just cephlad to insertion. Visualisation can be improved by positioning the arm in abduction and internal rotation. Depending on the preoperative examination one or both tendons can then be taken off the humerus and fully mobilized, there are commonly several posterior fascial bands that are released. The neurovascular

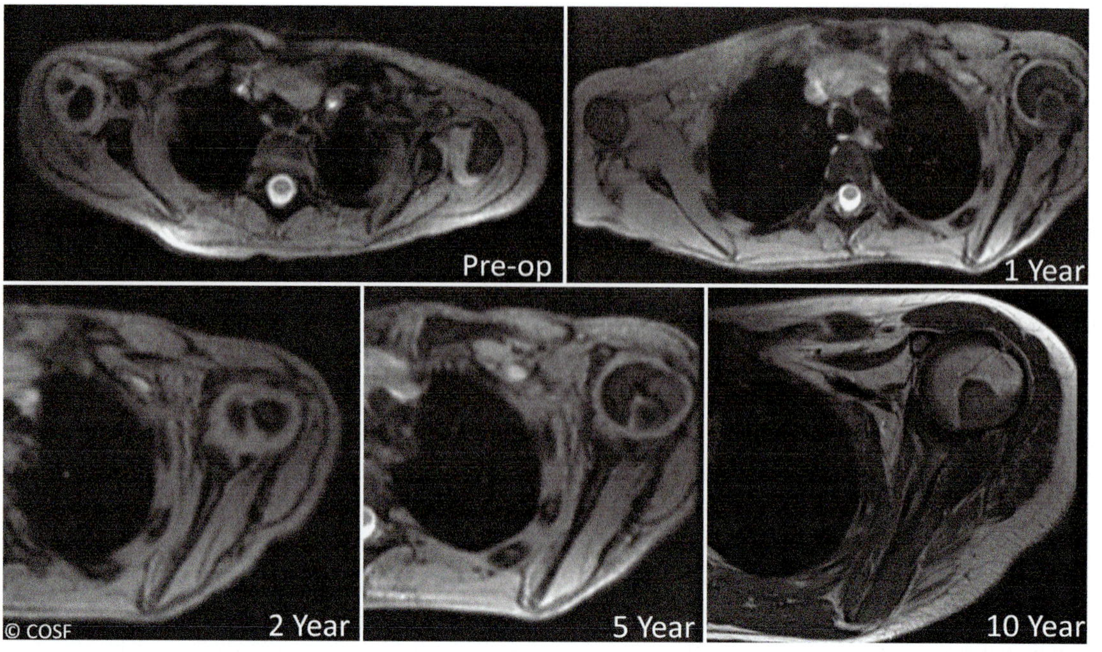

Fig. 29.6 Single patient longitudinal series of MRI scans following open reduction and tendon transfers, 10 year period of post-operative follow up. ©Children's Orthopaedic Surgery Foundation

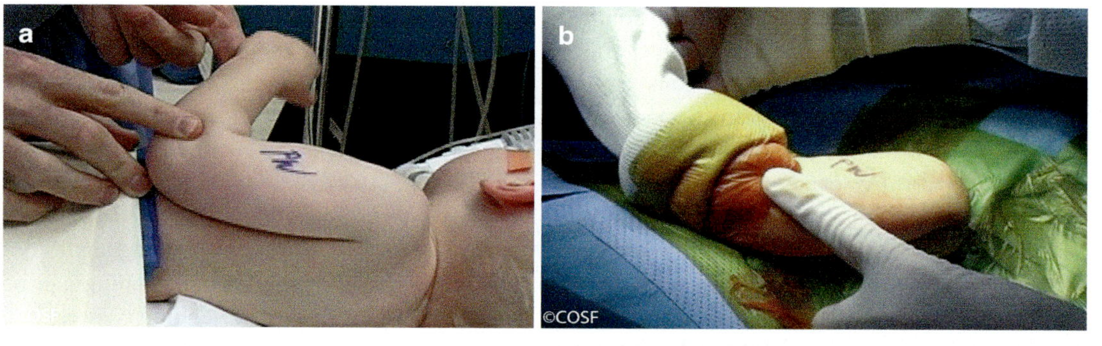

Fig. 29.7 (**a**) Lateral positioning using gel rolls or a bean bag and securing the patients pelvis with well-padded tape and (**b**) prepping and draping to ensure exposure maintained. ©Children's Orthopaedic Surgery Foundation

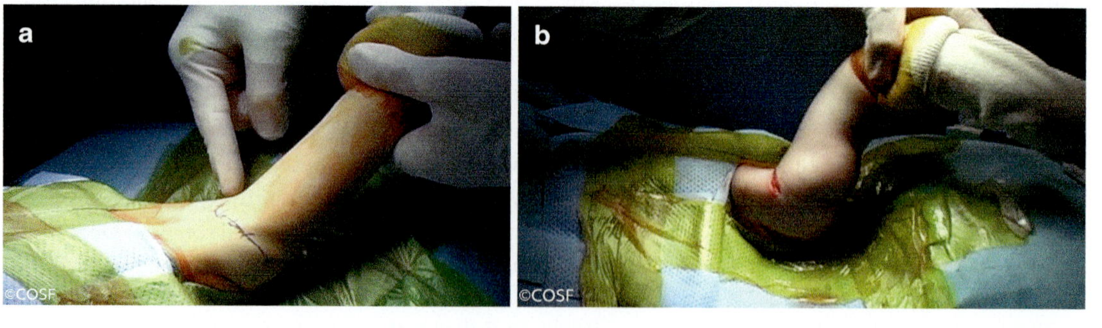

Fig. 29.8 Demonstration of the axillary incision location (**a**) and cosmesis within the skin fold (**b**). ©Children's Orthopaedic Surgery Foundation

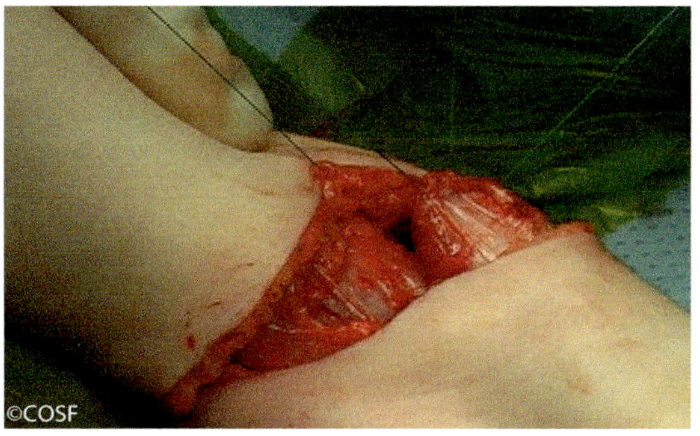

Fig. 29.9 Mobilisation of the conjoint teres major and latissimus dorsi tendons with inverted matress ethibond suture. ©Children's Orthopaedic Surgery Foundation

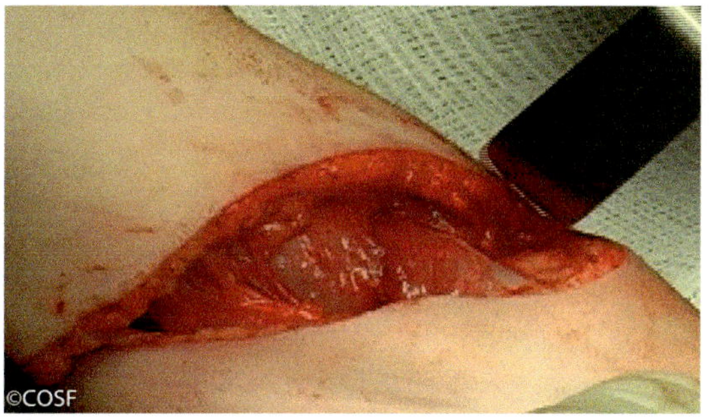

Fig. 29.10 Clinical photograph showing the tendon transfer position after fixation to the tuberosity and rotator cuff. ©Children's Orthopaedic Surgery Foundation

pedicle to the latissimus is at risk with injudicious mobilization and should be protected. Ethibond is placed into the free tendon ends in an upside down matress suture (Fig. 29.9).

Next the interval between the deltoid and triceps is developed. This is for passage of the tendon transfer. A digit, peanut or freer is passed up into the subacromial space and a subacromial decompression performed, freeing adhesions. In this same interval if there is residual tightness of the scapulohumeral angle then a fascial lengthening of the triceps can be performed. This also further decompressed the axillary nerve.

Once the tendons have been mobilized attention is returned to the joint reduction and the external rotation range of motion assessed in abduction and adduction. Back in the anterior interval, posterior to the pectoralis major tendon and anterior to the plexus the subscapularis can be partially released near its musculotendinous junction if additional external rotation is required particularly in the adducted position. Alternatively a subscapularis slide from the scapular body can be performed. The goal is 90 degrees of external rotation in the abducted position and 30 degrees in the adducted position. Over release of the subscapularis can lead to internal rotation weakness.

If the range of motion is still not adequate or the joint not reduced with the extra articular releases under direct visualization, a capsulotomy can performed from anteroinferiorly while protecting the labrum and the humeral head. Release continues until the humeral head is reduced into the glenoid, care must be taken to not over reduce the joint and cause anterior subluxation.

The Latissimus and teres tendons are then passed into the deltoid triceps interval while protecting the axillary nerve and sewn into the greater tuberosity (Fig. 29.10). A capsular plication can be performed whilst sewing in the transfer if capsular redundancy is noted or joint instability persists. Joint stability is again assessed including the position of reduction and any abduction contracture. The wounds are closed in layers.

The patient is then carefully positioned on the spica table, whilst maintaining the reduction and placed in a shoulder spica cast in a safe position of adduction and external rotation of about 30 degrees. The forearm is in a supinated position. Care is taken to pad all neurovascular structures, bony prominences and protect the skin and allow for proper respiratory and dietary function.

The patient remains in the cast for 1 month and then returns to clinic for removal of the cast and commencement of therapy.

Glenoid Osteotomy

Glenoid osteotomy is reserved for patients with more advanced glenoid deformity where joint reduction and rebalancing is not expected to result in remodelling. When a glenoid osteotomy should be performed is not well defined, although best indications appear to be older patients and those with more deformity who are less likely to remodel with open reduction and joint rebalancing. How much deformity and at which ages the remodelling potential is diminished requires further study. Glenoid osteotomy procedures can be divided into redirectional and reshaping osteotomies. Both have shown improved external rotation. Dodwell [30] showed good early results with a glenoid anteverting osteotomy combined with tendon transfers and Di Mascio [31] published similar outcomes using a glenoplasty technique without tendon transfer. These procedures carry a high degree of surgical complexity and long-term comparison to humeral derotation osteotomy is needed.

Clinical Pearls: BPBP Management

- Neurological reconstruction in those under 12 months (neurolysis, nerve repair and nerve transfers)
- Botulinium toxin plus spica to prevent internal rotation contracture
- Contracture release and/or tendon transfers to restore external rotation power
- Anteverting glenoid osteotomy and/or derotation humeral osteotomy for secondary skeletal deformities

TECHNIQUE: Glenoid Osteotomy

Glenoid osteotomy is commonly combined with open reduction and tendon transfers of the shoulder in BPBP. If being performed as a combined procedure, the glenoid osteotomy is performed after anterior release and mobilization of the latissimus and teres major tendon transfer and prior to placement of the tendon transfers.

The posterior limb of the incision used for the tendon tranfers (either axillary or posterior longitudinal) can be extended proximally and curved medially to along the scapular spine.

Wide subcutaneous flaps are elevated at the level of the fasica. The deltoid is elevated off the scapular spine using subperiosteal dissection and retracted laterally. This allows visualisation of the infraspinatus and teres minor and protects the axillary nerve. The interval between infraspinatus and teres minor is developed, this is more readily found medially and then developed laterally. Between 25 and 75% of the infraspinatus insertion is elevated and tagged for later repair allowing access to the underlying shoulder capsule and joint. A capsulotomy is performed to allow direct visualisation of the joint, which is commonly biconcave with a posterior pseudoglenoid. There is commonly redundant capsule present. Dissection is next taken superiorly and inferiorly in a subperiosteal plane on the posterior glenoid, 1 cm medial to the glenoid rim, to allow retractors to be placed superiorly and inferiorly around the glenoid neck. By remaining subperiosteal the suprascapular nerve is protected.

The osteotomy is then outlined and the anterior joint palpated to assist with orientation of the osteotomy. A freer elevated can be introduced into the joint to assist with this orientation.

A corticocancellous bone graft is harvested from the scapular spine prior to making the osteotomy, so as to minimise the number of manipulations of the osteotomy required. Osteotomes are used to create the osteotomy 1 cm medial to the posterior glenoid rim aiming to remain medial to the palpated anterior rim. The osteotomy is carefully wedged open and the graft impacted to maintain correction. The graft should be intrinsically stable and does not require fixation in young children. Bone wax is placed into the graft donor site. A posterior capsulorraphy is performed and the infraspinatus tendon repaired. Range of motion, particularly internal rotation, should be checked during posterior repair to avoid over tightening of the posterior capsulorraphy and infraspinatus.

At this point the latissimus and teres major transfers may be completed and then the deltoid repaired to the scapular spine using transosseous sutures. A layered closure of the subcutaneous tissues and skin is performed followed by a shoulder spica cast in approximately 30 degrees of external rotation and 30 degrees of abduction. We routinely obtain a CT scan on postoperative day 1 to check graft placement and correction (Fig. 29.11).

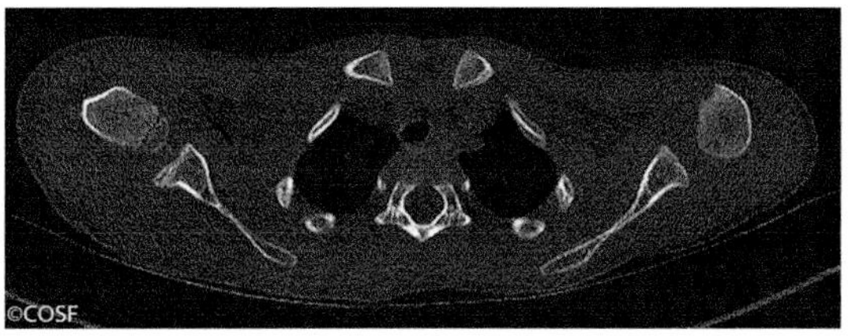

Fig. 29.11 CT scan post operatively showing correction of glenoid version. ©Children's Orthopaedic Surgery Foundation

Salvage Procedures

Humeral Osteotomy for Internal Rotation Contracture

Humeral osteotomy has been shown to improve global shoulder function in patients that are not suitable for joint reconstructive procedures. Waters [32] showed an average correction was 64° (range, 35°–90°) and mean Mallet classification score improvement from 13 to 18 ($p < 0.01$).

It is most commonly performed for patients with persistent internal rotation contracture and advanced glenohumeral joint deformity. Less commonly it is indicated to treat an external rotation positioning which may result as an outcome of treatment. Derotational osteotomies will-change the position of the functional arc and care must be taken to ensure that the patient can still bring their hand to their mouth, abdomen and perineum. An arc of at least 100 degrees is desired. Although exacerbation of the glenohumeral incrongruence with derotation is a theoretic risk is has not been shown to be of a functional concern. Humeral osteotomies for internal rotation contracture can be performed proximally, either above or below the deltoid insertion, or distally in the supracondylar region.

TECHNIQUE: Humeral External Rotation Osteotomy

The patient is positioned in a modified beach chair position with the entire shoulder girdle including the scapula and the entire involved left upper limb visualized and manipulated in a stable fashion. The scapula is stabilised on the bed so as to ensure accurate positioning and examination throughout the procedure.

Exam under anesthesia is undertaken assessing arc of rotation in the adducted position. Ability to reach the midline at the mouth, umbilicus and perineum. The total arc is preferably greater than 100 degrees. The planned correction is then determined, usually about 70 degrees in most cases.

Sterile prepping and draping is completed. A curvilinear incision with a slight medial distal curve is carried out, centered over the deltoid insertion, so as to allow for linear alignment after derotation of the distal fragment of the humerus. Skin and subcutaneous flaps are elevated. The cephalic vein is identified and protected. The deltopectoral interval is opened and subperiosteal dissection is carried out proximally between the deltoid insertion and the pectoralis major insertion. Distally the brachialis is split in line with its fibres. Homan retractors are placed around the humerus with particular care to stay within the periosteal sleeve so as to protect the radial nerve posteriorly as well as the musculocutaneous nerve adjacent. Marking of the bone is then carried out for the transverse osteotomy just above the deltoid insertion. Marking the bone linearly for the desired degree external rotation of osteotomy is also carried out with osteotomes and Bovie. A 70 degree correction is commonly planned and this in a yound adolescent is commonly the width of a small fragment semitubular plate.

Double stacked 6 hole semitubular plates are commonly used however the implant size should be appropriate for the size of the bone and for desired fixation in a particular patient. At least 2 proximal screws should be placed prior to performing the humeral osteotomy, this keeps control of the proximal articular side fragment. The screws are then removed. With care taken to stay within the periosteal sleeve and protect the soft tissues using Homan retractors, an oscillating saw osteotomy is performed under low velocity with irrigation so as to avoid osteonecrosis. After completion of the osteotomy, the plate was reapplied proximally with the 2 screws but not in a tight fashioning manner.

Rotation coinciding with marking the bone is carried out. Compression technique is utilized

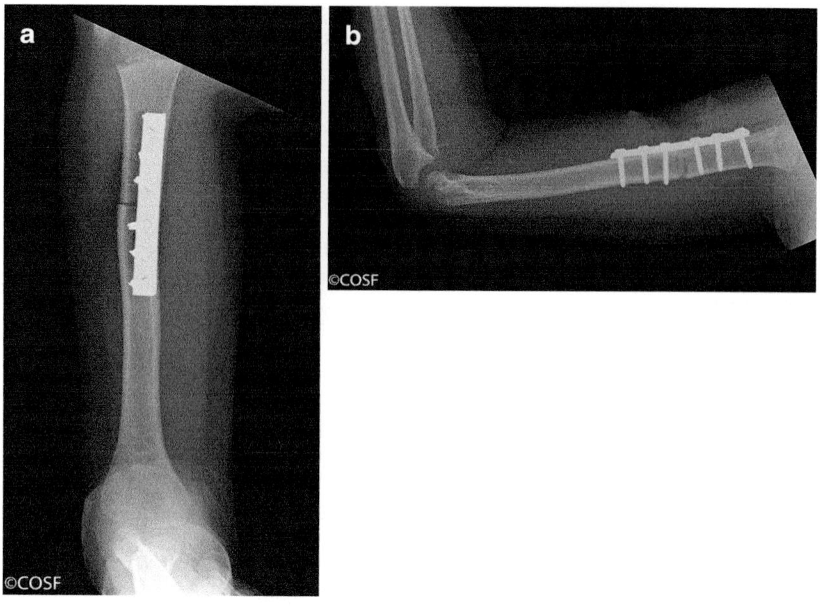

Fig. 29.12 Flat plate radiographs performed intraoperatively to confirm metal ware position. ©Children's Orthopaedic Surgery Foundation

and the plate is held to the bone with appropriate bone clamps. Once an initial screw is placed then check is made to ensure that the desired rotation has been achieved and the patient can reach midline still in terms of mouth, abdomen and perineum. Some varus can be allowed for a patient with a Putti sign due to an abduction contracture.

A flat plate radiograph is performed to ensure the desired alignment of the plate, screws and osteotomy (Fig. 29.12).

After irrigation, the wound is closed in layers with the periosteum followed by subcutaneous closure and subcuticular closure.

A sling a swathe is most commonly utilised however on occasion a spica cast may be required, particularly in younger children. Full time immobilisation is for 6 weeks and activity restricted for 3 months.

Scapular Procedures

Salvage procedures on the scapular and clavicle are less commonly utilized. Some advocate ostectomy of the superomedial border of the scapular with or without osteotomy of the acromion and clavicle; however, widespread use has not yet been published.

Facioscapulohumeral Dystrophy

Introduction

Facioscapulohumeral muscular dystrophy (FSHD) is the third most common hereditary disease of muscle and is unique in as much as it affects the shoulder girdle to a greater extent than other inherited muscular dystrophies. FSHD has an incidence of 1 in 20,000. Within the disorder there is a great degree of clinical and genetic variability [33]. The most common inheritance pattern is autosomal dominant, however some individuals show digenic inheritence [34].

Clinical Presentation and Investigation

Initial presentation most commonly involves the facial and periscapular muscles with lower extremity involvement being a later finding. The onset of weakness can occur in infancy however is most common in the second decade, and may on occasion only be seen in later adult life. Life expectancy is not usually affected however the condition is gradually progressive. There is commonly a marked asymmetry from side to side in the degree of weakness and variability of expression within families.

Although weakness is the most common finding, many patients present with pain [35].

Shoulder dysfunction occurs primarily due to periscapular muscle weakness with relative preservation of the deltoid and rotator cuff. The Horwitz manoeuvre is particularly helpful in the assessment of patients with FSHD as it portents the potential benefit of surgical stabilization of the scapular. The Horwitz manoeuvre is performed by manually fixing the scapula to the thorax and then observing an increase in shoulder forward flexion and abduction.

Genetic testing is available and should be performed in conjunction with a geneticist. Results must be interpreted in association with the clinical presentation. Additional investigation including EMG and MRI to investigate for alternate causes when genetic testing is inconclusive may also be indicated, aiming to exclude central, cervical, brachial plexus and isolated long thoracic nerve palsy as a cause for the patient's presentation.

Management of The Shoulder

Non-Operative Intervention

Initial management should consist of physical therapy. Therapy should work to maximize the strength of the affected and unaffected musculature. Physical exertion is not known to affect the progression of disease like it can in other muscular dystrophies. Occupational therapy can assist with managing activities of daily living.

Operative Intervention

Patients unable to maintain function with physical therapy and with a positive Horwitz manoeuvre may be candidates for surgical management. Options include both soft tissue and fusion procedures.

Historically soft tissue transfers to confer increased scapular stability were utilized and short-term results were promising; however, unlike patients with an isolated long thoracic nerve palsy, patients with FSHD continued to progress with their weakness and lost the benefit of the surgical procedure over time.

Current recommendation for patients undergoing surgical management is a scapulothoracic fusion. Scapulothoracic fusion aims to stabilize the scapula in a functional position by achieving a solid fusion between the posterior rib cage and the medial border of the scapula. In this position the rotator cuff and deltoid musculature have a stable base against which to function.

Several different techniques have been described; these tend to vary by the use of graft and fixation method [36–39].

Clinical Pearls: FSHD

- Horwitz manoeuvre to assess whether will benefit from scapula stabilising procedure
- Because FSHD is a progressive disorder, scapulothoracic fusion better than soft tissue procedures

TECHNIQUE: Scapulothoracic Fusion

The patient requires endotracheal intubation and on most occasions a Foley catheter due to the potential prolonged duration of the procedure. Standard perioperative antibiotics are administered.

Positioning is prone and a spinal operating table being most versatile. The patient is prepared and draped to allow intraoperative assessment of both shoulders. The entire back and the ipsilateral posterior iliac crest included in the field for the harvest of autogenous bone graft if desired. Allograft corticocancellous chips of bone can also be used. The operative limb is draped free allowing for intraoperative manipulation. The arm should be positioned so that the medial border of the scapula is in the desired retracted position and parallel to the spine. Extreme care should be taken to ensure that all bony prominences are padded, breasts and genitalia free and there is no undue tension on neurovascular structures.

A longitudinal incision is utilized midway between the spinous processes and the medial border of the scapula. Skin and subcutaneous flap should be extensively mobilized with dissection being carried down to the medial border of the scapula.

First the trapezius is taken off as a single layer and mobilized with 2-0 Ethibond sutures maintaining continuity of the layer. The distal aspect of the spinal accessory nerve is protected.

The Rhomboids are taken off the medial border of the scapular and similarly mobilized and tagged, reflecting them towards the midline. Next the Supraspinatus and infraspinatus are mobilized from their origin and retracted laterally. The posterior surface of the medial border is now exposed. Next the serratus anterior and subscapularis need to be released from the under surface of the medial border of the scapula. Dissection is carried in a subperiosteal plane (Fig. 29.13). The medial and central portion of these two muscles needs to be excised so as to allow the scapula to oppose to the medial border of the scapula to the thoracic cage (Fig. 29.14). Completely clearing all the soft tissues between the ribs and the under surface of the scapula is an important step in obtaining a solid fusion.

The most medial portion of the scapular spine is commonly resected using a rongeur so as to allow plate apposition. A 7-hole small fragment DCP plate (or plate appropriate in size to match the patient anatomy) is contoured to the medial scapular border.

Next attention is turned to the preparation of the ribs. Most commonly the scapular will overly the third through sixth ribs posterior. Sequentially a horizontal incision is made in the posterior periosteum of the rib and then subperiosteal elevation performed circumferentially around the rib. Curved rib periosteal elevators can be most useful for this step. Remaining subperiosteal will ensure that the

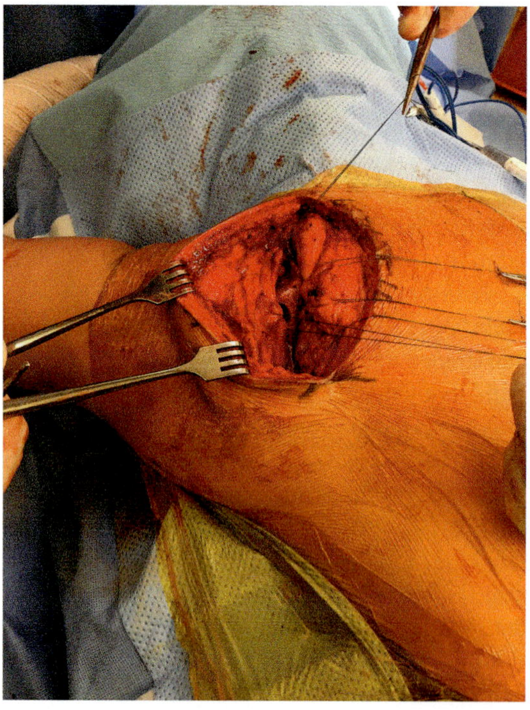

Fig. 29.13 Approach with mobilization of medial and lateral muscular envelopes. ©Children's Orthopaedic Surgery Foundation

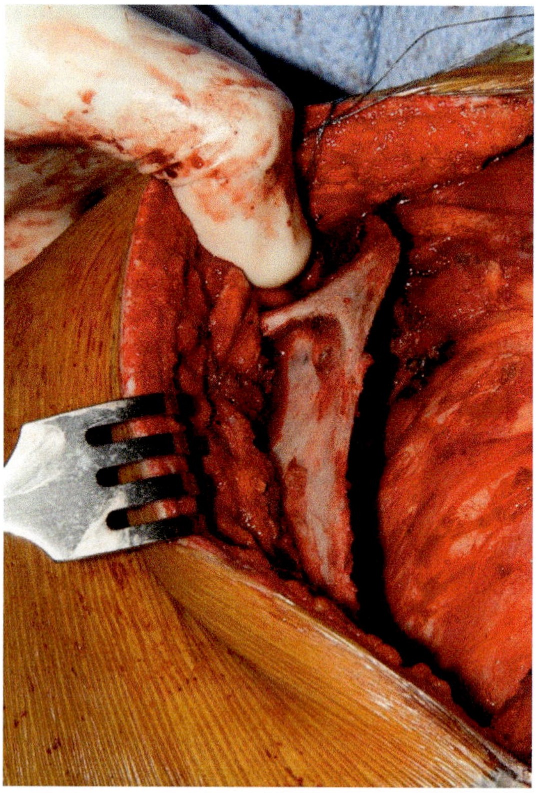

Fig. 29.14 Excision of medial aspect of subscapularis and serratus anterior. ©Children's Orthopaedic Surgery Foundation

neurovascular bundle running along the inferior aspect of the rib is elevated and protected. The parietal pleura is directly deep and at risk for penetration with resultant pneumothorax. Care must be taken not to plunge during elevation. Double stranded 16 or 18 gauge Luque wire is passed around each rib. Once all wires are passed the wound may be filled with saline and the anaesthetist performs a valsalva manoeuvre to check for pneumothorax. A burr is used to gently decorticate the posterior rib and under surface of the scapula (Fig. 29.15). The scapula is quite thin and thus, gentle use of the bur is needed to create bleeding bone but not penetrate the scapula. Meticulous technique is required to avoid osteonecrosis with irrigation and frequent cleaning of the flutes.

Posterior iliac crest graft is harvested through a separate incision if desired. A large volume of cancellous graft can be harvested through this approach.

The plate is then placed along the medial border of the scapula and drill holes made through the holes in the plate corresponding to the underlying ribs (Fig. 29.16). One end of the double stranded Luque wire is passed through the drill hole and plate and once all wires passed provisional wire tightening occurs. The position of the scapula should be at 25 degrees of forward inclination and 20–30 degrees of abduction (slightly closer to the midline superiorly). Once this has been checked then the graft is placed between the ribs and scapula and final tightening performed (Fig. 29.17). A Jet-X wire tightener may be used. Tightening can lead to a loss of the anterior inclination and should be mindfully avoided. Final position is checked and shoulder motion affirmed. Wires

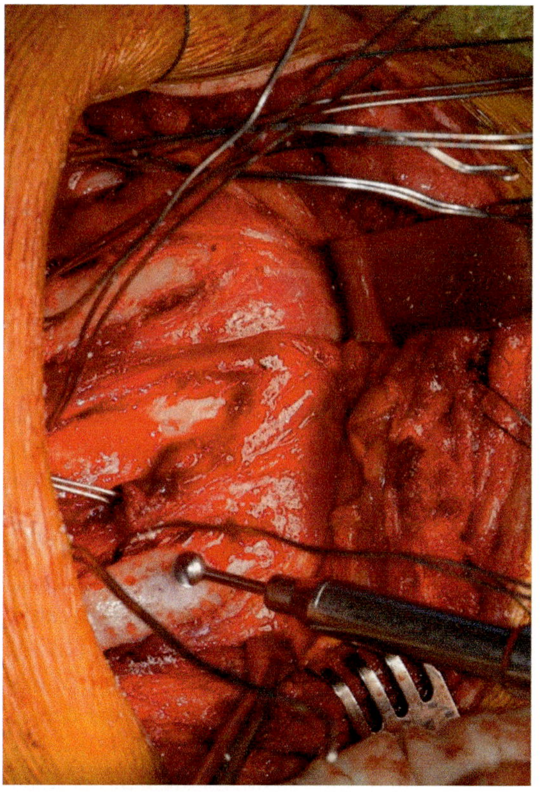

Fig. 29.15 Decortication of the posterior aspect of the ribs after placement of the Luque wire. ©Children's Orthopaedic Surgery Foundation

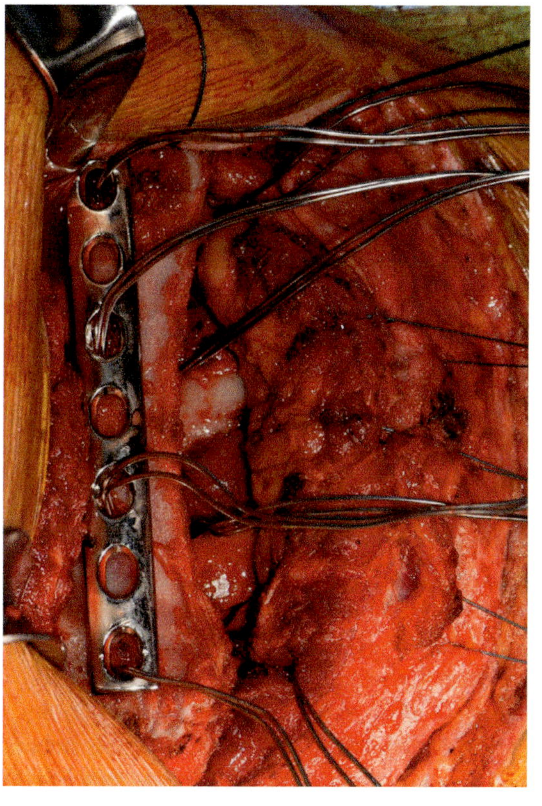

Fig. 29.16 Placement of the plate and passing of the Luque wires, prior to tightening. ©Children's Orthopaedic Surgery Foundation

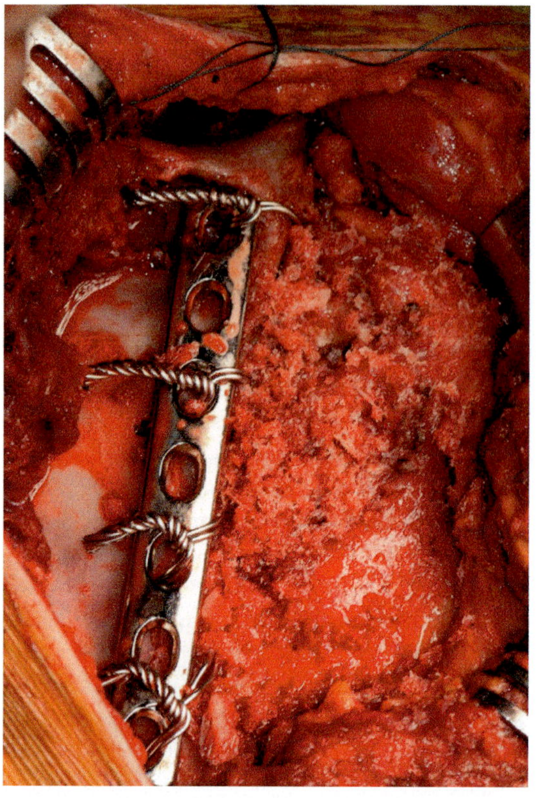

Fig. 29.17 Placement of the graft and final positioning of the tightened wires. ©Children's Orthopaedic Surgery Foundation

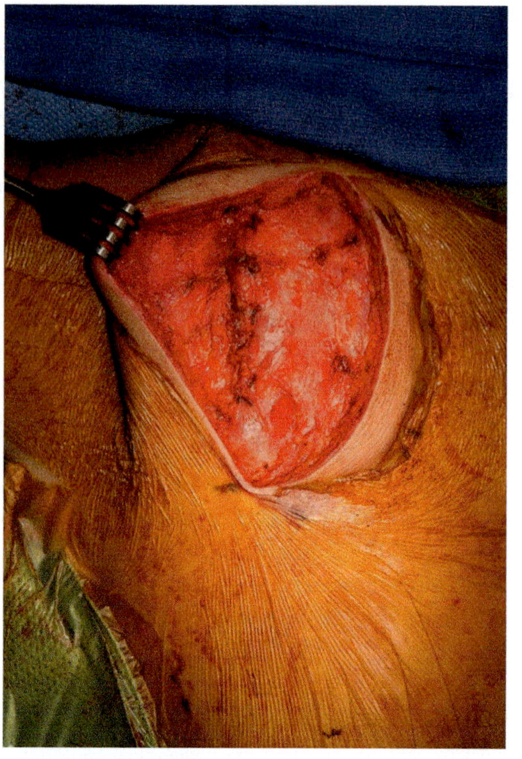

Fig. 29.18 Closure of the anatomic muscular envelope to minimize plate and wire prominence. ©Children's Orthopaedic Surgery Foundation

are cut and turned to avoid prominence. After irrigation, the muscular layers are closed with the Ethibond suture previously placed so that the rhomboids, infraspinatus, supraspinatus and trapezius are all repaired (Fig. 29.18). Subcutaneous and subcuticular closure then obtained.

A sling and swathe, Gunslinger brace or shoulder spica may be used for postoperative immobilisation, dependent on patient age, personality, and durability of fixation achieved.

A chest x-ray should be performed in recovery to assess for pneumothorax. Full time immobilisation is utilized for 6 weeks so as to achieve fusion. Maintaining distal musculature is important due to the underlying weakness that FSHD patients have. Rehabilitation should be commenced as soon as possible. Solid fusion takes up to 3 months (Fig. 29.19).

Cerebral Palsy

Management of the shoulder in patients with cerebral palsy rarely occurs in isolation. The typical upper extremity deformity is that of shoulder internal rotation, elbow flexion, forearm pronation, wrist flexion with ulnar deviation, thumb-in-palm and finger swan neck or clenched fist deformities.The central nervous system injury will determine the peripheral manifestations. The majority of patients will present with spasticity; however, dystonia can be significant and affect both the postural deformity and the outcome of surgical care. Treatment with peripheral surgery will not overcome the central deficits and the family and patient must understand this.

Treatment always starts with non-operative interventions. Postural retraining for shoulder abduction during gait, stretching pectoralis major and latissimus dorsi with or without the assistance

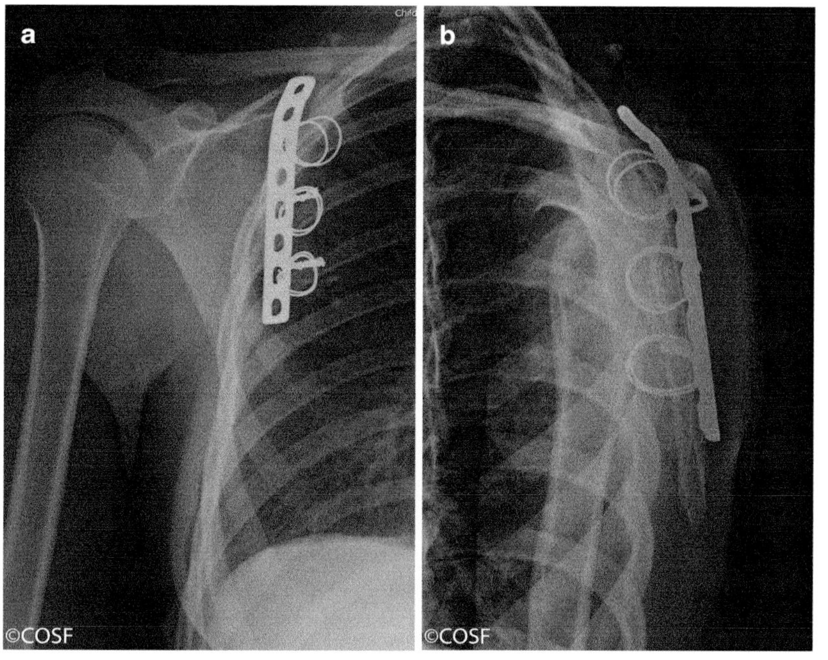

Fig. 29.19 Final radiographs (different patient to clinical example) showing position of the scapular and hardware following fusion. (**a**) AP projection (**b**) Lateral projection. ©Children's Orthopaedic Surgery Foundation

of botulinum. It should be noted that there are natural changes in tone and posture with growth and development and that dynamic positioning will be affected by this.

Surgery around the shoulder girdle is reserved for those refractory to other measures and is not commonly required. Surgical procedures for the shoulder fall into three main categories, soft tissue releases, osteotomies, and joint stabilizations. They may be aimed at improving postural positioning, active reach, or hygiene and dressing. Hygiene and difficulty with dressing is by far the most common surgical indication.

Soft tissue releases for postural position may include elevation of the deltoid insertion for abduction posturing, pectoralis major and lattisimus fractional lengthening for improved shoulder abduction/external rotation. It is more common with long standing internal rotation postural contracture (as occurs most commonly in hemiplegic patients) or external rotation contracture (more common in dystonia) to perform a derotational humeral osteotomy, although this is again uncommon. The surgical technique has previously been described in the section on brachial plexus birth palsy.

The most common indication for shoulder surgery in patients with cerebral palsy is in quadriplegic patients for contracture release for improved hygiene and dressing function. This can also include patients with axillary skin breakdown due to the tight contracture. It is anticipated that release of the pectoralis will achieve 30–45 degrees of increased abduction and latissimus adds an additional 30 degrees [40]. There are times where this is necessary for prone positioning for a spinal fusion in these more severely involved patients.

Very occasionally shoulder arthrodesis may be indicated in severe recurrent instability of the shoulder, this is particularly so in patients with dystonia and athetosis where soft tissue stabilizations are likely to fail.

Clinical Pearls: Cerebral Palsy

- Surgery indicated to improve washing / dressing / hygiene
- Soft tissue release of latissimus dorsi and/or pec major to relieve internal rotation / adduction contracture
- Derotation osteotomy for fixed contractures
- Glenohumeral arthrodesis occasionally indicated for painful chronic instability

TECHNIQUE: Pectoralis Major and Latissimus Dorsi Release for Shoulder Abduction

This operation is most commonly performed in conjunction with other procedures in the upper extremity and the entire arm should be prepped and drape freely. A hand table may be utilised however commonly the degree of contracture necessitating release means an assistant will be required to hold the arm whilst the surgeon operates in the tight space of the axilla.

An anterior axillary fold incision is made over the pectoralis major tendon. The skin is sharply incised, and cautery used through the subcutaneous tissues. The inferior border of the tendon is identified and then traced up proximally on both the superficial and deep surfaces, the cephalic vein at the proximal end of the tendon is protected. Once the tendon is isolated with a large hemostat it may be completely divided using cautery under direct vision. Complete release should ensued and then a gentle manipulation performed. The wound irrigated with normal saline and haemostasis checked and then closed in layers. Dermabond and an occlusive dressing aids with post operative hygiene.

If additional abduction is required then a posterior axillary skin fold incision can be made and the latissimus dorsi tendon isolated and divided as described above for the pectoralis major.

Gentle passive stretching is instituted immediately postoperatively.

Arythrogryposis

Arthrogryposis refers to a heterogeneous group of conditions with the common manifestation of multiple joint contractures and can be divided into three predominant subtypes: amylopalsia, distal and syndromic. Distal and syndromic subtypes will not be covered in this chapter as the need to address the shoulder is uncommon.

Amyloplasia presents with a typical posture of the upper extremities, the shoulders are adducted and internally rotated, elbows extended, wrists flexed and ulnarly deviated and the fingers stiff [41]. These deformities are accompanied by variable but usually present lower extremity involvement.

Most children with amyloplasia are of above average intelligence and will rely on their upper extremities for function and independence. The goals in treatment must aim to facilitate functional independence. They will commonly require bimanual use and passive range of motion to achieve this function. A comprehensive care plan should plan treatment for both upper extremities to encompass maximizing hand position and elbow range of motion in particular passive flexion for bimanual hand function. The muscular development around the shoulder girdle is lacking to a variable degree and patients will utilize what they have. It is uncommon to have sufficient donors to perform active tendon transfers and joint release procedures will not restore function due to the lack of motors units. In order to place the hands to allow them to come together for function, external rotation humeral osteotomies may be required. A resting position of 30–45 degrees of internal rotation will allow this [42]. The osteotomy can be performed proximally, especially when deltoid function is present as this can improve it's lever arm, or distally. Caution should be exercised and distal osteotomies avoided concurrently with elbow releases due to competing rehabilitation needs.

Conclusion

Shoulder surgery in neuromuscular conditions affecting the upper extremity should always be performed with consideration to the entire limb and underlying cause. The natural history and functional goals of the patient and family will often determine the most appropriate course of treatment. A multidisciplinary approach is always preferable including allied physicians and therapists.

References

1. Foad SL, Mehlman CT, Ying J. The epidemiology of neonatal brachial plexus palsy in the United States. J Bone Joint Surg Am. 2008;90(6):1258–64. https://doi.org/10.2106/JBJS.G.00853.
2. Wall LB, Mills JK, Leveno K, et al. Incidence and prognosis of neonatal brachial plexus palsy with and without clavicle fractures. Obstet Gynecol. 2014;123(6):1288–93. https://doi.org/10.1097/AOG.0000000000000207.
3. Waters PM, Smith GR, Jaramillo D. Glenohumeral deformity secondary to brachial plexus birth palsy. J Bone Joint Surg Am. 1998;80(5):668–77.
4. Pearl ML, Edgerton BW, Kon DS, et al. Comparison of arthroscopic findings with magnetic resonance imaging and arthrography in children with Glenohumeral deformities secondary to brachial plexus birth palsy. J Bone Joint Surg. 2003;85(5):890–8. https://doi.org/10.1097/01241398-198411000-00006.
5. Hoeksma AF, Steeg Ter AM, Dijkstra P, Nelissen RGHH, Beelen A, de Jong BA. Shoulder contracture and osseous deformity in obstetrical brachial plexus injuries. J Bone Joint Surg. 2003;85-A(2):316–22.
6. Fairbanks HAT. A lecture on birth palsy: subluxation of the shoulder-joint in infants and young children. Lancet. 1913;181(4679):1217–23., ISSN 0140-6736. https://doi.org/10.1016/S0140-6736(00)52017-0.
7. Dunkerton MC. Posterior dislocation of the shoulder associated with obstetric brachial plexus palsy. J Bone Joint Surg Br. 1989;71(5):764–6.
8. Torode I, Donnan L. Posterior dislocation of the humeral head in association with obstetric paralysis. J Pediatr Orthop. 1998;18(5):611–5.
9. Kim HM, Galatz LM, Das R, Patel N, Thomopoulos S. Musculoskeletal deformities secondary to neurotomy of the superior trunk of the brachial plexus in neonatal mice. J Orthop Res. 2010;28(10):1391–8. https://doi.org/10.1002/jor.21128.
10. Nikolaou S, Peterson E, Kim A, Wylie C, Cornwall R. Impaired growth of denervated muscle contributes to contracture formation following neonatal brachial plexus injury. J Bone Joint Surg Am. 2011;93(5):461–70. https://doi.org/10.2106/JBJS.J.00943.
11. Crouch DL, Hutchinson ID, Plate JF, et al. Biomechanical basis of shoulder osseous deformity and contracture in a rat model of brachial plexus birth palsy. J Bone Joint Surg Am. 2015;97(15):1264–71. https://doi.org/10.2106/JBJS.N.01247.
12. Li Z, Ma J, Apel P, Carlson CS, Smith TL, Koman LA. Brachial plexus birth palsy-associated shoulder deformity: a rat model study. J Hand Surg. 2008;33(3):308–12. https://doi.org/10.1016/j.jhsa.2007.11.017.
13. Einarsson F, Hultgren T, Ljung B-O, Runesson E, Fridén J. Subscapularis muscle mechanics in children with obstetric brachial plexus palsy. J Hand Surg Eur Vol. 2008;33(4):507–12. https://doi.org/10.1177/1753193408090764.
14. Pöyhiä TH, Nietosvaara YA, Remes VM, Kirjavainen MO, Peltonen JI, Lamminen AE. MRI of rotator cuff muscle atrophy in relation to glenohumeral joint incongruence in brachial plexus birth injury. Pediatr Radiol. 2005;35(4):402–9. https://doi.org/10.1007/s00247-004-1377-3.
15. Waters PM, Monica JT, Earp BE, Zurakowski D, Bae DS. Correlation of radiographic muscle cross-sectional area with glenohumeral deformity in children with brachial plexus birth palsy. J Bone Joint Surg. 2009;91(10):2367–75. https://doi.org/10.2106/JBJS.H.00417.
16. Narakas AO. The treatment of brachial plexus injuries. Int Orthop. 1985;9(1):29–36.
17. Curtis C, Stephens D, Clarke HM, Andrews D. The active movement scale: an evaluative tool for infants with obstetrical brachial plexus palsy. J Hand Surg. 2002;27(3):470–8.
18. Michelow BJ, Clarke HM, Curtis CG, Zuker RM, Seifu Y, Andrews DF. The natural history of obstetrical brachial plexus palsy. *Plast Reconstr Surg*. 1994;93(4):675–80. -discussion 681
19. Mallet J. Obstetrical paralysis of the brachial plexus. II. Therapeutics. Treatment of sequelae. Results of different therapeutic technics and indications. *Rev Chir Orthop Reparatrice Appar Mot*. 1972;58(Suppl 1):192–6.
20. Vathana T, Rust S, Mills J, et al. Intraobserver and interobserver reliability of two ultrasound measures of humeral head position in infants with neonatal brachial plexus palsy. J Bone Joint Surg Am. 2007;89(8):1710–5. https://doi.org/10.2106/JBJS.F.01263.
21. Zhang S, Ezaki M. Sonography as a preferred diagnostic tool to assess shoulder displacement in brachial plexus palsy. J Diagn Medica Sonography. 2008;24(6):339–43. https://doi.org/10.1177/8756479308326087.
22. Bauer AS, Anderson R, Lucas JF, Heyrani N, Kalish LA, James MA. Ultrasound screening for posterior shoulder dislocation in infants with brachial plexus birth palsy. J Hand Surg. 2016;41(9):S34–5. https://doi.org/10.1016/j.jhsa.2016.07.064.
23. Donohue KW, Little KJ, Gaughan JP, Kozin SH, Norton BD, Zlotolow DA. Comparison of ultrasound and MRI for the diagnosis of Glenohumeral dysplasia in brachial plexus birth palsy. J Bone Joint Surg Am. 2017;99(2):123–32. https://doi.org/10.2106/JBJS.15.01116.
24. Verchere C, Durlacher K, Bellows D, Pike J, Bucevska M. An early shoulder repositioning program in birth-related brachial plexus injury: a pilot study of the sup-ER protocol. Hand (NY). 2014;9(2):187–95. https://doi.org/10.1007/s11552-014-9625-y.
25. Little KJ, Little KJ, Zlotolow DA, et al. Early functional recovery of elbow flexion and supination following median and/or ulnar nerve fascicle transfer in upper neonatal brachial plexus palsy. J Bone Joint Surg Am. 2014;96(3):215–21. https://doi.org/10.2106/JBJS.L.01405.

26. Tse R, Marcus JR, Curtis CG, Dupuis A, Clarke HM. Suprascapular nerve reconstruction in obstetrical brachial plexus palsy: spinal accessory nerve transfer versus C5 root grafting. Plast Reconstr Surg. 2011;127(6):2391–6. https://doi.org/10.1097/PRS.0b013e3182131c7c.
27. Ezaki M, Malungpaishrope K, Harrison RJ, et al. Onabotulinum toxinA injection as an adjunct in the treatment of posterior shoulder subluxation in neonatal brachial plexus palsy. J Bone Joint Surg. 2010;92(12):2171–7. https://doi.org/10.2106/JBJS.I.00499.
28. Waters PM, Bae DS. Effect of tendon transfers and extra-articular soft-tissue balancing on glenohumeral development in brachial plexus birth palsy. J Bone Joint Surg Am. 2005;87(2):320–5. https://doi.org/10.2106/JBJS.C.01614.
29. Pearl ML, Edgerton BW, Kazimiroff PA, Burchette RJ, Wong K. Arthroscopic release and latissimus Dorsi transfer for shoulder internal rotation contractures and Glenohumeral deformity secondary to brachial plexus birth palsy. J Bone Joint Surg. 2006;88(3):564–74. https://doi.org/10.2106/JBJS.D.02872.
30. Dodwell E, O'Callaghan J, Anthony A, et al. Combined glenoid anteversion osteotomy and tendon transfers for brachial plexus birth palsy early outcomes. J Bone Joint Surg Am. 2012;94(23):2145–52. https://doi.org/10.2106/JBJS.K.01256.
31. Di Mascio L, Chin K-F, Fox M, Sinisi M. Glenoplasty for complex shoulder subluxation and dislocation in children with obstetric brachial plexus palsy. J Bone Joint Surg Br. 2011;93(1):102–7. https://doi.org/10.1302/0301-620X.93B1.25051.
32. Waters PM, Bae DS. The effect of derotational humeral osteotomy on global shoulder function in brachial plexus birth palsy. J Bone Joint Surg Am. 2006;88(5):1035–42. https://doi.org/10.2106/JBJS.E.00680.
33. Statland J, Tawil R. Facioscapulohumeral muscular dystrophy. Neurol Clin. 2014;32(3):721–8–ix. https://doi.org/10.1016/j.ncl.2014.04.003.
34. Lemmers RJLF, Tawil R, Petek LM, et al. Digenic inheritance of an SMCHD1 mutation and an FSHD-permissive D4Z4 allele causes facioscapulohumeral muscular dystrophy type 2. Nat Genet. 2012;44(12):1370–4. https://doi.org/10.1038/ng.2454.
35. Jensen MP, Hoffman AJ, Stoelb BL, Abresch RT, Carter GT, McDonald CM. Chronic pain in persons with myotonic dystrophy and facioscapulohumeral dystrophy. Arch Phys Med Rehabil. 2008;89(2):320–8. https://doi.org/10.1016/j.apmr.2007.08.153.
36. Diab M, Darras BT, Shapiro F. Scapulothoracic fusion for facioscapulohumeral muscular dystrophy. J Bone Joint Surg Am. 2005;87(10):2267–75.
37. Goel DP, Romanowski JR, Shi LL, Warner JJP. Scapulothoracic fusion: outcomes and complications. J Shoulder Elb Surg. 2014;23(4):542–7. https://doi.org/10.1016/j.jse.2013.08.009.
38. Twyman RS, Harper GD, Edgar MA. Thoracoscapular fusion in facioscapulohumeral dystrophy: clinical review of a new surgical method. J Shoulder Elb Surg. 1996;5(3):201–5.
39. Cooney AD, Gill I, Stuart PR. The outcome of scapulothoracic arthrodesis using cerclage wires, plates, and allograft for facioscapulohumeral dystrophy. J Shoulder Elb Surg. 2014;23(1):e8–e13. https://doi.org/10.1016/j.jse.2013.04.012.
40. Domzalski M, Inan M, Littleton AG, Miller F. Pectoralis major release to improve shoulder abduction in children with cerebral palsy. J Pediatr Orthop. 2007;27(4):457–61. https://doi.org/10.1097/01.bpb.0000271320.10869.d1.
41. Bamshad M. Arthrogryposis: A Review and Update. *J Bone Joint Surg Am*. 2009;91(Suppl 4):40. https://doi.org/10.2106/JBJS.I.00281.
42. Ezaki M. Treatment of the upper limb in the child with arthrogryposis. Hand Clin. 2000;16(4):703–11.

Paediatric Shoulder Instability

30

Mattthew F. Nixon and Allen Stevenson

Anatomy and Basic Science

Physis

The proximal physis of the humerus produces 80% of longitudinal growth by endochondral ossification at its metaphyseal diaphyseal junction. Its blood supply via the physeal vessels allows the removal of chondrocyte degenerate, the mineralisation of the cartilage matrix and transport of osteoblasts. The end result being the formation of lamellar bone [1]. The physis is undulating and the medially aspect lies within the reflection of the joint capsule and thus is classed as intraarticular at this point. As a result, osteomyelitis can progress to septic arthritis and vice versa. The proximal humeral physis closes between 14–17 years in girls and 16–18 years in boys (Tanner Whitehouse). It also changes shape from a gentle arch to a pyramid shape from infancy to maturity [2].

The physis becomes weaker as growth velocity increases particularly just prior to puberty. Thus they are more prone to injury at this time. Various mechanisms such as traction, direct impact, pathological process (cyst, tumour, infection) and repetitive stress.

M. F. Nixon (✉) · A. Stevenson
Department of Orthopaedic Surgery,
Royal Manchester Children's Hospital, Manchester, UK
e-mail: matthew.nixon@nhs.net;
rastevenson@doctors.org.u

Skeletal Maturity

The shoulder girdles' final stages of post-natal development involve the coalescence of multiple secondary ossification centres within the scapula, humerus and clavicle. The humeral head ossification centre is the first radiologically visible centre appearing at 6 months. The greater tuberosity then appears at 1–3 years and the lesser tuberosity at 4–5 years. The coalescence of the tuberosities occurs between 6–7 years [3, 4]. These studies however are based on x-ray and cadaveric studies. Variation in development rates and the presence of multiple ossification centres in each of the constituent parts of the shoulder girdle can therefore make radiological interpretation challenging [5].

More recently the development of the proximal humerus has been described in terms of MRI appearance [2]. These studies have not shown any significant difference in the pattern or timing of development but do offer a "road map" to differentiate between normal development and pathology.

Ossification of the scapula can be divided into the body (1 ossification centre which appears at 8 weeks in utero), medial and inferior borders (each having 1 ossification centre which appears at 14–20 years), coracoid (has 2 ossification centres which appear at 12–18 months), acromium (3 ossification centres appear at 14–20 years) and glenoid (has 4 ossification centres which appear

I. A. Trail et al. (eds.), *Textbook of Shoulder Surgery*, https://doi.org/10.1007/978-3-319-70099-1_30

at 10–11 years). The most clinically important of these are (1) the glenoid which appears at approximately 10 years old and can in the presence of an injury appear to be a Bony Bankart lesion, (2) the acromion which appears at 14–20 years and may resemble a fracture.

The skeletally immature only make up 1–5% of all glenohumeral dislocations [6–10]. A systematic reviews have shown the rate of recurrent instability after glenohumeral dislocation is highest in skeletally mature adolescents (92–95%) compared to skeletally immature adolescents (44–66%) [11, 12].

Healing Potential and Relative Weakness

It is well known that the healing potential in children is greater than in the adult population however the extent of difference of this effect in regard to shoulder pathology in children is not evident in the published literature. There are examples of conditions such as osteochondritis, in which a skeletally immature patient has a significantly better outcome than those of the adult population. It is difficult to extrapolate this to shoulder instability but a factor that should always be considered when developing new treatments.

The presence of the physis in the proximal humerus results in an area of lower tensile strength. Biomechanics testing has shown that that Young's modulus of elasticity of the physis is as much as ten times smaller than that of cortical bone. Fractures of the proximal humerus in the adolescent are therefore significantly more common than dislocations. Age and anatomical position within the physis have also been shown to influence Young's modulus. Some cadaveric studies have shown that the tensile side of the physis is up to 40% stiffer than the compressive side. The ultimate tensile strength and tangential strength has been shown to be same across the physis. It is important to adapt reduction techniques in children to avoid excessive applied force through the physis due to the increased risk of Salter Harris type fractures. Recommended reduction techniques employ gradual sustained inline traction and avoid rotation of the shoulder to reduce the risk of fracture.

The joint capsule attaches to a more lateral position on the glenoid in younger children. This relationship is not fully understood in regard to its effect on the dislocation rate but may be an important factor, as younger children are more likely to sustain a capsular rupture than an avulsion injury.

Classification

As in adults, shoulder instability in children is usually classified according to the Stanmore triangle in one of three ways, with room for overlap. The three categories of instability are I – traumatic, II – atraumatic structural and III – muscle patterning/non-structural. In addition, there are a number of developmental causes of shoulder instability, usually neuromuscular in origin that are unique to children that do not fit into this system, which we classify as type 4 instability. A patient can sit anywhere within the triangle and fall into one, two or three categories. It is therefore necessary that each patient is assessed and managed individually (Fig. 30.1).

Normally the cause of a type I injury would be caused by an external insult to the shoulder such as a fall, playing contact sports or collision with another object e.g. road traffic collision

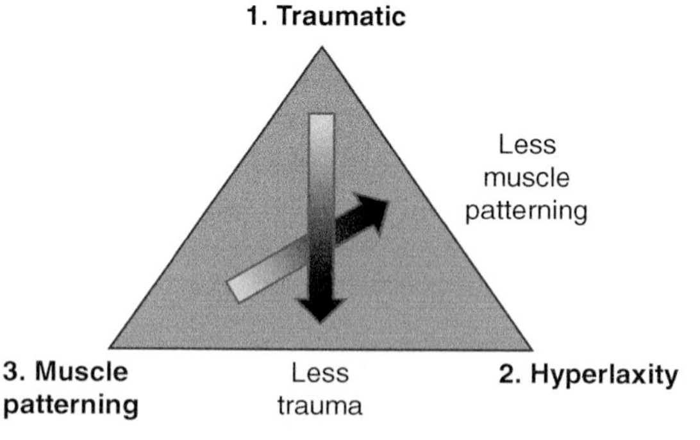

Fig. 30.1 The stanmore triangle of shoulder instability

(RTC) and the impactive force through which seatbelts posteriorly drive the shoulder girdle. This leads to a higher incidence of male: female type I shoulder instability, this type of instability comes with a high risk of damage to the surrounding labrum, cartilage and musculature. This would require diagnostic imaging to confirm a tear, surgery and then physiotherapeutic rehabilitation [13].

Type II shoulder instability would account for someone with a high degree of hyperlaxity, scoring >5/9 on the Beighton Score, or someone who has a known connective tissue disorder such as Marfan's. The risk is higher in females than males in this case and treatment is via diagnostic imaging to check for joint congruency and then either surgery to tighten the joint capsule or just physiotherapy for example core control and rotator cuff strengthening as well as proprioceptive retraining [14].

Type III shoulder instability accounts for those that have generalised muscle weakness and carries an equal weighting of 50% to male and female predisposition, either due to deconditioning or global muscle weakness. Physiotherapy is the core management for this type of instability, occasionally supplemented with botulinium toxin to temporarily break a dominant muscle patterning problem. This is backed up by [15] who state that approximately 50% of unstable shoulders can be treated solely with physiotherapy, therefore by utilising the multi-disciplinary team to its fullest and triaging of the patients effectively can lead to early intervention by the correct teams.

Type IV instability is due to an external neuromuscular disorder causing an imbalance of forces around the shoulder. These disorders may be due to upper motor neurone problems (such as cerebral palsy, lower motor neurone (such as brachial plexus injuries), both of which typically cause an adduction and internal rotation contracture leading to posterior shoulder dislocation, and muscular dystrophies (such as FSHD), which principally effect the scapulothoracic joint.

Epidemiology

In a study evaluating the aetiology of 100 consecutive paediatric instability patients, 9% had polar type 1 instability (a further 19% had mixed pattern but including type 1), 2% had polar type 2 instability (with a further 23% having mixed pattern type 2), 22% had polar type 3 (with a further 25% having mixed pattern type 3) and 33% being type 4, neuromuscular origin.

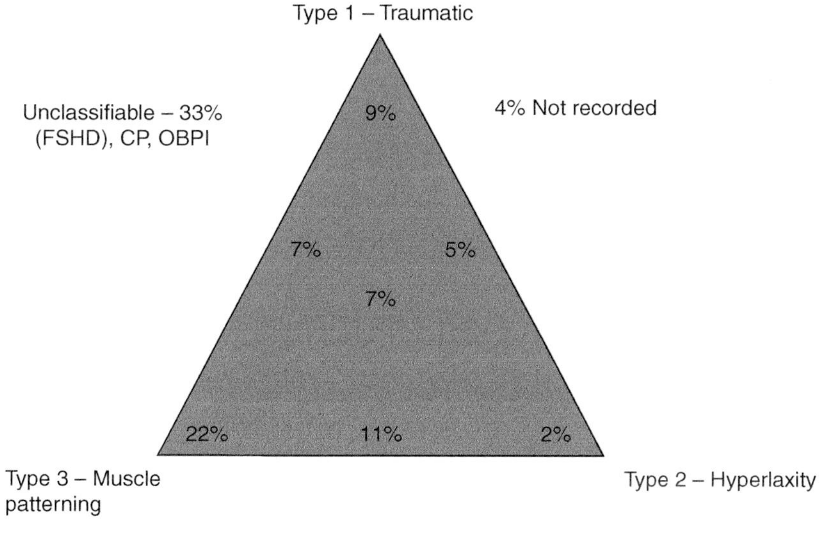

Type 1 instability is more common in boys, type 2 in girls, and types 3 and 4 roughly equally distributed between sexes

Assessment

Presentation

Acute traumatic instability presents in a similar fashion to adults and may require manipulation under sedation/anaesthesia to successfully reduce. Atraumatic instability (due to hyperlaxity or muscle patterning problems) may also present with an acute painful subluxation which may be difficult to reduce to maintain reduction. This may become chronic in nature requiring multiple hospital visits and multiple 'failed' manipulations. This can lead to prolonged time being spent in hospital and lead to secondary psychosocial problems. In alternative scenarios primary psychosocial problems can lead to somatisation of their symptoms and repeated hospital presentations of painful subluxation may be the presenting feature. Atraumatic instability may also present with secondary adaptive problems such as scapula winging, a snapping scapula or non-specific pain. Developmental neuromuscular instability presents with painful or painless stiffness in the joint with secondary adaptive mechanism to maintain a functional range of movement (for example in FSHD swing movements enable shoulder abduction, and in brachial plexus injuries, hyper mobility of the scapulothoracic joint compensate for contractures and stiffness in the glenohumeral joint). These often present with winging of the scapula and movement within an abnormal arc. As the majority cases of paediatric shoulder instability are due to multiple pathologies, understanding the aetiology and performing a systematic assessment is vital for proper management.

Assessment

A careful, systematic assessment is needed to determine the aetiology of paediatric shoulder instability. As the majority of cases of paediatric instability are multi-factorial, each aetiology of instability needs to be assessed and managed accordingly, as summarised in Table 30.1.

Traumatic Instability

Epidemiology

Polar Type 1 (structural) instabilitycan be acute, persistent or recurrent. It is secondary to trauma to the capsulolabral structures of a previously

Table 30.1 Clinical signs and symptoms of shoulder instability

	Traumatic	Hyperlaxity	Muscle patterning	Other
History	History of contact sport	History of bruising/bleeding disorder Mitral valve pathology Known connective tissue disorder	Pain or clicking in the shoulder Sport related specific muscle group over conditioning	Brachial plexus injury Cerebral palsy Family history of muscular dystrophy (such as FSHD)
Examination	Signs of structural pathology (anterior/ posterior labral tears, SLAP or LHB lesion)	Beighton score 5–9 Skin hyperlaxity Stretch marks Ghent criteria for Marfans	Core instability Scapula winging Infra-spinatous lag/ weakness Snapping scapula Spasm or over activity of one muscle group	Systemic features of neuromuscular problems (spasticity, facial weakness) Fixed or dynamic shoulder instability
Investigations	Radiographs MRI Arthroscopic findings	Referral to rheumatology for assessment. Genetic testing	Neurophysiology	Neurophysiology Muscle biopsy Genetic testing

normal glenohumeral joint. The paediatric population is susceptible to the same pattern of injury as in adults, however in the skeletally immature, avulsion injuries are possible. There is a distinct division in the literature between those who have reached skeletal maturity and those that have not. This occurs earlier in females than males, however the published articles have reached consensus on 14 years of age as a cut off for maturity. This also happens to be the average age of presentation for paediatric patients with instability.

Polar type 1: is more common in the adolescent than the paediatric population due to factors related to skeletal maturity.

Overall dislocation rate in paediatric/adolescent population:

- 4.7% rate in skeletally immature [16]
- 20% of dislocations occur between the age of 10–20 years of age [10]
- 2% in those under 10 years old

Distribution of shoulder dislocation by type

- Polar type 1: 13%
- Polar type 1 with mixed pattern: 9%

Pathology

Bankart's Lesion: Soft Tissue

Bankart's lesions make up 90% of the pathology in the adult anterior traumatic glenohumeral dislocation population. In the paediatric/adolescent cases, Nixon et al. showed a differing distribution of pathology. Anterior labral injuries of various types were present in only 61% of cases with 16% having posterior labral injury, 16% had SLAP lesion and the remaining 7% suffering from other pathology.

Perthes' Lesion

This is a tear to the anterior inferior labrum, whilst remaining attached to the periosteum of the anterior glenoid. It may remain in an anatomical position but it has become de-functioned and no longer offers stability to the IGHL. This results in ongoing instability and may be difficult to diagnosis on MRI and arthroscopy due to fibrosis.

Anterior Labroligamentous Periosteal Sleeve Avulsion (ALPSA) Lesion

The capsulolabral complex is avulsed from the glenoid on a periosteal sleeve. This lesion has a higher healing potential than a soft tissue Bankart lesion but may heal in a displaced position leading to medial displacement and inferior translation of the inferior glenohumeral ligament (IGHL). Thus, resulting in ongoing instability.

Humeral Avulsion of the Glenohumeral Ligament (HAGL) Lesion

More common in young males playing contact sports. Found to be a risk factor for recurrent dislocations in adolescents treated conservatively [17].

Treatment

Outcomes of Non-Operative Treatment

In the skeletally immature (<14 years old) the current standard treatment is non-operative. However, the evidence is of low quantity and quality with significant heterogeneity. Conservative treatment consists of immobilsation and analgesia with a course of physiotherapy. In those Ochs et al. [8] studied, in which acute traumatic anterior glenohumeral dislocation was treated conservatively in a population of 32 patients with an average age of 14.5 years, it was found that the recurrence rate was 92%, other studies have found that the recurrence rate in this group ranges from 75–100% [7, 10, 16, 17, 18] although there was variation in the age grouping between the studies. There is an unacceptably high re-dislocation rate in those treated conservatively that are ≥14 years old but in the patient population <14 years old the same conclusions cannot be drawn from the current literature. Hence conservative treatment has become popular. There is one article on surgery in this age group by Kraus et al. [19] who performed arthroscopic Bankart's repair on 5 first time dislocators with an average age of 11 years old, with a 0% re-dislocation at 2 years. Further research is required to clarify the optimal treatment strategies for the <14 years old patients.

The HAGL lesion has been suggested as a risk factor for recurrent dislocation in the primary conservative group. This was shown in a conservatively managed group in which 3/14 patients treated conservatively developed recurrent dislocations and all 3 where found to have a HAGL lesion [20].

Outcomes of Surgery

The most common primary outcome measure in the published literature on operative treatment for paediatric traumatic shoulder dislocation is re-dislocation. Return to sport is the major secondary outcome measure of interest. Arthroscopic capsulolabral repair is the most frequently performed surgery in recent articles however, there are some earlier studies in which the Laterjet procedure was the surgical treatment of choice. No common outcome measurement tool has been employed in these retrospective case control studies. As yet there is no randomised control trials and currently there is no core outcome set for paediatric shoulder instability.

When reviewing the literature, the age groupings for the studies varies. In general, the recurrence rate after arthroscopic capsulolabral repair is significantly lower than conservative treatment on patients between 13–18 years old. Lampert et al. [22] and Gigis et al. [23] have concluded that for those over 14 years old the re-dislocation rate after conservative management is unacceptably high and advocate primary arthroscopic stabilisation (Tables 30.2 and 30.3).

Review Summary of Literature on Management

Zaremski et al. [24] performed a meta-analysis of the literature and found that in the >14 years old paediatric population, that the rate of re-dislocation after a primary dislocation treated conservatively was 72.3%, the rate of re-dislocation of primary dislocators treated with surgery was 13.2% and re-dislocation was 22.3% for those who failed conservative treatment and later underwent surgical stabilisation [22]. This was based on small numbers (54 patients) due to the failure of many studies to meet the inclusion criteria for meta-analysis. The highest rate of re-dislocation after arthroscopic stabilisation has been found to be in those taking part in sports involving overhead activity (water polo, 40%) or contact (rugby 33.3%) [24].

Longo et al. also performed a systematic review and a quantitative synthesis of the literature in 2016 in patients less than 18 years of age [25]. Due to the poor research quality of the available literature 85% of articles failed to reach the inclusion criteria. However, 705 shoulders where included in their article (only 21 of which were in an isolated group of skeletally immature patients). They reported that of those treated conservatively for primary traumatic shoulder dislocation the re-dislocation rate was 71.3% and in the surgically treated category the re-dislocation rate was 17.5% (p-value <0.00001). The quantitative synthesis showed very low heterogenicity between the studies meaning that almost all the studies reported consistently. Due to the overlap of age groups and the low numbers in the isolated under 14 years old group, they were unable to draw conclusions on the skeletally immature but surgery clearly showed a lower re-dislocation rate in the under 18 years old population.

Re-Dislocation Rate After Surgical Repair

There is limited literature related to recurrence in the paediatric population post arthroscopic Bankart's repair. However, in the adult population, a meta-analysis of outcomes of arthroscopic Bankart's repair in 1781 adult patients showed recurrent instability of around 11% at 11 years [26], and 28% at 17 years [27]. Several studies have shown a significantly higher re-dislocation rate in the paediatric population (15% in the first year, 31% over 3 years and 21% at 63 months [25]. This higher rate is similar to recurrence rates reported in other high-risk groups (8–21% in army recruits or young adult athletes), [28–31].

It is difficult to draw firm conclusions from the small published series, but it is hypothesised that the two reasons for the high recurrent dislocation rate are generalized adolescent joint hyperlaxity and a desire to return to high-level contact sports.

Treatment should be tailored to match each patient's pathology and desire to return to contact sports. Hyperlaxity and capsular tears should be assessed in all patients and, where present, a cap-

Table 30.2 Recurrence rate after surgical treatment for paediatric traumatic shoulder dislocation

Article (year)	Surgical intervention	Average age (years)	Recurrence rate after surgery (%)	Recurrence rate after conservative treatment	Population (n)	Follow up (years)
Lampert et al. [22]	ABR and OBR	14.5	14.3	96	2 surgery 27 Gilchrist Bandage	1
Jones et al. [62]	ABR	15	12.5	100	2 surgery 14 sling	2
Kraus et al. [19]	ABR	11	0	n/a	5 Surgery	2
Castagna et al. [26]	ABR	16	21.5	n/a	65	5.2
Gigis et al. [23]	ABR	16.7	13.2	70.4	65	3
Khan et al. [34]	Open Latarjet	14.1 operative 13.7 non-operative	2	56	28 surgery 25 sling	9.7 8.3
Shymon et al. [63]	ABR vs OBR	16.5	ABR 24 OBR 14	n/a	ABR 71 OBR 28	2.4 5.5
Nixon et al. [4]	ABR	16.8	26	n/a	61	1.8

Modified from Longo et al. [25]

Table 30.3 Conservatively management of traumatic paediatric shoulder instability outcomes

Article (year)	intervention	Average age (years)	Recurrence rate after conservative treatment (%)	Population (n)	Follow up (years)
Postachini et al. [64]	Sling 4 weeks	15.5	92 (>14 years) 33 (<14 years)	25 3	7.1
Roberts et al. [65]	1 week sling	16.3	76.7	133	3.125

sular shift shoulder be performed as a part of the labral repair [32]. Ahmed et al. [32] routinely performed a capsular shift and had a lower recurrence rate.

Glenoid and humeral bone stock should be routinely assessed preoperatively using cross-sectional imaging. In cases of purely soft-tissue injury, we would advocate an arthroscopic Bankart's repair, but counsel the patient about the higher than reported rate of recurrence, particularly if they return to contact sports. In cases of significant glenoid or humeral erosions (bony glenoid defect or engaging Hill–Sachs lesion), we would consider performing a Latarjet coracoid transfer procedure. As this is a more robust stabilization, it may also be a reasonable primary procedure in patients keen to return to contact sports in the absence of bony erosions. Long-term studies suggest that the Latarjet procedure has a lower rate of recurrent dislocation than arthroscopic stabilization in the adult populations (13 vs. 28%, $P = 0.02$) [33] and one study in the paediatric population showed a lower re-dislocation rate of 2% (n = 28) with an average of 14.1 years [34]. This procedure is also effective as a salvage procedure after failed arthroscopic stabilization [35].

Conclusion: Traumatic Instability

From the literature, we can say that a skeletally mature paediatric patient with a first-time traumatic dislocation needs a focused clinical history and examination for signs and symptoms of hyperlaxity, in conjunction with an MRI scan to identify intraarticular injury. Surgery should be offered if surgically amenable lesions are identified owing to the significantly lower re-dislocation rates reported by meta-analysis. Due to the lack of published literature in the skeletally immature patients firm conclusions cannot be drawn.

Atraumatic Hyperlaxity Instability

Epidemiology

Generalised joint laxity is normal in paediatric population, however polar type 2 instability is relatively uncommon type in the paediatric population. It more commonly presents as a mixed pattern with type 3 muscle patterning or type 1 traumatic instability. There are associated co-morbidities and the risk of life threatening complication from surgery with some of the causes of joint hypermobility that any surgeon planning to treat these patients surgically need to appreciate, and also be aware that shoulder or other joint instability may be the presenting symptom of these conditions.

It has been reported that between 4.6–27.5% of children are hypermobile (dependant on the cut off threshold, previously a Beighton score >4 was used and resulted in the upper range prevalence of 27.5% but more recently this has been changed to a score of >6 = 4.6%). Joint pain in the absence of pathological findings is often attributed to hypermobility related joint pain. There is a significantly higher prevalence in females (5.4F:1M) and those not of Caucasian ethnicity [36]. Tobias' study looked at hyper mobility as a predictor of subsequent joint pain in 2901 paediatric participants in the ALSPAC cohort. There was a 4.6% prevalence of hypermobility at an average age of 13.8 years with moderately troublesome shoulder pain reported in 9.5% of these participants with an odds ratio of 1.68 [95% confidence interval1.04, 2.72] when measured at 4 year follow up. Hypermobility defined as a Beighton score >6 is therefore a risk factor for shoulder pain in adolescences. It is also a risk factor for recurrent dislocation in adults [37] but there is little in the literature regarding its effect on the prevalence on shoulder instability in the paediatric population.

Pathology

Connective tissue changes its characteristics as children reach skeletal maturity. These are thought to be some of reasons for the lower risk of recurrent dislocations in the skeletally immature paediatric population. The ratio of type 3 to type 1 collagen is higher in those <18 years old. Type 3 collagen is soluble and subtler, whereas type 1 collagen is insoluble and forms cross links as a result it is tougher and less flexible. Type 3 collagen production slows with age and type 2 collagen replaces it. This conversion happens at a predictable rate and patients can be chronological aged by this from collagen analysis via a skin biopsy. A recent study has shown the diameter of fibrillin in the collagen of patients with recurrent shoulder instability is smaller than the control group. As yet its significance requires further research to quantify.

General Approach to Management of Shoulder Instability in Hyperlaxity

Patients with hyperlaxity associated with a traumatic lesion should be approached in the same fashion as those patients with instability and no history of hyperlaxity. Arthroscopic stabilisation appropriate to the lesion and direction of instability. The Latarjet procedure has been shown to have long-term results in the presence of a glenoid rim defect [38].

Non-Operative Management

The mainstay of treatment is physiotherapy focusing on dynamic stability and proprioception. Many of these patients will have a reduction of their symptoms at skeletal maturity and prolonged physiotherapy is advised [39]. Outcomes of physiotherapy in this group is good to excellent. Physiotherapy needs to be delivered by a dedicated specialist paediatric physiotherapist with a specialist interest to obtain the best results and should be over a course of at least 1 year.

Operative Management

Indication for surgical intervention in the skeletally immature patient is limited. Surgery should not be considered until prolonged conservative management (at least 1 year) with specialist physiotherapy has failed to improve the patient's shoulder instability. It is advised that each patient prior to surgery has a psychological assessment as surgical outcomes are worse in those with co-commitment emotional or psychological disorders.

Then principle of surgery is to augment the primary stabilisers. This is achieved by direction specific capsular re-tensioning. It is therefore imperative that the direction of instability is accurately identified and the corresponding capsule then tightened. There is little in the literature regarding the surgical management of multidirectional instability in the paediatric population. The principals of treatment are however thought to be the same as that of the skeletally mature.

Open Capsular Shift

Vavken et al. reported a case series of 18 adolescent patients that underwent open capsular shift for recurrent shoulder dislocation on a background of hyperlaxity or Ehlers-Danlos syndrome after failed conservative treatment [39]. They found that 87% had an improvement of symptoms however there was a 47% recurrence of instability rate. The quality of evidence is poor and prone to selection biases thus making robust conclusions difficult to draw. The literature on open capsular shift in the adult population with hyperlaxity is more encouraging with success rates ranging from 80–95% at up to 10 years follow-up [39].

Arthroscopic Capsular Shift

The results of arthroscopic capsular shift are good in the evidence available (level III and IV) in the adult population. However, the only published article on its use in paediatric patients is a case report in which an 10 years old girl with recurrent instability after failed conservative treatment, had good results at 12 months with an arthroscopic capsular shift [41]. It is impossible to draw conclusions from the available literature on the safety and long-term outcomes of performing this procedure in the skeletally immature patient. There is a need for high level research before it's widespread use can be recommended.

Arthroscopic Capsular Plications

Greiwe et al. published a case series on arthroscopic capsular plication in adolescents with voluntary dislocation [42]. With good to excellent outcomes in all 10 patients and no recurrence of instability symptoms at a mean of 31 months. Rolfes et al. performed a systematic review of the eligible adult literature on arthroscopic capsular plication and found 4 studies with short term success rates ranging from 91–100% [43].

Capsular Shrinkage

A systematic review and meta-analysis [43] showed a lower success rate of capsular shrinkage versus arthroscopic plication (76.5% vs 91%) in 8 studies. An earlier review by Johnson et al. in 2010 concluded that arthroscopic capsular shrinkage resulted in unacceptable risk and recurrence in the adult population [39]. No evidence for its use in the paediatric population has been published.

Osteogenesis Imperfecta (OI)

Pathology

This is an inherited condition resulting in the production of abnormal Type 1 collagen. Ninety percent have a mutation of COL 1A1 and COL 1A2 leads to abnormal collagen cross linking and results in production of abnormal collagen and a reduction in collagen secretion. This results in reduced physeal and periosteal osteoid production. There are autosomal dominant milder forms (I & IV) and autosomal recessive severe forms (II & III). Four further types have later been added to the Sillence classification but these do not have type 1 collagen mutations. The mutations are often de novo.

Common Presentations

In milder cases the patient may present with multiple fractures. Olecranon avulsion fracture is a common first presentation and should be investigated further. The frequency of fracture slows with age and normally stops after puberty. In severe cases the fractures may present at birth and may be fatal. With recurrent fractures long bone deformity is common and may result in a Saber shin deformity, bowing and coax vara. Ligamentous laxity is a feature in OI patients and 65% have upper limb hypermobility which may be the only presenting feature in type 1 and 4. Type 1 patients have been shown to have a significantly higher risk of shoulder and elbow dislocation.

Diagnosis

Diagnosis in most cases is by family history, clinical examination along with characteristic radiological findings. Laboratory tests such as ALP are often within normal limits and new tests like urinary deoxypyridinoline are not specific enough. In equivocal cases, other tests including skull radiographs looking for a wormian bone (an extra puzzle piece like bone between the parietal and occipital bone within the lamboidal suture), biopsy of skin for collagen analysis, iliac crest bone biopsy looking for increased remodelling and decreased cancellous bone volume and fibroblast culture to analyse collagen production. DNA analysis for the specific mutation can also be used.

Typical radiographic signs are flaring, cupping and splaying. The reason for cupping is due to hypophospotaemia resulting in reduced apoptosis in the zone of calcification of the physis (Rubin classification: hypoplastic physeal dysplasia).

Systemic Treatment

Bisphosphonates have been shown to reduce pain and fracture rate, improve ambulation, increase cortical diameter and cancellous bone volume. They need to be avoided around time of osteotomies due to increased non-union rate.

Bone marrow transplant has shown approximately a third increase in whole body bone mineral content by 3 months post-transplant in a cohort of 3 patients. Further research is required to evaluate its efficacy.

These treatments do not have any effect on the collagen and therefore reduce the risk of fracture but do not improve the hyperlaxity.

Management of Shoulder Dislocation in OI

- There is no published literature on specific management of dislocations in OI patients, however the rate of fracture dislocation is thought to be higher and reduction should be performed with sustained inline traction and ideally under Image Intensifier control in theatre. Optimal management of recurrent dislocation is unclear.
- Patients with OI have higher risks of surgery as they can develop basal invagination which presents with apnoea, ataxia and myelopathy. This can be in their teenage years and imaging of their cervical spine prior to general anaesthesia is recommended. They also have a higher incidence of malignant hyperthermia, aortic regurgitation and mitral valve prolapse.

Ehlers-Danlos Syndrome

Pathology

Ehlers-Danlos syndrome (EDS) is a group of 11 inherited connective tissue disorders, 4 of which results in ligamentous laxity and hypermobility. Hypermobility type is the most prevalent form with classical type making up 90% of the EDS cases. Currently this is the only type that has no genetic diagnostic test therefore clinical criteria are relied on to diagnosis new cases [44, 45]. Six of the types have been shown to have collagen defects the remaining types have enzyme deficiencies or metabolic disturbances involved with collagen synthesis.

Presentation

The most common presenting Orthopaedic problem is pain and instability of the knee followed by back and shoulder. Stern et al. showed that of the 31.2% of cases presenting with shoulder pain and instability with only 20.3% having suffered a glenohumeral dislocation [46]. The rate of dislocation of any joint in patients with EDS rises with age and has been shown to be as high as 96% in the adult population with EDS. It can also cause gait disturbances and an increased risk of falls. In children, it has negative effects on the child's quality of life, the development of proprioception, muscle strength and psychosocial skills [47].

PROMs have shown that suffers from EDS have lower physical, psychosocial and functional scores than suffers of Rheumatoid Arthritis [48] (Table 30.4).

Diagnosis

Diagnosis of Ehlers Danlos syndrome is made according to the Brighton criteria with any one of the following:

- 2 MAJOR criteria
- 1 MAJOR and 2 minor criteria
- 4 minor criteria
- 2 minor criteria and a first degree relative with the diagnosis.

MAJOR	Beighton score of >4 Arthralgia for longer than 3 months in 4 or more joint
Minor	Beighton score 1–3 Arthralgia >3 months in 1–3 joints or back pain. Spondylosis, spondylolysis/ spondylolisthesis Dislocation/subluxation in more than one joint or in one joint in multiple occasions. Marfanoid habituds Skin striae, hyperextensibility, abnormal scarring Occular signs Hernia, uterine/rectal prolapse. Mitral valve prolapse

Brighton criteria for Ehlers Danlos syndrome diagnosis

Table 30.4 Described the various types of Ehlers-Danlos syndrome (Villefrance 1997). Identifying and typing the syndrome is particularly necessary if planning surgical intervention

Classical (90%)	Skin hyperextensibility, atrophic scarring, hypermobility and higher surgical complications. Type V procollagen is affected, AD inheritence. COL5 A1 & COL5 A2 mutation.
Others	Hypermobility, vascular, Arthrochalasia, Kyphoscoliotic, Dermatosparaxis Dermatosparaxis Associations with skin fragility, arterial and intestinal rupture, hip dislocation, muscle hypotonia.

Management

Treatment of Underlying Disorder

There are no widely accepted treatments for any of the types of Ehlers-Danlos. Prolotherapy and vitamin C supplements have been tried but with no good evidence of their benefits and there is no standard treatment for the underlying conditions.

General advice is to avoid contact sports and manual jobs, maintain fitness and muscle mass, physiotherapy to maintain range of movement and muscle patterning and genetic counselling. Joint dislocations should be reduced promptly to avoid complications. Splints and orthotics may help in certain joint dislocations.

There are no RCTs on the pain management of EDS patients and their needs may be complex and require specialist pain team input.

Relevance to Shoulder Instability

There is evidence that paediatric patients suffering from Ehlers-Danlos have a 31.2% prevalence of shoulder instability [46] with 20.3% of these patients suffering dislocation of the glenohumeral joint. These figures are not as high as conventional teaching suggests. Physiotherapy should be the main stay of treatment in these patients, with few requiring surgery. Inferior capsular shift has been shown to decrease pain and increase stability and function [40, 49] and open inferior capsular shift remains the gold standard for recurrent shoulder instability that has failed. Care should be taken if surgery is planned to be performed in those suffering from vascular type. Impaired wound healing in a feature of all types of ED syndrome due to fibroblast defects etc. conservative treatment. There is a lack of literature on the treatment of this population and they should be treated as those with hyperlaxity taking into account the risks mentions.

Marfan's Syndrome

Pathology

Marfan's syndrome is a autosomal dominant connective tissue disorder in which fibrillin production is abnormal with a 30% sporadic mutation rate of the FBN1 gene.

Fibrillin is a glycoprotein excreted by fibroblasts that polymer chains which forms the insoluble scaffold of elastin in the form of a microfibril. Fibrillin microfibrils within elastin is integral in maintaining the integrity of the extracellular matrix and connective tissues. It imparts important structural properties to vessel walls, lungs, ligaments, cartilage, the bladder and the extracellular matrix. Dysfunction of the microfibrils leads to the loss of elastin ability to resist repetitive stress and thus leads to increase strain of the connective tissue.

The most common initial Orthopaedic manifestation in Marfan's syndrome is scoliosis followed by ligament laxity resulting in sprains of the ankle. Shoulder instability is more common in patients with Marfan's syndrome. As their height is beneficial in sports that requires overhead activity such as basketball and volleyball, this subgroup have a significantly higher risk of instability. Albeit most patients are asymptomatic with characteristic appearance. These include long thin limbs (dolichtostenomelia), long thin digits (arachnodactyly) and a large arm span. The condition has association with: dural ectasia, superior lens dislocation, scoliosis, pertrusio acetabuli, res planus, ligamentous laxity and shoulder, finger and patella dislocation.

Diagnosis

Walker's test:	thumb and index finger overlap when grasping the contralateral wrist.
Steinberg's test:	tip of the thumb extends beyond the little finger when adducted across the palm and enclosed in a closed fist.

- Classification
  - In 2010 Ghent revised his original criteria from 1996:

Points for systemic score:	
Wrist AND thumb sign	3 points (wrist OR thumb sign = 1 point)
Pectus carinatum deformity	2 points (pectus excavatum or chest asymmetry = 1 point)
Hindfoot deformity	2 points (plain pes planes = 1 point)
Dural ectasia	2 points
Protrusio acetabuli	2 points
Pneumothorax	2 points
Reduced upper segment/lower segment ratio AND increased arm/height AND no severe scoliosis	1 point
Scoliosis or thoracolumbar kyphosis	1 point
Reduced elbow extension = 1	1 point
Facial features (3/5) (dolichocephaly, enophthalmos, downslanting palpebral fissures, malar hypoplasia, retrognathia)	1 point
Skin striae (stretch marks) = 1	1 point
Myopia >3 diopters	1 point
Mitral valve prolapse 1/4	1 point

Diagnostic of scores	
In the absence of a family history of MFS:	
	Aortic root USS Z-score ≥2 AND ectopia lentis
	Aortic root USS Z-score ≥2 AND an FBN1 mutation
	Aortic root USS Z-score ≥2 AND a systemic score of >7 points
	Ectopia lentis AND an FBN1 mutation with known aortic pathology
In the presence of a family history of MFS (as defined above):	
	Ectopia lentis
	Systemic score of ≥7
	Aortic root USS Z-score ≥2

Treatment

Shoulder

Physiotherapy and activity modification are the main stay of treatment for instability. Acute dislocations should be reduced promptly. The use of Entonox is contraindicated due to the risk of spontaneous pneumothorax. In children, the use of IV ketamine is an excellent means of conscious sedation.

There is one case report on recurrent dislocation in patients with Marfan's syndrome treated surgically with arthroscopic inferior capsular shift. A common finding in arthroscopy of the Marfanoid shoulder with recurrent instability was a grossly abnormal capsule in the mid anterior aspect [50, 51]. The posterior surface of subscapularis muscle was clearly visible and the capsule had migrated inferiorly. The outcome of arthroscopic capsular shift in this patient was excellent with no instability at 18 months and a good range of movement.

Any patient in which Marfan's syndrome is suspected an Echo should be obtained to screen for aortic dilation prior to considering surgery.

Conclusion: Atraumatic Hyperlaxity Instability

Surgery should only be considered in a symptomatic patient after failure of a compliant yearlong specialist physiotherapy program. There is insufficient literature to draw firm conclusions on the type of surgery but a pragmatic approach is required. Arthroscopic capsular plication or shift reports the best outcomes from the very limited literature. One should be aware and exclude potentially life-threatening co-morbidities associated with systemic connective tissue disorders prior to surgery.

Muscle Patterning Instability

Introduction

Muscle patterning instability is secondary to a disorganisation in the normal sequential recruitment of the muscles around the shoulder girdle in active movement. This results in a mixed pattern of abnormal over and under contraction of both the large scapulothoracic muscle groups combined with the suppression of the rotator cuff. The pathophysiology is unclear but certain features are seen. These include capsular dysfunction with no evidence of structural damage, no history of trauma and cases are often bilateral. The abnormal patterning is assumed to be the same in the adult population as the paediatric and in special adult shoulder clinics the incidence of type III instability is approximately 45% [52] in the paediatric equivalent clinics, type III instability has been shown to be the most common type making up 22% of instability cases and 18% of the mixed type cases.

Pathology

EMG studies have demonstrated that in type 3 the cuff is unable to be selectively recruited due to weakness in core stability which then leads to aberrant contractions of the larger shoulder girdle muscles such as the deltoid and latisimus dorsi [53]. Recent EEG studies have shown increased cortical activity in those with type 3 instability. Whether this is a cause or effect and the significance is unknown.

Presentation

Scapulothoracic Dyskinesis

The scapulothoarcic joint is formed by the anterior surface of the scapula and the posterior rib cage. Normal alignment and function is essential for the optimal function of the shoulder joint. Scapular dyskinesis is a general term for abnormal scapular positioning during shoulder movement. There are many causes and they are not specific to glenohumeral instability. The causes can be driven by the acromioclavicular or glenohumeral joints, dysplasia of the skeletal structures (such as clavicle fracture malunion), neurological causes (e.g. Cervical radiculopathy, long thoracic nerve injury) or painful conditions such as glenohumeral instability.

The most common result of scapular dyskinesis is passive or dynamic protraction of the scapula, resulting in suboptimal shoulder function.

Scapular Winging

The scapula can translate as well as rotate at the scapulothoracic joint. As the shoulder is abducted the centre of rotation of the scapula moves. From its resting position the upper and lower trapezius and serratus anterior muscles are the initiators of rotation. The centre of rotation moves as the scapula rotates and the scapulothoracic joint allows rotation and translation.

If there is weakness in the either of these two major rotators, mal-positioning of the scapulothoracic joint may result, presenting clinically as winging. There are two types of winging related to the position of the medial scapular border and the muscle group involved.

Weakness of the serratus anterior muscle results in an increased distance between the inframedial border of the scapula and the thorax and medial winging. The upper and lower trapezius still exerts medial translation and rotation to the scapulothoracic joint but the serratus anterior is unable to hold the scapula against the posterior rib cage. When there is weakness of the trapezius the superior border of the scapula no longer has a medialising force and thus it translates laterally and inferiorly. The scapular spine then tilts away from the midline superiorly, and lateral winging occurs. The type of winging can be distinguished by the position of the medial border of the scapula and the medial aspect of the scapular spine.

Position of the Scapula Spine

Medial winging: medial border is vertical, medial aspect of the scapular spine moves upwards and medially.

Lateral winging: superior medial border is tilted away from the midline. Medial aspect of the scapular spine moves downwards and laterally.

Medial winging is the most common type of winging in the paediatric population and can be related to recurrent instability [54, 55], pain, brachial plexus injuries, repetitive stretch in overhead sporting activities, direct compression from contact sports, muscle patterning and postural issues. In regard to recurrent instability the severity of winging has been shown to be proportional to the number of episodes of instability.

Snapping Scapula

This term is used to describe a range of conditions that result in the disturbance of smooth scapulothoracic movement. It can be secondary to osteochondroma, fibrosis, scapulothoracic dyskinesis or poor posture. The symptoms vary. Crepitus and dyskinesis may or may not be painful. The underlying cause can often be difficult to diagnosis and the main stay of treatment is conservative, once malignancy and underlying space occupying lesions has been excluded [56]. In contrast to the adult population where trauma is the cause in 70% of cases [57] the most common cause of snapping scapula in children is overuse followed by trauma then osteochondroma [57]. A CT is the imaging modality of choice to differentiate between structural and non-structural pathology. This is indicated if there is no improvement with anti-inflammatories [58]. There is no direct association in the literature between snapping scapula syndrome and glenohumeral instability. However scapular dyskinesis can be as a result of a snapping scapula and there have been some links between snapping scapula and hypermobility.

Psychosocial Factors

Painful, recurrent shoulder subluxations/dislocations may be the presenting symptom of primary psychological problems (somatisation), or the disruption it can cause may lead to secondary psychological problems. Voluntary subluxation in adults was reviewed by Rowe et al. and he classified them into (1) Significant emotional problems and using it as a psychological defence and (2) no significant psychological or social disorder [58]. Voluntary dislocation usually starts in childhood or adolescents after minor injury. Despite the number of dislocations, the patients do not sustain intra-articular damage. It has been associated with hypermobility in approximately 65% of cases [59]. We advocate routine screening to be performed by the patient's physiotherapists, spending time with the patient and gaining their trust, allowing them to have the opportunity to speak in the absence of their parents. Early referral for psychiatric evaluation is recommended in voluntary dislocators, as those with co-commitment psychiatric disorders respond poorly to any modality of treatment. In our experience identifying a clear underlying psychosocial trigger is relatively rare, but they are able to help with coping strategies for painful episodes.

There are few published articles on the psychological factors influencing behaviour in multi-directional shoulder instability paediatric patients. A measured and open approach is required to try and identify any non-organic contributing factors. Only by doing this can the overall requirements of the patient be met. At times, the type of presentation and their sheer frequency may result in an inconsistent approach from emergency and on call staff. In difficult cases a plan should be set in place to aid front line staff to management these types of dislocations appropriately and most frequently without any intervention. Patient education is important with clear documentation about the aetiology and management goals. This can be taken with the patient should they present to the emergency department to minimise unnecessary radiographs, manipulations and admissions.

Specific Assessment

Shoulder abduction requires multiple groups of muscles to work in synchrony along the kinetic chain. The large glenohumeral joint abductors cannot function if the humeral head is not held appropriately in the glenoid, and this requires the glenoid to held stably and this in turn requires a stable spine and pelvis. We therefore breakdown the assessment into three muscle groups:

Intrinsic Shoulder Muscles

(Supraspinatus, Infraspinatus, Teres minor and Subscauplaris).

These will show weakness and inhibition, in particular infraspinatous. Underactivity of infraspinatous is commonly seen in posteroinferior instability, and often demonstrates a lag. When recruited prior to shoulder abduction improved stability is often demonstrated.

Extrinsic Shoulder Muscles

These are divided into superficial (Deltoid, Latisimus dorsi, Trapezius and Pectoralis major) and deep (Rhomboid major, levator scapulae).

These may demonstrate under or over activity. Pectoralis major, anterior deltoid and latissimus dorsi often go into spasm and over fire, whereas serratus anterior and the lower trapezius are often underactive. The latter may be demonstrated by pronounced winging when testing external rotation power with the arm adducted.

Core Stability Muscles: may show weakness.

The groups that contribute to posture and core stability are divided into:

Major: Erector spinae, pelvic floor, abdominals.

Minor: Latissimus Dorsi, Gluteus maximus and trapezius.

TEST: unilateral hip bridge endurance test. The patient maintains the pelvis and hips in a neutral position in a single leg bridge position with one leg planted and one leg extended and their arms across the chest, for as long as possible. Greater than 20 s equates to good core stability. This has been shown to correlate best to lab based methods [60].

Management

Core strengthening and improvement of postural tone are the initial priorities of the rehabilitation program. This can lead to the relaxation of the extrinsic muscles who's over activity in turn inhibit the action of the rotator cuff. Normalisation of the glenohumeral joint position allows recruitment of the intrinsic muscles. If core strength and posture are normalised and over activity of the extrinsic muscles are still an ongoing problem then specific muscle relaxation exercises need to be the focus of treatment. If these fail then a multidisciplinary approach should be taken to identify the over active muscle clinically or via EMG studies. In some circumstances when painful spasms associated with prolonged shoulder subluxations persist, an ultrasound guided botulinum toxin injection can relax an overactive muscle, and in our experience the benefits of this can significantly outlast the pharmacological effect of the toxin. In general, we recommend avoiding systemic muscle relaxants as there is usually a mismatch of muscle under and over activity. In particular, the undesired inhibition of the intrinsic stabilisers seen with systemic muscle relaxants can have an adverse effect.

If there is failure of conservative management and in the absence of a structural abnormality, there is rarely a surgical option. Carefully targeted botulinium toxin may break a cycle of muscle overactivity and surgical management of associated hyperlaxity (such as with capsular shrinkage or plication) are occasionally indicated. There is a porosity of literature on the long term follow up of paediatric patients with type III shoulder instability. However, if symptoms continue, patients should be helped with life style modification, coping strategies and a clear plan of management for other healthcare providers in respect to acute management of further dislocations. The patient should be shown methods of self-reduction and be advised to avoid attendance to Accident and Emergency if possible. The risk of somatisation (manifestation of psychological distress by the presentation of bodily symptoms) in chronic dislocations is higher in children and the average age for somtatic symptoms is 14.6 years [61] with the most common symptom being pain. In any patient with chronic dislocation and inconsistent symptoms, psychiatric review should be sought.

Other Paediatric Shoulder Instability

There are other causes of instability in children that are neuromuscular in origin and their sub types, assessment and management are the topic of another chapter.

References

1. Trueta J, Amato VP. The vascular contribution to osteogenesis. III. Changes in the growth cartilage caused by experimentally induced ischaemia. J Bone Joint Surg Br. 1960;42-B:571–87. PubMed PMID: 17533673.
2. Kwong S, Kothary S, Poncinelli LL. Skeletal development of the proximal humerus in the pediatric population: MRI features. AJR Am J Roentgenol. 2014;202(2):418–25. https://doi.org/10.2214/AJR.13.10711. PubMed PMID: 24450686.
3. Ogden JA, Conlogue GJ, Jensen J. Radiology of the postnatal skeletal development: the proximal humerus. Skelet Radiol. 1978;2:153–60.
4. Caffrey J. Pediatric x-ray diagnosis. 8th ed. Chicago: Year Book Medical Publishers; 1972. p. 434–43.
5. Zember JS, Rosenberg ZS, Kwong S, Kothary SP, Bedoya MA. Normal skeletal maturation and imaging pitfalls in the pediatric shoulder. Radiographics. 2015;35(4):1108–22. https://doi.org/10.1148/rg.2015140254. PubMed PMID: 26172355.
6. Asher MA. Dislocations of the upper extremity in children. Orthop Clin North Am. 1976;7(3):583–91. PubMed PMID: 958684.
7. Hovelius L. Anterior dislocation of the shoulder in teen-agers and young adults. Five-year prognosis. J Bone Joint Surg Am. 1987;69(3):393–9. PubMed PMID: 2434509.
8. Marans HJ, Angel KR, Schemitsch EH, Wedge JH. The fate of traumatic anterior dislocation of the shoulder in children. J Bone Joint Surg Am. 1992;74(8):1242–4. PubMed PMID: 1400553.
9. Rowe CR. Anterior dislocation of the shoulder: prognosis and treatment. Surg Clin North Am. 1963;43:1609–14. PubMed PMID: 14090208.
10. Rowe CR. Prognosis in dislocations of the shoulder. J Bone Joint Surg Am. 1956;38-A(5):957–77. PubMed PMID: 13367074.
11. Olds M, Donaldson K, Ellis R, Kersten P. In children 18 years and under, what promotes recurrent shoulder instability after traumatic anterior shoulder dislocation? A systematic review and meta-analysis of risk factors. Br J Sports Med. 2016;50(18):1135–41. https://doi.org/10.1136/bjsports-2015-095149. Epub 2015 Dec 23. Review. PubMed PMID: 26701925.
12. Zaremski JL, Galloza J, Sepulveda F, Vasilopoulos T, Micheo W, Herman DC. Recurrence and return

to play after shoulder instability events in young and adolescent athletes: a systematic review and meta-analysis. Br J Sports Med. 2016. pii: bjsports-2016-096895. https://doi.org/10.1136/bjsports-2016-096895. [Epub ahead of print] PubMed PMID: 27834676.
13. Bottoni CR, Wilckens JH, Deberardino TM, D'Alleyrand JC, Rooney RC, Harpstrite JK, Arciero RA. A prospective, randomized evaluation of arthroscopic stabilization versus nonoperative treatment in patients with acute, traumatic, first-time shoulder dislocations. Am J Sports Med. 2002;30(4):576–80. PubMed PMID: 12130413.
14. Jakobsen BW, Johannsen HV, Suder P, Søjbjerg JO. Primary repair versus conservative treatment of first-time traumatic anterior dislocation of the shoulder: a randomized study with 10-year follow-up. Arthroscopy. 2007;23(2):118–23. PubMed PMID: 17276217.
15. Cools AM, Witvrouw EE, Declercq GA, Danneels LA, Cambier DC. Scapular muscle recruitment patterns: trapezius muscle latency with and without impingement symptoms. Am J Sports Med. 2003;31(4):542–9. PubMed PMID: 12860542.
16. Wagner KT Jr, Lyne ED. Adolescent traumatic dislocations of the shoulder with open epiphyses. J Pediatr Orthop. 1983;3(1):61–2. PubMed PMID: 6841604.
17. Nixon MF, Keenan O, Funk L. High recurrence of instability in adolescents playing contact sports after arthroscopic shoulder stabilization. J Pediatr Orthop B. 2015;24(3):173–7. https://doi.org/10.1097/BPB.0000000000000135. PubMed PMID:25569537.
18. Ochs BG, Rickert M, Schmelzer-Schmied N, Loew M, Thomsen M. Post-traumatic shoulder instability in adolescence. Orthopade. 2005;34(2):152–8. German. PubMed PMID: 15480544.
19. Kraus R, Pavlidis T, Dongowski N, Szalay G, Schnettler R. Children and adolescents with posttraumatic shoulder instability benefit from arthroscopic stabilization. Eur J Pediatr Surg. 2010;20:253–6.
20. Cordischi K, Li X, Busconi B. Intermediate outcomes after primary traumatic anterior shoulder dislocation in skeletally immature patients aged 10 to 13 years. Orthopedics. 2009;32(9). pii: orthosupersite.com/view.asp?rID=42855. https://doi.org/10.3928/01477447-20090728-34. PubMed PMID: 19750998.
21. Deitch J, Mehlman CT, Foad SL, Obbehat A, Mallory M. Traumatic anterior shoulder dislocation in adolescents. Am J Sports Med. 2003;31(5):758–63. PubMed PMID: 12975198.
22. Lampert C, Baumgartner G, Slongo T, Kohler G, Horst M. Traumatic shoulder dislocation in children and adolescents. Eur J Trauma. 2003;29:375–8.
23. Gigis I, Heikenfeld R, Kapinas A, Listringhaus R, Godolias G. Arthroscopic versus conservative treatment of first anterior dislocation of the shoulder in adolescents. J Pediatr Orthop. 2014;34(4):421–5. https://doi.org/10.1097/BPO.0000000000000108. PubMed PMID: 24172677.
24. Zaremski JL, Galloza J, Sepulveda F, Vasilopoulos T, Micheo W, Herman DC. Recurrence and return to play after shoulder instability events in young and adolescent athletes: a systematic review and meta-analysis. Br J Sports Med. 2016;pii:bjsports-2016-096895. https://doi.org/10.1136/bjsports-2016-096895. [Epub ahead of print] PubMed PMID: 27834676.
25. Longo UG, van der Linde JA, Loppini M, Coco V, Poolman RW, Denaro V. Surgical versus nonoperative treatment in patients up to 18 years old with traumatic shoulder instability: a systematic review and quantitative synthesis of the literature. Arthroscopy. 2016;32(5):944–52. https://doi.org/10.1016/j.arthro.2015.10.020. Epub 2016 Feb 23. Review. PubMed PMID: 26921126.
26. Castagna A, Delle Rose G, Borroni M, Cillis BD, Conti M, Garofalo R, Ferguson D, Portinaro N. Arthroscopic stabilization of the shoulder in adolescent athletes participating in overhead or contact sports. Arthroscopy. 2012;28(3):309–15. PubMed PMID: 22130494.
27. Harris JD, Gupta AK, Mall NA, Abrams GD, McCormick FM, Cole BJ, Bach BR Jr, Romeo AA, Verma NN. Long-term outcomes after Bankart shoulder stabilization. Arthroscopy. 2013;29(5):920–33. Feb 5. Review. PubMed PMID: 23395467.
28. Hovelius L, Vikerfors O, Olofsson A, Svensson O, Rahme H. Bristow-Latarjet and Bankart: a comparative study of shoulder stabilization in 185 shoulders during a seventeen-year follow-up. J Shoulder Elb Surg. 2011;20(7):1095–101. PMID: 21602067.
29. DeBerardino TM, Arciero RA, Taylor DC, Uhorchak JM. Prospective evaluation of arthroscopic stabilization of acute, initial anterior shoulder dislocations in young athletes. Two- to five-year follow-up. Am J Sports Med. 2001;29(5):586–92. PubMed PMID: 11573917.
30. Larrain MV, Montenegro HJ, Mauas DM, Collazo CC, Pavón F. Arthroscopic management of traumatic anterior shoulder instability in collision athletes: analysis of 204 cases with a 4- to 9-year follow-up and results with the suture anchor technique. Arthroscopy. 2006;22(12):1283–9. PubMed PMID: 17157726.
31. Wheeler JH, Ryan JB, Arciero RA, Molinari RN. Arthroscopic versus nonoperative treatment of acute shoulder dislocations in young athletes. Arthroscopy. 1989;5(3):213–7. PubMed PMID: 2775396.
32. Ahmed I, Ashton F, Robinson CM. Arthroscopic Bankart repair and capsular shift for recurrent anterior shoulder instability: functional outcomes and identification of risk factors for recurrence. J Bone Joint Surg Am. 2012;94(14):1308–15. PubMed PMID: 22810402.
33. Hovelius L, Saeboe M. Neer award 2008: Arthropathy after primary anterior shoulder dislocation--223 shoulders prospectively followed up for twenty-five years. J Shoulder Elb Surg. 2009;18(3):339–47. PubMed PMID: 19254851.

34. Khan A, Samba A, Pereira B, Canavese F. Anterior dislocation of the shoulder in skeletally immature patients: comparison between non-operative treatment versus open Latarjet's procedure. Bone Joint J. 2014;96-B(3):354–9. https://doi.org/10.1302/0301-620X.96B3.32167. PubMed PMID: 24589791.
35. Schmid SL, Farshad M, Catanzaro S, Gerber C. The Latarjet procedure for the treatment of recurrence of anterior instability of the shoulder after operative repair: a retrospective case series of forty-nine consecutive patients. J Bone Joint Surg Am. 2012;94(11):e75. https://doi.org/10.2106/JBJS.K.00380. PubMed PMID:22637215.
36. Tobias JH, Deere K, Palmer S, Clark EM, Clinch J. Joint hypermobility is a risk factor for musculoskeletal pain during adolescence: findings of a prospective cohort study. Arthritis Rheum. 2013;65(4):1107–15. PubMed PMID: 23450628.
37. Altchek DW, Warren RF, Skyhar MJ, Ortiz G. T-plasty modification of the Bankart procedure for multidirectional instability of the anterior and inferior types. J Bone Joint Surg Am. 1991;73(1):105–12. PubMed PMID: 1985978.
38. Burkhart SS, De Beer JF, Barth JR, Cresswell T, Roberts C, Richards DP. Results of modified Latarjet reconstruction in patients with anteroinferior instability and significant bone loss. Arthroscopy. 2007;23(10):1033–41. Erratum in: Arthroscopy. 2007 Dec;23(12):A16. Criswell, Tim [corrected to Cresswell, Tim]. PubMed PMID: 17916467.
39. Johnson SM, Robinson CM. Shoulder instability in patients with joint hyperlaxity. J Bone Joint Surg Am. 2010;92(6):1545–57. https://doi.org/10.2106/JBJS.H.00078. Review. PubMed PMID: 20516333.
40. Vavken P, Tepolt FA, Kocher MS. Open inferior capsular shift for multidirectional shoulder instability in adolescents with generalized ligamentous hyperlaxity or Ehlers-Danlos syndrome. J Shoulder Elb Surg. 2016;25(6):907–12. PubMed PMID: 26775746.
41. Martetschlaeger F, Kircher J, Magosch P, Lichtenberg S, Habermeyer P. Arthroscopic stabilization of antero-inferior shoulder instability with concomitant hyperlaxity in a 10-year-old girl. Obere Extremitat. 2010;5(4):229–33.
42. Greiwe RM, Galano G, Grantham J, Ahmad CS. Arthroscopic stabilization for voluntary shoulder instability. J Pediatr Orthop. 2012;32(8):781–6. https://doi.org/10.1097/BPO.0b013e31826b6ee1. PubMed PMID: 23147620.
43. Rolfes K. Arthroscopic treatment of shoulder instability: a systematic review of capsular plication versus thermal capsulorrhaphy. J Athl Train. 2015;50(1):105–9. https://doi.org/10.4085/1062-6050-49.3.63. Epub 2014 Oct 20. Review. PubMed PMID: 25329347; PubMed Central PMCID: PMC4299727.
44. Levy HP. Ehlers-Danlos syndrome, hypermobility type In: Pagon R, Adam M, Ardinger H, Bird TD, Dolan CR, Fong C, et al, editors. Gene reviews [Internet]. Seattle: University of Washington, Seattle; 1993–2016. http://www.ncbi.nlm.nih.gov/books/NBK1279/.
45. Beighton P, De Paepe A, Steinmann B, Tsipouras P, Wenstrup RJ. Ehlers-Danlos syndromes: revised nosology, Villefranche, 1997. Ehlers-Danlos National Foundation (USA) and Ehlers-Danlos Support Group (UK). Am J Med Genet. 1998;77:31–7.
46. Stern CM, Pepin MJ, Stoler JM, Kramer DE, Spencer SA, Stein CJ. Musculoskeletal conditions in a pediatric population with Ehlers-Danlos syndrome. J Pediatr. 2017;181:261–6. https://doi.org/10.1016/j.jpeds.2016.10.078. Epub 2016 Nov 28. PubMed PMID: 27908650.
47. Scheper MC, Engelbert RH, Rameckers EA, Verbunt J, Remvig L, Juul-Kristensen B. Children with generalised joint hypermobility and musculoskeletal complaints: state of the art on diagnostics, clinical characteristics, and treatment. Biomed Res Int. 2013;2013:121054. PubMed PMID: 23971021; PubMed Central PMCID: PMC3736514.
48. Rombaut L, Malfait F, De Paepe A, Rimbaut S, Verbruggen G, De Wandele I, Calders P. Impairment and impact of pain in female patients with Ehlers-Danlos syndrome: a comparative study with fibromyalgia and rheumatoid arthritis. Arthritis Rheum 2011;63(7):1979–1987. https://doi.org/10.1002/art.30337. PubMed PMID: 21391202.
49. Aldridge JM 3rd, Perry JJ, Osbahr DC, Speer KP. Thermal capsulorraphy of bilateral glenohumeral joints in a pediatric patient with Ehlers- Danlos syndrome. Arthroscopy. 2003;19:E41.
50. Rodeo SA, Suzuki K, Yamauchi M, Bhargava M, Warren RF. Analysis of collagen and elastic fibers in shoulder capsule in patients with shoulder instability. Am J Sports Med. 1998;26(5):634–43. PubMed PMID: 9784809.
51. Gomes N, Hardy P, Bauer T. Arthroscopic treatment of chronic anterior instability of the shoulder in Marfan's syndrome. Arthroscopy. 2007;23(1):110.e1–5. Epub 2006 Sep 20. PubMed PMID: 17210441.
52. Malone AA, Jaggi A, Calvert PT, et al. Muscle patterning instability—classification and prevalence in reference shoulder service. In: Norris TR, Zuckerman JD, JJP W, Lee QT, editors. Surgery of the shoulder and elbow: an international perspective. Illinois: American Academy of Orthopaedic Surgeons; 2006. Section 7.
53. Morris AD, Kemp GJ, Frostick SP. Shoulder electromyography in multidirectional instability. J Shoulder Elb Surg. 2004;13(1):24–9. PubMed PMID:14735069.
54. Ogston JB, Ludewig PM. Differences in 3-dimensional shoulder kinematics between persons with multidirectional instability and asymptomatic controls. Am J Sports Med. 2007;35(8):1361–70. Epub 2007 Apr 9. PubMed PMID: 17420507.
55. Illyés A, Kiss RM. Kinematic and muscle activity characteristics of multidirectional shoulder joint instability during elevation. Knee Surg Sports Traumatol

Arthrosc. 2006;14(7):673–85. Epub 2005 Dec 14. PubMed PMID: 16362361.
56. Warth RJ, Spiegl UJ, Millett PJ. Scapulothoracic bursitis and snapping scapula syndrome: a critical review of current evidence. Am J Sports Med. 2015;43(1):236–45. https://doi.org/10.1177/0363546514526373. Epub 2014 Mar 24. Review. PubMed PMID: 24664139.
57. Pearse EO, Bruguera J, Massoud SN, Sforza G, Copeland SA, Levy O. Arthroscopic management of the painful snapping scapula. Arthroscopy. 2006;22(7):755–61. PubMed PMID: 16843812.
58. Haus B, Nasreddine AY, Suppan C, Kocher MS. Treatment of snapping ScapulaSyndrome in children and adolescents. J Pediatr Orthop. 2016;36(5):541–7. https://doi.org/10.1097/BPO.0000000000000486. PubMed PMID: 25887839.
59. Rowe CR, Pierce DS, Clark JG. Voluntary dislocation of the shoulder. A preliminary report on a clinical, electromyographic, and psychiatric study of twenty-six patients. J Bone Joint Surg Am. 1973;55(3):445–60. PubMed PMID:4703200.
60. Butowicz CM, Ebaugh DD, Noehren B, Silfies SP. Validation of two clinical measures of core stability. Int J Sports Phys Ther. 2016;11(1):15–23. PubMed PMID: 26900496; PubMed Central PMCID: PMC4739044.
61. Mullick MS. Somatoform disorders in children and adolescents. Bangladesh Med Res Counc Bull. 2002;28(3):112–22. PubMed PMID: 14509383.
62. Jones KJ, Wiesel B, Ganley TJ, Wells L. Functional outcomes of early arthroscopic bankart repair in adolescents aged 11 to 18 years. Erratum in: J Pediatr Orthop. 2007;27(2):209–13. 2007 27(4):483.
63. Shymon SJ, Roocroft J, Edmonds EW. Traumatic anterior instability of the pediatric shoulder: a comparison of arthroscopic and open bankart repairs. J Pediatr Orthop. 2015;35(1):1–6. https://doi.org/10.1097/BPO.0000000000000215.
64. Postacchini F, Gumina S, Cinotti G. Anterior shoulder dislocation in adolescents. J Shoulder Elb Surg. 2000;9(6):470–4.
65. Roberts SB, Beattie N, McNiven ND, Robinson CM. The natural history of primary anterior dislocation of the glenohumeral joint in adolescence. Bone Joint J. 2015;97(B4):520–6. https://doi.org/10.1302/0301-620X.97B4.34989.

Part VIII

Miscellaneous

Nerve Problems Around the Shoulder

31

Chye Yew Ng, Dominic Power, and Sohail Akhtar

Introduction

The brachial plexus has an intimate anatomical relationship to the shoulder girdle. As the plexus travels from the cervical spine towards the arm, the nerve trunks divide into anterior and posterior divisions, beneath the clavicle. The plexus divisions then form the cords just medial to the coracoid process. The cords split further to form the terminal branches as the nerves travel across the axilla. The cords and certain terminal branches are particularly vulnerable to injury due to their intimate relationship to the shoulder girdle. Natural tether points and the mobility of the shoulder joint render the nerves susceptible to traction injury and rupture. Following trauma, the nerves may be compressed by haematoma, displaced fracture fragments or dislocations. The trend towards internal fixation of fractures, the development of interventional arthroscopy and the rise in shoulder arthroplasty has been associated with higher rates of iatrogenous nerve injury.

C. Yew Ng (✉) · S. Akhtar
Wrightington Hospital, Wigan, UK
e-mail: nerve@wwl.nhs.uk

D. Power
University Hospitals Birmingham NHS Foundation Trust, Birmingham, UK

Nerve Injuries Following Trauma

Clavicle Fracture

Clavicle fractures most commonly occur in young males between 15 and 24 years old [1]. The commonest mechanisms of injury were fall from standing height or bicycle accidents. Displaced midshaft fractures accounted for the majority of cases and were the most frequently operated fractures [1]. The occurrence of acute nerve injury as a direct result of clavicle fractures appears to be rare. In a consecutive series of 1000 clavicle fractures over a 6-year period, no case of acute nerve injury was reported [2]. However, case reports of displaced fragments causing direct injury to the retroclavicular plexus have been published, highlighting this exceptional but potentially serious risk [3–5].

There is now a trend towards plating of displaced clavicle fractures [6]. The surgeon needs to be aware of the proximity of neurovascular structures to the clavicle when plating a fracture. The supraclavicular nerves cross the clavicle in the lateral two-thirds supplying sensation to the upper chest. The nerves are prone to injury through traction, direct injury during the exposure of the clavicle or post-operative scar tether and irritation where they cross the anterior edge of the clavicle plate. In a series of 63 clavicle platings, numbness of the upper chest following clavicle fixation was identified in 55% of patients

I. A. Trail et al. (eds.), *Textbook of Shoulder Surgery*, https://doi.org/10.1007/978-3-319-70099-1_31

[7] although this may be reduced using a mini open technique [8]. Irritation of tethered nerves may necessitate plate removal and relocation of the neuromata proximal to the scar. The plexus is at its closest to the clavicle at the lateral three-fifths point of the clavicle, with a mean distance of 13 mm only [9]. Likewise, the subclavian vessels are most at-risk between the medial quarter and the midpoint of the clavicle [10]. The mean distance of the subclavian artery and vein from the middle of the clavicle was 17 mm and 12 mm respectively, but can be as close as 5 mm [11]. However the relationships may change with movements and trauma, which could imply an even closer distance.

Due to subspecialisation, organisation of fracture services and referral pathways, there is often a delay between injury and surgery. During delayed fixation, especially between 2 and 4 weeks after injury, the plexus are particularly vulnerable to iatrogenous injury [12]. Jeyaseelan et al. reported 21 patients who sustained injury to the brachial plexus following delayed fixation of clavicle fractures, over a 11-year period in a regional peripheral nerve injury (PNI) unit [12]. The patients typically present with neuropathic pain and paralysis postoperatively, which should prompt an urgent referral to the local specialist unit. The C5/C6 nerves, upper trunk, lateral cord and suprascapular nerve were the most commonly damaged nerves. The universal finding at exploration was tethering of the nerve to the undersurface of the clavicle by scar tissue at the site of fracture. Apart from plating, injury to the brachial plexus could similarly occur following intramedullary nailing of clavicular fractures [13]. Traction that occurred during reaming had been postulated to be the mechanism of nerve injury.

When nerves are implicated in clavicle fractures, the symptoms are usually delayed and could be due to costo-clavicular compression by hypertrophic callus formation, non-union, mal-union or subclavian pseudoaneurysm [14–17]. In an operative series of 23 clavicular non-unions over a 11-year period, 7 patients were found to have neurological dysfunction [16]. Two were noted to have neurological symptoms at the time of original injury while five were due to delayed local compression on the brachial plexus by the non-union. There were additional four patients who had dynamic symptoms consistent with thoracic outlet syndrome [16].

Surgeons who undertake surgery for clavicular fractures, whether for acute fixation or delayed reconstruction, should anticipate potential distortion of local anatomy due to the trauma and secondary scarring. When faced with complex cases such as medial fractures, mal-union, non-union and revision cases, preoperative CT or MR angiogram is recommended to delineate the relationship of the neurovascular structures to the clavicle. During surgery, the risk to the plexus can be reduced by careful and thorough release of the tissues from the undersurface of the clavicle before mobilising the fracture fragments [12, 18]. Furthermore, one has to avoid shortening of the clavicle during fixation as this may lead to narrowing of the space between the clavicle and the first rib, thus resulting in secondary thoracic outlet syndrome (TOS) [12]. Following clavicular fracture surgery, beware of unremitting pain, motor paralysis and/or sensory loss, as this may signify brachial plexopathy and the palsy need not be complete. Prompt referral to the local brachial plexus service is recommended.

Shoulder Dislocation or Fracture-Dislocation

In shoulder dislocations, anterior is the commonest direction of displacement of the humeral head. The infraclavicular plexus, as it travels from superomedial to inferolateral direction in relation to the coracoid process, is thus subject to traction force exerted by the humeral head. It is comprehensible that the point of maximal displacement occurs in the midst of trauma before the recoil of the humeral head by the attached muscles. The potential impact on the plexus is multifactorial. The injury factors include the energy transfer, as reflected by the mechanism of injury, the duration of dislocation (before the head is reduced thus relieving pressure on the plexus), and associated fracture with its fragment and haematoma that may contribute to on-going insult on the nerves. The patient factor relates to the inherent susceptibility of the nerves to traction injury and their regenerative potentials.

Involvement of the supraclavicular plexus is rare unless there has been significant trauma to the head and neck. Diagnostic confusion regarding the level of injury is common when there is infraclavicular plexus involvement because on initial examination it may appear as though the suprascapular nerve is also involved suggesting the injury is at the level of the upper trunk or even avulsion of the upper plexus. Careful examination will detect contraction of the supraspinatous muscle and confirm that the pathology is likely a concomitant rotator cuff tear rather than a more proximal nerve injury. The presence of dorsal scapular nerve and long thoracic nerve functions will confirm integrity of the upper plexus in such challenging cases.

The reported incidences of nerve injuries following glenohumeral dislocation range from 15% to 48% [19–21]. The axillary nerve is most commonly, and often most severely, injured with rates of isolated axillary nerve injury reported between 3.3% and 40% [19, 20] and there appears to be an increasing predisposition in those over 60 years of age [22].

Hems and Mahmood reported on a series of 101 infraclavicular plexus injuries and defined four common pathological patterns [23] (Table 31.1). The commonest pattern was an anterior glenohumeral dislocation associated with injury to the axillary nerve and the ulnar nerve, which was identified in 55% of patients. This is typically seen in the low-energy falls in the elderly and axillary nerve rupture in this group is rare (3.6%).

The authors' experience of closed glenohumeral dislocations and nerve injuries is similar. Isolated axillary nerve palsy is the commonest pattern, followed by axillary nerve and medial cord; medial and posterior cords; posterior cord in isolation and lastly, the least frequent but the most severe pattern is a three-cord injury.

Management of Nerve Injuries Associated with Shoulder Dislocation

Neurological deficits should be documented before prompt closed reduction using adequate analgesia and relaxant. Following reduction, a thorough repeat neurovascular examination of the limb should be undertaken. Any abnormal findings are accurately documented. Glenohumeral dislocations associated with injury to the infraclavicular plexus are usually managed non-operatively. Surgery is indicated in open injuries, in high-energy injuries associated with vascular disruption, in locked dislocation of the shoulder and in cases where there is deterioration under observation or no recovery in the expected timeframe. A static Tinel's sign on repeat examination and the development of neuropathic pain are signs of nerve rupture or development of a neuroma-in-continuity. Early exploration of such cases is warranted with intra-operative neurophysiology assessment to guide resection and autologous nerve grafting.

The associated nerve injuries are likely to be due to traction and of mixed nature. The severity of the nerve lesion could vary depending on the energy transferred, duration of dislocation, and intrinsic susceptibility of the individual to nerve injury. A period of observation and serial exami-

Table 31.1 Patterns of injury to the infraclavicular brachial plexus of 101 patients (age range 14–89 years old) who presented to the Scottish National BPI Service from 1997 to 2009

Patterns of injury	No	Characteristics
Anterior glenohumeral dislocation	55	Axillary & ulnar nerves most commonly injured Axillary nerve ruptured in 2 (4%)
Axillary nerve injury, without known dislocation	20	Nerve ruptured in 14 (70%)
Displaced proximal humeral fracture	15	Prompt reduction is required Arterial injury in 6 (3 repaired)
Hyperextension of the arm	11	All cases explored Musculocutaneous nerve disruption in 10

Hems and Mahmood [23]

nations over the initial 6–8 weeks are recommended. If there is early clinical sign of recovery, this signifies a favourable nerve lesion and conservative management is continued. However, if there is no recovery in terms of resolution of pain and/or motor/sensory improvement, nerve conduction studies and EMG are organised and referral to a specialist brachial plexus service is recommended. Spontaneous recovery beyond this timescale is still possible but early referral would give the nerve specialist an opportunity to monitor the clinical progress and to build a rapport with the patient who may eventually need to undergo a major plexus exploration.

The accuracy of the initial neurological examination is critical and allows useful prognostic information to be provided at the subsequent specialist review. Neurological deterioration following reduction, the development of neuropathic pain or loss of pulses should prompt immediate further investigation. The risk of nerve entrapment is low. However excessive force applied for reduction, delays to reduction or repeated attempts at reduction may result in further traction injury to the plexus. Pain and loss of pulse may be associated with a vascular injury and a false aneurysm or haematoma may compress the plexus. In such cases emergency angiography should be followed by exploration, decompression and vascular repair. Ideally the neural and vascular reconstructions are performed in the same setting by the appropriate specialists.

Delayed presentation of shoulder dislocation with a dense neurological injury should be reduced under general anaesthesia with neuromuscular paralysis. The surgeon should be prepared to perform an open reduction of the shoulder if necessary. Further delay transferring the patient to a brachial plexus service is not warranted. There is a higher rate of axillary nerve injury with shoulder dislocations not reduced within 12 h [24], with some evidence to suggest that those, who present with an associated nerve lesion and are reduced greater than 2 h following injury, are less likely to recover within 6 months than those with nerve injuries who are reduced promptly [25].

The isolated axillary nerve palsy usually recovers spontaneously. Neurapraxic injury will recover spontaneously and completely by 8 weeks. Higher-grade continuity lesions with axonotmesis will typically demonstrate some evidence of re-innervation at 3 months. In such patients, the muscle wasting is severe. Recovery of sensation at the axillary badge area may confirm physical continuity of the nerve but it does not preclude a partial injury. Deep deltoid muscle tenderness usually predates visible muscle contraction by 4 weeks and electromyography at 3–4 months may demonstrate evidence of polyphasia and motor unit potentials confirming neural continuity and ongoing recovery. The absence of neurophysiological evidence of recovery at this stage should prompt surgical exploration with a view to reconstruction of a rupture or neuroma-in-continuity with interposition autologous nerve grafting [26–28]. Delayed presentation beyond 6 months may be better treated using a distal nerve transfer reconstruction technique. A triceps motor branch is used to bypass the axillary nerve lesion and direct coaptation to the axillary nerve or the anterior division provides a source of motor axons close to the motor innervation point (Fig. 31.1) [29]. However the jury is still out regarding the relative merits of nerve grafting versus nerve transfer given the comparable outcomes from retrospective case series and the lack of randomised controlled trial [30, 31].

Persistent deficit of the musculocutaneous nerve beyond 3 months without evidence of re-innervation of biceps on electromyography should prompt exploration and neurolysis of the musculocutaneous nerve. Ruptures or neuroma-in-continuity without distal function should be grafted using autologous nerve. Late diagnosis or proximal lesions may be treated with distal nerve transfer. If medial cord function is preserved a transfer of a motor fascicle from the ulnar nerve can be transferred to the motor branch to brachialis as an adjunct to the proximal reconstruction for biceps restoration [32].

Persistent posterior cord dysfunction without clinical evidence of recovery in triceps at 3 months and no neurophysiological evidence of re-innervation should prompt exploration with a

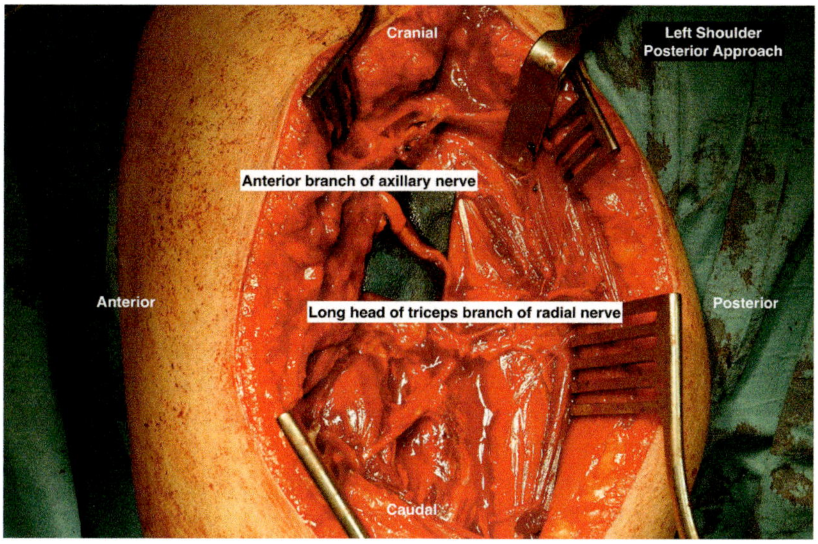

Fig. 31.1 Posterior view of a left shoulder showing the radial nerve (long head of triceps branch) transfer to the anterior branch of the axillary nerve (Bangkok transfer)

view to nerve graft reconstruction. In such cases the axillary nerve should be grafted as the salvage nerve transfer of a triceps motor branch is not available. The re-innervation distances are such that recovery of useful wrist and digit extension is not always possible. In such cases in the presence of an isolated posterior cord injury, early distal reconstruction using nerve transfers may be considered. Redundant flexor digitorum superficialis motor nerve branches may be transferred to the extensor carpi radialis motor branch and flexor carpi radialis and palmaris longus motor branches may be transferred to the posterior interosseus nerve distal to the supinator branches in the proximal volar forearm [33]. Late presentation or failed posterior cord graft may be treated with tendon transfers (*as per* for high radial palsy).

Management of medial cord injury is challenging. The re-innervation distances are long and early nerve grafting for ruptures or neuroma-in-continuity may provide some function in the proximal flexor carpi ulnaris and the flexor digitorum profundus. However, recovery of the ulnar-innervated intrinsics is typically poor. In such cases there are no good distal nerve transfer options and salvage reconstruction using tendon transfers is usually offered when recovery has plateaued after 18 months.

Scapular Fracture

Scapular fracture typically occurs as a result of high-energy injury and it may be associated with other injuries to the head, spine or chest. The clinician should be vigilant for any associated neurovascular injuries which could have devastating effects on the patient's outcome. Scapulothoracic dissociation represents an extreme end of periscapular trauma which could be potentially life threatening. In those with combined skeletal and neurologic injuries, the management is best undertaken in specialist units with the appropriate skillsets in order to offer comprehensive treatment.

Proximal Humerus Fracture

Fractures of the surgical neck of the humerus are common and typically low-energy injuries. Axillary nerve injury is rare. Higher energy injuries are associated with more significant fracture displacement and soft tissue disruption. Rupture of the axillary neurovascular bundle is typified by a large haematoma and significant pain. Axillary nerve should be formally explored and the fracture should be internally fixed at the same time. The surgeon who undertakes the procedure ideally should be prepared to graft the axillary nerve injury if necessary. If local expertise is not available, the fracture may be stabilised and the patient can be reviewed in outpatients at the regional peripheral nerve service with a view to axillary nerve reconstruction or later distal nerve transfer. Any neurological deterioration should prompt early transfer to a unit where the plexus can be explored and definitive fracture stabilisation performed.

Rarely the humeral shaft may displace medially to the subcoracoid area and in such cases neurovascular injury is commonplace. Attempts at closed realignment should be avoided. In such cases the humeral shaft fragment may become locked within the brachial plexus cords and attempt at traction and reduction may worsen the neurovascular injury. Vascular imaging is required if there is clinical evidence of impaired vascularity or extensive haematoma. The patient should be transferred emergently to a unit where orthopaedic trauma, vascular surgery and brachial plexus surgery are available. Open reduction and fracture fixation or shoulder arthroplasty can then be performed at the same time as neurovascular reconstruction.

Nerve Injuries Following Surgery

The occurrence of nerve injury during shoulder surgery is dependent on the type of procedure, the surgical approach and the experience of the surgeon. Surgical causes may be due to positioning, traction, misplacement of arthroscopic ports, retraction or direct surgical injury [34]. The incidence of neurological injuries for arthroscopic shoulder surgery ranges between 0.2% and 3% with transient paraesthesia reported in 10–30% of procedures [35]. For open procedures, nerve injuries are reported in 1–2% of patients undergoing rotator cuff surgery, 1–4% undergoing arthroplasty surgery and 1–8% undergoing instability surgery [36]. The majority of these injuries are reported as minor cutaneous nerve injuries and transient conduction block to the brachial plexus [34] although permanent neurological injuries do rarely occur.

Open Surgery

The anterior course of the axillary nerve is vulnerable in open anterior stabilisation procedures and may become tethered by sutures. The anterior division of the axillary nerve courses around the neck of the humerus under the deltoid muscle approximately 5 cm distal to the lateral edge of the acromion. It is particularly vulnerable during deltoid-split approach or mini-open procedures for proximal humeral fractures.

The supraclavicular nerves are vulnerable during lateral clavicle fracture fixation or stabilisation procedures for chronic instability at the acromioclavicular joint. The plexus is vulnerable during lateral clavicle stabilisation surgery when there is reconstruction of the coracoclavicular ligaments. During reverse shoulder arthroplasty, the anterior glenoid screw placement is critical in order to avoid anteromedial penetration, which could lead to direct plexus injury by a drill or screw irritation. The suprascapular nerve is at risk during mobilisation of the rotator cuff for massive cuff tear repair. When plating the proximal humerus, the musculocutaneous nerve is at risk of irritation from shaft screw that is too long (Fig. 31.2a, b).

Nagda et al. performed intraoperative continuous nerve monitoring during 30 cases of shoulder arthroplasty and noted frequent significant drop of nerve signals during glenoid and humeral preparations [37]. Removal of soft tissue retractors alone did not restore the nerve signals, but it was only after the limb was re-positioned to neutral that normal nerve signals resumed. The study is important in highlighting the excessive traction force that could be placed on the plexus with extreme positioning of the limb that is sometimes necessary with shoulder arthroplasty. In order to minimise such risk, the period of sustained hyperextension of the arm should be kept to the minimum.

A high index of suspicion of an iatrogenous nerve injury should be considered in cases where the patient reports significant neuropathic pain in the immediate post-operative period. Commonly shoulder surgery is performed with adjunctive regional anaesthesia and therefore post-operative

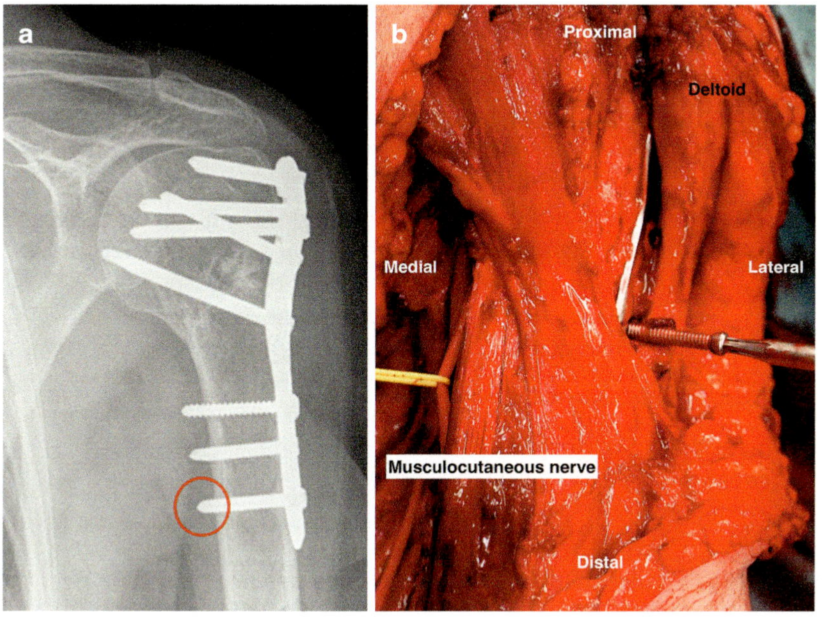

Fig. 31.2 (**a**) Radiograph of a well-reduced and well-healed proximal humerus fracture which had been treated with plating. The patient however suffered with paraesthesia and allodynia in the ipsilateral lateral antebrachial cutaneous nerve dermatome for 3 years following surgery. There was no weakness in elbow flexion. Note the length of the shaft screws. (**b**) Intraoperative image of nerve exploration and plate removal. The musculocutaneous nerve had been isolated with a loop and the distal shaft screw was found to be irritating the nerve (without causing obvious injury). The neuropathic symptoms resolved after the plate was removed

paralysis or weakness is typically overlooked or erroneously contributed to the nerve block. Should there be any clinical concern, prompt referral to a peripheral nerve specialist is recommended.

Arthroscopic Surgery

The shoulder joint is especially suited to arthroscopic techniques due to its size and mobility. Iatrogenous nerve injury may result from patient positioning, traction or direct nerve injury during instrumentation. The standard portals are positioned to avoid injury to the neurovascular structures and the rates of complications are low. A cadaveric study has identified, of 12 commonly used portals the 5 o'clock portal carries the highest theoretical risk of injury being located just 15 mm from the axillary nerve. The central posterior, anterior superior, anterocentral, anteroinferior, posterolateral, anterolateral and lateral portals are all more than 20 mm from a major neurovascular structure and the risk of injury is therefore lower [38]. Operator inexperience, swelling and extravasation of irrigation fluids can increase the risk of portal malposition with the attendant risks of inadvertent nerve injury and contribute to nerve compression.

Developments in instrumentation have extended the scope of reconstruction possibilities for a variety of pathologies, both intra-articular and extra-articular, using an arthroscopic technique. These procedures may be technically demanding and are uncommon resulting in a shallow learning curve. Endoscopic lateral clavicle stabilisation carries a risk of injury to the infraclavicular brachial plexus medial to the coracoid and the supraclavicular nerves over the lateral third of the clavicle [39, 40]. Endoscopic suprascapular nerve release simplifies what is a challenging open procedure, but carries a risk of direct trauma to the nerve or incomplete decompression [41].

The arthroscopic Latarjet procedure for instability carries a theoretical risk of injury to the musculocutaneous nerve and to the axillary nerve. Rates of injury may be higher in patients with aberrant neurovascular abnormalities including musculocutaneous nerve entrapment within the coracobrachialis tendon, resulting in a tether point creating traction on repositioning of the coracoid tip [42]. In practice the rate of nerve injury is low and a series of 83 identified only one transient injury to the axillary nerve [43].

Posterior Triangle Neck Surgery and Spinal Accessory Nerve

Spinal accessory nerve (SAN) has a superficial course and is particularly vulnerable during surgery at the posterior triangle of the neck, with lymph node biopsy being the commonest cause of this iatrogenous injury [44–46]. When injured, it leads to trapezius wasting which will manifest clinically as pain, droopy shoulder and restricted abduction. Other clinical signs include lateral scapular winging (on wall-press test), prominent medial border of scapula (on resisted active external rotation test [47]), and inability to extend arm against gravity when lying prone (‘*superman sign*’).

Despite the well-described anatomy and function of the SAN, injury to the nerve still appears to remain under-recognised. In a series of 111 cases of SAN lesions, only 14 were diagnosed by the operating surgeons [45]. Patients with the injury are often referred to the shoulder surgeon or physiotherapist, but the referrers have failed to recognise that the shoulder complaints are in fact manifestation of trapezius weakness.

EMG is crucial in confirming denervation changes in the trapezius muscle. Involvement of the sternocleidomastoid muscle would suggest a more proximal localisation of the nerve lesion, near the base of skull. MRI will show supplementary information of trapezius atrophy, when compared to the contralateral side.

Exploration of the SAN is generally indicated for pain relief, establishing extent of injury and nerve reconstruction. Depending on the intraoperative findings, nerve surgery may be in the form of neurolysis, nerve repair, nerve grafting, nerve transfer or direct muscular neurotisation [44, 45, 48]. Satisfactory results of nerve repair have been reported as long as three and a half years after the injury [45], implying a reasonable window of opportunity for neural reconstruction, provided the injury has been duly recognised. For the delayed cases or those following failed neural reconstruction, triple-tendon transfer (a modification of Eden-Lange procedure) has been shown to be effective at restoring the stability of the scapulothoracic articulation and shoulder function [49].

Nerve Injuries Following Anaesthesia

Regional anaesthetic blocks are commonly used in shoulder surgery in isolation or as an adjunct to general anaesthesia enabling many procedures to be performed in an ambulatory setting and improving peri-operative pain management. There is a small risk of significant nerve injury associated with regional anaesthesia which is estimated at 1:10,000 and may be due to direct intraneural injection, direct fascicle injury from the bevelled needle tip, extrinsic compression due to high volume injection in tight fascial spaces, haematoma compression or ischaemic neuropathy from injury to or compression of the vasa nervorum. Transient paraesthesia or paralysis from a prolonged conduction block are more common and the incidence is reported at around 8% [36]. The rate of complications may be reduced by using ultrasound guidance, nerve stimulation and low-volume nerve blocks in awake patients.

When shoulder surgery is conducted with interscalene block anaesthesia, the all-cause complication rate has been reported to have a 10-day prevalence of 14% dropping to 0.9% at 6 months [50]. Fredrickson et al. reported a 3.5% neurological complication rate with symptoms in 10 patients out of 659 resolving within 1 month and 13 resolving between 1 and 6 months [51]. Just over a third of the neurological injuries were attributed to blocks in Fredrickson's series whilst the majority of the high transient neurological complications were attributed to non-block related causes including traction and operative positioning [51].

The variation in complication rates is dependent upon how nerve injury is defined [52], the study design, the thresholds for reporting and duration of follow-up [53]. Attribution of a nerve injury to an anaesthetic block or to intra-operative traction is sometimes impossible and may explain the range of reported nerve injuries in the literature. Patients should be carefully examined in the post-operative clinic to ensure that there is no neurological deficit. Significant nerve injury as opposed to a transient conduction block is typified by pain and there is usually a positive Tinel's sign at the site of injection. This should be recorded, the anaesthetist notified and the patient referred for specialist nerve review.

The interscalene block has a higher rate of complications than the more laterally placed supraclavicular block, which is usually sufficient for most shoulder surgery. The medial approach carries a risk of direct phrenic nerve injury and temporary phrenic nerve blockade may compromise respiratory function in the post-operative period. The interscalene block involves injection of local anaesthetic into a tight interscalene space and there is a risk of medial displacement along the nerve root to produce a high cervical epidural blockade. Permanent quadriplegia has been reported as a consequence of interscalene anaesthesia [54].

Neuralgic Amyotrophy/Parsonage-Turner Syndrome

Neuralgic amyotrophy (NA) or Parsonage Turner syndrome refers to a clinical syndrome characterised by acute onset of pain around the shoulder girdle lasting from hours to 2 weeks, followed by paralysis of individual or multiple muscles of the upper limb [55, 56]. The acute pain usually subsides or is replaced by a dull ache as the paralysis appears. At times, there is also patchy numbness in the arm. There is often, but not always, a precipitant event and a subsequent latency period of several days before the onset of pain. The commonly quoted inciting events include viral illness, trauma, surgery and vaccination. However, it could occur without an apparent prodrome. The condition is believed to be mediated by an immune process but definitive evidence to prove the theory is lacking.

The syndrome covers a myriad of clinical presentations with single or multiple nerves involvements. The location of the presumed neuritis could be at the peripheral nerve, brachial plexus, spinal root or even the spinal cord. The most commonly involved nerve is the long thoracic nerve which leads to serratus anterior palsy and scapular winging. Other nerves that have been implicated include suprascapular, axillary, spinal accessory, musculocutaneous, posterior and anterior interosseous nerves.

Historically a benign natural history of the condition is assumed with spontaneous resolution in the majority of cases but it could take up to 2 years or longer. However van Alfen and van Engelen, in a prospective series of 246 NA cases, reported persisting pain and paresis in approximately two-thirds of patients who were followed for more than 3 years [57]. In another report of 89 patients with NA, about a quarter to a third of the group reported significant long-term pain and fatigue, and half to two thirds still suffered impairments in daily life, at an average follow-up of 2 years after onset [58].

While NA remains a clinical syndrome without a definitive test, investigations with neurophysiology (particularly EMG), radiology and select blood tests are recommended for exclusion of other conditions that could mimic the presentation. In a prospective series of 60 patients presenting with neurological disorders to a specialist shoulder clinic, NA was found not to be the commonest final diagnosis [59], thus highlighting the importance to consider other differential diagnosis. Myopathic conditions, such as fascioscapulohumeral dystrophy

(FSHD) has a wide spectrum of clinical presentation and one could present with unilateral scapular winging without obvious facial features. The diagnosis however can be confirmed with genetic testing. Other rarer muscular disorders may require muscle biopsy for confirmation. Hourglass-like constriction of the peripheral nerve, presentation of which can mimic NA, is an unusual condition that is becoming increasingly recognised as a potential cause of peripheral nerve palsy [60]. The constrictions could be visualised with the aid of high-resolution ultrasound scan and if identified, primary nerve surgery is recommended [61, 62]. It remains speculative whether the hourglass constriction is the direct result of inflammation and whether it could be attributable for NA cases that fail to recover spontaneously.

The mainstay of treatment for NA are physiotherapy and analgesia. The role of steroid remains controversial. If administered at the early stage of the condition, steroid may shorten the period of initial pain [63]. Except from those who show spontaneous signs of recovery within 6–9 months of onset, this group of patients may demand the attention of surgeon, neurologist, physiotherapist, neurophysiologist and musculoskeletal radiologist. For those who fail to recover in the predicted timeframe, there is emerging role for nerve surgery (neurolysis and nerve transfer). For the recalcitrant cases, tendon transfers are salvage surgical options.

Entrapment Neuropathy

Due to the complex anatomical arrangement of nerves passing from the neck and then around the shoulder before entering the arm, there is considerable potential for compression of these nerves by a number of anatomical structures. The anatomical structures may be congenitally abnormal, diseased by degeneration, or distorted by trauma or tumours. Regardless of the aetiology, the symptoms are related to compression of the nerve. This underlines the difficulty in clinical diagnosis, particularly in view of the proximal location of the compression. Patients may complain of a variety of symptoms from nonspecific pain to localised alterations in sensation.

Thoracic Outlet Syndrome

Thoracic outlet syndrome describes a group of symptoms that occur secondary to compression of nerves and/or blood vessels in their path from the base of the neck into the axilla. The thoracic outlet is defined anatomically by the scalene muscles, the first rib and the clavicle. The brachial plexus, subclavian artery and subclavian vein run through three important spaces, as they travel from the upper mediastinum to the axilla, namely interscalene triangle, costoclavicular space and subpectoral space, where compression could occur.

It may be over simplistic to state that diagnosis is purely from marrying together of symptoms and physical signs but in reality, in a clinical setting the diagnosis is usually considered only after exclusion of other conditions. Pain is often the most common symptom and the localisation of the pain can span from the neck to the shoulder and into the arm. Other than pain, patients also complain of alteration in sensation. Overall, neurogenic thoracic outlet syndrome account for approximately 90% of cases [64].

Other than nerve symptoms, physical signs and symptoms related to vascular disturbance may also be encountered but they are generally less commonly seen. Subtle skin discolouration or venous congestion may be seen in some cases. In view of the mobile nature of the thoracic outlet the volume within the space is not constant and as such the symptoms are usually intermittent. This adds to the diagnostic challenges as any investigation utilised must be able to adjust for the dynamic nature of the compression. Specific clinical examination tests such as Roos test utilise this concept of the dynamic volume changes. Roos test is very sensitive for thoracic outlet syndrome and is positive if symptoms are triggered within a minute when the shoulder is held at 90 degrees of abduction whilst the elbow is held in 90 degrees of flexion and the patient repeatedly opens and closes the hand [65].

The causes of thoracic outlet syndrome can be divided into four broad and sometimes interchangeable groups:

1. Congenital variations – This may be bony variations such as a cervical rib or a prolonged transverse process. Fibrous anomalies such as abnormal intercostal bands are only discovered intraoperatively.
2. Post traumatic – This may be due to isolated trauma or repetitive injuries. This is thought to be related to injury of the scalene muscles resulting in muscle fibrosis and shortening [66].
3. Acquired – This represents the most commonly presenting cause of symptoms. These are seen in certain professions who are exposed to repetitive movements or abnormal prolonged posture hold (the arms being held in a raised position) such as hairdressers, barbers and assembly lines workers or neck flexed in roles requiring computer screen use [65, 67].
4. Space occupying lesions – tumours

Imaging utilised includes chest x-ray or inlet view to look for a cervical rib. CT and/or MR angiogram (with the arms in abduction) are employed to identify any positional compression of the neurovascular structures, in addition to excluding abnormal space occupying lesions. Although it is operator dependent, dynamic duplex scanning may be a useful adjunct to diagnosis. Nerve conduction studies and EMG are often normal in the majority of patients, but these studies are helpful in the exclusion of other compression neuropathies. EMG changes that show chronic denervation of the small muscles of the hand may act as a pointer to the condition. Nerve conduction studies that demonstrate abnormalities in the medial antebrachial cutaneous nerve is also a specific pointer for the condition [68].

Decision-making on treatment will be dependent on severity and cause of the condition. The two treatment modalities available are physiotherapy and surgical intervention. Muscle bellies may adapt to develop shortened muscle resting lengths changes because of repeated or constant abnormal posture. Physiotherapy focuses on stretching the shortened muscles and on strengthening the lower scapular stabilisers [69, 70]. This approach will adjust the dimensions of the thoracic outlet by addressing muscle imbalances around the shoulder girdle that may result in a reduction of the space and subsequent nerve impingement and vascular obstruction. Preventative measures such as work place adjustments can be simple but effective means at reducing the likelihood of symptoms in those predisposed to the condition.

Surgical intervention should only be considered as first line treatment if there is a rapid or severe onset of nerve or vascular specific symptoms or if there is evidence of a space-occupying lesion in the thoracic outlet. Informed consent before surgery is particularly important as the severity of the potential complications sets it apart from other nerve decompression procedures. Severe and potentially disastrous complications may result from collateral damage to the structures in the vicinity, including pleura, subclavian artery or vein, thoracic duct and brachial plexus. The aim of surgery is to increase the volume of the thoracic outlet by removal of offending structures. This commonly involves removing the first rib and the scalene muscles as well as a cervical rib if it is present. Exposure of these structures is through either a supraclavicular or an axillary approach [71]. A supraclavicular approach allows for scalenectomy as well as a cervical rib excision whereas 1st rib excision is better suited to an axillary approach. Less invasive surgical procedures are more targeted and are appropriate for very specific cases such as a purely neurogenic thoracic outlet syndrome. If symptoms are recreated by pressure on the coracoid then tenotomy of the pectoralis minor muscle has been shown to be effective [72].

Suprascapular Nerve Entrapment

The suprascapular nerve takes its origin from the superior trunk (C5, C6) of the brachial plexus. It goes on to innervate the supraspinatus and infraspinatus muscles. As the nerve leaves the neck aiming for its target muscles, it has to take a path around the superior edge of the scapula through the suprascapular notch following which it gives off its branch to the supraspinatus muscle. The remaining nerve then passes through a further bony canal around the base of the spine of the scapula in the spinogleoid notch to reach the infraspinatus muscle. The nerve is thus prone to compression from abnormal pressure build up within these bony channels. Degenerative changes around these bony channels are responsible for abnormal pressure build up whether that be from a ganglion [73, 74] or thickening of the ligament.

Symptoms of compression to either one or both of the branches of the nerve relate to dysfunction of the muscles in question and if prolonged, also visible wasting. Pain is related to how distal the compression is located. A distal lesion that purely affects the infraspinatus muscle may not be associated by pain [75]. Symptoms are predominantly from entrapment at the suprascapular notch and less so at the spinoglenoid notch [76].

Diagnosis is confirmed by EMG and MRI scan can provide guidance as to the potential cause of the compression, particularly if there is a ganglion cyst encroaching into the suprascapular notch. Evidence of disease located at the suprascapular notch should be treated by decompression of the suprascapular notch whether via an open or arthroscopic approach. Should symptoms and tests that suggest that the site of the pathology to be at the spinoglenoid notch then these only need treatment if there are MRI signs of a ganglion causing compression. Symptoms without the presence of a ganglion often recover completely without surgery [75, 77].

Quadrangular Space Syndrome

A much less common presentation of nerve entrapment around the shoulder is quadrangular space syndrome. The quadrangular space is an anatomical aperture made up of the teres minor muscle superiorly, the teres major muscle inferiorly, the humeral shaft laterally and the long head of the triceps medially. The aperture allows for the passage of the axillary nerve and the posterior humeral circumflex artery (PHCA). Both of these structures are prone to compression by fibrous bands that most commonly develop secondary to repetitive trauma or by space-occupying lesions such as ganglions or rarely tumours. It may occasionally result from a single episode of trauma. The condition was first described by Cahill and Palmer, referring to patients who complained of pain that was poorly localised around the shoulder, who had well-localised tenderness over the quadrangular space and who had non-dermatomal paraesthesia on clinical examination [53]. Deltoid weakness and reduced shoulder abduction may be present [54]. Diagnosis is confirmed with an arteriogram performed with the arm abducted that demonstrates compression of the PHCA.

Physiotherapy is recommended and surgical decompression is reserved for those with persistent and intrusive symptoms. The space is exposed via a posterior approach with retraction of the deltoid muscle, long head of the biceps and teres minor muscle. A fascia between the teres muscles is divided to expose the axillary nerve and the vascular bundle. Any visible fibrous bands are divided and a neurolysis of the axillary nerve is performed [54].

Long Thoracic Nerve Entrapment

The long thoracic nerve (LTN) is responsible for innervating the serratus anterior muscle, which is a key stabiliser of the scapula. Apart from the serratus anterior, other key muscles that contribute to this stabilisation include the rhomboids and the trapezius. This control of the scapula on the ribcage is essential in the complex dynamics needed for a good shoulder range of movement. Dysfunction of the scapulothoracic stabiliser muscle results in the clinical sign of winging of the scapula. Weakness related to LTN dysfunction results in medial translation of the scapula along with rotation of the inferior angle of the scapula towards the midline.

The LTN takes its origin from the C5, C6 and C7 nerve roots. The nerve follows the brachial plexus lying just posterior to it as it passes from the neck into the axilla. The C5 and C6 contributions typically pass through the scalenus medius muscle (which is a potential entrapment point) and form an upper trunk while the C7 contribution passes around the scalenus muscles and joins the upper trunk near the axilla [78]. From the axilla, the nerve courses down the chest wall slightly posterior to the mid-axillary line, lying superficial to the serratus anterior, but deep to a fascial layer. This final part of the nerve path can be as long as 22–24 cm.

Dysfunction of the LTN results in a spectrum of symptoms ranging from cosmetic concern of the prominent scapula through to varying degrees of restriction of shoulder movement. Pain can be problematic and it is usually localised to the medial scapular border. In addition, patients may complain of symptoms which are in fact due to secondary shoulder impingement.

Multiple potential nerve entrapment points have been described, including scalenus medius muscle [79], a fascial band from the inferior brachial plexus [80], and tributary from the thoracodorsal vessel (so-called crow's foot lesion) [81, 82]. Other authors had proposed that the angulation of the LTN over the second rib [79, 83], and repetitive stretching of the nerve between the fixed points of the scalenus medius and serratus anterior to be the cause of nerve palsy [84]. Due to its relatively superficial location and long path, the nerve is vulnerable to direct trauma, sporting injuries, and even the use of crutches [85, 86]. It is also at risk of iatrogenous injury from any thoracic or axillary surgeries [87].

EMG by a skilled neurophysiologist is essential in the diagnosis of LTN palsy. Advanced imaging with MR neurography may allow visualisation of the involved nerve. The major differential diagnoses of entrapment neuropathy include neuralgic amyotrophy and myopathic disorders. In clinical practice, the distinction may not always be obvious. As such, involvement of a neurologist in the overall management is recommended.

A trial period of conservative treatment with physiotherapy is recommended. In those with persistent nerve palsy (beyond 9–12 months), exploration of the LTN may be considered. Neurolysis of the LTN may be performed at the supraclavicular region [88–90] or at the thoracic part [82, 91] or combined [92–94]. Nerve transfers using donor fascicles from medial pectoral nerve or thoracodorsal nerve have also been utilised with encouraging results [92–95]. If there is persistent scapular winging following nerve surgery, transfer of the sternal head of the pectoralis major tendon to the inferior angle of the scapula can be considered [96, 97].

Tumours

Peripheral nerve tumours are rare but may present within the brachial plexus or terminal branches. Many are asymptomatic but large tumours or tumours located at anatomical constriction points may cause nerve compression resulting in pain, weakness and sometimes sensory symptoms. Extra-neural tumours may also present in a similar way with symptoms attributable to nerve compression. Large atypical lipomata may track along the brachial plexus posterior to the clavicle and restrict shoulder movement. These rare presentations may mimic cuff pathology and impingement [98].

The main consideration for the shoulder surgeon is to consider this rare diagnosis when the clinical presentation is atypical. Swelling in the posterior triangle, supraclavicular or infraclavicular fossae, palpable masses or the presence of Tinel's sign over the brachial plexus should prompt further investigation with imaging of the brachial plexus and its branches.

Conclusion

The intimate anatomical relationship of nerves around the shoulder girdle and the multitude of potential pathologies present a unique challenge to the healthcare professional when a nerve palsy occurs. Trauma to the shoulder girdle may cause insult to the nerves, in addition to fractures and ligamentous injuries. The advent of arthroscopy, the maturing of arthroplasty and the increasing trend towards internal fixation of fractures over the last few decades have also seen the rise in iatrogenous nerve injuries. Other than external injury, there are also a number of potential points of abnormal compression of nerves around the shoulder which may present with a variety of symptoms. Identifying the site of compression requires directed history taking and examination as well as carefully selected investigations. In addition, neuromuscular conditions may manifest as shoulder complaints thus presenting initially to the shoulder clinic. The potential complexity of the condition demands a sound understanding of anatomy and a systematic approach to establishing the aetiology and localisation of a nerve palsy. With increasing subspecialisation of surgical training, effective inter-specialty communication becomes ever more important. The optimal management of a nerve palsy around the shoulder girdle may thus require close collaboration of shoulder surgeon, peripheral nerve surgeon, neurologist, neurophysiologist, radiologist and physiotherapist.

References

1. Kihlström C, Möller M, Lönn K, Wolf O. Clavicle fractures: epidemiology, classification and treatment of 2 422 fractures in the Swedish Fracture Register; an observational study. BMC Musculoskelet Disord. 2017;18(1):82. https://doi.org/10.1186/s12891-017-1444-1.
2. Robinson CM. Fractures of the clavicle in the adult: epidemiology and classification. J Bone Jt Surg. 1998;80(3):476–84. https://doi.org/10.1302/0301-620X.80B3.8079.
3. Rumball KM, Da Silva VF, Preston DNCC. Brachial-plexus injury after clavicular fracture: case-report and literature review. Can J Surg. 1991;34:264–6.
4. Barbier O, Malghem J, Delaere O, Vande Berg B, Rombouts JJ. Injury to the brachial plexus by a fragment of bone after fracture of the clavicle. J Bone Joint Surg Br. 1997;79(4):534–6. https://doi.org/10.1302/0301-620X.79B4.7552.
5. Lin C-C, Lin J. Brachial plexus palsy caused by secondary fracture displacement in a patient with closed clavicle fracture. Orthopedics. 2009;32(10):769–71. https://doi.org/10.3928/01477447-20090818-24.
6. Canadian Orthopaedic Trauma Society. Nonoperative treatment compared with plate fixation of displaced midshaft clavicular fractures. A multicenter, randomized clinical trial. J Bone Joint Surg Am. 2007;89(1):1–10. https://doi.org/10.2106/JBJS.F.00020.
7. Wang L, Ang M, Lee KT, Naidu G, Kwek E. Cutaneous hypoesthesia following plate fixation in clavicle fractures. Indian J Orthop. 2014;48(1):10–3. https://doi.org/10.4103/0019-5413.125478.
8. Beirer M, Postl L, Crönlein M, et al. Does a minimal invasive approach reduce anterior chest wall numbness and postoperative pain in plate fixation of clavicle fractures? BMC Musculoskelet Disord. 2015;16(1):128. https://doi.org/10.1186/s12891-015-0592-4.
9. Lo EY, Eastman J, Tseng S, Lee MA, Yoo BJ. Neurovascular risks of anteroinferior clavicular plating. Orthopedics. 2010;33(1):21. https://doi.org/10.3928/01477447-20091124-09.
10. Galley IJ, Watts AC, Bain GI. The anatomic relationship of the axillary artery and vein to the clavicle: a cadaveric study. J Shoulder Elb Surg. 2009;18(5) https://doi.org/10.1016/j.jse.2009.01.021.
11. Sinha A, Edwin J, Sreeharsha B, Bhalaik V, Brownson P. A radiological study to define safe zones for drilling during plating of clavicle fractures. Bone Joint J. 2011;93-B(9):1247–52. https://doi.org/10.1302/0301-620X.93B9.25739.
12. Jeyaseelan L, Singh VK, Ghosh S, Sinisi M, Fox M. Iatropathic brachial plexus injury: A complication of delayed fixation of clavicle fractures. Bone Joint J. 2013;95-B(1):106–10. https://doi.org/10.1302/0301-620X.95B1.29625.
13. Ring D, Holovacs T. Brachial plexus palsy after intramedullary fixation of a clavicular fracture. A report of three cases. J Bone Jt Surg Am. 2005;87(8):1834–7. https://doi.org/10.2106/JBJS.D.02919.
14. Miller DS, Boswick JA. Lesions of the brachial plexus associated with fractures of the clavicle. Clin Orthop Relat Res. 1969;64:144–9.
15. Della Santa D, Narakas A, Bonnard C. Late lesions of the brachial plexus after fracture of the clavicle. Ann Chir Main Memb Super. 1991;10(6):531–40. https://doi.org/10.1016/S0753-9053(05)80325-4.
16. Jupiter JB, Leffert RD. Non-union of the clavicle. Associated complications and surgical management. J Bone Joint Surg Am. 1987;69(5):753–60. http://www.ncbi.nlm.nih.gov/pubmed/3597476
17. Hansky B, Murray E, Minami K, Korfer R. Delayed brachial plexus paralysis due to subclavian pseudoaneurysm after clavicular fracture. Eur J Cardiothorac Surg. 1993;7(9):497–8.
18. Clitherow HD, Bain GI. Major neurovascular complications of clavicle fracture surgery. Shoulder Elb. 2015;7(1):3–12. https://doi.org/10.1177/1758573214546058.
19. Atef A, El-Tantawy A, Gad H, Hefeda M. Prevalence of associated injuries after anterior shoulder dislocation: a prospective study. Int Orthop. 2016;40(3):519–24. https://doi.org/10.1007/s00264-015-2862-z.

20. Visser CP, Coene LN, Brand R, Tavy DL. The incidence of nerve injury in anterior dislocation of the shoulder and its influence on functional recovery. A prospective clinical and EMG study. J Bone Joint Surg Br. 1999;81(4):679–85. https://doi.org/10.1302/0301-620X.81B4.9005.
21. te Slaa RL, Wijffels MPJM, Brand R, Marti RK. The prognosis following acute primary glenohumeral dislocation. J Bone Jt Surg Br. 2004;86(1):58–64. https://doi.org/10.1302/0301-620X.86B1.13695.
22. Gumina S, Postacchini F. Anterior dislocation of the shoulder in elderly patients. J Bone Joint Surg Br. 1997;79(4):540–3. http://www.ncbi.nlm.nih.gov/pubmed/9250734
23. Hems TEJ, Mahmood F. Injuries of the terminal branches of the infraclavicular brachial plexus patterns of injury, management and outcome. J Bone Joint Surg Br. 2012;94-B(6):799–804. https://doi.org/10.1302/0301-620X.94B6.28286.
24. Toolanen G, Hildingsson C, Hedlund T, Knibestol M, Oberg L. Early complications after anterior dislocation of the shoulder in patients over 40 years. An ultrasonographic and electromyographic study. Acta Orthop Scand. 1993;64(5):549–52. http://www.ncbi.nlm.nih.gov/pubmed/8237322
25. Kosiyatrakul A, Jitprapaikulsarn S, Durand S, Oberlin C. Recovery of brachial plexus injury after shoulder dislocation. Injury. 2009;40(12):1327–9. https://doi.org/10.1016/j.injury.2009.05.015.
26. Mikami Y, Nagano A, Ochiai N, Yamamoto S. Results of nerve grafting for injuries of the axillary and suprascapular nerves. J Bone Joint Surg Br. 1997;79(4):527–31. https://doi.org/10.1302/0301-620X.79B4.7481.
27. Bonnard C, Anastakis DJ, Narakas AO. Isolated and combined lesions of the axillary nerve: A review of 146 cases. J Hand Surg Eur Vol. 1997;22(1 suppl):38. https://doi.org/10.1016/S0266-7681(97)80245-8.
28. Okazaki M, Al-Shawi A, Gschwind CR, Warwick DJ, Tonkin MA. Outcome of axillary nerve injuries treated with nerve grafts. J Hand Surg Eur Vol. 2011;36(7):535–40. https://doi.org/10.1177/1753193411406477.
29. Leechavengvongs S, Witoonchart K, Uerpairojkit C, Thuvasethakul P. Nerve transfer to deltoid muscle using the nerve to the long head of the triceps, part II: a report of 7 cases. J Hand Surg Am. 2003;28(4):633–8. https://doi.org/10.1016/S0363-5023(03)00199-0.
30. Wolfe SW, Johnsen PH, Lee SK, Feinberg JH. Long-nerve grafts and nerve transfers demonstrate comparable outcomes for axillary nerve injuries. J Hand Surg Am. 2014;39(7):1351–7. https://doi.org/10.1016/j.jhsa.2014.02.032.
31. Kircher MF, Shin AY. A comparison of outcomes of triceps motor branch–to–axillary nerve transfer or sural nerve interpositional grafting for isolated axillary nerve injury. Plast Reconstr Surg. 2016:256–64. https://doi.org/10.1097/PRS.0000000000002368.
32. Oberlin C, Béal D, Leechavengvongs S, Salon A, Dauge MC, Sarcy JJ. Nerve transfer to biceps muscle using a part of ulnar nerve for C5–C6 avulsion of the brachial plexus: Anatomical study and report of four cases. J Hand Surg Am. 1994;19(2):232–7. https://doi.org/10.1016/0363-5023(94)90011-6.
33. Davidge KM, Yee A, Kahn LC, Mackinnon SE. Median to radial nerve transfers for restoration of wrist, finger, and thumb extension. J Hand Surg Am. 2013;38(9):1812–27. https://doi.org/10.1016/j.jhsa.2013.06.024.
34. Carofino BC, Brogan DM, Elhassan BT, Bishop AT, Spinner RJ, Shin AY. Iatrogenic nerve injuries during shoulder surgery: a series of 27 cases. J Hand Surg Am. 2011;36:6. https://doi.org/10.1016/S0363-5023(11)60006-3.
35. Marecek GS, Saltzman MD. Complications in shoulder arthroscopy. Orthopedics. 2010;33(7):492–7. https://doi.org/10.3928/01477447-20100526-15.
36. Boardman ND, Cofield RH. Neurologic complications of shoulder surgery. Clin Orthop Relat Res. 1999;368:44–53. http://www.ncbi.nlm.nih.gov/pubmed/10613152
37. Nagda SH, Rogers KJ, Sestokas AK, et al. Neer Award 2005: peripheral nerve function during shoulder arthroplasty using intraoperative nerve monitoring. J Shoulder Elb Surg. 2007;16(3 suppl) https://doi.org/10.1016/j.jse.2006.01.016.
38. Meyer M, Graveleau N, Hardy P, Landreau P. Anatomic risks of shoulder arthroscopy portals: anatomic cadaveric study of 12 portals. Arthroscopy. 2007;23(5):529–36. https://doi.org/10.1016/j.arthro.2006.12.022.
39. Boutsiadis A, Baverel L, Lenoir H, Delsol P, Barth J. Arthroscopic-assisted acromioclavicular and coracoclavicular ligaments reconstruction for chronic acromioclavicular dislocations: Surgical technique. Tech Hand Up Extrem Surg. 2016;20(4):172–8. https://doi.org/10.1097/BTH.0000000000000142.
40. Flinkkilä T, Heikkilä A, Sirniö K, Pakarinen H. TightRope versus clavicular hook plate fixation for unstable distal clavicular fractures. Eur J Orthop Surg Traumatol. 2015;25(3):465–9. https://doi.org/10.1007/s00590-014-1526-9.
41. Yamakado K. Quantification of the learning curve for arthroscopic suprascapular nerve decompression: An evaluation of 300 cases. Arthroscopy. 2015;31(2):191–6. https://doi.org/10.1016/j.arthro.2014.08.029.
42. Freehill MT, Srikumaran U, Archer KR, McFarland EG, Petersen SA. The Latarjet coracoid process transfer procedure: alterations in the neurovascular structures. J Shoulder Elb Surg. 2013;22(5):695–700. https://doi.org/10.1016/j.jse.2012.06.003.
43. Athwal GS, Meislin R, Getz C, Weinstein D, Favorito P. Short-term complications of the arthroscopic latarjet procedure: a North American experience. Arthroscopy. 2016;32(10):1965–70. https://doi.org/10.1016/j.arthro.2016.02.022.
44. Kim DH, Cho Y-J, Tiel RL, Kline DG. Surgical outcomes of 111 spinal accessory nerve injuries. Neurosurgery. 2003;53(5):1106–13. https://doi.org/10.1227/01.NEU.0000089058.82201.3D.

45. Camp SJ, Birch R. Injuries to the spinal accessory nerve: a lesson to surgeons. J Bone Joint Surg Br. 2011;93(1):62–7. https://doi.org/10.1302/0301-620X.93B1.24202.
46. Park SH, Esquenazi Y, Kline DG, Kim DH. Surgical outcomes of 156 spinal accessory nerve injuries caused by lymph node biopsy procedures. J Neurosurg Spine. 2015;23(4):518–25. https://doi.org/10.3171/2014.12.SPINE14968.
47. Chan PK, Hems TE. Clinical signs of accessory nerve palsy. J Trauma. 2006;60(5):1142–4. https://doi.org/10.1097/01.ta.0000174718.83440.75.
48. Maldonado Andres A, Spinner RJ. Lateral pectoral nerve transfer for spinal accesory injury. J Neurosurg Spine. 2017;26:112–5. https://doi.org/10.3171/2016.5.SPINE151458.
49. Elhassan BT, Wagner ER. Outcome of triple-tendon transfer, an Eden-Lange variant, to reconstruct trapezius paralysis. J Shoulder Elb Surg. 2015;24(8):1307–13. https://doi.org/10.1016/j.jse.2015.01.008.
50. Borgeat A, Ekatodramis G, Kalberer F, Benz C. Acute and nonacute complications associated with interscalene block and shoulder surgery: a prospective study. Anesthesiology. 2001;95(4):875–80. https://doi.org/10.1097/00000542-200110000-00015.
51. Fredrickson MJ, Kilfoyle DH. Neurological complication analysis of 1000 ultrasound guided peripheral nerve blocks for elective orthopaedic surgery: a prospective study. Anaesthesia. 2009;64(8):836–44. https://doi.org/10.1111/j.1365-2044.2009.05938.x.
52. Jeng CL, Torrillo TM, Rosenblatt MA. Complications of peripheral nerve blocks. Br J Anaesth. 2010;105(Suppl(3)):i97–107. https://doi.org/10.1093/bja/aeq273.
53. Bruce BG, Green A, Blaine TA, Wesner LV. Brachial plexus blocks for upper extremity orthopaedic surgery. J Am Acad Orthop Surg. 2012;20(1):38–47. https://doi.org/10.5435/jaaos-20-01-038.
54. Benumof JL. Permanent loss of cervical spinal cord function associated with interscalene block performed under general anesthesia. Anesthesiology. 2000;93(6):1541–4.
55. Parsonage MJ, Turner JW. Neuralgic amyotrophy; the shoulder-girdle syndrome. Lancet. 1948;1(6513):973–8.
56. Turner JW, Parsonage MJ. Neuralgic amyotrophy (paralytic brachial neuritis); with special reference to prognosis. Lancet. 1957;273(6988):209–12.
57. Van Alfen N, Van Engelen BGM. The clinical spectrum of neuralgic amyotrophy in 246 cases. Brain. 2006;129(2):438–50. https://doi.org/10.1093/brain/awh722.
58. van Alfen N, van der Werf SP, van Engelen BG. Long-term pain, fatigue, and impairment in neuralgic amyotrophy. Arch Phys Med Rehabil. 2009;90(3):435–9. https://doi.org/10.1016/j.apmr.2008.08.216.
59. Clarke CJ, Torrance E, McIntosh J, Funk L. Neuralgic amyotrophy is not the most common neurologic disorder of the shoulder: a 78-month prospective study of 60 neurologic shoulder patients in a specialist shoulder clinic. J Shoulder Elb Surg. 2016;25(12):1997–2004. https://doi.org/10.1016/j.jse.2016.04.005.
60. Pan Y, Wang S, Zheng D, et al. Hourglass-like constrictions of peripheral nerve in the upper extremity: a clinical review and pathological study. Neurosurgery. 2014;75(1):10–22. https://doi.org/10.1227/NEU.0000000000000350.
61. Nakashima Y, Sunagawa T, Shinomiya R, Ochi M. High-resolution ultrasonographic evaluation of "hourglass-like fascicular constriction" in peripheral nerves: a preliminary report. Ultrasound Med Biol. 2014;40(7):1718–21. https://doi.org/10.1016/j.ultrasmedbio.2013.12.011.
62. Wu P, Yang JY, Chen L, Yu C. Surgical and conservative treatments of complete spontaneous posterior interosseous nerve palsy with hourglass-like fascicular constrictions: a retrospective study of 41 cases. Neurosurgery. 2014;75(3):250–7. https://doi.org/10.1227/NEU.0000000000000424.
63. Van Alfen N, Van Engelen BGM, Hughes RAC. Treatment for idiopathic and hereditary neuralgic amyotrophy (brachial neuritis). Cochrane Database Syst Rev. 2009;3 https://doi.org/10.1002/14651858.CD006976.pub2.
64. Thompson RW, Driskill M. Thoracic outlet syndrome: neurogenic. In: Cronenwett J, Johnston K, editors. Rutherford's vascular surgery. 7th ed. Philadelphia: Elsevier; 2010. p. 1878–98.
65. Novak CB, Mackinnon SE, Patterson GA. Evaluation of patients with thoracic outlet syndrome. J Hand Surg Am. 1993;18(2):292–9. https://doi.org/10.1016/0363-5023(93)90364-9.
66. Ellison DW, Wood VE. Trauma-related thoracic outlet syndrome. J Hand Surg Br. 1994;19(4):424–6.
67. Barton N, Hooper G, Noble J, Steel W. Occupational causes of disorders in the upper limb. BMJ. 1992;304(6822):309–11.
68. Seror P. Medial antebrachial cutaneous nerve conduction study, a new tool to demonstrate mild lower brachial plexus lesions. A report of 16 cases. Clin Neurophysiol. 2004;115(10):2316–22. https://doi.org/10.1016/j.clinph.2004.04.023.
69. Novak CB, Collins ED, Mackinnon SE. Outcome following conservative management of thoracic outlet syndrome. J Hand Surg. 1995;20A(4):542–8. https://doi.org/10.1016/S0363-5023(96)80388-1.
70. Novak CB. Conservative management of thoracic outlet syndrome. Semin Thorac Cardiovasc Surg. 1996;8(2):201–7. http://www.ncbi.nlm.nih.gov/pubmed/8672574
71. Leffert RD. Complications of surgery for thoracic outlet syndrome. Hand Clin. 2004;20(1):91–8. https://doi.org/10.1016/S0749-0712(03)00084-2.
72. Vemuri C, Wittenberg AM, Caputo FJ, et al. Early effectiveness of isolated pectoralis minor tenotomy in selected patients with neurogenic thoracic outlet syndrome. J Vasc Surg. 2013;57(5):1345–52. https://doi.org/10.1016/j.jvs.2012.11.045.

73. Ganzhorn R, Hocker J, Horowitz M, Switzer H. Suprascapular-nerve entrapment. J Bone Jt Surg Am. 1981;63(3):492–4.
74. Fehrman DA, Orwin JF, Jennings RM. Suprascapular nerve entrapment by ganglion cysts: a report of six cases with arthroscopic findings and review of the literature. Arthroscopy. 1995;11(6):727–34. https://doi.org/10.1016/0749-8063(95)90118-3.
75. Ferretti A, De Carli A, Fontana M. Injury of the suprascapular nerve at the spinoglenoid notch. The natural history of infraspinatus atrophy in volleyball players. Am J Sports Med. 1998;26(6):759–63. https://doi.org/10.1177/03635465980260060401.
76. Kiss G, Komar J. Suprascapular nerve compression at the spinoglenoid notch. Muscle Nerve. 1990;13(6):556–7. https://doi.org/10.1002/mus.880130614.
77. Steiman I. Painless infraspinatus atrophy due to suprascapular nerve entrapment. Arch Phys Med Rehabil. 1988;69(8):641–3.
78. Bertelli JA, Ghizoni MF. Long thoracic nerve: anatomy and functional assessment. J Bone Joint Surg Am. 2005;87(5):993–8. https://doi.org/10.2106/JBJS.D.02383.
79. Horwitz MT, Tocantins LM. An anatomical study of the role of the long thoracic nerve and the related scapular bursae in the pathogenesis of local paralysis of the serratus anterior muscle. Anat Rec. 1938;71(4):375–85.
80. Hester P, Caborn DNM, Nyland J. Cause of long thoracic nerve palsy: a possible dynamic fascial sling cause. J Shoulder Elb Surg. 2000;9(1):31–5. https://doi.org/10.1016/S1058-2746(00)90007-7.
81. Cuadros CL, Driscoll CL, Rothkopf DM. The anatomy of the lower serratus anterior muscle: a fresh cadaver study. Plast Reconstr Surg. 1995;95(1):93–7.
82. Maire N, Abane L, Kempf JF, Clavert P. Long thoracic nerve release for scapular winging: clinical study of a continuous series of eight patients. Orthop Traumatol Surg Res. 2013;99(6 suppl) https://doi.org/10.1016/j.otsr.2013.07.010.
83. Warner JJ, Navarro RA. Serratus anterior dysfunction. Recognition and treatment. Clin Orthop Relat Res. 1998;349:139–48.
84. Hamada J, Igarashi E, Akita K, Mochizuki T. A cadaveric study of the serratus anterior muscle and the long thoracic nerve. J Shoulder Elb Surg. 2008;17(5):790–4. https://doi.org/10.1016/j.jse.2008.02.009.
85. Wiater JM, Flatow EL. Long thoracic nerve injury. Clin Orthop Relat Res. 1999;368:17–27. https://doi.org/10.1097/00003086-199911000-00004.
86. Murphy MT, Journeaux SF. Long thoracic nerve palsy after using a single axillary crutch. Clin Orthop Relat Res. 2006;447:267–9. https://doi.org/10.1097/01.blo.0000205880.27964.a3.
87. Kauppila LI, Vastamäki M. Iatrogenic serratus anterior paralysis: long-term outcome in 26 patients. Chest. 1996;109(1):31–4.
88. Disa JJ, Wang B, Dellon AL. Correction of scapular winging by supraclavicular neurolysis of the long thoracic nerve. J Reconstr Microsurg. 2001;17(2):79–84. http://www.ncbi.nlm.nih.gov/pubmed/11310753
89. Nath RK, Lyons AB, Bietz G. Microneurolysis and decompression of long thoracic nerve injury are effective in reversing scapular winging: long-term results in 50 cases. BMC Musculoskelet Disord. 2007;8 https://doi.org/10.1186/1471-2474-8-25.
90. Schippert DW, Li Z. Supraclavicular long thoracic nerve decompression for traumatic scapular winging. J Surg Orthop Adv. 2013;22(3):219–23.
91. Le Nail LR, Bacle G, Marteau E, Corcia P, Favard L, Laulan J. Isolated paralysis of the serratus anterior muscle: surgical release of the distal segment of the long thoracic nerve in 52 patients. Orthop Traumatol Surg Res. 2014;100(4S) https://doi.org/10.1016/j.otsr.2014.03.004.
92. Tomaino MM. Neurophysiologic and clinical outcome following medial pectoral to long thoracic nerve transfer for scapular winging: a case report. Microsurgery. 2002;22(6):254–7. https://doi.org/10.1002/micr.10046.
93. Ray WZ, Pet MA, Nicoson MC, Yee A, Kahn LC, Mackinnon SE. Two-level motor nerve transfer for the treatment of long thoracic nerve palsy. J Neurosurg. 2011;115(4):858–64. https://doi.org/10.3171/2011.5.JNS101615.
94. Noland SS, Krauss EM, Felder JM, Mackinnon SE. Surgical and clinical decision making in isolated long thoracic nerve palsy. Hand (N Y). 2017. https://doi.org/10.1177/1558944717733306.
95. Novak CB, Mackinnon SE. Surgical treatment of a long thoracic nerve palsy. Ann Thorac Surg. 2002;73(5):1643–5. https://doi.org/10.1016/S0003-4975(01)03372-0.
96. Elhassan B. Pectoralis major transfer for the management of scapula winging secondary to serratus anterior injury or paralysis. J Hand Surg Am. 2014;39(2):353–61. https://doi.org/10.1016/j.jhsa.2013.11.016.
97. Elhassan BT, Wagner ER. Outcome of transfer of the sternal head of the pectoralis major with its bone insertion to the scapula to manage scapular winging. J Shoulder Elb Surg. 2015;24(5):733–40. https://doi.org/10.1016/j.jse.2014.08.022.
98. Graf A, Yang K, King D, Dzwierzynski W, Sanger J, Hettinger P. Lipomas of the brachial plexus: a case series and review of the literature. Hand (N Y). 2017. https://doi.org/10.1177/1558944717735946. [Epub ahead of print].

Tumours of the Shoulder

32

Roger M. Tillman and Scott Evans

In general, the upper limb is involved by bone and soft-tissue neoplasms one-third as often as the lower limb. Despite this, the shoulder remains a common site for primary bone sarcomas as well as metastatic disease. Loss of function in the upper limb affects the ability of the patient to remain self-caring, and any improvement in function may therefore provide significant overall cost-benefit to the community despite the initial cost of surgery and implants.

Primary bone sarcomas, including Ewing's sarcoma and osteosarcoma predominantly in children and adolescents, and chondrosarcoma in adults, commonly affect the proximal humerus and scapula. Upper limb soft-tissue sarcomas also tend to have a propensity for the shoulder girdle. The complex anatomy of the shoulder normal girdle affords the patient a remarkable degree of freedom of movement, however it can raise site-specific issues related to surgery in this area, particularly in relation to preserving stability.

Forequarter amputation was the standard surgical treatment modality for bone sarcomas affecting the shoulder girdle up until the mid to late 20th century. Over the past 30 years limb salvage surgery for mailignant tumours has become more commonplace. This is due principally to improvements in cross-sectional imaging, which allows a more detailed assessment of the relationship between the tumour and the adjacent neurovascular structures. Furthermore, there have been significant advances in surgical technique and implant design such that forequarter amputation is now only rarely required.

The resection and reconstruction of tumours of the shoulder girdle consists of three basic components:

1. Surgical resection of the tumour following oncological principles.
2. Reconstruction of the skeletal defect.
3. Soft-Tissue Reconstruction

The goal of all shoulder girdle resections is to excise the tumour with a safe or acceptable surgical margin, whilst providing a stable shoulder to preserve as much function as possible, both to the shoulder itself, and the upper limb in general. Preservation of the neurovascular structures (if possible whilst still maintaining surgical margins) is therefore a primary concern. Forearm and hand function in particular are critically important in enabling independent living.

The aim of this chapter is to provide an overview of the surgical options of reconstruction of the shoulder girdle after tumour resection.

R. M. Tillman, FRCS, FRCS Orth (✉)
S. Evans, FRCS, FRCS Orth
Consultant Orthopaedic Oncologist, ROH, Birmingham, UK
e-mail: roger.tillman@nhs.net

I. A. Trail et al. (eds.), *Textbook of Shoulder Surgery*, https://doi.org/10.1007/978-3-319-70099-1_32

Anatomic Considerations

The shoulder girdle and proximal humerus is a complex anatomical area that is closely related to vital neurovascular structures. It is important to be able to assess the proximity and involvement of key structures when assessing a patient with a bone sarcoma affecting the shoulder girdle to determine the feasibility of limb salvage surgery. The proximal humeral metaphysis is the usual site of involvement, with variable extension into the diaphysis and epiphysis. The epiphyseal growth plate can act as a barrier to tumour extension in the skeletally immature patient. The shoulder joint relies almost entirely on the soft tissues for stability. Unlike the hip joint, the glenoid socket is shallow and the rotator cuff and deltoid contain the humeral head but the ligaments and muscles may be resected during tumour surgery to achieve adequate margins. Reconstruction is possible, but wound healing and proximal migration of the retained femoral head are issues.

If a wide surgical resection can be obtained safely, whilst maintaining the major neurovascular structures, the patient should be spared an amputation. Even if one of the major nerves must be resected, the patient can often retain significant function, particularly if the remainder of the limb is normal.

Pre-operative Evaluation

A careful history and detailed physical examination are important means of assessing a patient with a potential neoplastic disease affecting the shoulder girdle. Most patients will present with non-mechanical pain, which is often associated with swelling. It is common for the range of motion of the shoulder to be adversely affected, particularly if the tumour has grown into the joint. The distal neurovascular function of the entire the limb should be assessed, especially the axillary, musculocutaneous and radial nerves as these are often involved the most.

Plain radiographs and MRI of the shoulder should be obtained. Chest radiographs, chest CT and whole body isotope bone scintigraphy should be part of routine distal staging.

A biopsy is important to determine a histopathological diagnosis and is crucial in the staging process. Biopsies can be performed open or percutaneously but should be in line with the planned definitive surgical approach. The deltopectoral incision, in all its modifications, is the workhorse approach to the proximal humerus and shoulder girdle. A biopsy of the proximal humerus can be incorporated within the deltopectoral groove thereby making resection of the biopsy tract during subsequent definitive surgery easier.

Biopsies of the scapula are more difficult than the humerus. A posteriorly based biopsy approach should be undertaken to obtain tissue for analysis and, as with any biopsy, it should be sited along the intended site of incision for resection. Surgeons must, therefore, be familiar with all extensile approaches involving the shoulder girdle in order to access the scapular, clavicle and chest wall.

Types of Resection

Today, 90% of patients with primary bone sarcomas can be treated with limb-sparing surgery. Indeed, nowadays the indications for resection of the proximal humerus can be extended to patients with metastatic carcinoma, in particular those with renal or thyroid carcinoma, who can expect good disease-free survival in isolated metastases.

General contraindications to resection include:

- Significant involvement of the neurovascular bundle. Patients with extensive metastatic disease either from a primary bone sarcoma or carcinoma
- Patients with a limited life span
- Patients in whom other, non-surgical modalities, such as radiotherapy, may be more appropriate, for example, metastatic carcinoma to the clavicle or scapula.

Fortunately most tumours of the proximal humerus are separated from the anterior vessles by the subscapularis and short head of biceps. The three major cords of the brachial plexus follow the brachial artery and vein. Therefore, in general, if the vessels are thought to be involved, it is also likely the brachial plexus is involved. It may be necessary to sacrifice branches of the brachial plexus to achieve an adequate resection margin. Axillary nerve resection is usually required if a partial or total scapular excision is to be performed. The musculocutaneous and radial nerves are rarely involved. Resection of the radial nerve creates a bigger functional deficit for patients than resection of the musculocutaneous nerve, but this is not an indication for amputation. A forequarter amputation or shoulder disarticulation should be considered if major functional loss or a close margin, with an increased risk of local recurrence, is anticipated from a limb sparing resection.

Pre-operative evaluation through clinical examination and appropriate cross-sectional imaging can determine if a tumour is involving the chest wall. A limb salvage procedure may still be possible even if the shoulder girdle tumour does involve the chest wall, however, the degree of chest wall resection, and the possible involvement of adjacent neurovascular structures, determine the requirement for amputation.

Resection Techniques

Limb-salvage surgery around the shoulder girdle is technically more demanding than a forequarter amputation. The surgical techniques for non-amputative resection of the shoulder girdle have evolved with time. This coincides with improvements in surgical understanding of the complexities of resection and subsequent reconstruction, along with advances in cancer care and survival in general. With regards to bone sarcomas in particular, all patients will be considered for neoadjuvant and adjuvant chemotherapy along recognized international protocols. The use of such chemotherapy regimes, along with other adjuvant modalities, such as, radiotherapy in certain, sensitive cases, has greatly improved patient's long-term survival.

Malawer (1991) [1] proposed a surgical classification system for tumour resections involving the shoulder girdle. The system has six categories:

Type 1: Intra-articular proximal humeral resection
Type 2: Partial scapular resection
Type 3: Intra-articular total scapulectomy
Type 4: Extra-articular total scapulectomy and humeral head resection
Type 5: Extra-articular humeral and glenoid resection
Type 6: Extra-articular humeral and total scapular resection

The six categories describe the bony segments that are resected during surgery. Each type is further sub-divided into A or B, where A indicates the abductor mechanism is preserved and B indicates the abductor mechanism is resected. In general, type A resections are intra-articular, and type B resections are extra-articular. The abductor mechanism is inevitably resected if there is extra-osseous extension of the tumour of the proximal humerus.

A variety of different incisions have been described and can be employed to access the shoulder girdle. In order to provide as much access as possible the arm, shoulder girdle, base of the neck, anterior chest wall to the midline, posterior chest wall to the midline and flank up to the iliac crests should be prepared and draped accordingly.

One has to be aware that tumour resections often require an extensile approach. The utilitarian, extensile incision to access all of the shoulder girdle begins posteriorly, just inferior to the tip of the scapula, and ascends proximally over the scapula towards the acromion and then descends distally along the deltopectoral groove. If required, horizontal limbs can be added to this workhorse incision to access the medial clavicle or axilla. Large fasciocutaneous flaps are raised after performing the desired skin incision.

The type of resection required will dictate if all or part of this approach is necessary.

The anterior component of the incision is used if a tumour needs to be resected from the proximal humerus, proximal arm or axilla. The main neurovascular bundle of the upper limb needs to be adequately exposed and protected. The pectoralis major should be tagged, reflected from its humeral insertion and retracted medially. The coracoid origin of the conjoined tendon (short head of biceps and coracobrachialis) and the insertion of the pectoralis minor may also need to tagged and reflected. The deltoid may also need to elevated from its insertion and the rotator cuff may or may not be spared depending on whether the resection is intra- or extra-articular. The posterior part of the utilitarian incision is used for resections involving the scapula.

Type I Resection

An intra-articular resection of the proximal humerus is known as a Type I resection. This is the resection of choice for primary tumours involving the proximal humerus that have not invaded the shoulder joint and for metastatic tumours with extensive destruction. If the abductor mechanism can be salvaged the resection is termed IA. However, it is not uncommon for most high-grade proximal humerus sarcomas to have an extra-osseous component that is directly beneath or in contact with the deltoid. If this is the case, all or part of the deltoid will have to be included with the resection (IB resection).

Type II Resection

An extra-articular resection of the scapula is known as a type II resection. The most common resection involves the scapula inferior to its spine. As sufficient scapula and shoulder musculature is often maintained, reasonable shoulder function can be retained without the need for reconstruction. It is usually performed for low-grade bony malignancies or for small high-grade lesions. A type II resection may also be used to resect a soft-tissue sarcoma that invades the medial scapula. Rarely a limited chest wall resection may be required to achieve a negative margin.

Type III

An intra-articular resection of the whole of the scapula is a type III resection. It is the resection of choice if the tumour involves so much of the scapula that a total scapulectomy is the only way to achieve adequate surgical clearance or if any retained part of the scapula would be nonfunctional. Soft-tissue sarcomas that invade the scapula and primary osseous malignancies that do not invade the glenohumeral joint are the main indications for a type III resection.

Type IV

An extra-articular resection of the scapula including the glenohumeral joint, humeral head and the distal end of the clavicle, is known as a type IV resection. Classically, this en-bloc resection is also known as a Tikhoff-Linberg procedure. The indications for this resection include any high–grade osseous sarcoma originating within the scapula that extends to within the glenohumeral joint or invades the rotator cuff. Invasive soft-tissue sarcomas may also require this type of resection.

Type V

An extra-articular resection of the humerus including the glenohumeral joint, part of the scapula and distal clavicle is known as a type V resection. The scapula resection involves a transection through the scapular neck, medial to the coracoid. This is best achieved with an oscillating saw and completed carefully with a sharp osteotome. The shoulder abductors and axillary nerve are frequently sacrificed.

Type VI

An extra-articular resection of the proximal humerus, entire scapula and distal clavicle is known as a type VI resection. It is an uncommon resection and is usually reserved for extensive sarcomas of the proximal humerus that traverse the shoulder joint and invade the scapula.

Reconstruction Following Resection

The level of resection performed determines the type of defect that requires reconstruction. Endoprostheses are more commonly used in the UK for limb reconstruction following resection of musculoskeletal malignancies. Biological reconstructions using allografts and allograft composites have also been described.

Flail

The easiest reconstructive option following resection is to leave the shoulder flail. The humerus is suspended from the axial skeleton by repairing the remaining musculature to the remaining clavicle and chest wall. Tenodesis techniques can be used to ensure adequate muscle envelope and soft tissue tension is achieved, for example, the coracobrachialis can be sutured to the remaining clavicle and the deltoid can be repaired to the trapezius and long head of biceps. It is usual for the upper limb to be supported in a sling for a number of weeks to ensure the soft tissues heal, whilst encouraging elbow, forearm and hand motion.

Allograft Reconstruction

This type of reconstruction offers a biological solution to the defect created by the resection and maybe more appropriate in younger patients. After careful scrutiny of the plain radiographs and cross-sectional imaging to determine the level of resection an appropriately sized humeral allograft is selected preoperatively. The allograft does not have to be an exact size match but poor anatomical matching of both size and shape between the graft and the defect can alter the joint kinematics and load distribution, leading to bone resorption or joint degeneration.

An allograft reconstruction offers the possibility of attaching the remaining soft tissue muscles directly to the graft. Osteoarticular allografts can be utilized to reconstruct one side of the joint, while maintaining the uninvolved side of the joint. Furthermore, following resection, the graft can be fashioned to allow maximal direct bone-to-bone contact between the graft and the remaining host bone. Once the proper rotation has been established the construct is fixed using a compression plate to promote suitable osteosynthesis. Biomechanical and biological complications can occur including graft fractures, graft resoprtion, cartilage degeneration, joint instability, and delayed or non-bone union.

A proximal humeral allograft prosthetic composite (APC) combines the standard osteoarticular allograft reconstruction with a humeral endoprosthesis. This can add some surgical difficulty but it eliminates the risk of surgical neck fracture and degeneration of articular cartilage seen with osteoarticular grafts. Most APCs combine a standard humeral endoprosthesis cemented into a humeral allograft, which is fixed to the host bone with a plate. Long stem humeral endoprostheses are also described using an intramedullary fixation method to fix the allogaft to the host bone. Reverse polarity arthroplasty can also be used in those patients whose rotator cuff has to be resected or in those patients little function from any remaining rotator cuff.

APC reconstruction is a complex and demanding procedure. It requires meticulous attention to detail in order to restore length, rotation, and soft-tissue tension, as well as to obtain satisfactory bone contact and adequate stability at the graft-host junction.

Endoprosthetic Replacement of the Proximal Humerus

An endoprosthetic replacement of the proximal humerus is the most common reconstruction method used following resection of proximal humeral tumours. Modular systems are readily available making reconstruction relatively straightforward, but custom implants are usually essential in skeletally immature patients and for short fixation segments where the resection level is distal, i.e. close to the elbow.

An anterior delto-pectoral approach is advised, and previous surgical scars should be excised if this is deemed necessary by the MDT. It is usually possible to preserve the cephalic vein which can be dissected free and retracted medially or laterally.

If the deltoid and rotator cuff muscles can be safely retained they should be sutured to the implant to maintain as much shoulder abduction as possible. A variety of synthetic, tubular mesh grafts can be applied to the implant and used to anchor sutures when reconstructing the muscular envelope around the endoprosthesis. Shoulder abduction will not be possible when the rotator cuff and deltoid are sacrificed with the resection. However, an endoprosthesis provides a means of suspending the upper limb from the remaining shoulder girdle and can provide a stable base to perform other upper limb movements. An endoprosthetic replacement also allows the maintenance of a relatively normal shoulder contour, a benefit that patients find aesthetic more acceptable than a flail limb.

The stability of the endoprosthesis is dependent upon humeral head size, correct component orientation and length, and the repair of the remaining soft tissues following resection. Obtaining a stable shoulder can be difficult when the rotator cuff and capsule have been resected. A synthetic mesh graft can be used to augment the repair. The proximal part of the graft is sutured to the remaining glenoid and the distal part is fashioned to envelope the endoprostheses with humeral head passing through the graft. The graft is anchored distally by suturing it onto itself. The remaining muscles can then be sutured directly to the graft to maintain as much function as possible and stabilize the joint. A muscle flap, such as latissimus dorsi, is suggested in cases where radical muscular resection is required, for example, if a total deltoid excision is required. Providing a healthy muscular cover for the endoprosthetic implant can reduce the risk of infection, maintain as much function as possible and improve stability.

Proximal migration of the femoral head can also be a problem where the deltoid has been largely resected and some loss of length in the humerus should be accepted to avoid this occurring, particularly in adults.

Expandable endoprosthetic replacements can be used in the very young. A general recommendation is to ensure as much length as possible is obtained at the time of initial implantation as subsequent lengthenings can be complicated by radial nerve palsy (rare) and shoulder instability (more frequent).

Improvements in component design and implantation technique have seen the development of components utilizing a reverse geometry proximal humeral reconstruction. The use of a reverse geometry implant has the theoretical advantage of improved function in those patients with severe rotatory cuff deficiency. Costs are greater, and the long term results of reverse shoulder implants in tumour surgery remain unclear. No convincing benefit from the use of reverse shoulder technology in tumours has yet been proven.

On rare occasions the upper limb may be salvaged even if the entire humerus needs to be resected. A total humeral endoprosthetic reconstruction requires a surgical technique that combines proximal and distal humeral resections. The author recommends an anterior delto-pectoral approach proximally and a posterior approach with triceps turn down distally. This gives the optimum exposure.

Endoprosthetic Replacement of the Scapula

A scapular prosthesis can be considered following a type III or IV resection if a significant proportion of the periscapular musculature remains after resection, in particular, the trapezius, deltoid, rhomboids and latissimus dorsi. The prosthesis aims to avoid the instability seen following a flail shoulder resection. In addition, implanting a scapular total shoulder endoprosthetic replacement can, in some cases, maintain a relatively normal shoulder contour. The arm, forearm and hand can act as more functional unit as the shoulder girdle is more stable with a scapular implant. Maximal strength and length of contracture can be maintained by preserving a more normal length.

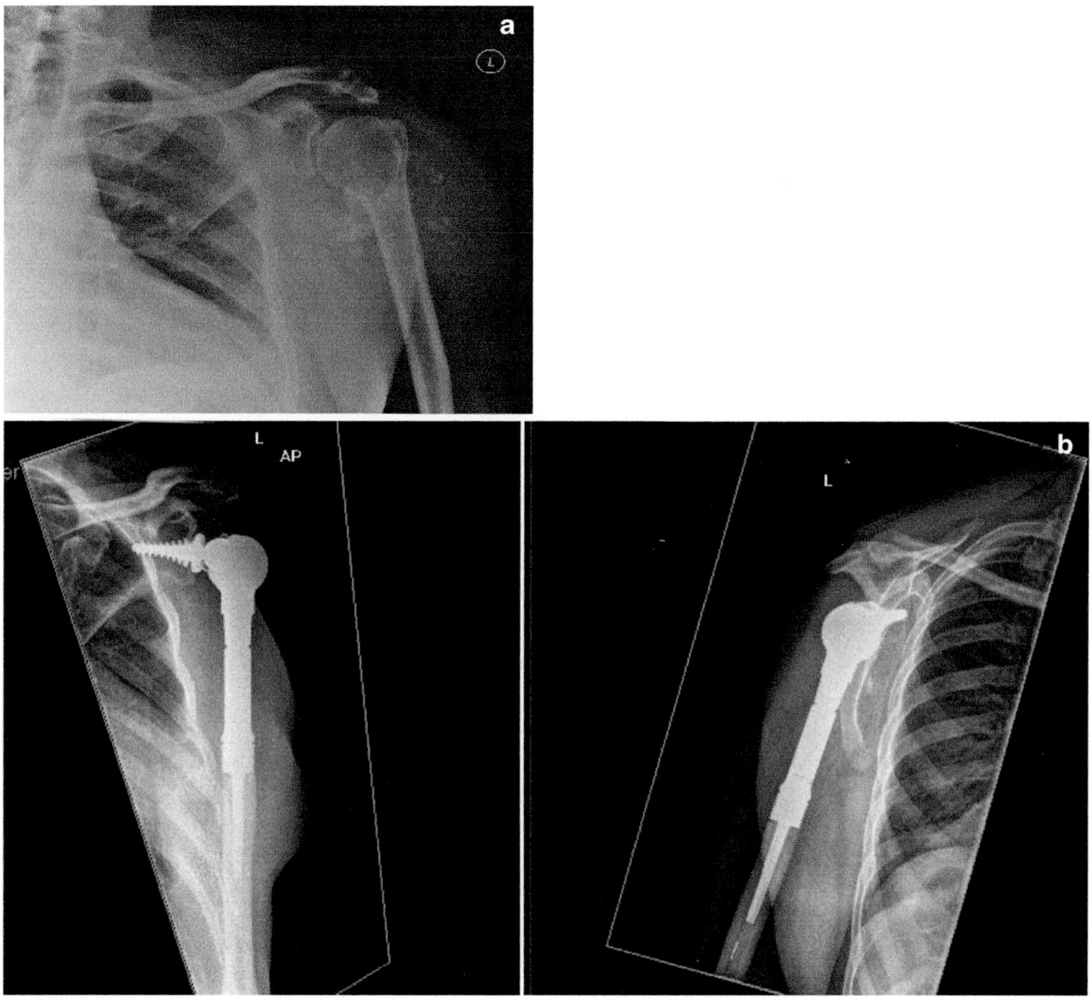

Fig. 32.1 (**a**) Pre-op. LEFT proximal humerus, high grade chondrosarcoma. (**b**) Post-operative reconstruction, modular endoprosthesis with Bailey-Walker total joint replacement

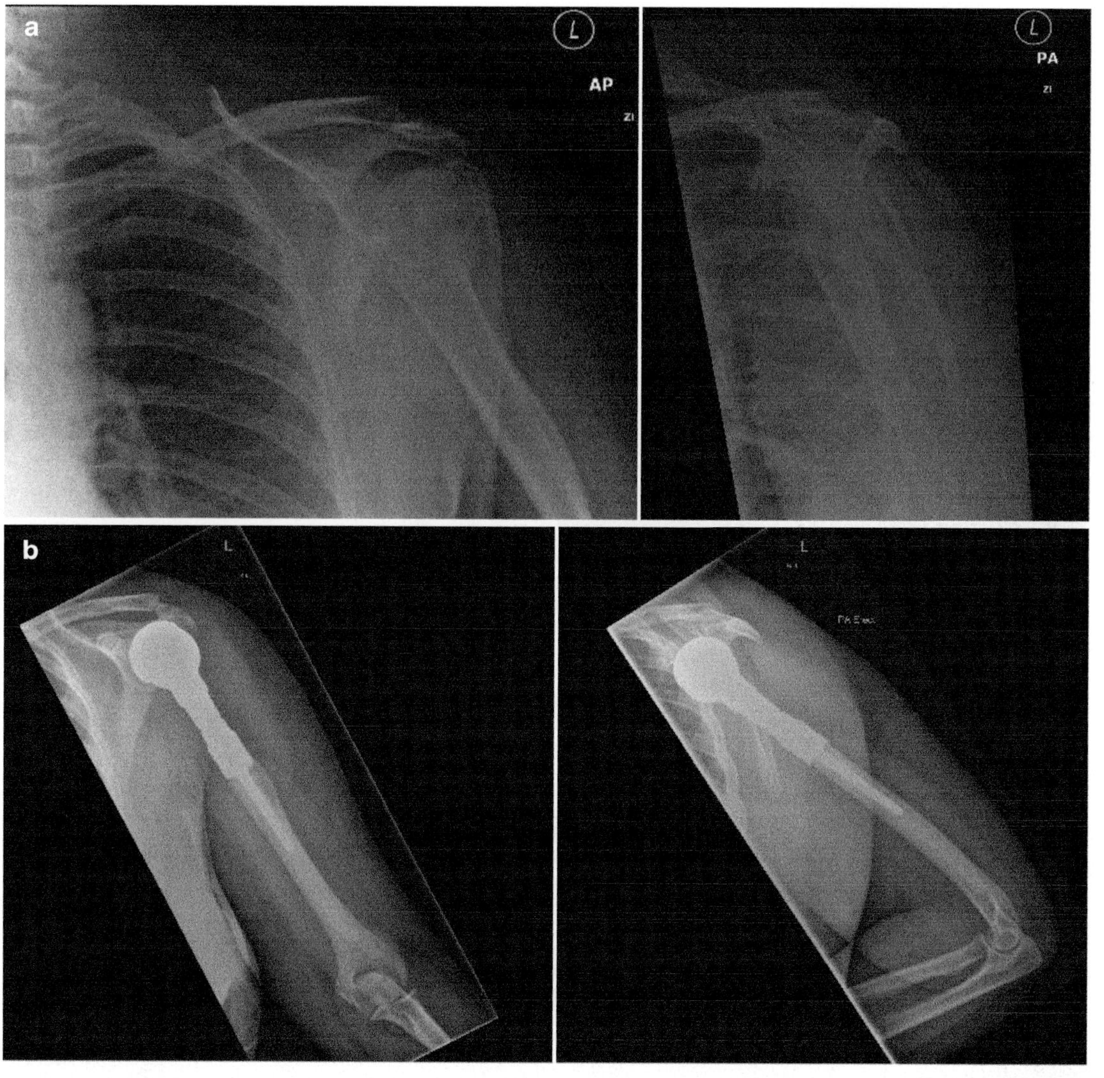

Fig. 32.2 (**a**) Pre-operative; chondrosarcoma, Left proximal humerus with pathological fracture. (**b**) Post-operative proximal humeral hemiarthroplasty

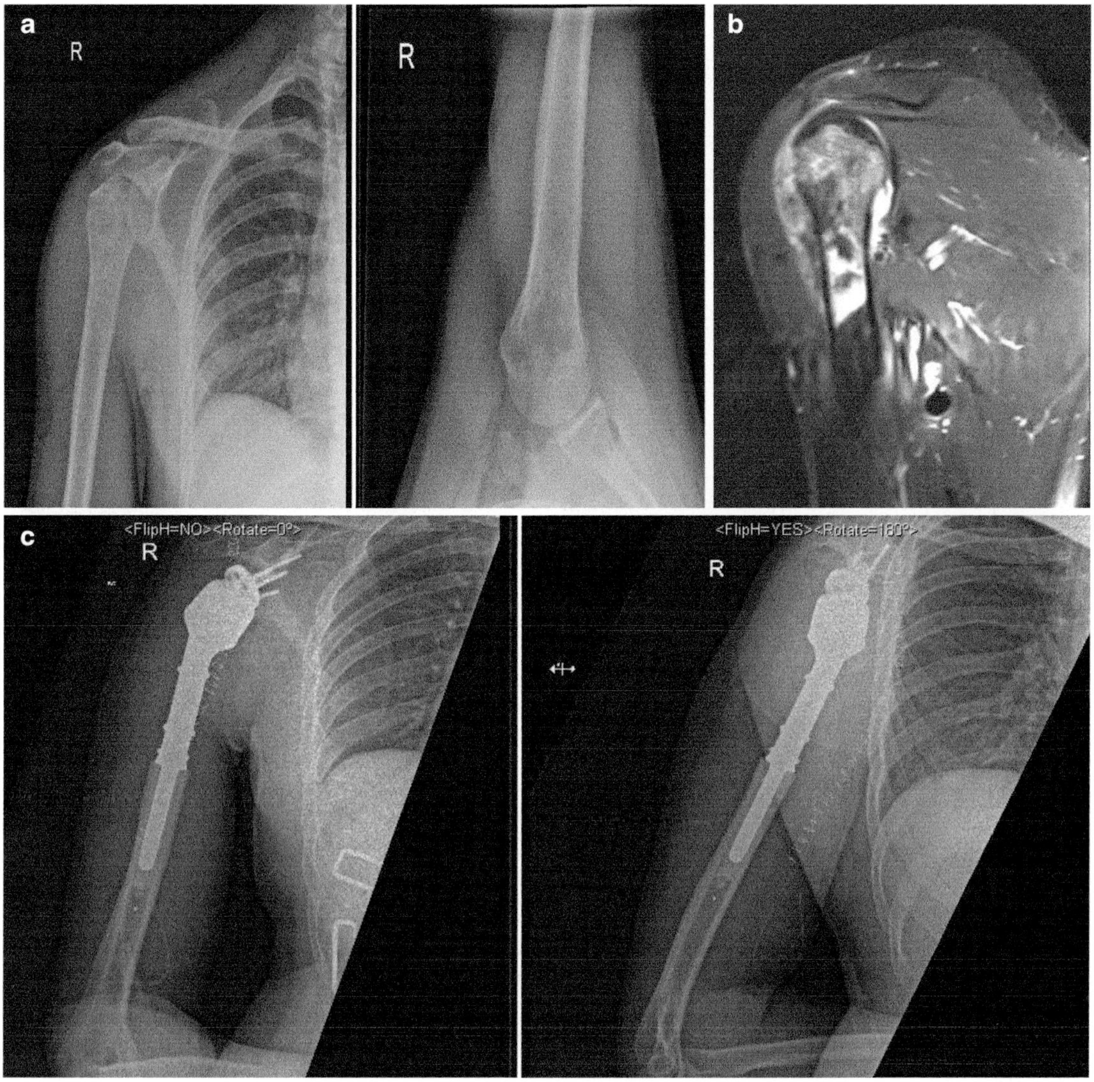

Fig. 32.3 (**a**) Pre-operative plain radiographs showing osteosarcoma. (**b**) Pre-operative STIR sequence MRI; osteosarcoma. (**c**) Post-operative proximal humeral endoprosthesis with reverse polarity shoulder joint

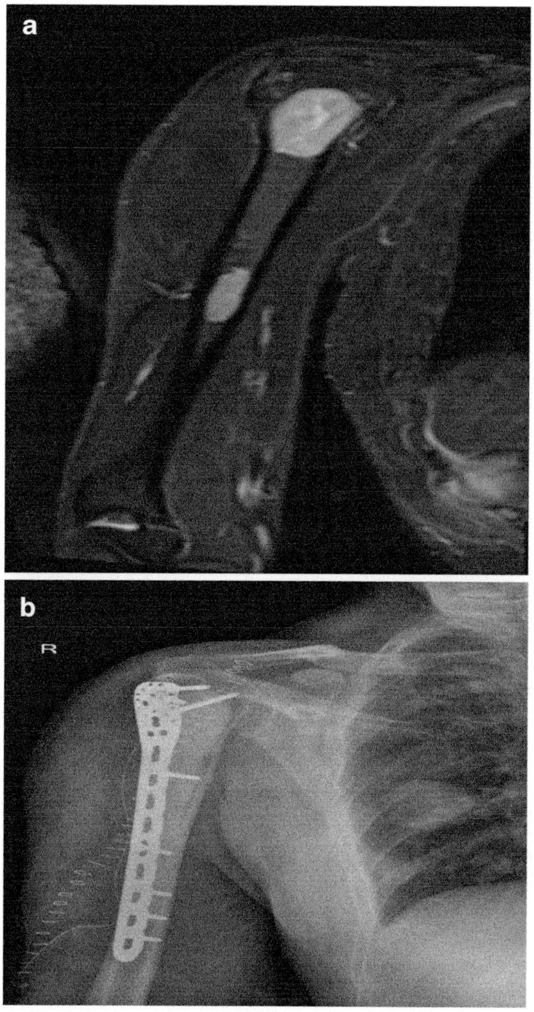

Fig. 32.4 (**a**) Pre-operative MRI of the RIGHT upper limb; metastatic salivary gland carcinoma. (**b**) Post-operative plain radiographs; curettage, cementation and plating of metastatic salivary gland carcinoma RIGHT humerus

The implant is manufactured according to CT scan images, and is designed to closely match the size and shape of the original scapula. Numerous holes are provided for soft-tissue reattachment. The implant ideally has large fenestrations that reduce the weight and to promote the development of scar tissue to enhance stability. Hydroxyapatite coated implants have been used to reduce the possibility of metallosis from abrasion.

The glenohumeral part of the implant can be varied according to the design requirement but generally consists of a reverse geometry constrained humeral prosthesis (Fig. 32.1, 32.2, 32.3, 32.4, and 32.5).

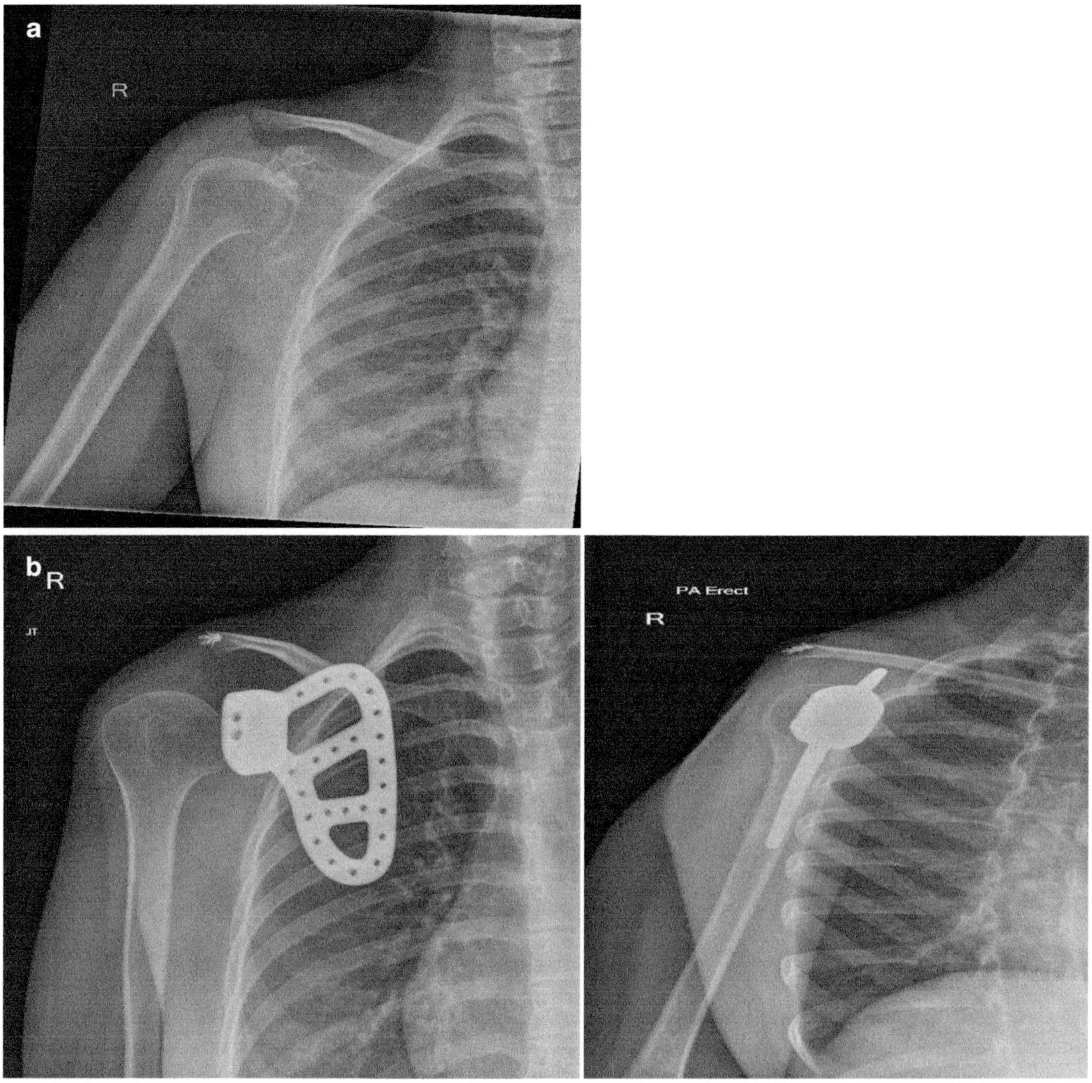

Fig 32.5 (**a**) Pre-operative X-ray showing desmoplastic fibroma of the Right scapula. (**b**) Post-operative right total scapular replacement with prosthesis following resection for desmoplastic fibroma of bone

Reference

1. Malawer MM. Tumors of the shoulder girdle. Technique of resection and description of a surgical classification. Orthop Clin North Am. 1991;22(1):7–35.

Infection of the Shoulder Joint

33

Aravind Desai, Pratima Khincha, Robert Nelson, and Puneet Monga

Introduction

Shoulder joint infection is a challenging problem. Shoulder infection can occur both in the native joint as well as following joint replacement. A delay in the diagnosis usually equates to a poor outcome of this condition. The principles of management, like in any other joint infection compromise of eradication of the infection, pain relief and restoration of the joint movement [1].

Long term sequel of shoulder joint infection are devastating and often results in poor functional outcome. Furthermore, the joint infection places a huge physical, financial and care burden on the patient, family and accountable organization. Reducing the economic burden of treating shoulder infections depends on developing clinical practice guidelines and incentivizing innovations in infection prevention [2].

A. Desai, MBBS, MS, MRCS, FRCS Tr and Orth
North Lincolnshire and Goole NHS Foundation Trust, Scunthorpe General Hospital, Scunthorpe, UK

Hull Yorkshire Medical School, University of Hull, Hull, UK

Sheffield Medical University, Sheffield, UK

P. Khincha
Pennine Acute Hospital NHS Trust, Manchester, UK

R. Nelson
Wrightington, Wigan and Leigh NHS Foundation Trust, Wigan, UK

P. Monga, MBBS, MS, DNB, MRCS, FRCS, MD (✉)
Upper Limb Unit, Wrightington Hospital, Wigan, UK

Edge Hill University, Ormskirk, UK

University of Salford, Salford, UK

Native Joint Infection

Septic arthritis of the shoulder joint is rare [3] and relatively uncommon (approximately 3% of all joint infections) [4]. Cleeman et al. [5] reported associated co-morbidities and risk factors such as diabetes mellitus, rheumatoid arthritis, immunosuppressive drugs and tumours in 87% of the patients with septic arthritis in their cohort. It is indeed very unusual to come across native joint infection in otherwise healthy adults. The diagnosis of such an infection should indeed trigger an investigation into the potentially associated co-morbidities. A vast majority of septic shoulders can be related to Haematogenous spread (up to 55%), although previous Steroid injections (33–35%) and Intra articular procedures (11–15%) comprise the iatrogenic etiology.

Diagnosis

The classic clinical features of a joint infection include pain, restricted range of movements (ROM), swelling (with or without redness), and

I. A. Trail et al. (eds.), *Textbook of Shoulder Surgery*, https://doi.org/10.1007/978-3-319-70099-1_33

Table 33.1 Severe shoulder pain of sudden onset – differential diagnosis

Infection
Calcific Tendinitis
Adhesive capsulitis
Parsonage Turner Syndrome
Tumours

systemic symptoms such as fever. The patients may present with a feeling of malaise or being unwell. There may be a history of recent sore throat, chest infection or dental infection. Differential diagnosis of sudden onset severe shoulder pain should be considered carefully (Table 33.1). One needs to be aware that occasionally infection can be present even in the absence of "classic" features. A high degree of suspicion must be maintained.

The diagnosis is made by taking a detailed history including any risk factors and enquiries related to other foci of infection. Physical examination should include assessment of range of movement. Imaging studies include plain radiographs to exclude other pathology such as calcific tendonitis, fractures and tumours. Ultrasonography of the shoulder is useful to assess fluid collection in the joint and is especially useful to exclude a collection. In modern medical practice MR Imaging is very commonly used to aid diagnosis. It would pick up fluid collection, bone oedema, osteomyelitis and abscess formation. Technetium Bone scan may be used is children to diagnose osteomyelitis, when an MR may not be practical.

It is very useful to perform laboratory tests such as white cell count, CRP and ESR. Raised counts not only help in making a diagnosis but also serves as a useful method of monitoring progress. Aspiration of the shoulder joint under ultrasound control is often requested and may confirm the diagnosis. Although urgent gram stains are very specific when positive, they have a poor sensitivity. Hence, even with negative gram stains but a high index of clinical and biochemical suspicion, one must consider the diagnosis of the shoulder infection. Positive cultures are gold standard for diagnosis but may only be available after 48 h and hence cannot be awaited before instituting treatment.

Management

Septic arthritis represents an absolute indication for urgent surgical intervention, to prevent irreversible local changes and possible mortality [6]. Septic arthritis can be managed both by open/arthroscopic washout and debridement or combination of both in recalcitrant cases. Arthroscopic technique is minimally invasive, less morbid and effective as compared to open debridement. An average of 2–4 operations (reoperation rate of 26–50%) may be needed to eradicate the infection and thorough debridement [7]. Non-operative management may be indicated in patients having a high risk of surgery and needle aspiration may be used as an alternative option in such situations.

Along with surgical debridement, isolation of causative organism is highly desirable in the eradication of the infection. Fluid analysis and tissue sample for culture and sensitivity (extended cultures for *propionibacterium*) is integral part of the management of the condition. *Methicllin sensitive Staphylococcus aureus* is the most common causative organism (40–87%), followed by *Methicillin resistant Staph aureus* (MRSA) (9–17%) and *Propionibacterium acnes (P. acnes) and others* (1–3%). A multidisciplinary approach guided by the microbiologists is essential in management of these patients as most often they require long-term antibiotics up to 6 weeks.

Complications

Untreated septic arthritis of the shoulder is a life threatening condition. Septicemia from joint infection may lead onto mortality if there is delay in diagnosis or treatment, particularly in immunocompromised patients. Delayed diagnosis or inadequate treatment may lead to long-term sequalae such as bone and cartilage destruction, rotator cuff damage, osteonecrosis, secondary arthritis and ankylosis of the joint [1].

> **Clinical Pearl**
> Shoulder infection may not present with "classic" symptoms and signs and a high degree of suspicion is necessary.

Infection After Surgery

Postoperative infection can occur after both open and arthroscopic surgery and the rate of infection after shoulder surgery is relatively low, ranging from 0.4% to 5% [8]. It is a serious cause of patient morbidity and increase in health care expenditures. Postoperative infections can be difficult to diagnose, eradicate and treat with patients often having poorer outcomes than their matched counter parts who have uncomplicated courses [9]. Up to 50% of patients with postoperative shoulder infection have the associated risk factors (Table 33.2) [11]. Finally, hair follicles and sebaceous glands of the axillary fossa facilitate the development of bacteria and thus increase the risk of infection of the surgical site [12].

The commonest organisms implicated in infection after shoulder surgery are *Staphylococcus aureus, coagulase-negative Staphylococcus* and *Propionibacterium acnes.*

Propionibacterium acnes (P. acnes) is a gram positive anaerobic bacillus commonly isolated from flora of face, chest and axilla. Once considered as an inconsequential skin flora, it has emerged now as a major pathogen in Periprosthetic Shoulder Infection (PSI) which is difficult to diagnose and eradicate. Patel et al. [13] demonstrated greater rate of colonisation of *P. acnes* in men and particularly more in the axilla as compared to hip and knee.

Table 33.2 Risk factors associated with post-operative shoulder infection

General factors:
Diabetes mellitus,
Rheumatoid arthritis,
Obesity,
Renal or liver failure,
Chemotherapy,
Immunosuppressive drugs,
Intrarticular steroid injections
Intra venous drug abuse.
Limb specific risk factors:
Haematoma formation after surgery,
Increase in dead space,
Revision surgery,
Previous surgical procedures of the shoulder (3–5% higher risk),
Arthroplasty for trauma (3% increase risk) and
Cuff tear arthropathy (6% greater risk) [10]

P. acnes has been isolated in infections of primary shoulder arthroplasty in 16% of cases and in up to 21% cases of revision arthroplasty [14]. Common anti-bacterial preps used in the operating may not provide sufficient efficacy for skin eradication compared to other common skin flora [15]. Infective and inflammatory blood markers have poor sensitivity and specificity for detecting *P. acnes* infection, hence the diagnosis of this infection is difficult and challenging for the treating surgeon [16]. Extended cultures up to 14 days may be required to isolate the organism [17].

Several authors have recommended the use of two or more combination of antibiotics in order to prevent emergence of resistant strains and also for the treatment of polymicrobial infections [16].

In the following sections we discuss Periprosthetic Shoulder Infection (PSI), post-arthroscopy shoulder infection and infection following trauma surgery respectively.

Clinical Pearl
Post operative shoulder infection with *P. acnes* is challenging to identify, interpret and manage.

Periprosthetic Shoulder Infection (PSI)

PSI is one of the most dreaded postoperative complications after shoulder arthroplasty. The incidence of infection after primary shoulder arthroplasty ranges from 0.4% to 3% and for revision surgery ranges from 3% to 15% [18]. As the number of primary shoulder arthroplasties has increased, so has the subsequent number of patients requiring revision arthroplasty for the treatment of infection [8]. The UK National Joint Registry recorded 'infection' as the indication in 12% of revision shoulder operations in 2013. It may be classified variously (Table 33.3).

The clinical presentation of PSI is generally nonspecific. Pain is one of the commonest presenting symptom (86%) in patients with PSI. Other signs include: discharging sinus (44%), stiffness (35%), Erythema (35%), localised collection (32%), fever and chills (10–20%) [19].

Table 33.3 Classification of Periprosthetic Shoulder Infection (PSI)

Based on etiology:	Intraoperative wound contamination
	Haematogenous spread
Infection can be either:	Superficial or deep
Based on duration:	Acute (Within 6 weeks after surgery)
	Late (After 6 weeks)

Once PSI is suspected a complete diagnostic workup is mandatory including laboratory evaluation including Full blood count (peripheral leukocyte count and neutrophil count usually normal) CRP and ESR. One needs to remember that often these tests are not elevated in case of *P. acnes* infection. If serological tests are normal, the decision to aspirate a shoulder with suspected prosthetic joint remains largely based on the judgement of the evaluating surgeon. Synovial fluid WBC Count of >50,000cells/mm3 with more than 75% polymorphonuclear (PMN) cells or even direct germ visualisation are suggestive of infection [20].

New synovial fluid biomarkers like Alfa-defensin 1 and IL-6 are reported to be more specific and sensitive in detecting PSI [21]. Their role in detecting shoulder infection is currently controversial and perhaps unclear. Intraoperative culture is the gold standard diagnostic test for PSI. Gram stain and cultures for aerobes, anerobes, fungi and mycobacteria along with extended/prolonged cultures (3–4 weeks) for *P. acnes* are recommended. Histopathology examination of the tissues is a useful adjunct to diagnosis although not as specific as culture. A minimum of 4–6 intraoperative periprosthetic samples should be studied (2 from joint tissues, 2 from prosthetic bone interface and 2 from medullary canal and bone). More than five PMN cells per high power field suggest infection if noted in at least 2 samples [20]. Implant Sonification is a new technique involving study of the retrieved implants and the biofilm. It is more sensitive than intraoperative tissue specimens.

Radiographs may reveal lucent lines around bone metal/bone-cement interface, medial calcar erosion, tuberosities resorption and osteolysis (seen in subacute/chronic infections) (Fig. 33.1). CT and/or MRI with metal artifact reduction protocols may be useful in certain cases and are more useful in planning revision/reconstructive surgery. Radionucleotide scans: (Tc99/In111-labelled WBC Scan) are useful for diagnosis but have a high false positive rate.

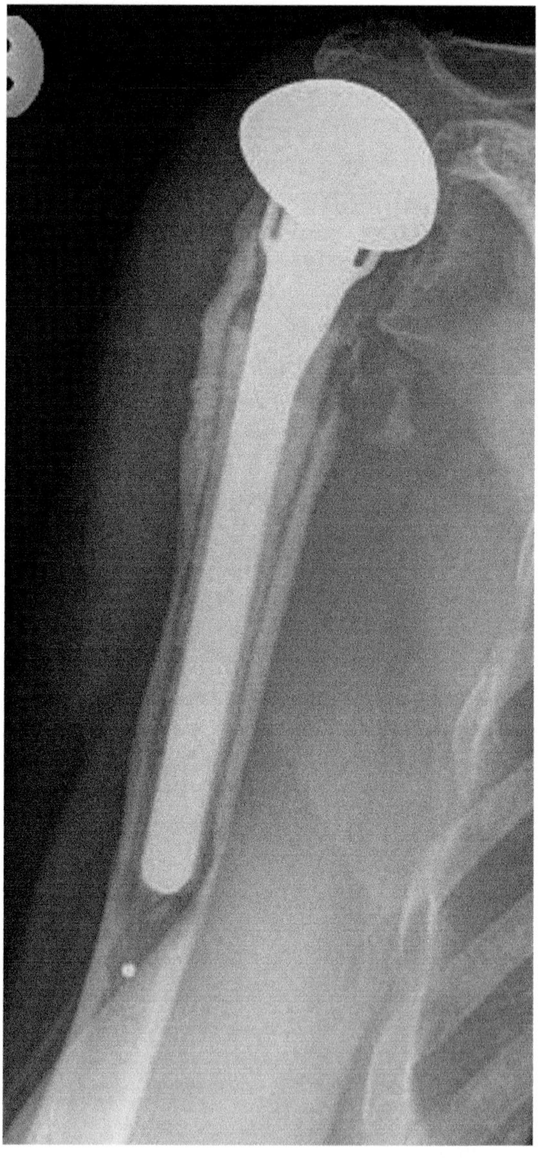

Fig. 33.1 X-ray appearance of chronic peri-prosthetic infection in a 56 year female patient demonstrating lucency around the cement, cavitation around the distal cement restrictor and periosteal reaction

Never-the-less they are useful for their negative value to exclude infection on cases of diagnostic conflict.

Management

The primary goal of treating shoulder sepsis in PSI is the elimination of the infection and restoring the function of the shoulder joint.

Treatment options are based on type of infection, duration, virulence of organism, patient co-morbidities, associated risk factors, expectations, soft tissue and bony integrity. The treatment strategies available to the physician are:

(a) *Debridement, Antibiotic and Implant retention (DAIR):*

In cases with acute infection with early diagnosis (<6 weeks of primary surgery), when the organism has been identified and if prosthesis is stable, PSI can be managed with thorough open debridement, polyethylene exchange (if possible) and appropriate antibiotic cover. There is little data available in the outcomes of this approach and some studies have reported poor results with up to 50% recurrence rates with this approach [19].

(b) *Single stage Revision:*

One stage revision is not as popular as the staged revision surgery. The procedure involves thorough debridement, removal of the prosthesis and implantation of an exchange definitive prosthesis in a single stage. On one hand this procedure offers advantages of being a single procedure with less morbidity, less soft tissue and bone loss and cost effectiveness, however risks recurrence of infection. Few studies have reported satisfactory outcome in small group of patients who underwent single stage surgery for PSI [22, 23].

(c) *Two-stage revision:*

Two-stage revision is considered as gold standard procedure for managing deep PSI when infection is treated beyond the first few weeks of primary surgery (Fig. 33.2a–c). It has become the treatment of choice because of low rates of persistent infection and optimal outcomes. The procedure involves removal of all infected and necrotic tissues, bone, implant, cement and placement of temporary antibiotic impregnated cement spacer device in one stage. Subsequently the definitive prosthesis is implanted in the second stage. Antibiotic therapy as per culture and sensitivity are administered till inflammatory and infective markers are returned to normal levels. It is the authors' practice to obtain negative cultures before implantation of the definitive prosthesis. Staged revision offers an advantage of effective clearance of infection but means that the patient needs multiple procedures and it is associated with higher morbidity, expense, soft tissue and bony deficits. Success rates for infection clearance has been reported up to 90% at mean follow-up of 48 months using this approach [24].

(d) *Resection Arthroplasty:*

This procedure is generally considered for patients who are elderly, debilitated with low demands, higher risk of surgery and for patients with extensive soft tissue/bone loss. It provides eradication of infection, good pain relief but limited/poor function [25]. This is a relatively simple procedure and one can expect pain relief at the cost of poor functional outcome. Despite this procedure, up to 30% rate of recurrence of infection has been reported [24].

(e) *Suppressive Antibiotic therapy:*

Long term suppressive antibiotic therapy alone should only be considered for seriously ill patients with significant co-morbidities and unfit for surgery. Failure rates of 75% have been reported with this modality of treatment [26].

Clinical Pearl

In early peri-prosthetic shoulder infection, prosthesis retention may be considered. In Chronic PSI, two stage revision is currently gold Standard.

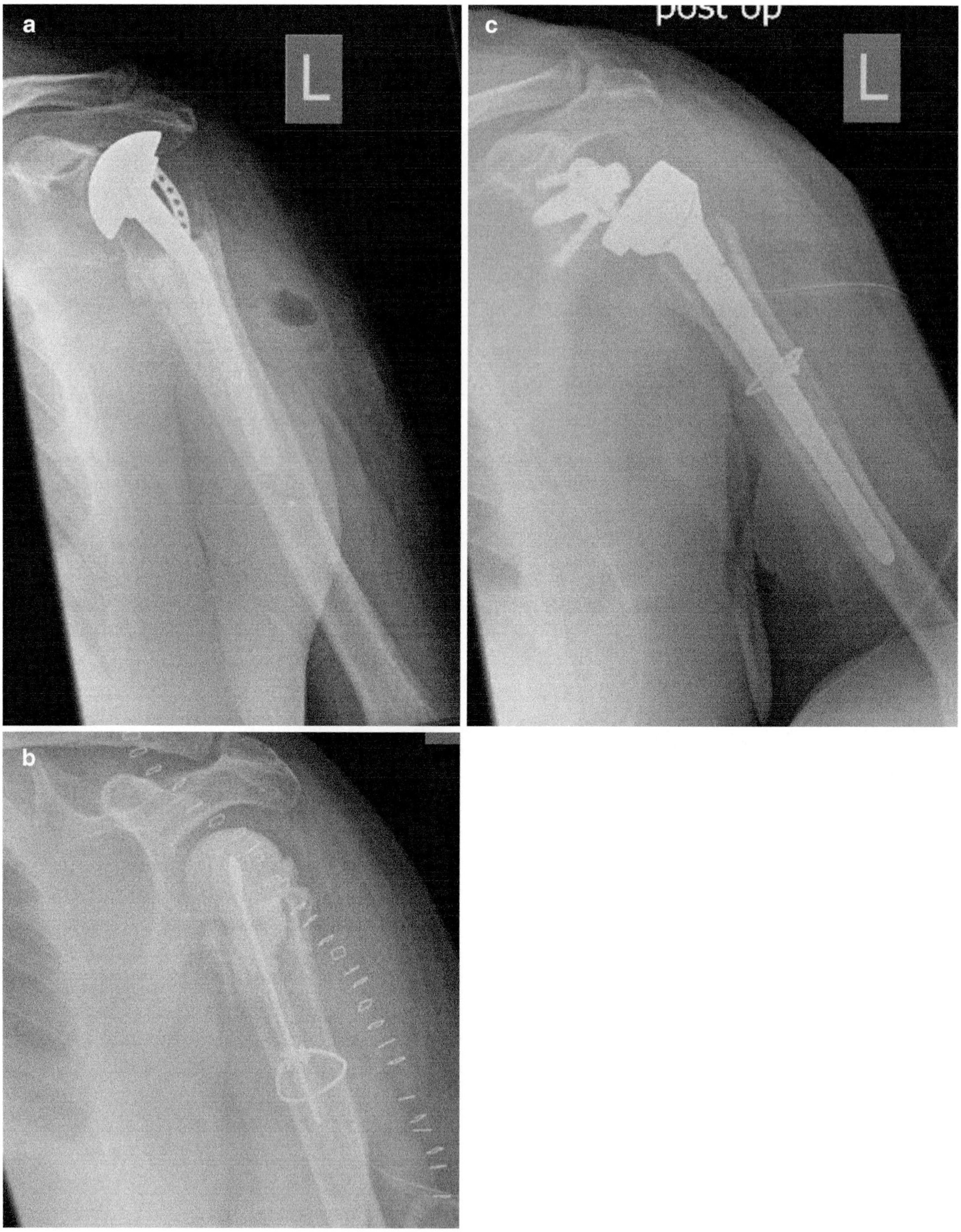

Fig. 33.2 (**a**) Radiograph of a 63 year male patient who developed infection following Hemiarthroplasty performed for a comminuted Proximal humeral fracture. (**b**) First Stage of two stage revision involved excision of implant, cement and cement restrictor. A Antibiotic laden space was introduced. Humeral osteotomy was necessary for thorough debridement and was secured using a single cable. (**c**) Second stage of 2-stage revision using a long stem reverse humeral component and a poly glenosphere

Post Arthroscopy Septic Arthritis

Deep infection after shoulder arthroscopic procedures is rare, with a reported prevalence of 0.3–3% [12] (Fig. 33.3a, b). However, the incidence is probably underestimated as *P. acnes* is often the causative organism. Arthroscopic cuff repair has a high incidence of infection amongst all procedures particularly in patients over 60 years of age and with prior surgery on the same shoulder [27]. There is a paucity of literature about infection secondary to instability procedures [12].

A high index of suspicion of infection and a thorough diagnostic workup as described earlier is necessary in patients presenting with unexplained pain, fever, painful effusion, systemic inflammation or positive culture of aspirate after arthroscopic procedures. Management consists of arthroscopic or open surgical debridements involving synovectomy, removal of all foreign material such as sutures and anchors and appropriate antibiotic cover as per the culture and sensitivity.

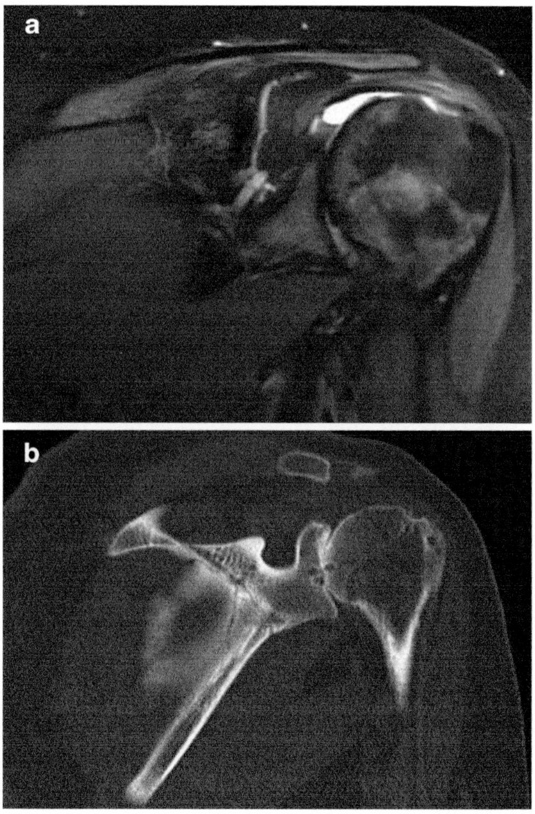

Fig. 33.3 (**a**) MRI Scan of a 46 year old patient demonstrating advanced Glenohumeral arthritis as a sequel to arthroscopy related infection. (**b**) CT Scan demonstrating loss of gleno-humeral joint space

Infection After Fracture fixation

Infection after open reduction and internal fixation of fracture fragments can be managed by the same principles of infection with arthroplasty procedures. Hence surgical debridement, antibiotics and implant retention is recommended in early post op infection with removal of implant at later stage after fracture healing. However, if there is evidence of deep infection with poor bone stability, implant removal and a two stage procedures should be considered. Non-union of the fracture and soft tissue loss are the main concerns along with avascular necrosis and arthritis of the shoulder joint in the long term.

Prevention of Infection in Shoulder surgery

Many factors have been examined in relation to prevention of orthopaedic infection. According to Hackett et al. [8], several studies have demonstrated that operating time, operating room traffic, duration of trays opened and wound irrigation have a role in the prevention of infection in shoulder surgery.

Hand washing has been reported as single most effective measure of minimising infection [28]. Both alcohol and chlorhexidine have proved to be more potent than povidone- iodine scrubs in reducing the infection [8]. In addition to hand washing, frequent glove changing has been found to significantly reduce the rate of surgical site infection [29]. Though several studies have reported that chlorhexidine to be more effective skin preparation agent, it still has minimal effect on eradication of *P. acnes* from the operative site. According to Sabetta et al. [30] and Chaung et al. [31], pre-operative topical application of benzoyl peroxide have shown decrease in rate of *P. acnes* culture positivity. Removal of axillary hair had higher total bacterial burden as compared to unclipped axillae [32]. Hence routine preoperative shaving of axillary area is not recommended prior to surgery. The relative risk of obtaining a positive *P. acnes* culture is twice as high with the anterolateral approach as with deltopectoral approach [33].

There have been no studies evaluating the role of prophylactic antibiotics in preventing infection following the shoulder surgery [8]. However, several studies of lower limb arthroplasty have clearly demonstrated the efficacy of pre and post-operative administration of antibiotics to prevent infection. Decisions regarding antibiotic type, delivery and duration should be made by a multi-disciplinary team on a case by case basis. The involvement of an experienced bacteriologist is mandatory. Isolation of the infecting organism and identification of sensitivities is critical [34]. Antibiotic loaded cement is more effective than standard cement in deep infection [35].

Clinical Pearl
A multipronged approach is necessary to prevent infection following shoulder surgery. Prophylactic antibiotics, theatre discipline, hand washing, meticulous surgical technique and involvement of microbiology team are key components to this approach.

Summary

Infection of the shoulder joint is a challenging situation both for the patient and treating surgeon, whether it occurs in the native joint or in the postoperative setting. Post-operative patients with this complication have inferior outcome as compared to those without infection. A high index of suspicion is necessary to diagnose this potentially devastating condition as early diagnosis and management has substantially better outcomes compared to delayed treatment. A multidisciplinary approach involving the microbiologist is key to achieve optimal outcomes.

References

1. Klinger HM, Baums MH, Freche S, Nusselt T, Spahn G, Steckel H. Septic arthritis of the shoulder joint: An analysis of management and outcome. Acta Orthop Belg. 2010;76:598–603.
2. Hackett DJ, Rothenberg AC, Chen AF, et al. The economic significance of Orthopaedic infections. J Am Acad Orthop Surg. 2015;23(Suppl):S1–7.
3. Leslie BM, Harries JMIII, Driscoll D. Septic arthritis of shoulder in adults. J Bone Joint Surg. 1989;71-A:1516–22.
4. Duncan SFM, Sperling JW. Treatment of primary isolated shoulder sepsis in the adult patient. Clin Orthop Relat Res. 2008;446:1392–6.
5. Cleeman E, Auerbach JD, Klingelstein GG, Flatow EL. Septic arthritis of the glenohumeral joint: a review of 23 cases. J Surg Orthop Adv. 2005;14:102–7.
6. Wick M, Muller EJ, Ambacher T, et al. Arthrodesis of shoulder after septic arthritis. Long-term results. J Bone Joint Surg. 2003;85-B:66–670.
7. Abdel MP, Perry KI, Morrey ME, et al. Arthroscopic management of native shoulder septic arthritis. J Shoulder Elb Surg. 2013;22:418–21.
8. Heckett DJ, Crosby LA. Infection prevention in shoulder surgery. Bull Hosp Joint Dis. 2015;73(Suppl 1):140–4.
9. Dines JS, Fealy S, Strauss EJ, et al. Outcomes analysis of revision total shoulder replacement. J Bone Joint Surg Am. 2006;88(7):1494–500.
10. Richards J, Inacio MC, Beckett M, et al. Patient and procedure specific risk factors for deep infection after primary shoulder artrhoplasty. Clin Orthop Relat Res. 2014;472(9):2809–15.
11. Toploski MS, Chin PY, Sperling JW, Cofield RH. Revision shoulder arthroplasty with positive intraoperative cultures: the value of preoperative studies and intraoperative histology. J Shoulder Elb Surg. 2006;15(4):402–6.
12. Saltzman MD, Marecek GS, Edwards SL, Klainov D. Infection after shoulder surgery. J Am Acad Orthop Surg. 2011;19(4):208–18.
13. Patel A, Calfee RP, Plante M, Fischer SA, Green A. Propinobacterium acnes colonization of the human shoulder. J Shoulder Elb Surg. 2009;18(6):897–902.
14. Kelly JD 2nd, Hobgood ER. Positive culture rate in revision shoulder arthroplasty. Clin Orthop Relat Res. 2009;467(9):2343–8.
15. Saltzman MD, Nuber GW, Gryzlo SM, Mareck GS, Koh JL. Efficacy of surgical preparation solutions in shoulder suregry. J Bone Joint Surg Am. 2009;91(8):1949–53.

16. Saper D, Caprio N, Ma R, Li X. Management of propionibacterium acnes infection after shoulder surgery. Curr Rev Musculoskeletal Med. 2015;8:67–74.
17. Dodson CC, Craig EV, Cordasco FA, et al. Propionbacterium acnes infection after shoulder arthroplasty: a diagnostic challenge. J Should Elbow Surg. 2010;19(2):303–7.
18. Mook WR, Garrigues GE. Diagnosis and management of periprosthetic shoulder infections. JBJS. 2014;96-A(11):956–65.
19. Sperling JW, Kozak TK, Hanssen AD, Cofield RH. Infection after shoulder arthroplasty. Clin Orthp Relat Res. 2001;382:2016–216.
20. Francsehini V, Chillemi C. Periprosthetic shoulder infection. Open Orthop J. 2013;7:243–9.
21. Frangiamore SJ, Saleh A, Kovac MF, Grosso MJ, Zhang X, Bauer TW, et al. Synovial fluid Interlukin-6 as a predictor of periprosthetic shoulder infection. J Bone Joint Surg. 2015;97:63–70.
22. Ince A, Seeman K, Frommelt L, Katzer A, Loher JF. One stage exchange arthroplasty for peri prosthetic infection. J Bone Joint Surg Br. 2005;87(6):814–8.
23. Cuff DJ, Virani NA, Levy J, et al. The treatment of deep shoulder infection and glenohumeral instability with debridement, reverse shoulder arthroplasty and postoperative antibiotics. J Bone Joint Surg. 2008;90(3):336–42.
24. Nelson GN, Davis DE, Namdari S. Outcomes in the treatment of periprosthetic joint infection after shoulder arthroplasty: a systematic review. J Shoulder Elb Surg. 2016;25:1337–45.
25. Rispoli DM, Sperling JW, Athwal GS, Schleck CD, Cofield RH. Pain relief and functional results after resection arthroplasty of the shoulder. J Bone Joint Surg Br. 2007;89(9):1184–7.
26. Coste JS, Reig S, Trojani C, Berg M, Walch G, Boileau P. The management of infection in the arthroplasty of the shoulder. J Bone Joint Surg Br. 2004;86(1):65–9.
27. Bauer T, Boisrenoult P, Jenny J-Y. Pos-Arthroscopy septic arthrtis: current data and practical recommendations. Orthop Traumatol Surg Res. 2015;101:s347–50.
28. Farrington RM, Rabindran J, Crocker G, et al. 'Bare below the elbows' and quality of hand washing: a randomised comparison study. J Hosp Infect. 2010;74(1):86–8.
29. Al-Maiyah M, Bajwa A, Mackeney P, et al. Glove perforation and contamination in primary total hip arthroplasty. J Bone Joint Surg Br. 2005;87(4):556–9.
30. Sabetta JR, Rana VP, Vadasdi KB, et al. Efficacy of topical benzyl peroxide on the reduction of *Propionibacterium acnes* during shoulder surgery. J Shoulder Elb Surg. 2015;24(7):995–1004.
31. Chaung MJ, Janccosko JJ, Mendoza V, Nottage WM. The incidence of *Propionibacterium acnes* in shoulder arthroscopy. Arthroscopy. 2015;31(9):1702–7.
32. Marecek GS, Weatherford BM, Fuller EB, Saltzman MD. The effect of axillary hair on surgical antisepsis around the shoulder. J Shoulder Elb Surg. 2015;24(5):804–8.
33. Hudek R, Sommer F, Kerwat M, et al. *Propionibacterium acnes* in the shoulder surgery: true infection, contamination or commensal of the deep tissue? J Shoulder Elb Surg. 2014;23(12):1763–71.
34. Pinder EM, Ong CY, Bale SR, Trail IA. Ten questions on prosthetic shoulder infection. Should Elb. 2016;8(3):151–7.
35. Nowinski RJ, Gillespie RJ, Shishani Y, et al. Antibiotic-loaded bone cement reduces deep infection rates for primary reverse shoulder arthroplasty: a retrospective, cohort study of 501 shoulders. J Shoulder Elb Surg. 2012;21(3):324–8.

History Taking and Clinical Assessment of the Shoulder

34

Simon Robinson, Nanette Oakes, and Shantanu Shahane

Introduction

A reproducible and accurate assessment of the shoulder is important before contemplating investigations and a treatment plan. In this chapter, we are describing our way of assessing the patient who presents with shoulder related symptoms. This chapter will include important history taking points and examining the shoulder. This is however not an exhaustive chapter on all the possible special tests, which can be used when performing a clinical assessment.

We will explain our system and thought processes and provide reasoning for our methods and the tests we have chosen.

Patient History

A number of diagnoses with regards to the shoulder can be made from a good history. There are certain diagnoses with classical symptoms that are age specific. In general, these can lead us to a provisional diagnosis before beginning the examination.

S. Robinson, MBChB, MRCS.Ed, FRCS (Tr&Orth.) (✉)
Wirral University Teaching Hospitals NHS Foundation Trust, Upton, Birkenhead, Wirral, UK
e-mail: simon.robinson21@nhs.net

N. Oakes, MSc (Adv. Physio), BSc (Physio)
S. Shahane, MS(orth), Mch(orth), FRCS(orth)
Chesterfield Royal Hospital, Calow, Chesterfield, Derbyshire, UK

Age (yrs)	
<20	Atraumatic instability, (hyperlaxity, Sprengel shoulder, Little Leaguer's shoulder)
<30	Labral lesion
30–50	Subacromial Impingement syndrome/ capsulitis
50–65	Rotator cuff tear
65–75	Glenohumeral joint arthritis
>75	Rotator cuff tear arthropathy

Our usual technique involves a general history from the patient and then focus in on salient shoulder specific symptoms. Our focused closed questions begin with age, hand dominance and occupation followed by enquiring about major medical problems (such as diabetes mellitus, hypertension, ischaemic heart disease and strokes). We then enquire if the patient is on anticoagulants and ask regarding history or family history of thrombosis. We next enquire about current medication (where appropriate) and note drug allergies.

Effect of the shoulder on the patient's occupation is detailed further. Enquires are made with regards to the nature of the job (manual/sedentary) and how the shoulder affects their work. We would also enquire about effect of shoulder symptoms on activities of daily living (ADL), sports and hobbies.

We then follow with open questions regarding the shoulder and enquire more specifically about points raised by the patient. We ask about pain,

I. A. Trail et al. (eds.), *Textbook of Shoulder Surgery*, https://doi.org/10.1007/978-3-319-70099-1_34

stiffness, weakness, range of movement, clicking and crepitus. Onset and duration of each symptom is elicited. Mechanism of injury (if traumatic) along with precipitating and relieving factors are discussed. If clicking is present and especially when assessing the younger patient, eliciting whether the click is painful or not and if it developed after trauma is important.

With regards to specific symptoms we find the below questions of use (grouped by symptom):

Instability:	Injury (how/when/multiple)
	Position of arm during injury
	Dislocations/subluxations (Number/ relocations without intervention or with medical intervention i.e. A&E/theatre +/− proof of dislocation)
	Exacerbating activities
	Previous interventions
Weakness:	Trauma/insidious onset
	Duration
Stiffness:	Pain
	Duration
	Diabetes
	Previously resolved
Radicular Symptoms:	Neck to past the elbow
	Character (Sharp/shooting/electric shock)
	Distribution
	Neck ROM
	Balance problems (Upper Motor Neuron [UMN] lesion)
Tumors/ Metastases:	Past history
	Family history
	Night pain and rest pain
	Systemic features (weight loss/Malaise)

Pain can classically be further broken down into **SOCRATES.**

Site	Cervical spine/Trapezius
	SCJ
	Ant shoulder (Biceps, Subscapularis, rotator interval)
	Lateral (Impingement/cuff tear)
	Deep inside (Labral pathology/SLAP)
	Superior (ACJ)
Onset	When did it start? Was it sudden or gradual? Has it worsened over time, plateaued or improved?
Character	Sharp? Stabbing? Aching? Burning?
Radiation	Where does it radiate to?
Associations	Any other signs or symptoms associated with the pain?
Timing	Does the pain follow a pattern?
Exacerbating/ relieving factors	Does anything change the pain?
Severity	(VAS: We score pain from 0 to 10 with 0 as no pain and 10 as most severe pain)

Previous treatment: categorized into Analgesia, steroid injections, physiotherapy & surgery.

Analgesia:	If the patient requires analgesia, (type and frequency).
Injections:	When? Where? Who gave them? How many? Did they make a difference? (how long for)
Physiotherapy:	When? By Whom? What did the physiotherapy actually involve? Did you comply with the physiotherapy? Did it improve your symptoms?
Surgery:	When? What surgery? Did it improve symptoms and if so for how long?

Physical Examination

A thorough history gives us a good idea as to the focus of our clinical examination. It is important to take verbal consent from the patient and expose the entire upper extremity including the neck and scapula.

We start our examination with screening of the cervical spine (including neurological examination) followed by standard "look, feel and move". After this, we group the more focused examination by pathology. We then examine for thoracic outlet syndrome, distal neuro-vascular status and finally assess joints above and below.

Inspection

The entire shoulder examination is performed with the patient in a standing position (except part of instability testing which needs a patient to ideally be in a lying posture). Also, we keep enough space for the examiner to walk around the patient and examine/observe the scapula as this forms an important part of shoulder examination.

We inspect from the front, back, side and in the axilla with the specifics of what we are looking for set out below:

Front Scars, ACJ and SCJ alignment, Clavicle mal union, Deltoid contour, long head of biceps rupture (Popeye sign)

Side Scars, deltoid shape / wasting

Back Scars, thoracic Kyphosis, Scapula (Winging, Muscle wasting), cuff wasting in supraspinous and infraspinous fossa

Axilla Scars (cervical rib excision), mass, lymphadenopathy

Clinical Pearl
In presence of a chronic postero-superior cuff tear, wasting of the infraspinous fossa is often seen earlier and is more evident. This is due to the coverage of supraspinous fossa by trapezius muscle, which masks supraspinatus wasting.

Palpation

We palpate as is clinically indicated and note the areas of specific discomfort. If a painful location has been found then palpating the area just once is all that is required. Specific areas that may be of diagnostic use are:

Sterno-clavicular joint (SCJ),
Clavicle (mal-union or non-union),
Acromio-clavicular joint (ACJ),
Greater Tuberosity, Codman's point [1] and the Bicipital groove.

SCJ and ACJ tenderness to palpation is usually a good indication of local degenerative process. A dislocated ACJ can be palpated for reducibility to differentiate between, Rockwood grade 3 and grade 4/5 dislocations [2].

Codman's point is 1 cm away from the insertion of the supraspinatus insertion. Local tenderness at this point can point to supraspinatus tendinopathy and possible impingement lesion. The Bicipital groove can be palpated anteriorly with the arm slightly externally rotated. Biceps is located deep within the anterior aspect of the shoulder and accurate assessment with palpation is difficult.

Range of Motion (ROM)

ROM decreases with age and is often higher in females. Forward elevation and abduction should be equal bilaterally. The dominant side often shows increased external rotation with the non-dominant side showing increase internal rotation and extension [3].

For ease and smoothness of the examination, we assess the ROM in the standing position. All movements are assessed actively and passively. Though individually variable, normal ROM is shown below [4]:

Flexion (forward elevation)	0–180°
Extension	0–60°
Abduction	0–180°
Adduction	0–30°
Internal rotation (IR)	0–70°
External rotation (ER)	0–90°

Clinical Pearl
Reduced external rotation in a non-traumatic setting can only indicate two potential clinical diagnoses. Either frozen (primary or secondary) or glenohumeral joint osteoarthritis.

The senior author's standard practice is to assess active flexion and abduction from the front (Figs. 34.1 and 34.2). Then assess for passive improvement in motion if deficit is noted. The next step is to assess ER with elbows tucked to the side (to eliminate forearm prono-supination from interfering with shoulder rotation) (Fig. 34.3). ER is the only motion that is performed only passively.

Next, functional internal rotation is assessed (Fig. 34.4). This is a composite movement including shoulder extension, shoulder IR, elbow flexion and thumb extension. This is often noted as the position of the thumb to reach the following landmarks; greater trochanter, sacroiliac joint, L3, T12, lower border of scapula and spine of scapula. It is more important to assess functional IR as opposed to true IR, which is simply internally rotating the arm (which is by the side of the shoulder). After assessing IR, the examiner stays standing at the back of the patient. We then ask the patient to forward flex and abduct the shoulder again to assess scapulo-thoracic rhythm. ROM of the symptomatic side is always compared to the opposite normal side.

Upon assessing shoulder abduction in the younger patient (and if the history correlates), asking about any clicking or grinding over the shoulder blade (in keeping with the snapping scapula) at this stage is of benefit. Crepitus maybe felt and further investigations warranted where appropriate.

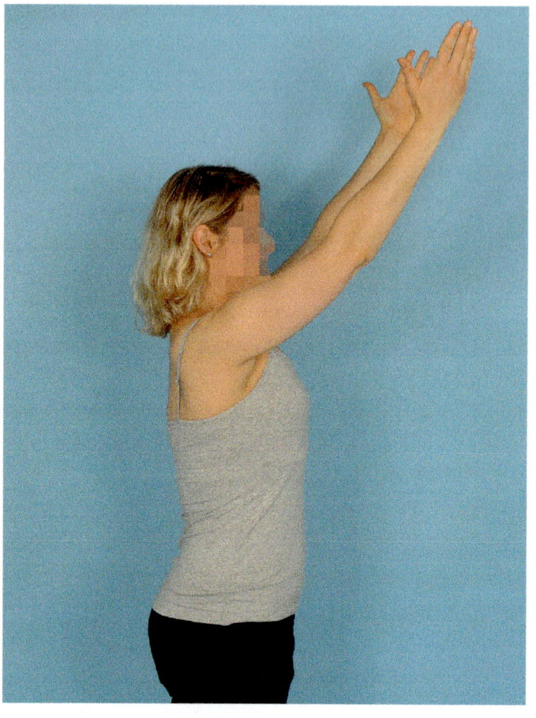

Fig. 34.1 Shoulder flexion

> **Clinical Pearl**
> Never forget to examine the shoulder from the back to assess scapulothoracic motion. Shoulder elevation is a composite of glenohumeral and scapulothoracic movements with the scapulothoracic joint contributing approximately one third.

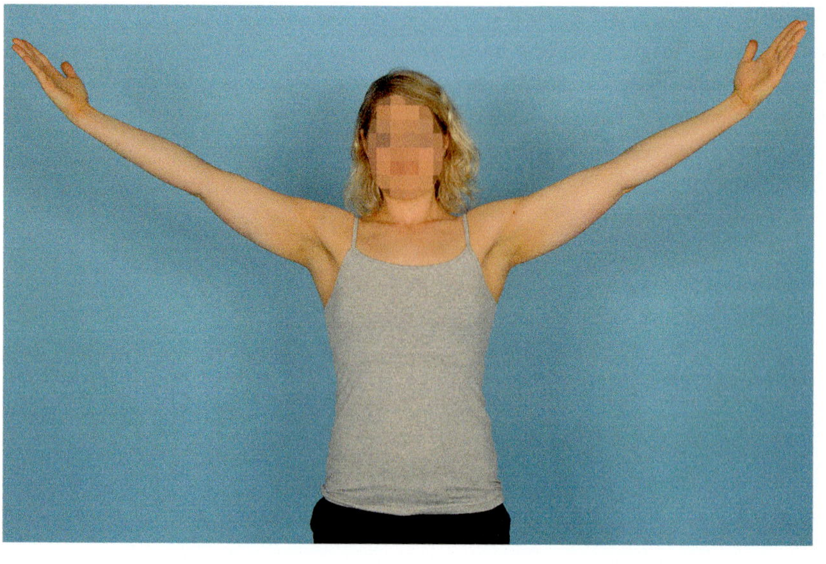

Fig. 34.2 Shoulder abduction

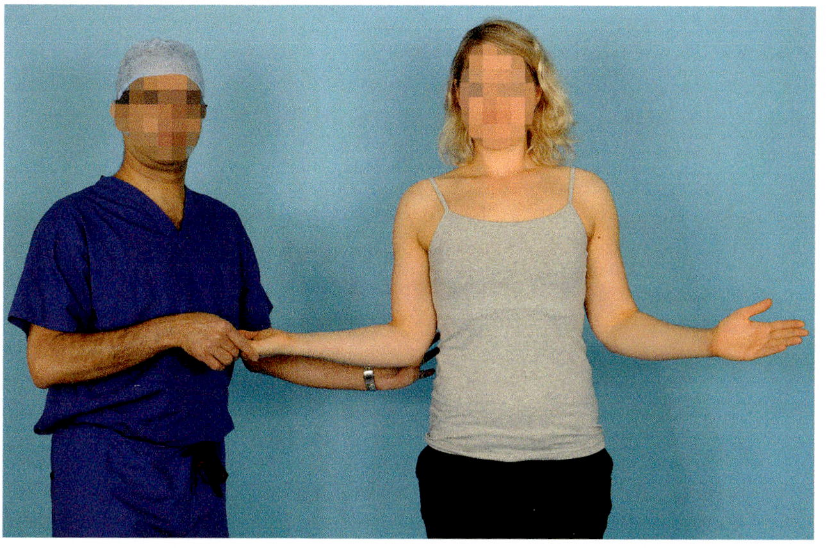

Fig. 34.3 Passive external rotation

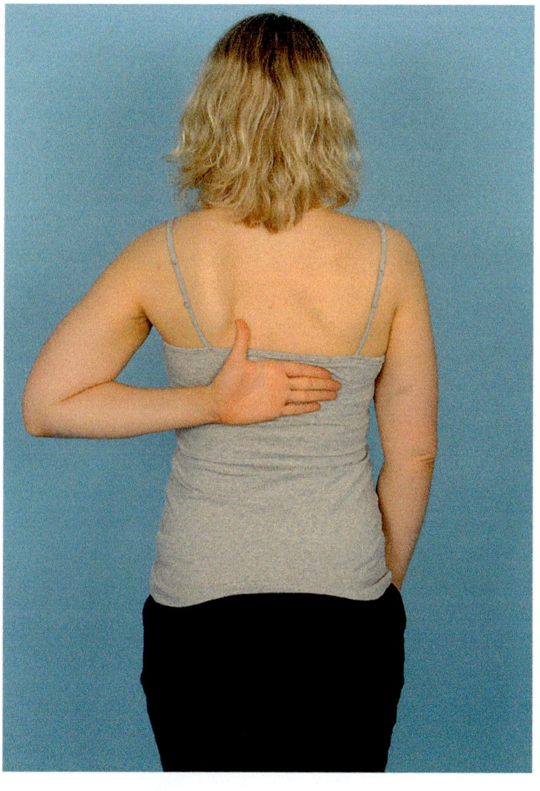

Fig. 34.4 Functional internal rotation

It is also the senior author's practice to perform the entire shoulder examination in front of a mirror. It allows him to assess patient facial features for pain while assessing the patient from behind.

Special Tests

No one single positive special test should be relied upon to reach a diagnosis but should be used in conjunction with other aspects of your assessment. A reliable history, an examination that correlates with this, a number of positive special tests and the appropriate investigations are often all needed to reach a firm diagnosis.

We divide the special tests we use into the below categories:

1. Impingement and ACJ
2. Rotator Cuff
3. Capsulitis and osteoarthritis
4. Disorders of the biceps including superior labral lesions (SLAP tear)
5. Instability
6. Thoracic outlet syndrome and the cervical spine

In this article, we shall not endeavor to describe all known tests to diagnose a certain pathology. We will only describe tests used by the senior author in his routine practice. Demonstration of all tests will be as if the patient's right shoulder is being examined.

Shoulder Impingement and the Acromioclavicular Joint

Shoulder impingement or subacromial impingement is a clinical syndrome where pain is elicited as the rotator cuff tendons/muscles pass through the subacromial space. Classically, there is a mid-range painful arc (60–120°) upon active shoulder elevation, more so than when performed passively. The painful arc is often in a higher range (160–180°) when involving acromioclavicular joint (ACJ) pathology.

We use two main special tests when assessing for impingement and the one for the ACJ.

Neer's Sign and Test

First mentioned in 1972 and formally published in 1983, Neer's sign describes pain at the anterior edge of the acromion on forced elevation [5]. We perform this in a standing position (was originally described being performed in a seated position). The examiner stabilizes the scapula with his left hand and passively elevates the affected arm in scapular plane. Pain during this maneuver is indicative of a positive result (Fig. 34.5).

Neer's Test Pain during Neer's Sign can be reproduced with a number of pathologies but Neer's test is then performed to help eliminate a number of these. If pain is eliminated or significantly reduced when reproducing the movement after injection of local anaesthetic in the subacromial space, the patient has had a positive result and diagnosis of impingement syndrome is confirmed [6].

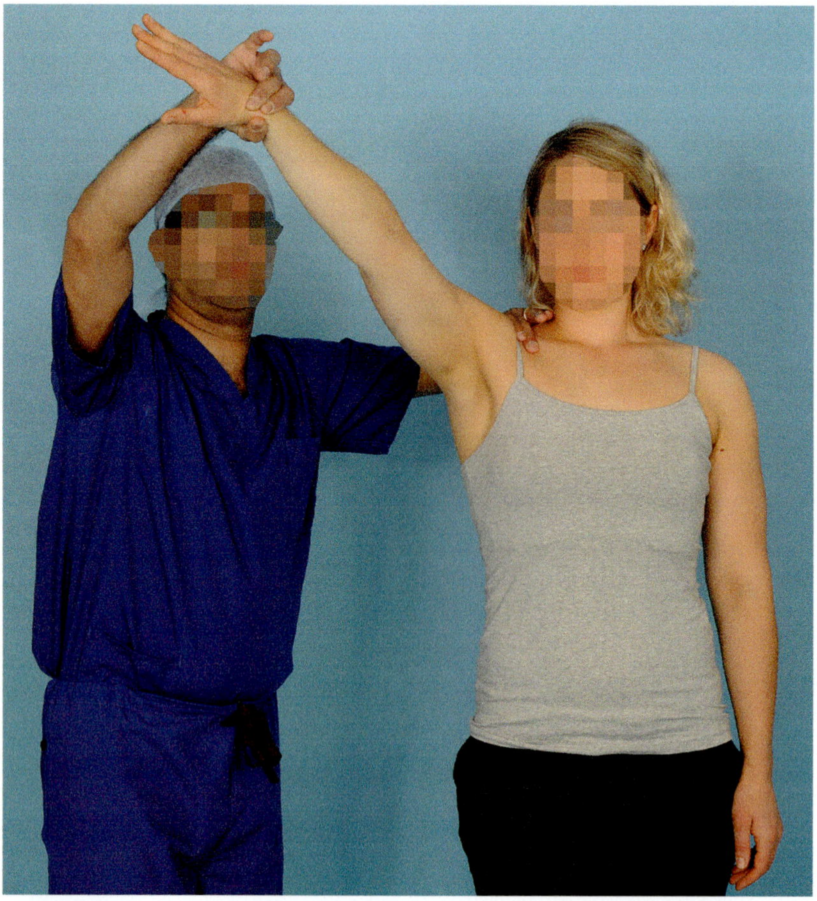

Fig. 34.5 Neer's sign

Hawkins' Test (Hawkins'-Kennedy Test)

Described in 1980 by Hawkins and Kennedy, this test involves forward elevating the shoulder to 90° (in scapular plane with the elbow at 90°) and forcibly internally rotating the shoulder [7]. Pain is indicative of a positive result (Fig. 34.6).

Scarf Test (Cross Body Adduction Stress Sign)

If the patient has pain on palpation of the ACJ along with high arc pain on shoulder elevation, then the scarf test is useful in confirming the site of the pain. This sign was first described in 1951 [8]. The shoulder is forward elevated to beyond 90° (high arc) and then adducted across the body (so the hand touches the opposite shoulder) (Fig. 34.7). Pain felt at the ACJ is indicative of ACJ pathology. It is often useful to ask the patient to pinpoint the exact area of pain with a single finger to ensure the patient is not complaining of pain elsewhere in the shoulder. This can be termed "The Single Finger test".

The senior author performs these three tests (Neer's, Hawkins and Scarf tests) in one sweeping motion.

Tests for Rotator Cuff

Here we test the supraspinatus, infrapsinatus and subscapularis routinely. If a massive cuff tear is suspected, then we will also test Teres Minor. There are many tests available when assessing the rotator cuff but we find the below tests the most reliable and reproducible in our hands.

> **Clinical Pearl**
> Beware that pain inhibition can mimic a rotator cuff tear. It is important to inject sub-acromial space with a local anaesthetic to reduce pain before examining rotator cuff for structural integrity.

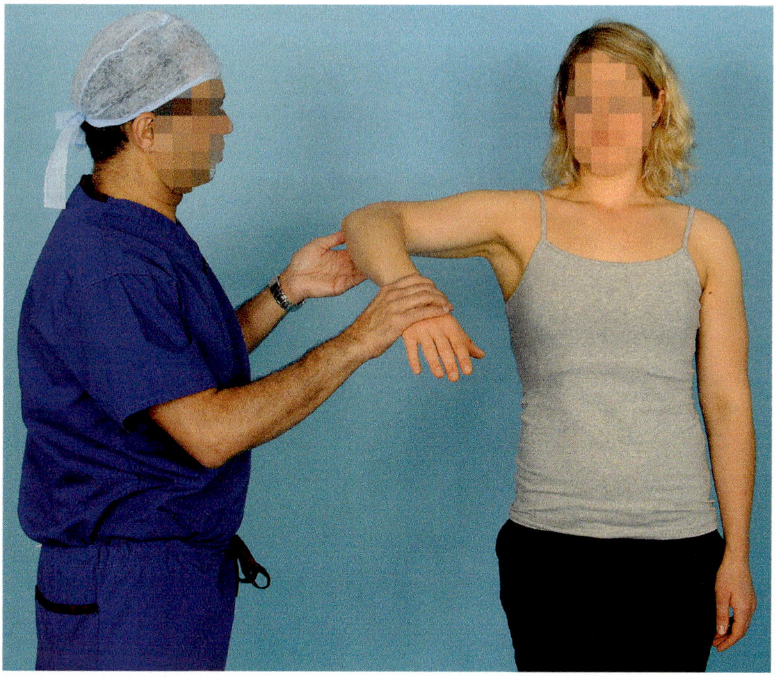

Fig. 34.6 Hawkins' test

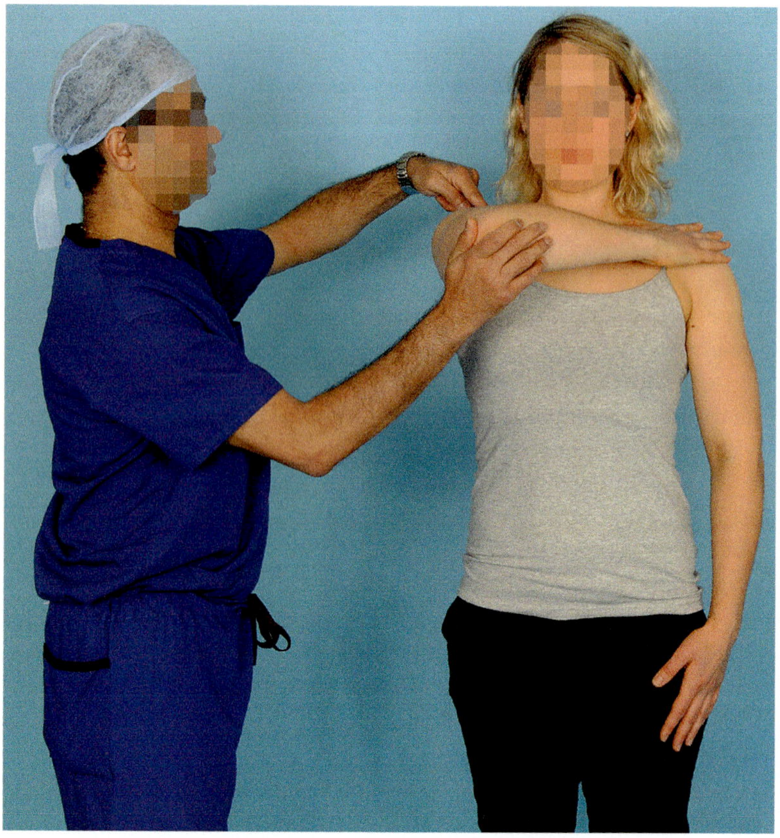

Fig. 34.7 Scarf test

There are two prerequisites before testing for cuff integrity. The shoulder needs to have a reasonable passive ROM to position the arm in positions needed to test the cuff and secondly, that pain should not inhibit the examination.

Supraspinatus: The Empty Can Test/ Jobe's Test

This was first described in 1982 and then more formally in 1983 when described as the 'supraspinatus test' [9, 10]. Deltoid strength is first assessed with the shoulder abducted to 90° in neutral rotation. The shoulder is then angled forward 30° (in scapular plane) and internally rotated, so the thumb points to the floor. We then push down on the arm just above the elbow (to eliminate triceps integrity giving a false negative result) and ask the patient to resist this action (Fig. 34.8). The test is most accurate when using weakness as your criteria for a positive result for a full thickness supraspinatus tear [11].

According to Itoi, the full can test (with the thumb pointing upwards) is slightly more accurate (75% Vs 70%). This is performed with 45° external rotation of the humerus whilst forward elevating the shoulder to 90° and resisting a downward force. According to Kelly, Kadrmas and Speer, this isolates the supraspinatus better than the Empty Can Test on EMG [12].

Empty can test is the senior author's preferred test to diagnose a full thickness supraspinatus tear. We believe it is important to separate the deltoid from interfering with supraspinatus strength testing. Complete elimination of deltoid from supraspinatus testing is not possible however the "Empty can test" places the supraspinatus at maximal mechanical advantage (IR creates a straight line of action for supraspinatus) and also creates maximal mechanical disadvantage for the deltoid (IR of shoulder moves the deltoid attachment too far medially to allow the deltoid to function as an effective unit).

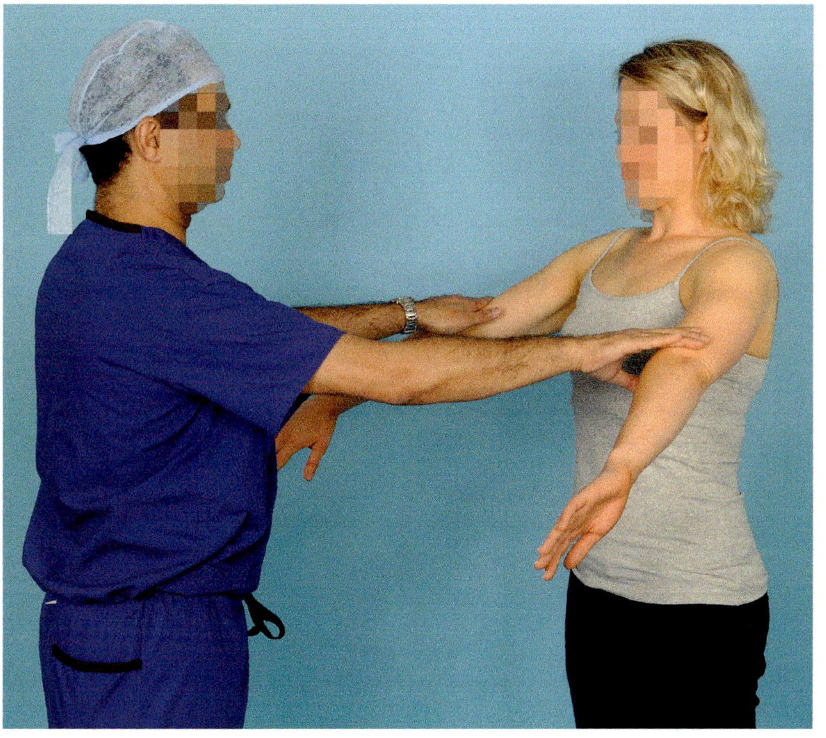

Fig. 34.8 Supraspinatus testing

Infraspinatus

Infraspinatus is the primary external rotator with the arm by the side of body. We start by assessing if the external rotation lag sign is present. Hertel described this in 1996 as a test of integrity of the supraspinatus and infraspinatus [13]. This can be performed sitting or standing. We perform this standing. We passively flex the elbow to 90°, elevate the shoulder 20° in the plane of the scapula and maximally externally rotate the shoulder. This is then decreased 5–10° and the patient is asked to hold this position. A loss of external rotation (arm falling internally) indicates a positive result and weakness of the superior cuff (External rotation Lag sign).

We then test the strength of Infraspinatus using the 'Infraspinatus strength test'. We keep the arm by the patient's side, passively flex the elbow to 90° and externally rotate the shoulder to just less than the maximal external rotation and ask the patient to hold that position whilst we push against the forearm to try and internally rotate the shoulder.

The examiner's other hand can be used to hold the elbow in at the side to attempt to isolate infraspinatus or can also be placed on the infraspinous fossa to assess contraction of the muscle. Merolla described this test nicely in 2010 [14] (Fig. 34.9).

Teres Minor

Teres minor is the prime external rotator of the shoulder in an abducted position. If the superior rotator cuff is weak, then assessing Teres Minor is of use. We support the arm at 90° of abduction in the scapular plane and with the elbow flexed to 90°. The shoulder is then maximally externally rotated. We then ask the patient to hold the shoulder in this position (Fig. 34.10). If the patient is unable to hold their arm in the position and the arm falls in IR, the test is positive. It is also described as postive 'Hornblower's sign'. This was first described by Arthuis in relation to obstetric brachial plexus paralysis [15]. A positive result has 100% sensitivity and 93% specificity for Goutallier grade 3/4 degeneration of Teres Minor on CT scan [16, 17].

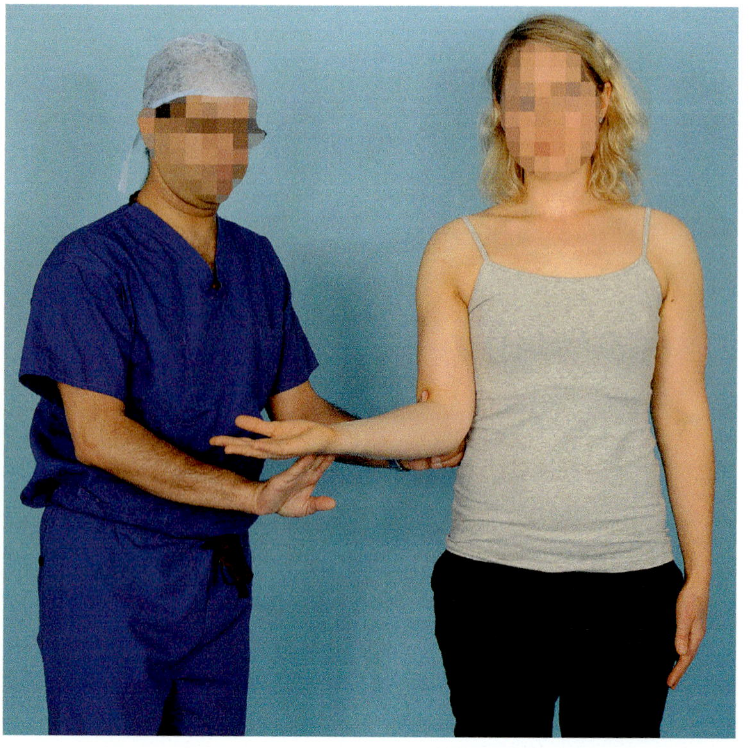

Fig. 34.9 Infraspinatus testing

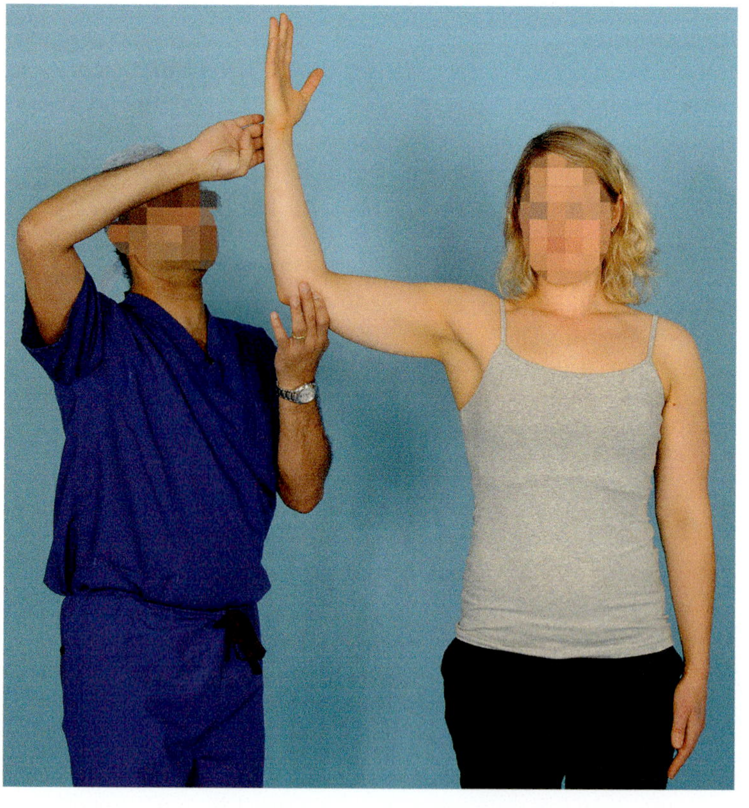

Fig. 34.10 Teres minor testing

Subscapularis

We perform a number of tests on subscapularis as some are more suited to some patients than others. We advise to start with the.

'Bear Hug Test' (BHT)

We start with this test, described by Barth, Burkhart and De Beer [18]. The patient is asked to place their hand on their opposite shoulder with the fingers extended (to prevent them from gripping the shoulder and giving a false negative result). They are then asked to prevent the examiner from lifting their hand off the shoulder (with an external rotation force) (Fig. 34.11). A difference of 20% strength (or more), but not pain, compared to the other side is a positive result.

Barth showed this test to be the most sensitive test for subscapularis as compared to the belly press (BPT) or the lift off test (LOT) (BHT 60%, BPT 40%, LOT 17%). The test however is slightly less specific (BHT 91.7%, BPT 97.9%, LOT 100%), making it ideal as a screening test, before evaluating the subscapularis further. The BHT is also said to be more likely to be positive with smaller tears of the subscapularis.

Lift Off Test (LOT)

If the patient can reach behind their back, we then perform the 'lift off test' [19]. In maximal internal rotation and shoulder extension, the subscapularis is maximally active [20]. We ask the patient to place their hand in the small of their back and lift it away from the body. If they can, then resistance is tested, ensuring that wrist flexion is not compensating for a weak subscapularis (Fig. 34.12). It can also be performed by the examiner passively bringing the patient's arm behind the body into maximal internal rotation (around the lower back region and pull it backwards away from the back). The result of this test is considered normal if the patient maintains maximum internal rotation after the examiner releases the patient's hand. The test is positive if the patient cannot maintain this position due to weakness of the subscapularis.

Belly Press Test (BPT)

If the patient cannot place their hand in the "lift off" position, then we use the 'Belly Press Test', again described by Gerber [21]. The patient is asked to place both hands on their abdomen and lift the elbows forwards and maintain that posi-

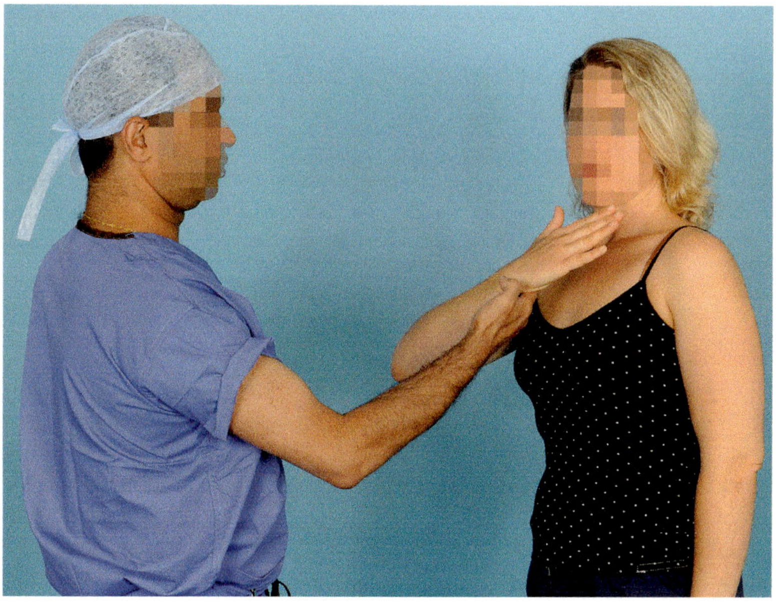

Fig. 34.11 Bear hug test

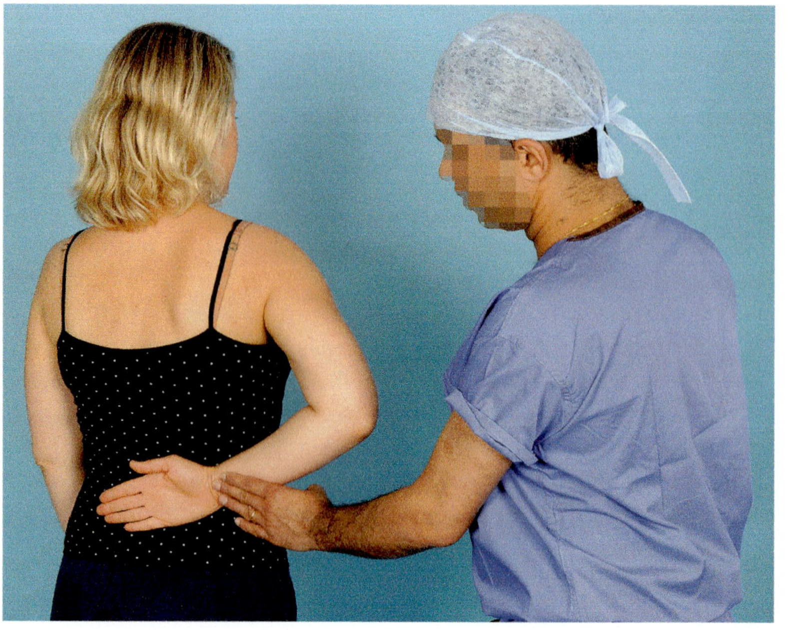

Fig. 34.12 Lift off test

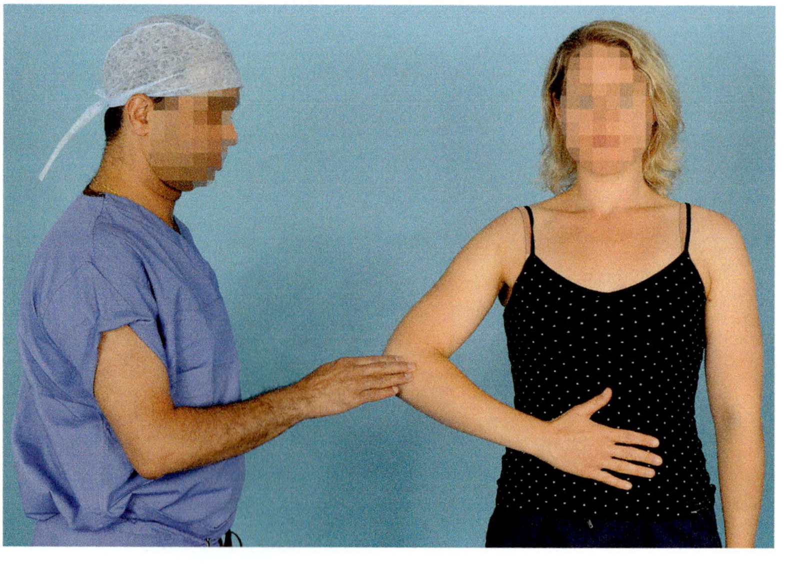

Fig. 34.13 Belly press test

tion. Examiner can apply pressure on the elbows from the front to assess strength. Again wrist flexion should be avoided to ensure a false negative result isn't recorded (Fig. 34.13).

Both of these tests (LOT & BPT) rely upon integrity of subscapularis in keeping the humerus internally rotated. If subscapularis is torn, while performing these tests, the humerus rotates externally and the patient is unable to perform lift off (in lift off test) and the elbow falls posteriorly (in belly press test), due to loss of fulcrum.

Tests for Disorders of the Proximal Biceps

O'Brien's Active Compression Test (for Diagnosis of SLAP Lesions)

Described in 1998, this test distinguishes between ACJ pathology and superior labral pathology [22]. He described this with the examiner standing behind the patient. We find it easier to perform standing to the front or the side. The patient forward flexes to 90°, adducts 15° and internally rotates the shoulder so the thumb points to the floor. The patient then resists downward pressure. The process is repeated with the thumb pointing laterally (externally rotating the shoulder). If the pain is reduced or diminished during the second part of the test, then the test is positive (Figs. 34.14 and 34.15). The test however may indicate ACJ or superior labral pathology. If the pain is located over the ACJ then the test is positive for ACJ pathology (again the single finger test is useful here). If the patient complains of a deep pain within the GHJ or a painful click, then the test is positive for superior labral pathology. O'Brien's series showed a sensitivity of 100% for both labral and ACJ pathology and specificities of 98.5% for the labrum and 96.6% for the ACJ. These results haven't been matched in further studies with sensitivities of 41–63% specificities of 73–95% [23, 24].

The first part of the test creates deep-seated pain in the shoulder in the presence of an unstable superior labral complex (SLAP lesion). As the biceps attachment proximally is unstable, the biceps tendon in the first part of the test has a "tendency to sublux" over the lesser tuberosity creating symptoms. The second part of the test (externally rotating the shoulder) relocates the biceps within the bicipital groove, thus reducing/abolishing symptoms (even in the presence of an unstable superior biceps anchor). The test is then classically said to be positive for a SLAP lesion.

Clinical Pearl

Pain over the ACJ whilst performing O'Brien's test may indicate ACJ arthritis and not a SLAP lesion.

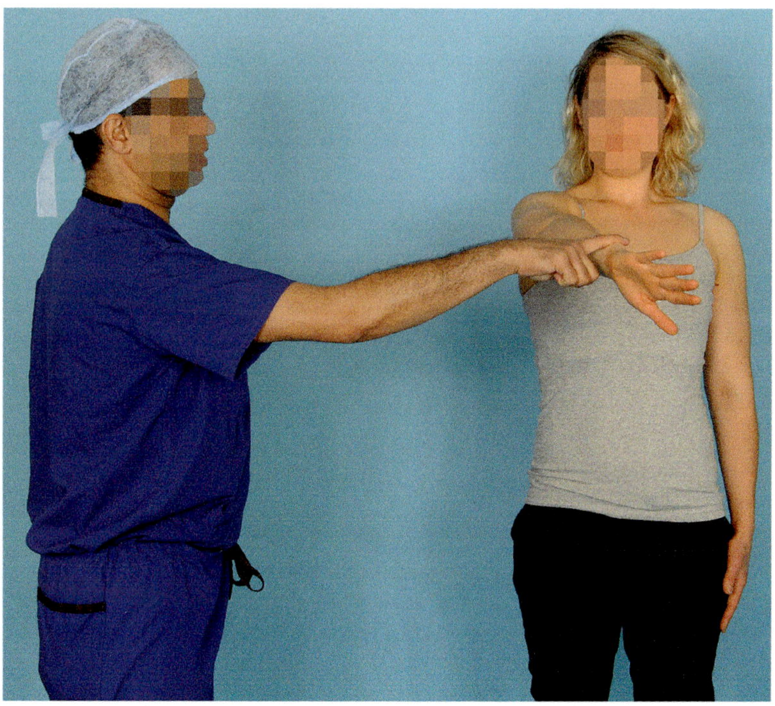

Fig. 34.14 O'Brien's test: shoulder internally rotated

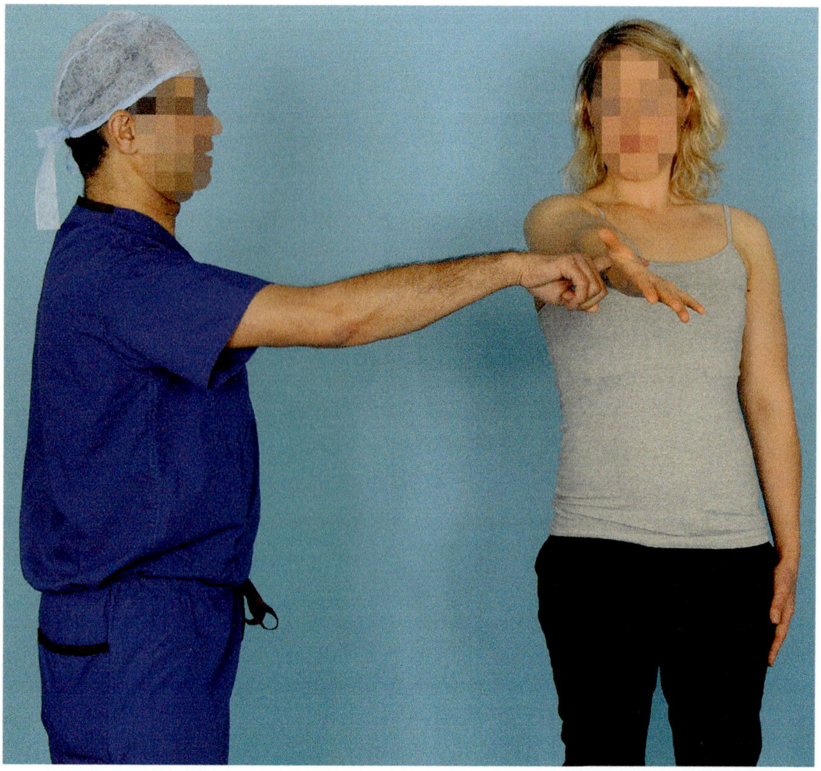

Fig. 34.15 O'Brien's test: shoulder externally rotated

Speed's Test

This test was first described by Speed for biceps tendonitis. The test involves positioning the upper extremity with 60° of shoulder elevation with full supination of the forearm and with the elbow completely extended. The examiner forcefully presses down on the patient's arm at the forearm. The patient attempts to resist the pressure of the examiner (Fig. 34.16). Alternatively, the patient attempts to forward flex the shoulder while the examiner resists. Pain over the anterior aspect of the shoulder is a positive result. This test is said to be positive in not only biceps tendonitis but also SLAP lesions and biceps avulsions. It has however been shown to be positive in a large number of shoulder pathologies. Bennett (1998) showed a specificity of 13.8%, a sensitivity of 90% in a prospective study looking at biceps/labral pathology [25]. Holtby and Razmjou (2004) however showed a specificity of 75% and a sensitivity of 32% [26].

Yergason's Test

There are variations described while performing this test. It was originally described in 1931 [27]. The patient's elbow is flexed and their forearm kept pronated. The examiner then holds their arm at the wrist. Patient is asked to actively supinate against resistance (Fig. 34.17). We describe a positive test as being when pain is reproduced in the bicipital groove area. Holtby and Razmjou (2004) showed results for Yergason's test with a specificity of 79% and a sensitivity of 43% [26].

Capsulitis (Frozen Shoulder) and Osteoarthritis

The main distinction between the two is the age group affected. Middle-aged patients (40–60 years) are more likely to suffer from a capsulitic shoulder as compared to an older patient (more than 60 years) being more likely to suffer from an arthritic shoulder.

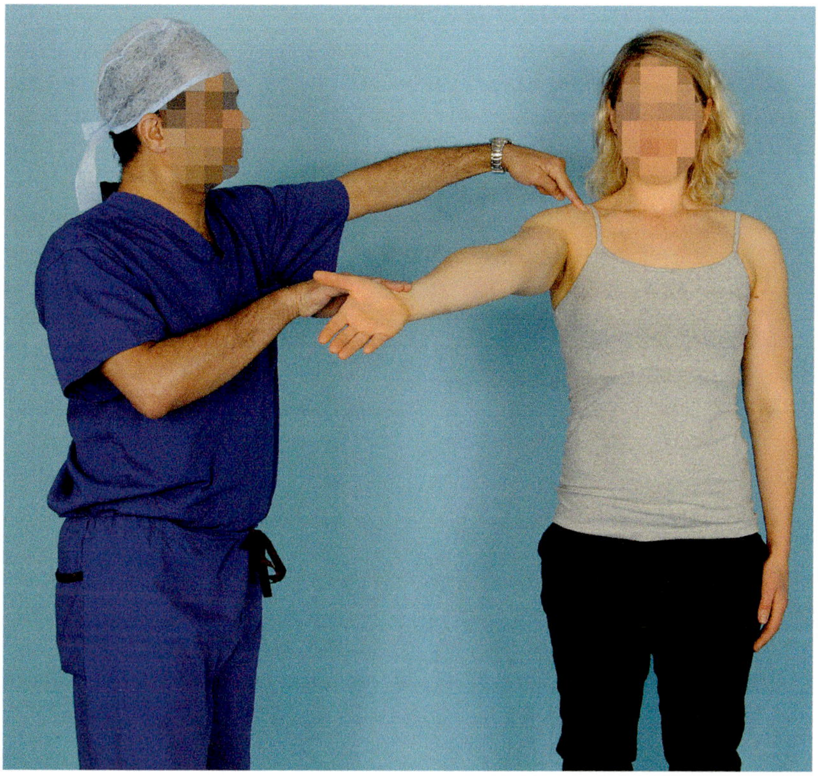

Fig. 34.16 Speed's test

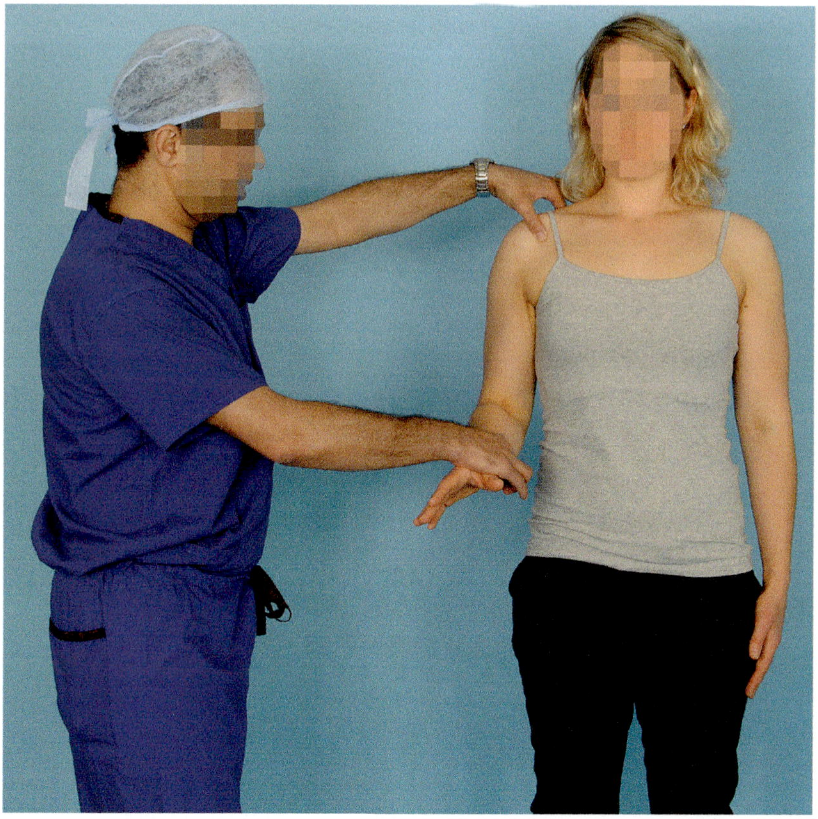

Fig. 34.17 Yergason's test

Clinically, both of these conditions exhibit reduced active and importantly, also passive ROM. The best technique to diagnose these two conditions is to attempt external rotation of the shoulder with the elbow flexed to 90° and the arm by the side of the body. Reduced passive external rotation on the pathological side indicates one of the above two diagnoses. The final distinction between the two is made on an X ray (which is normal in capsulitic shoulder and shows features of arthritis in an arthritic shoulder). Occasionally, crepitus is apparent on ROM in an arthritic shoulder.

Clinical Pearl

Whilst testing for apprehension/relocation for diagnosis of anterior instability, stabilisation of the scapula is essential to prevent thoracic external rotation. This test is therefore best done with the patient lying down (the couch stabilises the scapula). In the absence of a couch in the examination room, use a chair with back rest to stabilise the scapula before performing this test.

Instability

GHJ stability is defined as maintenance, or prompt return, of humeral head alignment within the glenoid fossa. This relies on coordination between static and dynamic components. This is mediated by the sensorimotor and proprioceptive systems via mechanoreceptors to the central nervous system [28]. Shoulder 'instability' can be defined as abnormal glenohumeral joint (GHJ) motion resulting in symptoms due to a variety of structural and non-structural causes which result in pain +/− subluxation or dislocation for the patient [29].

To understand shoulder instability, it is important to understand "The Stanmore Triangle". This was developed to help classify shoulder instability as a continuum of pathologies [30] (Fig. 34.18).

Stanmore Classification

Type I (traumatic, structural)
Type II (atraumatic, structural), usually associated with hyperlaxity
Type III (atraumatic, non-structural), usually associated with abnormal muscle patterning

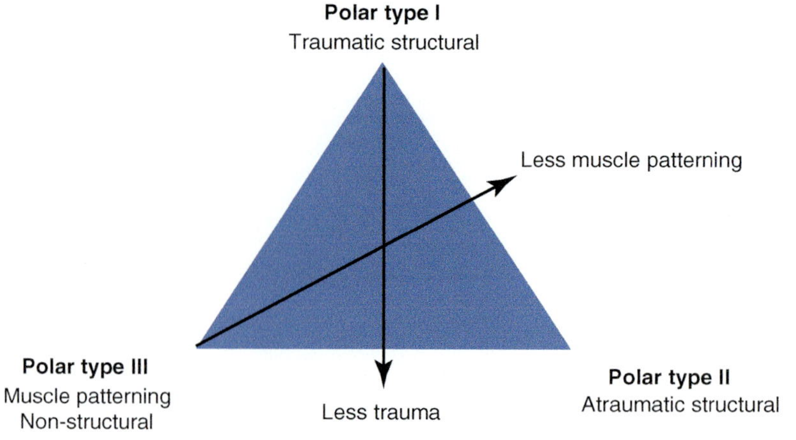

Fig. 34.18 Stanmore classification of shoulder instability

Eliciting clinical signs from patients suffering from this type of instability using specific 'tests' is not easy as often patients do not have polar type instabilities (e.g. purely Type I, II or III) but present as a combination (for example a type II instability that then goes on to develop abnormal muscle patterning as seen in type III).

Type 1: Traumatic Instability with Mostly a Structural Causation

Orthopaedic surgeons are mostly faced with this pathology when a patient presents with an acute traumatic event resulting in shoulder instability. It is usually unilateral with no muscle patterning pathology. Investigations often reveal a structural pathology such as a "Bankart and Hill-Sach's lesion". In a proportion of patients, these episodes of instability can become recurrent, more often than not needing surgical intervention.

The following clinical tests can be used to diagnose this condition.

Assessment of Structural Causes of Instability

When assessing a patient with instability, we first try and distinguish between laxity and instability. Laxity is mostly physiological and instability pathological. Laxity can sometimes predispose to instability. Initially we assess generalised laxity with the Beighton Hypermobility Score [31].

The threshold for joint laxity in a young adult, ranges from 4 to 6. A score above 6 indicates hypermobility (Table 34.1).

If the Beighton score is greater 6 it is also worth looking for skin hyperlaxity and asking about bleeding disorders to differentiate between benign joint hypermobility and a collagen disorder, such as Ehler-Danlos Syndrome or Marfan's (Heart valve surgery / lens dislocation). The "systemic score" can be performed to aid in the diagnosis of Marfan Syndrome if unsure.

Table 34.1 Beighton hypermobility score

Joint	Finding	Points
Left little (fifth) finger	Passive dorsiflexion >90°	1
	Passive dorsiflexion ≤90°	0
Right little (fifth) finger	Passive dorsiflexion >90°	1
	Passive dorsiflexion ≤90°	0
Left thumb	Passive dorsiflexion to the flexor aspect of the forearm	1
	Cannot passively dorsiflex thumb to flexor aspect of the forearm	0
Right thumb	Passive dorsiflexion to the flexor aspect of the forearm	1
	Cannot passively dorsiflex thumb to flexor aspect of the forearm	0
Left elbow	Hyperextends >10°	1
	Extends ≤10°	0
Right elbow	Hyperextends >10°	1
	Extends ≤10°	0
Left knee	Hyperextends >10°	1
	Extends ≤10°	0
Right knee	Hyperextends >10°	1
	Extends ≤10°	0
Forward flexion of trunk with knees full extended	Palms and hands can rest flat on the floor	1

We then assess the laxity of the shoulder.

1. The ability to externally rotate past 90° with the arm by the patient's side is often seen in lax shoulders (in the absence of a subscapularis tear). Both shoulders should be assessed and compared.
2. We then assess for the presence of a sulcus sign using the inferior sulcus test [32]. The patient can remain sitting or standing. Inferior traction is applied to the arm and the appearance of a sulcus just inferior to the lateral border of the acromion is assessed (Fig. 34.19). In lax patients, the result is

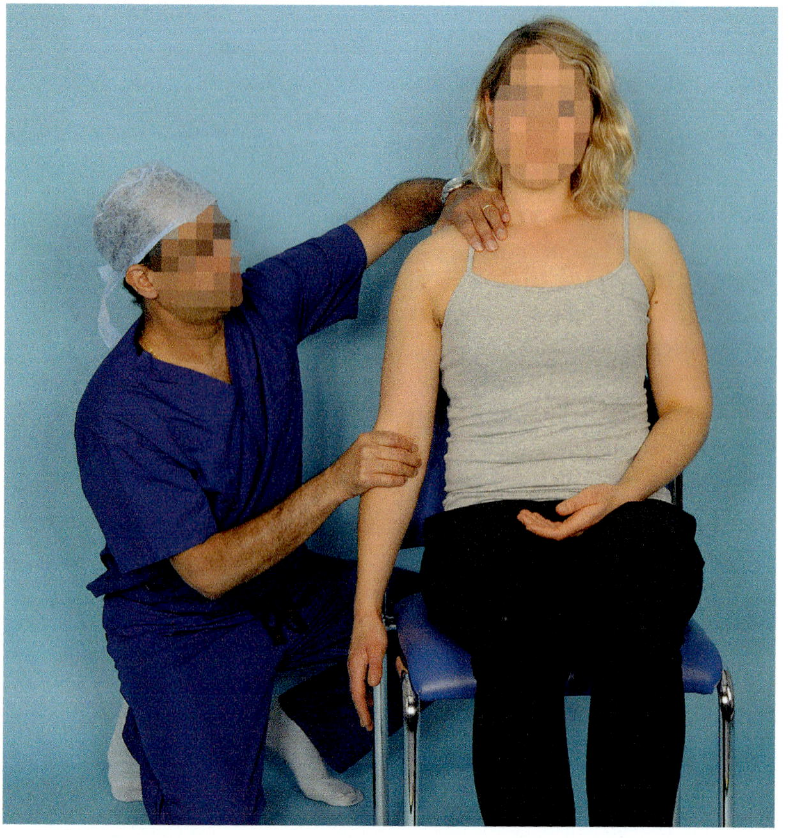

Fig. 34.19 Sulcus sign

usually similar bilaterally. Asking the patient if this sensation feels like their symptoms can be helpful.

The size of the sulcus may be recorded as Grade 1 (0–1 cm), Grade 2 (1–2 cm) and Grade 3 (>2 cm). The test should be repeated with the shoulder in maximal external rotation. This should tighten the superior glenohumeral ligament and rotator interval decreasing the amount of inferior laxity. If this doesn't and the result is unilateral, a lesion should be considered.

3. Gagey's Hyperabduction Test to assess inferior Glenohumeral joint complex laxity [33]. The scapula is stabilized with one hand and the examiner (who stands behind the patient) hyper abducts the shoulder until the scapula wants to move (Fig. 34.20). This measures the range of passive abduction of the glenohumeral joint with a positive result being over 105°.

We believe shoulder instability as being caused by structural and non-structural causes. The next section will cover tests to diagnose structural causes of shoulder instability.

Tests for Anterior Instability

1. Load and Shift Test described by Silliman and Hawkins [34]. The patient is sitting or supine and the arm is abducted 20°, forward flexed 20° and in neutral rotation. The GHJ is then loaded with an axial force. An anterior and then a posterior force are applied to the humerus (Figs. 34.21 and 34.22). The amount of translation is recorded along with symptoms of instability and apprehension. The translation can be graded using the same

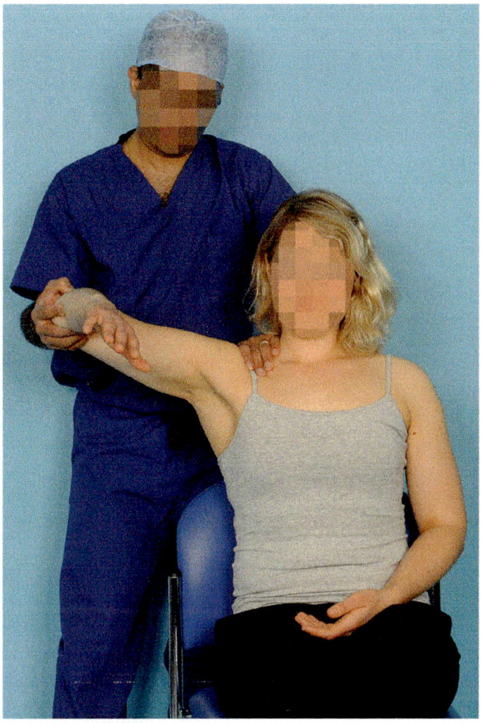

Fig. 34.20 Gagey's hyperabduction test

measurements as for the Sulcus Sign. The senior author does not routinely perform this test as it can be difficult to interpret this is muscular patients (common in this patient group).

2. Jobe's Apprehension-Relocation Test in the supine position [35]. We perform this test in four steps. Apprehension, Augmentation, Relocation and Release.

Apprehension

The shoulder is actively abducted to 90°, maximally externally rotated and the sensation of apprehension is assessed.

Augmentation

With this position maintained, an anterior force is exerted over the posterior aspect of proximal humerus to assess if apprehension increases.

Relocation

A posterior force is then applied over the humeral head (to relocate the subluxing humeral

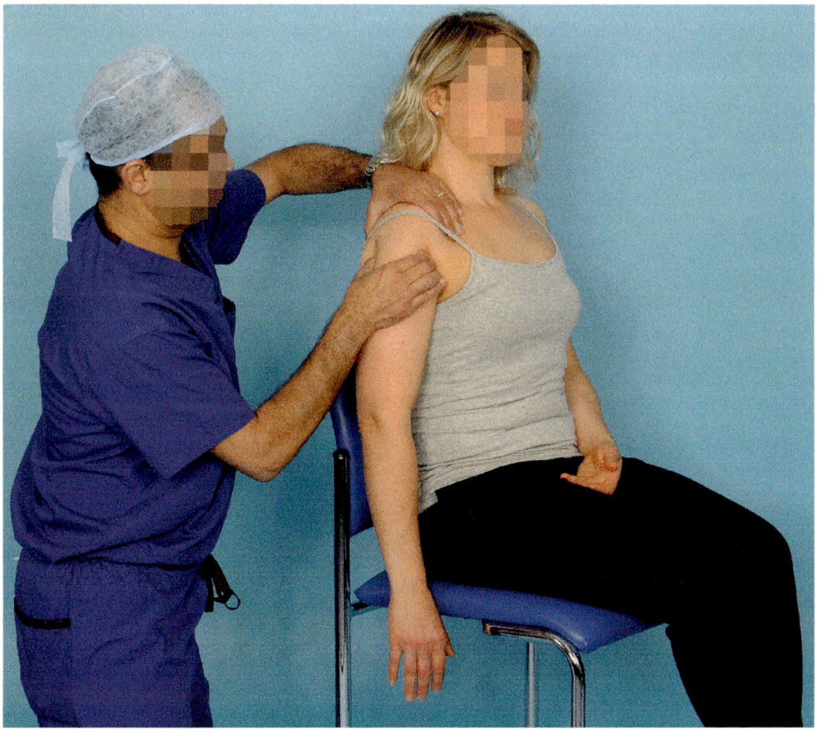

Fig. 34.21 Load and shift test sitting

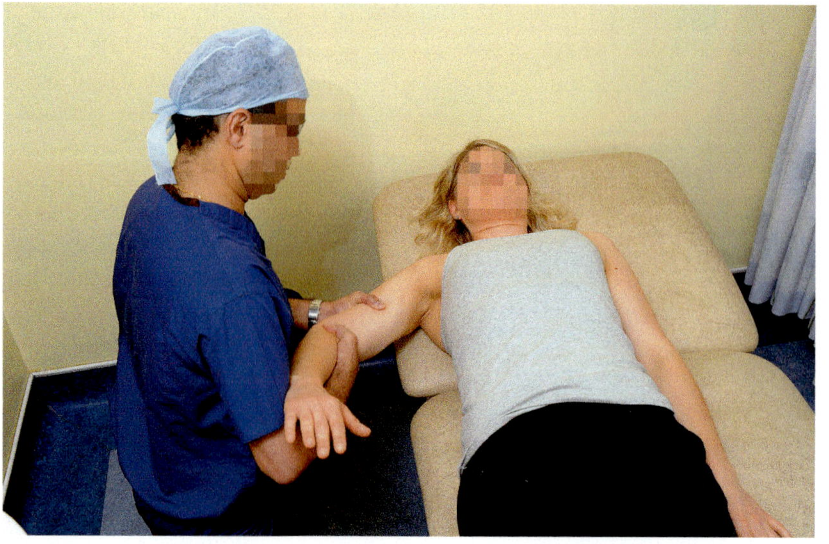

Fig. 34.22 Load and shift test supine

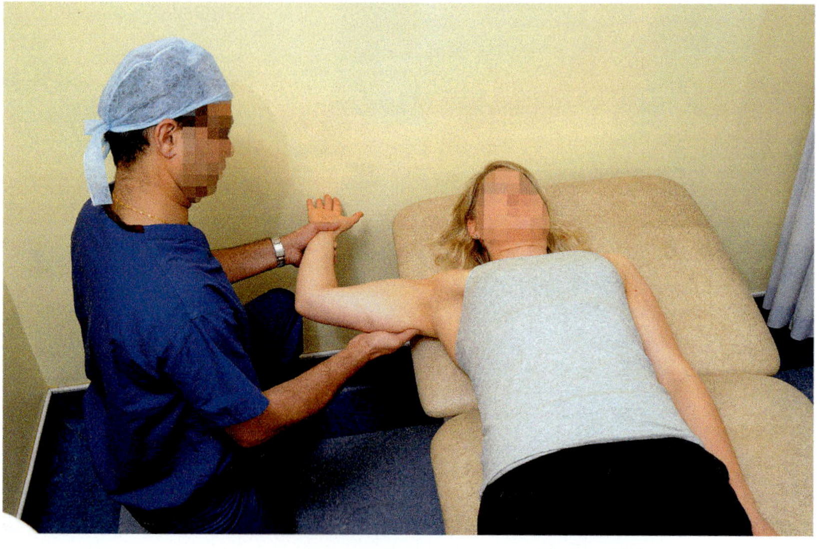

Fig. 34.23 Anterior instability: augmentation

head), which should decrease the feeling of apprehension/instability.

Release

We then release this posteriorly directed force and the patient experiences sudden increase in his instability symptoms (extreme care needs to be taken to not dislocate the shoulder during this maneuver). Figures 34.23, 34.24 and 34.25 demonstrate the steps for anterior instability testing.

When using apprehension (not pain) as a positive result, Speer (1994) showed the test to be 68% sensitive and 100% specific [36].

Tests for Posterior Instability

The Jerk Test and Kim's Test are our preferred tests to assess for posterior instability.

Jerk Test

The surgeon grasps the patient's scapula with one hand and the affected arm is held at 90° abduction and internal rotation. The examiner then grasps the elbow and axially loads the humerus in a proximal direction. The arm is moved horizontally across the body (adducted) (Figs. 34.26 and 34.27).

A positive result is indicated by a sudden clunk or pain as the humeral head slides/tries to

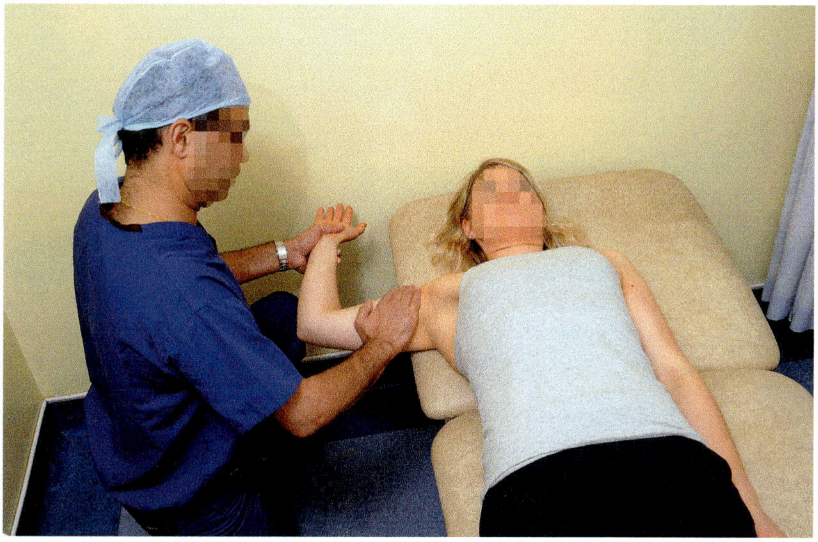

Fig. 34.24 Anterior instability: relocation

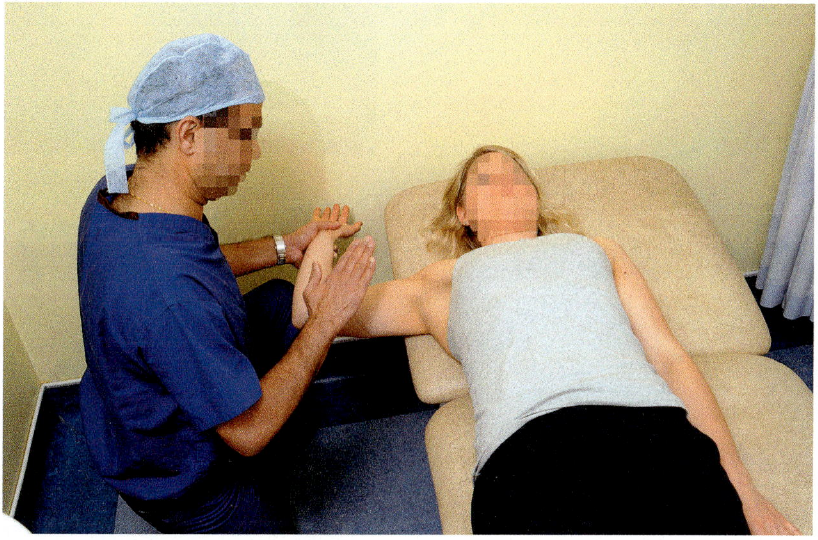

Fig. 34.25 Anterior instability: release

slide off the back of the glenoid. When the arm is returned to the original position, a second jerk may be observed, that of the humeral head returning to the glenoid. The sensitivity of this test is 73% and specificity 98% [37].

Kim's Test

In this test, the patient is in a sitting position. The arm is elevated to 90° of abduction and the examiner holds the elbow and lateral aspect of the proximal arm, and applies a strong axial loading force. The arm is then elevated 45° diagonally upward, and then a downward and backward force is applied to the proximal arm (Figs. 34.28 and 34.29). A sudden onset of posterior shoulder pain indicates a positive test result, regardless of accompanying posterior clunk of the humeral head. The sensitivity of the Kim's test was 80% and specificity was 94% [38].

Kim's test was more sensitive in detecting a predominantly postero-inferior labral lesion, whereas the jerk test was more sensitive in detecting a predominantly posterior labral lesion. The

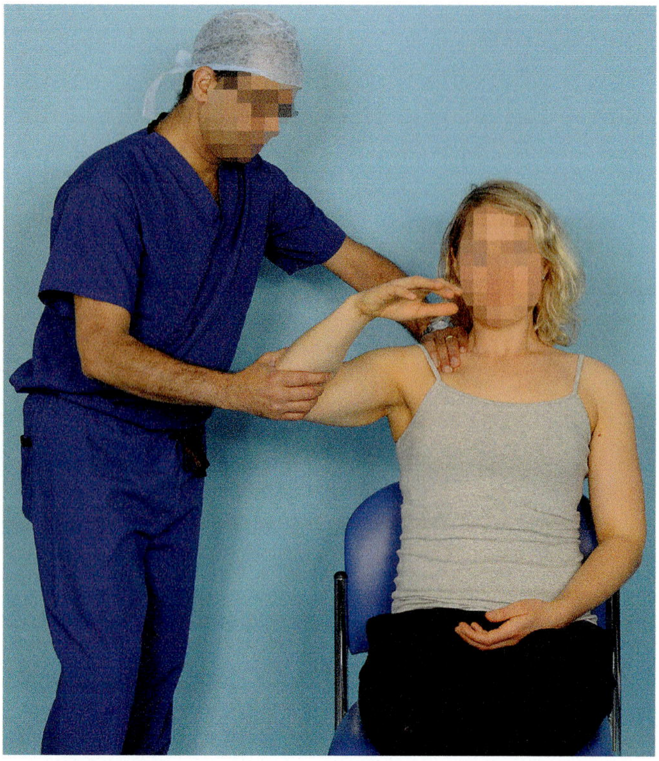

Fig. 34.26 Jerk test starting position

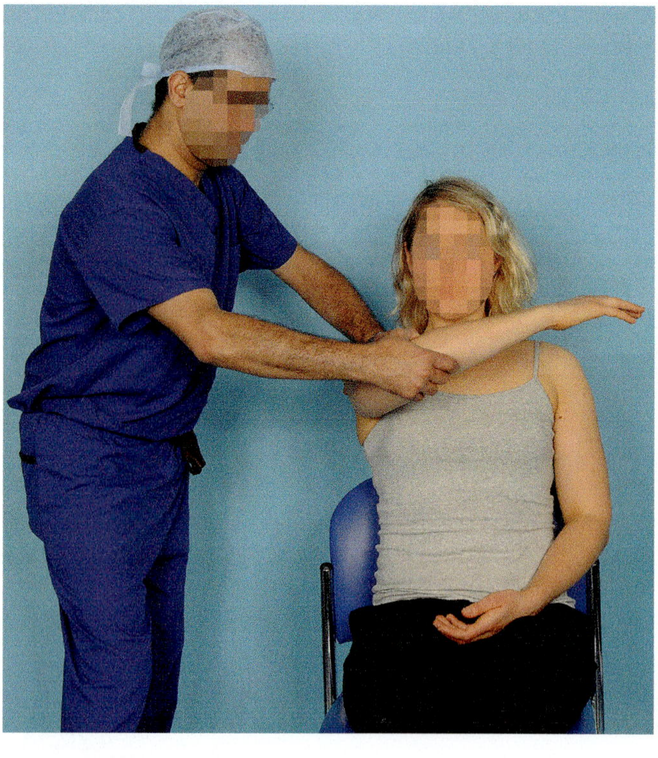

Fig. 34.27 Jerk test adducted position

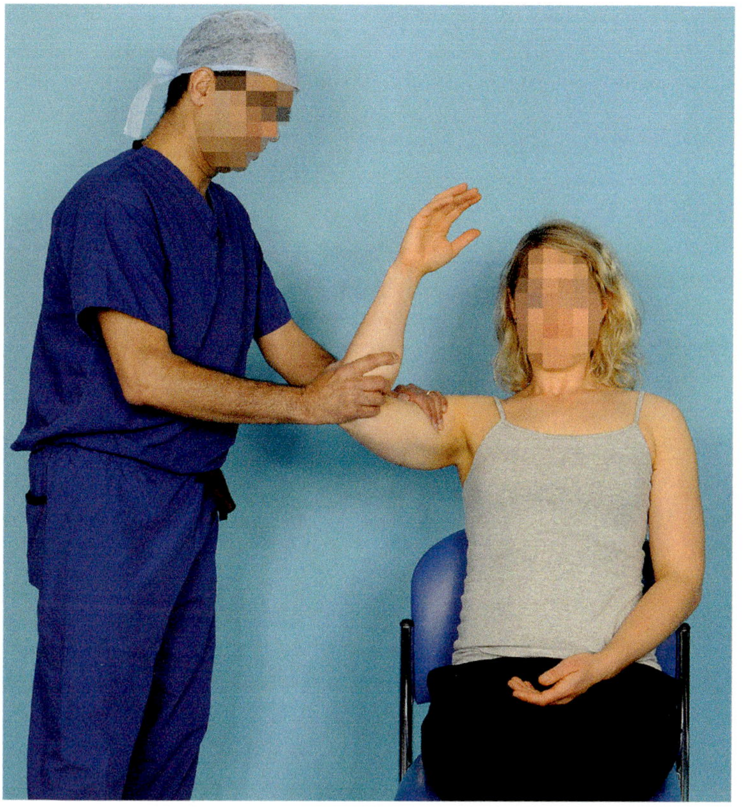

Fig. 34.28 Kim's test starting position

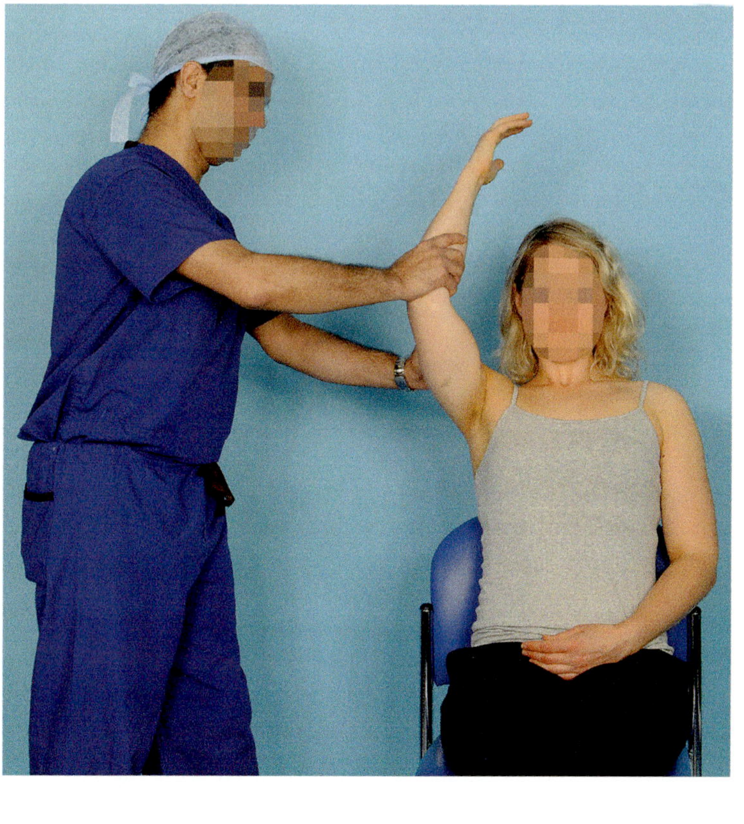

Fig. 34.29 Kim's test final position

sensitivity in detecting a postero-inferior labral lesion increased to 97% when the 2 tests were combined.

Type 2: Atraumatic Instability with Occasional Structural Causation – Includes 'Dynamic Shoulder Instability' in the Younger Patients

Shoulder assessment in non-structural pathology can be challenging. In most cases, problem solving involves making clinical decisions in ambiguous situations [39]. Diagnosing these "non-structural pathologies" should incorporate not only a combination of 'orthopaedic tests' previously described but also identify other contributory factors to a patient's symptom presentation, which are often multifactorial and complex in nature.

Our aim in this section is to identify some useful examination procedures for the orthopaedic clinician to utilise in the outpatient clinic setting to aid identification of patients who should be directed towards specialist physiotherapy management as surgical intervention in such patients is usually contraindicated [40]. These may not be the 'traditional' specialist tests which are designed to identify a single structural pathology but instead should enable the examiner to assess the patient in the context of presenting symptom, combined with subjective history and epidemiological knowledge [41].

The previous section has described in detail how to assess for patients presenting with structural shoulder pathology. This section aims to further build on this assessment of the shoulder.

There is a complex interaction between the structural (capsulo-labral complex, rotator cuff and congruency between the glenoid and humeral head) and non-structural elements (GHJ neuromuscular control including central and peripheral nervous system) which are pre-requisites for a stable shoulder [30].

These patients usually present with unilateral shoulder symptoms with no significant trauma but may describe minor and/or repetitive injuries. They often present with capsulo-ligamentous dysfunction and/or damage to the articular surfaces. They do not have marked abnormal patterning causing GHJ dislocation but they often exhibit reduced neuromuscular GHJ control resulting in subtle instability causing the so called 'dynamic impingement' [29].

Strength of the rotator cuff muscles can be assessed as previously described using orthopaedic tests. However, a recent systematic review concluded that although these tests have high sensitivity in reproducing shoulder symptoms, they have low specificity which greatly reduces their ability to diagnose specific structural pathology [42]. Tests for individual rotator cuff muscles lack specificity partly as they do not function as individual entities [43]. Furthermore, the highly innervated subacromial bursa has a central role in shoulder pain generation, and orthopaedic tests designed to assess individual muscles also will compress bursal tissue [44]. No combination of orthopaedic tests has emerged to date that are capable of accurately assessing rotator cuff and bursal pathology [45]. Furthermore, non-structural shoulder instability is usually the result of abnormal levels of shoulder muscle activation (neuromuscular control) and not a strength deficit, thus requiring a different method of assessment [46].

In response to this, alternative methods of shoulder assessment have been presented to modify a patient's symptoms through clinical examination that aids treatment and can be used as an adjunct to the orthopaedic tests previously described (for diagnosis of a structural shoulder pathology) [47]. The premise behind these procedures being that once a symptomatic movement is identified, a Symptom Modification Procedure or 'SSMP' is applied to correct it.

The main correctional procedures which will be highlighted as useful tests that are currently utilised by the authors in clinical practice [39].

1. The effect of thoracic posture and the scapula
2. The relationship between the humeral head and scapula

The effect of manual correction during an objective test performed by the therapist to the scapula/humeral head determines whether the 'assisted' position reduces the patient's symptoms and/or improves objective findings e.g. range of shoulder motion. Altered neuromuscular control of the scapula and humeral head are characteristics of non-traumatic shoulder instability and can led to a range of problems including pain, apprehension, 'impingement' and neuropathic symptoms [29]. Improvement in any of these through clinician facilitation is likely to confirm the presence of some of these characteristics and can be a helpful guide for therapist led shoulder rehabilitation [48].

If patient's objective tests fail to improve following a 'symptom modification procedure' in terms of reduced pain and/or increased range of motion, the examiner needs to consider if there are any underlying structural lesions which may be contributing to their clinical presentation and further investigations may be warranted [48].

Thoracic Posture and the Scapula

Some patients have been shown to have downwardly rotated scapulae with deficient in upward rotation [49]. This reduces the contact area between the humeral head and glenoid and results in excessive humeral head translation. This can cause pain due to subtle instability causing dynamic impingement [48].

The aim of these simple clinical procedures described below is to change the patient's symptoms by influencing shoulder biomechanics. If the clinician can influence a patient's symptoms positively then directed physiotherapy can be instituted.

Techniques

(a) **Active scapular shrug** – simply ask the patient to actively shrug their shoulder and whilst maintaining the position, repeat the painful motion e.g. shoulder flexion [50].

If pain is reduced or abolished, then weakness in the upper trapezius muscles could be partly responsible for the patient's symptoms.

Scapular dykinesia is characterised by a protracted, drooping and downwardly tilted scapula with reduced upward rotation [51]. The 'shrug' helps to facilitate scapular upward rotation and therefore potentially increase the sub-acromial space and reduce positive impingement signs (such as a painful arc) [50].

(b) **Manual assistance of the scapula into a 'corrected position'**:

Currently, there are various 'tests' described in the literature that essentially have the same purpose which is to manually facilitate/correct scapulothoracic motion in order to influence symptoms [52]. This can be collectively simplified as:

The Modified Scapula Assistance test (SAT)

The Scapula assistance test (SAT) was first described by Kibler (1998). If the scapula is downwardly rotated (or laterally tilted), clinician should facilitate manual upward rotation of the scapula through its correct motion plane [52]. This maneuver facilitates the force couple activity of the serratus anterior and lower trapezius muscles. Rabin et al. (2006) described a modified version of the SAT by assisting posterior tipping of the scapula in addition to assisted upward rotation to further facilitate scapular kinematic motion [53] (Figs. 34.30 and 34.31).

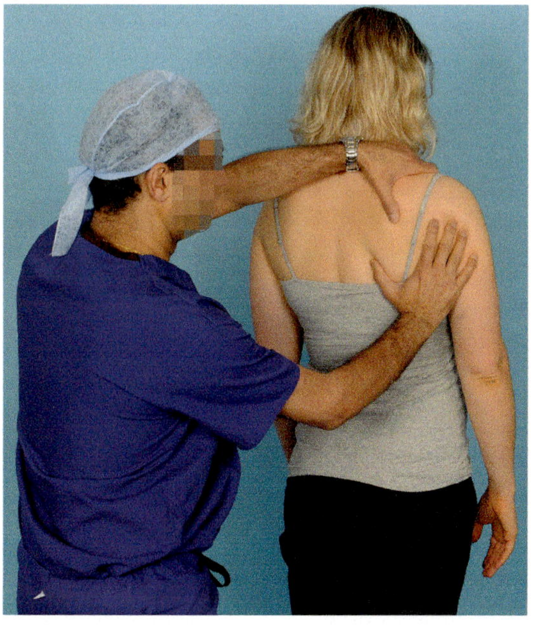

Fig. 34.30 Scapular assistance test starting position

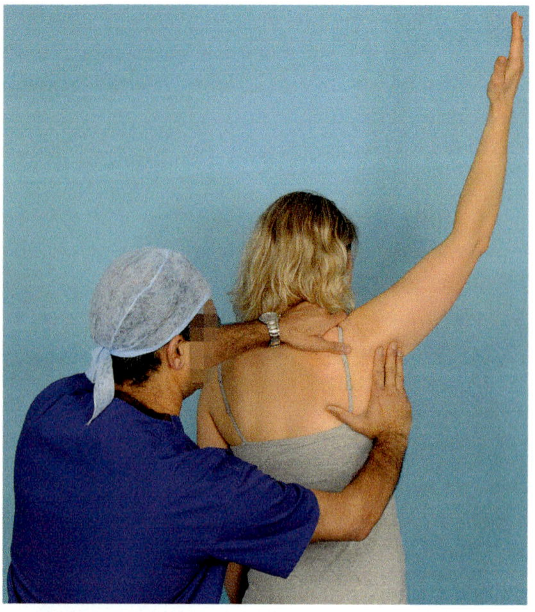

Fig. 34.31 Scapular assisitance test final position

Scapula Retraction Test (SRT)
This involves the clinicians palm of the hand stabilising the medial border of the scapula (if winging) into a position of retraction on the thorax, then maintaining this pressure to prevent medial border winging as the arm is elevated. If symptoms during movement are reduced or abolished with these maneuvers, then the patient would benefit from physiotherapy to address scapular control and rotator cuff strengthening prior to considering any surgical intervention [54] (Fig. 34.32).

(c) **Correction of thoracic kyphosis**
Simply correct the patient's thoracic kyphosis either by verbal instruction or gentle manual assistance, then re-test patient's painful movement [49]. Pronounced thoracic kyphosis can cause scapular protraction/tilt reducing the sub acromial space. Reduction in kyphosis has been shown to improve shoulder range of motion in symptomatic shoulders [55].

The Relationship Between the Humeral Head and Scapula

The aim of this manual correction technique is to influence the humeral head position in relation to the glenoid fossa. Weakness and/or reduced activation of the infraspinatus and supraspinatus muscles during shoulder flexion can result in excessive translation superiorly of the humeral head in the fossa [39, 56]. This leads to reduction in subacromial joint space and subsequent mechanical compression of the internal structures and has been observed in patients with subacromial impingement syndrome [56, 57].

Technique
A posteriorly (or anteriorly directed pressure) is gently applied by the clinician's hand as the patient raises their arm. A 'positive' response would be a patient reported reduced or abolished symptoms and/or increased range of motion [48]. A reduction in humeral head anterior/posterior glide is the result of manual facilitation to increase activity in the rotator cuff. This helps to increase the sub acromial space and thus reduce 'impingement' like symptoms [41, 57].

Positive results would also indicate that the patient may benefit from specific physiotherapy exercises to address GHJ neuromuscular control and activation / strengthening of the rotator cuff muscles [58].

Type III: Abnormal Muscle Patterning Causing Shoulder Instability

This type of non-traumatic shoulder instability is caused due to abnormal glenohumeral neuromuscular control affecting the shoulder muscles, mainly pectoralis major (PM), latissimus dorsi (LD), deltoid and the rotator cuff [46]. There is no structural damage to the articular surfaces. This is often bilateral and an associated underlying generalised joint hypermobility and / or excessive shoulder laxity [29].

Biomechanical as well as electromyography studies have highlighted that muscles can have both, a stabilizing and a destabilizing role within the shoulder, which can occur in the absence of structural damage. Konrad et al. (2006) illustrated in a cadaveric model, how increased forces in PM and LD increased anteriorly directed forces in end-range positions of the gleno humeral joint, resulting in decreased joint stability [59]. Infaspinatus and supraspinatus stabilise the GHJ when it is externally rotated in abduction and

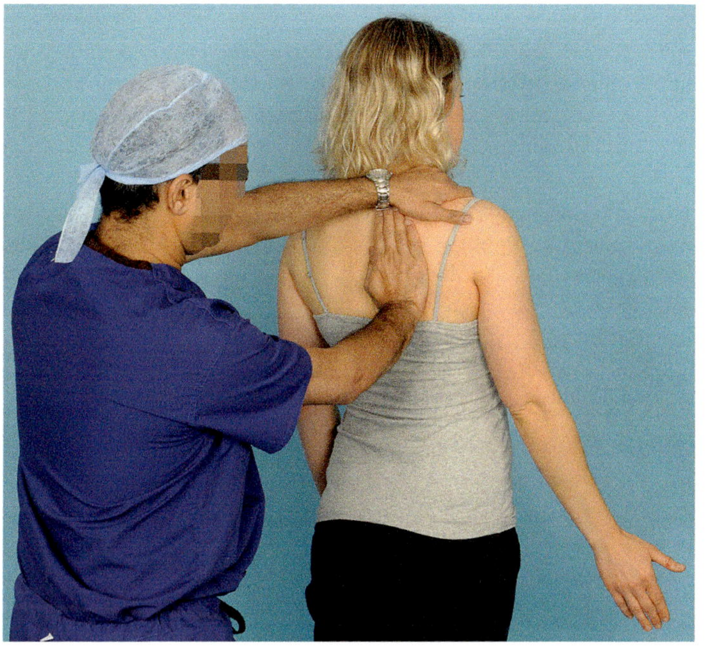

Fig. 34.32 Scapular retraction test

therefore deactivation of these muscles secondary to deficiencies in neuromuscular control could further compromise anterior shoulder stability [46, 60]. The rotator cuff acts as a unit to prevent unwanted humeral head translation and asynchronous patterns of activation are apparent in patients with MDI [46, 61].

Clinical Observation of Pectoralis Major Dominance

The arms are lifted in internal rotation and the clinician observes / palpates PM hyper activity. It is also useful to assess abnormal PM activation with active elbow flexion. Just ask that the patient flexes and extends their elbow joint and palpate/observe for inappropriate activation of the pectoralis major muscle. As a result of excessive activity of PM, there is an associated inhibition of infraspinatus, lower trapezius, serratus anterior and posterior deltoid resulting in GHJ instability [29]. PM was found to be more active in 60% of shoulders presenting with anterior instability [62]. Targeted therapy can be used to then treat this condition.

Clinical Observation for LD Dominance

The clinician observes for palpable activation of latissimus dorsi with GHJ flexion and/or lateral rotation in neutral shoulder position [29] The scapula will appear fixed with reduced upward rotation due to the resultant downward pull of the latissimus dorsi.

Side flexion of trunk to 'dominant side' with inability to stand on one leg is also a common feature of patients with LD dominance (often trunk will side flex more on symptomatic side as they fix to maintain trunk stability with their LD) [63]. LD was found to be more active in 81% of shoulders with anterior instability and 80% with posterior instability [62]. In asking a patient to 'step forwards and reach upwards' (through scaption) with both upper limbs, latissimus dorsi activity in some patients can be reduced by increasing postural muscle tone and increasing activation of the deep stabilizing muscles to allow upwards rotation of the scapula and improved glenohumeral joint positioning. This results in an improvement in range and quality of shoulder movement [29, 64].

Involuntary Posterior Positional Instability

This is defined as an involuntary instability caused by abnormal muscle action around the GHJ. It was first described by Huber & Gerber (1994) who first recognised that some dislocations had an involuntary component, which in the absence of any psychiatric disorder, often responded well to appropriate strengthening programmes [65].

Shoulder elevation often reveals as the primary abnormal movement pattern, with many patients commonly exhibiting posterior subluxation of the GHJ as the arm is raised. This is often the result primarily of under-activity of the external rotators (infraspinatus, supraspinatus, posterior deltoid) with some patients exhibiting over activity in the medial rotators, anterior deltoid and LD [66].

Patients often move their arms with the glenohumeral joint in internal rotation. A simple correction of this abnormal movement pattern is achieved by asking the patients to raise their arms in a position of external rotation, which can facilitate activation of the posterior rotator cuff and reciprocal inhibition of the internal rotators, resulting in normal movement patterns being achieved. Referral to a physiotherapist for further assessment and rehabilitation is recommended and surgery in these patients where structural pathology has been excluded, is contraindicated.

Assessment of Core Stability

Deficiencies in core stability may result in proximal muscle imbalances and should therefore be evaluated as part of a shoulder examination. No standard way has been described but one option is the 'single leg squat' or 'Corkscrew test' [67].

Test

The patient is asked to stand on one leg with no verbal cue, and perform a single leg squat. The clinician observes deviations such as trendelenburg posture or an external rotation of the standing limb indicating poor postural control and proximal core muscle weakness. Other indicators of poor core stability include the patient using their arms for balance, or motion in to an excessive flexed or rotated posture ('corkscrewing').

Cervical Spine and Thoracic-Outlet Syndrome "Neurological Assessment"

Cervical Spine

We inspect the alignment of the spine and observe skin condition for any cervical surgery scars. We palpate for tender spots followed by assessment of range of movement (ROM). This involves flexion/extension, rotation and lateral flexion (on either side). We observe if these movements cause pain around cervical spine or if they create any shooting pains, specifically past the elbow. If there is suspicion of the cervical spine being the pain source, then we would look for Lhermitte's sign and perform Spurling's test and assess for upper limb tension.

Lhermitte's Sign/Phenomenom First described in 1917 and popularised by Lhermitte [68]. A positive test occurs when an electrical sensation runs down the back or affected limbs upon neck flexion. It indicates a lesion or compression of the upper cervical spinal cord or lower brainstem.

Spurling's Sign/Test Passively slightly extend and laterally flex the cervical spine towards the symptomatic side. If further axial compression with the neck in this position reproduces the characteristic pain and radicular features on the same side the neck is tilted, then the sign/test is positive. This test is positive for cervical radiculopathy and is indicative of "pinching of the nerve root" with the maneuver [69] (Fig. 34.33).

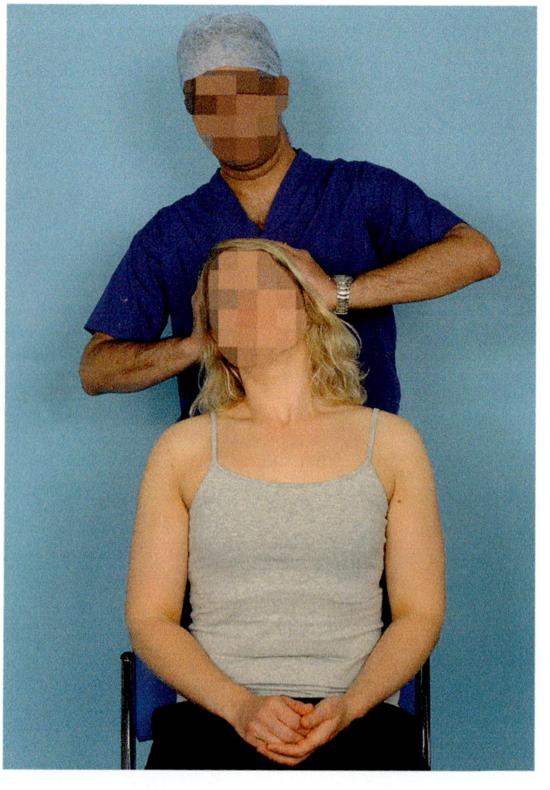

Fig. 34.33 Spurling's test

If any of the above are positive, a more targeted spine examination is required along with full neurological assessment.

Thoracic Outlet Syndrome (TOS) involves compression of the nerves, arteries or veins in the passageway from the lower neck to the axilla, with symptoms generally occurring with overhead activities. It can cause pain around the neck, shoulder, shoulder girdle as well as the upper back and into the hand. We use two main special tests to aid the diagnosis of TOS.

Adson's Test

This test was first described in 1927 and formally published in 1947 [70]. The patient is asked to rotate the head to the ipsilateral side with an extended neck along with abduction, external rotation and extension of the shoulder (Fig. 34.34). The patient is then asked to take a deep inspiration. A positive result is seen with the loss of radial pulse (or reduction in vigour of the pulse). However, a positive result may be seen in up to 50% of normal patients [71]. This maneuver reduces the sub-clavicular space and in the presence of a cervical rib/ fibrous band (or other such lesion), creates symptoms.

Roos' Test

This test was popularised by Roos in 1966 [72]. It is also called the "Hands Up" Test or EAST (Elevated Arm Stress Test) Test. It involves abducting and externally rotating the shoulders to 90° with elbows bent at 90°. The patient is then asked to flex and extend his fingers for up to 3 min. It is most useful in diagnosing neurogenic TOS with pain and paraesthesia occurring within 60 s in 94% of patients [73]. The same authors described a reduction or loss of radial pulse with this test but this was observed in only 24% of patients.

To complete shoulder examination, we advise assessment of distal neuro-vascular status, examination of ipsilateral elbow and hand and contralateral shoulder, elbow and hand.

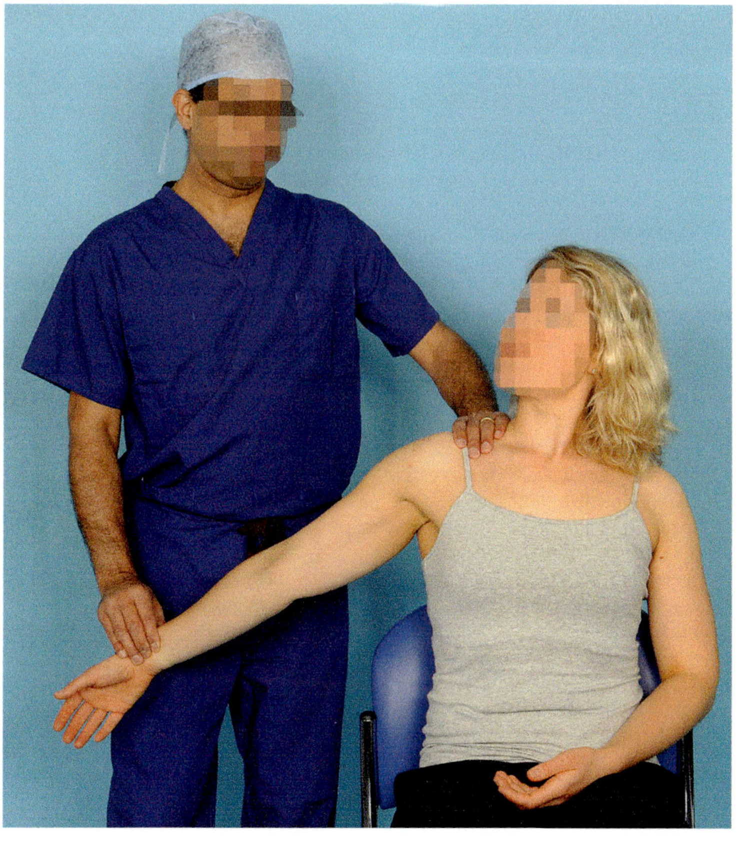

Fig. 34.34 Adson's test

Clinical Pearl

No one single positive special test should be relied upon to reach a diagnosis but should be used in conjunction with other aspects of your assessment. A reliable history, an examination that correlates with this, a number of positive special tests and the appropriate investigations are often all needed to reach a firm diagnosis.

References

1. Codman EA. The shoulder: rupture of the supraspinatous tendon and other lesions in and about the subacromial bursa. Chap 5. Boston: Thomas Todd; 1934. p. 123–77.
2. Williams GR, Nguyen VD, Rockwood CA. Classification and radiographic analysis of acromioclavicular dislocations. Appl Radiol. 1989;18:29–34.
3. Barnes CJ, Van Steyn SJ, Fischer RA. The effects of age, sex, and shoulder dominance on range of motion of the shoulder. J Shoulder Elb Surg. 2001;10(3):242–6.
4. American Academy of Orthopaedic Surgeons. Joint motion: method of measuring and recording. Chicago: American Academy of Orthopaedic Surgeons; 1965.
5. Neer CS II. Anterior acromioplasty for the chronic impingement syndrome in the shoulder: A preliminary report. J Bone Joint Surg. 1972;54A:41–50.
6. Neer CS II. Impingement lesions. Clin Orthop. 1983;173:70–7.
7. Hawkins R, Kennedy J. Impingement syndrome in athletes. Am J Sports Med. 1980;8(3):151–8.
8. McLaughlin HL. On the frozen shoulder. Bull Hosp Joint Dis. 1951;12:383–90.
9. Jobe FW, Moynes DR. Delineation of diagnostic criteria and a rehabilitation program for rotator cuff injuries. Am J Sports Med. 1982;10(6):336–9.
10. Jobe FW, Jobe CM. Painful athletic injuries of the shoulder. Clin Orthop. 1983;173:117–24.
11. Itoi E, Kido T, Sano A, Urayama M, Sato K. Which is more useful, the "full can test" or the "empty can test," in detecting the torn supraspinatus tendon? Am J Sports Med. 1999;27(1):65–8.
12. Kelly BT, Kadrmas WR, Speer KP. The manual muscle examination for rotator cuff strength. An electromyographic investigation. Am J Sports Med. 1996;24(5):581–8.
13. Hertel R, Ballmer FT, Lombert SM, et al. Lag signs in the diagnosis of rotator cuff rupture. J Shoulder Elb Surg. 1996;5:307–13.
14. Merolla G, De Santis E, Sperling JW, Campi F, Paladini P, Porcellini G. Infraspinatus strength assessment before and after scapular muscles rehabilitation in professional volleyball players with scapular dyskinesis. J Shoulder Elb Surg. 2010;19(8):1256–64.
15. Arthuis M. Obstetrical paralysis of the brachial plexus I. diagnosis: clinical study of the initial period. Rev Chir Orthop Reparatrice Appar Mot. 1972;58:124–36.
16. Goutallier D, Postel J-M, Bernageau J, Lavau L, Voisin M-C. Fatty muscle degeneration in cuff ruptures. Clin Orthop. 1994;304:78–83.
17. Walch G, Boulahia A, Calderone S, Robinson AH. The 'dropping' and 'hornblower's signs in evaluation of rotator-cuff tears. J Bone Joint Surg Br. 1998;80(4):624–8.
18. Barth JR, Burkhart SS, De Beer JF. The bear-hug test: a new and sensitive test for diagnosing a subscapularis tear. Arthroscopy. 2006;22(10):1076–84.
19. Gerber C, Krushell RJ. Isolated rupture of the tendon of the subscapularis muscle. Clinical features in 16 cases. J Bone Joint Surg Br. 1991;73:389–94.
20. Greis PE, Kuhn JE, Schultheis J, Hintermeister R, Hawkins R. Validation of the lift-off test and analysis of subscapularis activity during maximal internal rotation. Am J Sports Med. 1996;24(5):589–93.
21. Gerber C, Hersche O, Farron A. Isolated rupture of the subscapularis tendon. J Bone Joint Surg Am. 1996;78:1015–23.
22. O'Brien SJ, Pagnani MJ, Fealy S, McGlynn SR, Wilson JB. The active compression test: A new and effective test for diagnosing labral tears and acromioclavicular joint abnormality. Am J Sports Med. 1998;26:610–3.
23. Chronopoulos E, Kim TK, Park HB, Ashenbrenner D, McFarland EG. Diagnostic value of physical tests for isolated chronic acromioclavicular lesions. Am J Sports Med. 2004;32(3):655–61.
24. Guanche CA, Jones DC. Clinical testing for tears of the glenoid labrum. Arthroscopy. 2003;19(5):517–23.
25. Bennett WF. Specificity of the Speed's test: Arthroscopic technique for evaluating the biceps tendon at the level of the bicipital groove. Arthroscopy. 1998;8:789–96.
26. Holtby R, Razmjou H. Accuracy of the Speed's and Yergason's tests in detecting biceps pathology and SLAP lesions: comparison with arthroscopic findings. Arthroscopy. 2004;20(3):231–6.
27. Yergason RM. Supination sign. J Bone Joint Surg Br. 1931;13:160.
28. Myers JB, Wassinger CA, Lephart SM. Sensorimotor contribution to shoulder stability: Effect of injury and rehabilitation. Man Ther. 2006;11:197–201.
29. Jaggi A, Lambert S. Rehabilitation for shoulder instability. Br J Sports Med. 2010;44:333–40.
30. Lewis A, Kitamura T, Bayley JIL. Mini symposium: shoulder instability (ii). The classification of shoul-

der instability: new light through old windows! Curr Orthop. 2004;18:97–108.
31. Beighton PH, Horan F. Orthopedic aspects of the Ehlers-Danlos syndrome. J Bone Joint Surg (Br). 1969;51:444–53.
32. Neer CS II, Foster CR. Inferior capsular shift for involuntary inferior and multidirectional instability of the shoulder: a preliminary report. J Bone Joint Surg Am. 1980;62:897–908.
33. Gagey OJ, Gagey N. The hyperabduction test. J Bone Joint Surg Br. 2001;83:69–74.
34. Silliman JF, Hawkins RJ. Classification and physical diagnosis of instability of the shoulder. Clin Orthop Relat Res. 1993;291:7–19.
35. Jobe FW, Kvitne RS, Giangarra CE. Shoulder pain in the overhand or throwing athlete. The relationship of anterior instability and rotator cuff impingement. Orthop Rev. 1989;18(9):963–75.
36. Speer KP, Hannafin JA, Altchek DW, et al. An evaluation of the shoulder relocation test. Am J Sports Med. 1994;22:177–83.
37. Kim SH, Park JC, Park JS, Oh I. Painful jerk test: a predictor of success in nonoperative treatment of posteroinferior instability of the shoulder. Am J Sports Med. 2004;32(8):1849–55.
38. Kim SH, Park JS, Jeong WK, Shin SK. A novel test for posteroinferior labral lesion of the shoulder—a comparison to the Jerk test. Am J Sports Med. 2005;33(8):1188–92.
39. Lewis J. Rotator cuff related shoulder pain: assessment, management and uncertainties. Man Ther. 2016;23:57–68.
40. Malone AA, Jaggi A, Calvert PT, et al. Muscle patterning instability – classification & prevalence in reference shoulder service. In: Norris TR, Zuckerman JD, Warner JJ, Lee QT, editors. Surgery of the shoulder and elbow: an international perspective. Rosemont: American Academy of Orthopaedic Surgeons; 2006a. section 7.
41. Hegedus FJ, Wright AA, Cook C. Orthopaedic special tests and diagnostic accuracy studies: house wine served in very cheap containers. Br J Sports Med. 2017;51(22):1578–9.
42. Hegedus EJ, Goode AP, Cook CE, Michener L, Myer CA, Myer DM, et al. Which physical examination tests provide clinicians with the most value when examining the shoulder? Update of a systematic review with meta-analysis of individual tests. Br J Sports Med. 2012;46:964–78.
43. Clark JM, Harryman DT. Tendons, ligaments and capsule of the rotator cuff. Gross and microscopic anatomy. J Bone Joint Surg Am. 1992;74:713–25.
44. Ide K, Shirai Y, Ito H, Ito H. Sensory nerve supply in the human subacromial bursa. J Shoulder Elb Surg. 1996;5:371–82.
45. Lewis JS, Tennent TD. How effective are diagnostic tests for the assessment of rotator cuff disease of the shoulder? In: Evidence based sports medicine. 2nd ed. London: Blackwell Publishing; 2007. p. 327–60.
46. Barden JM, Balyk R, Raso VJ, Moreau M, Bagnall K. Atypical shoulder muscle activation in multidirectional instability. Clin Neurophysiol. 2005;116(8):1846–57.
47. Lewis JS. Rotator cuff tendinopathy / subacromial impingement syndrome: is it time for a new method of assessment? Br J Sports Med. 2009;43:259–64.
48. Watson L, Warby S, Balster S, Lenssen R, Pizzari T. The treatment of multidirectional instability of the shoulder with a rehabilitation programme: Part 1. J Shoulder Elb Surg. 2016;8(4):271–8.
49. Illyés Á, Kiss RM. Shoulder muscle activity during pushing, pulling, elevation and overhead throw. J Electromyogr Kinesiol. 2005;15:282–9.
50. Pizzari T, Wickham J, Balster S, Ganderton C, Watson L. Modifying a shrug exercise can facilitate the upward rotator muscles of the scapula. Clin Biomech. 2014;29:201–5.
51. Kibler WB, Sciascia A. Current concepts: scapular dyskinesis. Br J Sports Med. 2010;44:300–5.
52. Willmore EG, Smith MJ. Scapular dyskinesia: evolution towards a systems-based approach. Should Elb. 2016;8:61–70.
53. Rabin A, Irrgang JJ, Fitzgerald GK, Eubanks A. The Intertester reliability of the scapular assistance test. J Orthop Sports Phys Ther. 2006;36(9):653–9.
54. Roche SJ, Funk K, Sciascia A, Kibler B. Scapula dykinesis: the surgeon's perspective. J Shoulder Elb. 2015;7(4):289–97.
55. Bullock MP, Foster NE, Wright CC. Shoulder Impingement: the effect of sitting posture on shoulder pain and range of motion. Man Ther. 2005;10(1):28–37.
56. Reddy AS, Mohr KJ, Pink MM, Jobe FW. Electromyographic analysis of the deltoid & rotator cuff muscles in persons with subacromial impingement. J Shoulder Elb Surg. 2000;9:519–23.
57. Cholewinski JJ, Kusz PJ, Wojgechowski P, et al. Ultrasound measurement of rotator cuff thickness and acromiohumeral distance in the diagnosis of subacromial impingement syndrome of the shoulder. Knee Surg Sports Traumatol Arthrosc. 2008;16:408–14.
58. Horsley I, Herrington L, Hoyle R, Prescott E, Bellamy N. Do changes in hand grip strength correlate with shoulder rotator cuff function? J Shoulder Elb. 2016;8(2):124–9.
59. Konrad GG, Jolly JT, Labriola JE, McMahon PJ, Debski RE. Thoracohumeral muscle activity alters glenohumeral joint biomechanics during active abduction. J Orthop Res. 2006;24(4):748–56.
60. Itoi E, Newman SR, Kuechle DK, Morrey BF, An KN. Dynamic anterior stabilisers of the shoulder with the arm in abduction. J Bone Joint Surg. 1994;76(5):834–6.
61. Boettcher CE, Cathers I, Ginn K. The role of the shoulder muscles is task specific. J Sci Med Sport. 2010;13:651–6.
62. Jaggi A, Noorani A, Malone A, Cowan J, Lambert S, Bayley I. Muscle activation patterns in patients with recurrent shoulder instability. Int J Shoulder Surg. 2012;6:101–7.

63. Barrett C. The clinical physiotherapy assessment of non-traumatic shoulder instability. J Shoulder Elb. 2015;7(1):60–71.
64. Mcmullen J, Uhl T. A Kinetic Chain approach for shoulder rehabilitation. J Athl Train. 2000;35(3):329–37.
65. Huber H, Gerber C. Voluntary subluxation of the shoulder in children: a long-term follow up study of 36 shoulders. J Bone Joint Surg (Br). 1994;76(1):118–22.
66. Takwale VJ, Calvert P, Rattue H. Involuntary positional instability of the shoulder in adolescents and young adults. J Bone Joint Surg. 2000;82(5):719–23.
67. Kibler B, Press J, Sciascia A. The role of core stability in athletic function. Sports Med. 2006;36(3):189–98.
68. Lhermitte JJ, Bollak NM. Les douleurs à type décharge électrique consécutives à la flexion céphalique dans la sclérose en plaques. Un cas de la sclérose multiple. Rev Neurol. 1924;2:56–7.
69. Spurling RS, Scoville WB. Lateral rupture of the cervical intervertebral discs: a common cause of shoulder and arm pain. Surg Gynecol Obstet. 1944;78:350–8.
70. Adson AW. Surgical treatment for symptoms produced by cervical ribs and the scalenus anticus muscle. Surg Gynecol Obstet. 1947;85:687–700.
71. Gergoudis R, Barnes RW. Thoracic outlet arterial compression: prevalence in normal persons. Angiology. 1980;31:538–41.
72. Roos DB, Owens JC. Thoracic outlet syndrome. Arch Surg. 1996;93:71–4.
73. Sanders RJ, Haug CE. Thoracic outlet syndrome: a common sequela of neck injuries. Philadelphia: Lipppincott; 1991. p. 77.

35 Radiological Evaluation

David Temperley

Introduction

Radiological evaluation plays a major role in the assessment of shoulder trauma and in patients presenting with acute and chronic shoulder problems. This chapter will look at the major imaging modalities and assess their uses, advantages and disadvantages in specific clinical presentations.

Imaging investigation of the shoulder will often start with plain radiological examination. The indications for and radiological findings in ultrasound, MRI, MRI arthrogram, CT and nuclear medicine will be described in this chapter, along with the role of imaging in guiding therapeutic interventions.

Plain X-Ray

Plain x-ray of the shoulder is the most commonly performed imaging investigation in the initial assessment of the shoulder, whether in the context of acute trauma or patients presenting with chronic shoulder problems. An x-ray of the shoulder is of low cost and usually immediately available in the hospital setting. It is useful to assess or exclude common bony pathologies; fracture or dislocation in the context of acute trauma, and arthritis and degenerative changes in the patient presenting with chronic shoulder abnormalities. Plain x-ray does not generally allow assessment of the soft tissues, although calcification in soft tissues can readily be assessed, for example within the rotator cuff in calcifying tendonitis.

Three common views of the shoulder are performed; anteroposterior (generally with the shoulder externally rotated), lateral scapular 'Y-view', (where the coracoid and acromion form a Y shape with the blade of the scapula), and the axillary view (where the arm is abducted and the x-ray taken, generally, from inferior to superior).

Trauma

For a detailed description of shoulder trauma the reader should refer to appropriate chapters in the trauma section. The purpose of this section is to describe some of the radiographic difficulties in assessment of shoulder trauma.

Dislocation The most common anterior, subcoracoid dislocation is easily seen on standard radiographic analysis, including the AP view. Posterior dislocation, which occurs in less than 5% of cases, is more difficult to assess, as the humeral head may dislocate in a direct posterior position, with the result that the glenohumeral

D. Temperley, MB, MRCPI, FRCR (✉)
Department of Radiology, Wrightington Hospital, Wigan, UK
e-mail: david.temperley@wwl.nhs.uk

I. A. Trail et al. (eds.), *Textbook of Shoulder Surgery*, https://doi.org/10.1007/978-3-319-70099-1_35

space may appear to be preserved on the AP view. More commonly it overlaps the glenoid surface, or the glenohumeral joint space may appear widened. A hint to the presence of a posterior dislocation is the 'light bulb sign' where the contour of the greater tuberosity, normally seen on the AP view, is lost because of internal rotation leading to an oval-shaped 'light bulb' appearance (Fig. 35.1). In fixed posterior dislocations a ridge may be seen, representing the humeral head depression fracture caused by impaction by the glenoid [1].

Bony injuries associated with dislocation In anterior dislocation the glenoid rim and humeral head can both be fractured. Humeral head fractures typically form a wedge-shaped defect on the posterolateral surface of the humeral head due to impaction by the glenoid at the time of dislocation. This is known as the Hill-Sachs defect. These can be difficult to assess on plain x-ray, if small, due to not being seen in profile and also confusion with the normal shape of the greater tuberosity. A Bankart lesion is a tear of the glenoid labrum as a result of anterior humeral dislocation. Where this is accompanied by a bone defect, this is known as a bony Bankart fracture. Fractures of the glenoid rim can also be difficult to assess on plain x-rays. Assessment often requires CT scanning, where the bony Bankart defect can be measured in either degrees or percentage of the glenoid rim circumference. The bony and labral injuries associated with dislocation can be assessed with MRI arthrography, which will be discussed in the MRI section. In general, a defect of 20–25% of the glenoid surface is more likely to be associated with further dislocation [2]. Fractures of the scapula, in general, can be difficult to identify and assess on plain x-ray. This is due to the complexity of the shape of the bone, overlying structures, and difficulty in obtaining adequate x-ray views in the context of major trauma.

Proximal humerus fractures These are most commonly described according to the Neer classification [3]. This divides the upper humerus into 4 'parts'; the anatomic humeral head, the greater and lesser tuberosities and the humeral shaft. If a fracture fragment is fractured and displaced by more than 1 cm or 45°, this counts as a separate 'part'. Thus, fractures of the upper humerus could be 1, 2, 3 or 4 part fractures.

Post-traumatic osteolysis of the distal clavicle may occur as a result of acute or chronic repetitive trauma. This is thought to be associated with microfractures of the subchondral bone with osteolysis associated with chronic repetitive stress. In the early stage the x-ray may show distal clavicular osteopenia, followed by subtle ero-

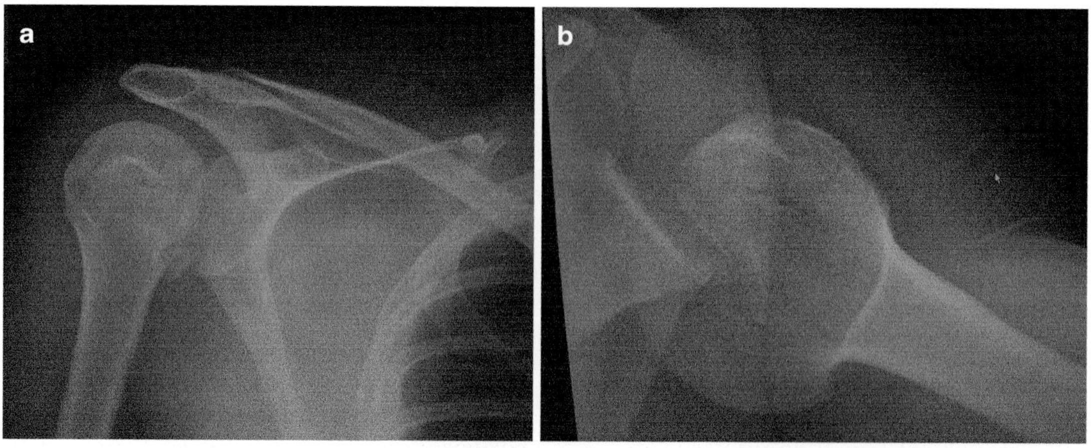

Fig. 35.1 AP (**a**) and axillary (**b**) views of the right shoulder. On the AP view the orientation between the humeral head and the glenoid is not clear, but the rounded 'light bulb' shape of the humeral head suggests the possibility of posterior dislocation, confirmed on the axillary view. There is an impaction fracture of the humeral head

sions which become larger, leading to tapering of the distal clavicle. MRI will show the erosive features with surrounding soft tissue and bone marrow oedema. The acromion side of the joint appears preserved [4].

Impingement and Rotator Cuff Tears

Impingement is a clinical diagnosis, and plain x-rays cannot visualise the rotator cuff; nevertheless secondary signs on plain x-ray can be useful.

Impingement in rotator cuff pathology is often associated with degenerative-type changes, including sclerosis and bony cyst formation, typically around the greater tuberosity. These tend to worsen with increasing severity of the rotator cuff disease. Acromioclavicular joint osteoarthritis should be observed; inferior osteophyte formation may be a cause of rotator cuff impingement.

When the rotator cuff tears and retracts the humeral head tends to displace superiorly into the space. This leads to a reduction in the distance between the humeral head and acromion which is normally around 10 mm. If the humeral head contacts the acromion, degenerative-type 'arthritis' may develop between the two bones. This will cause the acromion to mould to the shape of the humeral head. The glenoid and acromion thereby form an effectively continuous cavity; this process is known as acetabulisation. There is sometimes associated glenohumeral arthritis. In combination, these changes are known as 'rotator cuff arthropathy', and signify an inoperable rotator cuff tear [5] (Fig. 35.2).

Arthritis associated with massive rotator cuff tears has been classified according to severity [6]. This classification may have implication for disease progression and surgical outcome [7].

Classification of rotator cuff tear arthritis [6].

Grade 1. Preservation of subacromial space (greater than 6 mm)

Grade 2. Reduction of subacromial space (< 7 millimetres)

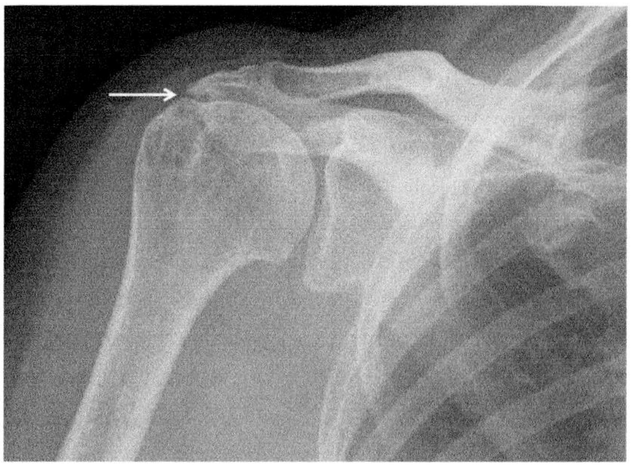

Fig. 35.2 Rotator cuff arthropathy. AP x-ray of right shoulder. There is elevation of the humeral head with reduction of the subacromial space (arrow). MRI (not shown) showed a massive full-thickness rotator cuff tear

Grade 3. Concave deformity of the undersurface of the acromion (acetabulisation)

Grade 4A. Associated glenohumeral arthritis without acetabulisation.

Grade 4B. Associated glenohumeral arthritis, with acetabulisation.

Grade 5. Rotator cuff arthropathy with osteonecrosis of the humeral head.

Certain anatomical variants have been associated with the development of impingement and rotator cuff disease. Such associations are not universally accepted, and are certainly not considered as being causative. The most commonly described association is with the shape of the undersurface of the acromion, as seen on the lateral scapular view, sagittal MRI sequence or sagittal CT reconstruction. Three acromion shapes were described by Bigliani in 1986 [8]; these are flat (type I), concave curve (type II) and an anterior acromion hook (type III). The type III acromion shape has been associated with impingement and rotator cuff tears, although not all authors have found such an association. A lateral down sloping acromion, as seen on the AP view, has also been associated with impingement. An unfused acromion, which is present in around 8% of the population, may be important as an additional cause of impingement and in surgical treatment, and should be observed when present.

Arthritis

Osteoarthritis Primary osteoarthritis of the glenohumeral joint is less common than in the hips and knees, but nevertheless is a significant clinical problem. As with other joints, the radiological features are of osteophyte formation, sclerosis of the joint surfaces and loss of cartilage, leading to reduction of joint space on the x-ray. When full-thickness cartilage loss occurs, sub articular cysts can occur which can lead to the erosion of the articular surfaces. Osteoarthritis of the acromioclavicular joint is more common, and can be associated with impingement and rotator cuff tears as described above.

Inflammatory arthritis The shoulder joint can be involved in inflammatoty arthritides, particularly rheumatoid arthritis. This is a multisystem disease of multifactorial cause, but autoimmune mediated. It most commonly involves the synovial joints, with inflammation of the synovium and consequent destruction of articular cartilage and bone, leading to loss of the joint spaces and erosion, with joint deformities in the later stages. In the shoulder, the glenohumeral joint can be involved, or erosions may be found in the humeral head away from the joint surface. The acromioclavicular joint is a common site of involvement with rheumatoid arthritis, leading to erosion typically of the lateral clavicle.

Crystal arthritis Crystals of mono sodium urate (gout), calcium pyrophosphate or hydroxyapatite may occur in or around the shoulder.

Gout Gouty arthritis is uncommon in the shoulder. Typical radiographic findings are of juxta-articular soft tissue swellings due to gouty tophi. Calcification of tophi is unusual. Intra-articular or juxta-articular erosions with overhanging edges are typical, and may be large.

Milwaukee shoulder is a specific but uncommon form of arthritis in the shoulder, first described in 1981. It typically occurs in elderly women and presents with pain and restricted movement. It is associated with hydroxyapatite crystals in or around the shoulder, although these are not necessarily causative. Initial x-ray may show findings of osteoarthritis, but the disease progresses rapidly with marked destruction of bone and soft tissue calcifications. Cross-sectional imaging, particularly MRI, will show complete rotator cuff tears and a large non-inflammatory effusion [9, 10].

Calcium pyrophosphate deposition disease may occur in the shoulder, although less commonly than in the knee or wrist. The cardinal radiological finding is of chondrocalcinosis; punctate or linear densities in fibrocartilage or hyaline cartilage. Arthritis may occur; typically findings similar to osteoarthritis, but often in unusual sites or distribution. This may lead to joint deformity. Diagnosis is by pathological finding of positively birefringent crystals in synovial fluid [11].

Septic arthritis As with septic arthritis in other joints, the x-ray will typically be normal in early stages of septic arthritis, and diagnosis should be made with microbiological analysis of joint fluid. With progression of untreated disease, there will be subarticular bony erosion and demineralisation with loss and subsequently destruction of the joint space.

Less common forms of arthritis and joint pathology The following conditions may present as or simulate arthritis in the shoulder. Typical radiological features are given [10].

Primary synovial chondromatosis This benign neoplastic process involves cartilaginous proliferation of the synovium. It typically occurs in three phases. In the early stage chondroid nodules develop in the synovium, which then become detached forming numerous loose bodies, and subsequently calcify or ossify. X-ray shows soft tissue swelling only, until the loose bodies calcify. Later, the loose bodies may be associated with joint erosion and osteoarthritis. MRI appearances depend on the stage of the disease; initially synovial proliferation will be seen, followed by numerous cartilaginous and subsequently calcified/ossified loose bodies. Typically the loose bodies are of similar size.

Pigmented villonodular synovitis This is a benign disease of synovial proliferation occurring in joints, bursae or tendon sheaths. Typically it presents in the third or fourth decades of life in most joints, but in an older age group in the shoulder joint. It is usually mono-articular. On imaging studies soft tissue swelling is present with bony erosions, typically on both sides of the joint, with sclerotic margins. MRI typically shows a lobulated mass which can be focal or diffuse. Multiple small haemorrhages occur, leading to haemosiderin deposition which shows as low signal on all sequences. Recurrent intra-articular haemorrhage occurs in relatively few conditions, so providing a useful diagnostic clue on MRI.

Haemophiliac arthropathy Osteoporosis secondary to synovial inflammation in the early stage, followed by bony erosion, joint space narrowing and changes similar to osteoarthritis. Epiphyseal overgrowth occurs when inflammation and hyperaemia persist in skeletally immature patients. On MRI, recurrent haemorrhages lead to haemosiderin deposition which is of low signal on all sequences and thus readily visible.

Neuropathic arthropathy In the shoulder, neuropathic arthropathy, also referred to as Charcot joint, is typically associated with syringomyelia. Early changes on x-ray may be similar to osteoarthritis, but the disease progresses with destruction and fragmentation of subchondral bone, deformity and sclerosis. Secondary fractures may occur, and MRI scanning and other cross-sectional imaging will show an effusion.

Calcifying Tendonitis

Calcifying tendonitis occurs when calcium hydroxyapatite crystals are formed within the rotator cuff tendons. The calcifications most commonly develop in supraspinatus, but not uncommonly in infraspinatus and subscapularis. The condition typically occurs in patients in their 40s or 50s and is self limiting with eventual spontaneous resorption of the calcification. However, it is painful and the symptoms may last for months or even years. X-ray shows sharply delineated calcification in the rotator cuff tendon (Fig. 35.3) which may become ill-defined and diffuse if the calcification ruptures into the overlying subacromial bursa.

Avascular Necrosis

Avascular necrosis of the humeral head is the second most common site after the femoral head. It is also known as osteonecrosis. It can

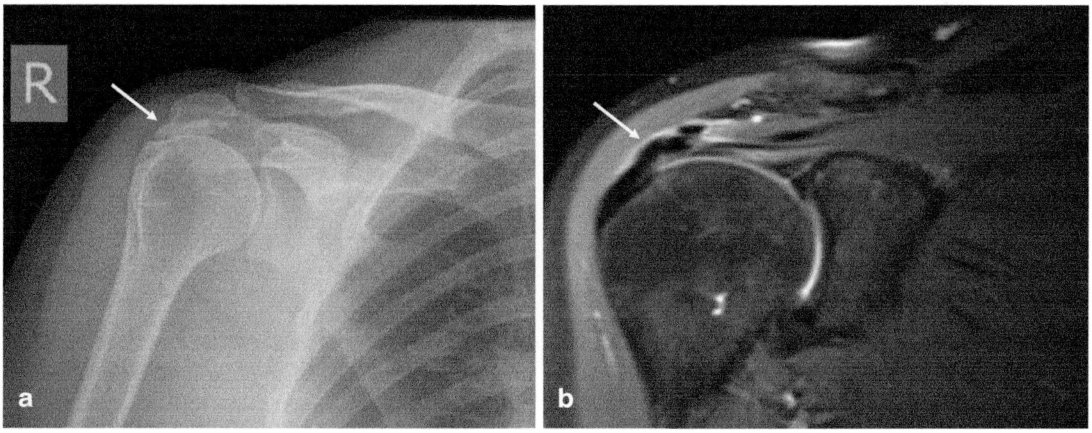

Fig. 35.3 AP x-ray (**a**) Oblique coronal fat-suppressed PD MRI (**b**) of the right shoulder. Large focus of calcification in the supraspinatus tendon due to calcifying tendonitis (arrow)

occur due to trauma or non-traumatic causes. In proximal humeral fractures, avascular necrosis is more likely with a greater degree of deformity (3 part or 4 part fractures), with fractures involving the anatomical neck, or if anatomical alignment is not achieved before healing. The commonest causes of non-traumatic avascular necrosis are steroid use and alcohol, and as with avascular necrosis in the hip, numerous other causes can be associated. Sometimes idiopathic cases are found without an obvious aetiological factor [12].

X-rays are initially normal. As the disease progresses, changes in bone density are seen, typically with subarticular radiolucency surrounded by a sclerotic line. This progresses to depression or fractures of the cortical surface. A thin linear fragment of subcortical bone may separate, known as the 'crescent sign'. This is followed by collapse of the humeral head, with secondary osteoarthritis developing as the final stage. MRI will show bone marrow oedema in the early radiologically normal stage. The avascular segment will then be demarcated from normal marrow by what is known as the 'double line sign' followed by depression and collapse of the humeral head as seen on x-ray [13].

Avascular necrosis has been classified according to a number of systems. The Steinberg staging system is summarised in brief as follows [14]:

Stage 0. Asymptomatic with normal imaging. Histological diagnosis only.
Stage I. Patient may be symptomatic. X-ray normal. MRI shows bone marrow oedema.
Stage II. Patient is symptomatic. X-ray shows osteopenia with marginal osteosclerosis. MRI is diagnostic and shows double line sign. Contour of humeral head is preserved.
Stage III. Imaging shows subchondral lucency and collapse with crescent sign.
Stage IV. Obvious flattening of the humeral head.
Stage V. Seclondary osteoarthritis.
Stage VI. Extensive destruction.

Adhesive Capsulitis

Also known as frozen shoulder, this condition is characterised by thickening and contraction of the shoulder joint capsule. It commonly occurs spontaneously, but can be post-traumatic and is 2–4 times more common in diabetics than the general population, and can be more severe in diabetics. It is self limiting, but symptoms can last for several years. The condition is divided into three stages.

- The painful 'freezing' stage, characterised by pain and increasing restriction of movement.
- The transitional 'frozen' stage, characterised by reduction in shoulder movement, where pain is less prominent.
- The thawing stage, characterised by gradual recovery and return of shoulder mobility.

X-rays are normal, and radiography will be performed to exclude other conditions. At arthrography (contrast injection under x-ray guidance) the volume of the shoulder joint will be reduced, particularly the axillary pouch. MRI may show thickening of the inferior glenohumeral ligaments and abnormal soft tissue thickening in the region of the rotator interval. However imaging is not diagnostic in this condition, and diagnosis relies on clinical features.

Hydrodilatation Treatment of adhesive capsulitis is discussed elsewhere, but includes an imaging guided technique known as hydrodilatation or arthrographic distension, in which contrast and saline are injected into the shoulder joint, generally under x-ray guidance, in order to distend the joint capsule. Steroid and local anaesthetic are usually injected during the procedure, which is followed by physiotherapy starting a few days afterwards. This procedure has been shown to be successful in improving pain and to a lesser extent movement in 70–90% in case studies (for example see reference 15, where the procedure is described). If hydrodilatation is not successful, or the condition recurs, the procedure can be repeated, or the patient can be considered for manipulation under anaesthetic or arthroscopic capsular release.

Systematic reviews have found insufficient high quality primary research to make conclusions about the cost-effectiveness of the procedure when compared with other treatments [16, 17].

Ultrasound

Principles of Ultrasound

Medical ultrasound uses high-frequency sound waves in order to gain diagnostic images from soft tissues. Sound is audible from frequencies of approximately 20–20,000 Hz. Ultrasound uses inaudible frequencies very much higher than this; typically from 2.5 to 18 MHz.

An electric current is applied to a piezoelectric crystal. This in turn vibrates and transmits oscillations of pressure (sound waves) into the tissues. These may be absorbed, reflected or scattered by the soft tissues. Most of the reflected or scattered waves are lost into the tissues, but some travel back to the transducer which vibrates in response. This vibration is converted back into an electrical current which is analysed to give an analogue picture. The property of the transducer crystal- converting electrical current to sound waves and back again- is called the piezoelectric effect.

Sound waves are reflected at interfaces of different impedance (impedance is the product of the physical density of the tissue and the speed of sound in the tissue). There are subtle differences in the impedance between soft tissues. As a result a little sound is reflected (but most transmitted) for example at the interface between fat and muscle or between muscle fibres. A little more sound is reflected from the next tissue interface and so on. The computer calculates depth by the time taken for the sound to return. As a result an image is built of the slice of tissue directly deep to the probe, and a three-dimensional picture obtained by sweeping the probe across the skin.

When the sound waves strike an interface between materials of very different impedance, for example soft tissue to bone, almost all of the sound is reflected, and therefore ultrasound cannot be used to assess bones or tissues that are occluded by bones, such as joint spaces. If there is no difference in impedance within a tissue no sound will be reflected; hence fluid appears 'anechoic' (or black).

Special Techniques in Ultrasound

Doppler Effect

This relies on the fact that in a moving substance (blood) the reflected surface will be successively closer or further away with each echo. The scanner computer translates this into colour, which is superimposed on the image. In musculoskeletal ultrasound the Doppler Effect is generally used to calculate the overall amount of blood flow, which is increased in inflammation (for example inflammatory arthritis) and infection.

Elastography

Diseased tissues are often harder or stiffer than normal tissues. Ultrasound can make use of the principal by applying pressure, either manual or by creating an ultrasonic shockwave. The elasticity or stiffness of the tissue can be measured by assessing how much this deforms the tissue. Thus a harder tissue, such as a tumour, can be distinguished from surrounding normal soft tissues, as it deforms or compresses less. The principal is similar to clinical palpation; a tumour is felt on applying pressure as it is harder and than surrounding tissues. In musculoskeletal ultrasound, elastography is currently a developing technology, and not in general standard use [18].

Use of Ultrasound in Assessing Shoulder Pathology

From the above it will be apparent that musculoskeletal ultrasound is useful for the assessment of muscles and tendons and also in the assessment of fluid collections including effusions. It is not useful for bony pathology and cannot fully visualise inside the shoulder joint. This means, for example, it can be used to assess the rotator cuff, but not a full examination of the glenoid labrum.

Impingement and Rotator Cuff Pathology

Assessment of patients presenting with impingement and pathology of the rotator cuff is the most common clinical indication for shoulder ultrasound. It is accurate in the assessment of full-thickness rotator cuff tears, and can visualise partial-thickness tears, although with less accuracy. Ultrasound is often performed when initial conservative management for impingement including physiotherapy has failed.

A practitioner learning to scan for shoulder pathology should undergo a specific training program, and some authorities define a particular number of cases scanned in addition to an assessment of proficiency. However, the basic scanning technique can be detailed here [19].

The practitioner may stand behind the seated patient, or can be sitting facing the patient. The patient is initially scanned with the elbow flexed and palm facing upwards. This brings the long head of biceps and bicipital groove directly anterior to the humeral head, and the biceps is scanned in this position. The arm is then externally rotated to examine the subscapularis, and then internally rotated, for example the hand placed behind the back, in order to bring the supraspinatus anteriorly. The infraspinatus is examined from behind with the arm adducted (placed on the opposite shoulder). Each tendon can be examined in the longitudinal and transverse planes. The acromioclavicular joint is then assessed for osteoarthritis and fluid. An examination of the supraspinatus and infraspinatus muscles can be made by observing them superior and inferior to the scapular spine respectively. It should be noted that ultrasound is not as accurate at assessing rotator cuff atrophy as MRI or CT. The patient can be scanned to assess for impingement by elevating the arm and watching the rotator cuff pass underneath the coraco-acromial ligament. A thickened subdeltoid bursa may be seen to 'bunch' as it passes under the ligament. However, impingement is a clinical diagnosis and the principal use of ultrasound in impingement is to assess for rotator cuff tears.

The normal rotator cuff tendons are seen in the longitudinal plane as a series of echogenic lines, showing the linear fibrillar structure of the tendon. This is a common appearance to tendons throughout the body.

Full-thickness rotator cuff tears are seen as defects in the rotator cuff tendon, most commonly supraspinatus, which extend across the full width of the tendon at least for a small area. In the acute traumatic rotator cuff tear there is often fluid outlining the defect. This is not usually the case in the chronic, degenerative rotator cuff tear. A small full-thickness tear will be seen because the sub-deltoid bursa dips into the tear defect leaving a concave bursal margin as compared to the normal convex margin. In massive rotator cuff tears the rotator cuff tendons may not be seen as they retract under the acromion. In this situation the tear could be overlooked if the operator mistakes normal deltoid for the retracted rotator cuff tendon. Rotator cuff tears are most commonly seen to involve supraspinatus, extending to infraspinatus and/or subscapularis when they become larger. A subscapularis tear may be seen in isolation; it is particularly important to identify subscapularis tears as they may change the surgical approach compared with the tear that involves supraspinatus only.

Partial-thickness tears can be identified as a defect which does not completely traverse the full-thickness of the rotator cuff tendon. In rotator cuff tendinopathy the tendon appears thickened and can present an amorphous appearance instead of the normal linear fibrillar structure.

Fluid collections and effusions associated with rotator cuff pathology are readily visualised, and can be identified in the subcoracoid bursa, biceps tendon sheath or subdeltoid bursa.

Ultrasound has been shown to be accurate in the assessment of full-thickness rotator cuff tears, with a sensitivity of 92% and specificity of 93% in a recent meta-analysis (Cochrane review, 2013) [20]. This is comparable to MRI. Ultrasound is less sensitive than MRI in the detection of partial-thickness rotator cuff tears, but with similar specificity. (Ultrasound: Sensitivity 52%, specificity 93%. MRI: Sensitivity 74%, specificity 93%).

Biceps Tendon Pathology

The long head of biceps tendon is examined as part of the rotator cuff ultrasound technique described above. It can easily be seen within the bicipital groove on the anterior aspect of the humeral neck. The normal tendon is visualised as an echogenic linear fibrillar structure. In tendinopathy the tendon becomes thicker and less echogenic, and fluid can be seen within the tendon sheath. When torn, the biceps tendon usually retracts inferiorly, below where the pectoralis major tendon crosses, and the torn biceps tendon end can usually be seen here when not identified within the bicipital groove. The intact biceps tendon can dislocate medially from the bicipital groove; and can be readily seen here if specifically sought.

Calcifying Tendonitis

As described above, ultrasound does not pass from soft tissues into bone due to marked differences in acoustic impedance. The same applies to calcification from any cause, and as a result the calcium hydroxyapatite found in calcifying tendonitis is easily visualised on ultrasound because almost all of the sound is reflected from the surface of the calcification. The symptoms, pathogenesis and stages of calcifying tendonitis will be described in a separate chapter. On ultrasound, calcifications are most commonly seen within the supraspinatus tendon, but can also occur within infraspinatus or subscapularis. Calcifications may be sharply delineated, typically seen with the 'chalky' calcification seen in the calcifying phase, with a softer and more amorphous appearance seen during the resorptive phase. Ultrasound can be used to guide a definitive treatment of calcifying tendonitis as described below.

Ultrasound Guided Injections

Ultrasound guidance is commonly used to help ensure correct placement of injections, typically corticosteroid and local anaesthetic, into the intended joint or tissue space. Many injections can be undertaken either blind or with ultrasound guidance, but ultrasound has been shown to ensure more accurate placement and better results [21]. The intended target is identified on ultrasound and, while holding the probe in one hand, the injection is made with the other. The needle is generally advanced obliquely along the plane of the ultrasound probe, so that the tip can be seen as it reaches its intended position. A diagnostic injection of local anaesthetic can now be made, or a therapeutic corticosteroid injection. Alternatively, an effusion or fluid collection can be aspirated for microbiological or biochemical analysis.

Commonly, the subacromial space, biceps tendon sheath or acromioclavicular joint are accessed in this way, while the glenohumeral space can be injected under ultrasonic or x-ray fluoroscopic guidance.

The suprascapular notch, which contains the suprascapular nerve, can readily be identified and accessed under ultrasound guidance. Injections around the suprascapular nerve are typically given to patients with painful rotator cuff arthropathy who are medically unfit for definitive surgery [22]. An injection of local anaesthetic and corticosteroid is given for diagnosis and temporary pain relief (suprascapular nerve block) or pulsed radiofrequency can be applied under ultrasound guidance to ablate the nerve and provide longer term pain relief [23].

As described above, the calcifying foci in calcifying tendonitis are readily identified on ultrasound. Under ultrasound guidance fluid (generally local anaesthetic) can be injected into the calcification and calcium containing fluid aspirated. After repeated aspiration most of the calcification can be removed with this technique. This procedure is known as barbotage. Alternatively, or if the aspiration is unsuccessful, the calcification can be needled (punctured on multiple occasions) in order to encourage natural resorption of the calcification and healing. An injection of corticosteroid and local anaesthetic is often given into the overlying subdeltoid bursa in order to suppress any inflammatory reaction caused by the needling. Treatment of calcifying tendonitis in this way has been shown to be significantly better than steroid injection alone, with over 70% improvement in pain [24]. The procedure can be repeated, but refractory cases may require surgery.

Advantages of ultrasound guided therapeutic procedures include

- Diagnostic assessment can be made at time of injection to exclude other conditions.
- Accurate placement of needle.
- Structures to be avoided (for example vessels) can easily be seen
- Outpatient procedure; general anaesthetic not required.
- Trauma to surrounding tissues is less than with surgery.
- Rapid recovery compared with surgery.
- Avoidance of ionising radiation.

Ultrasound in Other Conditions

Tumours Musculoskeletal soft tissue tumours around the shoulder, as elsewhere, can readily be assessed with ultrasound or magnetic resonance imaging. If a palpable lesion is most likely to be benign, ultrasound is appropriate to confirm the clinically suspected diagnosis. Ultrasound will accurately distinguish between cystic and soft tissue masses. Effusions, bursal fluid collections and ganglions can be distinguished and assessed. Ultrasound is also accurate in the assessment of superficial lipomas. If the mass is clinically concerning for malignancy the initial cross-sectional imaging should be with MRI, with early involvement of a centre that treats soft tissue tumours.

Infection Ultrasound is useful to assess for effusions or fluid containing abscesses which can be aspirated for diagnosis under ultrasound guidance.

Inflammatory arthritis Ultrasound will show effusions associated with the arthritis. Doppler assessment is useful to show increased blood flow signifying inflammation. Ultrasound in the diagnosis of inflammatory arthritis is most commonly performed of the hands and wrists rather than large joints.

Assessment of instability and labral tears The glenoid labrum is poorly and incompletely assessed on ultrasound; as a result MRI and MRI arthrography are commonly used for assessment of instability and labral tears.

Summary

Ultrasound is a useful diagnostic technique in shoulder pathology. It can be used in association with clinical assessment to provide a rapid diagnosis. The most common indications include diagnostic ultrasound for assessment of the rotator cuff and biceps tendons, and ultrasound guidance for therapeutic injections. The main disadvantages are its inability to assess bony and intra-articular pathology.

Magnetic Resonance Imaging

Introduction

Magnetic resonance imaging (MRI) provides the most comprehensive imaging assessment of shoulder pathology, and can assess a wide range of conditions. It provides useful information on bone, cartilage, tendon and muscle in rotator cuff pathology and instability/labral abnormalities. These are the two most common clinical indications where MRI is used [25].

Principles of MRI Imaging

In its most commonly used form, MRI only 'sees' protons (hydrogen nuclei). The patient is placed into a strong magnetic field. The quantum physics behind the behaviour of protons in the magnetic field is beyond the scope of this chapter (and most doctors!) However a basic understanding is helpful in image interpretation. The proton spins on an axis which 'wobbles', like a spinning top. This wobbling is known as precession. The proton is therefore acting like a tiny magnet. Normally, the proton axes are in a random orientation. Within the strong magnetic field of the MRI scanner, the protons align along the line of the magnetic field (the head to foot alignment of the patient), but continue to precess at random. A short electromagnetic pulse is applied to the patient. This is in the radiofrequency range; for a 1.5T magnet the frequency is around 64 MHz, just below the standard radio FM range. The protons respond by deflecting, so that the magnetic field becomes transversely rather than longitudinally orientated, and the precession, rather than being random is now in phase (the protons now precess together). When the radiofrequency pulse is removed the magnetic pulse recovers to its longitudinal orientation. This is known as T1 relaxation. In addition, the protons, precessing together under the influence of the radiofrequency pulse, start to go out of phase as they relax towards completely random precession. This is known as T2 relaxation. The T1 and T2 relaxation produce a signal, which is picked up electronically by the scanner and used to convert into an image.

By changing the timing of the radiofrequency pulses this scanner can pick up predominantly T1 or T2 signals, and thus T1 and T2- weighted MRI images are produced [26].

Protons in water, fat and different soft tissues have different T1 and T2 values, and therefore appear different on the MRI image. This inherent contrast resolution, distinguishing between different soft tissues, is the greatest advantage of MRI, particularly in musculoskeletal imaging.

T1 and T2-weighted images are different; with T1-weighting fluid and oedema (and thus many pathological processes) are of low signal (dark) while on T2-weighting fluid and oedema are of high signal (bright). Fat is of high signal on both, but can be suppressed either as an inherent part of the scan sequence (STIR sequence) or after the signal has been produced (fat suppression sequence).

Special Techniques in MRI Scanning

MRI Arthrography

Gadolinium has paramagnetic properties, and as a result diluted gadolinium shows high signal on T1-weighted images. In clinical practice chelated gadolinium compounds are used as gadolinium ions are toxic. Diluted gadolinium injected into a joint distends the joint and outlines the joint surfaces and cartilage, leading to accurate assessment of cartilage and labral tears. It should be noted that undertaking an MRI arthrogram turns a non-invasive examination into an invasive one.

Metal Artefact Reducing Sequences

Metal implants can safely be scanned with MRI, but produce a distortion of the surrounding magnetic field which can preclude accurate visualisation of surrounding structures. A number of simple physical alterations to the scan protocol (for example: using a lower strength magnet, thinner slices, increasing the bandwidth and particular sequences) will significantly reduce this artefact. Collectively, these changes are referred to as 'metal artefact reducing sequences' (MARS).

Advantages and Disadvantages of MRI imaging

Advantages

- Inherent contrast resolution between soft tissues. This enables assessment of ligamentous, tendon and muscle pathology which may not be available from other imaging modalities.
- Multiplanar imaging. MRI scans can be performed in any imaging plane; for example directly along the line of the supraspinatus tendon.
- Absence of ionising radiation.

Disadvantages

- Significant safety considerations for some patients; patients with pacemakers cannot in general be scanned, while claustrophobia may preclude scanning in some patients.

- Expensive compared with some other imaging modalities.
- Only hydrogen ions can be imaged. Therefore calcification and bone cortex do not return the signal (although bone marrow fat and oedema in the bone marrow are accurately imaged by MRI)

Scanning Technique

In shoulder MRI scanning multiple sequences are taken in different planes. In the shoulder, these sequences are typically in the axial plane, the coronal oblique plane (parallel to the supraspinatus tendon) and sagittal oblique (perpendicular to the coronal plane). Typically, 4 or 5 sequences are undertaken between the 3 planes. A standard MRI scan involves T1 and T2-weighted sequences, and also T2-weighted sequences with fat suppression. The coronal oblique plane is useful for assessing the supraspinatus tendon, while the sagittal plane is useful for assessing rotator cuff muscle bulk. The axial plane is best for visualising the anterior and posterior labrum, and the biceps tendon within the bicipital groove.

Clinical Uses of MRI

Impingement and Rotator Cuff Tears

MRI gives a comprehensive analysis of the shoulder and surrounding soft tissues in the patient presenting with impingement or suspected rotator cuff tear. Impingement cannot be imaged directly on a static MRI scan, but secondary effects of impingement, and in particular rotator cuff tears, are clearly visible and assessable. MRI will identify full-thickness and partial-thickness rotator cuff tears as defects in the rotator cuff, often filled with fluid. A full-thickness rotator cuff tear extends through the whole width of the tendon, at least for a small area, while a partial thickness rotator cuff tear will be seen as a defect which does not completely traverse the tendon. A massive rotator cuff tear is defined as a complete tear of at least two tendons. Rotator cuff tears most commonly involve the anterior supraspinatus tendon and extend into the subscapularis and/or infraspinatus. The subscapularis can be predominantly or exclusively torn. Massive rotator cuff tears are typically posterosuperior (supraspinatus and infraspinatus, and possibly teres minor) or anterosuperior (subscapularis and supraspinatus). Further progression will result in a tear of all three (or four) tendons. In larger rotator cuff tears the tendon end retracts towards the level of the glenohumeral joint. On MRI scanning the retracted tendon end can be clearly identified and the size of the defect estimated.

Assessment of Muscle Atrophy in Rotator Cuff Tears (Fig. 35.4)

Assessment and quantification of rotator cuff muscle atrophy and associated fatty infiltration of muscle fibres is important because, with greater degrees of atrophy, the torn tendons are less likely to be repairable, and repair is more likely to fail.

Fatty infiltration in the context of rotator cuff tears is graded using the Goutallier classification.

This grades the amount of fatty replacement of the muscle according to the following scale [27]:

Grade 0: Normal muscle.
Grade 1: Some fatty streaks.
Grade 2: Less than 50% replacement of muscle by fat.
Grade 3: 50% replacement of muscle.
Grade 4: Greater than 50% replacement of muscle by fat.

The classification was originally described in CT of the shoulder, but is applicable to MRI.

The degree of supraspinatus muscle atrophy can be quantified by comparing the percentage of occupation of the supraspinatus fossa by the supraspinatus muscle. This is measured on the oblique sagittal sequence, where the blade of the scapula, the root of the coracoid and the root of the acromion give a ‘Y’ shape. (Similar to the

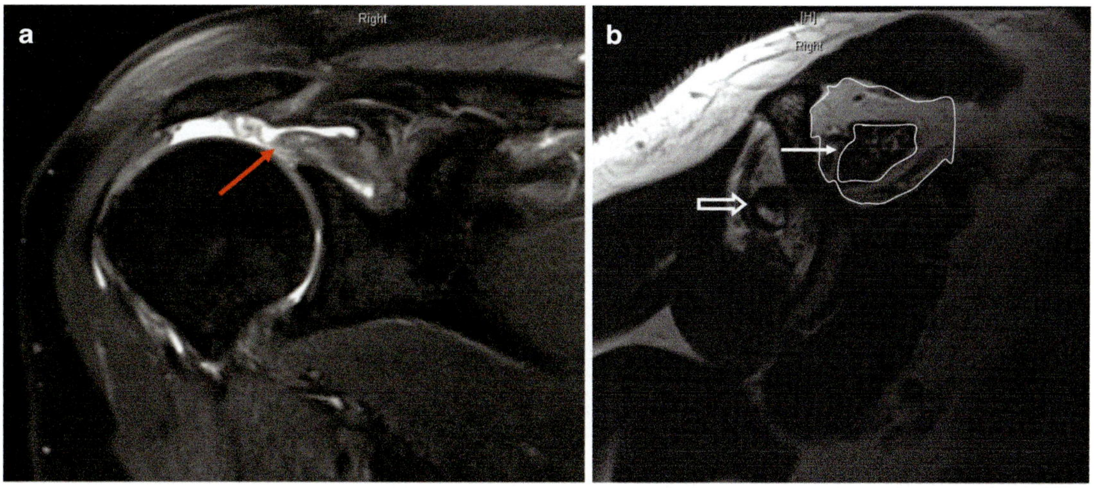

Fig. 35.4 MRI right shoulder. Proton density coronal oblique (**a**) and T2TSE oblique sagittal (**b**). Large full thickness supraspinatus tear with retraction (red arrow). Atrophy of the supraspinatus (arrow) and infraspinatus (open arrow) muscles. In (**b**) the occupation of the supraspinatus fossa by the supraspinatus muscle is around 25%, indicating severe atrophy (see text)

lateral scapular 'Y' view on x-ray.) The muscle should occupy most of the supraspinatus fossa, but with increasing atrophy will occupy a lesser percentage as the atrophied muscle is replaced by fat. Such atrophy of the supraspinatus can be classified using the Thomazeau classification [28]:

> Ratio of occupation of the supraspinatus fossa by the supraspinatus muscle.
> Stage I. Occupation ratio between 0.60 and 1.00—Normal or slightly atrophied.
> Stage II. Occupation ratio between 0.40 and 0.60—Moderate atrophy.
> Stage III. Occupation ratio less than 0.40—Severe atrophy (Fig. 35.4).

Biceps tendon pathology may occur alongside rotator cuff tears, or as a separate injury. Full-thickness long head of biceps tendon tears are identified on MRI; the tendon commonly retracts into the upper arm, just beyond where the pectoralis major crosses. Biceps tendinopathy, as with tendons elsewhere, causes thickening and increased signal within the normally low signal tendon. Fluid in the biceps tendon sheath can be seen, even in small amounts. Dislocation of the biceps tendon is often associated with subscapularis tears (Fig. 35.5).

MRI and ultrasound can both be used for assessment of the rotator cuff. Ultrasound affords a dynamic examination which can be performed as a continuation of clinical examination. Assessment of full-thickness rotator cuff tears is as accurate as with MRI scanning. MRI is more accurate in the assessment of partial-thickness tears, and is significantly better at assessing rotator cuff muscle atrophy. Underlying bony pathology can be assessed with MRI, but not ultrasound.

Cochrane review (2013) [20] shows sensitivity and specificity of 94 and 93% respectively for full-thickness tears on MRI. For partial-thickness tears the sensitivity and specificity values were 74% and 93% respectively. MR arthrography can also be used to assess for rotator cuff tears. While the images may give improved detail compared with plain MRI, the Cochrane review shows no significant advantage in sensitivity or specificity, and for this reason plain MRI is usually preferred.

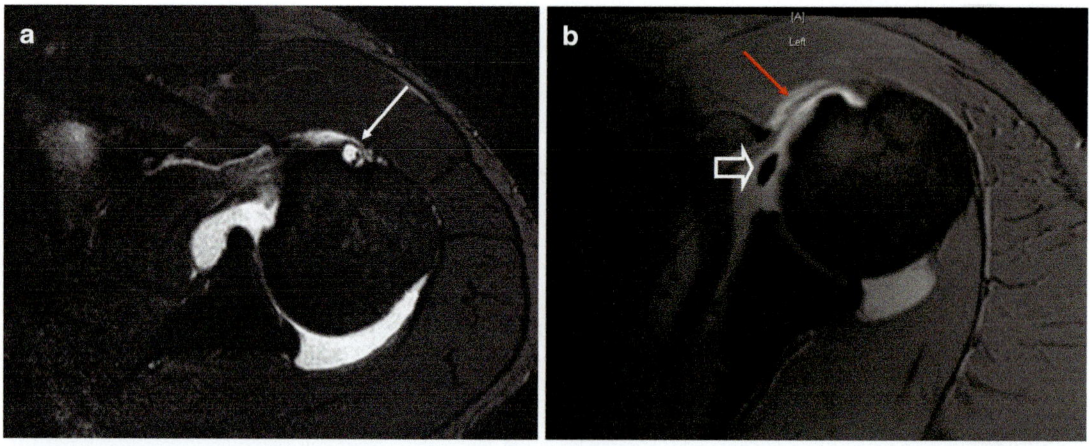

Fig. 35.5 Biceps tendon abnormalities. Gradient Echo axial slices through the left shoulder (different patients). In (**a**) the long head of biceps is torn, and is absent from the bicipital groove (white arrow). In (**b**) the long head of biceps is medially dislocated (open arrow). In addition, there is a tear of the subscapularis tendon (red arrow)

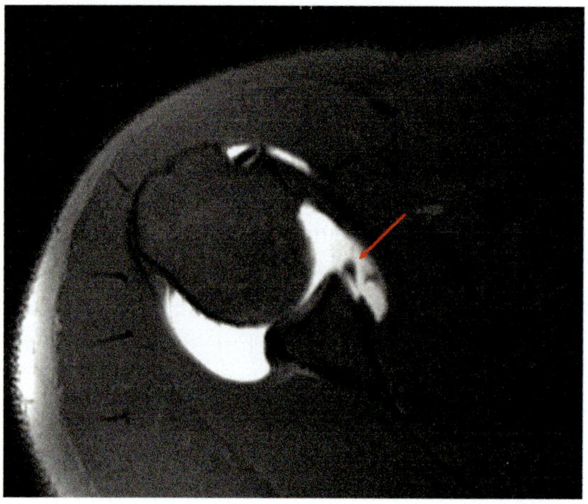

Fig. 35.6 T1 weighted axial section from an MRI arthrogram study in a patient who suffered a previous anterior dislocation. This shows a tear of the anterior labrum (arrow) known as a Bankart lesion

Instability and Labral Tears

Assessment of the glenoid labrum is significantly more sensitive and accurate when contrast is injected into the joint space before MRI scanning. (MRI arthrogram). This has two advantages; the joint is distended outlining the internal structures of the shoulder joint, for example articular cartilage, fibrocartilaginous labrum and glenohumeral ligaments (Fig. 35.6) [29]. In addition to tears of the anterior and posterior labral segments, tears of the superior labrum and superior labral/biceps complex (SLAP tears) can be assessed and described (Fig. 35.7). In addition the glenohumeral ligaments are much more clearly visualised on MRI arthrogram, and therefore tears of the superior glenohumeral ligament and the other structures in the rotator interval are preferentially assessed with MRI arthrography. For a description and pictorial review of the labral and ligamentous pathologies that can be seen on MRI arthrogram, see [30].

The variable anatomy of the labrum should be understood; a cleft can normally occur between the articular cartilage and superior labrum, and the anterosuperior segment may be completely separate leading to a foramen between the labrum and articular cartilage. The anterosuperior labral segment may be absent, in association with a thickened middle glenohumeral ligament. This is called the Buford complex. Knowledge of these anatomical variants is important in order to avoid diagnosing them as pathological tears [31].

Cysts developing in association with labral tears are known as paralabral cysts. These may extend superiorly, into the spinoglenoid notch, where they can compress the suprascapular nerve. This leads to weakness of the supraspinatus and infraspinatus muscles. Neuropathic degeneration of muscles on MRI presents initially as oedema (high signal on T2W scans) fol-

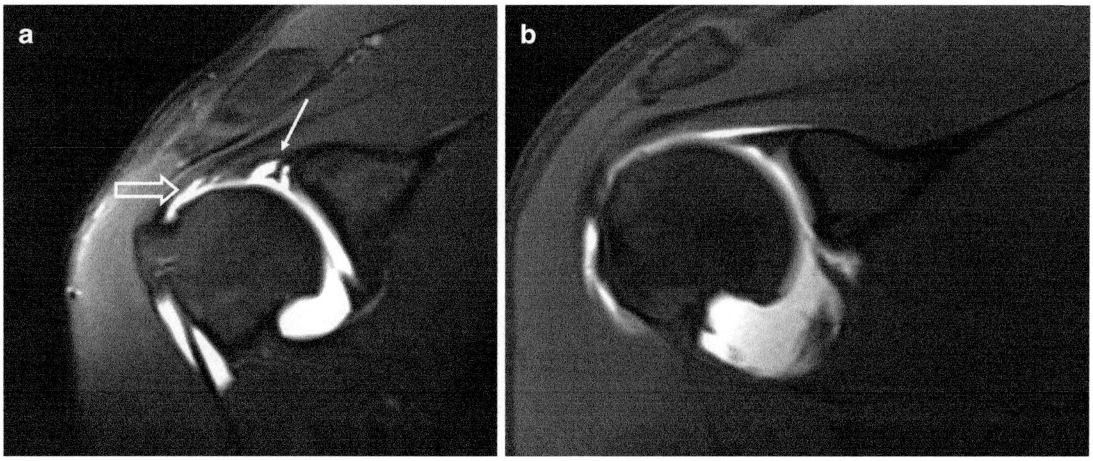

Fig. 35.7 MRI arthrogram. T1-weighted fat-suppressed coronal sequences at the level of the long head of biceps origin. (**a**) shows a superior labral tear (arrow). (**b**) for comparison shows a normal superior labrum. (**a**) also shows an articular surface partial thickness tear of the supraspinatus tendon (open arrow)

lowed by atrophy (Fig. 35.8). Alternatively, they may protrude inferiorly, compressing the axillary nerve leading to involvement of the teres minor and/or deltoid muscles.

Associated pathology can be as effectively assessed on MRI arthrogram as on MRI. Bone marrow abnormalities are readily seen, and rotator cuff tears identified. Undersurface partial-thickness rotator cuff tears may be better identified on MRI arthrogram than on MRI, although plain MRI is preferred for rotator cuff assessment as the examination is non-invasive.

The Use of MRI in Other Shoulder Conditions

- *Tumours*. MRI is used to diagnose, describe and characterise tumours around the shoulder joint. Bone and soft tissue tumours are readily assessed. In cases where a benign tumour or tumour-like condition is suspected, such as a lipoma or a cyst, ultrasound is sufficient to characterise the abnormality, but where a malignant tumour enters the differential diagnosis early MRI scan is indicated.
- *Infection*. MRI is useful in the assessment of bone or joint infection. The diagnosis of septic arthritis should be made by aspiration and microbiological analysis, but MRI will characterise the site and size of fluid collections, bone marrow involvement and bony destruction associated with septic arthritis and osteomyelitis (Fig. 35.9). MRI can also be used to help follow the progress of the infection during and after treatment. MRI will not distinguish between infected bone and surrounding reactive oedema, so the extent of the infection may be difficult to assess.
- *Arthritis*. MRI of the shoulder is not used to diagnose or characterise osteoarthritis or inflammatory arthritis, but in complex cases it may be useful to assess effusions, fluid collections and the degree of bony involvement.
- *Calcifying tendonitis*. The calcification in this condition is identified as a low signal focus within the rotator cuff tendon, which is also of low signal. It is therefore not the most sensitive diagnostic modality; both plain x-ray and ultrasound will more readily and confidently identify calcification (Fig. 35.3).
- *Adhesive capsulitis/frozen shoulder*. Imaging is not diagnostic in this condition, but MRI typically shows thickening of the inferior glenohumeral ligaments and soft tissue thickening in the region of the rotator interval.
- *Avascular necrosis*. See under 'Plain X-ray' section.

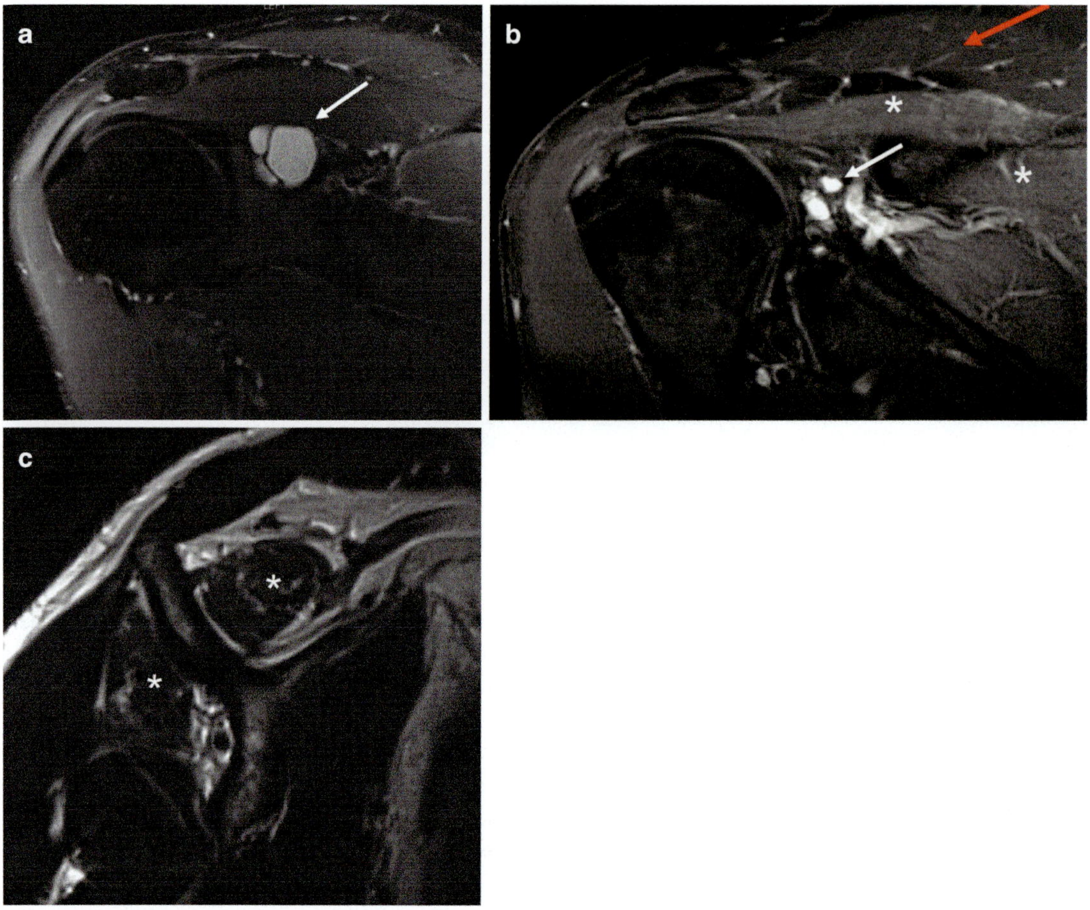

Fig. 35.8 Coronal oblique PD fat suppressed sections (**a**, **b**), different patients. T2TSE coronal (**c**). Both patients in (**a**) and (**b**) have paralabral cysts in the spinoglenoid notch (white arrows). In (**b**) there is oedema (increased signal) in the supraspinatus and infraspinatus muscles (asterisk) compared with the normal trapezius muscle (red arrow). (**c**) demonstrates atrophy of the two muscles

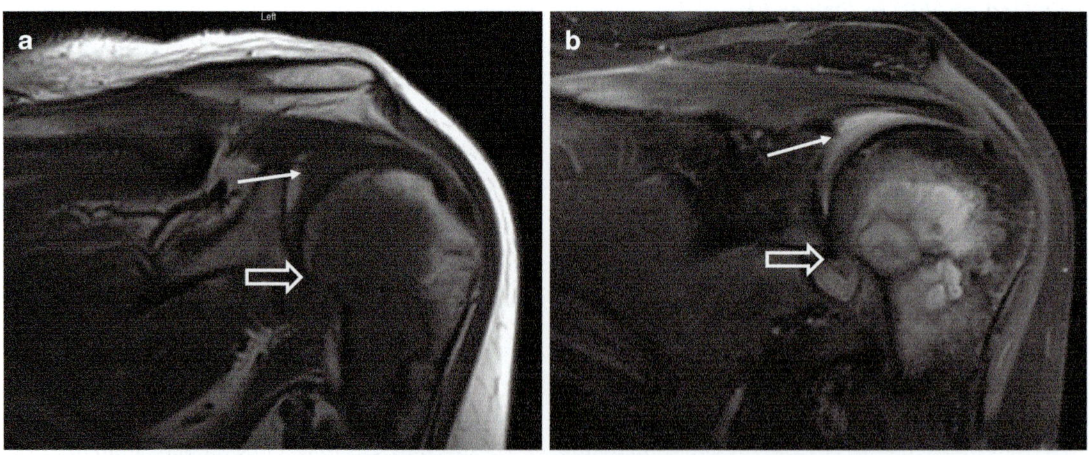

Fig. 35.9 MRI shoulder. Oblique coronal T1 (**a**) and fat-suppressed proton density (**b**) Joint effusion (arrow). Cystic changes in the upper humerus with cortical breach (open arrow) and surrounding marrow oedema in a patient with septic arthritis and osteomyelitis

- *Pigmented Villonodular Synovitis*. See under 'Plain X-ray' section.
- *Synovial Chondromatosis*. See under 'Plain X-ray' section.

Computed Tomography (CT)

CT is an x-ray based imaging modality. An x-ray tube is rotated around the patient. X-rays are either absorbed by the patient or transmitted to an array of detectors arranged in a circle around the patient. X-ray absorption is dependent on the physical density and atomic number of the tissue; therefore calcified tissues (bone) absorb more than air/gas with, in order of decreasing density, soft tissues, fluid and fat in the middle of the density range. As the tube rotates around the patient, the detectors pick up the transmitted radiation from all directions of the circular rotation. As a result the data can be mathematically reconstructed to produce a density number, known as a pixel, at each point. Thus an axial cross section or 'slice' is constructed, with each pixel represented by and number representing the density at that point. The density number is known as the Hounsfield number. This is named after Sir Godfrey Hounsfield who played a central role in the development of CT scanning in the 1960s and early 1970s. It sets air at −1000 HU and water at 0 HU. Typically, fat is around −100 HU, soft tissues +30 to 80 HU and cortical bone around +1000 HU. The Hounsfield numbers are visually displayed as a grey scale to give a two-dimensional axial section. The process is then repeated with successive slices building up a three-dimensional picture through the whole body or area of clinical interest. Modern multi-slice spiral CT scanners produce slices with an effective thickness of 0.5 or 1 mm; as a result the data can be reconstructed to give coronal, sagittal or oblique images with minimal loss of resolution. In addition, all of the information from the scan can be reconstructed to produce a shaded 3-D image [32].

In musculoskeletal radiology, CT utilises the large density difference between bone and other tissues, and is therefore useful in the assessment of bony pathology. The bony cortex and trabeculae are clearly and sharply visualised, and bony erosion, destruction and fractures can be readily assessed. On the other hand, the relatively low density difference between soft tissues makes CT less than ideal for assessment of soft tissue pathology, although administration of intravenous iodine based contrast will allow inflammatory lesions and tumours to be assessed where MRI is not available or contraindicated. Intra-articular contrast can be used to assess cartilage defects and labral tears as an alternative to MRI arthrography.

Clinical Uses of CT

Fractures

CT can be used to diagnose radiographically occult fractures. It should be noted, however, that completely undisplaced fractures can occasionally be missed on CT, but these will show on MRI as bone marrow oedema. The negative predictive value of CT in excluding a fracture is very high, but not 100% as it is on MRI. More commonly, CT is used to assess complex fractures for extent of the fracture, fracture fragment position, angulation and displacement. CT shows callus formation and developing bony trabecular union across a fracture line, and is therefore useful in the assessment of fracture healing where this is not clearly evident on plain x-ray.

Arthritis

CT gives an accurate and clear picture of joint surfaces, and can therefore assess joint space narrowing, subarticular erosion and bony destruction associated with inflammatory arthritis or osteoarthritis. CT is most commonly used to assess for glenoid bony erosion and bone loss prior to joint replacement surgery in order to ensure that there is sufficient remaining glenoid bone stock to take the glenoid replacement prosthesis (Fig. 35.10). It is also used to assess bone loss and loosening after joint replacement. See 'radiological considerations in shoulder prostheses' section below.

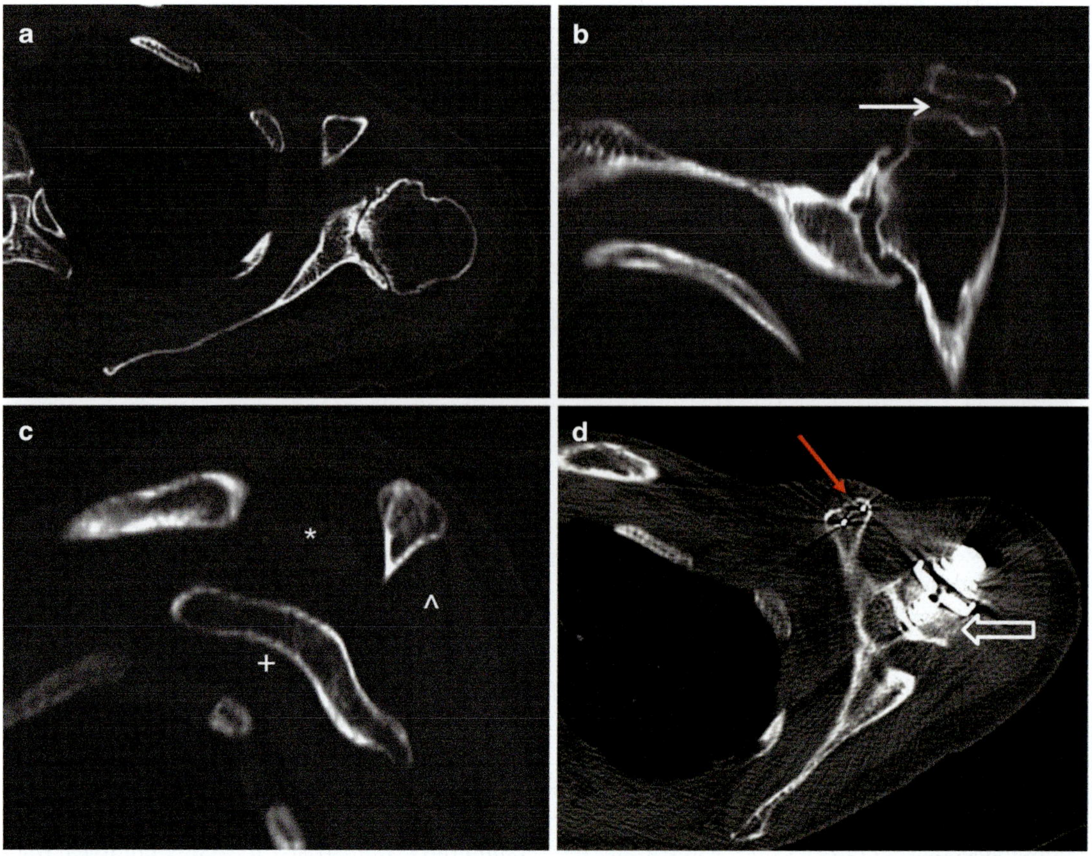

Fig. 35.10 CT left shoulder. 67-year-old female patient with OA of the glenohumeral joint (**a**). There is bony glenoid erosion, hence a bone graft was used at the time of joint replacement. Coronal reconstruction (**b**) shows loss of the subacromion space due to rotator cuff tear (arrow). Sagittal reconstruction (**c**) shows atrophy of supraspinatus (*), subscapularis (+) and infraspinatus (^). Post op axial CT (**d**) displays the reverse shoulder replacement and bone graft (open arrow) Tantalum balls were inserted to help assess post op glenoid displacement. See text. (Red arrow in **d**)

Classification of primary glenohumeral osteoarthritis Preoperative wear in the posterior part of the glenoid is common in osteoarthritis, and if not corrected at joint replacement surgery may lead to joint instability with subluxation and eventual glenoid component loosening. When the posterior glenoid is eroded or worn the humeral head displaces posteriorly because it is not supported by the deficient glenoid. Less commonly the wear and subluxation may occur in the anteriorly. The most commonly used classification of glenohumeral osteoarthritis is the Walch classification [33]; this is based on the degree of glenoid erosion and whether of the head of the humerus is centred or subluxed. The version given below is a 2016 modification of the original classification [34].

Type A. Humeral head is centred. (Distance between the centre of the humeral head and the centre of the glenoid are within 25% of the humeral head diameter).

A1. Minor erosion.

A2. Major central erosion. A line drawn across the glenoid transects the humeral head.

Type B. Humeral head is posteriorly subluxed.

B1. No bony erosion.

B2. Posterior erosion with biconcavity of the glenoid.

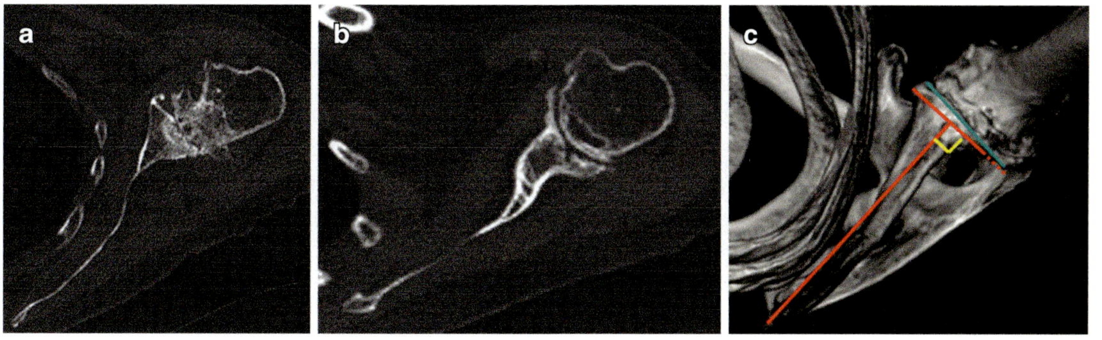

Fig. 35.11 (**a**) Glenohumeral osteoarthritis with posterior subluxation and glenoid erosion (type B2) (**b**). Glenohumeral osteoarthritis with centred humeral head and major central glenoid erosion (type A2). (**c**) Axially orientated CT 3-D reconstruction of case a. Measurements on (**c**) show calculation of glenoid version

B3. Posterior erosion and at least 15° retroversion or 70% posterior humeral head subluxation.

Type C. Dysplastic glenoid with at least 25° of retroversion

Type D. Glenoid anteversion or anterior subluxation of the humeral head.

Measurements are generally obtained on CT; to calculate glenoid version a 3-D reconstruction is often used due to imprecision when taking the scapular axis from a single axial slice [35] (Fig. 35.11).

Instability

Glenoid rim and humeral head fractures associated with dislocation can be clearly assessed and measured on CT scanning, as described in the x-ray trauma section.

In cases of instability, iodinated contrast can be given directly into the glenohumeral joint before CT scanning (CT arthrography). This outlines the articular cartilage and fibrocartilaginous labrum, giving a clear depiction of cartilaginous loss and tears. Thus labral and SLAP tears can be assessed on CT arthrography. The long head of biceps tendon can also be assessed as injected contrast extends into the bicipital groove, outlining the biceps.

MRI is generally the preferred technique for assessment of instability; however CT has the advantage of greater spatial resolution, and therefore giving a clearer depiction of articular cartilage and labral defects. It may also be preferred in the post-operative context, particularly if metallic anchors have been used, as the MRI scan may be degraded by the metalwork. CT will also provide better image of bony defects in the glenoid or humeral head [36].

Impingement and Rotator Cuff Tears

Plain CT cannot directly identify rotator cuff tears, and therefore assessment of rotator cuff pathology is carried out by ultrasound or MRI. However, CT can provide a clear assessment of rotator cuff muscle atrophy and fatty infiltration which may be useful if MRI is contraindicated. CT arthrography can accurately assess rotator cuff tears, including partial-thickness rotator cuff tears [37]; although MRI and ultrasound are preferred as they are non-invasive.

Other bony pathology

CT is the most sensitive technique to assess bony erosion or invasion from soft tissue tumours or infection.

The glenohumeral joint and scapula can be assessed in cases of dysplasia to look for glenoid area, depth and version.

Nuclear Medicine

In nuclear medicine techniques, a small amount of a radioactive substance is injected into the patient, usually bound to biologically active molecules. The gamma photons emitted by the radioactive substance are detected in a gamma camera. This consists of a flat sheet of sodium iodide, which exhibits a property called scintillation. In scintillation the gamma rays are absorbed, and the energy is re emitted in the form of light. This is detected and augmented using a photomultiplier tube. The resulting light flash can be detected and displayed in a two-dimensional image.

Traditionally, the most common form of nuclear medicine imaging in musculoskeletal radiology is the isotope bone scan. A technetium isotope (Tc99m) attached to methylene diphosphonate is injected. This is incorporated into sites of increased osteoblastic activity. Increased activity will be detected in bone tumours, infections, fractures, arthritis and other forms of increased metabolic activity such as Paget's disease. The technique is thus sensitive in detecting bony pathology, but not specific.

Imaging with 111Indium-oxine or more recently anti granulocyte scintigraphy using technetium labelled monoclonal antibodies provides a high degree of specificity in imaging osteomyelitis.

In patients presenting with chronic shoulder symptoms such as pain, weakness or instability nuclear medicine has been superseded by other imaging modalities, particularly MRI. However, white cells labelled scanning can be useful in the detection of occult bony and soft tissue infection.

Radiological Considerations in Shoulder Prostheses [38]

The use of shoulder joint replacement has increased rapidly in recent decades. It is the third most commonly replaced joint after hip replacement and knee replacement. The commonest indication for total shoulder replacement is osteoarthritis of the glenohumeral joint, but other indications include inflammatory arthritis, massive rotator cuff tears with rotator cuff arthropathy, avascular necrosis and complex proximal humeral fractures.

Preoperative considerations Total shoulder replacement can be 'anatomic' or 'reverse'. In anatomic shoulder replacement the normal ball and socket arrangement of the shoulder joint is maintained; with a convex humeral head and concave glenoid. The anatomic replacement requires an intact rotator cuff; otherwise the prosthetic humeral head will sublux superiorly into the space left by the rotator cuff. Reverse shoulder replacement is used when the rotator cuff is deficient, but requires an intact deltoid. Therefore, preoperative assessment may require radiological evaluation of the deltoid, rotator cuff tendons and rotator cuff musculature with MRI or ultrasound as described in the relevant sections.

The integrity and contour of the glenoid is an important preoperative consideration. If the glenoid is smooth and concentric, a hemiarthroplasty may be appropriate, while asymmetrical glenoid erosion, particularly when this leads to posterior glenoid tilt (retroversion), will predispose to complications following total shoulder replacement. If there is excessive glenoid erosion there may be insufficient remaining bone to implant the glenoid prosthesis. In this situation a glenoid bone graft may be required at the time of shoulder arthroplasty (Fig. 35.10), or a hemiarthroplasty may be appropriate. Accurate preoperative assessment of glenoid morphology generally requires CT scanning with two-dimensional and three-dimensional reconstructions as described in the CT section above.

Anatomic total shoulder replacement Prosthetic loosening is a common complication of total shoulder arthroplasty, and is much more common on the glenoid side than on the humeral side. As with joint replacements in other joints, a radiolucent line more than 1.5 mm thick, particularly if complete, is an indicator of loosening. As the loosening progresses, the prosthesis may tilt or even frankly dislocate. Plain x-ray assessment of the glenoid component is more difficult than on the humeral side, and as a result CT scanning is often used.

Anatomic shoulder replacement requires an intact rotator cuff, and post-operative rotator cuff tears will lead to loss of function of the prosthesis. The axial plain x-ray view should be assessed for anterior subluxation of the humeral head which may signify a subscapularis tear. Imaging of the rotator cuff is difficult in the post-operative context because of artefact from the metal replacement, but metal artefact reducing MRI techniques are available to give diagnostic images. Thus MRI is used along with ultrasound and sometimes CT arthrography.

Reverse total shoulder replacement
The most common complication in the early post-operative period is anterior dislocation; unlike anterior dislocations in the native or anatomic shoulder replacement, this occurs in the anterosuperior direction, and is caused by the unopposed action of the deltoid.

At a later stage, scapular 'notching' (erosion of the inferior glenoid due to impingement from the humeral prosthesis) is very common, and can be sufficient to undermine the glenoid prosthesis.

Infection Infection may occur after any implant. Imaging is difficult because of metal artefact which tends to degrade MRI and CT images and also in cases of indolent infection where imaging may be negative particularly in the initial stages. Infection may lead to bone destruction around the prosthesis, which can be assessed with x-ray or CT, and fluid collections and bone marrow oedema, which can be assessed with MRI. Standard technetium Tc99m bone scanning is sensitive to infection, but will be positive anyway in the first year after the operation. A positive scan is not specific to infection, and will also be present in non-infective loosening. Imaging of white cells with 111 indium-oxine or anti-granulocyte scintigraphy using technetium labelled monoclonal antibodies provides a high degree of specificity, although again may not be sensitive to low grade infections.

Periprosthetic fracture This can occur intraoperatively, or post operatively due to trauma. Post-operative traumatic fractures are more likely because of stress shielding. This occurs when the bone around the prosthesis becomes osteoporotic, and therefore weaker, as a result of removal of the stresses which normally occur. Fractures of the acromion are relatively common in patients who have had reverse arthroplasty.

Assessment of loosening with radiostereometric analysis (RSA) [39] Radiological assessment of loosening and consequent displacement of shoulder arthroplasty can be difficult. The glenoid component, which is by far the more common component to become loose, is poorly visualised on plain x-rays, and to some extent on CT scans due to artefact. Sub millimetre displacement or rotation of the glenoid component can be detected with radiostereometric analysis (RSA). During operation 1 mm metallic (tantalum) beads are inserted into the scapula (acromion, glenoid and coracoid) (Fig. 35.10). In the months or years after the operation radiographs are taken on a specially constructed RSA table in two planes. These are compared with similar x-rays taken immediately post-operatively. The x-rays are digitised and digitally analysed to detect tiny movements of the glenoid component with respect to the fixed tantalum balls. Using this method linear displacement of the order of 0.1–0.2 mm can be detected.

Conclusion

A number of imaging modalities are available in the investigation of shoulder trauma and in patients presenting with acute and chronic shoulder conditions. Radiological investigation will usually start with plain film radiography. Further investigation will typically involve ultrasound or MRI scanning, with CT and nuclear medicine useful for specific clinical indications. Injection of contrast into the shoulder joint followed by MRI or CT (MRI or CT arthrography) is the best method to assess the intra-articular cartilage, labrum and ligaments. Ultrasound or x-ray fluoroscopy guided interventions are often used to deliver pain relieving injections or curative therapies, such as hydrodilatation for adhesive capsulitis.

This chapter has assessed the different imaging modalities in turn, briefly discussed their scientific background and described the indications for their use and the imaging findings. The radiological investigation of common shoulder conditions has been discussed, particularly impingement and rotator cuff tears, and also instability and labral tears.

References

1. Sandstrom C, Kennedy S, Gross J. Acute shoulder trauma: what the surgeon wants to know. Radiographics. 2015;35(2):475–92.
2. Itoi E, Lee S-B, Berglund LJ, Berge LL, An K-N. The effect of a glenoid defect on anteroinferior stability of the shoulder after bankart repair: a cadaveric study. J Bone Joint Surg Am. 2000;82(1):35–46.
3. Neer CS. Displaced proximal humeral fractures. J Bone Joint Surg Am. 1970;52(6):1077–89.
4. Schwarzkopf R, Ishak C, Elman M, Gelber J, Strauss D, Jazrawi L. Distal clavicular osteolysis: a review of the literature. Bull NYU Hosp Jt Dis. 2008;66(2):94–101.
5. Nam D, Maak TG, Raphael BS, Kepler CK, Cross MB, Warren RF. Rotator cuff tear arthropathy: evaluation, diagnosis and treatment. J Bone Joint Surg Am. 2012;94(6):e34.
6. Walch G, Edwards TB, Boulahia A, Nové-Josserand L, Neyton L, Szabo I. Arthroscopic tenotomy of the long head of the biceps in the treatment of rotator cuff tears: Clinical and radiographic results of 307 cases. J Shoulder Elb Surg. 2005;14(3):238–46.
7. Hamada K, Yamanaka K, Uchiyama Y, Mikasa T, Mikasa M. A radiographic classification of massive rotator cuff tear arthritis. Clin Orthop Relat Res. 2011;469(9):2452–60.
8. Bigliani LU, Morrison DS, April EW. The morphology of the acromion and its relationship to rotator cuff tears. Orthop Transact. 1986;10:228.
9. Nguyen VD. Rapid destructive arthritis of the shoulder. Skelet Radiol. 1996;25(2):107–12.
10. Llauger J, Palmer J, Rosón N, Bagué S, Camins À, Cremades R. Nonseptic monoarthritis: Imaging features with clinical and histopathologic correlation. Radiographics. 2000;20(Suppl 1):S263–78.
11. Miksanek J, Rosenthal AK. Imaging of calcium pyrophosphate deposition disease. Curr Rheumatol Rep. 2015;17:20. https://doi.org/10.1007/s11926-015-0496-1.
12. Assouline-Dayan Y, Chang C, Greenspan A, Shoenfeld Y, Gershwin ME. Pathogenesis and natural history of osteonecrosis. Semin Arthritis Rheum. 2002;32(2):94–124.
13. Murphey MD, Foreman KL, Klassen-Fischer MK, Fox MG, Chung EM, Kransdorf MJ. From the Radiologic pathology archives imaging of Osteonecrosis: Radiologic-Pathologic correlation. Radiographics. 2014;34(4):1003–28.
14. Steinberg M, Hayken G, Steinberg D. A quantitative system for staging avascular necrosis. J Bone Joint Surg Br. 1995;77(1):34–41.
15. Quraishi NA, Johnston P, Bayer J, Crowe M, Chakrabarti AJ. Thawing the frozen shoulder: A randomised trial comparing manipulation under anaesthesia with hydrodilatation. J Bone Joint Surg Br Vol. 2007;89-B(9):1197–200.
16. Maund E, Craig D, Suekarran S, Neilson A, Wright K, Brealey S, Dennis L, Goodchild L, Hanchard N, Rangan A, Richardson G, Robertson J, McDaid C. Management of frozen shoulder: a systematic review and cost-effectiveness analysis. Health Technol Assess. 2012;16(11):1–264. https://doi.org/10.3310/hta16110.
17. Buchbinder R, Green S, Youd JM, Johnston RV, Cumpston M. Arthrographic distension for adhesive capsulitis (frozen shoulder). Cochrane Database Syst Rev. 2008;1:CD007005.
18. Gill R. The physics and technology of diagnostic ultrasound: a practitioner's guide. Abbotsford: High Frequency Publishing; 2012. ISBN: 9780987292100.
19. Moosikasuwan JB, Miller TT, Burke BJ. Rotator cuff tears: Clinical radiographic and US findings. Radiographics. 2005;25:1591–607.
20. Lenza M, Buchbinder R, Tagwoingi Y, Johnston RV, Hanchard NCA, Faloppa F. Magnetic resonance imaging, magnetic resonance arthrography and ultrasonography for assessing rotator cuff tears in people with shoulder pain for whom surgery is being considered (review). Cochrane Database Syst Rev. 2013;9:CD009020.
21. Soh E, Li W, Ong K, Chen W, Bautista D. Image-guided versus blind corticosteroid injections in adults with shoulder pain: A systematic review. BMC Musculoskelet Disord. 2011;12(1):137.
22. Harmon D, Hearty C. Ultrasound-guided suprascapular nerve block technique. Pain Physician. 2007;10:743–6.
23. Kane T, Rogers P, Hazelgrove J, Wimsey S, Harper G. Pulsed radiofrequency applied to the suprascapular nerve in painful cuff tear arthropathy. J Shoulder Elb Surg. 2008;17(3):436–40.
24. deWitte PB, Selten JW, Navas A, Nagels J, Visser CP, Nelissed RG, Reijnierse M. Calcific tendinitis of the rotator cuff: randomised controlled trial of ultrasound guided needling and lavage versus subacromial corticosteroids. Am J Sports Med. 2013;41(7):1665–73.
25. McNally EG, Rees JL. Imaging in shoulder disorders. Skelet Radiol. 2007;36:1013–6.
26. Pooley R. Fundamental Physics of MR Imaging. Radiographics. 2005;25(4):1087–99.
27. Goutallier D, Postel JM, Bernageau J, et al. Fatty muscle degeneration in cuff ruptures. pre-and post operative evaluation by CT. Clin Orthop Relat Res. 1994;304:78–83.
28. Thomazeau H, Rolland Y, Lucas C, Duval J-M, Langlais F. Atrophy of the supraspinatus belly assess-

ment by MRI in 55 patients with rotator cuff pathology. Acta Orthop Scand. 1996;67(3):264–8.
29. Magee T, Williams D, Mani N. Shoulder MR arthrography: which patient group benefits most? AJR. 2004;183:969–74.
30. Carroll J. Glenohumeral instability. Radsource MRI Web Clinic. September 2009.
31. De Maeseneer M, Van Roy F, Lenchik L, Shahabpour M, Jacobson J, Ryu K, et al. CT and MR Arthrography of the normal and pathologic anterosuperior labrum and labral-bicipital complex. Radiographics. 2000;20(Suppl 1):S67–81.
32. Mahesh M. The AAPM/RSNA physics Tutorial for residents. Radiographics. 2002;22(4):949–62.
33. Walch G, Badet R, Boulahia A, Khoury A. Morphologic study of the Glenoid in primary glenohumeral osteoarthritis. J Arthroplast. 1999;14(6):756–60.
34. Bercik MJ, Kruse K, Yalizis M, Gauci M-O, Chaoui J, Walch G. A modification to the Walch classification of the glenoid in primary glenohumeral osteoarthritis using three-dimensional imaging. J Shoulder Elb Surg. 2016;25(10):1601–6.
35. Petscavage JM, Ha AS, Chew FS. Current concepts of shoulder arthroplasty for radiologists: Part 1 Epidemiology, history, Preoperative imaging, and Hemiarthroplasty. Am J Roentgenol. 2012;199(4):757–67.
36. Zappia M, Negri G, Grassi S, Pecoraro C, Rotondo A. The CT-arthrography in the antero-inferior glenoid labral lesion: pictorial presentation and diagnostic value. Int J Shoulder Surg. 2008;2(1):7.
37. Omoumi P, Bafort A, Dubuc J, Malghem J, Vande Berg B, Lecouvet F. Evaluation of rotator cuff tendon tears: comparison of multidetector CT Arthrography and 1.5-T MR Arthrography. Radiology. 2012;264(3):812–22.
38. Lin DJ, Wong TT, Kazam JK. Shoulder Arthroplasty, from indications to complications: what the radiologist needs to know. Radiographics. 2016;36(1):192–208.
39. Nuttall D, Haines JF, Trail II. A study of the micromovement of pegged and keeled glenoid components compared using radiostereometric analysis. J Shoulder Elb Surg. 2007;16(3):S65–70.

Index

A

Abduction and external rotation (ABER), 123, 124
Abnormal muscle patterning, 580
  core stability, assessment of, 582
  involuntary posterior positional instability, 581, 582
  LD dominance, clinical observation, 581
  pectoralis major dominance, clinical observation, 581
Acetabulisation, 589
Acromial fracture, RSA, 314, 315
  conservative measures, 316, 318
  Crosby's classification, 315
  displaced, 316
  Levy's classification, 317
Acromioclavicular joint (ACJ) injuries, 557
  allograft, 49, 50
  anatomy, 457
  anterior-posterior plane stability, 45
  axillary view, 47
  bilateral zanca view, 47
  biological healing window, 49
  classification, 46
  clinical evaluation, 458
  clinical presentation, 47
  complications, 51, 52
  coracoacromial (CA) ligament, 49
  coraco-clavicular fixation, 48
  coracoid process transfer, 49
  deltotrapezial fascia, 49, 51
  distal clavicle resection, 49, 51
  epidemiology, 46
  high-grade dislocations, 49
  imaging and classification, 48, 458, 459
  intrinsic and extrinsic ligaments, 45
  ligament reconstruction, 48
  mechanism of injury, 458
  medial and lateral clavicle tunnels, 49, 50
  meniscus, 45
  non-surgical treatment, 459
  paediatric, treatment principles, 462
  passive and active restraints, 45
  postoperative management, 49, 51
  post traumatic osteoarthritis, 38
  primary fixation, 48
  soft tissue repair/reconstruction, 51
  superior-inferior stability, 46
  surgical treatment, 459, 461
  test, 560, 561
  type I and II sprains, 48
  type III dislocations, 48
Acromioclavicular joint osteoarthritis, 589
Acromio-clavicular ligaments, 46
Acromion, 462
Acromion fractures, 66
Acromioplasty, 152
Active Movement Scale (AMS), 474, 475
Acupuncture, 184
Adhesive capsulitis (AC), 592–593
  clinical conditions, 178
  definition, 174
  demographics, 174
  diagnosis
    arthrography, 183
    arthroscopy, 183
    laboratory studies, 182
    MRI, 182
    ultrasound, 182
  epidemiology, 174
  functional impairment, 180
  histochemical studies, 178
  histology, 177
  natural history
    duration of symptom, 181
    prognostic factors, 181
    recovery phase, 181
    resolution of pain, 181
  non-operative and operative treatment, 189
  pathology
    cytokines, 175, 176
    fibrotic changes, 177
    ICAM-1, 176
    TIMP's, 176, 177
  physical signs, 180
  primary, 175
  secondary, 175

I. A. Trail et al. (eds.), *Textbook of Shoulder Surgery*, https://doi.org/10.1007/978-3-319-70099-1

Adhesive capsulitis (AC) (*Cont.*)
stages, 180
surgical interventions
'ELM POPI' non-operative approach, 188
manipulation under anesthesia, 186
selective capsular release, 187, 188
treatment
acupuncture, 184
anti-inflammatories (NSAIDs), 183
corticosteroids injection, 183, 184
flow chart, 189
hydrodilatation, 185
intra-articular corticosteroids, 185
LLLT, 184
mobilisation, 184
oral steroid therapy, 184
prophylaxis, 183
suprascapular nerve block, 185
therapeutic exercise, 184
Adson's test, 583
Alfa-defensin 1, 548
Allograft prosthetic composite (APC), 537
Allograft reconstruction, 537
Alpha (α) angles, 475
Amyloplasia, 473, 490
Anaesthesia, 522, 523
Anatomical neck fractures, 63
Anatomical shoulder arthroplasty
age, 236
Charnley's low friction arthroplasty, 234
comorbidities, 237
complications, 240
design-related outcome factors, 240–241
fatty infiltration, 239
gender, 237
glenoid design
Aequalis multicentre group, 248
cemented glenoid component, 242, 243
clinical results, 244
failure rates, 244
Mayo experience, 244
metal-backed glenoid component, 243, 244
glenoid morphology, 239
hemi *vs.* total arthroplasty, 241
implant survival, 235
indication, 237
muscular atrophy, 239
osteoarthritis, 237
outcome measures, 235, 236
partial defects and small tears, 239
radiolucency lines, 235
registries, 235
rheumatoid arthritis, 237
surgeon-related outcome factors, 240
Anatomic shoulder replacement
age, 255
complication rate, 254
complications, 265
diabetes, 255
fractures and fracture sequelae, 256
glenoid, 256
glenoid component loosening, 257
glenoid erosion, 260, 261
hemi vs. total arthroplasty, 265
hepatitis C, 256
humeral component, loosening of, 263
implants, 256
infection, 264
instability, 261
medical comorbidities, 254
neurologic complications, 263, 264
obesity, 255
outcome, 254
perioperative transfusion, 256
periprosthetic fractures, 262, 263
rotator cuff failure, 261, 262
smoking, 255
uncemented glenoid components, 258
Anatomic stemless humeral prosthesis, 407
complications, 418
indications and contraindications, 408
postoperative management
phase 1, 416, 417
phase 2, 417
phase 3, 417
phase 4, 417
phase 5, 418
preoperative planning
biomechanical principles, 408
clinical findings, 409
instrument-based diagnostics, 409
medical history, 409
pathomechanics, 408
primary humeral osteoarthritis, course of, 408, 409
surgical technique
biceps tendon, tenodesis of long head, 410, 411
deltopectoral approach, 410
glenohumeral joint capsule, preparation of, 411
humeral component, implantation, 413–415
humeral head, preparation of, 411, 412
humeral head, resection, 412, 413
patient positioning, 410
subscapularis muscle, preparation of, 411
Anatomic total shoulder arthroplasty
addressing glenoid bone loss, techniques for, 338, 339
with asymmetric glenoid bone loss, 337
polyethylene augmented glenoid
biomechanical and computational data, 344
clinical outcomes, 343, 344
history and modern biomechanics, 339, 341–343
preoperative planning, 3D CT imaging for, 344, 345
Anchor peg' design, 215
Angulation, 61
Anterior humeral circumflex artery, 158

Anterior instability
augmentation, 574
release, 575
relocation, 575
Anterior labroligamentous periosteal sleeve avulsion (ALPSA) Lesion, 497
Anterior-posterior plane stability, 45
Anti-injury mechanism, 123
Apprehension-Relocation test, 123
Apprehensive Sulcus sign, 123
Arthrex Eclipse™, 256
Arthritis
crystals, 590
inflammatoty arthritides, 590
osteoarthritis, 590
septic arthritis, 590
Arthrographic distension, 592
Arthrography, 389
Arthrogryposis, 490
Arthroscopic capsular plications, 501
Arthroscopic capsular shift, 501
Arthroscopic capsulolabral repair, 498
Arthroscopic capsuloplasty, 125
Arthroscopic Latarjet procedure, 128, 522
Arthroscopic superior labrum anterior to posterior repair
complications, 169
failure of, 167
outcomes, 167
rehabilitation, 166
treatment, 163, 165
Arthroscopic surgery, nerve injuries, 521, 522
Articular surface geometry, 213
Atraumatic hyperlaxity instability
EDS (*see* Ehlers-Danlos syndrome (EDS))
epidemiology, 500, 501
Marfan's syndrome (*see* Marfan's syndrome)
non-operative management, 500
open capsular shift, 501
operative management, 500, 501
arthroscopic capsular plications, 501
arthroscopic capsular shift, 501
capsular shrinkage, 501
open capsular shift, 501
osteogenesis imperfecta (*see* Osteogenesis imperfecta (OI))
pathology, 500
Atraumatic instability, 496, 578, 579
active scapular shrug, 579
corrected position, 579
SAT, 579
SRT, 580
thoracic kyphosis, correction of, 580
thoracic posture and scapula, 579
Atypical lipomata, 527
Autografts, 197
Avascular necrosis, 591, 592
Axillary crease incision, 479
Axillary nerve, 465, 479
Axillary nerve palsy, 517, 518

B
Bankart lesion, 124, 125, 497
Baseplate design, 279
Bear hug test (BHT), 565
Beighton hypermobility score, 571
Belly press test (BPT), 565, 566
Benign neoplastic process, 590
Biceps tendon pathology, 599
Biceps tendon, tenodesis of long head, 410, 411
Biconcave glenoid, 354, 357
Biconcave glenoid deformity, 353
Bigliani-Flatow anatomic shoulder arthroplasty system, 354
Biomechanical body, 57
Biomechanical cadaveric study, 136
Biomet TESS™, 256
Biotenodesis screw technique, 165
Bisphosphonates, 502
Bone augmentation, shoulder arthroplasty in, 323
assessing glenoid bone loss, 323–325
bespoke options, 332, 333
bone graft, source of, 327, 328
bone grafting techniques, 326, 327
iliac crest, 328
iliac wing, 328–331
non bone grafting option, 331, 332
proposed algorithm, 333
standard anatomic glenoid, limits of, 325, 326
standard reverse glenoid, limits of, 326
Bone cysts, 465
Bone grafting techniques, 326, 327
Bone marrow transplant, 502
Bone preservation, 230
Bony avulsion, 199
Bony Bankart fracture, 588
Bony increased-offset reverse shoulder arthroplasty (BIO-RSA), 396
Botox, 478
Botulinum injections, 478, 479
Botulinum toxin, 12, 13, 478, 508
Brachial plexus, 19, 24, 37, 179, 367, 454, 455, 465, 469, 515, 516, 525, 527
Brachial plexus birth palsy, 473
aetiology and pathoanatomy, 474
botulinum injections with shoulder and spica casting closed reduction, 478, 479
botulinum toxin, 478
clinical assessment, 474, 475
clinical presentation, 474
glenohumeral joint reduction and rebalancing, 479
glenoid osteotomy, 481, 482
imaging, 475, 476
non-operative intervention, 477
open reduction and tendon transfers, 479–481
reinnervation, 477, 478
salvage procedures, 484
humeral external rotation osteotomy, 483, 484
humeral osteotomy, 483
splinting, 477

Brachial plexus injuries, 37, 469
Bristow-Latarjet technique, 127
British Elbow and Shoulder Society (BESS), 375
Buford complex, 600

C

Calcific tendinitis, 591, 595, 601
 acromioplasty, 152
 adhesive capsulitis, 152
 aetiology, 145
 associated medical conditions, 146
 clinical presentation, 146
 conservative management, 148
 ESWT, 149
 formative phase, 146
 greater tuberosity osteolysis, 153
 imaging, 147
 incidence, 145
 investigations, 147
 non-operative treatment, 150, 151
 ossifying tendinitis, 153
 pathogenesis, 145
 pathology, 146
 post-calcific phase, 146
 pre-calcific phase, 146
 radiographic classification, 147
 resorptive phase, 146
 resting phase, 146
 rotator cuff tears, 152
 rotator cuff tendon repair, 152
 subacromial injections, 148
 surgical technique, 151
 UGNB, 149
Calcium pyrophosphate deposition disease, 590
Campbell type D fracture, RSA, 312
Capsular arthrotomy, 187
Capsular shrinkage, 501
Capsule laxity, 126
Capsulitis, 568, 570
Cemented glenoid component, 242, 243
Cementing techniques, 216
Cementless metal-backed components, 216
Cephalic vein, 483
Cerebral palsy, 488–490
Cervical spine, 582
 Adson's test, 583
 Lhermitte's sign/phenomenom, 582
 Roos' test, 583
 Spurling's sign/test, 582
Charcot joint, *see* Neuropathic arthropathy
Charcot neuroarthropathy, *see* Neuropathic osteoarthropathy
Charnley's low friction arthroplasty, 234
Chlorhexidine, 551
Chondrosarcoma, 539
Chronic regional pain syndrome, 198
Circumflex scapular artery, 57
Clavicle fracture, 68, 453
 Allman classification, 20
 anatomy, 18, 19, 453
 clinical assessment, 455
 clinical evaluation, 454, 455
 clinical investigations, 25
 clinical presentation, 23–25
 complications, 457
  infection, 38
  intramedullary fixation, 39
  malunion, 35, 36
  neurovascular injuries, 37–38
  nonunion, 34
  plate fixation, 38, 39
  post traumatic osteoarthritis, 38
  refracture, 38
 Craig classification, 21
 displacement forces on, 454
 Edinburgh classification, 22–23
 embryology, 17, 18
 epidemiology, 20
 floating shoulder, 32
 function, 19
 history, 17
 imaging, 455
 lateral, 456
 lateral end
  coracco-clavicular screws, 31
  Kirschner wiring or K-wire fixation, 31
  plate fixation, 29
  suture and sling techniques, 30
 mechanism of injury, 454
 medial clavicle fractures, 456
 medial end, 31
 mid shaft, 456, 457
  intramedullary fixation, 28, 29
  non-operative treatment, 25–26
  operative treatment, 26–27
  plate fixation, 27
 nerve injuries, 515, 516
 non-surgical treatment, 456
 relative indications, 27, 33
 superior approach plating, 33
 surgical treatment, 456, 457
 treatment rationale, 33
Cobb elevator, 392
Codman's point, 557
Compression technique, 483
Computed tomography (CT)
 anatomic shoulder replacement, 607
 anatomic stemless humeral prosthesis, 409
 bony erosion or invasion, 605
 fatty infiltration, 605
 fractures, 603
 infection, 607
 instability, 605
 nuclear medicine techniques, 605
 osteoarthritis, 603
 periprosthetic fracture, 607
 preoperative considerations, 606
 primary glenohumeral osteoarthritis, 604
 radiostereometric analysis, 607

reverse total shoulder replacement, 607
rotator cuff muscle atrophy, 605
rotator cuff tears, 605
scapula fractures, 463
Computerized planning software, 421, 427
Constant score, 235, 236
Continuous Passive Motion (CPM), 71
Conventional double-row technique, 135
Convex-backed glenoid component, 214
Coracoacromial (CA) ligament, 49
Coracobrachialis
anatomy, 206
associated injuries, 207
clinical background, 206
clinical features, 207
investigations, 207
non-operative treatment, 207
operative treatment, 207
site of rupture, 206
Coraco-clavicular ligaments, 45
Coracoglenoidal notch, 56
Coracohumeral ligament (CHL), 159
Coracoid process fractures, 65
Coracoid process transfer, 49
Core Outcome Measures in Effectiveness Trials (COMET), 102
Core stability, assessment of, 582
Corticocancellous bone graft, 482
COSMIN checklist, 102
Crescent sign, 592
Crystal arthritis, 590
Cuff tear arthropathy (CTA), 288–290, 356
Cytokines, 175, 176

D
Da Vinci System, 81
Degenerative theory, 146
Delta design, 281
Delta prosthesis, 276
Deltoid
acute rupture, 203
anatomy, 202
anterior deltoid ruptures, 203
associated injury, 204
clinical features, 204
imaging modality, 204
non-operative management, 204
operative treatment, 204
partial or full thickness, 202–203
posterior deltoid ruptures, 203
spontaneous ruptures, 203
Deltoid tuberosity index (DTI), 77
Deltopectoral approach, 67
Deltopectoral interval, 483
DEXA method, 77
Dislocation, shoulder arthroplasty, 371
Displaced extraarticular fractures, 66
Displaced intraarticular fractures, 66
Distal clavicle resections, 49, 51
Distal musculature, 488
Drawer test, 124
Dysplastic retroverted glenoid, 357
Dystrophic calcification, 145

E
Eccentric humeral head component, 228
Ecchymosis, 199
Education, shoulder arthroplasty, 445
Ehlers-Danlos syndrome (EDS), 5
diagnosis, 503
pathology, 502
presentation, 502, 503
shoulder instability, relevance to, 503
underlying disorder, treatment of, 503
Elevated arm stress test (EAST), 583
Empty can test, 562
Endoprosthetic replacement, proximal humerus, 538
Entire glenoid fractures, 62
Entrapment neuropathy, nerve injuries, 524
LTN, 526, 527
quadrangular space syndrome, 526
suprascapular nerve, 525, 526
thoracic outlet syndrome, 524, 525
tumours, 527
Erb's palsy, 474
Ethibond, 481
Excessive humeral anteversion, 384
Extrinsic shoulder muscles, 507

F
Facioscapulohumeral muscular dystrophy (FSHD), 484, 523–524
non-operative intervention, 485
operative intervention, 485
presentation and investigation, 484, 485
scapulothoracic fusion, 485–489
Fatty infiltration, 605
FiberTape (Arthrex), 135
Fibrillin, 504
Fibrocartilaginous metaplasia, 146
Finite element analysis (FEA), 229, 281, 340
Floating Shoulder, 24, 32, 65
Foley catheter, 485
Formative phase, 146
Fracture fixation, 551
Fractures, shoulder arthroplasty, 369
Friedman method, 423
Frozen shoulder, *see* Adhesive capsulitis
Full-thickness rotator cuff tears, 594
Functional internal rotation, 559

G
Gagey's hyperabduction test, 572, 573
Generalised joint laxity, 500
Genetic testing, 485
Glenohumeral arthritis, treatment of, 337

Glenohumeral joint (GHJ), 373
arthroplasty, 383
capsule, preparation of, 411
reduction and rebalancing, 479, 480
stability, 570
Glenohumeral osteoarthritis, 233, 337, 354, 604, 605
Glenoid arthrosis, 386, 390, 399, 400
Glenoid bone deficiency, 122, 124, 340
Glenoid bone loss, anatomic TSA, 337
asymmetric, 337
techniques for, 338, 339
Glenoid component, rules for, 422
Glenoid component failure, 385, 386
Glenoid component loosening, shoulder arthroplasty, 375–377
Glenoid design
Aequalis multicentre group, 248
cemented glenoid component, 242, 243
clinical results, 244
failure rates, 244
Mayo experience, 244
metal-backed glenoid component, 243, 244
Glenoid erosion, 260, 261, 377, 378, 386
Glenoid fractures, 62, 63, 67, 69, 70, 311, 369
Glenoid morphology, 239
Glenoid osteotomy, 481–483
Glenosphere, 280, 281
inferior tilt of, 305
overhang of, 304
Global advantage modular prosthesis, 224
Gouty arthritis, 590
Grammont concept, 276, 277

H

Habermeyer stemless prosthesis, 225
Haematoma, 318
Haemophiliac arthropathy, 591
Hands Up test, 583
Hawkins' test, 561
Hemiarthroplasty, 81, 87, 88
glenoid arthrosis, RSA, 399, 400
native glenoid arthrosis after, 386, 390
proximal humeral fractures
complications, 93
outcomes, 90
Heterotopic ossification (HO), 179, 374
High-grade dislocations, 49
Hill-Sachs defect, 588
Horizontal glenoid deficiency, 352
Hornblower's sign, 563
Horner's syndrome, 474
Horwitz manoeuvre, 485
Humeral avulsion of the glenohumeral ligament (HAGL) Lesion, 497
Humeral bone loss, revision shoulder arthroplasty, 396
Humeral component, anterior dislocation of, 308
Humeral external rotation osteotomy, 483, 484
Humeral fracture, 309, 310, 312, 313
Humeral head
anatomic replacement, 224, 230
anatomical considerations, 225
cemented and uncemented humeral stems, 229
clinical outcome, 230
eccentric humeral head component, 228
finite element analysis, 229
glenoid access, 230
global advantage modular prosthesis, 224
global AP with increased variability, 224
Habermeyer stemless prosthesis, 225
head-shaft angle or inclination, 225, 227
humeral tray positioning, 229
inlay Grammont design and onlay design, 229
modularity, 228
Neer prosthesis, 223, 225
offset, 225, 227
preparation of, 411, 412
radius of curvature and shape, 225, 226
resection, 412, 413
resurfacing systems, 224, 225
reverse design prosthesis, 229
reverse shoulder replacement, 230
short stem, 224
shoulder prostheses, 225
soft-tissue balance, 230
stem length, 229
surgical consideration, 227
version of, 225, 226
Humeral osteotomy, 393, 483
Humeral shaft, 520
Humeral-sided capsular release, 391
Humeral stem loosening
from infected reverse arthroplasty, 370
shoulder arthroplasty, 377, 378
Hydrodilatation (HD), 185, 592
Hylamer ultra-high molecular weight polyethylene implant, 215

I

Iatrogenic injuries
brachial plexus, 37
vascular injury, 37, 38
Iatrogenous nerve injury, 520, 521
Iliac crest, 34, 295, 296, 326, 328, 394, 395, 485, 487
Iliac wing
baseplate, implantation of, 329
Bateman technique, 330
bone healing, 330
cancellous graft, quantity of, 331
defect, 329
femoral canal, reamer in, 330
K wire insertion and reaming of outer table, 329
novel technique, 330
procedure, 328
quality bone, thick column of, 328
swabs/retractors, 328
Impingement, 589
Inclination angle, 281

Infection
revision shoulder arthroplasty, 384, 387, 388
RSA, 318, 319, 397, 398
shoulder arthroplasty, 369, 370
shoulder joint, 545
complications, 546
diagnosis, 545, 546
after fracture fixation, 551
long term sequel, 545
management, 546, 549
native joint infection, 545
post arthroscopy septic arthritis, 551
PSI, 547–549
shoulder surgery, prevention, 551, 552
after surgery, 547
Inferior glenoid fractures, 62
Inflammatory arthritis, 293, 294
Infraclavicular plexus injuries, patterns of, 517
Infraspinatus, 563, 564
Inhibitors of matrix metalloproteases (TIMP's), 176
Instability
and Labral Tears, 600–601
revision shoulder arthroplasty, 384, 388
RSA, 398
Intercellular adhesion molecule 1 (ICAM-1), 176
Interclavicular ligament, 3
Interleukin-6 (IL-6), 548
Internal rotation contracture, 475, 483
Interscalene block, 523
Intraarticular biceps tendon, 157
Intra-articular corticosteroids, 185
Intramedullary fixation
advantages, 28
clinical results, 29
complications, 39
disadvantages, 28
methods, 28
mid shaft clavicle fracture, 28
Intra-operative fracture, 311
Intrinsic shoulder muscles, 507
Involuntary posterior positional instability, 581, 582
Irreparable massive cuff tear without osteoarthritis, 293
Irreparable tears
conventional double-row technique, 135
latissimus dorsi tendon transfer, 137
partial repair, 137
reverse total shoulder arthroplasty, 136
superior capsule reconstruction, 135, 136
suture-bridge technique, 135
teres major transfer, 137
trapezius tendon transfer, 137

J
Jerk test, 574, 576
Jobe's apprehension-relocation test, 573
Jobe's test, 562
Joint arthrosis, 22, 36, 441–443
Judet posterior approach, 67

K
Kim's test, 575, 577, 578
Kinesiophobia, 443
Kinetic chain, 447
Knotless technique, 164, 165

L
Lateral clavicle fractures, 29, 456, 520
Lateral end clavicle fracture
coracco-clavicular screws, 31
Kirschner wiring or K-wire fixation, 31
plate fixation, 29
suture and sling techniques, 30
Lateralized glenoid (LG) design, 279
Lateral pillar fractures, 65
Latissimus and teres tendons, 481
Latissimus dorsi (LD)
advantages, 201
associated injury, 199
clinical features, 199
complete tears, 199
dominance, 581
investigations, 199
non-operative treatment, 200
operative treatment, 200
site of rupture, 199
for shoulder abduction, 490
Laxity, 571
Lazurus method, 215
Lift off test (LOT), 565, 566
Light bulb sign, 588
Limb-salvage surgery, 535
Load and shift test, 123, 124, 573, 574
Locking plate open reduction and internal fixation
blunt Eva retractor, 85
Browne Deltoid Retractor, 85
deltopectoral approach, 85
Hohman retractor, 85
patient position, 85
reduction and fixation technique, 85
Long head of the biceps tendon (LHBT)
anatomy, 157
anterior humeral circumflex artery, 158
arthroscopic SLAP repair
complications, 169
failure of, 167
outcomes, 167
rehabilitation, 166
treatment, 163, 165
arthroscopy, 163
biomechanical studies, 160
electromyography studies, 160
function, 159, 160
history, 160
intraarticular biceps tendon, 157
MRI, 162
origin, 157, 158
osseous anatomy, 159
physical examination, 160, 161

Long head of the biceps tendon (LHBT) (*Cont.*)
SLAP tear, 157
soft tissue restraints, 159
sub-pectoral biceps tenodesis
complications, 169
fixation method, 165, 168
location, 168
outcomes, 168
pectoralis major, 164
rehabilitation, 167
unicortical button technique, 165, 166
superior labrum, 157
superior vs. inferior glenoid labrum, 158
sympathetic fibers, 158
tenotomy
complications, 169
outcomes, 167
rehabilitation, 166
treatment, 163, 164
ultrasound, 161, 162
x-ray, 161
Long thoracic nerve (LTN) entrapment, 526, 527
Lower motor neuron lesions, 179
Low-level laser therapy (LLLT), 184

M
Magnetic resonance imaging (MRI)
adhesive capsulitis/frozen shoulder, 601
advantages, 597
anatomic stemless humeral prosthesis, 409
arthritis, 601
avascular necrosis, 601
brachial plexus birth palsy, 476
calcifying tendonitis, 601
disadvantages, 597–598
impingement, 598
infection, 601
instability and labral tears, 600–601
metal artefact reducing sequences, 597
MRI arthrograph, 597
pigmented villonodular synovitis, 603
principles, 596
rotator cuff muscle atrophy, 598
rotator cuff tears, 598
scanning technique, 598
synovial chondromatosis, 603
tumours, 601
Mallet score, 475
Malunited clavicle fracture, 35, 36
Marfan's syndrome
diagnosis, 504
pathology, 503, 504
treatment, 505
Marginal dog-ear deformity, 135
Mason-Allen suture technique, 411
Matrix metalloproteases (MMPs), 176
Medial clavicle fractures, 456
Medial clavicular epiphysis, 453
Medial cord injury, 519
Medial end clavicle fractures, 31
Medialized glenoid (MG) design, 279
Medialized humerus (MH), 279
Medio-lateral displacement, 61
Metal artefact reducing sequences (MARS), 597
Metal augments, shoulder arthroplasty
anatomic, 354
bone loss assessment, 349, 350
horizontal glenoid deficiency, 352
indications, 352
limitations/complications, 361
metal-backed glenoid component, 352
PMA, 350, 351
primary anatomic, 351, 352
primary RSA, 356, 357
revision anatomic and RSA, 358–360
rheumatoid arthritis, 352
RSA, 356–358
surgical technique, 353, 354
Metalback convertible socket, 407
Metal-backed glenoid component, 215, 243, 244
Mid shaft clavicle fracture, 455–457
intramedullary fixation, 28, 29
non-operative treatment, 25–26
operative treatment, 26–27
plate fixation, 27
Milwaukee shoulder, 590
Minimal invasive plate osteosynthesis (MIPO) technique
complications, 92
locking plates, 87
outcomes, 89, 90
Modified Walch classification, 423
Modularity, 228
MRI, *see* Magnetic resonance imaging (MRI)
Multidirectional instability (MDI), 122, 123
Multi-disciplinary communication, 442
Multidisciplinary teams, 444, 445
Multiphasic theory, 145
Murley score, 236
Muscle patterning instability, 505
extrinsic shoulder muscles, 507
intrinsic shoulder muscles, 507
management, 507, 508
pathology, 505
psychosocial factors, 506, 507
scapula spine, position of, 506
scapular winging, 506
scapulothoracic dyskinesis, 505, 506
snapping scapula, 506
Musculocutaneous nerve, 518
Musculoskeletal soft tissue tumours, 596
Myofibroblasts, 177

N
National Surgical Quality Improvement Program (NSQIP), 265
Neer monoblock prosthesis, 223
Neer's sign, 560
Neer-Horowitz type IV fracture, 469

Neer-Horwitz classification, 467
Nerve injuries
  clavicle fractures, 515, 516
  entrapment neuropathy, 524
    LTN, 526, 527
    quadrangular space syndrome, 526
    suprascapular nerve, 525, 526
    thoracic outlet syndrome, 524, 525
    tumours, 527
  following anaesthesia, 522, 523
  following surgery, 520
    arthroscopic surgery, 521, 522
    open surgery, 520
    posterior triangle neck surgery and SAN, 522
  management of, 517–519
  neuralgic amyotrophy/Parsonage-Turner syndrome, 523, 524
  proximal humerus fracture, 519, 520
  scapular fracture, 519
  shoulder arthroplasty, 367, 368
  shoulder dislocation/fracture-dislocation, 516, 517
Neuralgic amyotrophy (NA), 523, 524
Neurapraxic injury, 518
Neurologic recovery, 477
Neurological injury, 316, 318
Neuromuscular shoulder reconstruction, 473
  arthrogryposis, 490
  brachial plexus birth palsy, 473
    aetiology and pathoanatomy, 474
    botulinum injections with shoulder and spica casting closed reduction, 478, 479
    botulinum toxin, 478
    clinical assessment, 474, 475
    clinical presentation, 474
    glenohumeral joint reduction and rebalancing, 479
    glenoid osteotomy, 481, 482
    humeral external rotation osteotomy, 483, 484
    imaging, 475, 476
    internal rotation contracture, humeral osteotomy for, 483
    non-operative intervention, 477
    open reduction and tendon transfers, 479–481
    reinnervation, 477, 478
    salvage procedures, 484
    splinting, 477
  cerebral palsy, 488–490
  FSHD, 484
    non-operative intervention, 485
    operative intervention, 485
    presentation and investigation, 484, 485
    scapulothoracic fusion, 485–489
Neuropathic arthropathy, 591
Neuropathic osteoarthropathy, 179
Neurovascular injuries
  acute injury, 37
  delayed injury, 37
  iatrogenic injury, 37
Noncemented metal-back glenoids, 216
Non-standard glenoid components, 215
Non-traumatic shoulder instability, 580
Notching, shoulder arthroplasty, 373
Nuclear medicine techniques, 605

O

O'Brien's test, 161, 567
Obesity, 255
Olecranon avulsion fracture, 501
Open capsular shift, 501
Open capsuloplasty, 125
Oral steroid therapy, 184
Osseointegration, 215
Osteoarthritis, 13, 14, 237, 568, 570
Osteogenesis imperfecta (OI)
  diagnosis, 502
  management, 502
  pathology, 501
  presentations, 501
  systemic treatment, 502
Osteopure, 396
Osteotomy, 412
Outcome measurement
  COMET, 102
  COSMIN checklist, 102
  orthopaedic research and audit, 101
  PROMS, 101–103
  PROQOLID, 102
  QALY, 103

P

Paediatric acromioclavicular injuries, 459, 460
Paediatric clavicle fractures, patterns of, 454
Paediatric shoulder instability
  anatomy and science
    healing potential and relative weakness, 494
    physis, 493
    skeletal maturity, 493, 494
  assessment, 496
  atraumatic hyperlaxity instability
    epidemiology, 500
    non-operative management, 500
    open capsular shift, 501
    operative management, 500, 501
    pathology, 500
  classification, 494, 495
  EDS
    diagnosis, 503
    pathology, 502
    presentation, 502, 503
    relevance to, 503
    underlying disorder, treatment of, 503
  epidemiology, 495, 496
  Marfan's syndrome
    diagnosis, 504
    pathology, 503, 504
    treatment, 505
  muscle patterning instability, 505
    management, 507, 508

Paediatric shoulder instability (*Cont.*)
pathology, 505
psychosocial factors, 506, 507
scapula spine, position of, 506
scapular winging, 506
scapulothoracic dyskinesis, 505, 506
snapping scapula, 506
osteogenesis imperfecta
diagnosis, 502
management, 502
pathology, 501
presentations, 501
systemic treatment, 502
presentation, 496
signs and symptoms, 496
traumatic instability, 497
ALPSA lesions, 497
Bankart's lesions, 497
HAGL lesions, 497
non-operative treatment, outcomes of, 497, 498
surgery, outcomes of, 498, 499
Paediatric trauma
AC joint injuries, 457
anatomy, 457
clinical evaluation, 458
imaging and classification, 458, 459
mechanism of injury, 458
non-surgical treatment, 459
paediatric, treatment principles, 462
surgical treatment, 459, 461
clavicle fractures, 453
anatomy, 453
clinical assessment, 455
clinical evaluation, 454, 455
complications, 457
imaging, 455
lateral, 456
mechanism of injury, 454
medial clavicle fractures, 456
midshaft, 456, 457
non-surgical treatment, 456
surgical treatment, 456
surgical treatment, indications of, 457
proximal humerus fracture, 464
anatomy, 464, 465
clinical evaluation, 465
complications, 469
imaging and classification, 466
mechanism of injury, 465
Neer-Horwitz classification, 466
non-surgical treatment, 467, 468
paediatric, clinical assessment, 465
surgical treatment, 468
scapula fracture, 462
anatomy, 462
clinical evaluation, 462, 463
imaging and classification, 463
mechanism of injury, 462
non-surgical treatment, 463
paediatric, treatment principles, 464
surgical treatment, 463, 464
Pain management, 446
Palpation, 557
Parsonage Turner syndrome, *see* Neuralgic amyotrophy (NA)
Partial-thickness tears, 594
Passive external rotation, 559
Patient Reported Outcome and Quality of Life Instruments Database (PROQOLID), 102
Patient reported outcome measurement systems (PROMS), 101–103, 236
Patient Reported Outcome (PRO), 102
Patient specific planning, 427, 431–435
Michaelangelos David's Scapula, 432
and patient-specific instrumentation, 427, 432–435
reverse shoulder arthroplasty, 429–431
total shoulder arthroplasty, 427–429
Patient-specific instrumentation, 421
assessment and plan, 432
history and physical exam, 431, 432
patient specific planning and, 427, 432–435
reverse shoulder arthroplasty, 429–431
total shoulder arthroplasty, 427–429
post-operative evaluation, 437
preoperative counseling, 435
reverse shoulder arthroplasty, 426, 427
total shoulder arthroplasty
CT retroversion, 425
Friedman method, 423
glenoid component, malpositioning of, 422–424
glenoid component positioning, 426
glenoid retroversion, 425
guidewire, 425
value, 431
Pectoralis major (PM) muscle
advantages, 199
anatomy, 195
associated injury, 197
clinical feature, 196
elderly patient group, 196
imaging modalities, 197
incidence, 196
incomplete rupture, 196
mechanism of rupture, 196
non-operative treatment, 197
operative treatment, 197, 198
young active, 196
Pectoralis major dominance, clinical observation, 581
Pectoralis major release, 490
Pegged polyethylene components, 216
Peripheral nerve tumours, 527
Periprosthetic fracture, 262, 263, 387, 607
revision shoulder arthroplasty, 390, 400
Periprosthetic radiolucent lines, 386
Periprosthetic shoulder infection (PSI), 547, 548
Physiotherapy, 443, 448, 505, 525, 526
Physis, 493
Pigmented villonodular synovitis, 591, 603
Platelet derived growth factor (PDGF), 175–176
Polar Type 1 (structural) instability, 496
Polyethylene augmented glenoid
biomechanical and computational data, 344
clinical outcomes, 343, 344

history and modern biomechanics, 339, 341–343
preoperative planning, 3D CT imaging for, 344, 345
Polyethylene glenoid components
alignment, 217
anchor peg design, 215
articular surface geometry, 213
cementing techniques, 216
convex-backed glenoid component, 214
humeral head positioning, 217
'in-line' peg design, 215
keel or pegs, 214
local factors, 213
metal-backed, 215
non-conforming, 213
non-standard, 215
osseointegration, 215
pegged prosthesis, 216
porous tantalum-backed, 216
positioning, 217
preparation, 216
radiolucencies, 215
radiostereographic analysis, 218
shape, 214
surgical technique, 218
in total shoulder arthroplasty, 213
Porous metal augments (PMA), 349–351
Porous tantalum-backed glenoid component, 216
Post arthroscopy septic arthritis, 551
Posterior cord dysfunction, 518
Posterior dislocation, 587
Posterior glenoid rim fractures, 62
Posterior humeral head displacement (PHHD), 475, 476
Posterior iliac crest graft, 487
Posterior triangle neck surgery, 522
Posterosuperior approach, 67
Post-surgical/post-traumatic stiffness (PTS), 173, 174, 178
Post-traumatic osteolysis, 588
Primary adhesive capsulitis, 175
Primary glenohumeral osteoarthritis, 604
Primary humeral osteoarthritis, course of, 408, 409
Primary shoulder osteoarthritis, 352
Primary synovial chondromatosis, 590
Processes fractures, 68
Proliferative acromial spurs, 131
Prophylaxis, 183
Propionibacterium acnes, 319, 384, 547
Protease inhibitors, 174
Proximal biceps
abnormal muscle patterning, 580
core stability, assessment of, 582
involuntary posterior positional instability, 581, 582
LD dominance, clinical observation, 581
pectoralis major dominance, clinical observation, 581
atraumatic instability, 578, 579
humeral head and scapula, 580
thoracic posture and scapula, 579, 580
capsulitis and osteoarthritis, 568, 570
cervical spine, 582
Adson's test, 583
Lhermitte's sign/phenomenom, 582
Roos' test, 583
Spurling's sign/test, 582
instability, 570
Jerk test, 574
Jobe's apprehension-relocation test, 573, 574
Kim's test, 575–578
load and shift test, 572
Stanmore classification, 570
structural causes, assessment of, 571
traumatic instability, 571
O'Brien's active compression test, 567
speed's test, 568
Yergason's test, 568
Proximal humeral allograft, 396, 397, 535, 537, 538
Proximal humeral deformity, 229
Proximal humeral fractures, 102, 292
AO/ASIF classification system, 78
bone quality, 77
clinical examination, 76
Codman/Neer classification, 78
conservative treatment
in elderly patients, 79, 80
protocol, 80
in young(er) and active patients, 80
epidemiology, 76
hemiarthroplasty, 87, 88
complications, 93
outcomes, 90
Hertel classification, 78
locking plate ORIF
blunt Eva retractor, 85
Browne Deltoid Retractor, 85
deltopectoral approach, 85
Hohman retractor, 85
patient position, 85
reduction and fixation technique, 85
mechanism of injury, 76
MIPO
complications, 92
locking plates, 87
outcomes, 89, 90
nonoperative treatment, 92
percutaneous fixation technique, 87
postoperative rehabilitation, 88
quantitative CT, 77
radiographic examination, 76
reverse total shoulder arthroplasty, 88
complications, 93, 94
outcomes, 90, 91
surgical treatment, 81, 82
surgical treatment
Da Vinci System, 81
hemiarthroplasty, 81
intramedullary nail, 81
locking plate, 81
non-locking plate, 80
percutaneous fixation, 81
treatment algorithm, 91
treatment strategy
for elderly patients, 83, 84
for younger and active patients, 82, 83

Proximal humerus, 534
Proximal humerus allograft
  preparation, 396
  secured with nice loops, 397
  step-cut, 396
Proximal humerus fracture, 169, 464, 588
  anatomy, 464, 465
  clinical evaluation, 465
  complications, 469
  imaging and classification, 466
  mechanism of injury, 465
  Neer-Horowitz type IV left, 467
  Neer-Horwitz classification, 466, 467
  nerve injuries, 519, 520
  non-surgical treatment, 467, 468
  paediatric, clinical assessment, 465
  surgical treatment, 468
  well-reduced and well-healed, 521
Putti sign, 475, 484

Q
Quadrangular space syndrome, 526
Quality Adjusted Life Years (QALY), 103

R
Radial nerve, left shoulder, 519
Radiological evaluation
  adhesive capsulitis, 592–593
  arthritis
    crystals, 590
    inflammatoty arthritides, 590
    osteoarthritis, 590
    septic arthritis, 590
  arthrographic distension, 592
  calcifying tendonitis, 591
  computed tomography
    anatomic shoulder replacement, 607
    bony erosion or invasion, 605
    fractures, 603
    infection, 607
    instability, 605
    nuclear medicine techniques, 605
    osteoarthritis, 603
    periprosthetic fracture, 607
    preoperative considerations, 606
    primary glenohumeral osteoarthritis, 604
    radiostereometric analysis, 607
    reverse total shoulder replacement, 607
    rotator cuff muscle atrophy, 605
    rotator cuff tears, 605
  dislocation, 587
  distal clavicle, 588
  haemophiliac arthropathy, 591
  Hill-Sachs defect, 588
  hydrodilatation, 592
  impingement, 589
  magnetic resonance imaging
    adhesive capsulitis/frozen shoulder, 601
    advantages, 597
    arthritis, 601
    avascular necrosis, 601
    calcifying tendonitis, 601
    disadvantages, 597–598
    impingement, 598
    infection, 601
    metal artefact reducing sequences, 597
    MRI arthrograph, 597
    pigmented villonodular synovitis, 603
    principles, 596
    rotator cuff muscle atrophy, 598
    rotator cuff tears, 598
    scanning technique, 598
    synovial chondromatosis, 603
    tumours, 601
  neuropathic arthropathy, 591
  pigmented villonodular synovitis, 591
  plain x-ray, 587
  primary synovial chondromatosis, 590
  rotator cuff arthropathy, 589
  trauma, 587
  ultrasound
    advantages, 596
    biceps tendon pathology, 595
    calcifying tendonitis, 595
    Doppler effect, 593
    elastography, 593
    fluid collections and effusions, 594
    full-thickness rotator cuff tears, 594
    impingement, 594
    infection, 596
    inflammatory arthritis, 596
    injections, 595
    instability and labral tear, 596
    musculoskeletal soft tissue tumours, 596
    partial-thickness tears, 594
    principles, 593
    shoulder pathology, 593
Radiolucency lines (RLL), 235
Radio Stereographic Analysis (RSA), 258
Radiostereometric analysis (RSA), 607
Range of motion (ROM), 557, 558
Reactive calcification, 145
Regional anaesthetic blocks, 522
Rehabilitation, shoulder arthroplasty, 441
  balances protection and enhancement, 441
  education, 445
  extrinsic factors, 443, 444
  factors affecting, 442
  intrinsic factors, 443
  movement and strength, 446
  multi-disciplinary communication, 442
  pain management, 446
  phases of, 444, 445
  pre-operative assessment, 442, 443
  return to function, recreational activities and sport, 447, 448
  surgeon/surgical considerations, 445, 446
Reinnervation, 477
Reparable tears
  arthroscopic vs. mini-open rotator cuff repair, 134
  clinical and anatomic outcomes, 133
  cyclic loading, 134

double-row *vs*. suture-bridge (transosseous-equivalent) repairs, 134
factors, 133
healing elements, 135
healing rate, 133
marginal dog-ear deformity, 135
margin-convergence and interval-slide techniques, 135
medial mattress stitches, 134
medial-row fixation, 134
single-row vs. double-row repairs, 134
suture-bridge procedure, 135
Resection arthroplasty, 319, 549
Resorptive phase, 146
Resting phase, 146
Resurfacing systems, 224, 225
Reverse geometry shoulder replacements, 371
Reverse shoulder arthroplasty (RSA), 421
metal augments, 357, 358
patient specific implants, 358
pre-operative planning, 359–360
primary indications, 356, 357
patient-specific instrumentation, 426, 427, 429–431
patient specific planning, 429–431
revision shoulder arthroplasty, 394–396
Reverse shoulder replacements (RSA), 301
acromial fracture, 314, 315
conservative measures, 316, 318
Crosby's classification, 315
displaced, 316
Levy's classification, 317
dislocation, 306–309
glenoid complications
disassembly, 312–314
glenoid fracture, 311
glenoid loosening, 312, 314
haematoma, 318
humeral fracture, 309, 310, 312, 313
indications, 301
infection, 318, 319
neurological injury, 316–318
procedure, 301
scapular notching, 302
anterior and posterior, 302
centre of rotation, lateralisation of, 303
glenoid erosion, Favard classification of, 302, 303
glenosphere, overhang of, 305
inferior overhang, 305
inferior tilt, 305
scapular neck, lateralisation, 304
Sirveaux classification of, 302
Reverse total shoulder arthroplasty (RTSA), 88, 136
clinical results, 297
cuff tear arthropathy, 288–290
fracture sequelae, 291–293
humeral stem, 291
inflammatory arthritis, 293, 294
irreparable massive cuff tear without osteoarthritis, 293
outcomes, 298
proximal humeral fractures
complications, 93, 94
outcomes, 90, 91
revision surgery, 295
shoulder hemi-arthroplasty or reverse prosthesis, 290
surgical treatment, 81, 82
unreconstructable or severe fracture dislocation, 290
upper humerus, 290
Reverse total shoulder replacement, 607
Revision shoulder arthroplasty, 383
complications, 400, 401
etiology, 384
glenoid component failure, 385, 386
hemiarthroplasty, native glenoid arthrosis after, 386
humeral component, 386
infection, 384
instability, 384
periprosthetic fractures, 387
rotator cuff insufficiency, 385
glenoid component, 399
hemiarthroplasty, glenoid arthrosis of, 399, 400
humeral component, 399
infection, 397, 398
instability, 398
periprosthetic fracture, 400
presentation, investigations and treatment options
glenoid component, 389
hemiarthroplasty, native glenoid arthrosis after, 390
humeral component, 390
implant loosening, 389
infection, 387, 388
instability, 388
periprosthetic fractures, 390
rotator cuff insufficiency, 388, 389
rotator cuff insufficiency, 398, 399
surgical technique
glenoid component, removal of, 393
humeral bone loss, 396
humeral component, removal of, 392, 393
pre-operative planning, 390, 391
surgical exposure, 391
to anatomic, 393, 394
to RSA, 394–396
Revision surgery, 295
Rheumatoid arthritis, 237, 352, 354, 357
Rhomboids, 486
Rocking horse phenomenon, 372, 375, 385, 422
Rockwood classification, 458–460
Roos' test, 583
Rotator cuff
arthropathy, 589
injury, shoulder arthroplasty, 368
shoulder
BHT, 565
BPT, 565, 566
empty can test/Jobe's test, 562
infraspinatus, 563
LOT, 565
Teres minor, 563
test, 561

Rotator cuff deficiency, 371, 372
Rotator cuff insufficiency
  revision shoulder arthroplasty, 388, 389
  RSA, 398, 399
Rotator cuff muscle atrophy, 598, 605
Rotator cuff tears
  causes, 131
  conservative treatment
    natural history, 132
    occupational therapy, 132
    physical therapy, 132, 133
    subacromial injection, 132
  epidemiologic study, 131
  imaging, 131
  irreparable tears
    conventional double-row technique, 135
    latissimus dorsi tendon transfer, 137
    partial repair, 137
    reverse total shoulder arthroplasty, 136
    superior capsule reconstruction, 135, 136
    suture-bridge technique, 135
    teres major transfer, 137
    trapezius tendon transfer, 137
  muscle degeneration, 137, 138
  reparable tears
    arthroscopic vs. mini-open rotator cuff repair, 134
    clinical and anatomic outcomes, 133
    cyclic loading, 134
    double-row *vs.* suture-bridge (transosseous-equivalent) repairs, 134
    factors, 133
    healing elements, 135
    healing rate, 133
    margin-convergence and interval-slide techniques, 135
    medial mattress stitches, 134
    medial-row fixation, 134
    single-row vs. double-row repairs, 134
    suture-bridge procedure, 135
  SEVERE degeneration/retraction, 137, 138
  signs, 131
  tendon degeneration, 137, 138
  tendon retraction, 137, 138
Rotator cuff tendon repair, 152

S
Salter-Harris II fracture, 4
Scapula assistance test (SAT), 579
Scapula fractures, 65, 462
  anatomy, 462
  clinical evaluation, 462, 463
  imaging and classification, 463
  mechanism of injury, 462
  non-surgical treatment, 463
  paediatric, treatment principles, 464
  surgical treatment, 463, 464
Scapular assistance test, 579, 580
Scapular body fractures, 64, 65, 68
Scapula retraction test (SRT), 580
Scapular fractures
  anatomy
    bone, 56, 57
    muscles, 57
    nerves and blood vessels, 57
  classifications
    anatomical neck fractures, 63
    anterior glenoid rim, 62
    combined fractures, 66
    coracoid process fractures, 65
    entire glenoid, 62
    glenoid fractures, 62, 63
    inferior angle of scapula, 66
    inferior glenoid, 62
    lateral pillar fractures, 65
    posterior glenoid rim, 62
    scapula, 65
    scapular body fractures, 64, 65
    scapular neck fractures, 62, 64
    scapular spine, 65
    spinal pillar fractures, 64, 65
    superior angle of scapula, 66
    superior glenoid fractures, 62
    surgical neck fractures, 63
    trans-spinous neck fractures, 64
  clinical examination
    palpation, 59
    patient medical history, 59
    peripheral innervation and vascularity, 59
    range of motion, 59
    visual assessment, 59
  complications
    non-operative treatment, 71
    operative treatment, 71
  epidemiology, 57, 58
  imaging method
    angulation, 61
    CT examination, 60, 61
    fragment displacement, 61
    GPA angle, 61
    medio-lateral displacement, 61
    radiology, 59
    translation, 61
  indication, 66
  injury mechanism, 58
  nerve injuries, 519
  non-operative management, 67
  operative treatment
    clavicular fractures, 68
    deltopectoral approach, 67
    glenoid fractures, 69, 70
    implants, 67
    Judet posterior approach, 67
    posterosuperior approach, 67
    processes fractures, 68
    scapular body fractures, 68
    scapular neck fractures, 68
  postoperative treatment, 68
  treatment, 66
Scapular neck fractures, 62, 64, 68

Scapular notching, 302
anterior and posterior, 302
centre of rotation, lateralisation of, 303
glenoid erosion, Favard classification of, 302, 303
glenosphere, overhang of, 305
inferior overhang, 305
inferior tilt, 305
scapular neck, lateralisation, 304
Sirveaux classification of, 302
Scapular retraction test, 581
Scapular spine fractures, 65
Scapular winging, 506
Scapula spine, position of, 506
Scapuloaxial system, 57
Scapulobrachial system, 57
Scapulothoracic dynamics, 45
Scapulothoracic dyskinesis, 132, 505, 506
Scapulothoracic fusion, 485–488
Scarf test, 561, 562
Secondary adhesive capsulitis, 175
Septic arthritis, 590
Serratus anterior (SA) muscle
anatomy, 205
associated injury, 205
clinical features, 205
investigation, 205
non-operative treatment, 206
operative treatment, 206
site of rupture, 205
in young active patients, 205
Shoulder
assessment of, 555
patient history, 555, 556
inspection, 556, 557
pain, 556
palpation, 557
physical examination, 556
ROM, 557, 558
symptoms, 556
test, 559
treatment, 556
proximal biceps
capsulitis and osteoarthritis, 568, 570
instability (*see* Proximal biceps, instability)
O'Brien's active compression test, 567
speed's test, 568
Yergason's test, 568
rotator cuff, 561
BHT, 565
BPT, 565, 566
empty can test/Jobe's test, 562
infraspinatus, 563
LOT, 565
Teres minor, 563
test, 559
Hawkins' test, 561
Neer's sign and, 560
scarf test, 561
Shoulder abduction, 490, 558
Shoulder arthroplasty (SA), 367, 421, 422, 441
bone augmentation in, 323
assessing glenoid bone loss, 323–325
bespoke options, 332, 333
bone grafting techniques, 326, 327
bone graft, source of, 327, 328
iliac crest, 328
iliac wing, 328–331
non bone grafting option, 331, 332
proposed algorithm, 333
standard anatomic glenoid, limits of, 325, 326
standard reverse glenoid, limits of, 326
glenoid component loosening, 375–377
glenoid erosion, 377, 378
heterotopic ossification, 374
humeral stem loosening, 377, 378
implant specific complications
notching, 373
rotator cuff deficiency, 371, 372
stiffness, 373, 374
intraoperative complications
fractures, 369
implant malpositioning, 368, 369
nerve injuries, 367, 368
rotator cuff injury, 368
metal augments
anatomic, 354
bone loss assessment, 349, 350
horizontal glenoid deficiency, 352
indications, 352
limitations/complications, 361
metal-backed glenoid component, 352
PMA, 350, 351
primary anatomic, 351, 352
primary RSA, 356, 357
revision anatomic and RSA, 358–360
rheumatoid arthritis, 352
RSA, 356–358
surgical technique, 353, 354
postoperative complications
dislocation, 371
infection, 369, 370
rehabilitation, 441
balances protection and enhancement, 441
education, 445
extrinsic factors, 443, 444
factors affecting, 442
intrinsic factors, 443
movement and strength, 446
multi-disciplinary communication, 442
pain management, 446
phases of, 444, 445
pre-operative assessment, 442, 443
return to function, recreational activities and sport, 447, 448
surgeon/surgical considerations, 445, 446
VTE, 374, 375
Shoulder dislocation/fracture-dislocation, 516, 517
Shoulder dysfunction, 485
Shoulder flexion, 558
Shoulder girdle, 534

Shoulder instability
arthroscopic capsuloplasty, 125
biomechanics, 122
Bristow-Latarjet technique, 127, 128
clinical evaluation, 123, 124
conservative treatment, 124, 125
imaging, 124
multidirectional instability, 122, 123
Stanmore classification of, 570
treatment, 124
unidirectional, 122
Shoulder joint infection, 545
complications, 546
diagnosis, 545, 546
after fracture fixation, 551
long term sequel, 545
management, 546, 549
native joint infection, 545
post arthroscopy septic arthritis, 551
PSI, 547–549
shoulder surgery, prevention, 551, 552
after surgery, 547
Shoulders reverse arthroplasty
baseplate design, 279
glenosphere, 280, 281
Grammont concept, 276–278
humeral component, 283
inclination angle, 281
lateralized centre of rotation, 280, 281
principles, 276
rotator cuff-deficient shoulder, 275
Shoulder stiffness, *see* Stiff shoulder
Significant nerve injury, 523
Simple Shoulder Score, 236
Simple Shoulder Test (SST), 236
Single Assessment Numeric Evaluation (SANE) rating, 162
Single stage revision, 549
Skeletal maturity, 493, 494
Snapping scapula, 506
Soft tissue contractures, 446
Sonography, 409
Speed's test, 160, 161, 568, 569
SpeedBridg, 135
Spica cast, 478, 484
Spinal accessory nerve (SAN), 522
Spinal pillar fractures, 64, 65
Spinoglenoid notch, 56
Splinting, 477
Spurling's test, 582
Standard anatomic glenoid, 325, 326
Standard reverse glenoid, limits of, 326
Stanmore classification, 570
Stanmore triangle, 494
Staphylococcus epidermidis, 319
Steinberg's test, 504
Sternoclavicular joint (SCJ), 557
anatomy, 3, 4
anterior and posterior, 3
disc injuries, 13, 14
elevation/depression, 4
examination, 4–6
history, 4–6
osteoarthritis, 13, 14
pathologies, 15
retraction/protraction, 4
rotation, 4
stabilizers, 3, 4
type I traumatic structural group
acute symptoms, 8
clavicular malunion, 12
closed reduction, 10
complications, 8
CT scan, 9
hamstring tendon graft, 11
lethal complications, 11
management, 9, 10
mechanism of injury, 7
medial physeal clavicle fractures, 11, 12
open reduction, 10, 11
posterior dislocation, 6, 8–10
traumatic subluxations, 6
type II atraumatic structural group, 6, 12
type III muscle patterning group, 7, 12, 13
Stiff shoulder, 373, 374 *See also* Adhesive capsulitis
heterotopic ossification, 179
lower motor neuron lesions, 179
neuropathic osteoarthropathy, 179
post-surgical/post-traumatic stiffness (PTS), 174, 178
post-surgical/traumatic stiffness, 173
range of motion, 174
upper motor neuron lesions, 179
Streptococcus pyogenes, 361
Subchondral plate, 325
Subcoracoid dislocation, 587
Sub-pectoral biceps tenodesis
complications, 169
fixation method, 165, 168
location, 168
outcomes, 168
pectoralis major, 164
rehabilitation, 167
screw technique, 165
unicortical button technique, 165, 166
Subscapularis muscle, preparation of, 411
Sulcus circumflexus, 57
Sulcus sign, 572
Superior capsule reconstruction, 135, 136
Superior glenohumeral ligament (SGHL), 159
Superior glenoid fractures, 62
Superior shoulder suspensory complex (SSSC), 32
Superior-inferior stability, 46
Suppressive antibiotic therapy, 549
Supraclavicular nerves, 520
Suprascapular artery, 57
Suprascapular nerve, 57
Suprascapular nerve block (SSNB), 185

Suprascapular nerve entrapment, 526
Suprascapular nerve transfer, 478
Suprascapular notch, 462
Supraspinatus test, 562, 563
Surgery, nerve injuries, 520
  arthroscopic surgery, 521, 522
  open surgery, 520
  posterior triangle neck surgery and SAN, 522
Surgical neck fractures, 63
Suture-bridge technique, 135
SwiveLock, 135
Synovial chondromatosis, 603
Synovial fibroblasts, 177

T
Tendon transfers, 479, 481
Tenotomy
  complications, 169
  outcomes, 167
  rehabilitation, 166
  treatment, 163, 164
Teres major (TM)
  anatomy, 201
  associated injury, 201
  clinical features, 201
  complete ruptures, 201
  investigation, 201
  non-operative treatment, 202
  operative treatment, 202
  partial TM rupture, 201
  site of rupture, 201
Teres minor, 563
Thoracic kyphosis, correction of, 580
Thoracic outlet syndrome (TOS), 516, 524, 525, 583
Thromboembolism, 374
Tightrope technique, 30
Tinel's sign, 523, 527
Toronto Test Score (TTS), 474
Total shoulder arthroplasty (TSA), 301, 421
  patient-specific instrumentation, 427–429
    CT retroversion, 425
    Friedman method, 423
    glenoid component, malpositioning of, 422–424
    glenoid component positioning, 426
    glenoid retroversion, 425
    guidewire, 425
  patient specific planning, 427–429
Trabecular Metal wedge, 355
Trabecular Titanium™, 351
Transforming growth factor-B (TGFb1), 175
Translation, 61
Translation-Rotation-Elevation osteotomy, 276
Trans-spinous neck fractures, 64
Traumatic instability, 571
  ALPSA lesions, 497
  Bankart's lesions, 497
  epidemiology, 497
  HAGL lesions, 497
  non-operative treatment, outcomes of, 497, 498
  surgery, outcomes of, 498, 499
Trunion, 413
Tumours, 527
Tumours of shoulder
  allograft reconstruction, 537
  anatomic considerations, 534
  pre-operative evaluation, 534
  proximal humerus, endoprosthetic replacement of, 538
  reconstruction, following resection, 537
  resection and reconstruction, 533
  resection techniques, 535, 536
    type I, 536
    type II, 536
    type III, 536
    type IV, 536
    type V, 536
    type VI, 537
  resection, types of, 534, 535
  scapula, endoprosthetic replacement of, 539, 540, 542, 543
  tenodesis techniques, 537
Tuning-fork instrument, 392
2D computer scapula model, 307
Two-stage revision, 549, 550
Type I resection, 536
Type II resection, 536
Type III resection, 536
Type IV resection, 536
Type V resection, 536
Type VI resection, 537

U
Ultrasound (US)
  advantages, 596
  biceps tendon pathology, 595
  brachial plexus birth palsy, 475
  calcifying tendonitis, 595
  Doppler effect, 593
  elastography, 593
  fluid collections and effusions, 594
  full-thickness rotator cuff tears, 594
  impingement, 594
  infection, 596
  inflammatory arthritis, 596
  injections, 595
  instability and labral tear, 596
  musculoskeletal soft tissue tumours, 596
  partial-thickness tears, 594
  principles, 593
  shoulder joint infection, 546
  shoulder pathology, 593
Uncemented glenoid components, 258
Unicortical button technique, 165, 166
Unidirectional traumatic instability, 122
Upper extremity deformity, 488

Upper extremity injuries, 102
Upper limb trauma
  outcome measurement
    COMET, 102
    COSMIN checklist, 102
    orthopaedic research and audit, 101
    PROMS, 101–103
    PROQOLID, 102
  outcome scoring systems, 101, 103–104
  pain or associated symptoms, 101
  response fatigue, 102
Upper motor neuron lesions, 179

V
Vascular injury, 37, 38
Voluntary dislocation, 507

W
Walch classification, 337, 338
Walker's test, 504
Waters' Classification, 476
Wright Simplicity™, 256

X
X-ray, anatomic stemless humeral prosthesis, 409

Y
Yergason's sign, 160, 161
Yergason's test, 568, 569

Z
Zimmer Sidus™, 256

Printed by Printforce, the Netherlands